PRINCIPLES OF
HEALTH CARE ETHICS

PRINCIPLES OF
HEALTH CARE ETHICS

Edited by

RAANAN GILLON BA (PHILOSOPHY) MB BS FRCP (Lond)

General Medical Practitioner; Director, Imperial College Health Service;
Visiting Professor of Medical Ethics,
St Mary's Hospital Medical School/Imperial College,
London University; Editor, Journal of Medical Ethics

Assistant Editor:

ANN LLOYD BA

JOHN WILEY & SONS

Chichester · New York · Brisbane · Toronto · Singapore

Other Wiley Editorial Offices

John Wiley & Sons, Inc., 605 Third Avenue,
New York, NY 10158-0012, USA

Jacaranda Wiley Ltd, 33 Park Road, Milton,
Queensland 4064, Australia

John Wiley & Sons (Canada) Ltd, 22 Worcester Road,
Rexdale, Ontario M9W 1L1, Canada

John Wiley & Sons (SEA) Pte Ltd, 37 Jalan Pemimpin #05-04,
Block B, Union Industrial Building, Singapore 2057

Library of Congress Cataloging-in-Publication Data

Principles of health care ethics / edited by Raanan Gillon; assistant
  editor, Ann Lloyd.
      p.   cm.
    Includes bibliographical references and index.
    ISBN 0 471 93033 4 (cloth)
    1. Medical ethics.
    [DNLM: 1. Bioethics. 2. Ethics, Medical. W 50 P957]
  R724.P69 1993
  174'.2—dc20
  DNLM/DLC
  for Library of Congress   92-23746
                                                             CIP

British Library Cataloguing in Publication Data

A catalogue record for this book is available from the British Library

ISBN 0 471 93033 4

Typeset in 10/12pt Palatino by Photo·graphics, Honiton, Devon.
Printed and bound in Great Britain by Bookcraft (Bath) Ltd.

Contents

Contributors

Terrence F. Ackerman PhD	Professor and Chairman, Department of Human Values and Ethics, College of Medicine, The University of Tennessee, 956 Court Avenue, Suite B324, Memphis, Tennessee 38163, USA
Brenda Almond	Professor of Moral and Social Philosophy and Director of the Social Values Research Centre, University of Hull, Hull HU6 7RX, UK
Garland D. Anderson MD	Professor and Chairman, Department of Obstetrics and Gynecology, University of Texas Medical Branch, Galveston, Texas 77550, USA
David Armstrong	Department of General Practice, UMDS, Guy's Hospital, London Bridge, London SE1 9RT, UK
Michael Baum ChM FRCS	Professor of Surgery, Royal Marsden Hospital, Fulham Road, London SW3 6JJ, UK
Tom L. Beauchamp	Professor of Philosophy, Joseph and Rose Kennedy Institute of Ethics, Georgetown University, Washington DC 20057, USA
Sir Douglas Black MD FRCP	President, Institute of Medical Ethics; Past President, Royal College of Physicians; The Old Forge, Duchess Close, Whitechurch, nr Pangbourne, Reading, Berkshire RG8 7EN, UK
Sophie Botros	Lecturer in Medical Ethics, Centre of Medical Law and Ethics, King's College, Strand, London WC2R 2LS, UK
The Reverend Dr Kenneth M. Boyd	Research Director and Scottish Director, Institute of Medical Ethics; 1 Doune Terrace, Edinburgh EH3 6DY, UK

Peter R. Braude BSc, MB, BCh, MA, PhD, MRCOG, DPMSA — Professor and Chairman, Department of Obstetrics and Gynaecology, 6th Floor, Ward Block, St Thomas' Hospital, London SE1 7EH, UK

Bob Brecher BA PhD — Principal Lecturer in Philosophy, School of Historical and Critical Studies, University of Brighton, Falmer, Brighton, Sussex BN1 9PH, UK

Howard Brody MD PhD — Director, Center for Ethics and Humanities in the Life Sciences; Professor, Family Practice and Philosophy, Michigan State University, A-108 East Fee Hall, East Lansing, Michigan 48824, USA

Andrew Bush MD MRCP — Senior Lecturer in Paediatric Respiratory Medicine, Royal Brompton National Heart and Lung Hospital and National Heart and Lung Institute, Sydney Street, London SW3 6NP, UK

Alastair V. Campbell — Professor of Biomedical Ethics and Director of the Bioethics Research Centre, University of Otago, POB 913, Dunedin, New Zealand

K. Danner Clouser — University Professor of Humanities, Pennsylvania State University College of Medicine, The Milton S. Hershey Medical Center, 500 University Drive, PO Box 850, Hershey, Pennsylvania 17033, USA

Rebecca J. Cook JD LLM — Associate Professor (Research), Faculty of Law, University of Toronto, 78 Queens Park, Toronto, Canada M5S 2C5

Panagiota Dalla-Vorgia Dr Med. Sc. — Assistant Professor, Department of Hygiene and Epidemiology, University of Athens, Medical School, Goudi, Athens 115 27, Greece

Alison Davis — 35 Stileham Bank, Milborne St Andrew, Blandford Forum, Dorset DT11 0LE, UK

Bernard M. Dickens PhD LLD — Barrister (England); Barrister and Solicitor (Ontario); Professor of Law, Faculty of Law, University of Toronto, 78 Queens Park, Toronto, Canada M5S 2C5

Jack Dowie MA (NZ), PhD (ANU) — Senior Lecturer in Social Sciences, The Open University, Milton Keynes MK7 6AA, UK

R.S. Downie MA BPhil FRSE — Professor of Moral Philosophy, Department of Philosophy, University of Glasgow, Glasgow, G12 8QQ, UK

Len Doyal — Senior Lecturer in Medical Ethics, Department of Human Science and Medical Ethics, The London and St Bartholomew's Medical Colleges, Turner Street, London E1 2AD, UK

H. Tristram Engelhardt Jr PhD MD — Professor, Department of Medicine, Baylor College of Medicine; Professor, Department of Philosophy, Rice University; Adjunct Research Fellow, The Institute of Religion; Member of the Center for Ethics, Medicine and Public Issues, Baylor College of Medicine, One Baylor Plaza, Houston, Texas 77030, USA

Donald Evans BA PhD — Director, Centre for Philosophy and Health Care, University College, Swansea SA2 8PP, UK

Martyn Evans BA PhD — University College Fellow, Centre for Philosophy and Health Care, University College of Swansea, Swansea SA2 8PP, UK

Anne Fagot-Largeault PhD MD — Université de Paris-X, Département de Philosophie, 200 Avenue de la République, 92001 Nanterre Cedex, France

John Finnis LLB (Adelaide) DPhil (Oxon) FBA — Professor of Law and Legal Philosophy, Oxford University; Fellow and Tutor, University College, Oxford, UK

Anthony Fisher OP BA (Sydney) LLB (Sydney) BTheol (Melbourne) — Blackfriars, St Giles, Oxford OX1 3LY, UK

R.E. Florida PhD — Associate Professor, Department of Religion, Brandon University, Brandon, Manitoba, Canada R7A 6A9; Visiting Professor Mahidol University, Bangkok, Thailand

R.S. Frey — Professor of Philosophy, Bowling Green State University, Bowling Green, Ohio 43403-0222, USA

K.W.M. Fulford DPhil MRCP — Consultant Psychiatrist and Research Fellow, Green College, Oxford, UK

S.H. Furness BA PhD — The Former Vicarage, Whissendine, Oakham, Rutland LE15 7HG, UK

Tina N. Garanis MA — Lawyer, Department of Public and Administrative Health, Athens School of Public Health, 196 Alexandras Avenue, Athens 115 21, Greece

Bernard Gert

Eunice and Julian Cohen Professor for the Study of Ethics and Human Values, Dartmouth College, Hanover, New Hampshire 03755, USA

Grant Gillett

Associate Professor in Medical Ethics, Bioethics Research Centre, Medical School, University of Otago, PO Box 913, Dunedin, New Zealand

Raanan Gillon BA (Philosophy) MB BS FRCP (Lond)

General Medical Practitioner; Director, Imperial College Health Service; Visiting Professor of Medical Ethics, St Mary's Hospital Medical School/Imperial College, London University; Editor, *Journal of Medical Ethics*

Luke Gormally LicPhil

Director, Linacre Centre for Health Care Ethics, 60 Grove End Road, London NW8 9NH, UK

Paul Goulden FRC Anaes

Consultant Anaesthetist, Dewsbury District Hospital, UK

Philip Graham FRCP FRCPsych

Consultant Paediatrician, The Hospital for Sick Children, Great Ormond Street, London WC1N 3JH, UK

The Most Reverend and Right Honourable John Habgood

Archbishop of York, Bishopthorpe Palace, Bishopthorpe, York YO2 1QE, UK

Richard M. Hare FBA

Graduate Research Professor of Philosophy, University of Florida, Gainesville, FL 32611, USA; White's Professor of Moral Philosophy Emeritus, University of Oxford, UK

John Harris

Professor of Applied Philosophy and Research Director of the Centre for Social Ethics and Policy, University of Manchester, Oxford Road, Manchester M13 9PL, UK

K. Zaki Hasan MB FRCP FCPS (Pak)

Dean and Professor of Behavioural Sciences, Baqai Medical College, 35-G/VI, PECHS, Karachi 75400, Pakistan

Michael Henderson

49 Bakers Road, Church Point, New South Wales 2105, Australia

Henk A.M.J. ten Have MD PhD

Professor of Medical Ethics, Department of Ethics, Philosophy and History of Medicine, Faculty of Medical Sciences, Catholic University of Nijmegen, Postbus 9101, 6500 HB Nijmegen, The Netherlands

Roger Higgs MBE MA FRCP FRCGP	Professor of General Practice and Primary Care, King's College School of Medicine and Dentistry, Bessemer Road, London SE5 9PJ, UK
Jeremy Holmes MRCP FRCPsych	Consultant Psychiatrist/Psychotherapist, Department of Psychiatry, North Devon District Hospital, Raleigh Park, Barnstaple, Devon EX31 4JB, UK
Bernard Hoose	Heythrop College, University of London, Kensington Square, London W8 5HQ, UK
Tony Hope PhD MRCPsych	Consultant Psychiatrist and Leader of the Oxford Practice Skills Project, The Medical School, University of Oxford, Oxford OX3 9DU, UK
Joan Houghton BSc	Deputy Director, Cancer Research Campaign Clinical Trials Centre, Rayne Institute, 123 Coldharbour Lane, London SE5 9NU, UK
Charlotte Humphrey	Department of Public Health and Primary Care, Royal Free School of Medicine, London, UK
Jennifer Jackson	Director, Centre for Business and Professional Ethics, Leeds University, Leeds LS2 9JT, UK
Bryan Jennett CBE MD FRCS	Professor, Department of Neurosurgery, Institute of Neurological Sciences, The Southern General Hospital, Glasgow G51 4TF, UK
Albert R. Jonsen	Professor of Ethics in Medicine, Department of Ethics, School of Medicine, University of Washington, Seattle, Washington 98195, USA
Peter Kasenene BA DipEd MA PhD	Senior Lecturer and Head of Theology and Religious Studies, University of Swaziland, Kwaluseni Campus, P/Bag Kwaluseni, Swaziland, Southern Africa
Justice Michael Kirby AC CMG	President of the Court of Appeal of New South Wales, Supreme Court, GPO Box 3, Sydney NSW 2001, Australia
M.H. Kottow MA(Soc) MD	Professor of Ophthalmology, University of Chile, Santiagó, Chile, South America
David Lamb BA PhD	Reader in Philosophy, Department of Philosophy, University of Manchester, Oxford Road, Manchester M13 9PL, UK

Sandra D. Lane RN PhD MPH — Assistant Professor, Department of Anthropology, Case Western Reserve University, 10900 Euclid Avenue, Cleveland, Ohio 44106-7125, USA

John M. Last MD DPH FRACP FRCPC FFCM FACPM — Editor, *Annals RCPSC*; Emeritus Professor of Epidemiology and Community Medicine, Faculty of Medicine, University of Ottawa; Health Sciences Centre, 451 Smyth Road, Ottawa, Ontario, Canada K1H 8M5

Richard Lindley PhD — Solicitor; formerly Lecturer in Philosophy, University of Bradford, UK

Leonora Lloyd — National Abortion Campaign, Wesley House, 4 Wild Court, London WC2R 5AU, UK

Ernst Luther Dr ScPhil — Professor and Head of Department, Martin-Luther-Universität Halle/Wittenberg, Bereich Medizin, Abt Ethik und Geschichte d-medizin, PSF 302, Halle 0-4090, Germany

R.I. McCallum CBE MD DSc FRCP FRCP(E) FFOM — Emeritus Professor of Occupational Health and Hygiene, University of Newcastle upon Tyne; Honorary Consultant in Occupational Medicine, Institute of Occupational Medicine, Roxburgh Place, Edinburgh EH8 9SU, Scotland, UK

Robert J. Maxwell — Chief Executive, The King's Fund, 14 Palace Court, London W2 4HT, UK

Maurizio Mori — Editor Bioethica Revista Interdisciplinare; Secretary, Consulto di Bioethica; Coordinator, Bioethics Group of Politeia; Via XI Febbraio 25, 26100, Cremona, Italy

J A Muir Gray MD FRCP (Glas) MRCGP FFCM — Specialist in Public Health Medicine, Oxford Regional Health Authority, Old Road, Headington, Oxford OX3 7LF, UK

Rabbi Julia Neuberger — Chair, Camden and Islington Community Health Services NHS Trust; Vice-President, Patients' Association; 36 Orlando Road, London SW4 0LF, UK

R.H. Nicholson MA BM BCh DCH — Editor, *Bulletin of Medical Ethics*, 31 Corsica Street, London N5 1JT, UK

Astrid Norberg RN PhD — Professor, Department of Advanced Nursing, Umeå University, Box 1442, S-901 24 Umeå, Sweden

Patrick Nowell-Smith	Honorary Vice-President, Voluntary Euthanasia Society and Past President, World Federation of Right-to-Die Societies; 5 Thackley End, 119 Banbury Road, Oxford OX2 6LB, UK
Magne Nylenna MD	Editor-in-Chief, *Journal of the Norwegian Medical Association*, Fjellveien 5, Lagåsen, N-1324, Norway
Edmund D. Pellegrino MD	John Carroll Professor of Medicine and Medical Ethics and Director, Center for the Advanced Study of Ethics, Georgetown University, Washington DC 20057, USA
Anthony J. Pinching DPhil FRCP	Professor of Immunology, St Bartholomew's Hospital Medical College, West Smithfield, London EC1A 7BE, UK
Ronald H. Preston DD (Oxon)	Emeritus Professor of Social and Pastoral Theology, University of Manchester, 161 Old Hall Lane, Manchester M14 6HJ, UK
Povl Riis MD FRCP	Professor, Physician in Chief, Herlev University Hospital (University of Copenhagen), Herlev Ringvej 75, 2730 Herlev, Denmark
Christobel M. Saunders MB BS FRCS	Clinical Research Fellow, Academic Department of Surgery, Royal Marsden Hospital, Fulham Road, London SW3 6JJ, UK
Dame Cicely Saunders OM DBE FRCP	Chairman, St Christopher's Hospice, 51–59 Lawrie Park Road, Sydenham, London SE26 6DZ, UK
Dr Viola Schubert-Lehnhardt	Martin-Luther-Universität Halle/Wittenberg, Bereich Medizin, Abt Ethik und Geschichte d-medizin, PSF 302, Halle 0-4090, Germany
Mary J. Seller PhD DSc	Reader in Developmental Genetics, Department of Medical and Molecular Genetics, Paediatric Research Unit, Prince Philip Research Laboratories, 7th and 8th Floors, Guy's Tower, Guy's Hospital, London SE1 9RT, UK
Robert A. Sells	Director, Renal Transplant Unit, Royal Liverpool University Hospital, Prescot Street, Liverpool L7 8XP, UK
G.I. Serour FRCOG, FRCS	Professor of Obstetrics and Gynaecology, Director, International Islamic Center for Population Studies and Research, Al-Azhar University, 11851 PO Box 1894, Cairo, Egypt

Elliot A. Shinebourne MD FRCP	Consultant Paediatric Cardiologist, Royal Brompton National Heart and Lung Hospital and National Heart and Lung Institute, University of London, Sydney Street, London SW3 6NP, UK
Elizabeth Snowden SRN BEd (Hons)	Research Assistant, Institute of Population Studies, University of Exeter, Hoopern House, 101 Pennsylvania Road, Exeter EX4 6DT, UK
Robert Snowden BA PhD DSA	Professor of Family Studies, Sociology Department, Institute of Population Studies, University of Exeter, Hoopern House, 101 Pennsylvania Road, Exeter EX4 6DT, UK
Carol Mason Spicer MA	Managing Editor, *Kennedy Institute of Ethics Journal*; Lecturer, Philosophy Department, Georgetown University, Washington DC 20057, USA
T.L.S. Sprigge	Professor of Philosophy, University of Edinburgh, David Hume Tower, George Square, Edinburgh EH8 9JX, UK
John M. Stanley PhD	Edward F. Mielke Professor of Ethics in Medicine, Science and Society; Director, Lawrence University Program in Biomedical Ethics, PO Box 599, Appleton, Wisconsin 54912, USA
Avraham Steinberg MD	The Center for Medical Ethics, The Hebrew University–Hadassah Medical School, and Department of Paediatrics, Shaare Zedek Medical Center, POB 3235, Jerusalem 91031, Israel
Dr Harry Stopes-Roe	155 Moor Green Lane, Moseley, Birmingham B13 8NT, UK
Carson Strong PhD	Associate Professor, Department of Human Values and Ethics, University of Tennessee, 956 Court Avenue, Suite B324, Memphis, Tennessee 38163, USA
Marianne Thoresen MD PhD	Neonatal Research Fellow, The National Hospital, 0027 Oslo 1, Norway
Yannis Tountas MD MPH	Assistant Professor of Social Medicine, University of Athens, Medical School, 24 Dimokritou Street, Athens 106 73, Greece

Robert M. Veatch PhD — Director and Professor of Medical Ethics, Kennedy Institute of Ethics; Professor, Philosophy Department and Medical Center, Georgetown University, Washington DC 20057, USA

Sir David Weatherall FRS — Honorary Director, Institute of Molecular Medicine, University of Oxford, John Radcliffe Hospital, Oxford OX3 9DU, UK

A Whitelaw MD FRCP — Associate Professor of Neonatology, The National Hospital, 0027 Oslo 1, Norway

Kevin William Wildes SJ MA MDiv — Managing Editor of the *Journal of Medicine and Philosophy*, Center for Ethics, Medicine and Public Issues, Baylor College of Medicine, One Baylor Plaza, Houston, Texas 77030, USA

Alan Williams — Professor of Economics, Centre for Health Economics, University of York, Heslington, York YO1 5DD, UK

Jenifer Wilson-Barnett — Professor of Nursing Studies, King's College, Chelsea Campus, 522 Kings Road, London SW10 0UA, UK

Henrik R. Wulff MD — Professor of Clinical Theory and Ethics, Consultant Physician, Herlev University Hospital, 2730 Herlev, Denmark

Preface: Medical Ethics and the Four Principles

RAANAN GILLON BA (PHILOSOPHY), MB, BS, FRCP (Lond)

*General Medical Practitioner; Director, Imperial College Health Service;
Visiting Professor of Medical Ethics, St Mary's Hospital Medical School/
Imperial College, London University; Editor, Journal of Medical Ethics*

Why this enormous book? It was conceived of two parental motives. The first was to provide a collection of papers accessible to English-speaking health care workers internationally, introducing the wide range of issues that comprise health care ethics from a wide variety of perspectives—a variety that was more international, multidisciplinary and less predominantly American bioethical, than earlier collections. The second motive was a desire to invite each writer at least to consider in his or her contribution a common moral theme—notably that of the four *prima facie* principles of health care ethics and their scope of application, developed by Beauchamp and Childress (1) and used and enthusiastically promoted in my own book (2), originally published as a series in the *British Medical Journal*. I asked the writers to refer to this underlying theme either by using it and or by criticising it. In this way I hoped that the book would acquire an additional 'sub-plot', and that the uses and limitations of the four principles plus scope approach would emerge. To what extent this has happened the reader will judge—but certainly the breadth and depth of analysis, description and insight offered by this volume's many authors has educated me. While I offer counter-arguments in Chapter 28 against those of their arguments that reject the four principles approach, the reader has an opportunity to confront the pros and cons—while browsing in the rich and varied pastures of health care ethics.

Since Beauchamp's opening chapter in this volume is substantially concerned with rebutting some of the philosophical objections that have been made against the four principles plus scope approach (and are made by some of the contributors to this book), and because a short summary might assist the reader who is unfamiliar with it and reluctant at this stage to consult the original source, I offer this introduction—my own potted account of the four principles and their scope from my perspective as a philosophically trained practising medical practitioner, with apologies to its originators for any unacceptable deviations from their own model. Interested readers are also referred to use of the model to analyse a particular case in general medical practice (3).

In brief, the four principles plus scope approach claims that whatever your personal philosophy, politics, religion, moral theory or life stance, you will find no difficulty in committing yourself to four *prima facie* moral principles plus a concern for their scope of application. Moreover these four principles plus attention to their scope of application can be seen to encompass most if not all of the moral issues that arise in health care (I am increasingly inclined to believe that the approach can, if sympathetically interpreted, be seen to encompass *all* moral issues, not merely those arising in health care). The principles are respect for autonomy, beneficence, non-maleficence and justice. 'Prima facie', a term introduced by the English philosopher W. D. Ross, means that the principle is binding unless it conflicts with another moral principle—if it does then you have to choose between them. The four principles approach does not claim to provide a method for doing so—a source of much dissatisfaction to those who suppose that ethics can be boiled down to a set of prioritised rules such that once the relevant information is fed into the algorithm (or computer) out will pop The Answer. What the principles plus scope approach *can* provide is a common set of moral commitments, a common moral language, and a common set of moral issues to be considered in particular cases, before coming to your own answer, using your preferred moral theory or other approach to choosing between these principles when they conflict (various different approaches are advocated in this book).

RESPECT FOR AUTONOMY

Autonomy—literally self rule, but probably better summarily described as deliberated self rule—is a special attribute of all moral agents, including ourselves. It involves deciding for ourselves on the basis of deliberation; sometimes it also involves intending to do things as a result of those decisions; and sometimes it involves going ahead and doing those things so as to implement the decisions (what I have previously described as autonomy of thought, of will or intention, and of action). Respect for autonomy is the moral obligation to respect the autonomy of others *in so far as such respect is compatible with equal respect for the autonomy of all potentially affected*. Respect for autonomy is also sometimes described, in Kantian terms, as treating others as 'ends in themselves' and never merely as means, one of Kant's formulations of his 'categorical imperative'.

In health care, treating people as ends, or respecting their autonomy, has many *prima facie* implications. It requires us to consult them and to obtain their agreement before we do things to them—hence the *prima facie* obligation to obtain informed consent from patients before we do things to try to help them. The *prima facie* obligation of medical confidentiality is another implication of respect for people's autonomy: it is not that people have any general obligation of confidentiality—but health care workers explicitly or implicitly *promise* their patients and clients to maintain the secrets they confide in them as confidential. Keeping promises is a way of respecting people's autonomy, for an aspect of running one's own life depends on being able to rely on the promises others make to one—thus people infringe our self rule or autonomy if they break their promises to us. (It is also true that without such promises of confidentiality patients are far less likely to divulge the often highly private and sensitive information that is needed for their optimal care—so not only does maintaining confidentiality respect patients' autonomy—it also increases the likelihood of our being able to benefit them). Respect for autonomy also requires us not to deceive each other, (except in circumstances where deceit is contextually agreed to be permissible), for non-deceit is part of the implicit agreement between moral agents when they communicate with each other. They organise their lives on the assumption that people will not deceive them; their ability to do so— their autonomy—is infringed if they are deceived. Respect for autonomy even requires us to be on time for appointments we make—for again promise-keeping is involved (agreeing an appointment is a kind of mutual promise-making) and breaking the appointment is breaking the promise.

Among the practical skills that respect for autonomy requires from health care workers is the ability to communicate well with patients and clients—including most importantly listening (and not just with the ears) as well as telling (and not just with the lips or word processor). Only through good communication will it generally be possible to give patients adequate information about any proposed intervention and find out from them their views about its desirability. Note, too, that only through good communication is it possible to discover when patients do *not* want a lot of information (for example *some* patients do not want to be told about a bad prognosis, or to be involved in deciding which of a variety of treatment options to have, preferring to leave such decision-making to their doctors). Respecting such decisions is also respecting a patient's autonomy, just as giving patients information that they do want is respecting their autonomy (and in practice, in my experience, most patients given the opportunity want more not less information, and do want to be involved in decision-making about their medical care).

Respect for autonomy is one of the themes that permeates very many of the contributions to this book, but of particular relevance are those by Engelhardt and Wildes, Furness, Cook, Dickens, Downie, Neuberger, Veatch and Mason Spicer, Kirby, Higgs, Holmes and Lindley, the two chapters by Fulford and Hope, Gray, Nowell-Smith, and Seller.

BENEFICENCE AND NON-MALEFICENCE

Whenever we try to benefit others we inevitably risk harming them—so in the context of health care, which is committed to benefiting others, it is essential to consider the principles of beneficence and non-maleficence together. (It is nonetheless important to retain the two principles as separate ones, precisely for those circumstances in which we have or acknowledge no obligation of beneficence to others—for we will still have obligations not to harm them). Thus the traditional moral obligation of medicine is to provide net benefit to patients, with minimal harm—beneficence in the context of non-maleficence. In order to achieve these moral objectives health care workers are committed to a wide range of *prima facie* obligations. First we need to ensure that we actually *can* provide the benefits we profess (hence, professional) to be able to provide. Hence the need for rigorous and effective educational and training programmes, both before and throughout our professional lives. We also need to make sure that what we are offering actually constitutes net-benefit for patients—and not just for patients in general but for the *particular* patients concerned. Interestingly in order to do so we must once again respect the patient's autonomy. What constitutes a net benefit for one patient may be a net harm for another (a blood transfusion to save our lives may constitute a net benefit for most of us—but for committed Jehovah's Witnesses it will constitute an overwhelmingly harmful assault: a radical mastectomy may constitute a prospective net benefit for one woman with breast cancer, while for another the perceived destruction of an aspect of her feminine identity may be so harmful that it cannot be outweighed by the prospect even of extending her life expectancy). Thus assessment of *how much* benefit and how much harm a proposed intervention will provide will turn to a large extent on the perceptions of the patients concerned.

As well as needing to be clear about how much harm and benefit we will produce, the obligation to provide net-benefit to patients also requires us to be clear about the role of *risk* and *probability* in making our assessments of harm and benefit. Clearly a very low probability of a very large harm, say death or major disability, is of less moral importance in the context of non-maleficence than is a very high probability of such harm: equally obviously a very high probability of major benefit, say cure of a life-threatening disease, is of more moral importance in the context of beneficence than is a very low probability of such benefit. Once such obvious points are acknowledged the need becomes equally obvious for empirical information about the probabilities of the various harms and benefits that may result from proposed health care interventions. In order to find out such information, and in order more generally to try to ensure that we provide net benefit to patients with minimal harm, we need to do effective medical research, so that too is a *prima facie* moral obligation. However, the obligation to produce net benefit also requires us to be clear (and to make clear) *whose* benefit and *whose* harms are likely to result from a proposed intervention. This moral scope problem is of especial importance in the context of medical research and also in the context of 'population medicine'—issues that are addressed by various contributors, including Henderson, Saunders Baum and Houghton, Jennett, Ackerman, Last, Garanis Tountas and Dalla-Vorgia, and McCallum.

One moral concept that has in recent years gained currency in health care is that of 'empowerment'—doing things to help patients and clients be more in control of their health and health care. Sometimes this is even proposed as a new moral obligation. On reflection, however, I think that empowerment is essentially action that combines the two moral obligations of beneficence and respect for autonomy so as to help patients in ways that not only respect but also enhance their autonomy. It is autonomy-enhancing beneficence. Pinching's contribution is particularly interesting in this context.

JUSTICE

The fourth *prima facie* moral principle is justice, often regarded as synonymous with fairness, and reasonably summarised as the moral obligation to act on the basis of fair adjudication between competing claims. For practical purposes I have found it useful to subdivide obligations of justice into three categories; justice as fair distribution of scarce resources (distributive justice), justice as respect for people's rights (rights-based justice), and justice as respect for morally acceptable laws (legal justice). Equality is at the heart of justice, of whichever category, but as Aristotle argued so long ago (4), equality is not all there is to justice, for in a variety of ways people may be unjustly treated if they are treated equally. The important thing, he argued, was to treat equals equally, and to treat unequals unequally, in proportion to the morally relevant inequalities. People have argued ever since—and continue to argue—about what are the morally relevant substantive criteria for regarding and treating people as equals and for regarding and treating them as unequals. These are issues of continuing vigorous moral, religious, philosophical and political debate and we are no closer to agreement than we were in 1985 when I wrote 'I have not yet discovered a way to give consistent moral priority to any of these substantive criteria . . . . (and I do not really expect to do so)' (2).

A wide variety of alternative approaches exist, of which several are outlined in this book (including Hare on a utilitarian approach, Williams on economics and a quality-adjusted-life-years approach, Engelhardt and Wildes on a libertarian approach, Luther and Schubert-Lehnhardt on Marxist approaches, Doyal on a needs-based approach, Dickens on legal approaches, Dowie on a decision-analytic approach, Almond on a rights-based approach, Maxwell on a health-care-management approach and Jennett on a multifaceted-medical-professional approach. The variety of these approaches to justice affords good evidence of the lack of substantive agreement in this area.

Pending such agreement health care workers need to tread warily, for we have no special justification for imposing our own personal or professional views about justice on others. We certainly need to recognise and acknowledge the competing moral concerns. For example, in the context of resource allocation there are conflicts between the following common moral concerns: to provide sufficient health care to meet the needs of all who need it; when this is impossible, to distribute health care resources in proportion to the extent of people's health care needs; to allow health care workers to give priority to the needs of *their* patients; to provide equality of access to health care; to allow people as much choice as possible in the selection of their health care; to maximise the benefit produced by the available resources; to limit the demands on the purses of those who provide those resources, whether as tax-payers or as subscribers to health insurance schemes. All these criteria for just allocation of health care resources have moral justifications (and there are other candidates too), and not all can simultaneously be fully met.

Similar moral conflict arises in the other two categories, rights-based justice and legal justice.

The best moral strategy that I have been able to devise for myself as a health care worker in the context of these complex dilemmas of justice is first to distinguish those dilemmas in which *I* am required to decide from those in which the decision is organisational, professional or societal. For decisions that I must make myself, my first objective is to exclude decisions that simply have no moral basis or justification. Pursuit of my own self-interest (for example by accepting bribes from patients, hospitals or drug manufacturers) is not a just or morally acceptable basis for allocation of scarce health care resources or for any other category of justice. Nor is action that disadvantages patients on the basis of personal preference or prejudice (we mere mortals almost certainly can't avoid *having* personal preferences and prejudices—but we can at least try very hard to ensure that these do not unjustly affect our patients). Nor is it my role as a doctor to punish patients—so withholding antibiotics from smokers who do not give up smoking, or refusing to refer for specialist assessment heavy drinkers with alcohol-induced liver damage, or patients who regret the tattoos they earlier chose for themselves, on the grounds that 'they brought it on themselves, they have only themselves to blame', is not a just or morally acceptable basis for *my* rationing medical resources in the course of my clinical practice. (If I want such criteria to be introduced into the rationing process I have the same rights as any other citizen to use the democratic process to try to persuade society of their merits). So far as positive allocation decisions go, I have no doubt that I ought not to waste the resources at my disposal. So if a cheaper medication can be expected to produce as much benefit as a more expensive one, I ought to prescribe the cheaper one. Cost and its team mate opportunity cost are *moral* issues, central to distributive justice. On the other hand if I believe that an expensive medication is clearly and significantly better for my patient than a cheaper alternative, and I am allowed to prescribe it, then I believe that I should do so. (Here I am giving priority to my obligation to benefit my patient over my obligation in distributive justice to save costs, even though those saved resources might produce more benefit for others than they will for my patient. Again I recognise that society, through its democratic processes, may legitimately decide to prevent me from having the choice of prescribing the expensive alternative).

I ought to respect patients' rights. For example, my possible disapproval of the life-style of a patient would not be a morally acceptable justification for refusing to provide a certificate of sickness—in the UK if he or she is unable to work because of sickness he or she has *a right* to such a certificate, and I should provide it. On the other hand I have no special privilege as a health care worker to create rights for my patients. For example, while I might think that all my unemployed patients should receive sickness benefit, they only have a *right* to receive it if they are unable to work as a result of sickness; and I only have a right to sign sickness benefit certificates if such is the case.

I ought to obey morally acceptable laws. Thus even though I may disapprove of breaking my patient's confidences, if he or she has one of a variety of infectious diseases I am legally obliged to notify the relevant authorities. (Of course I may believe that the law is morally unjustified, in which case I am *morally* entitled to break the law. But I shall have to be clear that this gives me no legal entitlement to break the law, and I shall have to be prepared to face the legal consequences of disobeying it. And I shall have to distinguish clearly in my mind about what exactly I mean by a morally unjustified law. I would argue—though here merely suggest—that it is the processes whereby laws are enacted that confer moral legitimacy, not the content of the laws. Thus if a law is enacted through a democratic—and hence fundamentally autonomy-respecting—political system that represents conflicting views within its population, and whose law-making system is committed to certain moral values—for convenience representable under the rubric of the four principles—then I believe that that law is morally acceptable, and *prima facie* we are morally required to obey it).

For those decisions about justice that are organisational, professional or societal my role in determining them should only be that of a member of the relevant organisation, profession, or society. Thus using this strategy it is morally consistent to pursue at different levels objectives that are themselves mutually inconsistent. My 'medical directorate' in my hospital may have legitimately excluded the use of a particularly expensive medication. As a member of that organisational group I may have argued in favour of its use in special cases but my arguments, having been heard, have been rejected. It is morally proper for me to accept the directorate's decisions, and to act accordingly even when faced as a clinician with the exceptional case in which the expensive medication would have been preferable, and even though I continue to believe that the patient would benefit from the more expensive but proscribed medication. It is *also* morally legitimate for me to point to such cases ('shroud waving') when exercising my political role as a member of a democratic society and, for example, arguing the case for more resources to be put into health care rather than, say, defence.

We are still feeling our way even at the level of making explicit what the competing moral concerns of justice are. Meanwhile it is important to be particularly wary of apparently simple solutions to what for at least 2500 years have been perceived as highly complex problems. For example, in the context of distributive justice, populist solutions, as in Oregon, USA (5), and technical economists' solutions as with the costed QALY system (6), are tempting in their definitiveness and relative simplicity—but they fail to give value to the wide range of other potentially relevant moral concerns. Until there is far greater social agreement and indeed understanding of these exceedingly complex issues, I believe that it is morally safer to seek gradual improvement in our current methods of trying to reconcile the competing moral concerns—to seek ways of 'muddling through elegantly' as Hunter advocates (7), rather than to be seduced by systems that seek to convert these essentially moral choices into apparently scientific numerical methods and formulae. As Calabresi and Bobbitt suggested in the '70s, rationing of scarce life-prolonging and health-enhancing resources often involves 'tragic choices'—choices between people, choices between values. Societies adopt strategies to minimise the destructive effect of such choices, including the strategy of changing those strategies as they become increasingly unpopular (8). To pursue a metaphor of Calabresi's, in pursuing justice we are like a juggler trying to keep too many balls in the air, but whose audience is not prepared to let any one ball stay on the ground for long. Like the juggler we must do our best to improve our juggling skills so as to keep more balls in the air for more of the time, and so as to avoid letting any ball stay on the ground for too long; but like the juggler too we must, I believe, simply accept that in contexts of *competing and mutually incompatible claims*; not all the balls can always be in the air—there will always be some on the ground. Nor, in practical terms, should we be surprised that some people will always be dissatisfied even after justice has been done—for by definition not everyone's claims can be met.

SCOPE

We may agree on our substantive moral commitments, we may agree about our *prima facie* moral obligations in terms of respect for autonomy, beneficence, non-maleficence and justice, and yet we may still disagree, perhaps radically, about their scope of application. That is, we may disagree radically about to what or to whom we owe these moral obligations. Interesting and important theoretical issues are outstanding in regard to the scope of each of the four principles. It seems clear that we cannot owe a duty of beneficence to everyone and everything that could be benefited: so who or what do we have a moral duty to benefit? And *how much ought* we to benefit them? While it is reasonably clear that we have a *prima facie* obligation not to harm everyone (ie that the scope of non-maleficence is universal) who and what *count* as 'everyone'? Similarly, even if we agree that the scope of the principle of respect for autonomy is universal, encompassing all autonomous agents, just who or what *counts* as an autonomous (or adequately autonomous) agent? And in the context of justice, who or what falls within the scope of our obligation to distribute scarce resources fairly? (Is it everyone in the world? Future people? Just people in our own countries? Who?) And who or what have rights? (Do plants have rights? Does the environment have rights? Does a work of art have rights? Do animals have rights? And if so, *which* animals, what rights?). Conversely, against whom may holders of rights claim the correlative moral obligation? And while the scope of (morally acceptable) laws at first may seem fairly clear (those whom the lawmakers properly encompass within the scope of their laws!), what constitutes 'properly' in this context? Much philosophical and other reflection and research is required to clarify answers to these broad questions.

Fortunately for health care workers some of these issues of scope have been clarified for them by virtue of their special relationship with their patients or clients. In particular the controversial issue of who falls within the scope of beneficence—i.e. whom do we owe a duty to benefit?—is answered unambiguously for at least one category of people; all health care workers have a moral obligation to benefit their patients and or clients: that is, patients or clients fall within the scope of the duty of beneficence of their health care workers. This fact is established by the personal and professional commitments of the health care professionals themselves and of their organisations (they all *profess* a commitment to benefit their patients and clients, and to do so with minimal harm); and this commitment is underwritten by the societies within which they practise, both informally, and formally through legal rules and regulations that define the *duties of care* (i.e. duties of beneficence with minimal harm) of health care professionals. Many of the chapters in the second section of this book address issues of scope arising in the context of health care relationships.

Two issues of scope are of particular practical importance for health care workers. The first is the question: Who falls within the scope of the *prima facie* principle of respect for autonomy? The second is: what is the scope of the widely acknowledged 'right to life'—who, and indeed what, has a 'right to life'? Obviously only autonomous agents can fall within the scope of the principle of respect for autonomy—one simply cannot respect the autonomy of a boot or a slug, nor of anything else that is not autonomous. But who or what *counts* as an autonomous agent? When we disagree about whether or not to respect the decision of a girl of fourteen to take the oral contraceptive pill, we are in effect disagreeing about the scope of application of the principle of respect for autonomy: (Yes, fourteen-year-olds are adequately autonomous to have their deliberated decisions on such medication respected v. no, they are not). Similar questions about the scope of respect for autonomy arise in other paediatric contexts, in care of the severely mentally ill or impaired, and in care of the elderly when those elderly are severely mentally impaired, as by dementia. Some patients clearly do not fall within the scope of respect for autonomy—newborn babies, for example, are not autonomous agents—for autonomy requires the capacity to deliberate. But seven-year-olds usually can deliberate—to a degree. How much capacity for logical thought and deliberation, and what other attributes are required for somebody to be an 'adequately autonomous agent'? (Possible candidates include: an adequately extensive and accurate knowledge base—including that provided by experience and perception—upon which to deliberate; an ability to conceive of and reflect about oneself over time, past and future; an ability to reason hypothetically—'what if?' reasoning; an ability to defer gratification for oneself as an aspect of one's self rule; and sufficient will power for self rule.)

However these philosophical questions are answered, in the context of health care it is increasingly acknowledged that the autonomy of even quite young children and of quite severely mentally impaired patients ought *prima facie* to be respected unless there are good *moral* reasons not to do so. Moreover those reasons will be highly context-relative—a young child, or a severely mentally impaired patient, may not be adequately autonomous to have decisions to reject an operation respected—but be entirely adequately autonomous to decide what food to eat or clothes to wear. Where patients are not adequately autonomous for their decisions to be respected, if those decisions appear to be against their interests, important issues arise about who should be regarded as 'proper proxies' to make decisions on their behalf, and on what criteria. The importance of societal involvement in clarifying such issues, whether formally through law or more informally, emerges in various chapters addressing these issues directly or obliquely, including those by Graham, Holmes and Lindley, Fulford and Hope, Muir Gray, Norberg and Dame Cicely Saunders. In addition a helpful international discussion on proxy decision-making in the context of forgoing life-prolonging treatment is to be found in the Appleton Conference document (9).

The second important practical issue of scope concerns the universally acknowledged 'right to life'. Who or what has this right to life? To answer the question it is of course important to be clear about what is meant by 'right to life'. Specifically, is it simply the right not to be unjustly killed; or is it that plus a right to be maintained alive? The scope of the first right will clearly be greater than the scope of the latter (i.e. we have moral obligations not to kill all people; we have obligations to keep alive only some people). Even in the context of the first sense of 'right to life'—a right not be unjustly killed—there is still a question of scope; for while it is clear that all *people* fall within its scope, do (non-human) animals have a right to life—and if so, which sorts of animal? (In this context see the last two chapters by Sprigge and Frey on the use of animals in biomedical experimentation). And what do we mean by 'people' in this context? It is in response to this latter question that much debate—often extremely acrimonious—arises in health care ethics over the right to life of human embryos, fetuses, newborn babies (born at various stages of fetal development), and at the other end of the spectrum, patients who are permanently unconscious and even those who are brain dead. Various chapters in this book address these issues, including those by Mori, Finnis, Lloyd, Fagot-Largeault, Strong and Anderson, Whitelaw and Thoreson, Davis, Harris, Nowell-Smith, Gormally, Braude, Lamb and M Evans.

It is salutary to reflect that these contentious issues are not about the content of our moral obligations—about what those obligations *are*—but rather about to whom and what we owe them, i.e. they are questions about the scope of our agreed moral obligations. They are questions about which there are reasoned and carefully argued but deeply conflicting views. Disagreement, for example, about the permissibility of research on human embryos or about the permissibility of abortion, does not reflect intractable moral relativism, or irresoluble disagreement about our moral obligations to each other. Rather it reflects philosophical and or religious disagreement about what we mean by each other—about the attributes of human embryos and fetuses and consequently about whether they fall within the scope of our agreed moral obligation not unjustly to kill each other. It is disagreement about which we can, do and should argue rationally and vigorously. It is *not* disagreement that justifies accusing all those who disagree with us of bad faith or incompatible moral standards. Rather, it is disagreement about *the scope* of our shared moral commitment to the principles of respect for autonomy, beneficence, non-maleficence and justice; moreover it is disagreement that, at least in principle, is open to resolution within a shared moral commitment.

This preface would be incomplete without my thanks to all who have participated in the project. Most important of all, of course, are the many contributors who have combined to produce a collection of enormous range, variety and intellectual stimulation. My particular thanks to my Assistant Editor, Ann Lloyd, without whose unflagging determination and hard editorial work this volume would never have been published.

REFERENCES

1. Beauchamp T, Childress J, 1989. *Principles of biomedical ethics*, 3rd ed. Oxford University Press, New York, Oxford.
2. Gillon R, 1985, and subsequent reprints. *Philosophical medical ethics*. Wiley, Chichester.
3. Gillon R, 1989. Ethics in a college health service. In: Dunstan G R, Shineborne E A, eds, 1989. *Doctors' decisions—ethical conflicts in medical practice*. Oxford University Press, Oxford, New York.
4. Aristotle. Nichomachean ethics, Book 5 and Politics, Book 3, Chapter 9.
5. Klein R, 1991. On the Oregon trail: rationing health care—more politics than science. *British Medical Journal*, **302**: 1–2.
6. Williams A, 1993. Economics, society and health care ethics. This volume, Chapter 71, p. 829.
7. Hunter D J, 1993. Rationing dilemmas in health care. NAHAT (National Association of Health Authorities and Trusts), *Research Paper No 8*. NAHAT, Birmingham.
8. Calabresi G, Bobbitt P, 1978. *Tragic choices*. Norton, New York.
9. Stanley J, ed., 1992. The Appleton International Conference: Developing guidelines for decisions to forgo life-prolonging medical treatment. *Journal of medical ethics*. **18** (3): (supplement).

PART I

APPROACHES TO APPLIED HEALTH CARE ETHICS

1

The 'Four-principles' Approach

*Professor of Philosophy, Joseph and Rose Kennedy Institute of Ethics,
Georgetown University, USA*

This essay presents and supports the four-principles approach to health care ethics that Jim Childress and I developed almost two decades ago (1). The principles included in the framework are:

1. Beneficence (the obligation to provide benefits and balance benefits against risks).
2. Non-maleficence (the obligation to avoid the causation of harm).
3. Respect for autonomy (the obligation to respect the decision-making capacities of autonomous persons).
4. Justice (obligations of fairness in the distribution of benefits and risks).

Rules for health care ethics can be formulated by reference to these four principles, together with other moral considerations, although these rules cannot be straightforwardly *deduced* from the principles, because additional interpretation and specification is needed. Such rules include rules of truth-telling, confidentiality, privacy and fidelity, as well as more specific guidelines pertaining to problems such as physician-assisted suicide, informed consent, withdrawing treatment, using randomized clinical trials.

In the four-principles approach, moral principles in their bare form as principles are little more than abstract rallying points for reflection. Principles are starting, foundational points in health care ethics, not solely sufficient or final appeals. The four principles, as well as rules such as 'Don't kill' and 'Tell the truth', do not give us much more information about how to lead our lives than such admonitions as 'Be competent' or 'Act virtuously'. All skeletal moral norms must be embedded in and then interpreted for specific contexts; that is, there must be some means to clothe them with a specific content that develops their meaning, implications, complexity, limits, exceptions, and the like.

In the first section I motivate the analysis of the four principles by arguing that some of the principles have played an important historical role, whereas

Principles of Health Care Ethics. Edited by Raanan Gillon.
© 1994 John Wiley & Sons Ltd

others came into prominence because of distinctively modern problems. In the second section I connect the principles to models of moral responsibility in medicine. In the third section I discuss the normative character of principles, particularly their status as *prima-facie* moral principles. Then, in the fourth section, I discuss some recent criticisms of the four-principles approach to health care ethics, especially those who refer to the account as *principlism* and reject it altogether. In the penultimate section I discuss the need to interpret and specify these principles for particular contexts, and also the need for a method known as 'reflective equilibrium'. Finally, in the Conclusion, I connect the previous five sections to the thesis that there is no canon of principles for biomedical ethics.

I cannot here engage in extended philosophical argument about the meaning and commitments of these principles. Instead, I try to express why principles are important and why these particular principles provide a useful, but not canonical, framework for health care ethics.

THE FRAMEWORK AND ITS ROOTS IN HEALTH CARE

Recent systematic and theoretical work in health care ethics tends to converge to the conclusion that moral responsibility in medicine ideally should be conceived in terms of fundamental principles, rules, rights, and virtues. Many controversies in health care ethics turn on the precise moral content of these guidelines, as well as on how much weight they have in particular contexts, how conflicts among the notions are to be handled, and how to specify their precise significance for particular circumstances.

Some moral guidelines seem to be best framed as rules, others as standards of virtue, others as rights, and others as principles. Although rules, rights, and virtues are unquestionably of the highest importance for health care ethics, I believe principles provide the most comprehensive starting point, for reasons I shall try to make clear as we proceed. Other principles may be relevant to moral judgement. Nothing in the four-principles approach makes a claim to have assembled the only worthwhile listing of relevant principles.

The justification for choosing the particular four moral guidelines I am defending is in part historical—that is, some of the principles are deeply embedded in medical traditions of health care ethics—and in part that the principles point to an important part of morality that has been traditionally neglected in health care ethics but now needs to be placed at the foreground. To defend these claims I shall first briefly discuss some aspects of the history of health care ethics.

Throughout the centuries the health professional's obligations, rights, and virtues, as found in codes and learned writings on ethics, have been conceived through professional commitments to shield patients from harm and provide medical care, expressed in ethical terms as fundamental obligations of non-maleficence and beneficence. Medical beneficence has long been viewed as the proper goal of medicine, and professional dedication to this goal has been viewed as essential to being a physician.

The principle of beneficence expresses an obligation to help others further their important and legitimate interests by preventing and removing harms; no less important is the obligation to weigh and balance possible goods against the possible harms of an action. This principle of beneficence potentially demands more than the principle of non-maleficence because it requires positive steps to help others, not merely the omission of harm-causing activities.

The principle of non-maleficence has long been associated in medicine with the injunction *primum non nocere*: 'Above all [or first] do no harm'. This maxim has been mistakenly attributed to the Hippocratic tradition, but the Hippocratic corpus does proclaim both a duty of non-maleficence and a duty of beneficence; together they carve out a conception of medical ethics in which the overriding principle is acting for the patient's best medical best interest (2,3). This Hippocratic tradition was carried forward from medieval to modern medicine as an ideal of moral commitment and behavior.

From the perspective of the English-speaking world it was British physician Thomas Percival who furnished the first well-shaped doctrine of health care ethics. Easily the dominant influence in both British and American health care ethics of the period, Percival argued that non-maleficence and beneficence fix the physician's primary obligations and triumph over the patient's rights of autonomy in any serious circumstance of conflict:

> To a patient...who makes inquiries which, if faithfully answered, might prove fatal to him, it would be a gross and unfeeling wrong to reveal the truth. His right to it is suspended, and even annihilated; because, its beneficial nature being reversed, it would be deeply injurious to himself, to his family, and to the public. And he has the strongest claim, from the trust reposed in his physician, as well as from the common principles of humanity, to be guarded against whatever would be detrimental to him....The only point at issue is, whether the practitioner shall sacrifice that delicate sense of veracity, which is so ornamental to, and indeed forms a characteristic excellence of the virtuous man, to this claim of professional justice and social duty (4).

Like the Hippocratic physicians, Percival moved from the premise of the patient's best medical interest as the proper goal of the physician's actions to descriptions of the physician's proper deportment, including traits of character such as benevolence and sympathetic tenderness that maximize the patient's welfare.

Percival's work served as the pattern for the American Medical Association's (AMA) first code of ethics in 1847. Many passages were taken verbatim from his book. But much more than Percival's language survived in America: his beneficence-based viewpoint on ethics gradually became the creed of professional conduct in the United States. Beneficence and non-maleficence became through his delineations the landmark principles that gave shape to health care ethics. These two principles remained until very recently the most prominent values in the major writings on medical ethics in the patient–physician relationship.

In recent years, however, the idea has emerged—largely from writings in law and philosophy—that the proper model of the physician's moral responsibility should be understood less in terms of traditional ideals of medical benefit, and more in terms of the rights of patients, including autonomy-based rights to truthfulness, confidentiality, privacy, disclosure and consent, as well as welfare rights rooted in claims of justice. These proposals have jolted medicine from its traditional preoccupation with a beneficence-based model of health care ethics in the direction of an autonomy model, as well as into a confrontation with a wider set of social concerns.

The principle of respect for autonomy is rooted in the liberal western tradition of the importance of individual freedom, both for political life and for personal development. 'Autonomy' and 'respect for autonomy' are terms loosely associated with several ideas, such as privacy, voluntariness, choosing freely, and accepting responsibility for one's choices.

Finally, *the principle of justice* is really many principles about the distribution of benefits and burdens, not a single principle. Several distributive theories of justice have been put forth, and to a limited extent these theories give us anchors in health care ethics. To cite one example, an egalitarian theory of justice implies that if there is a departure from equality in the distribution of health care benefits and burdens, such a departure must serve the common good and enhance the position of those who are least advantaged in society.

Of course there are other theories of justice than the egalitarian theory. For example, utilitarian theories emphasize a mixture of criteria so that public utility is maximized, comparable to the way public health policy has often been formulated in western nations. In the distribution of health care utilitarians see justice as involving trade-offs and balances. In devising a system of public funding for health care the utilitarian believes we must balance public and private benefit, predicted cost savings, the probability of failure, the magnitude of risks, etc. Under this theory a just distribution of the benefits and burdens of research is to be determined by the utility of research to all affected by the research.

The arrival of a new health care ethics emphasizing autonomy rights and justice-based rights is not surprising, in light of recent social history. It seems likely that both increased legal interest and increased ethical interest in the professional–patient relationship and in a variety of topics of social justice are but instances of a new civil-rights orientation that various social movements of the past 30 years introduced. The issues raised by minority rights, women's rights, the consumer movement, and the rights of prisoners, the homeless, and the mentally ill often included health care components such as reproductive rights, rights of access to abortion and contraception, the right to health care information, access to care, and rights to be protected against unwarranted human experimentation.

One result of these developments has been to introduce both confusion and constructive change into medicine and health care institutions, which continue to struggle with unprecedented challenges to their authority in the control and treatment of patients. Several justice-based controversies in contemporary public policy have added to the confusion in the attempt to determine what is fair or owed when scarce medical resources must be rationed, or when third parties have interests and rights in the treatment or non-treatment of an individual.

These problems in health care ethics cannot be addressed here. The point of this section has simply been to explain the background and motivation for the acceptance of four moral principles.

MODELS AND THEIR UNDERLYING PRINCIPLES

I spoke above of 'models' of health care ethics (or of responsibility in providing health care). These are philosophically loaded ideas that give shape to what is only inchoate and unsystematically formed in the history of medical practice and health care ethics.* The 'autonomy model' refers to the view that responsibilities to the patient of disclosure, confidentiality, privacy, and consent-seeking are established primarily (perhaps exclusively) by the moral principle of respect for autonomy. The conflict between this principle and the principle of beneficence, of course the mainstay behind the beneficence model, can be expressed as follows: the physician's responsibilities are conceived in terms of the physician's primary obligation to provide medical benefits. The management of information is therefore understood in terms of the management of patients ('due care') generally. That is, the physician's primary obligation in handling information and in making recommendations is understood in terms of maximizing the patient's medical benefits, not in terms of respecting the patient's autonomous choices.

The central problem of authority in these discussions has become whether an autonomy model of medical practice should be given practical priority over the beneficence model, and whether even some combination of the two is adequate to address many problems of social justice to which health care finds itself inextricably linked. Major conflicts of value occur between autonomy and beneficence. For example, some health care professionals will accept a patient's refusal as valid, whereas others will ignore the fact that no consent has been given, and so try to 'benefit' the patient through a medical intervention. The difference between these two models can be understood in terms of the underlying principled justifications at work. The premise that authority rests with patients or subjects should be justified, according to proponents of the autonomy model, *not* by arguments from beneficence to the effect that decisional autonomy by patients enables them to survive, heal, or otherwise improve their own health, but solely by the principle of respect for autonomy. Similarly in research settings, a proponent of the autonomy model holds that requiring the consent of subjects must be based on the principle of respect for autonomy, and never solely on the premise that consent protects subjects from risks.

Both respect for autonomy and beneficence are valid moral principles, and both are of the highest importance for health care ethics. I shall return momentarily to the problem of how to handle conflicts between the two principles.

THE NORMATIVE NATURE OF PRINCIPLES

Principles in the four-principles approach should be conceived neither as rules of thumb nor as absolute prescriptions. Rather, they are *prima facie*: they are always binding *unless* they conflict with obligations expressed in another moral principle, in which case a balancing of the demands of the two principles is

---

* See ref. 5, esp. pp. 26–27.

necessary. In this event, further specification is required of the precise commitments of the guidelines for the special circumstance(s). Which principle overrides in a case of conflict will depend on the particular context, which is likely to have unique features.

This method of 'overriding' duties by other duties might seem precariously flexible, as if moral guidelines in the end lack mettle and mainstay. But this is a misunderstanding. It is true that in ethics, as in all walks of life, there is no escape from the exercise of judgement in circumstances of uncertainty; but not just any judgement will be acceptable. For an infringement of a moral principle or rule to be justified the infringement must be necessary in the circumstances, in the sense that there are no morally preferable alternative actions that could be substituted, and the form of infringement selected must constitute the least infringement possible.

RECENT CRITIQUES OF PRINCIPLISM

Not everyone agrees that these four principles, or any principles, provide the best framework for health care ethics. Some have severely criticized the four-principles approach as a 'mantra of principles', meaning that the principles have functioned for some adherents like a ritual incantation of norms repeated with little reflection or analysis. The most sustained and best-argued attack on principle-based ethics has come from K. Danner Clouser and Bernard Gert in a critique of 'principlism' (6), a term they use to designate all theories that rely on a plural body of potentially conflicting *prima facie* principles (but especially ours and William Frankena's).

In particular, Gert and Clouser bring the following accusations against our four-principle system: (1) the 'principles' are little more than checklists or headings for lists of values worth remembering, and so the principles have no deep moral substance and do not produce directive guidelines for moral conduct; (2) principle analyses fail to provide a theory of justification or a theory that ties the principles together so as to generate clear, coherent, specific rules, with the consequence that the principles and so-called derivative rules are *ad hoc* constructions without systematic order; (3) these *prima facie* principles must often compete in difficult circumstances, yet the underlying account is unable to decide how to adjudicate the conflict in particular cases and unable theoretically to deal with a conflict of principles.

I do not deny that these are important problems, worthy of the most careful and sustained reflection in moral theory. I do deny, however, that Clouser and Gert—or anyone else who uses either a principle-based or rule-based theory (as they do)—have surmounted the very problems they list for our four-principles approach. The primary difference between what Childress and I call principles and they call rules is that their rules tend (as they point out) to have a more directive and specific content than our principles, thereby superficially seeming to give more guidance in the moral life. But we have pointed out this very fact since our first edition (in 1979). We have always accepted specific rules, not merely principles, as essential for health care ethics. There is also not more and not less normative content between their rules and our rules; not more and not less direction in the moral life. It is true that principles order and classify more than they lay down directive moral law, and therefore principles do have more of a 'heading'-like character, but what we say about rules is noticeably similar to what Clouser and Gert say about rules, and with a similar content.

The principles Childress and I defend are not constructed with an eye to eliminating possible conflicts among the principles, because no system of guidelines could reasonably anticipate the full range of conflicts. No set of principles or general guidelines can provide mechanical solutions or definitive procedures for decision-making about moral problems in medicine. Experience and sound judgement are indispensable allies.

So far as I can see, the major difference between our theory and the Clouser/Gert approach has nothing to do with whether principles or rules are the primary normative guides in a theory, but rather with several aspects of their theory that I, at least, would reject. First, they assume that there is or at least can be what they call a 'well-developed unified theory' that removes conflicting principles and consistently expresses the grounds of correct judgement—in effect, a canon of rules that expresses the 'unity and universality of morality'. They fault us heavily for believing that more than one kind of ethical theory can justify a moral belief. They insist that to avoid relativism there can only be 'a single unified ethical theory', and that there cannot be 'several sources of final justification' (ref. 6, pp. 231–232). These are all claims that I would reject, although there is no space to engage in such tussles here.

I must now bring this discussion of Gert and Clouser's criticism to a conclusion, in order to deal with two problems that grow out of their criticisms. First, a major problem in health care ethics, for our critics as well as for us, is how to interpret and make more specific the principles and rules in the system—so as to give them more determinative content for practice and help in the resolution of particular problems. I will sketch a solution to this problem in the next section. Second, Gert and Clouser say that

> In formulating theory we start with particular moral judgments about which we are certain, and we abstract and formulate the relevant features of those cases to help us in turn to decide the unclear cases (ref. 6, p. 232).

This is precisely the model Childress and I have supported since the first edition. I will also discuss this problem of methodology in the next section.

THE NEED FOR SPECIFICATION AND REFLECTIVE EQUILIBRIUM

The philosopher G. W. F. Hegel properly criticized Immanuel Kant for developing a moral theory of 'empty formalism' that preached obligation for obligation's sake, without any power to develop what Hegel called an 'immanent doctrine of duties'. He thought all 'content and specification' in a living code of ethics had been replaced by abstractness in Kant's account (7). The four-principles analysis has been similarly accused,* and I believe the criticism does rightly

---

* In addition to Clouser and Gert (6), see Toulmin (8), pp. 31–39.

point to a serious gap in contemporary health care ethics. Every ethical theory, and indeed morality itself, contain regions of indeterminacy that need to be reduced through further development of principles, augmenting them with a more specific moral content.

Here is an example of the problem: if non-maleficence is the principle that we ought not to inflict evil or harm, this principle does little to give specific guidance for the moral problem of whether active voluntary euthanasia can be morally justified. If we question whether physicians ought to be allowed to be the agents of euthanasia, we again get no real guidance. Although abstract guidelines provide relevant considerations, they must be developed into concrete action-guides, taking into consideration such factors as efficiency, institutional rules, law, clientele acceptance, and the like. That is, in addition to abstract principles there must be mediating rules that translate an ethical theory into a practical strategy and set of meaningful guidelines for real-world problems involving demands of efficiency, political procedures, legal constraints, uncertainty about risk, and the like.

In light of indeterminacy at the heart of principles, I follow Henry Richardson (9) in arguing that the specification of principles and related rules involves a filling in of details so as to overcome apparent moral conflicts. The process of specification is the progressive, substantive delineation of principles, pulling them out of abstractness and making them into concrete rules.

The following is a simple example of specification. The principle 'doctors should always* put their patients' interests first' has long been advanced as foundational for medical ethics. But suppose the only way to advance the patient's interest is to act illegally by purchasing a kidney from someone who needs the money. It hardly follows from the principle of patient-priority that a physician should act illegally by purchasing or using someone's organ. The original principle needs specification so as to give better, more fully stated moral advice. We might start on this project by replacing the principle of patient-priority, in its spare form, with the following more concrete rule: 'physicians should place their patients' interests first using all means that are both morally and legally acceptable'.

This principle itself will need further specification in other circumstances of conflict; in fact, progressive specification usually must take place, gradually eliminating the dilemmas and circumstances of conflict that the abstract principle itself has insufficient content to resolve. All moral norms are, in principle, subject to such further revision and specification. The reason, as Richardson nicely puts it, is that 'the complexity of the moral phenomena always outruns our ability to capture them in general norms'.

There are, however, tangled problems about the best method to use in order to achieve specification, and how we know whether any particular proposed specification is justified. The model of analysis for reaching specification and justification in health care ethics that Childress and I have long used is that of

---

* Richardson (9), p. 294. ('Always' in this formulation should perhaps be understood to mean 'in principle always'; specification may, in some cases, reach a final form.) For an example of elementary specification (but not so called) using the four-principles approach, see Raanan Gillon (10).

a dialectical balancing of principles against other encountered moral considerations, in an attempt to achieve general coherence and a mutual support among
the accepted norms. As Joel Feinberg suggests, moral reasoning is analogous to
the dialectical process that occurs in courts of law. If a legal principle commits
a judge to some unacceptable judgement, the judge needs to modify or
supplement the principle in a way that does the least damage to the judge's
beliefs about the law. Yet, if a well-founded principle demands a change in a
particular judgement, the overriding claims of consistency with precedent may
require that the judgement be adjusted, not the principle. Sometimes both
judgements and principles need revision (11).

One method of special importance for the specification of principles is
'reflective equilibrium', a method formulated by John Rawls for use in general
ethical theory. It views the acceptance of principles in ethics as properly
beginning with our 'considered judgements', those moral convictions in which
we have the highest confidence, and which we believe to have the lowest level
of bias. The goal of reflective equilibrium is to match, prune, and develop
considered judgements and principles in an attempt to make them coherent. We
start with the paradigms of what is morally proper or morally improper. We
then search for principles that are consistent with these paradigms and consistent
with each other (12).

'Considered judgements' is in effect a technical term referring to 'judgements
in which our moral capacities are most likely to be displayed without distortion'.
Examples are judgements about the wrongness of racial discrimination, religious
intolerance, and political conflict of interest. But, as Rawls puts it, considered
judgements occur at all levels of generality in our moral thinking: 'from those
about particular situations and institutions through broad standards and first
principles to formal and abstract conditions' (13). Widely accepted principles of
right action (moral beliefs) are thus taken, as Rawls puts it, 'provisionally as
fixed points', but also as 'liable to revision'.

By using reflective equilibrium, general ethical principles and particular
judgements can be brought into equilibrium. From this perspective, moral
thinking is like other forms of theorizing in that hypotheses must be tested,
buried, or modified through experimental thinking. A specified principle, then,
is acceptable in the system if it heightens the mutual support of the guidelines
in the system that have themselves been found acceptable using reflective
equilibrium.

CONCLUSION

Health care ethics is often said to be an 'applied ethics', but this metaphor may
be as misleading as it is helpful. There is no such thing as a simple 'application'
of a principle so as to resolve a complicated moral problem. It is no less
misleading to suggest that those who engage in ethical theory can produce all
relevant moral guidelines or crank out conclusions that immediately follow from
principles. Ethical theory using principles invites us to reason through our moral
dilemmas and offers some ways of doing so. But general ethical theory has long

contained within its own fabric a sustained body of controversies, and it needs careful development to serve the needs of health care ethics.

Among the advantages of 'principlism' is that it disavows the idea that there is a single ultimate principle of ethics or some rules that are either absolute or that receive a priority ranking. The four-principles approach supports a method of content-expansion into more specific normative rules, rather than a system layered in terms of priorities among rules. In this respect the four principles are the point at which the real work begins, rather than a system of norms ready-to-hand for reaching moral conclusions of concern in health care. Moreover, it is insupportably optimistic to think we will ever attain a fully specified system of norms for health care ethics.

Not surprisingly, the four-principles approach rejects the view that there is a canon for bioethics, including a canon of four principles. There is no scripture, no authoritative interpretation of anything analogous to scripture, and no authoritative interpretation of that large mass of judgements, rules, standards of virtue, and the like that we often collectively sum up by use of the word 'morality'. Nonetheless, much work in health care ethics and in ethical theory is an attempt to articulate basic, pre-existing values with a philosophical sophistication and polish that provides a solid basis for the specification of norms. This is the most that can reasonably be expected of general philosophical ethics.

REFERENCES

1. Beauchamp. T. L. and Childress, J. F. 1989. *Principles of biomedical ethics*, 3rd edn. Oxford University Press, New York.
2. Jones, W. H. S. 1923. *Hippocrates*, vol. 1, p. 165. Harvard University Press, Cambridge, MA.
3. Jonsen, A. R. 1977. Do no harm: axiom of medical ethics. Pp. 27–41, *in* Spicker, S. F. and Tristram Engelhardt, jr, H. (Eds), *Philosophical and medical ethics: its nature and significance*. Reidel, Dordrecht.
4. Percival, T. 1803. *Medical ethics; or a code of institutes and precepts, adapted to the professional conduct of physicians and surgeons*, pp. 165–166. S. Russell, Manchester.
5. Beauchamp, T. L. and McCullough, L. 1984. *Medical ethics*. Prentice Hall, Englewood Cliffs, NJ.
6. Clouser, K. D. and Gert, B. 1990. A critique of principlism. *Journal of Medicine and Philosophy* **15**: 219–236. See also Chapter 22, this volume.
7. Hegel, G. W. F. (trans. T. M. Knox) 1942. *Philosophy of right*, pp. 89–90, 106–107. Clarendon Press, Oxford.
8. Toulmin, S. 1981. The tyranny of principles. *Hastings Center Report* **11**.
9. Richardson, H. S. 1990. Specifying norms as a way to resolve concrete ethical problems. *Philosophy and Public Affairs* **19**: 279–310.
10. Gillon, R. 1986. Doctors and patients. *British Medical Journal* **292**: 466–469.
11. Feinberg, J. 1973. *Social philosophy*, p. 34. Prentice Hall, Englewood Cliffs, NJ.
12. Rawls, J. 1971. *A theory of justice*, pp. 20ff., 46–49, 195–201, 577ff. Harvard University Press, Cambridge, MA.
13. Rawls, J. 1974–5. The independence of moral theory. *Proceedings and Addresses of the American Philosophical Association* **48**: 8.

2

Clinical Ethics and the Four Principles

ALBERT R. JONSEN

Professor of Ethics in Medicine, University of Washington, USA

Modern biomedical ethics, or bioethics, came into being as a distinct discipline during the seventh decade of the twentieth century. Scholars from moral philosophy and moral theology began to consider the ethical problems that had begun to appear as modern scientific medicine moved from the laboratory to the bedside. During the 1960s several prominent examples caught the attention of these scholars. In 1961 the techniques that made possible chronic hemodialysis for patients suffering from end-stage renal disease led to a widely publicized problem: how could the very limited resources for hemodialysis be made available to the large number of persons whose lives depended on admission to the program. In Seattle, Washington, where the technique was developed, a committee of laypersons was formed to decide 'who should live, who should die'. Several years later the advent of heart transplantation in South Africa stimulated debate about how far society should go in the effort to save life and about the definition of death. In the early 1970s, in the United States and in Great Britain, cases in which medical science had employed experimental methods on human subjects without consent and sometimes with disastrous consequences came to light (1).

Events such as these not only aroused public interest and indignation, but stimulated the curiosity of scholars whose disciplines, moral philosophy and moral theology, were by definition devoted to the analysis of ethical problems. However, neither discipline was, in the 1970s, well equipped to take up these new questions. Moral philosophy had become, during the previous 100 years, a highly theoretical field. In the Anglo-American philosophical world, scholars rarely discussed practical questions; they debated the meaning (or meaninglessness) of such terms as 'good', 'right', and 'ought'. Moral theologians, while more interested in practical questions, worked from premises that were embedded in theological doctrines not widely shared outside their faiths and denominations.

Principles of Health Care Ethics. Edited by Raanan Gillon.
© 1994 John Wiley & Sons Ltd

Thus, in the 1970s, the newborn discipline of bioethics was primarily a scholarly interest without a method.

If, however, the scholars' interest was to produce something more than discussion of the issues, some commonly accepted method for analysis had to be found. Scholars attempted to bring pieces from their familiar disciplines that appeared to suit the nature of the problems. Thus, utilitarianism, the dominant theory in moral philosophy, seemed to suit the problem of allocation of scarce resources. However, it was quickly noted that utilitarianism, which takes as its sole principle the greater good of the greater number, appeared to conflict with an ancient principle of medical ethics, namely, 'be of benefit to your patients and do them no harm or injustice'. Similarly, utilitarian theory might justify unconsented research that could benefit future patients, but again the medical imperative 'do no harm' seemed to prohibit this. Also, there was at that time a vivid interest in the rights of individuals, particularly of minorities. That interest had a philosophical correlate in the concept of autonomy that, in different forms, had inspired such important philosophers as John Stuart Mill and Immanuel Kant. At the same time, doctors were perplexed by an affirmation of their patient's autonomy, since they inherited a long ethical tradition that directed them to act in their patient's best interests, even if that meant contradicting the patient's wishes. Finally, questions of social justice, vigorously debated in the society, resuscitated a buried philosophical interest in the nature of justice. Again, it was apparent that the philosophical doctrines of justice, which are concerned with the common good and the distribution of burdens and benefits within a society, could conflict with the fiduciary duty of doctors, which required them to seek the welfare of their patients. Thus, the early encounter between philosophical doctrines and the traditions of medical ethics raised questions about compatibility.

Still, out of this ferment of ideas, philosophers and theologians interested in bioethical problems began to distill several principles. In their first published form, in *The Belmont Report: ethical guidelines for the protection of human subjects of research*, issued by the US National Commission for the Protection of Human Subjects of Biomedical and Behavioral Research in 1978, a triad of principles was mentioned: respect for autonomy, beneficence/non-maleficence, and justice (2). The simplicity and suitability of this triad impressed many scholars and, as a result, it found its way into the growing literature about biomedical ethics. It also became a useful format for education about ethics in health care, and was commonly used in the lectures and courses for practitioners that were offered in increasing numbers throughout the United States. Quickly, the original triad of principles was split into quadruplicate, since it seemed philosophically rational and pedagogically practical to separate non-maleficence and beneficence as distinct principles. Thus, as the 1980s opened, biomedical ethics had at least one of the essential elements of a true discipline, namely, an agreed set of principles for the analysis of its proper problems (3).

An agreed set of principles provided some consistency in bioethics: around them could coalesce the variety of particular considerations that scholars and commentators had been raising about the ethical problems of modern health care. However, bioethics appeared to be more than the speculative reflection on these problems. It also had a very practical side: the problems being discussed by the scholars involved real persons who were ill and real persons who were providing care. The somewhat speculative problem of how best to allocate a scarce medical resource, such as dialysis, touched single sick individuals, their doctors, nurses and families. Decisions had to be made about what ought to be done. Bioethics, then, was practical philosophy.

The term 'clinical ethics' came into being in the early 1980s as a response to this practical side of bioethics (4). This term captured the growing sense among practitioners of health care that the decisions they made daily in their clinical work had an ethical dimension. They had always known this in a vague, general way, since medicine and nursing have long proclaimed that they were professions with a responsibility, as Hippocrates stated centuries ago, 'to benefit the sick and do them no harm'. However, in the circumstances of contemporary health care it was not always easy to know what would benefit and how to avoid harm. Modern technology could produce physiological results with an almost unfailing regularity: a ventilator, for example, can maintain oxygen levels compatible with continued life for months, even years. However, it is not always clear that those incessant effects are benefits: suppose the patient whose breathing is maintained is in a state of irreversible coma? Indeed, might not the effect be a harm? Considerations of this sort pushed their way into the consciences of providers of care. They began to ask questions that they hoped the bioethicists could answer, but clearly the answers would have to be clinically relevant, that is, able to be applied in the circumstances of this or that particular case.

For centuries, philosophers have realized that there exists a wide gap between theory and practice, between speculation and decision, between principle and action. That perennial realization was and still is expressed in the phrase, 'In principle...' that often prefaces a noble statement that must be modified or compromised 'in practice'. Bioethicists acknowledged this problem and became concerned about the construction of methods that would bridge the gap. They hoped that their invocation of principles could be supplemented by counsel that practitioners might carry into their decisions. Some bioethicists suggested that 'clinical ethics' was a kind of 'casuistry', the name for a once-respected but now disdained form of thinking through moral problems that focused on the circumstances of particular cases (5).

WHAT IS A MORAL PRINCIPLE?

Of course, if the perennial problem of the gap between principle and practice is to be solved, the meaning of principle needs to be clarified. Again, philosophers have discussed this question interminably and it will never be definitively answered. Among the many points of view, however, a few common points can be found and they will be summarized here. It seems clear that human beings, wherever and whenever found, manifest what is called 'normative behavior', that is, they describe certain behaviors as good and right and other behavior as bad or wrong; they praise persons who practice the former while blaming and punishing those who perform the latter. The great diversity of descriptions of right and wrong in different cultures does not negate, indeed, it reinforces the universality of normative behavior or, in a more common term, morality.

Judgements of right and wrong can be made about particular behaviors or practices only if certain standards are commonly understood and appreciated in a society. These standards are the norms against which particular actions, practices and institutions are judged. The norms are usually stated as imperatives, that is, as statements that explicitly or implicitly contain the concept 'ought or ought not to be done'. These statements can be rather specific, such as 'you ought to assist a blind person to cross the street', or can be expressed in quite general terms, 'there is a moral obligation to assist those in need'. Philosophers tend to call the more specific norms, 'rules', and the more general ones 'principles'. It is obvious that human intercourse involves a great multitude of such norms. Sociologists and anthropologists describe them at length. Philosophers disagree over whether they can or should be reduced to system. They disagree even more strongly over the origins, foundations and justifications for these norms. Despite these theoretical debates, the inevitability and the importance of norms is manifest: we cannot conceive of human society without them.

One way to think about the role of moral principles is to reflect on the origin of the word 'principle' itself. It derives from the Latin, *'principium'*, which means 'beginning, starting place'. However, the Latin word itself reflects a deeper meaning. It is a composite of *'primum'*, 'first' and *'capere'*, 'take', which suggests something that takes first place: the word *'princeps'*, or 'prince' is from the same root. Thus, a principle is a statement that takes first place in some discourse, whether it be about physics, economics or ethics. It takes first place in several senses. It allows one to start thinking through the details of a problem or to relate those details back to a foundation. It also rules the process of thinking: as the various details are raised it allows one to rule in the relevant and rule out the irrelevant. It keeps the discourse on track so that the conclusion can be recognized as an answer to the problem raised. In an important way, reasoned thought is principled thought.

When the realm of discourse is ethics or morality, the process of thinking must terminate in a moral judgement, that is, a judgement that this action or policy is right or wrong and this or that ought to be done. Thus, the movement of moral thinking must somehow find its way between principles and decisions. However, in moral discourse the problem under discussion will frequently be about which of several principles should prevail. It is not always clear that one of several competing principles has priority. Further, in moral discourse, problems are not at all like the elegantly clean lines of a mathematical problem. They are rather messy concoctions of many details, some salient, others obscure, but all calling for attention. A moral problem is rather like a detective story in which the details, the facts of the case, are crucial. The great detectives of fiction rarely invoke principles; they stalk clues. At the end, however, they can, sometimes with wondrous ingenuity, relate the clues to principle. Thus, the problem of clinical ethics is how to view the principles in the light of the multiple details of particular cases.

HOW DO THE PRINCIPLES FUNCTION IN RESOLVING CLINICAL–ETHICAL PROBLEMS?

The mere invocation of principles does little to resolve actual problems. The understanding of principles is essential. However, even understanding the definition and the limits of principles will not resolve problems. It is frequently suggested that one must learn to apply principles to problems. The term 'apply', however, is rather misleading. It suggests that a clear line of reasoning can lead from the principle, once understood, to the resolution of a practical problem. In actuality, moral reasoning is considerably more intricate. Every moral problem is enmeshed in a multitude of circumstances, that is, the concrete setting of time, place, differing persons and their roles, institutional policies, etc. Similarly, every moral problem involves not a single principle, but several, even many, norms that compete for attention. Moral reasoning must weave its way through this intricacy of multiple circumstances and norms.

We have suggested that moral principles are starting and ruling points for this passage. Even this suggestion may be rather misleading. Moral thinking need not have, and probably rarely has, its temporal beginning with the invocation of a principle. Rather, we actually begin with the perception of a variety of circumstances that seem to pose some sort of obstruction to the ordinary course of decision and action that we might take in relatively similar situations. Our habitual pattern of decision and action is disrupted and we say 'wait, what should we do now?' or, in the more formal language of the moral philosopher, 'what ought to be done?'

A Case

Mr A, a 62-year-old carpenter, has been seen by his doctor for several years for emphysema, which has become quite severe. In the last year he had to be hospitalized twice for severe exacerbations of his disease but had not required ventilatory support. He is divorced, has a grown son and two daughters and has been living with a female companion for six years. He has been a heavy smoker since his teens, but quit four years ago. In June of this year he was admitted to the hospital with pneumonia. When a chest X-ray is taken, a coin lesion of the left lung is noted. A biopsy is ordered and, during its performance, Mr A suffers a pneumothorax and is intubated. He experiences cardiac irregularities. The biopsy is positive for adenocarcinoma. Mr A is informed that he has lung cancer. His doctor explains his condition and prognosis and, in the course of the discussion, asks Mr A if he desires to be resuscitated if he suffers cardiac arrest. If not, the doctor will write a do not resuscitate (DNR) order. Mr A indicates that he wants resuscitation. Within a week, Mr A develops symptoms consistent with adult respiratory distress syndrome (ARDS). He becomes obtunded and is no longer able to communicate. Renal function deteriorates and dialysis is indicated. His doctor confers with Mr A's female companion and recommends that dialysis not be initiated. She concurs in that recommendation. However, Mr A's son and daughter strongly insist that everything be done. They recall his refusal of the DNR order and state that he was a strong man and a fighter who would want to live, even if it meant fighting cancer. What ought to be done now?

In this case there are a variety of contingent features: the age and occupation of the patient, his particular medical problems, his history of smoking, his marital status, the opinion that he expresses about his care and the opinions of his companion and children. We might also add that, as a veteran of the United States Navy, Mr A receives his medical care from the Veterans Administration. This health care system is fully supported by the federal government and its health care providers are government employees. It is the only American health care system that resembles the National Health Service in Great Britain. Features such as these will change from case to case. Any real case will have a vast number of such contingent features, so that the story might be expanded almost *ad infinitum*. The complexity and multiplicity of circumstances are daunting to anyone who attempts to answer the questions posed by the case. Some are led to assert that, since every case is unique, no general response can be given to a moral question. The question 'is it right to initiate dialysis' can be answered, they say, with the response 'it depends on the circumstances'.

This is not a satisfying answer, since the question is 'on what circumstances?' and 'how does it depend?' Such an answer may be a claim that only the personal, private intuition and feeling of the respondent can answer the question. On the other hand, others will say that an answer depends on clear reasoning from principles, such as those we have discussed above. However, in most cases that raise ethical issues, the problem is caused by the apparent collision of several principles. Thus, it is not enough to reason from principles; it is necessary to sort out what principle prevails in the apparent conflict.

In the above case several principles vie for attention. The principle of respect for autonomy appears in the expression of the patient's wishes, the preferences of his family and the opinion of the doctor. Whose autonomy should be respected? Why? The principles of beneficence and non-maleficence lurk in the patient's medical condition and the forms of treatment that might be used to manage it. Yet, to what extent can those forms of treatment benefit the patient? Might not some be more harmful than beneficial? So, as we move from the clear intellectual air of principles to the foggy obscurity of cases with their multiple circumstances, we need more specific guidance than the principles themselves can provide.

Moral principles are not unlike the skymarks used in celestial navigation: a position is determined and a course marked by continual reference to fixed points, sun, stars, planets. At the same time the navigator must look, not only to the skymarks, but to any visible landmarks and to the wind and waves. Thus, while the principles provide an indispensable general guiding direction, other features of the problem must be taken into consideration as the passage from moral question to moral answer is navigated. Pilots rarely depend solely on celestial navigation. They usually have charts made by those who have preceded them, and that give them a general sense of position and of geographical setting. Similarly, the clinical case has not only its panoply of general principles and its multiplicity of contingent circumstances. It has constant features, present in every clinical encounter, that can be charted and to which those who must navigate the course of a particular case can refer.

All clinical encounters, that is, particular cases of medical care, have four constant features: medical indications, patient preferences, quality of the patient's life and contextual features (4). These constant features or topics provide reference points to which both the principles and the circumstances can be related. 'Medical indications' refers to the fact that a medical encounter is initiated by a person who experiences certain symptoms suggestive of illness and who seeks, or is brought, to someone who has the ability to understand those symptoms and to deal with the disease that may underlie them. Medical indications are the facts about the patient's pathophysiology that require diagnosis and treatment. The topic of medical indications is loosely related to the principle of beneficence, since the question to be asked is 'how can the human good called health be maintained or restored?'

The second topic, patient preferences, refers to the fact that in every medical encounter a person requests, directly or through another, assistance. In so doing patients express preferences about how they hope to be helped and with what results. They may also express limitations on help. Their preferences reflect certain understandings and attitudes that may, or may not, correspond to the reality of their medical situation. If the patient is unable to express preferences due to immaturity or mental incapacity, the question arises about the standards for surrogate determinations in that patient's behalf. The principle of autonomy is associated with the topic of patient preferences, since the question is 'to what extent should a patient's preferences determine the nature and extent of their care?'

The third topic, quality of life, suggests that the episode of illness takes place within the larger setting of a patient's life as a whole. The illness itself may bring pain and discomfort but pass quickly. It may, on the other hand, leave serious deficits that will limit the ability of the person to function well. Judgements about quality of life are made by the persons who live that life. Still, in medical care, persons may not be able to make such judgements at crucial moments and others may make them in their behalf. The question arises about the criteria that should be used when others are placed in this position. This also recalls the principle of beneficence/non-maleficence, since the question is 'what states of living are to be considered good or bad and to what extent are others obliged to produce them by interventions?'

Finally, the fourth topic, contextual features, refers to the fact that medical encounters, while intensely personal, take place within a social setting. Other parties are involved: families, caretakers, administrators, policy-makers. Social institutions provide resources, financing, training, support, legal systems, etc. All of these have interests that must be served. This raises the question of justice which is so difficult to accommodate to the care of the sick. The principle of justice asks the relevant question, 'to what extent and under what conditions do the interests of other parties supersede the interests of the patient?'

The particular case is approached through these constant features or topics. The question that incites ethical reflection, 'what should we do now?' has arisen, as we mentioned above, from some obstacle that looms in the way of the habitual path of activities, just as a reef might appear in the path of a sail boat. The obstacle in Mr A's case appears at the point where the doctor recommends to Mr A's family that dialysis not be initiated. This might have been, in the doctor's mind, the ordinary course of good care, since he judges that Mr A has a lethal disease that has reached a terminal stage, namely, his ARDS, overlaid on his chronic obstructive lung disease. He also thinks that the prospects of lung cancer would be best avoided if the patient is allowed to die now, rather than linger. In this his thinking follows, although he will not explicitly refer to them, the principles of beneficence and non-maleficence. He judges that, given these circumstances, the patient would be benefited by an early death and that further treatment would be harmful. Indeed, he may judge, given the prognosis for ARDS, that further treatment would be useless.

This ordinary course of judgement, guided by beneficence and non-maleficence, is interrupted by the insistence of son and daughter that Mr A receive all available treatment. They explicitly cite his refusal of a DNR order as evidence that he would want aggressive care. They are, in so doing, invoking the principle of respect for autonomy. They discount, as Mr A's companion does not, any consideration of the quality of Mr A's life, should he survive this episode and live to experience the effects of his lung cancer.

Although no one has raised the question of the costs and use of resources for Mr A, it might be raised quite reasonably by someone who is responsible for these matters. Mr A who, as a veteran, is entitled to government-subsidized medical care, is absorbing considerable resources in money, time, energy and space. While even this considerable expenditure is but a tiny fraction of the enormous budget of the Veterans Administration (as it would be of the National Health Service), each similar case adds up to considerable sums. In a time of constrained budgets, cases such as Mr A's cannot be disregarded. Further, in the particular hospital where he is lodged, Mr A is utilizing space and services that might be more profitably directed to other patients whose prospects are better. Thus, a question of justice is raised.

The particular facts of this case, viewed in the context of the four constant topics of all clinical encounters, allow us to interpret the four principles. We prefer the word 'interpret' rather than 'apply' because we see the relevance and the limits of the principles in and through the facts of the case and the topics. One popular metaphor that is heard when a moral problem is discussed is the metaphor of 'weighing'. It is said 'we must weigh the importance of various principles in order to discover their priority'. This, too, is misleading. Principles do not, we think, having anything like weight. Indeed some principles, such as respect for autonomy, are more important than others, say politeness or punctuality, but at the highest levels, such as autonomy or beneficence, the principles are presumably of equal importance. A better metaphor would refer to the weighing of the circumstances of the case. The circumstances, the facts in the case, are weighed in the balance or scales of the principles. Some facts will be placed in the pan of the principle of autonomy, others in the counterbalancing pan of the principle of beneficence. (Admittedly, the metaphor breaks down when our scale has more than two pans; still, let it serve as best it can.) The principles are given weight by the circumstances.

In Mr A's case many of the facts in the topic of medical indications will be piled on the pan of beneficence/non-maleficence. An objective review of medical indications will reveal that modern technological medicine has very little to offer Mr A. The various goals of medicine, such as restoration of health and maintenance of function, are very unlikely to be achieved. The countervailing expressions of Mr A's preferences are piled on the pan of respect for autonomy. They are, given these circumstances, quite light. Mr A cannot in fact be asked his preferences about dialysis and other life-sustaining circumstances. His only known preference is about another procedure, namely DNR. His children are interpreting, on the basis of that expression, and on what they think of their father's values. In addition, the expectation of future quality of life and the utilization of resources, while not explicitly mentioned, can be factored into this equation. When all the circumstances are weighed, it appears that the scale is tipped towards beneficence and non-maleficence. In this setting beneficence is not a commanding principle since intervention cannot attain health benefits for Mr A. On the other hand, the possibility of maleficence, by sustaining a life that will be of miserable quality, is real. The case is ethically resolved by following the doctor's recommendation that treatment be forgone and Mr A's companion's acquiescence in that recommendation.

Others may view this case differently. However, they will do so because they see circumstances in a somewhat different light. For example, someone may judge that the prospects for quality of life, should he survive this episode, may not be so bad, or that the preference about DNR should be interpreted as a preference about aggressive care in general. Nevertheless, the ultimate judgement about what should be done will flow from an interpretation of the principles in light of the circumstances and constant topics of clinical care. Principles alone do not lead to ethical decisions; decisions without principles are ethically empty.

REFERENCES

1. Rothman, D. 1991. *Strangers at the bedside.* Basic Books, New York.
2. National Commission for Protection of Human Subjects of Biomedical and Behavioral Research. 1978. *The Belmont Report: ethical guidelines for the protection of human subjects of research.* Department of Health, Education and Welfare, Washington, DC.
3. Beauchamp, T. L. and Childress, J. F. 1979. *Principles of biomedical ethics.* Oxford University Press, New York.
4. Jonsen, A., Siegler, M. and Winslade, W. 1983. *Clinical ethics.* Macmillan, New York (3rd edn, McGraw-Hill, 1992).
5. Jonsen, A. and Toulmin, S. 1988. *The abuse of casuistry.* University of California Press, Berkeley, CA.

3

The Four Principles and their Use: the Possibilities of Agreement between Different Faiths and Philosophies

RONALD H. PRESTON, DD (OXON)

Emeritus Professor of Social and Pastoral Theology in the University of Manchester, UK

The peoples of the world are of great cultural and religious diversity. Yet modern means of communication have brought them in touch with one another as never before. If they are to hold together they need to have some common ethical understanding and commitment, and the effort to find such a basis is a first priority. Pope John XXIII (in his encyclical *Pacem in Terris*, 1963) attempted it in the area of international relations with his four bases of political society, truth, justice, charity and freedom. More recently Hans Küng, the well-known Roman Catholic theologian from the University of Tübingen, has written a vigorous tract for the times on a theme with three imperatives. 'No human life together without a world ethic for the nations; no peace among the nations without peace among the religions; no peace among the religions without dialogue among the religions' (1). It is in this setting that we must see the explosion of discussions in medical ethics, sparked off by the greater powers of human intervention in the treatment and prevention of human diseases and physical failures, of which the advent of cardiac transplants and the problems of rationing scarce resources in the case of renal dialysis may be taken as heralds. So there has come the emphasis on the four principles—respect for autonomy, beneficence, non-maleficence and justice—which is a main theme of this book. In this chapter I am concentrating on two issues. (a) Whether there is, or can be, a common agreement between different faiths and philosophies on these principles and (a connected point), how far if they are agreed upon they will be interpreted in the same way. (b) How they can be used in practice in dealing with particular

Principles of Health Care Ethics. Edited by Raanan Gillon.
© 1994 John Wiley & Sons Ltd

cases, and how far we can expect agreement on that. I shall not discuss what the various religions and philosophies make of the four principles; other chapters do that. But I will make one or two references to the Christian tradition. The discussion is basically concerned with issues in moral philosophy; and any theology of the human person has an explicit or implicit moral philosophical position.

SCEPTICISM

Those for whom questions of medical ethics are of urgent and practical professional concern and who, when presented with the four principles, think them relatively straightforward and indeed basic, may be surprised at the amount of scepticism there is in the 'western' world at present on the matter. I take the influence of Alasdair MacIntyre as an example, because he has written three books in the past decade on the themes of fundamental moral disagreements in that world, all of them very influential, not least because they are so vigorously and clearly expressed.* After considering his influence on the debate we will consider what there is to be said for a different view.

The more extreme position which many have gathered from MacIntyre is that there are irreconcilable moral disagreements in our world because we have lost a common vocabulary in which to communicate intelligibly with one another; we have no common standard by which such moral disagreements can be comprehended and measured. Even if we use the same terms it does not mean that we use them in the same sense, or are talking about the same thing. It used to be thought that humans could in principle distance themselves from their personal and cultural backgrounds, traditions and commitments, and agree on the basis of an abstracted, uncommitted rationality to some absolutely certain ethical propositions. Since, however, it is impossible thus to stand outside one's milieu in a kind of disembodied rationality, there is no possibility of a rational resolution of differing ethical stances. So we are reduced to the kind of relativism which holds that ethical judgements are, minimally, a purely personal ethical stance (commonly called emotivism) or, more strongly, are what one is prepared to act on oneself and recommend others to do the same (commonly called prescriptivism). Lacking, therefore, any common basis we are at the mercy of the manager, or the therapist, or the bureaucrat. In such a perspective the four principles have little significance.

MacIntyre is not in fact as extreme as this. He suggests that the traditions of moral reasoning which have been eroded by the acids of pluralism in the modern world have each had flaws which it is in their own interests to correct. He asks whether they have enough in common to hold out the possibility of fruitful intellectual interchange between them. In doing so they will each have to pay attention to, and give some account of, their rivals. To be able to bridge the ethical gaps between them the proponents of each will have to take on the task of what is equivalent to learning a 'second first language'. It will be as if

---

* See refs 2–4; a solid response to the first of these is Stout (5).

an English person might set out to learn French or Japanese so thoroughly as to be able to think in it as spontaneously as in his or her first language.

However, as we shall see, the task may not be as far-reaching as MacIntyre suggests. The appeal of the more extreme variant of his positions is due to the increasingly widespread appreciation of the conditioning factors in human life and thought, which has undermined a previous rather simple rationalism. (It should be noted that conditioning factors are not to be thought of as *determining* factors, though this is not the occasion to explore the difference.) Simple rationalism (which derives particularly from the eighteenth-century Enlightenment) is an excessive trust in the power of human reason to control and direct human affairs from an independent, unconditional stance. It needs to be differentiated from rationality, which recognizes the conditionality of all human experience (6). Another way of putting it is to say that, since Marx, we have come to understand much more the ideological elements in human thought and actions. But that is not to deny that in principle we can partially, though not completely, transcend them, and that an element of 'interest-free' thought and action is possible for us (7). The realization of this leads to a less pessimistic view of the possibilities and difficulties of human understanding in ethical matters across religious, cultural and philosophical boundaries than that of MacIntyre. So we are led back to the four principles.

People, or to confine myself to my own experience, British people, are fond of discussing ethical issues. If, for instance, a preacher deals with one in a sermon the hearers will be so attentive that one could hear the proverbial pin drop. Vigorous ethical arguments can quickly be developed over a pint in a 'pub'. There will be voluble disagreements, and probably no resolution of the arguments but only an agreement to disagree. Nevertheless the participants will not be arguing past one another in mutual incomprehension. There will be a substratum of common ground, part articulate, part not. Indeed total disagreement in ethics is impossible without living in a solipsistic universe. Moreover, the advocates of different views will almost always imply, or assert, that the conclusions they reach are not just a matter of their personal idiosyncrasy or their social or cultural position, but have a certain objectivity about them. If I say 'Hitler was an evil man' I do not mean that he does not appeal to me but he might to you, or to someone else; I mean that he *was* an evil man, and everyone else should think so too. Anyone who denies an element of objectivity in their moral judgements and is prepared to accept in theory their totally conditioned nature will soon be found passing moral judgements in the clear tones of one who thinks they do have an element of objectivity about them. One used to find, at a time when there were self-consciously 'pure' Marxists around, those who maintained that there was no such thing as objective morality short of the classless communist society, and before that only a class morality, that it was a position impossible to maintain consistently. Soon they were found making moral judgements which clearly implied a more universal validity. Also they cut off the bough on which they sat. If speaking the truth meant saying what in a given situation they judged would favour the cause of the coming workers' revolution, others found before long that there was no necessary correspondence between what they said and what they thought, and the basis of human communication with them was removed. Human life together then becomes impossible, and the procedure was self-defeating.

This means that human reason is not totally dissolved in a cultural milieu, and that there are common features of, and common conceptions of, human nature over and above its expression in particular religions, cultures and traditions. It means that one can appeal to the experience that every person has of growth and development in relation to other persons, from infancy to old age. This accords with classical Christian faith which teaches that human persons have the capacity by the use of their reason to differentiate between the true and the false in matters of fact and, in matters of morals, to recognize a difference between good and evil, right and wrong, and to know that they should follow what they judge to be right and shun what they judge to be wrong in particular cases. (This does not suggest, of course, that they will always do this in practice, or agree among themselves about what is right and wrong, or not make serious misjudgements from time to time.)

When in this context we talk of human reason we mean more than an understanding of the basic laws of logic, such as the principle of non-contradiction. We also mean more than being consistent and comprehensive within a particular standpoint. We mean that there are broad criteria of rationality and ethical discernment which are relatively independent of particular religious and ideological traditions. This is to claim that certain moral virtues have an objective basis, a certain universalism. That is the claim made for the four principles.

Moreover they need to be fostered in communities which promote a commitment to them. If they are merely taken for granted human beings will be less prone to stand by them under pressure. This is particularly so in view of the 'free-rider' problem. This is the person who flouts them on the assumption that others will stand by them. This is hit off by one of Groucho Marx's quips, 'Sure, justice and fair dealing are the foundation of human life: if you can fake that you've got it made.' In the last resort only a moral answer can be given to the question 'Why be moral?' A basic human morality can be supported by such arguments as: (a) it ought to be followed because all humans are basically alike in sharing a common rationality; or (b) it ought to be followed because they are all of the same species. (The moral relations of humans to other species or inanimate nature is a further question.) These are based on a secular humanist faith which says that because there is no God and humans are alone in the world they ought to stand by it, and by one another. Religious faiths say that humans are not alone in the world and have further reasons for standing by a basic human morality such as is expressed in the four principles. The Christian faith, for instance, says that not only are humans created in 'God's image', but through the work of Jesus Christ have been restored when the image was marred. The point is that human beings are not shut up in mutually incomprehensible traditions of moral and doctrinal belief, but in traditions which can, for partly overlapping and partly different reasons, support the basic morality expressed in the four principles (8). It is not that there will not be exceptions to this here and there in the world, nor that there will not be a spectrum of attitudes to them; but within the spectrum there will be a certain 'family resemblance' (to use a phrase of the twentieth-century philosopher Wittgenstein) on which one can build.

This human morality will stress such virtues as truth-telling, promise-keeping, courage and natural justice (one is not judge in one's own cause). It goes further to the widespread, but not complete, agreement that slavery is evil, so is apartheid, so is the abuse of children. In some matters there is disagreement between whose who agree on this basic human morality on what is the proper human way of behaving in accordance with it. Abortion is an example. How far is the prohibition of abortion an inhuman restriction? Or how far is the desire for abortion an inhuman attitude? The proponents of both positions want to adopt a properly human stance. (At what point the conceptus is to be given a fully human status is a subsidiary issue in the debate.)

A certain type of society is needed if this common morality is to flourish. It is obviously consistent with what we would call a liberal democracy; equally clearly a totalitarian society which does not admit of dialogue is not a congenial milieu for it. However, such a society may not in fact deny it, even if it allows only one form of religious or ideological backing for it. So that certain what we might call 'fundamentalist' forms of religion can support it. Engelhardt has explored the basis for a moral framework within which public policy in medical decision-making can be made, when the public moral perceptions may have very different roots: Catholic, Protestant, post-Catholic, post-Protestant, Enlightenment, post-Enlightenment, post-modernist, to say nothing of ethnic minorities (9). Not only must these traditions respect one another, but they must also explore the nature of the common morality we have been discussing, and why it must be supported. For there must be some common ground to hold society together. Sheer force will not do; or not for long. Nor is it enough to respect all opinions and leave it at that. Some convictions must be held in common, and some must be ruled out. There must be some limits. For instance, what should be the attitude of the State to a Jehovah's Witness who refuses to allow her child to have a blood transfusion?

The concern of the State must be to foster the kind of structure of family, working and community life which promotes good human relationships. Trusting relationships in infancy and in childhood nurture in the home and school, and humane and just structures in working and in civic life, together with vigorous voluntary organizations, are a source of commitment to the common morality and the common good, as well as to the finer graces which go beyond that. An authoritarian society is a handicap to this. The psychological roots of moral discernment are important, even though it is not determined by them (10). Just as it is possible to be a saint in the slums (and that is no defence of the slums), so it is possible to exhibit rational moral discernment in spite of bad interpersonal relations and social structures (and that is no reason for tolerating either of them). Once again, to be conditioned is not to be determined.

THE FOUR PRINCIPLES

We return to the four principles. They clearly are based on the concept of rational personhood, the characteristics of which, and the grounds for the defence of which, I have already mentioned. However, there are problems with respect to their meaning and application which must be mentioned. For one thing they may conflict. So one has to ask whether there is a hierarchy among them. For instance, respect for autonomy is clearly a key one, but not the only one, even in the case of competent patients. In the case of children (and in many cases of mental handicap) the question of proxy consent arises. Alderson argues (11) that it will require a deep confidence between parents, between parents and medical experts and, in the case of older children, between the child and both the parents and the medical experts. This confidence goes beyond the four principles into an empathy which is close to what in the Christian vocabulary is called *agape*, or love. Indeed the four principles can each of them lead a long way. Justice, for instance, in this context relates not to criminal justice, but to commutative justice (between persons), which derives from the affirmation of the status of each human being, the possible grounds for which have already been discussed. This affirms the uniqueness of each person and their fundamental equality in status; and will go on to affirm that they should not only be allowed to exercise control over their lives in terms of their basic convictions (which brings in the respect for autonomy), but also that they should have enough resources to be able in practice to do so. Hence concern for justice will lead to a particular concern for those who are disadvantaged in terms of economic resources, and therefore of economic power. All of these four principles have therefore to be considered in a social context, and thus benevolence and non-maleficence to the common good. Issues of community care bring this sharply before us.

We still have to ask how these principles can be used in practice in moral reasoning, in this case in medical ethics concerned with particular cases. It is not a simple matter. It is not a procedure where timeless moral principles are applied deductively to a changing human scene. The verbal expression of the principles may not change, but in the course of time the understanding of their range and depth does. Also the way a case is described requires care. For instance, if the four principles are held to involve a 'reverence for [human] life', and from that it is deduced that murder is wrong, further questions arise. Is every killing to be called murder? If not, murder is the term for killings we abhor. Which killings are to be included in this category? If we call practically every case of abortion murder (as some do), we are incorporating an evaluative term into the description of the act. Or if we go back one stage, and bring abortion under the principle of 'respect for the person' (as being directly implied in the principle of autonomy), we have to ask, as I have already suggested, such questions as (a) when in the process of conception, growth in the womb, and birth is the full status and protection which we ascribe to a person to operate; (b) what do we do when the claims of the life of one person conflict with those of others?

If it is desired to bring each case under the four principles is there a fixed hierarchy among them? Since there can be only one principle which admits of no exceptions, can we arrange these four in a scale of weightage when, in a particular case, the principles conflict with one another? Surely not. That would be too static a picture of human life. Rather, we have to use our power of reasoning discernment, singly and collectively, to evaluate the priorities among the principles in each case. It is not a one-way movement from principle to a particular case, but a reciprocal relation where each influences and illuminates the other. New situations, new cases arise; a new awareness of cultural pluralism may strike us. This influences our selection of significant data as we bring it alongside our previous understanding of the range and depth of the principle to see how they bear on the new case.

This is in fact how decisions are usually made in medical ethics. It is in accord with the best traditions of casuistry as it developed in the Christian tradition. Casuistry is the art of resolving particular cases in the light of basic moral insights and principles. It got a bad name in the seventeenth century through the attack of Pascal on much current practice (12). It seemed a sophisticated means of evading moral responsibility, rather than thinking out the best way of discharging it. To some extent the mud still sticks. But whether the word is used or not the practice is essential, whether in moral philosophy or moral theology. Philosophers have had to go beyond preoccupation with the meaning of moral words and the logical properties of rules and principles, and to work at a method for resolving particular cases. Theologians likewise have to go beyond quoting basic commandments, like the ten of the Old Testament, or Jesus' summing up of them into two (love of God and one's neighbour). They need to show how to move from them to particular cases. The way the best casuists clarified a case was not by the direct application of a principle. They started with a clear-cut case, for instance one which practically everyone agreed should be called murder, and then considered other ones with varying circumstances, and then a particular case, asking how far it differed from the clear-cut case, and common deviations from the clear-cut case. Then they considered what were the priorities among agreed principles in this particular case. 'Circumstances alter cases' was the formula (13). To repeat, this is in fact how the great explosion of discussion on cases in medical ethics has usually been carried on. Those involved have found that principles and the data of cases react reciprocally on one another. It has, for instance, been a fairly common experience that agreement could be reached on what it was best to do in a particular case by those who had difficulty in agreeing on the precise statement of principles.

This will raise in many minds the question of certitude in moral judgements. Many people, both religious and secular, expect certitude in judgements in particular cases, or long for it. They think there is a defect in themselves or in their religious or ideological position if it does not provide one. A few cases are clear-cut; but the great majority are subject to varying degrees of ambiguity. Yet if one is a member of a community which takes moral judgements seriously, and which is concerned to develop corporately powers of discerning moral reason, there is no reason why we should not make competent moral judgements, especially if we are willing openly to learn from experience, and are not afraid to face challenging new cases. That is why the recent explosion in medical ethics, and the generally responsible way in which it is being handled, is so welcome. Attention to the four principles and how they are used in practical reasoning on particular cases is a good example of what I mean.

REFERENCES

1. Küng, H. 1991. *Global responsibility: in search of a new world ethic.* English translation, SCM Press, London.
2. MacIntyre, A. C. 1981. *After virtue: a study in moral theory.* Duckworth, London.
3. MacIntyre, A. C. 1988. *Whose justice? Which rationality?* Duckworth, London.
4. MacIntyre, A. C. 1991. *Three rival versions of moral enquiry: encyclopaedia, genealogy and tradition.* Duckworth, London.
5. Stout, J. 1988. *Ethics after Babel: the languages of morals and their discontents.* Beacon Press, Boston, Mass.
6. Oakeshott, M. J. 1962. *Rationalism in politics and other essays.* Methuen, London (enlarged edition Liberty Press, Indianapolis, 1990).
7. Eagleton, T. 1991. *Ideology: an introduction.* Verso, London.
8. Mitchell, B. G. 1980. *Morality, religious and secular: the dilemma of the traditional conscience.* Clarendon Press, Oxford.
9. Engelhardt, H. T. Jr, 1991. *Bioethics and secular humanism: the search for a common morality,* SCM Press, London.
10. Kitwood, T. 1990. *Concern for others.* Routledge, London.
11. Alderson, P. 1990. *Choosing for others.* Oxford University Press, London.
12. Pascal, B. 1967. *Lettres provinciales 1656.* English translation, Penguin, London.
13. Jonsen, A. R. and Toulmin, S. 1988. *The abuse of casuistry: a history of moral reasoning.* University of California Press, Berkeley, Los Angeles and London.

4

Theology and the Four Principles: A Roman Catholic View I

JOHN FINNIS, LLB (ADELAIDE), DPHIL (OXON), FBA

Professor of Law and Legal Philosophy, Oxford University; Fellow and Tutor, University College, Oxford, UK

ANTHONY FISHER, OP, BA (SYDNEY), LLB (SYDNEY), BTHEOL (MELBOURNE)

Blackfriars, Oxford, UK

THE TRUE CONTEXT OF THE FOUR PRINCIPLES

'The four principles of bioethics' have their rational basis and truth only within the wider set of moral principles. Outside that context they demarcate a rather legalistic ethic while also, paradoxically, providing labels for rationalizing almost any practice.

Morality's principles (including 'the four') can be recognized by anyone following reason's guidance, undeflected by distracting emotion, prejudice or convention. They are matter for moral philosophy. But reason's full implications, and morality's practical applications, are well understood only when full account is taken of the human situation. And our human predicament and opportunities include some realities adequately and reliably revealed only by the life and teachings of Jesus Christ, through the Church's scriptures and tradition. All moral principles are thus matters also for doctrine, faith, and theology. They are guides to a life which befits human nature, responds to the divine calling, and prepares people for eternal life in God's family. They educate conscience, shape virtues, and make possible wise decisions in particular cases.

Principles of Health Care Ethics. Edited by Raanan Gillon.
© 1994 John Wiley & Sons Ltd

What is it reasonable to do? What choices 'make sense', are 'good', 'fair', 'right'? Moral philosophy begins its answer with two basic features of human persons. We are responsible, i.e. can deliberate rationally and make free choices (1) (see also ref. 2, pp. 11–12; ref. 3, p. 137) and nothing short of a happiness and flourishing in which we might share can give our choices rationally sufficient point (4).

Freedom

When tempted, for example to fabricate or steal some experimental results, we see through excuses like 'only following orders', or 'my upbringing' or 'I'm slave to my passions'. In judging oneself or others culpable, or in thinking 'if only I'd...', one recognizes one's freedom to choose and to choose rationally. Inherited characteristics, upbringing, present restrictions and pressures, all can influence but none need eliminate the demand to choose, to adopt one proposal for action (or inaction) in preference to others. *Autonomy* (self-rule) is less a principle than a fact.

Free choosing is self-making and self-telling (5): choices shape and express one's life and moral identity ('character'). Choices last: they continue affecting who one is, at least until one makes some contrary choice. Some big choices commit one to a certain relationship; but each of my morally significant choices actualizes and limits me, and orients me (and everyone to whom my choice tacitly speaks as an 'example') towards similar future choices. Each such choice thus has implications far deeper and wider than the external behaviour and states of affairs which were its direct object and outcome (see ref. 3, pp. 139–144, 153). Morality takes account of all this.

Integral Human Fulfilment

No-one finds real happiness in sheer pleasurable experience, independent of worthwhile accomplishment. Happiness (including its joys) is personal completeness or harmonious wholeness, something achievable only along with and through other people. An *integral* human fulfilment, answering to all of one's reasonable desires, would be the happiness and flourishing of all human persons and their communities (see ref. 6, pp. 281–284; ref. 7, pp. 79–81). Authentic morality is not social convention, nor a law supported by threats and prizes, nor a key to egoistic self-fulfilment. It articulates what is involved in being rationally interested (without sub-rational restrictions or deflections) in integral human fulfilment (see ref. 8, pp. 121–131).

Morality

Morality's guidelines for making one's choices fully reasonable all make more specific the most general and foundational moral principle: that one should will those and only those possibilities whose willing is compatible with integral human fulfilment (see ref. 8, pp. 121–131).

The various aspects of this fulfilment provide the real *reasons for* all human actions: these are such basic human goods as life and health, knowledge, skills, friendship, practical reasonableness, and religion (see ref. 9, pp. 59–99). None of these basic human goods is a mere means to any of the others; all are equally fundamental and intrinsically good (ref. 8, pp. 106–110; ref. 7, pp. 54–56). Fully realized and actualized in all human lives, they would constitute integral human fulfilment, total human happiness. What sorts of choices are incompatible with that?

Various sorts. Choices shaped by egoism or partiality are not open to *integral* human fulfilment. So one basic moral principle is the Golden Rule: 'In everything, do to others as you would have them do to you' (Mt 7.12). This is central to *justice*. Moral philosophers speak of 'universalizability'. Common speech talks of fairness. In the Old Testament it was formulated along with *non-maleficence*: 'And what you hate, do not do to anyone' (Tob 4.15). Jesus extended the Old Testament formulation so as to link it also with *benevolence*: 'You shall love your neighbour as yourself' (see Mt 7.12 and 22.40).

Still, there are principles of non-maleficence distinct from the Golden Rule. Blood feuds, for example, need not be unfair, but are immoral. For acting on hostile feelings towards oneself or others cannot be in line with a will to integral human fulfilment. Respect for the dignity of persons—treating them always as ends in themselves and never as mere means—involves more than treating them fairly.

Positive feelings, too, can motivate one to do evil—to destroy, damage or impede an instantiation of some basic human good. Such choices are often defended as the greater good, or lesser evil. But though many comparisons of values and disvalues are possible, any comparison which hopes to guide moral judgement by an overall 'weighing' of the goods and evils at stake in morally significant options is always made by feelings, not rational commensuration. Such 'calculations' can only be rationalizations. Choices to 'do evil', in the sense just defined, willy-nilly play favourites among instantiations of basic human goods, just as in violating the Golden Rule one plays favourites among persons. No such choice is compatible with a will towards integral human fulfilment. Moral philosophy thus clarifies and justifies the common sayings: 'The end does not justify such means', 'Never treat anyone as a mere means', 'Do not do evil that good may come'.

Moral philosophy articulates other strategic moral principles, and identifies the virtues or character-traits which facilitate a life in line with all these guidelines for a conscientious openness to integral human fulfilment. But here we turn, instead, to note some implications of the additional data made available to conscience by revelation.

Christian Moral Life

In these wider and deeper perspectives, integral human fulfilment is no mere 'ideal of reason' for the critique of a will distorted (rather than supported) by feelings. Instead it is a reality which, by virtue of God's promise and grace, can begin in this life and extend into the completed kingdom and family of God (see ref. 10, pp. 115–140, 459–476). In restating Christian hope, the Second Vatican

Council indicated the intrinsic relationship between every morally good act, done in God's friendship, and the life of heaven. Even when defeated by events in this world, good works and dispositions are 'material' which God has promised to raise up into a city which will last for ever (see ref. 11, paras 38–39; ref. 12, para. 47).

Thus the most fundamental moral principle of openness to integral human fulfilment becomes: 'Love the Lord your God, and your neighbour as yourself' (cf. Lev 19.18; Deut 6.5; Mt 19.19, etc.), and 'Seek first the Kingdom' (Mt 6.33). Morality identifies not arbitrary laws and rewards, but sets us on the way to the ultimate happiness of communion with God's Trinitarian self, through living lives worthy of children of God the Father, of siblings and members of Christ the Son, and of temples of the Holy Spirit (Mt 12.50; Jn 1.12; 1 Cor 6.19; Eph 2.21; 4.1; Phil 2.15, etc.). Human nature's unity and dignity, and the permanence of the principles (the moral 'natural law' as clarified and supplemented by the revealed 'divine law') articulating conditions for its integral fulfilment, are guaranteed by Christ's sharing that nature with every human person, past, present and future, and by his having come once-for-all as teacher and saviour (see ref. 13, pp. 24–28).

Moral teachings, like other matters of faith, can be definitively and thus by divine assistance infallibly taught. This authoritative distillation of the tradition can be by explicit definitions by a Pope or a general Council, as in the Council of Trent's teaching against polygamy and divorce. Or it can be by the concurrence, at some point in time, of the bishops, agreeing in teaching something as a moral truth to be definitively held (see ref. 14, pp. 258–312) as in the teaching against adultery, abortion and indeed any direct killing of the innocent. Such teachings, like others authoritatively proposed by the Church's magisterium, either restate or consistently unfold implications of Christ's very firm moral teaching, e.g. against divorce and remarriage, and his reassertion of the morality of the Ten Commandments (see Mt 19: 18–20) (see ref. 13, pp. 6–9). Thus they trace the implications of a free commitment to a way worthy of our earthly–heavenly calling, and befitting a human nature shared and redeemed by Jesus.

The Witness of Christ

Care for the sick, the weak, the suffering and the sinful was a principal focus of Jesus' life. A healing ministry taking many communal forms—monastic pharmacies, hospitals, nursing homes, hospices and nurses' training run by religious orders, lay faithful committed to health care as their vocation, sacramental and other pastoral care for the sick, reflection on medical ethics— fulfils the vocation to be a servant of humankind and mediator of God's healing power: true beneficence.

But pain and death will not be eliminated in this life. Suffering must be faced head-on, against the pervasive temptation to demand an immediate technological 'fix' for every discomfort, and to marginalize those who suffer so that the rest can withdraw undisturbed. Faith recalls the profounder possibilities for good occasioned by illness and pain: for the sufferer, re-evaluation, conversion, growth in virtue, setting things right with God and other persons; for onlookers, compassion and selfless behaviour (see ref. 15, pp. 47–49, 197–199). The crucified God gives new significance to these redemptive qualities of suffering; contemplation of the cross and uniting onself with Christ's passion make possible greater endurance, assist in our redemption (see e.g. Rom 8.17–18), and overcome temptations to a false beneficence and delusive mercy.

The Resurrection, too, has implications for bioethics. It recalls the eternal destiny of the moral agent who has only one life in which to choose for or against God; it discourages a therapeutic obstinacy born of secular despair of an afterlife; it demands that we respect the person's dignity to the end, and give special pastoral as well as medical care to the dying; and it requires that we honour even the symbol of that dignity, the corpse: their mortal remains.

SOME FALSE CONTEXTS FOR MORAL DISCOURSE

Moral principles tend to lose their meaning and their rational warrant when they are announced (as by Beauchamp and Childress (16)) as if plucked out of the air, a 'moral code' akin to civil law or club rules to be strictly applied, compromised or 'balanced'. A bioethics with such oracular 'foundations' overlooks the true basis for a *rational* (and thus, too, a Christian) ethics (17–19) as set out in the first section of this chapter. Such a bioethic is legalistic and fails, we think, to meet the contemporary challenges to morality in health care. These challenges include:

1. Using the prevalence of bioethical controversy to 'validate' denials of moral responsibility or a relativized or privatized morality ('what's right for me might not be right for you', 'I don't want to impose my moral beliefs on people', 'I can do whatever I please as long as I don't hurt anyone else', etc.). Slavery and genocide, even when 'controversial' or vigorously defended, were not thereby made right.

2. Appeals to conscience as self-validating. To violate one's conscience by choosing options one believes wrong is indeed immoral, even when one is actually mistaken in judging them wrong (20) (see also ref. 10, pp. 73–96). But it is also immoral to leave one's conscience uneducated, settling serious moral questions by mere preferences or private 'intuitions'. For conscience is simply one's ability to know moral truth, recognize objective moral standards, and bring them to bear in practical judgements about particular options—an ability dependent for its proper use (as is every other intellectual capacity) on willingness to learn, attention to relevant data, self-discipline, and the help of a morally decent culture.

3. Dreams of a 'value-free', 'objective', 'scientific' bioethic, as opposed to 'moralizing', 'judgemental', 'religious' or 'interfering' bioethics. Supposedly 'objective' principles like 'scientific progress should be allowed to continue unencumbered' are as value-laden as other ethical approaches. To call one's preferred ethic 'value-free' or one's principles of deliberation 'scientific' simply prepares one to shirk justifying them and to pursue uncritically whatever one's feelings or environment happen to favour.

4. Subjection to the 'technological imperative': that whatever we can do, we inevitably will, and should or rightly may. The illogicality of deeming all technological advances justified and good is not well disguised by tagging opponents 'backward' or 'fearful'.
5. Consequentialist misconceptions of beneficence and denials of true non-maleficence. Claims that any means can be justified by a sufficiently good end are unreasonable, as we show on pp. 37–38 below. They also contradict the western medical–ethical tradition (with its absolutes such as 'never kill, or exploit, your patients'), the political–legal tradition of inalienable and inviolable human rights, and the moral *tradition* of most Christian churches (with their constant teachings against doing evil for the sake of good—cf. Rom 3.8—and against every direct killing of the innocent) (21).

Take *in-vitro* fertilization (IVF) as one example (among many!) of all these conflicting ethical voices. 'Value-free' technological imperativists might say: this technology is available, its application is 'inevitable', so go ahead. Relativists: it's for the individual couple or their doctors or their society to decide. Legalists: the law of beneficence requires it (or: this holy book forbids it). Consequentialists: though not the best way to have a child, it is the only way for some, and on balance is good (or: it will lead to Brave New World and on balance is bad).

A better approach (22,23), recognizes that not all ways of supplying good desires are truly open to integral human fulfilment; some ethical principles cannot rationally be compromised. More specifically, human life must not be intentionally destroyed or damaged, even in its earliest stage. And the radical equality of parents and child is wrongly contradicted when the child is brought into being precisely as a product of mastery over materials. Nor can there be any genuinely rational 'balancing up' of IVF's bad effects (such as the disjunction of the life-giving and love-giving dimensions of marital intercourse, the enslavement and destruction of many embryos, the dangers to the women and children, etc.) with the good ones (giving a childless couple a child, new scientific knowledge, income and kudos for the scientist): for these values and disvalues are all so basically different. There remain also the self-making aspects of such choices. Acting as master of the destiny of tiny human beings, choosing to manipulate or kill some for whatever purposes, disintegrating human sexuality and parenting, all will mould us as certain kind of people and sway our future attitudes and choices in many, perhaps all, our activities. The Catholic moral judgement against all laboratory reproduction of human beings (24) is, then, considered and definite; it is not a 'law' or a 'ban' but a rational judgement about moral truth, drawing on an understanding of the human realities which is enriched by revelation.

Still, while it thus draws on a wider and deeper context of principle, it can also be taken as a conclusion about what, in this matter, truly is beneficent and just, and what is maleficent and unjust because imposing, in the name of parental or scientific autonomy, new forms of human domination and subjection. So, against this background, we offer a few further observations on 'the four principles'.

BENEFICENCE

Health care's traditional vocation (object and responsibility) has been: promote the good health of your patients and cure (or prevent) their illnesses. Though serving other basic benefits too—knowledge, skill, community between patient and professional, practical reasonableness, etc.—health care has as its primary rationale the basic human good of life. 'Life' here includes health, the well-integrated, harmonious functioning of a living being of an organic, sentient and rational nature.

Health care often calls for 'calculation', to find the most efficient cure, palliation, management, etc., the best proportion of likely therapeutic benefits to burdens. In relation to each available therapy one considers various factors; some are objective though partly indeterminable (prognosis, likely and possible side-effects, costs, etc.); some are subjective (the patient's fears, ability to cope with pain, own assessment of benefits and burdens, etc.).

This kind of assessment need involve no 'end justifies the means' ethic (consequentialism). The best-known consequentialism, 'utilitarianism', exists in many incompatible forms, but all assert something like: choose what seems most likely to maximize good and minimize bad effects. Lately, some Catholic bioethicists have proposed various hybrids of consequentialism with classical Christian morality. 'Situation ethics', for instance, counsels choosing whatever, in the particular 'situation', seems most humane or loving or in line with 'faith instinct' (see ref. 25, p. 243). 'Proportionalism' (in its main forms) bids us seek the option promising to maximize the balance of 'premoral' goods (such as lives, health, contentment) over premoral evils (such as deaths, sickness, sadness) (26–29).

Such approaches have been refuted at length elsewhere (30,31) (see also ref. 6, pp. 238–272; ref. 3, pp. 80–135 and ref. 13, pp. 13–24, 93–101). They all fallaciously assume that because some rational comparisons of value are possible, therefore it is possible, at least in principle, to make a determinate rational comparison of the goods and bads anticipated in options. Extrapolating rashly from what is (at least logically) possible in a technical, cost–benefit problem with a single definite goal, they all gratuitously suppose a similar logical possibility in moral deliberations, which involve an open horizon, many different benefits and harms, and one's whole stance towards integral human fulfilment.

True beneficence, then, will not be so narrowly focused on 'foreseeable consequences' that it overrides questions of means and intentions (which have implications and consequences that only divine providence can adequately foresee, master and dispose).

NON-MALEFICENCE

Primum non nocere ('first of all, do no harm') was a classic first principle of medical (and other) ethics. As the Hippocratic oath puts it: 'I will use treatment to help the sick to the best of my ability and judgement, but I will never use it to injure or wrong them.' But what is harm, what is wrong?

In the first section of this chapter we sketched the rational basis for such traditional formulae as: 'The end does not justify the means', 'Never treat anyone as a mere means', 'Do not do evil that good may come'. It is always wrong to choose to destroy, damage or impede an instance of a basic human good for the sake of some ulterior end. That good provides *a* reason against such a choice, and because that good cannot rationally be 'outweighed', that choice will be not merely against *a* reason but against *reason*.

In health care practice three forms of maleficence are common: (a) lying, (b) killing and (c) mutilation.

Lying

In lying, one expresses outwardly, and tries to get others to accept, something at odds with one's inner self. One thus divides one's inner and outer self, contrary to one's own self-integration and authenticity, and impedes or attacks the real community that truthful communication would foster, even when deception seems very desirable. So, though telling the whole truth (or even *telling* anything at all) is quite often destructive or heartless, lying is always wrong.

Killing

Someone who brings about death, intending to do so as an end or as a means (and whether by action or deliberate omission), is said to kill 'directly'. (Causing death only as a side-effect, however predictable, is 'indirect' killing.) The *direct taking of innocent human life* always violates the principle of maleficence and is always wrong (32) (see also ref. 6, pp. 297–319). (Some but not all indirect killings, too, violate the principles of justice and non-maleficence.) Whether in abortion, eugenic prenatal testing and selection, embryo experimentation and non-therapeutic genetic engineering, infanticide of the handicapped, assisted suicide or euthanasia, direct killing always demeans both victim and perpetrator, invites further 'therapeutic' killing, and violates the divine trust given us in human life.

'Quality of life' decisions to deal with certain persons on the basis that they are 'better off dead', because their life 'is of no benefit' or has no (or a negative) value are notoriously arbitrary and elastic. They also, and inevitably, violate either the principle of non-maleficence, or a principle of justice (or both). Even the very reduced and deficient life of the irreversibly comatose is an instance of a basic human good; it is the very existence of a unique person, who can still be harmed, e.g. by being subjected to indignities. A decision to discontinue feeding and hydrating may be either direct killing (as a means to relieve others of burdens created by the patient's continued existence) or, if motivated solely by desire to avoid the burdens of *feeding and hydrating*, an abandonment which could be just only in circumstances of emergency or poverty rarely if ever found in modern western society (33,34).

Of course there may be good *therapeutic* reasons for withholding or withdrawing some treatments. Their continued use may be futile, i.e. of no therapeutic value. Or they may impose a burden (such as pain, indignity, risk, cost, etc.) which those concerned feel is out of proportion to the benefit gained. Here the health care worker does not indulge in arbitrary 'quality of life' decision-making, but rather makes a (sometimes difficult) therapeutic judgement about the helpfulness or not of the proposed medical treatment in dealing with the patient's illness. On this basis some treatments will be medically indicated and morally required ('ordinary'); others will be optional ('extraordinary'); and still others will be contraindicated (and immoral) (35–37).

Mutilation

Respect for persons and the good of life includes respect for their physical, psychological and spiritual integrity. Non-maleficence forbids mutilation, even when consented to (e.g. to facilitate begging, preserve choristers' voices, or prevent conception). For example, sterilization chosen in order to prevent conception is, at best, a bad means to a good ulterior end, an act of well-motivated but morally confused maleficence. For in no way does sterility as such truly benefit anyone; it only facilitates sexual intercourse—a distinct act in and through which some benefit is expected—by excluding conception. Even when well-motivated, every choice directly to impair a function involves an intention to damage a basic human good, and is always wrong.

But it can be morally good and even obligatory to remove a part of the body when this removal, of itself, protects or promotes health, and one does not intend the detriment to function as a means to any end, but only accepts it as a side-effect. For example, an infected limb or non-vital organ may rightly be amputated or excised when that is necessary to prevent the infection from doing great harm to the whole body. Even a healthy part may be removed if doing so has natural consequences which are necessary for the health of the whole body and cannot be effected in another, less detrimental way.

Donating parts of one's remains after death damages no human good, and can rightly be done to benefit another or others—provided, of course, that death is properly established and there is proper respect for grieving relatives and staff. Donating blood typically involves no harm and very little risk, is permitted by the principles of non-maleficence and can be recommended or even required by the principles of beneficence. The live donation of an organ (e.g. a cornea), when the benefit to another will be secured only and precisely by detracting from the functioning of the donor (e.g. the donor's depth vision), is a bad means to a good end, and always wrong. But the live donation of an organ (e.g. a kidney) can be right, even though it involves some risk of future detriment to function; for here the potential loss of function is not part of one's chosen means but only an accepted side-effect.

These distinctions are often explained by Catholic moralists by reference to a 'principle of totality': mutilation is morally permissible when necessary for the good of the whole body (38) (see also ref. 15, pp. 36–43, 194–196). But that principle is no more than the application, in a particular context, of the quite general considerations which determine when there is and is not a choosing of evil for the sake of good. Catholic moralists, during the past 200 years or so, often discussed those considerations under the headings of the 'principle of double effect'. But that principle (39,40) (which is misrepresented in many works, e.g. ref. 16, pp. 127–134), is reducible, on analysis, to two propositions: (a) neither as an end nor as a means may one choose to destroy, damage or impede any instance of a basic human good; (b) a result of a choice is not a chosen means merely because it is foreseen as a probable or certain result, but because it is part of the proposal which one shaped in deliberation and adopted in that choice. The analysis of chosen actions, to establish what one is and is not really intending, can be difficult and delicate. It affords much opportunity for rationalization and self-deception. But it is eminently a matter for rational reflection and discussion. It is also a matter on which, for salient conclusions about the morality of some specific types of choice, one can look to the Church's authoritative wisdom.

AUTONOMY

Ideals of autonomy today contain much that is unacceptable. They often involve or promote a dream of absolute self-sufficiency, independent of God, community, reason and reality. Social authority is seen as a necessary evil for limiting social conflict, but ideally one should be free to do as one pleases, adopting one's own lifestyle and conception of fulfilment. 'Privacy' and 'my right to my body', in the context of such ideas, veil a hardening of hearts against human beings for whose very existence one is responsible. Conscience is considered a private internal voice with authority to judge without too much regard for reality, truth and wisdom. The ideal of autonomy woven of these strands, though widely felt to be self-evident, is but the distorted shadow of a truth clarified by revelation: every human person has the dignity of one redeemed by Christ, and none is properly the slave or instrument of another's purposes. So the greatest of Catholic moralists have made the cornerstone of their ethics this proposition: mature human persons, having free will, image God principally by being rational masters of their own acts (see ref. 20, prologue; ref. 10, pp. 41–72).

Properly understood, then, the principle of autonomy is an acknowledgement of both the radical equality of all human beings, and the inalienable responsibility of all who can choose to make their choices open to integral human fulfilment.

We have mentioned one way in which that radical equality is denied (in IVF). Here is another: well-intentioned lying. Those who lie to their patients manipulate them. Very often they overconfidently judge what they cannot know: that the one they try to deceive cannot deal with reality, cannot make good use of the freedom that only truth can give, and will not suspect or even detect the deception, with a consequent loss of trust. By their impact on freedom and fostering of mistrust, supposedly helpful lies often do great, although unintentional, harm.

As to each individual's inalienable responsibility: the primary duty of health care is one's responsibility to look after oneself, physically, psychologically and spiritually—to treat one's health as one of the 'talents' entrusted by God to one's stewardship. In seeking and consenting to the needful help of others one cannot repudiate one's personal responsibility or grant them authority to do more than one can responsibly ask. Interventions by health care professionals which do not respect the proper directions of a patient fail to respect the patient as (like all human beings) the health care worker's radical equal.

We shall not here repeat the still generally sound norms of the health care professions concerning respect for patients, informed consent, nurturing of trust, confidentiality of records, and so forth. Instead we express a fear. Unhinged from its true ethical context the principle of autonomy (often reduced to the right to 'privacy' or 'to choose') soon may become the principal formula for rationalizing the extermination of many sick and handicapped persons, young and old. For if non-maleficence is re-interpreted so as to allow assisted suicide and voluntary euthanasia in the name of autonomous 'self'-liberation from a burdensome life, it doubtless will soon be held that those who *cannot* (and in many cases *never* did or could) give their consent to it should not thereby be deprived of their equal 'privacy right' to liberation from burdensome life. The 'right' will be exercised 'on their behalf' by someone who will choose for them the death which, it will thus be presumed, they would have (or should have) chosen had they been capable of choice. A false 'principle of autonomy' could thus be the constitutional and ethical vehicle for the profound injustice of a 'beneficent' maleficence, ridding the community of many lives deemed 'not worth living' (*lebensunwertes Lebens*).

JUSTICE

There are two senses of 'justice' (ref. 9, pp. 161–197). As fairness, justice is a principle distinguishable from beneficence and non-maleficence. As respect for all the rights of others, justice is a principle which includes beneficence, non-maleficence and true autonomy. Here, then, we add only a few points.

Concern for the common good—'love of neighbour', or 'solidarity'—requires fellow-feeling, genuine self-giving, joint effort with others to promote the flourishing of all, encouragement and support for the efforts of others. Health care certainly requires joint effort and deliberate coordination, at various levels of institutions, communities and governments. But true autonomy requires that larger communities should assist smaller ones, not absorb them—this is the principle of 'subsidiarity'—just as smaller ones should help individuals to help themselves. Governments should assist with resources, coordination and encouragement, but not take charge of all the functions of smaller groups where (given suitable freedom and assistance) those smaller groups could direct and perform these functions (see ref. 9, pp. 146, 159, 164; ref. 41, para. 41).

Justice supports neither centralized control of all aspects of health care (a violation of subsidiarity), nor leaving health care, a fundamental right (see ref. 42, para. 19.5), to the whim of 'market forces' (which violates solidarity). As we have the right to expect the help of others, so we have the reciprocal duty to help others in need of health care, whether through our taxes, insurance payments, or provision of personal care. A system of health care violates the Golden Rule (I must presume) if I would think that system unfair were I (or someone I loved) in the weakest position in the community. The world's material resources are *given* to all humankind, for the needs of all, and so while private property is often a requirement of justice, the needs of others establish duties on the part of those who have more than they need towards those who have less than they need—in health care as in other basic human needs (ref. 11, para. 69; ref. 12, para. 42; ref. 41, para. 31).

Special care for the (materially and/or spiritually) poor, underprivileged, powerless and desperate is something the Church considers itself called upon to give ('the preferential option for the poor') (ref. 41, para. 57). Among the various just regimes of health care distribution which are possible in a community (ref. 15, pp. 112–144), the Christian will prefer ones which give special care to the most needy and defenceless.

Mercy calls us to go beyond (without violating) the principles of justice and non-maleficence in healing every form of evil (ref. 10, pp. 644–646). Is 'mercy killing' (euthanasia) the truly compassionate way to treat those in severe pain or incurable illness or coma? Or to distribute finite health resources? Compassion means wanting the best for others, having empathy with them in their suffering, and seeking positively to assist by acts of mercy in keeping with their dignity. Far from contributing to 'death with dignity', support for euthanasia promotes a culture which whispers to the old and infirm 'Your condition is intolerably undignified. You would be better off dead. We would be too, if you were dead. You may even have a duty to acquiesce in being killed.' Thus false views of mercy and justice can conspire to institute a 'beneficent' maleficence, injustice, and the ultimate negation of autonomy (43).

REFERENCES

1. Boyle, J. M., Grisez, G. and Tollefsen, O. 1976. *Free choice: a self-referential analysis.* Notre Dame University Press, Notre Dame and London.
2. Grisez, G. and Shaw, R. 1988. *Beyond the new morality: the responsibilities of freedom,* 3rd edn. University of Notre Dame Press, Notre Dame.
3. Finnis, J. 1983. *Fundamentals of ethics,* Clarendon Press, Oxford.
4. Finnis, J. 1984. Practical reasoning, human goods and the end of Man. *Proceedings of the American Catholic Philosophical Association* 58: 23–36 (also in *New Blackfriars* 1985; **66**: 438–451).
5. McCabe, H. OP. 1969. *What is ethics all about?* Corpus Books, Washington DC.
6. Finnis, J., Boyle, J. and Grisez, G. 1987. *Nuclear deterrence, morality and realism.* Oxford University Press, Oxford and New York.
7. Grisez, G. and Shaw, R. 1991. *Fulfilment in Christ: a summary of Christian moral principles.* University of Notre Dame Press, Notre Dame and London.
8. Grisez, G., Boyle, J. and Finnis, J. 1980. Practical principles, moral truth, and ultimate ends. *American Journal of Jurisprudence* 32: 99–151 at 121–131.
9. Finnis, J. 1980. *Natural law and natural rights.* Clarendon Press, Oxford.
10. Grisez, G. 1983. *The way of the Lord Jesus,* Vol. I: *Christian moral principles.* Franciscan Herald Press, Chicago.
11. Vatican Council II. 1975. *Gaudium et spes.* (Pastoral constitution on the Church in the modern world, 7.12.65), *in* Flannery, A., OP (Ed.). *Vatican Council II: The conciliar and post conciliar documents,* pp. 903–1001 and 937–938. Scholarly Resources, Wilmington; Dominican Publications, Dublin.
12. John Paul II, Pope. 1987. *Sollicitudo rei socialis.* Encyclical for the twentieth anniversary of populorum progressio (30.12.87). Libreria Editrice Vaticana, Vatican City.
13. Finnis, J. 1991. *Moral absolutes: tradition, revision, and truth.* Catholic University of America Press, Washington, DC.

14. Ford, J. C., SJ, and Grisez, G. 1978. Contraception and the infallibility of the ordinary magisterium. *Theological Studies* **39**: 258–312 (also in Ford, J. C., SJ, Grisez, G., Boyle, J., Finnis, J. *et al.* 1988. *The teaching of Humanae vitae: a defense.* Ignatius Press, San Francisco).
15. Ashley, B. M., OP, and O'Rourke, K. D., OP. 1989. *Healthcare ethics: a theological analysis*, 3rd edn. Catholic Health Association, St Louis.
16. Beauchamp, T. L. and Childress, J. F. 1989. *Principles of biomedical ethics*, 3rd edn, Oxford University Press, New York.
17. Hauerwas, S. 1974. *Vision and virtue.* Fides, South Bend.
18. Hauerwas, S. *et al.* 1981. *Truthfulness and tragedy.* University of Notre Dame Press, Notre Dame, IN.
19. MacIntyre, A. 1985. *After virtue: a study in moral theory*, 2nd edn. Duckworth, London.
20. Aquinas, T. *Summa theologiae.* 1a.2ae, q. 19, a. 5–6; trans. in Gilby, T., OP (Ed.). 1965. *St Thomas Aquinas, Summa theologiae*, vol. 18, *Principles of morality*, pp. 18–27. Eyre and Spottiswoode, London.
21. Grisez, G. 1970. *Abortion: the myths, the realities, and the arguments.* Corpus Books, New York.
22. Fisher, A. OP. 1989. *IVF: the critical issues.* Collins Dove, Melbourne.
23. Catholic Bishops' Joint Committee on Bioethical Issues. 1983. *In vitro fertilisation and public policy.* Catholic Media Office and Joint Committee on Bioethical Issues, Abingdon.
24. Congregation for the Doctrine of the Faith. 1987. *Donum vitae. Instruction on respect for human life in its origin and on the dignity of procreation* (22.2.87). Catholic Truth Society, London.
25. Rahner, K. SJ. *Theological investigations*, vol. 9. Crossroad Press, New York.
26. Hoose, B. 1987. *Proportionalism: the American debate and its European roots.* Georgetown University Press, Washington, DC.
27. McCormick, R. A. 1973. *Ambiguity in moral choice.* Marquette University Press, Milwaukee.
28. McCormick, R. A. 1985. *Health and medicine in the Catholic tradition.* Crossroad, New York.
29. McCormick, R. A. and Ramsey, P. (Eds). 1978. *Doing evil to achieve good.* Loyola University Press, Chicago.
30. Grisez, G. 1978. Against consequentialism. *American Journal of Jurisprudence* **23**: 21–72.
31. Kiely, B., SJ. 1985. The impracticability of proportionalism. *Gregorianum* **66**: 655–686.
32. Pius XII, Pope. 1944. Address to the St. Luke Union of Italian Physicians (12.11.1944). Discorsi e radio-messaggi 1944; 6:191; quoted in *Congregation for the Doctrine of the Faith* (see ref. 35, p. 452). *Declaration on procured abortion* (18.11.74).
33. Grisez, G. 1990. Should nutrition and hydration be provided to permanently unconscious and other mentally disabled persons? *Linacre Quarterly* **57**: 30–43.
34. May, W. E. 1987. Feeding and hydrating the permanently unconscious and other vulnerable persons. *Issues in Law and Medicine* **3**: 203–217.
35. Sacred Congregation for the Doctrine of the Faith. 1982. *Jura et bona (Declaration on euthanasia)*, 5.5.80, in Flannery, A., OP, (Ed.). *Vatican II*, vol. 2: *More postconciliar documents*, pp. 510–518. Costello Publishing, New York.
36. Linacre Centre. 1982. *Euthanasia and clinical practice: trends, principles and alternatives.* Linacre Centre for the Study of the Ethics of Health Care, London.
37. Pollard, B. 1989. *Euthanasia: should we kill the dying?* Mount Press, Sydney.
38. Gallagher, J., CSB. 1984. The principle of totality: man's stewardship of his body, *in* McCarthy, D. G. (Ed.) *Moral theology today: certitudes and doubts*, pp. 217–242. Pope John Center, St Louis.
39. May, W. E. 1978. Double effect, principle of, *in* Reich, W. (Ed.) *Encyclopedia of bioethics.* Macmillan, New York.
40. Boyle, J. M. 1980. Toward understanding the principle of double effect. *Ethics* **90**: 527–538.

41. John Paul II, Pope. 1991. *Centesimus annus.* Encyclical on the hundredth anniversary of rerum novarum, 1.5.91. Middlegreen: St Paul Publications.
42. John Paul II, Pope. 1981. *Laborem exercens.* Encyclical on human work, 14.9.81. London: Catholic Truth Society.
43. Grisez, G. and Boyle, J. M. 1979. *Life and death with liberty and justice: a contribution to the euthanasia debate.* University of Notre Dame Press, Notre Dame and London.

5

Theology and the Four Principles: A Roman Catholic View II

BERNARD HOOSE

Heythrop College, London, UK

It is all too easy to make statements which imply absolute norms for human behaviour, norms which apply always and everywhere, regardless of circumstances, intentions and likely consequences. Such absolutist speech is commonly used by parents when addressing children. Thus we find young Albert being told that he must never do 'that' again. The world of adulthood, however, is often quite complex, and 20 years later Albert may find that the morally right thing to do in a particular situation is precisely 'that' which his mother told him never to do again. He discovers that the word 'never' in his mother's command should not be taken too literally, although the command certainly functions as a rough guideline for behaviour most of the time. Other examples of 'absolute-sounding' guidelines are: 'never harm anybody' and 'doctors should always protect people from harm'. We need little experience to discover that sometimes we can help people only if we cause some damage to their bodies and/or inflict some kind of pain upon them. We also see that, in some situations, if we use up expensive and rare resources to protect a certain person from harm, we leave other people, whom we could have helped if we had not used up those resources, exposed to even greater harm. These examples serve to illustrate problems attached to the principles of beneficence, non-maleficence and justice. Whilst admitting these difficulties, some may feel that the principle of autonomy is a quite different matter. A norm demanding respect for the autonomy of patients, they might say, is more than just a rough guideline. Even here, however, there are problems of interpretation. What does such respect involve when a doctor or other person involved in health care is dealing with an infant, a drug addict or a person bent on suicide?

I imagine that all Christians, as well as many non-Christians, would uphold

---

Principles of Health Care Ethics. Edited by Raanan Gillon.

the importance of the principles of autonomy, beneficence, non-maleficence and justice in health care ethics. All, however, would have to admit that there are problems attached to their application, and that the principles often conflict with each other in particular cases. It may be claimed that such problems are of a purely philosophical nature. We would, I think, be foolish, however, to ignore the contributions that particular religious groups, such as, for instance, Christianity, can make to debates involving the good of human beings. Schools of philosophical thought, moreover, have grown up within certain branches of Christianity, and that is certainly true of Roman Catholicism.

AUTONOMY OF THE PERSON

In all branches of Christianity respect for the autonomy of the individual is high on the list of priorities. This is hardly surprising, given the belief that we are all children of God, created in his image and likeness. The belief that the Holy Spirit—God him/herself—can dwell in one's very personality only serves to reinforce the call for such respect. As David C. Thomasma puts it: 'All persons are seen as sacramental, that is, extensions of God in human history. Each person is a created presence of God.' A little further on he adds: 'One loves the person, not only as a person but as a presence of God' (1). The respect called for is much more than respect for autonomy (or 'self-rule'), but it certainly includes it. All those involved in the health care professions should, therefore, respect their patients' rights to self-determination, and should ensure that those patients are supplied with all the information necessary for the decisions they need to make about treatment of their illnesses. It goes without saying that they should also respect their patients' need for confidentiality, truth and privacy. Promises they make to patients, moreover, should not be lightly broken. We might add that prudence counsels that promises be not too lightly made.

Also under the heading of respect for persons, however, we find the demands of the principles of beneficence, non-maleficence and justice and, in particular cases, the demands of these various principles can be in competition with each other. Much of what has been written by Roman Catholic moral theologians in recent years concerns the problems involved in such clashes between values and/or principles which are intended to protect values. Many of the main points of debate will arise as we discuss the demands of beneficence and non-maleficence.

BENEFICENCE AND NON-MALEFICENCE

Beauchamp and Childress distinguish these two principles by putting the prevention and removal of evil or harm, as well as the promotion of good, under the heading of beneficence, and taking non-maleficence to mean 'not inflicting evil or harm' (2). Raanan Gillon, moreover, points out that our *prima facie* duty to non-maleficence is general in that it encompasses all other people, whilst our duty to beneficence is more specific, applying only to some people, although he is quick to add that it does not follow from this that avoiding doing harm takes priority over beneficence (see ref. 3, p. 81). Such distinctions are useful but, of course, they do not suffice to solve the problem of how to balance the various harms and benefits involved in a particular case against each other.

All our actions have more than one effect. Sometimes when we try to achieve something good a far from negligible evil effect also results. To establish whether or not the evil effect can be justified in such cases, it has been common for many years in Catholic circles to employ the principle of double effect. This principle states that the evil effect may be justified if all four of the following conditions are fulfilled:

1. the act performed is good in itself.
2. the good effect does not result from the evil effect.
3. the person acting intends only the good effect.
4. there is a proportionate reason for causing the harm.

To illustrate the application of the principle let us take the case of a pregnant woman with a cancerous uterus. Given the well-known attitude to abortion within the Roman Catholic Church, could a hysterectomy be justified in such a case? If we take the act to be a surgical operation to save the woman's life, and if we can assume that the surgeon's intention is only that of saving the woman's life, conditions (1) and (3) are, it seems, fulfilled. The second condition is also satisfied because saving the woman's life does not depend upon the death of the fetus, which is merely a tragic side-effect. Clearly, in view of the fact that the woman's life is in danger, and there is no way in which the life of the fetus can be saved in this case, there is a proportionate reason for the death of the fetus, and thus we have the fulfilment of the fourth condition. The expression 'indirect abortion' is sometimes used to describe such cases. Similarly, in cases of ectopic pregnancy where the embryo is forming in the Fallopian tube, the principle of double effect has been employed to justify excising the tubes and thereby again causing an indirect abortion.

In all that we have said so far everything may seem very clear and tidy, but in recent years a certain amount of dissatisfaction with the principle of double effect has been expressed. For instance, questions have been raised about the possibility of curing the problem of an ectopic pregnancy such as that described above by removing the embryo whilst leaving the tube intact. Could such an abortion be justified by the principle of double effect? Some would say that it could not, because the act directly performed would be an abortion, and the good effect, the saving of the woman's life, would depend upon the removal and, therefore, the death of the embryo. However, to suggest that the death of the embryo could be justified if the surgeon were willing to cause more harm by excising the tube involved seems ridiculous. Not surprisingly, a good deal of rethinking has gone on in Catholic circles concerning this principle in recent years, although there are still some, it would seem, who continue to use it in its traditional form.

One of the thinkers involved is Germain Grisez. He discusses the problem of having to choose 'between removing a nonviable ectopic embryo and allowing the pregnancy to continue, with a definite threat to the mother's life and little hope for the embryonic child's survival'. In choosing to remove the embryo, he says, one would not necessarily be choosing to kill it. 'The embryo's death is not a means and is in no way helpful to solving the problem. Rather one can make this choice—to remove the ectopic embryo—simply to remove its threat to the mother's life, accepting the embryonic child's certain death only as an inevitable side effect.' Grisez goes on to say that apparent conflicts like this one arise because of the way in which certain acts are conventionally classified. We need to classify them in another way. He illustrates this using the case of killing an attacker, which could be reclassified, he suggests, as stopping a violent attack (4). Now, according to Grisez's own moral theory, a direct attack on life is impermissible. It would seem, therefore, that here he is putting the emphasis on the agent's intention in order to establish that the act directly performed is not evil. Some others would say that such reclassification based on the agent's intention would be insufficient. It has traditionally been taught and is surely still generally accepted that, when attacked, one should use no more violence than is necessary. Obviously, in the heat, uncertainty and panic of the moment, questions about how much violence is too much can seem purely academic. However, if you know that someone is about to slap you across the face, stabbing him or her with a bread knife in order to stop the attack is clearly unjustifiable, in spite of the fact that your act can be classified as 'stopping a violent attack'. In other words, one needs a proportionate reason for the harm which results from one's actions. Thus we find numerous Catholic moral theologians saying that, whilst it is important to know the object of the action, its justification still depends upon whether or not the harm in the various aspects of the act and in its consequences is disproportionate to the good.

It is sometimes said that whoever was responsible for the formulation of the principle of double effect was obviously influenced by St Paul's teaching that evil should not be done in order that good may come of it (Rom. 3.8). A number of the so-called revisionist moral theologians we have been discussing have pointed out, however, that, in his use of the term 'evil' in this passage, Paul is obviously referring to morally wrong acts. Not all evils are moral evils or moral wrongs. Pain and frustration of any kind may be regarded as evils, but they are not in themselves moral evils, and it does not follow that, merely because one or more of these evils exists in a particular case, a moral wrong has been done. Such evils have traditionally been described as physical evils. In much recent literature we find them referred to as 'ontic evils', 'premoral evils' and 'non-moral evils'. Thus we can say, without fear of contradicting St Paul, that a surgeon may inflict such ontic evils as pain and mutilation upon a patient in order that good may come about, provided, of course, that the ontic evils involved do not outweigh the ontic goods. This same kind of thinking is applied by revisionist moral theologians, who are sometimes referred to as proportionalists, to cases of abortion like those described above.

It is sometimes claimed that the premises for the principle of double effect are to be found in Thomas Aquinas' discussion of self-defence (see, for instance, ref. 5). We would have to indulge in a very complicated and unusual use of language, however, if we set out to demonstrate that people defending themselves do not bring about the good of saving their lives *by means* of the ontic evil of killing, or at least hurting, their attackers. Like Grisez, Thomas says that the way in which a moral act is to be classified depends upon what is intended by the person acting. It is legitimate, he says, for a person to intend to save his or her life. Nevertheless, an act of self-defence may still be vitiated if it is not proportionate to the end intended. In short, Aquinas holds that it is legitimate to indulge in violent defence provided the defender intends only the good of self-preservation and uses no more force than is required to achieve that end. It follows that, if the degree of force required results in the assailant's death, the killing is justified (6).

References to intention in such discussions can be very confusing at times because the word has various shades of meaning. It is evident that, when a surgeon cuts away a part of a patient's body, he or she fully intends to do so, but there is undoubtedly some sense in trying to classify the act in accordance with what the operation as a whole is aimed at. Only thus can we know whether we are talking about a surgical operation to improve the patient's lot in some way or a mere act of mutilation. Both Aquinas and present-day proportionalists, however, insist that such classification is not enough. There must be proportion, they say, between the harms and benefits involved. Moreover, say the proportionalists, the fact that the good is brought about through an ontic evil (in this case, mutilation) does not suffice to make the act wrong.

It is clear, then, how these authors deal with the principles of beneficence and non-maleficence, but I should hasten to emphasize, in case this is not already clear, that they also take autonomy into account. Any overriding of a person's autonomy involves ontic evil. A certain patient's demands, however, regarding his or her self-determination may, in a particular instance, conflict with the principles of beneficence and non-maleficence. This could be the case, for instance, with a child. Health care professionals, on the other hand, should beware the danger of overriding the child's rights too easily.

A number of critics have said that it is hard to distinguish these revisionist moral theologians from utilitarians. If these critics were correct, the proportionalists might be expected to encounter insuperable problems in trying to accommodate the principle of justice. Utilitarianism can be described, in what we might call its classical form, as the doctrine that a person should, in all situations, perform that action among those available which will produce the greatest amount of good for the greatest number of people. W. D. Ross pointed out some years ago, however, that justice is concerned, not with the production of a maximum of good, but with the right distribution of it (7).

JUSTICE

The alarm thus raised, however, is very much a false one. The proportionalists would surely have no difficulty in regarding an unfair allocation of resources (a problem regarding distributive justice) as an ontic evil. The same could be said with regard to a lack of equity in exchanges between individuals or groups (problems regarding commutative justice). Similarly, not permitting people to participate in the production of society's goods would involve ontic evil. All such evils would have to be taken into account in the proportionalists' scheme of things.

There are on occasions conflicts between what we might call 'justice issues' and the demands of the principles of autonomy, beneficence and non-maleficence. It is sometimes claimed, for instance, that a doctor is obligated only to his or her patient, or that the interests of his or her patient should always come first. However, as Beauchamp and McCullough point out,

> 'The best interests of my patient come first' is not absolute. It is a rebuttable presumption that must sometimes give way to the principle, 'The interests of third parties come first.' Although there is no well-developed *model* of moral responsibility to third parties, any adequate account of the physician's moral responsibilities must accommodate interests of parties such as the family, health care institutions, medical education and research, future generations of patients, employers, the local community and the state. For each, a range of conflicts is present for the physician. Some forms of conflict are best resolved in favor of the patient, others present genuine dilemmas, and still others are best resolved in favor of the third party (8).

We could, for instance, take the case of a doctor whose patient's best interests would be served by the employment of an extremely rare and expensive piece of equipment for a very long period of time, although the same piece of equipment could be used to effect much more rapid cures in several patients of other doctors. Some people, following W. D. Ross, would see such problems in terms of clashes between or among *prima facie* duties, and, in some way or other would have to compare those *prima facie* duties in order to decide which is their real duty. The Catholic revisionist theologians referred to above would compare the various ontic goods and evils involved.

Although there is a good deal of variety among the theories of justice which are available, there is at least some general agreement among the various schools of thought regarding the usefulness, at least in the sphere of distributive justice, of a basic principle taken from Aristotle's writings. This principle states that equals should be treated equally and that unequals should be treated unequally in accordance with their relevant inequalities (9). As Raanan Gillon points out, the reason why this principle remains so widely accepted is that it has little substantive content (see ref. 3, p. 88). Which inequalities should count and how they should be calculated are matters for debate and have been for centuries. Regarding distributive justice, some scholars have advanced arguments, for example, in favour of distributing material goods, privileges, honours, services, etc. according to merit. Some have said that they should be distributed according to need, and others have argued in favour of leaving things largely to market forces. It could, of course, be argued that all should be given an equal share but, in the world as we know it, a policy of that kind would surely be unfair. It is probable that many people would suffer as a result of such a distribution or allocation, whilst many others would not need, merit or perhaps even want much of what they were given.

In order to understand the thought of many Catholic scholars in this sphere it is useful to turn for a moment from specifically medical issues to the development of social teaching within that Church, including papal encyclicals on social issues since the publication of Leo XIII's *Rerum novarum*. Although various developments and even changes have taken place, Karen Lebacqz notes that 'the Catholic tradition on social teachings is rooted in three basic affirmations: 1) the inviolable dignity of the human person, 2) the essentially social nature of human beings, and 3) the belief that the abundance of nature and of social living is given for all people' (10). These three affirmations can, of course, be shown to be biblically based. A brief glance at some of the biblical background should therefore be useful at this point. Israel was a community, and giving help to one's brothers and sisters to the best of one's ability was very much part of the covenant with God. Relationships were of immense importance. Indeed, as John R. Donahue puts it:

> In general terms the biblical idea of justice can be described as *fidelity to the demands of a relationship*. In contrast to modern individualism the Israelite is in a world where 'to live' is to be united with others in a social context either by bonds of family or by covenant relationships. This web of relationships—king with people, judge with complainants, family with tribe and kinfolk, the community with the resident alien...—constitutes the world in which life is played out (11).

Maintaining law and justice, says Th. C. Vriezen, meant taking care that true relations were not disturbed and that each person's integrity was fully protected. Every relation was truly humane. Thus, although equality was not recognized in every sense, even slaves were not to be regarded as commodities, but as human beings. They were to be admitted to the cult and were to share in the Sabbath rest (12).

Having read various documents from the Catholic tradition, on the subject of justice, David Hollenbach found a good deal there about the importance of relationships:

> What is *due* to a person or a group is to be determined by the kinds of relationships which shape and influence the life and action of that person or group. Human dignity—the fact that human beings are not things or mere means—always exists *within* these various concrete relationships. The justice or injustice of these relationships is to be judged in terms of the way they promote human dignity by enhancing mutuality and genuine participation in community or, put negatively, by the way they abuse human dignity by reifying persons and excluding or marginalizing them from the relationships without which humanity withers (13).

There is, of course, much here that is relevant to the ethics of health care. One thing I would like to highlight, however, is the call to recognize the needs of the stranger, who may be all too easily dismissed as a 'third party' or 'someone on the waiting list', a person I do not know. This is a person with whom, through our shared humanity, I do have a relationship. Perhaps that relationship calls for precedence to be given to a stranger's needs in a particular case. Perhaps it calls in a more general way for us to play our part in altering structures and habitual practices in the world of health care which cause some people—for the most part strangers to us—to be excluded or marginalized in some way.

CLARIFICATIONS AND CONFLICTS

We have already had reason to note that cases of conflict among the principles of autonomy, beneficence, non-maleficence and justice are not always easy to resolve. Something that can complicate matters even more is the possibility that the meaning a particular therapy has for a patient is not obvious to the health care professionals involved. Such factors should not be too easily categorized as being of importance only in the world of psychiatry and psychotherapy. Psychological factors are surely always a large part of the healing process in any branch of health care. The main point I wish to make here, however, is the fact that the meaning of certain kinds of therapy can vary so much from patient to patient as to lead to different conclusions in different cases of conflict. In a recently published article the present writer discussed the ethics of enhancement genetic engineering. I took up the case of Joseph Merrick (otherwise known as the elephant man). Merrick, it would appear, was a victim of the hereditary disease neurofibromatosis. Obviously, therefore, he was in need of much more than enhancement therapy. The point I wished to make, however, was that an enormous percentage of his suffering was directly attributable to his ugliness. The question therefore arises, if it were possible, through genetic engineering, to considerably improve the lot of a person whose appearance was grotesque, would we not be justified in doing so (14)? The same question could be asked about other forms of enhancement therapy. Now, one hears it said sometimes that treatment which is aimed merely at beautifying clients is not a serious matter for health care professionals and that it should not even be classified as therapy. Moreover, even if one can safely assume that the doctors and nurses who indulge in such practices fulfil the requirements of the principles of autonomy and beneficence, there could be a clash with the requirements of justice if the resources being utilized were needed by people with 'real problems'. Clearly, however, improving the appearance of somebody who is even a good deal less ugly than Merrick could be accurately described as dealing with a real problem, and, indeed, a serious one. We should add, of course, that sufficient attention should be given to the principle of non-maleficence. In some cases of enhancement therapy there would seem to be a considerable risk of inflicting a far from negligible degree of harm upon the patient. With regard more specifically to enhancement genetic engineering, our present general lack of knowledge would seem to call for extreme caution.

In some cases of apparent conflict the problem can be caused by the meaning that particular actions or things have, not for the patient, but for those concerned with the patient's health care. Take, for instance, the case of a terminally ill patient whose life is being prolonged because, says the doctor in charge of the case, it is his job to preserve life. Some people might say that justice demands that expensive and rare resources being used in this case should be released for use elsewhere. There is a conflict here only if there is a serious possibility that the patient in question can be expected to benefit in some way from the treatment. Let us suppose that the only 'benefit' is keeping the patient alive. The problem here lies in seeing life as an absolute value. Within Christianity life is certainly valued as a basic good but, in the words of Richard McCormick, it is 'a good to be preserved precisely as the condition of other values. It is these other values and possibilities that found the duty to preserve life and that also dictate the limits of this duty' (15). If, then, the patient can be kept alive, but only in a permanent vegetative state through the use of these rare and expensive resources, what benefit is to be gained? The patient's life is prolonged merely in order that he or she may stay alive for a longer period than would have otherwise been the case. Of course, if the patient is conscious but in extreme pain, and the prolongation of his or her life will merely result in the prolongation of agony, and if that patient wants to be allowed to die, all four principles could be attacked by a doctor who ignores the patient's wishes. In other words, such a case would not really involve conflict between principles.

Weighing ontic goods and evils against each other is not always an easy matter. Not the least problem is the apparent incommensurability of those goods and evils. Often they are not quantifiable and, therefore, mathematics is of no use at all in the 'calculations'. It has been pointed out on numerous occasions, however, that humans have to be much more than mere computers. Throughout our lives we have to make choices between competing goods or values. In the field of morality we have to struggle to find the most human solutions to the problems that face us. It is not an easy task, but taking in the fruits of accumulated wisdom and fine-tuning our sensitivities will certainly help.

Having said all this, it is useful to add something which is not obviously covered by the four principles. The integrity of those involved in health care must not be ignored by their superiors, their patients or themselves, and here, notwithstanding what we have said above, the meanings which actions and things have for them are of enormous importance. Nobody should be forced to do something which is against his or her conscience. This principle has been highlighted regarding the subject of abortion, but it should also be taken into account in other spheres in which certain people could perform certain actions only by doing violence to their own moral integrity.

REFERENCES

1. Thomasma, D. C. 1987. The basis of medicine and religion: respect for persons. Pp. 290–291, in Lammers S. E. and Verhey, A. (Eds) *On moral medicine. Theological perspectives in medical ethics.* William B. Eerdmans, Grand Rapids, MI.
2. Beauchamp, T. L. and Childress, J. F. 1989. *Principles of biomedical ethics,* pp. 122–123. Oxford University Press, Oxford.
3. Gillon, R. 1985. *Philosophical medical ethics.* John Wiley & Sons, Chichester.
4. Grisez, G. 1983. *Christian moral principles,* Vol. 1 of *The way of the Lord Jesus,* pp. 298–299. Franciscan Herald Press, Chicago, IL.
5. Gula, R. M. 1989. *Reason informed by faith. Foundations of Catholic morality,* p. 270. Paulist Press, New York.
6. Aquinas, T. *Summa theologiae,* II–II, q.64, a.7.
7. Ross, W. D. 1951. *Foundations of ethics,* p. 319. Oxford University Press, Oxford.
8. Beauchamp, T. L. and McCullough, L. B. 1984. *Medical ethics. The moral responsibilities of physicians,* p. 164. Prentice-Hall, Englewood Cliffs, NJ.
9. Aristotle, *Nichomachean Ethics,* Book 5.
10. Lebacqz, K. 1986. *Six theories of justice,* p. 67. Augsburg, Minneapolis, MN.
11. Donahue, J. R. 1977. Biblical perspectives on justice. P. 69, in Haughey, J. C. (Ed.) *The faith that does justice.* Paulist Press, New York.
12. Vriezen, Th. C. 1970. *An outline of Old Testament theology,* pp. 389–390. Basil Blackwell, Oxford.
13. Hollenbach, D. 1977. Modern Catholic teachings concerning justice. P. 213, in Haughey, J. C. (Ed.) *The faith that does justice.* Paulist Press, New York.

14. Hoose, B. 1990. Gene therapy: where to draw the line. *Human Gene Therapy*, 302–303.
15. McCormick, R. A. 1981. *How brave a new world? Dilemmas in bioethics*, p. 345. SCM Press, London.

6

An Anglican View of the Four Principles

THE MOST REVEREND AND RIGHT HONOURABLE JOHN HABGOOD

Archbishop of York, UK

The Anglican Communion is a worldwide family of episcopal churches, all of which trace their origin to the post-Reformation Church of England. It now consists of 27 autonomous provinces, covering most countries of the world and, as might be expected from its association with colonial expansion, is found in greatest strength in Commonwealth and ex-Commonwealth countries, and in the United States. The Archbishop of Canterbury acts as a focus of unity, but he has no actual jurisdiction over any province other than his own. The 600 or so Anglican Diocesan Bishops meet every 10 years to confer together on a wide variety of theological and practical matters, but this gathering, known as the Lambeth Conference, has only advisory powers. Given this loose structure, it is not surprising to find different parts of the Communion sometimes expressing divergent views on a variety of topics, including some ethical issues. It is not possible, therefore, to describe clearly and unequivocally the Anglican approach, say, to some problem in medical ethics, and this limitation must be borne in mind in any essay which purports to speak for the whole of Anglicanism.

Nevertheless the different provinces share a similar family inheritance, there are many common traditions, and there is a distinctive Anglican style, which has persisted more or less strongly from the Reformation period. During the sixteenth and seventeeth centuries the Church of England defined its character as being a Reformed Catholic Church, rather than a purely Protestant or Catholic one, and this attempt to hold catholicity and reform in balance has characterized it, and the churches which have grown from it, ever since.

One aspect of this balance, of special significance for the subject of this essay, has been the recognition that the sources of moral authority, no less than the sources of theology, are complex and are not to be reduced to a single principle. Anglican churches appeal for guidance to Scripture, tradition and reason. Scripture is the definitive witness to the events which lie at the heart of Christian faith, and in particular to the life, death and resurrection of Jesus Christ.

Principles of Health Care Ethics. Edited by Raanan Gillon.
© 1994 John Wiley & Sons Ltd

Tradition is the accumulated wisdom of the church in interpreting and responding to those events. And reason, which includes ordinary human experience, entails reflection on both Scripture and tradition in the light of the best available contemporary knowledge. This three-fold structure has given Anglican thought a flexibility and an openness to learning which some have regarded as its chief glory, and others as its chief weakness.

The emphasis on reason has also entailed a readiness to enter into dialogue with secular ethics. Though Anglicans would certainly want to emphasize the distinctiveness of Christian ethical insights, in the field of health care as in other fields, they are also happy to recognize large areas of common ground with other religious or non-religious ethical traditions. It is easy for them to acknowledge that there are basic truths about human life and behaviour, into which religion may offer a deeper insight, but which remain recognizably true whether they are approached from a religious perspective or not. This belief in universal moral principles, somehow given in the nature of things, underlay the medieval development of the concept of Natural Law. Protestant thinking has on the whole rejected this, preferring to locate morality always in the context of Biblical revelation and a personal response to God. Anglicanism, on the other hand, has tended to adhere to it, but to develop it along lines rather different from traditional Roman Catholicism.

There is thus a predisposition within Anglicanism to look favourably on the idea of there being certain identifiable basic principles in health care ethics, which may not encapsulate all that a Christian might want to say, but which can provide an appropriate framework for practical ethics in a pluralist society. In fact the Anglican moral tradition can go further than this, in that one of its greatest exponents, Joseph Butler, himself rooted his moral thinking in a set of principles which in some respects bear a striking resemblance to those advocated in this book. It may be instructive, therefore, to use Butler as a benchmark for comparison, and also as an indicator of where his, and similar statements of principle, in the end prove inadequate.

Butler's moral thinking was set out in a series of 15 sermons delivered to members of the judiciary in the Rolls Chapel in 1726. They were, in other words, addressed to those bearing responsibility in public life, and though they are clearly Christian sermons they have been mainly valued as superb and pioneering examples of moral psychology. Butler explored with enormous insight the complexity, contradictoriness and diversity of human affections and aversions. Human nature is not simple, he said, nor are the situations in which human beings find themselves. A morality, therefore, which engages with the way people actually are, cannot be reduced to a single formula but must itself be complex and must reckon with human life, not in the abstract, but in its totality and in its total environment.

Thus far Butler acknowledges, as this book does, the intricacy, variety and particularity of moral problems. But the significance of this is not simply that people and circumstances are different and that decisions have to be made about individual cases. There is for him a religious dimension in this act of recognition, in that coming to terms with the complexity of human nature as it is actually given, is in itself an occasion of moral growth. A moral decision can turn into an act of self-discovery. And if what is discovered is the inherent ambivalence of human dispositions, this can itself reveal unsuspected depths in human existence.

Health care decisions which try to take account of particular circumstances may not often be viewed in this rather exalted light. If Butler is right, however, and if the complexity of human life, far from being an awkward complication for the would-be moralist, is a key to moral understanding, then the process of health care decision-making must itself carry moral significance. The care and attention given the actualities of an individual case may have more to say to both patient and doctor than the contents of the decision. And if the application of general principles detracts from this concreteness then a vital opportunity for personal moral growth may have been lost.

Nevertheless the general principles are necessary. Butler's were consonant with what he already knew of human nature. In addition to the multitude of 'affections and aversions' which make up the complexity of human nature, he identified three major springs of action—'cool self-love', 'benevolence', and 'conscience'.

Cool self-love, or enlightened self-interest as it is now more usually called, enables human beings to look beyond their immediate impulses and to plan for longer-term goals with the aim of maximizing happiness. Most people, for most of the time, pursue cool self-love. To be lacking in self-love is often to be mentally ill, whereas to be consumed by self-love is to become intolerable to other people. Cool self-love entails following the demands of actual human nature, but with a degree of distance and detachment which avoids slavery to them.

Benevolence looks outwards and controls affections and aversions towards others. It is an attitude of mind, and one of Butler's most insistent claims is that it is natural to human beings. Whatever its origins might be there is for him a kind of luminous self-evidence in the belief that human beings *do* care about each other, as well as in the belief that they ought to. In today's world, unfortunately, it may not be as luminous to everybody as it was to Butler and his contemporaries. Nevertheless it is still striking to observe how often we describe those who seem to lack all benevolence not merely as wicked, but as less than human.

Butler saw no ultimate conflict between cool self-love and benevolence. A world in which people care about each other is one in which the interests of each are more likely to be satisfied. He also brilliantly observed how the deliberate pursuit of happiness invariably fails to achieve it, whereas the practice of benevolence, while seeming often to be against self-interest, may lead to greater happiness as a kind of long term by-product.

In all this it has to be remembered that Butler was preaching to a relatively secure and complacent society, which in any case believed that everything was providentially ordered by God, and was therefore not inclined to look for ultimate conflict in its moral principles. It has to be asked in the twentieth century whether the same orderliness prevails in a society where not-so-cool self-love and barely enlightened self-interest have assumed such large proportions. It also has to be asked whether in such a society benevolence will seem so natural. These are questions to which we must return in assessing the adequacy of the four principles.

By 'conscience' Butler meant the capacity for moral reflection. It is not some esoteric faculty, but it does somehow represent the claim of goodness on a human life, and the discomfort arising from a mature assessment of how far one has met the claim. In religious terms conscience is frequently referred to as the voice of God, but this does not imply that such a voice is readily accessible without strenuous efforts to learn what God might actually be saying. In secular terms conscience can be seen as the guardian of moral integrity. On the whole people know when they have disregarded their own internalized moral values.

It thus follows, as Butler saw, that in any hierarchy of principles conscience must be supreme. This does not mean that it must always be directly operative. To regard all action as conscience-driven would be to turn everything into a duty, with depressing results. In fact the best conscience is one which has little occasion to make its presence felt. But when conscience is needed, most characteristically when other principles are in conflict, then its judgements have unique authority. To deny the deliverances of conscience in these circumstances is to deny what makes us moral beings.

So much for Joseph Butler, later to be Bishop of Durham, a seminal Anglican thinker, not much regarded these days, but still relevant, I suggest, in the search for a public morality which is Christian-based yet accessible to a much wider constituency. I turn now to ask how the four principles compare with his insights, and whether there is anything to be learnt from him about them.

RESPECT FOR AUTONOMY

'Respect for autonomy' needs some careful unpacking. The idea that individuals can somehow be a law to themselves belongs very much to the heady stage of Enlightenment enthusiasm, when it was believed that an overthrow of authority by reason was the answer to all human problems. Despite this optimism, the autonomous individual 'captaining his soul and mastering his fate' remained much more bound by his environment, and much more dependent on other people, than extreme advocates of autonomy cared to admit. Complete autonomy is a nonsense, just as unbridled individualism is the negation of morality. Much of the moral disintegration of the twentieth century can be traced to the belief that ethical principles are in the last resort self-chosen, and that it is a necessary feature of the freedom and dignity of human life that this should be so.

Such a belief is incompatible with Christianity. In fact it is fundamental to most religious interpretations of life that individuals are not free to make such ultimate choices with impunity, but that there are conditions inherent in the nature of things under which alone true freedom is possible. Human life flourishes, in other words, not in total independence, but in fruitful interdependence with realities which lie outside it. The same point can be made in Christian language by saying that human freedom and dignity lie not in the individual self, but in the self's relationship with God.

Autonomy, therefore, is not a concept which fits easily in a Christian context. There are less extreme interpretations of it, however, which Christians ought to welcome, and which Butler would have found no difficulty in identifying with his own thinking. To respect the autonomy of other people may mean simply to respect their integrity as free and responsible individuals, capable of making decisions about their own futures, and capable of growth as persons in exercising that freedom and accepting the consequences of it. To respect their autonomy in this sense may also mean respecting their interests and treating them on the assumption that they know best what those interests are, and are better acquainted than others with all the particularities of their lives. To respect autonomy may also mean to respect conscience, especially when conscience is understood as an expression of a person's integrity. Conscience may lead people to do all sorts of strange things because it has to be formed through teaching, and not all teaching is conducive to wise behaviour. But if a person's moral integrity is at stake, however strange it may seem to an observer, it deserves *prima facie* respect. The attitude of Jehovah's Witnesses to blood transfusion is an obvious example. In short, respect for autonomy may in many circumstances be little different in practice from respect for persons.

The difference may become important, though, and even crucial, when the word 'persons' is seen to carry an overtone of relationship with others, which the word 'autonomy' seems to deny. 'A woman's right to choose', say, in the case of a proposed abortion is an assertion of autonomy—'my right to do what I like with my own body'—which looks and feels a good deal less convincing when expressed in terms of respect for persons. Which persons? All those involved, or just one of them? And in what sense, if any, is the fetus a person to whom respect, albeit perhaps not as overriding as that due to the mother, is also due?

Discussions in Anglican churches on abortion have generally reflected this hesitancy, an unwillingness to be polarized, a recognition that what is at stake is more than a mere matter of human choice, and a desire to take proper account of the actual complexity of individual human circumstances.

Euthanasia provides another example of a topic on which Christian thought has almost universally been suspicious of over-zealous claims about autonomy. Good medical practice has rightly made consent one of the main criteria in the decision about what treatment may or may not be given. On this basis there is a strong case for saying that patients may refuse life-prolonging treatment when it is clear that no substantial benefits can be expected from it and when life itself has become too burdensome. But active euthanasia entails more than this. It is an assertion of personal autonomy which actually requires another person to take life. It is not merely consenting to die but actively procuring one's own death, and most religions have condemned it on these grounds. If there are limits to autonomy, if there are God-given boundaries which restrain its unbridled exercise, then surely they must lie here, in the continued acceptance of the gift of life itself.

To apply the criterion of respect for persons to such circumstances is to arrive at a somewhat different answer. Personal life is not a solitary possession, and even the most isolated and lonely individual is related to others through the mere fact of existence as a fellow human being. To treat such a person as disposable, or for such persons to think of themselves as disposable, subtly affects the way in which everyone else regards human worth. The persons to be respected, in other words, are not just those who, for whatever reasons, wish to die, but also all those others who in various ways, some great some minuscule, will receive ripples from their death. The perceptions of a social group, and the expectations of its members, depend enormously on what kinds of action are publicly legitimated.

The tendency of the concept of autonomy to focus attention on the isolated individual may also further reinforce a bias which is already inherent in health care. For fully understandable reasons traditional medicine has tended to concentrate on the needs of individual patients. In fact to give and accept treatment is to enter into a kind of personal one-to-one contract, and for many purposes such a limitation of the horizon does no harm. This model ignores, however, the way in which a multiplicity of individual decisions, each of which may be justifiable in individual terms, may create a social context which puts undesirable pressure on those involved to seek a particular answer to their problems. Each person may be able to make a case for their own abortion, for instance, but an accumulation of such cases may generate an atmosphere of abortion-mindedness in which the individual decision whether to abort may be skewed by social pressure. Recent discussion on sex selection raises similar problems. Worldwide advocacy of such selection on the grounds of a couple's supposed autonomous right to choose may seem entirely appropriate to individuals distressed by their own family imbalance. But the larger picture has to reckon, for example, with recent figures from a Bombay hospital in which sex selection has been carried out by amniocentesis and abortion, and where it is claimed that out of 8000 such abortions all but one were girls.

The principle of respect for autonomy clearly has to have a social dimension and to be linked with the principle of justice. This may help to restrain some of the worst excesses practised in its name. In contrast the traditional Christian emphasis on the dignity and rights of persons, and the respect due to them, retains what is valuable in the concept of autonomy, but without its bias towards individualism, and for this reason has generally been preferred by the churches.

BENEFICENCE AND NON-MALEFICENCE

These two concepts belong together, and as basic principles of health care there can hardly be much argument about them. Indeed, doing good and avoiding harm are fundamental to almost every system of ethics, particularly in the realm of public policy. Even Butler, though far from a precursor of utilitarianism, stressed the relationship between moral principles and their actual consequences in terms of human well-being. Morality makes sense by satisfying the real needs of human nature. But what truly makes for human well-being may not be easy to discern, and this is where Butler's perceptiveness as a moral psychologist is a useful reminder that stating principles is only the first step on a long road of moral analysis.

He also saw that even at the level of general principles it is necessary to set some limits on the pursuit of well-being, which he expressed by saying that benevolence has to be kept 'within the bounds of justice and veracity'. 'Justice' we shall consider later. The need for 'veracity' can alert us to the danger of benevolence slipping into sentimentality, or into that over-protectiveness towards others, which in the end robs them of their dignity. Perhaps in this respect benevolence runs fewer risks than beneficence. Wishing to do well which does not actually turn into doing well is merely a drastically truncated virtue. But doing well which is not firmly rooted in wishing well can easily become insensitive to the actual needs of its recipients. Without a truthful relationship between giver and receiver beneficence can simply impose good on others irrespective of what they think is good for themselves. C. S. Lewis's oft-quoted remark comes to mind here: 'She's the sort of woman who lives for others— you can always tell the others by their hunted expression.'

Oppressive beneficence of this order is not unknown in health care. Doctors and nurses and hospital regimes which deskill their patients may do so on the grounds that 'doctor knows best'. Sometimes this temptation is intensified by the enormous difficulty of knowing what is actually for the best, and the horrendous consequences of getting it wrong. Is it best, for example, for individuals and for society at large, that HIV testing should be as widespread as possible, and that its results should be known to the individuals concerned? Questions like these can be answered only in a relationship of trust and truthfulness between doctors and patients, and that can be built up only by the kind of benevolence which is prepared to listen as well as to act.

MALEFICENCE

'Maleficence' ought not to be a problem in a system devoted to the care of others. The main issues arise, I suspect, in those uncertain areas surrounding the beginning and the ending of life. What justification can there be for destroying a developing embryo? or for refusing to operate on a horribly deformed neonate? or for arranging the formal termination of a life to suit the needs of a transplant? or for undertaking clinical research which may be painful, or even dangerous, to those who will not themselves benefit from it?

Maleficence, if it is to be identified in any such cases, is certainly not the result of malevolence, and in this respect it is not the mirror-image of beneficence. Harm in these circumstances is usually the by-product of good intentions, perhaps misdirected, perhaps not. In the end the judgements which have to be made are not about beneficence or maleficence at all, but about the nature of persons, and about the relationships of trust which can subsist between them.

This is not to deny the reality of evil. Any system can contain corrupt and evil people, and any person can be driven by corrupt and evil motives. A Christian appraisal of a set of ethical principles must at some point ask how far they take account of the reality of such evil, and the less dramatic human propensity to mean well and still to get things wrong. 'Non-maleficence' is a helpful warning that, although within health care the majority of harm done to people is inadvertent or incidental, sometimes it is more than this. An ethical system needs some firm defences against violations of the dignity and rights of persons. Just as in public life a broadly consequentialist style of ethical thinking needs to be tempered by a Kantian insistence on some basic moral absolutes, and just as in Butler's ethics all other considerations are subject to conscience interpreted as the voice of God, so in the ethics of health care the bottom line is respect for persons, a claim which for Christians is buttressed by the belief that all human persons are children of God. To know that there is such a bottom line which is more than a mere matter of opinion, affords protection against those forms of maleficence which are deliberate.

JUSTICE

'Justice', like beneficence, is an element in most ethical systems, and proves equally hard to define. Presumably in the context of health care questions of justice centre mainly on the distribution of resources. Butler, as we have seen, prescribed benevolence 'within the bounds of justice', and must have had in mind the dangers of partiality which are all too evident in the way benevolence is frequently exercised. 'Favourite charities' are a case in point. Butler was also conscious that it is impossible to love humanity at large or to do good to everybody in general, and therefore drew on the phrase 'love your neighbours', i.e. those who 'come under your immediate notice', as the most simple, practical and scriptural way of exercising impartial benevolence. The fact that he advocated this in a society marked by flagrant inequalities between rich and poor without drawing attention to them must be counted against him. But there is wisdom in trying to spell out the implications of justice on a manageable scale and in face-to-face encounters, provided that the wider scene is not forgotten.

Decisions about the allocation of resources in health care narrow down eventually to decisions which have to be made about individual patients. There are, of course, wider issues at stake in a centrally funded health care system. In Britain the accessibility of the National Health Service to all, and equality of treatment within it, are regarded by many as prime indicators of social justice. Planners face the impossible task of supplying more and more expensive forms of treatment on an equitable basis and within a limited budget. Attempts to assign priorities, to assess the relative values of, say, heart transplants and hernia operations, to get the balance right between cure and care, between remedial treatment and health education, constantly run into the problems of rivalries between specialties, different perceptions of what health care is, and above all the lack of any agreed criteria by which to judge. In the past the National Health Service usually managed to escape from such dilemmas by spending more money.

There may therefore be the germ of an ethical idea, overlaid maybe by excessive emphasis on market forces, in trying to push decision-making away from global planners, and more in the direction of those most closely involved. Justice as an abstract idea can be too blunt an instrument to shed much light on global policies, though it is needed as a constant reminder that the welfare of the population as a whole must never be forgotten. But the approach to justice which emphasizes the need for participation by people in the decisions which affect them, may lead to a kind of equity arising out of a growing consensus about what is fair. To know the cost of one's own treatment, for example, may seem to introduce a mercenary element into medicine which is undesirable in itself and puts pressure on the most conscientious. But the gradual dissemination of such knowledge within a particular community of care, and public discussion of the difficult choices which have to be faced, may help to form expectations along more realistic lines, and may gradually increase that vitally necessary understanding and trust between doctors and patients, to which I have already referred.

Local face-to-face attempts to act justly are all of a piece with Butler's insistence on the actual complexity of the human scene, and the need to concentrate on particulars. This is a theme which has been very characteristic of Anglican ethical thinking in the 265 years since he wrote. And this is my excuse for devoting so much space to an ethical thinker from such a different age.

Modern Anglican ethics has retained this empirical pragmatic slant. It has remained receptive towards secular knowledge, while trying to keep a firm hold on a few basic theological truths. Its favourite method during the past 50 years has been the interdisciplinary working party, bringing together a variety of appropriate kinds of expertise in the expectation that light will emerge from well-informed and Christianly-oriented minds as they grapple with concrete issues. Sometimes such discussion, as for example on the issues surrounding *in vitro* fertilization, succeeds only in displaying the wider dimensions of a problem. But it would be typical of Anglicanism to regard this as preferable to retreating into a one-sided over-simplification. Deeper understanding emerges as truths are held in tension, and progress in ethical thinking may involve a stage of conflict as a means of sharpening up the choices which ultimately may have to be made. Sometimes agreements are expressed in terms of 'middle axioms', a name given widely to accepted principles which are not so general as to be vacuous nor so specific as to be limited in their use. The four principles on which this book is based could be thought of as appropriate middle axioms for health care though, as I have indicated, I have strong reservations about the first of them.

A fully Christian ethical approach, however, cannot be content simply with principles, or middle axioms. Some ethical problems, as we have seen, contain a strong element of theological interpretation and religious insight. Where is the line to be drawn between fully personal life, and something less than personal? The authority undergirding some prohibitions, notably against the taking of life, more often than not gains its force from religion. The tendency to stress the social implications of individual choices can in the end be traced back to an understanding of persons as always persons-in-relationship, which itself carries strong echoes from a Trinitarian belief in God. Ethical systems may wear secular clothes but they have frequently had religious up-bringings.

There are other aspects of ethics to which the religious dimension is still more central—indeed, paramount. Failure, for instance. Admitting and coping with failure is an essential feature of health care, as it is of the rest of life, but it is difficult in a formal ethical system to give space for the bewilderment, frustration and recrimination which frequently attend difficult decisions. To live with the promise of forgiveness and to wait for the renewal of hope can provide a supportive context in decision-making for which no amount of subtle analysis can substitute. But such thoughts take us beyond the subject of this essay which is intended to be about views, rather than about the inwardness of the life of faith. Nevertheless in the actual exercise of ethics, the life of faith is primary.

7

A Jewish Perspective on the Four Principles

Avraham Steinberg, MD

The Center for Medical Ethics, The Hebrew University–Hadassah Medical School and Department of Pediatrics, Shaare Zedek Medical Center, Jerusalem, Israel

THE FOUNDATIONS OF JEWISH LAW

Halakhah is the generic term for the whole legal system of Judaism, embracing all the laws, practices and observances. Orthodox Jews consider the Halakhah, in its traditional form, to be absolutely binding.

The source of Halakhah is divine revelation. To the basic corpus of biblical law were added rabbinic enactments and decrees. The sources of authority in Halakhah are composed of different elements: (a) the written law, a composition of 613 positive and negative commandments of Sinaic origin, which are included in the books of the Pentateuch; (b) the oral law, which includes the interpretation of the written law transmitted in its entirety with its details and minutiae at Sinai, as well as logical deductions, and also rabbinical decrees, customs, as well as positive and negative enactments.

PRINCIPLES OF JEWISH MEDICAL ETHICS

Jewish medical ethics, in the sense of normative Jewish law and philosophy applied to practical medical issues, is characterized by and distinguished from secular medical ethics in its range, in its methods of analysis, in its endpoint, and in its principles.

With respect to the *range*—Jewish medical ethics deals with all the diverse universal ethical problems in medicine, but also includes 'pure' Halakhic topics related to the practice of medicine. From the standpoint of Judaism, these topics—which are normative, religious laws and customs—are as important as the classic, universal ethical issues.

With respect to the *methods of analysis*—the mode of discourse and the

Principles of Health Care Ethics. Edited by Raanan Gillon.
© 1994 John Wiley & Sons Ltd

cognitive background pertaining to Jewish medical ethics is based on the ancient sources of the Bible, the Talmud, and the vast literature of codification and responsa. Any medical issue in medicine is analysed according to the foundation of Halakhah, much in the same way as any other issue in life is being analysed, when a Halakhic problem arises.

With respect to the *endpoint*—Judaism, like other religions and secular legal systems, gives finite and decisive answers to the ethical issues posed to the decisors, although the solutions are not always accepted by all members of the community. Dispute-resolution mechanisms are built into the Halakhic system so that final decisions can be reached. The Jewish model of decision-making in medicine is composed of a triad: the *physician*, who has the obligation to treat the patient and to recommend to him the best medical advice; the qualified *rabbi*, who is required to solve any ethical or legal problem that may be encountered by either the patient or the physician; and the *patient*, who has the obligation to seek medical help, and has the autonomy to choose his medical and Halakhic advisers, and to decide on matters that do not involve either medical or ethical expertise, or in specific, precisely defined quality-of-life situations, as will be discussed below. Since the most qualified person makes the decisions relevant to his expertise, this triad should be able to reach the best solution to any complex medical and ethical issue concerning any individual case on its own merits and according to its specific circumstances. This model causes a great measure of the patient's autonomous decisions to be abdicated to those who are best qualified to make the decision. This model should be viewed as a predetermined free and voluntary choice of individuals to abdicate their power of decision-making to others, as part of an ideological way of life.

With respect to the *underlying principles*—these certainly include the four principles under discussion in this volume. However, many other Jewish moral and legal principles and rules have significant bearing upon the practice of medicine. Obviously they cannot be described in detail in this chapter. It is, however, worthwhile to mention a few basic suppositions, which have a significant modifying power over the four principles:

1. Judaism subscribes to commitments, obligations, duties and commandments, commonly shared by all observant Jews, rather than to rights and pure hedonism. A rights ethic is a minimalistic ethics, sanctioning any individual's wish and conduct, as long as it does not disturb the peaceable community. This approach disregards, or at least minimizes, other socially shared values. By contrast, Jewish ethics subscribes to moral self-fulfilment through the obedience to moral–religious norms and requirements.

2. Judaism, in general, favours a casuistry approach, rather than zealous adherence to general principles. Hence, each case is dealt with on its own merits, depending heavily on the specific and individual circumstances. A vast Halakhic literature of responsa has been developed due to this particular approach. In the medico-ethical sphere this approach is particularly pertinent, because of the great variety of specific circumstances, which undoubtedly have significant influence on the decision-making process.

3. Judaism, in general, is opposed to absolutizing any single precept; rather a

golden path, a middle way, is always advocated and favoured. No principle is construed as one that always overrides all other principles. Rather, any principle can compete with any other for priority in a particular case. Therefore, when conflicting values in practical medicine are encountered, each patient must be considered individually, and a solution is reached depending on the specific clinical and ethical circumstances. This is, obviously, done within the general framework of Halakhic rules and regulations.

4. The principal aim of studying ethics and Jewish law is to act accordingly, not merely to engage in intellectual exercise or academic analysis.

5. The physician–patient relationship is viewed as a covenant, which does not provide for the notion of freely contracting individuals. There is an obligation upon a physician always to extend his help to those in need of his/her services: 'The Torah gave permission to the physician to heal; moreover, this is a religious precept and is included in the category of saving life; and if the physician withholds his services it is considered as shedding blood' (1). According to Judaism, the physician is viewed as God's messenger in healing people in need.

6. Judaism views the seeking of medical attention by the patient as a moral imperative. Moreover, man is obligated to exercise prudence in preserving health. No-one has the right to refuse medical treatment deemed necessary and effective by competent opinion. The obligation to be healed sets aside most biblical commandments and takes precedence over the patient's wishes even if his desire not to be healed is based upon his desire to fulfil a religious commandment. If it is necessary to desecrate the Sabbath on his behalf and he wishes to be stringent and not allow it, he should be forced to accept the proposed treatment, because such a man is a pious fool. Such an approach is not an act of piety but an act of suicide. If a patient does not do whatever is required to save his life, he is considered as a shedder of his own blood.

7. Human life is sacrosanct and of supreme worth. It constitutes one of the most important principles in Judaism, and is regarded by some Jewish scholars as being of infinite value. Hence any precept, whether religious or ethical, is automatically suspended if it conflicts with the interests of human life, the exceptions being only idolatry, murder and adultery. Every human life is equal; therefore, to kill a decrepit patient approaching death constitutes exactly the same crime of murder as to kill a young, healthy person who may still have many decades to live. Every life is equally valuable and inviolable, including that of criminals, prisoners and the physically or mentally defective. It should be pointed out that the value of human life as a major principle has been lately deliberately omitted by many secular medical ethicists.

THE FOUR PRINCIPLES

The importance of the four principles on a *prima facie* basis is certainly recognized in Judaism. The problematic issue, however, pertains to decisions of *prioritization*, namely in cases of conflict between these principles—Which should override? Under what conditions? Who decides?

These are the real concerns, not the substantive philosophical definitions of any of the principles in isolation, or in purely academic circumstances. The answers to these questions from the Jewish standpoint depend on many variables, including the relative moral–legal weight of each of the principles, other relevant principles and rules as enumerated above, and the case-by-case specific circumstances.

AUTONOMY

The range and the application of the notion of autonomy constitutes one of the most significant differences between current secular and Jewish medical ethics, as will be pointed out below. In western culture the principle of autonomy has been promoted to one of the most important and overriding moral principles.

The relevance of autonomy in health care decisions is undeniable. However, a zealous and unconciliatory interpretation of the right to autonomy has been severely criticized even in a pluralistic, secular society. These criticisms are particularly strong from the Jewish standpoint. It is, therefore, pertinent to cite some of the disagreeable aspects of the notion of autonomy, as stipulated by Pellegrino and Thomasma (2). They suggest that the practical question in clinical decisions is not whether or not we have a right to autonomy; we most certainly do. Rather, the question focuses on the proper exercise of autonomy. Do we have a right to exercise autonomy when the decision we wish to make is not morally good? Are we free to make morally wrong decisions? Have we lost a common consensus on morals to such a degree that there is no longer any community of values? Are there any other values in common other than autonomy? By promoting autonomy to the extreme overriding power, are we not promoting a degradation of moral life and principles? Does this approach not educate to amoral or even immoral life? Can a society survive such radical pluralism in which there are no longer any shared values? Moreover, an extreme interpretation of autonomy may contribute to a serious educational gap in neglecting to promote the requirements for personal duty and social responsibility.

Most current secular ethicists, however, admit that the principle of autonomy should be a relative one. The question is: how much, when, and by whom should it be restricted.

According to the Jewish viewpoint there is a combination of human free choice together with divine providence, which is a form of predeterminism. According to this theory, God determines the rules and actions in the universe and supervises human deeds, but there exists a definite and extensive range of human freedom of mind. This approach differs from certain other philosophies and theological principles, which either ascribe absolute predeterminism or absolute free choice. The Jewish approach is concisely summarized by the Talmudic sages: 'All is foreseen, but the choice is given' (3). This idea was further elaborated upon by the Talmudic sages and extended by the medieval Jewish philosophers and legalists. Maimonides, for instance, states that every person can choose to be good or evil, with no divine predeterminism. Maimonides and other Jewish scholars realized, however, the inherent religious conflict between human freedom and God's knowledge and providence. Various ways to reconcile between these opposing ideas were proposed, and several attempts were undertaken to assess the quantitative input of each of them into a given action or behaviour. These deliberations, however, are beyond the scope of this paper. The Jewish point of view on this matter can be summarized in the following way: human behaviour and actions are *neither* absolutely free *nor* absolutely predetermined; rather, they are *both* free and determined, in a relative admixture.

Thus, Judaism acknowledges the ability of freedom of the mind. Indeed, the very approval of medicine in normative Jewish law is based on the rejection of absolute determinism. Hence, the engagement in medical practice is permissible, and even required, disclaiming the notion that by doing so one is abrogating God's wishes and deeds.

However, the mere fact that one is *able* to exercise free will does not give him/her necessarily the *right* to do so. In fact, generally, most moral principles take precedence over autonomy, unless they are very ambiguous, or significant autonomous considerations exist in the particular case. Hence, in Jewish philosophy, the right to execute autonomous decisions has significant restrictions and limitations.

Indeed, autonomy as a concept of *respect for others* is highly valued and demanded in Jewish thought. However, Judaism ascribes to a high order of *personal* moral conduct, which obligates the individual and society. Autonomous decisions that do not comply with the required moral standards are overridden by higher moral values, as determined by Jewish law. Therefore, Judaism restricts the notion of autonomy to actions that are morally indifferent.

Observant Jews live their lives according to rules and regulations of the Jewish laws laid down in the Bible, the Talmud and the later codifiers and interpreters. Hence, in any case of dispute or moral concern, it is within the mode of life of observant Jews to abdicate their personal and individual wishes and to conduct themselves according to what is right or wrong in Jewish legal–moral terms.

Moreover, according to strict Jewish rules the required norms and conducts can even be imposed upon the individual, although rules and regulations exist as to when and how such coercion is administered.

In medical situations that involve ethical conflicts, the solution should be based upon the appropriate Jewish law which governs both the physician and the patient. According to Jewish law the physician is obligated to heal and the patient is obligated to seek healing. Therefore, the medical treatment is occasionally not determined by the desire and consent of the patient but by objective facts.

The autonomy of the patient, however, is preserved in certain medical situations:

1. If the suggested treatment is not proven to be efficacious, or if the treatment is clearly futile, or if the treatment is a matter of dispute amongst the experts— the patient has the right to refuse the initiation of such treatments.
2. If the treatment entails great suffering, or significant complications—the patient has the right to refuse such treatment.
3. If there are several equally effective medical options and one option is

preferred because of non-medical reasons, i.e. limited resources, or value-based causes—the patient has the right to refuse such an option.

NON-MALEFICENCE–BENEFICENCE

Jewish law is divided into two major components: positive and negative precepts concerning the relationship between man and God; positive and negative precepts concerning the interrelationship between fellow men and between individual and society. The two principles of non-maleficence and of beneficence constitute a major part of the latter group of commandments. They are not optional, nor merely praiseworthy; rather, they are composed of definite moral–legal duties and requirements. All four elements of William Frankena's definition of non-maleficence–beneficence (4), namely not to inflict evil or harm, to prevent evil or harm, to remove evil, and to do or promote good—are clearly defined as positive duties in Judaism.

NON-MALEFICENCE

Harm or injury is interpreted in Jewish law in a very broad range, including injury to body, to soul, to reputation, to property and to privacy.

Judaism distinguishes between harm produced intentionally or unintentionally. Precise definitions are available as to what constitutes an intentional or an unintentional deed, and under what circumstances.

Several biblical statements, and numerous biblical and rabbinic laws and regulations, affirm the great importance placed in Judaism to avoid harm, either by actions—whether by commission or by omission—or by words, or even by thoughts. One of the outstanding affirmations of this viewpoint is the following: 'What is hateful to you, do not do unto your neighbour, that is the whole Torah, while the rest is the commentary thereof; go and study it' (5).

There are precise and exact rules and regulations which define the requirements, their limitations, and priority decisions—when to overrule, to waive, or to cancel specific regulations—depending on the particular circumstances.

In medical situations the requirement upon a physician is to help and heal, but never to use his knowledge to harm or to injure anyone. Moreover, health care professionals are required to be experts, and to keep up with the best standards of knowledge and skills, in order to minimize any potential damage of necessary medical intervention (6).

As opposed to secular ethics, the Jewish perspective of non-maleficence includes not only a prohibition to harm others, it also prohibits harmful actions against oneself. Every person is commanded to watch over his/her own health and life and is obligated to avoid self-harm, injury, or suicide. Hence, preventive medicine, both as positive measures and as negative ones, is considered in Judaism as a moral–legal duty. In the Pentateuch it is stated: 'Duly take heed to yourself, and keep your soul diligently' (7); 'Take you, therefore, good heed unto yourselves' (8). From these and other scriptural phrases the Talmudic sages (9) and later decisors deduced the obligation to protect our bodies from harm and danger. Maimonides (10) and Karo (11) write: 'The sages prohibited many things because they involve danger to life. Whoever disregards these things and their like and says: "I will place myself in danger; what concern is this to others?", or "I am not particular about such things"—disciplinary flogging is inflicted upon him. But he who is careful about these matters will receive great blessing.'

Suicide is absolutely forbidden, and strongly condemned in Jewish law.

BENEFICENCE

To benefit a fellow-man is considered to be one of the most important positive precepts in Judaism. It is not optional; it is commandable. Beneficence and altruism are promoted over mere non-maleficence.

Several biblical statements and specific laws attest to the great importance attributed in Judaism to beneficence. The Talmudic sages and later Jewish codifiers have further elaborated upon this principle, and exemplified various items of required behaviour in this respect:

1. 'Love thy neighbour as thyself' (12), which is interpreted as a requirement to love and to respect others, as much as one would wish it to be done to oneself. According to one of the Talmudic sages, this is the essence of the whole Torah (13).
2. 'Thou shalt not stand against the blood of thy neighbour' (14), which is exemplified by the Talmudic sages (15) as saving a drowning person, or saving a person that is being chased by robbers or by beasts. There is a positive duty to save a fellow-man, even if it requires spending money or is associated with significant inconvenience, or even when a minimal risk to the rescuer is involved. However, if the rescuer is at a substantial risk of loss or damage, he is not required to do the act, and occasionally he is even prohibited from doing so (16).
3. 'And thou shalt do that which is right and good in the sight of the Lord' (17). Since God is described as acting in ways of beneficence, mercy and passion, the human being is required to imitate God in this respect (18).
4. 'Before a blind man thou shalt not put a stumblingblock' (19), which is interpreted in a figurative form, with a broader meaning not to mislead others or not to provide unfair advice.
5. 'Let the honour of your fellow-man be as dear to you as your own' (20).

In the patient–physician relationship the notion of beneficence is strongly emphasized in the requirement of a physician to treat and to assist every patient. The patient–physician relationship is considered as a covenant, rather than a contract. Hence, the physician is duty-bound to treat any patient for his benefit.

JUSTICE

There is no justice theory that is free of moral problems, and there is no one theory that is approved by all philosophers. The acceptance of any justice theory which justifies any degree of unequal treatment of people inevitably affects other spheres of social policy in significant ways.

Philosophically, the principle of justice has several meanings. Currently, justice is generally considered in terms of distribution, namely the proper distribution of social benefits and burdens. Recent literature on distributive justice has even further restricted the notion to considerations of fair economic distribution. This is the major perception of the concept as related to current medico-ethical dilemmas.

In Jewish thought, justice is paired with mercy, grace, charity, truth, trust, peace, fairness and integrity; thus, many values are consistently associated with justice, as its components or products, and there is no one clear definition of this term.

Distributive justice is essentially a procedural principle, i.e. how to do things, while Jewish outlook of justice is essentially substantive, i.e. what human life should be like. This view of justice is concerned with the full enhancement of human and social life.

Justice is considered to be one of the most important moral values in Judaism. In the Bible, great emphasis is put on the notion of justice, i.e. 'Justice justice shall ye pursue' (21); the commandments of God to men are essentially for the purpose of the establishment of justice in the world (22).

However, what defines true justice according to Judaism is not always what seems to be the case in contemporary human mind; these concepts of justice are changeable and transitional, dependable upon cultural perspectives, and upon individual and societal needs. According to Judaism, men fulfil the purpose of justice by acting in accordance with God's laws and in other ways set forward by the Sages that imitate the divine quality of justice; hence, the rules of justice are deep-rooted and firmly established.

Judaism recognizes that the ideal of absolute equality is untenable, and inherent inequalities are unavoidable—'For the poor shall never cease out of the land' (23). This fact, however, should never justify discrimination; on the contrary—'Therefore I command thee, saying, thou shalt open thine hand wide unto thy brother, to thy poor, and to thy needy' (23). Differential treatment between unequals is justified only in very restricted and well-characterized circumstances.

In medical conditions, triage decisions are primarily decided according to the following rules: first come, first served is the basic rule; if two patients present simultaneously—the one who is in greater medical danger takes priority; if both are equal in their medical needs—a hierarchy based on social worth is stipulated.

CONCLUSION

The four principles are part and parcel of the Jewish moral and legal system. However, there are basic and extensive differences between Jewish and secular philosophy in their definition, their moral validity, their scope, and their prioritization, as described throughout this chapter.

REFERENCES

1. Karo's Shulchan Aruch, *Yore Deah* 336:1.
2. Pellegrino, E. and Thomasma, D. C. 1988. *For the patient's good.* Oxford University Press, New York.
3. Mishnah Avot 3:15.
4. Frankena, W. K. 1973. *Ethics*, 2nd Ed. Prentice Hall, Englewood Cliffs.
5. Babylonian Talmud, Tractate Shabbat 31a.
6. Karo's Shulchan Aruch, *Yore Deah* 336:1.
7. Deuteronomy 4:9.
8. Deuteronomy 4:15.
9. Babylonian Talmud, Tractate Berachot 32b.
10. Maimonides' Mishneh Torah, Rotzeach U'Shmirat Ha'Nefesh 11:4–5.
11. Karo's Shulchan Aruch, end of Choshen Mishpat.
12. Leviticus 19:18.
13. Jerusalem Talmud, Tractate Nedarim 9:4.
14. Leviticus 19:16.
15. Babylonian Talmud, Tractate Sanhedrin 73a.
16. Responsa Radvaz, part 3, no. 1052.
17. Deuteronomy 6:18.
18. Babylonian Talmud, Tractate Shabbat 133b.
19. Leviticus 19:14.
20. Mishnah Avot 2:10; Maimonides' Mishneh Torah, Deot 6:3.
21. Deuteronomy 16:20.
22. Psalms 119:137–144.
23. Deuteronomy 15:11.

8

Islam and the Four Principles

Professor Dr G.I. Serour, FRCOG, FRCS

*Professor of Obstetrics and Gynaecology, Director, International Islamic
Center for Population Studies and Research, Al-Azhar University; Clinical
Director of the Egyptian I.V.F. & E.T. Center, Cairo, Egypt*

In any learned profession, to set specific standards of conduct, which guide the behaviour of its members, it is important to adhere to a code of ethics. Medicine has enjoyed high standards, and these have been the hallmark of the good doctor and a safeguard of the patient's welfare since its earliest recorded history. Since time immemorial, medicine as a profession has been accorded a place of the highest order, and those who practise it have been held as bearing a holy responsibility (1). The first existing documents that dealt with medical ethics are the Egyptian papyri (from about the sixteenth century BC); they outlined methods of knowledge, attitude and practice, to do with, for instance, establishing diagnosis, making decisions about whether to treat, and what therapy is appropriate. As long as doctors followed the rules they were held non-culpable should the patient die. On the other hand, if doctors transgressed, tried a new form of treatment, and the patient died, they might lose their own lives. Medicine developed in Mesopotamia in parallel with its growth in Egypt. Hammurabi, one of the great kings of Babylon, set surgical fees according to the social status of the patient and established punishment for poor technical performance. Both Egyptian and Babylonian societies issued rules and sanctions to control the activities of doctors and surgeons (2).

Medical ethics are based on the moral, religious and philosophical ideals and principles of the society in which they are practised. It is therefore not surprising to find that what is ethical in one society might not be ethical in another society. It is mandatory for practising doctors and critics of conduct to be aware of such backgrounds before they make their judgement on different medical practice decisions. According to each society's condition the ethical attitude of the individual may be coloured by the attitude of the society which reflects the interest of the theologians, legislators, sociologists, economists, doctors, ethicists, demographers, family planning administrators and policy-makers. Ethical discourse is necessary for any society to form its responses to any scientific or

Principles of Health Care Ethics. Edited by Raanan Gillon.
© 1994 John Wiley & Sons Ltd

medical innovation (3). Responsible policy-makers in the medical profession in each country have to decide on what is ethically acceptable in their own country, guided by the international guidelines which should be tailored to suit their own society (3). Truly ethical conduct consists of personal searching for relevant values that lead to an ethically inspired decision.

Those for whom religion is important, and it is so for Muslims, need to distinguish between medical ethics and humanitarian considerations on the one hand, and religious teachings and national laws on the other hand. The doctor is always concerned about the legal basis of his acts and that they are undertaken on the basis of ethical precepts. He should always keep clear the distinctions and potential conflicts between legal and ethical duties. What is legal might not be ethical. Law rarely establishes positive duties such as beneficence. On the contrary professional medical ethics makes beneficence a primary obligation (4).

THE FOUR ETHICAL PRINCIPLES IN MEDICINE

There are four characteristics of the twentieth century, namely civilization, progressive secularization of the legislation of a worldwide society, the accelerated progress of technology and science, and the increasingly complex interdependence of human beings. The vast development of communication systems and methods of transportation, and worldwide migration have made such interdependence not only limited to one society or country but rather regional and even global in its nature. What occurs in one society is rapidly reflected in other societies not only in the same region, but also in different countries all over the world.

The four principles of ethics as known today are autonomy, beneficence, non-maleficence, and justice. Autonomy incorporates respect for the individual's freedom of choice. It involves autonomy of competent persons and protection of those incapable of autonomy. The latter prevents the abuse of the powerless within a community such as the mentally defective and institutionalized persons, such as occupants of hospital charity beds or prisoners. One classic formulation of this principle, in John Stuart Mill's *On Liberty*, is that individuals should be able to choose freely what they will do, unless or until their actions cause serious harm to others or seriously limit others' liberty (5). Beneficence upholds others' welfare. Non-maleficence is the duty not to do harm to other persons. Justice, which the law claims primarily to serve, involves distributive justice and corrective justice. Distributive justice is concerned with the fair allocation of burdens and benefits, while corrective justice is concerned with the compensation of the wrong act. Victims of the wrong act may be identified as individuals, or as members of a population group (6).

In cultures that are powerfully directed by religious principles and precepts, a role exists for secular legislation. Religion shapes the transcending principles of law in many countries. Laws usually try to accommodate ethical choices of conduct and try not to compel conduct on those who consider it unethical (4).

There are tensions between autonomy, beneficence, non-maleficence, and justice—the basic rules of bioethics. They are not mutually exclusive; they must be balanced (7). Ethical norms are guidelines. The context must influence the moral judgement. Ethics and morality are valid only when individuals can act freely. When there is a conflict among these four principles of ethics, some would give precedence to one of them. In broad terms one principle always takes precedence over the other three. For utilitarians the principles of beneficence and non-maleficence are always uppermost. The libertarians always give precedence to the principle of respect for autonomy, while the egalitarians give precedence to the principle of justice.

However, the law historically and more recently has been used not only to deny justice, but also to deny respect for persons and to be used maleficently. It is noteworthy that the determination of whether the law in general, or an individual law in particular, is just, is a matter for political, social and individual determination. Such determination may be made in accordance with whether ethical principles are considered to have been properly applied (8).

To these four principles of bioethics a last one may be added; that is the human person should not be subject to commercial exploitation.

ISLAMIC BACKGROUND

Islam is a faith which had over 1.225 billion adherents worldwide in the year 1990, and with the present rate of population growth this figure is expected to increase to 2.5 billion in the year 2020 (9). Islam is a comprehensive system that regulates the spiritual as well as civil aspects of individual and communal life. It has brought with it the fundamentals that are consistent with demands of the soul and body. It aims to develop the unique personality of the individual, and a distinct culture for the community, based on Islamic ideals and values. The teaching of Islam covers all fields of human activity, spiritual and material, individual and social, educational and cultural, economic and political, national and international (10).

Instructions which regulate everyday activity of life, to be adhered to by good Muslims, are called Sharia'. The primary sources of Sharia' in chronological order are the Holy Qur'an; the very word of God, the Sunna and Hadith (which is the authentic tradition and sayings of the Prophet Mohamed developed by jurists over time), the unanimous opinion of Islamic scholars or Aimma (Igmaah) and finally analogy (Kias) which is the intelligent reasoning by which to rule on events the Qur'an and Sunna did not mention, by matching against similar or equivalent events already ruled on. The secondary sources of Sharia' include Istihsan, which is the choice of one of several lawful options, not necessarily the most popular, as more suitable in a given situation, views of the Prophet's companions, current local custom, if lawful, public welfare, and finally rulings of previous divine religions, unless replaced or modified by Islamic rulings.

If an instruction on a certain issue is mentioned in Qur'an, it is the one which should be followed. Sunna is resorted to if the issue is not mentioned in Qur'an. The opinion of Aimma is the source of Sharia', if the issue is not mentioned in either Qur'an or Sunna. Finally religious leaders can decide the Sharia' for issues not mentioned in Qur'an, Sunna or by Aimma simply by analogy.

The Sharia' is therefore not rigid or fixed except in a few legislations such as worship, rituals and codes of morality. It leaves latitude to adapt to emerging situations in different eras and places. It can accommodate different honest opinions as long as they do not conflict with the spirit of its primary sources, and are directed to the benefit of humanity (10). The Sharia' classifies all human actions without exception into one of five categories, namely obligatory, recommended, permitted, disapproved but not forbidden, and absolutely forbidden. Even if the action is forbidden, it may be undertaken if the alternative would cause harm. Also what is forbidden today may become allowed in the future, if science proves that the alternative would be harmful to the human being.

The development of the science of Fiqh (jurisprudence) resulted in the establishment of certain guiding principles to help to drive rulings. There are several examples which show the role of Fiqh, such as: harm should be removed, the choice of the lesser of two harms, and the public interest takes priority over enjoying benefits. The goals of Sharia' can be summarized in the preservation and protection of self (life, health, procreation, etc.), mind (prohibition of alcohol, drugs; freedom of thought, etc.), religion (freedom of faith, non-compulsion in religion, rituals of worship, etc.), ownership (sanctity of private ownership, legitimate commercial relationships, prohibition of stealing, fraud and usury, etc.) and honour (purity, marriage and laws of family formation, chastity, prohibition of adultery, etc.) (11).

An example in health care to clarify how instructions to Muslims are formulated is family planning. No Quranic text explicitly forbids prevention of conception. The sayings of the Prophet Mohamed allowed some of his followers to practise 'withdrawal' (12). Most scholars of the Prophet's tradition 'Hadith' agree that permission was granted. Religious judges do not object to contraception so long as the methods are used within its teachings, prescribed by trustworthy doctors and cause no harm (13–16). By analogy, methods of contraception available today which were not available at the time of Prophet Mohamed would be permitted, provided they cause no harm and prevent conception temporarily (13–16).

Another example is medically assisted procreation (MAP). It was not mentioned in the primary sources of Sharia', namely Qur'an, the Sunna and Hadith, or by Aimma. However, these same sources have affirmed the importance of marriage, family formation and procreation (17–21). Also in Islam adoption is not acceptable as a solution to the problem of infertility (22). Treatment of the infertile couple is therefore encouraged and becomes a necessity (23). Many modalities of MAP as it is practised in many of the western societies do not comply with the social, cultural and religious background of the Muslim countries. As Qur'an and Sunna did not refer to MAP, the opinion of religious scholars would be the reliable reference in this matter. Since marriage is a contract between the wife and husband during the span of their marriage, no third party intrudes into the marital functions of sex and procreation. A third party is not acceptable whether providing an egg, a sperm or a uterus. If a marriage contract has come to an end because of divorce or death of the husband, MAP cannot be performed on the female partner even using the sperm from the former husband (23–29).

ETHICAL PRINCIPLES IN ISLAMIC SHARIA'

The primary sources of Sharia', namely the Qur'an, Sunna and sayings of Muslim scholars, have stressed the four universally accepted principles of ethics throughout Islamic history. The Islamic Sharia' has also given attention to the principle of protection of the human subject against commercial exploitation. In the next section of this chapter reference will be made to different verses of the Holy Qur'an. As it is extremely difficult to translate such verses, and in order not to deprive the English-speaking reader from enjoying such important references, an attempt has been made to give the overall meaning of such verses to the best of the author's knowledge. For the exact meaning of these verses the reader is referred to the original verses.

The Principle of Autonomy

The principle of autonomy implies respect for the person. Islam aims at the creation of a lofty human life where both the will and the thought are free, where every individual feels free and independent and is not mastered by anyone else and is powered by none other than the supreme creator of the universe. Several verses of the Holy Qur'an clearly indicate this. Here, Almighty God has said what translates as:

> And we have honoured mankind and carried them on land and across the sea and made them earn the good and preferred them tremendously to many of what we created (30).

When God created mankind, He made him/her in the best and most wonderful bodily form:

> O man, what has seduced you from thy Lord, the most beneficent? Him, who created you, fashioned you in due proportion and gave you a just bias; in whatever form He wills, does he put you together (31).

In another version

> We have created man on the best mould (32).

As a sign of respect to mankind the Qur'an has given importance not only to mankind's form but also to his/her spirit.

> They ask you concerning the spirit. Say the spirit by command of my Lord; of knowledge, only a little is communicated to you (33).

After creating him/her in the best form, Almighty God made him/her the master of all that He created to enjoy all and properly use all for his benefit and welfare.

> God who created heavens and earth, and sent down rain from the sky which brings out fruits to feed you, and made the ships subject to you to sail in the sea by His command, and the rivers also He has made subject to you. And he has made subject to you the sun and the moon, both diligently pursuing their courses, and the night and day has He also made subject to you, and has given you all that you asked of Him, and if you count God's favours to you, you will not be able to include them all. Man is given up to injustice and ingratitude (34).

Even though Allah has created the body and the spirit of mankind and subjected all that He created for his/her service, yet as an important sign for the respect of autonomy, He leaves the choice to him/her, to take his/her own decisions. A guide for the right decision is provided but the final decision on which action to take is left for the person him/herself.

> And thus have We, by Our command, sent inspiration to thee: Thou knewest not before what was Revelation, and what was Faith; but We have made the Qur'an a Light, wherewith We guide such of Our servants as We will; and verily thou dost guide men to the Straight Way (52)(35)

> The Way of God, to Whom belongs whatever is in the heavens and whatever is on earth. Behold how all affairs tend towards God! (53).

Respect for the person in Islam has also been indicated in several sayings of the Prophet Mohamed (peace be upon him). The Prophet has said:

> The first thing God created was mind. With the mind He takes, gives, rewards and punishes (36).

When the Prophet was asked by his wife Aisha about the basis of evaluation of people in the world, He said the mind, and in the thereafter He said the mind. When she asked, 'Is it not by their deeds?', He said: 'O Aisha, did they not *act*, except with as much as Almighty God has given them of mind?' (37).

Respect for the person in Islam is not only restricted to the living human being but also extends to the fetus before it is born. A woman came to the Prophet Mohamed and confessed that she was guilty of adultery. She had an illegitimate pregnancy. She was asking for purification according to the rules of Islam. The Prophet told her not to return till she had delivered her baby. She came after delivery, with her baby, to the Prophet, asking him to apply the rule of legislation on her again. The Prophet asked her to go away until her baby ceased fostering. The Prophet did not carry out the punishment till the child became independent. This event clearly shows the importance which Islam has given to the respect of the fetus, the newly born and the adult. None is punished for the sins of others.

As a sign of respect for the person Islam has given a great value to thinking, learning and informed consent even in worship. No-one can blame the Muslim for his opinions and decisions as long as it is in the right way and does not cause harm to other people or himself. The Prophet Mohamed said: 'No worship is equal to thinking and contemplation' (38).

The Holy Qur'an says 'Behold! in the creation of heavens and the earth, and the alteration of night and day, there are indeed signs for men of understanding' (39).

The Prophet said, distinguishing between those who read, think and understand and those who do not: 'Woe betide those who read and do not contemplate' (40). He also said: 'One hour thinking is better than a night of worship' (41).

Islam has stressed the right of studying and seeking knowledge. It makes it essential for every Muslim, whether male or female. Islam distinguishes between the learned and non-learned. It also stresses the importance of relaying the knowledge to others and teaching others. The Qur'an says:

> Say, are those equal, those who know and those who do not know? Is it those who are embued with understanding that receive admonition? (42).

The most important indication of how much importance Islam has given to learning and respect for the person is that the first verses in the Qur'an revealed to the Prophet, urged people to study and teach. The Qur'an says:

> Proclaim! (or read) in the name of your Lord who created man out of a mere clot of congealed blood. Proclaim! and thy Lord is most bountiful. He who taught the use of the pen, taught man that which he knew not (43).

It is not therefore surprising that Islam, which ordered thinking, learning and teaching, would maintain autonomy and respect for the person in its beliefs and religion. It considers the belief of the imitator to be wrong and not valid. The believer should consent and be convinced and not just be an imitator. It maintains the right of belief and religion and forbids compelling anyone to believe what he is not convinced of. The Qur'an, addressing the Prophet, says:

> It is not required of you to set them on the right path. But God sets on the right path whom He wills whatever of good you give benefits your own souls and you shall only do seeking the face of God. Whatever good you do, shall be rendered back to you and shall not be dealt with unjustly (44).

Almighty God, addressing his Prophet Mohamed, also said: 'If your Lord wanted, all people in the world would have become believers. Do not oblige people to be believers' (45).

The Principles of Beneficence and Non-maleficence

These two principles have been mentioned in a large number of verses in the Qur'an and Hadith. Also the literature is very rich with the sayings of scholars endorsing such important issues. The Qur'an has encouraged doing good and even ordered it. Almighty God has said: 'Whatever good you do, the Lord knows of it' (46). Almighty God encourages Muslims not only as individuals but also as a nation to do good, as He says: 'Be a nation which calls for good' (47). He also indicates that if one does good one is rewarded with good.

> Then shall anyone who has done an atom's weight of good see it and anyone who has done an atom's weight of harm shall see it (48).

Instructions to do good have been mentioned in several Hadith of the Prophet Mohamed. These were restricted not only to doing good for other human beings but extended also to animals, plants and the environment. The Prophet said: 'The Muslim makes no implementation or planting which results in feeding of a human being, an animal or a bird for which he gets no reward till the day of hereafter' (49). The Prophet said that one might avoid punishment for bad deeds in the hereafter even by planting a date (50).

Instructions to do good in Islam are extended even to the casual meeting of people with each other, and not necessarily involving the deeds. The Prophet Mohamed, addressing Abou Zar, one of his companions, said: 'You should not devalue the good deed whatever it is; even meeting your brother with a welcoming face, counts' (51).

The principle of not doing harm has been mentioned in the Qur'an and by the Prophet Mohamed in several verses. These principles were stated very strongly, not as advice but as an order from God to be followed by people. Almighty God has encouraged doing good and not doing harm, as the Qur'an says:

> God commands justice, doing good, and liberality to kith and kin. He forbids all shameful deeds, injustice and rebellion. He instructs you, that you may receive admonition (52).

In another verse Almighty God says:

> And those who annoy (do harm to) male and female believers undeservedly, bear a calumny and a glaring sin (53).

The Prophet Mohamed also stressed the principle of not doing harm in several of his sayings. He said:

> Don't sever relations, don't plot, don't hate, and don't envy each other, and be brothers in worship (54).

Islam not only encourages and orders beneficence and non-maleficence in deeds, but has extended this to ensuring that one's deeds do not harm the feelings of others. The Prophet Mohamed said: 'One should not harm one's neighbour with the smell of one's food vessel' (55). This means that one should care for the feelings of one's neighbours and should not let the neighbour feel hurt or uncomfortable through the smell of one's food, as the neighbour may not be able to afford to buy his family similar food. Also, Prophet Mohamed said: 'The Muslim is the one who saves the Muslims the harm of his tongue and his hand' (56).

The instruction to do good and not to do harm is not restricted in Islam only to human beings, but it also extends to animals. Prophet Mohamed said that a woman entered Hell for the sake of a cat she imprisoned till death. She neither fed the cat nor offered her a drink, nor set her free to feed herself from the land (57). Also the Prophet mentioned in one of his sayings that Allah had forgiven a man who filled his shoes with water from a well, to help a very thirsty dog to drink, and told his companions that they would be rewarded for doing good to all living creatures (58).

The Principle of Justice

The principle of justice is very clear in Islam. It has been stressed in many verses of the Holy Qur'an and Hadith of the Prophet Mohamed. Also the sayings and deeds of the companions of the Prophet and the scholars have always indicated the importance of justice as an essential principle in Islam.

Almighty God clearly said: 'And for the unjust, no supporter' (59). Almighty God has ordered us to do just as mentioned in the Holy Qur'an (52). The statement in that verse was at a level of an order, and not merely advice. In another verse of the Holy Qur'an, Almighty God said: 'Do justice, God likes just people' (60).

Human rights were recognized by Islam before the world came to know about the issue. Islam has recognized that man has his rights to obtain and enjoy, but also his duties to fulfil. It also clearly indicated that these rights are not a grant from anybody, however high his social status or rank. Islam guarantees justice for all people. The Prophet Mohamed said:

> O people! Your God is only one God and your father is one. There is no superiority for Arab over non-Arab, and no superiority of non-Arab over Arab, nor red over black or black over red except by piety. The most favourite to Allah is he who fears him (61).

Emphasizing this fact the Prophet Mohamed, in another saying, said that people are as equal as teeth in the toothcomb, and superiority comes only through good deeds and piety (62).

Islamic instruction for justice was restricted not only to relations between members of the society, but was also extended to relations between the governor and his people and between members of the same family. The Prophet Mohamed said:

> People rewarded by being in heaven are three: a just and correct governor, a merciful kind-hearted man to all relatives, and a dignified Muslim (63).

In another version Prophet Mohamed said:

> Seven will be under the protection and shade of God in a day when there is no shade except His. The first is a just governor (64).

The Prophet Mohamed also ordered justice between members of the same family, and condemned injustice between brothers, as reported by Numan Ibn Basheer. He warned people that injustice is a reason for punishment in the hereafter. He said: 'Avoid injustice, injustice is darkness in the hereafter' (65). He also said: 'God tolerates the unjust for some time, but when they go far he punishes them' (66).

The Prophet also advised Muslims not only to be just but also to ensure that justice is taking place and that members of the society are getting their share of food, money, love and care. He said: 'He who is fed while his neighbour is suffering from hunger is not a believer' (67).

Islam encourages Muslims to make orphans feel happy and to provide for their needs, as they are the members of the society who are more likely to suffer the bitterness of life. Islam considers money as a gift from God, and man is only responsible for its just distribution in society, with a place for the rich and the poor according to the amount and quality of work they perform. This ensures a society that flourishes with love, happiness, sympathy, kindness and fraternity.

The principle of liberty has been observed in Islam. It prohibited slavery and urged masters to set free their slaves. The Holy Qur'an says:

> O Mankind! Reverence your Guardian-Lord, Who created you from a single person, created, of like nature, his mate, and from them twain scattered like seeds countless men and women; Reverence God, through Whom ye demand your mutual rights, and reverence the wombs that bore you: for God ever watches over you (68).

The principle of prevention of human exploitation has also been addressed in Islam. Islam forbids exploitation of members of the society by other members. This was clearly indicated in the Holy Qur'an in Sura Al-Ahzab (53).

Also in a prophetic tradition, one day the Prophet was asked what is the most important matter in Islam? He replied: 'Not to abuse Muslims either in words or deeds' (69).

From the above description it is clear that Islam is the religion of humanity. It is the tolerant religion which secures man's happiness. What all Islam is about is summarized in the very clear message from God to his Prophet Mohamed, mentioned in the Holy Qur'an, which says: 'We have sent you for none else but a mercy for all creatures' (70). The prophetic tradition also emphasizes this fact. The companions of Prophet Mohamed asked him, what is best in Islam? He replied: 'To feed and greet whom you know and whom you do not know' (71).

THE ETHICAL PRINCIPLES IN OLD ISLAMIC MEDICAL PRACTICE

Islamic medical practice has for a long time followed what today we know of as medical ethics. It is true that all four main principles had not been observed simultaneously. This is reflected in the different disciplines and oaths which were developed for Muslim doctors throughout Islamic history.

Hippocratic ethics, especially the oath, are incorporated into the teachings of Muslim doctors as well as Christian and Jewish doctors. The Hippocratic oath clearly indicated the two principles of beneficence and non-maleficence. The oath, which every practising doctor had to swear before he practised, stated:

> The regimen I adopt shall be for the benefit of the patients, to the best of my power and judgement, not for their injury or for any wrongful purpose. . . . I will not give a deadly drug to anyone though it be asked of me, nor will I lead the way such council, and likewise, I will not give a woman a pessary to produce abortion (1).

Moses Maimonides, who was an Egyptian scholar and doctor and the private doctor to Saladin the Great (AD 1135–1204) developed an oath and prayers. His oath clearly stated the two principles of beneficence and non-maleficence. It stated:

> I shall use my professional skills to help in achieving the objectives of all living creatures to live in peace, and him to perfect his ego . . . I swear to fight through my work so as to reduce danger, noise, attempts at impairment of purity of earth, air and water pollution and fight destruction of natural beauty, mineral elements and wildlife.

The oath extended the two principles of beneficence and non-maleficence to the environment and did not restrict it to human beings (72).

Abil Hassan Ibn Radwan, who was an Egyptian scientist and doctor 500 years ago, advised that a doctor should distinguish himself by seven virtues. He included the three principles of beneficence, non-maleficence and justice among these virtues. He stated that the doctor should have a stronger drive to serve his patient than his desire to obtain payment (beneficence). His desire to treat the poor should be greater than his desire to treat the rich. He should treat his enemy with good intention just as he would do with a friend (justice). The doctor should refrain from taking advantage of knowledge obtained through visiting the homes of his patients. He should be trustful and never prescibe a deadly medicine or inform others about it, or prescribe a drug which aborts a fetus (non-maleficence) (72).

The medical oath which was adopted on the occasion of the opening of the medical school in Cairo during the reign of the founder of the modern Egypt, Mohamed Aly Pasha, (AD 1806–1848) included the three principles of beneficence, non-maleficence and justice. It stated that the doctor should be keen to preserve the conditions of honour, help and doing good in his practice (beneficence). The doctor should serve the poor free of charge and should not overcharge his patient (justice). The doctor should not use his profession in doing harm, should never prescribe a poison and should not give a harmful or abortion-inducing drug to a pregnant woman (non-maleficence) (72).

THE ETHICAL PRINCIPLES IN CONTEMPORARY ISLAMIC MEDICAL PRACTICE

The ethics of contemporary Islamic medical practice are based on the instructions of the Islamic Sharia', the ethical guidelines developed throughout history by earlier doctors and scholars, and on the additions of religious leaders and leading doctors, which were necessary as a result of the accelerated progress of technology and science and the marked development of medical bioengineering. In Islamic societies contemporary medical practice is shaped by the interaction of legal regulation, professional responsibilities, personal moral decisions and ethical principles. Such interaction is reflected in the oath to which the graduate doctor swears to adhere before he/she embarks on medical practice. The long-held Hippocratic ethics, during the past two decades, could not withstand the challenge of the complex ethical problems evolving because of many factors, namely scientific advances and technology, civil rights, public education, the effect of law and economics on medical practice and the heterogeneity of many societies. Such heterogeneity has become a reality because of worldwide immigration and migration movements which the past two decades have witnessed. Consequently, it is not surprising that the past two decades have witnessed much greater changes in medical ethics than in the entire history of medical ethics. The four main ethical principles have been recently extensively incorporated in the medical oaths of several Islamic countries. Egypt, as an example of Muslim countries, is a Muslim country with a highly medicalized society in which research assumes considerable importance, and where a great deal of it is conducted. In 1984 there was one doctor for every 770 people (73). There are 11 medical schools with over 2900 faculty members and 7900 doctors studying for advanced degrees; at least 15 governmental and private research institutes carry out health-related research (74). Thousands of students from Egypt, as well as from many other Muslim countries, study and graduate from these 11 faculties every year. These doctors swear the oath developed by the Egyptian Medical Syndicate before they embark on medical practice. The oath includes three ethical principles, namely beneficence, non-maleficence and justice (72). It states that the doctor will protect human life in all its stages, and in all conditions and circumstances. He will do his utmost to rescue it from death, disease, pain and anxiety (beneficence). He will strive in the pursuit of knowledge, and harness it for the benefit of mankind and not for mankind's harm (non-maleficence). He will extend his medical care to the near and far, to the virtuous and the sinner and to friend and enemy (justice).

The oath of the Muslim doctor, accepted by the First International Conference on Islamic Medicine, held in Kuwait in 1981 and published by the Islamic Medical Organization, Kuwait, in 1982, included the main four ethical principles, namely autonomy, beneficence, non-maleficence and justice (72). It stated that the doctor will respect people's dignity and their privacy, and will not disclose their secrets (autonomy). The doctor will protect human life in all its stages, in all circumstances and conditions, and will do his utmost to rescue it from death, disease, pain and anxiety (beneficence). The doctor will strive in the pursuit of knowledge and harness it for the benefit of mankind and not for mankind's harm (non-maleficence). He will extend his medical care to the near and the far, to the virtuous and the sinner and to friend and enemy (justice).

The oath of the Muslim doctor adopted by the Islamic Medical Society of North America included the four main ethical principles (72). It clearly indicated that the medical profession is a sacred profession which deals with the human mind, dignity and life, all of which should be greatly respected (autonomy). It also stated that the doctor will sacrifice his life for the service, love, and mercy of mankind (beneficence). The doctor will adhere to the instructions of Islamic Sharia' and will not kill or hurt a human being (non-maleficence). The doctor will offer his medical care to poor and rich, to cultured and illiterate, to Muslim and non-Muslim, and to white and black (justice).

Recently interest in bioethics has emerged in the Muslim world; although not on a wide scale, it has certainly started. This is indicated by the appearance of some articles in the Muslim world in literature dealing with this topic (1,3,11, 26,28,29).

ETHICAL PRINCIPLES AND MEDICAL RESEARCH

The rapid expansion of scientific knowledge has made medical research a top priority for the practising doctor. Though scientific excellence may be one of the objectives of medical research, the patient's health is always the doctor's first consideration. It is not therefore surprising that adherence to ethical principles in medical research involving the human subject is just as important as it is in therapeutic medical practice.

Though therapeutic medical practice in Islamic countries had paid attention in one way or another to the main ethical principles, medical research had neglected these principles to some extent. It is not uncommon to come across unethical biomedical research conducted in Muslim countries. The essence of the problem is not that the doctors do not care about their patients but that they have placed the value of 'scientific knowledge' and the pursuit of high-technology medicine above the welfare of the research subjects (75). The scarcity of research ethics committees to review this research before it is conducted on human subjects, and scientific journals' ethics committees to review these papers before they are published, for the protection of individuals from potential harm, has played a role in the appearance of some scientific papers which did not adhere to ethical principles (77–80). To fill this gap, the International Islamic Center for Population Studies and Research, Al-Azhar University, Cairo—in collaboration with the Ford Foundation and the WHO Special Program of Research Development and Research Training in Human Reproduction (HRP) Geneva, with the support of several other organizations—held the first International Conference on Bioethics in Human Reproduction Research in the Muslim World during the period 10–13 December 1991, with the participation of about 200 doctors, demographers, lawyers theologians, sociologists, ethicists, policy-makers and representatives of international organizations from all over the world. A proposed guideline on *Bioethics in Human Reproduction Research in the Muslim World,* based on the presentations, discussions and recommendations of this meeting, is in publication (72). In this document the four ethical principles of autonomy, beneficence, non-maleficence and justice have been observed for those conducting research in human reproduction on human subjects. Although these guidelines have observed the social, cultural and religious background of Muslim societies, they adhere to the framework of internationally accepted guidelines proposed by the WHO and the Council for the International Organization of Medical Science (CIOMS) in 1982 (76), taking into consideration the marked development which has occurred in the field of human reproduction and medically assisted procreation. It is hoped that this new guideline will be adopted by the different universities, health and research institutes in the different Muslim countries.

PRACTICAL APPLICATION OF ETHICAL PRINCIPLES IN HEALTH CARE IN ISLAM

As Islam places great importance on the family, its formation and the protection of its integrity, medical innovation in the Muslim world should serve and protect family life as it is perceived in the Islamic tradition. Human reproduction, or family formation, in its very early stages, is directly connected to human sexual relationships and deals with human cells, whether eggs or sperm, *in vivo* or *in vitro*. Therefore, as far as Muslims are concerned, human reproduction could be said to be the most sensitive issue in health care; the attitude of Islam towards the application of ethical principles in this area is most illustrative. Islamic teachings and instructions imply that children are God's gift, marriages should be fertile and children should be of a high quality, and properly maintained and educated. Permanent prevention of a couple's conception, or abortion, are unacceptable unless pregnancy endangers a woman's life or health, or results in a seriously handicapped child. Third-party intervention in sexual relationships or conception is not allowed. Thus the gametes of strangers are not available to a couple, and surrogacy is not permitted. Genetic coherence and integrity are important in Islam, and repeated consanguineous unions are discouraged.

The following review is an illustration of the application of the ethical principles to mankind in Islam starting from early intrauterine life, passing through life, and ending at the immediate post-mortem phase.

The principle of non-exploitation of human beings makes it unethical to subject Muslim individuals to research unless it is directed to that individual's benefit and is expected to improve his therapy and alleviate his sufferings.

If the pregnant woman is exposed to any type of research or therapy it is unethical if this research or therapy exposes the unborn fetus to any hazards or risks. The informed consent of the couple, or at least the mother, who is considered the guardian of the unborn child, should be obtained before conducting any type of research or therapy on the pregnant mother.

When a woman gets married it is ethical for the treating doctor to postpone conception, should the couple wish it, by prescribing a suitable method of contraception other than sterilization or termination of pregnancy. However, if pregnancy is known to endanger the health or life of the mother, or would result in a seriously handicapped child, it becomes unethical not to sterilize the woman or terminate the pregnancy if she wishes it. When the woman wants to space and plan her pregnancies it is unethical for the treating doctor not to offer her a suitable method of contraception. If she has had sufficient pregnancies, and further pregnancies become associated with risks for her physical or psychological health, it is unethical for the doctor to withhold surgical contraception or termination of pregnancy from her. It is equally unethical for the doctor to refrain from informing the patient of all the implications of the procedure and to fail to obtain her informed consent in advance.

On the other hand if the marriage proves to be infertile it becomes unethical to withhold a MAP service from the couple if it is indicated. However, it is unethical not to inform the couple of the results of the procedure and its implications. It is just as unethical if mixing of eggs or sperm is performed in order to improve the results. It is unethical to transfer the embryos of one couple to the uterus of another woman (23–29).

Sometimes diseases, whether benign or malignant, develop in the genital tract; it then becomes unethical not to remove the genital organs if this is indicated medically for the sake of the health of wife or husband. Although such procedures would lead to castration of the spouse, it is totally ethical to do this. If an organ essential for the life of an individual stops functioning, it is ethical to replace it via organ donation from another person, provided the procedure is non-commercial and does not involve exploitation of the human subject, neither the donor nor the recipient (72,81). When the person grows old and becomes weak, helpless and sick, it is unethical to leave him/her unattended or for him/her not to be helped by his/her sons and daughters (82). Finally, when the person dies, it is unethical to leave the deceased unattended or to deal with him/her without respect (83). The Prophet said: 'Breaking the bones of the dead is as sinful as breaking the bones of the living person' (84).

One may conclude from this chapter that Islam is a religion which has given great importance to what are known today as the ethical principles of autonomy, beneficence, non-maleficence and justice. Also it is a flexible religion, adaptable to the necessities of life, and what is unethical in one situation or at one time may become ethical in another situation or at another time.

REFERENCES

1. Badran, I. G. 1988. Knowledge, attitude and practice, the three pivots of excellence and wisdom. A place in the medical profession. *Journal of the Egyptian Medical Association* **71**: 463–490.
2. The American College of Physicians 1989. Ethics Manual; Part 1: History; the patient, other physicians. *Annals of Internal Medicine* **111**: 245–252.
3. Serour, G. I. 1991. Antiprogestins: ethical issues. Paper presented at the International Symposium on Antiprogestins, Dhaka, Bangladesh, 7–8 October.
4. Dickens, B. M. 1992. Guidelines on the use of human subjects in medical research. Pp. d190–201, in Serour, G. I. (Ed.) *Proceedings of the First International Conference on Bioethics in Human Reproduction Research in the Muslim World*, 10–13 December 1991, Cairo, IICPSR.
5. Kempers, R. D. (Ed.) 1990. The Ethics Committee of the American Society. Ethics and the new reproductive technologies. *Fertility and Sterility* **53** (Suppl. 2): 17S-22S.
6. Cook, R. J. 1992. Ethical and legal aspects in women's reproductive health research. Pp. 140–156, in Serour, G. I. (Ed.) *Proceedings of the First International Conference on Bioethics in Human Reproduction Research in the Muslim World*, 10–13 December 1991. Cairo IICPSR.
7. Barzelatto, J. Ethical and legal considerations in women's reproductive health research. Pp. 63–67, in Bankowski, Z., Barzellato, J. and Capron, A. M. (Eds) *Ethics and human values in family planning, conference highlights, papers and discussion*. XXII CIOMS Conference, Bangkok, Thailand, 19–24 June 1988, Council for International Organizations of Medical Sciences (CIOMS), Geneva.
8. Fathalla, M. 1988. The health care system, the seven sins. *Proceedings of the XIIth World Congress of Gynecology and Obstetrics*, Rio de Janeiro, Vol. 1, 3.
9. Omran, A. 1990. UN Data on demography of the Islamic World. Paper presented at the International Conference on Islam and Population Policy, 19–24 February. Jakarta and Lhokseumawe, Indonesia.
10. Serour, G. I. 1991. Research findings on the role of religion in family planning, 1991. Paper presented at the IPPF Regional Conference, 23–24 October, 1991, Cairo, Egypt.
11. Hathout, H. 1992. Islamic origination of medical ethics. *In* Serour, G. I. (Ed.) *Proceedings of the First International Conference on Bioethics in Human Reproduction Research in the Muslim World 10–13 December, 1991*. Cairo, IICPSR.
12. Hadith Shareef, reported by Musalaam.
13. Gad El Hak, A. G. H. (His Eminence). 1984. Islam and birth planning. *Population Sciences*, IICPSR, **2**: 40–45.

14. Gad El Hak, A. G. H. (His Eminence). 1992. Family planning and Islamic Sharia'. *Gynecological problems in the legacy of Islam*, pp. 135–141. IICPSR.
15. Tantawi, M. S. (His Eminence). 1988. *Birth planning and Islamic Sharia'*. Dar El Iftaa, Cairo, Egypt.
16. El-Ghazali, M., Ibn, H. Al-Azhar, In Ihia Ulum El Din. (1269 A.H.) Vol. II: 45, Cairo, Egypt.
17. Holy Qur'an, Sura Al-Shura 42:49–50.
18. Holy Qur'an, Sura Al-Nahl 16:72.
19. Holy Qur'an, Sura Al-Ra'd 13:38.
20. Hadith Shareef, reported by Abou Daoud.
21. Hadith Shareef, reported by Bukhary and Musalaam.
22. Holy Qur'an, Sura Al-Ahzab 32:4–5.
23. Gad El Hak A. G. H. (His Eminence). 1980. Dar El Iftaa, Cairo, Egypt, (1225) 1:115:3213-3228.
24. Proceedings of 7th Meeting of the Islamic Fikh Council on I.V.F. & E.T. and A.I.H., Mecca. 1984. *Kuwait Siasa Daily Newspaper*, March.
25. Kattan, I. S. 1991. *Islam and contemporary medical problems*. Edited by Abdel Rahman A. El-Awadi. Organization of Islamic Medicine, 365–374.
26. Serour, G. I., Aboulghar, M. A. and Mansour, R. T. 1990. *In vitro* fertilization and embryo transfer: ethical aspects in techniques in the Muslim World, 1990. *Population Sciences*, IICPSR, **9**: 45–53.
27. Serour, G. I., Aboulghar, M. A. and Mansour, R. T. 1991. *In vitro* fertilization and embryo transfer in Egypt. *International Journal of Gynecology and Obstetrics* **36**: 49–53.
28. Serour, G. I. 1992. Medically assisted procreation. Dilemma of practice and research in the Muslim World. Pp. 234–242, in Serour, G. I. (Ed.) *Proceedings of the First International Conference on Bioethics in Human Reproduction Research in the Muslim World*, 10–13 December 1991. Cairo, IICPSR.
29. Aboulghar, M. A., Serour, G. I. and Mansour, R. T. 1990. Some ethical and legal aspects of medically assisted reproduction in Egypt. *International Journal of Bioethics* 1: 265–268.
30. Holy Qur'an, Sura El-Israa 17:70.
31. Holy Qur'an, Sura Al-Infitar 82:6-8.
32. Holy Qur'an, Sura Al-Teen 95:4.
33. Holy Qur'an, Sura Al-Israa 17:85.
34. Holy Qur'an, Sura Ibrahim 14:32-34.
35. Holy Qur'an, Sura Al-Shoura 42:52-53.
36. Hadith Shareef, reported by Tabrany.
37. Hadith Shareef, reported by Tarmazy.
38. Hadith Shareef, reported by Aly Ibn Abou Taleb.
39. Holy Qur'an, Sura Aali Omran 3:190.
40. Hadith Shareef, reported by Ibn Haban.
41. Hadith Shareef, reported by Abbas Ibn El Dardaa.
42. Holy Qur'an, Sura Al-Zumor 39:9.
43. Holy Qur'an, Sura Al-Alak 96:1-5.
44. Holy Qur'an, Sura Al-Bakara 2:272.
45. Holy Qur'an, Sura Younis 10:99.
46. Holy Qur'an, Sura Al-Bakara 2:215.
47. Holy Qur'an, Sura Al-Omran 3:104.
48. Holy Qur'an, Sura Al-Zalzala 99:7-8.
49. Hadith Shareef, reported by Anas.
50. Hadith Shareef, reported by Adie Ibn Hatem.
51. Hadith Shareef, reported by Musalaam.
52. Holy Qur'an, Sura Al-Nahl 16:90.
53. Holy Qur'an, Sura Al-Ahzab 33:58.
54. Hadith Shareef, reported by Anas. Agreed upon.*
55. Hadith Shareef, mentioned by Gaber and reported by Musalaam.

56. Hadith Shareef, reported by Abdullah Ibn Amr Ibn Elass.
57. Hadith Shareef, reported by Ibn Omar. Agreed upon.*
58. Hadith Shareef, reported by Boukhary.
59. Holy Qur'an, Sura Al-Heg 22:71.
60. Holy Qur'an, Sura Al-Hegrat 49:9.
61. Hadith Shareef, mentioned by Omar Ibn El-Khattab, reported by Imam Ahmed.
62. Hadith Shareef, the Prophet's address at Heg El-Wadah. Agreed upon.*
63. Hadith Shareef, reported by Musalaam.
64. Hadith Shareef, reported by Abi Huraira.
65. Hadith Shareef, reported by Gaber.
66. Hadith Shareef, mentioned by Riad El-Saleheen. Agreed upon.*
67. Hadith Shareef, mentioned by Omar, reported by Imam Ahmed.
68. Holy Qur'an, Sura Al-Nesa 4:1.
69. Hadith Shareef, reported by Bukhary.
70. Holy Qur'an, Sura Al-Anbia 21:107.
71. Hadith Shareef, reported by Musalaam.
72. Serour, G. I. (Ed.) 1992. *Proceedings of the First International Conference on Bioethics in Human Reproduction Research in the Muslim World*, 10–13 December 1991, Cairo, IICPSR.
73. World Bank. 1990. *World development report. 1990: Poverty*, p. 232. Oxford University Press, Oxford.
74. Wahab, Y. 1989. Egypt: Country report on the present status of health research for development. Unpublished manuscript.
75. Lane, D. S. 1992. Research bioethics in Egypt. Personal communication with Serour, G. I. and unpublished manuscript, Ford Foundation, Cairo, Egypt.
76. WHO and CIOMS. 1989. Proposed international guidelines for biomedical research involving human subjects. A joint project of the WHO and the Council for international organizations of medical sciences. CIOMS, Geneva, 1989.
77. Fathalla, M. 1992. Ethics in medical research. Pp. 173–182, *in* Serour, G. I. (Ed.) *Proceedings of the First International Conference on Bioethics in Human Reproduction Research in the Muslim World*, 10–13 December 1991. Cairo, IICPSR.
78. Serour, G. I. 1992. Ethical concerns. Pp. 13–19, *in* Serour, G. I. (Ed.) *Proceedings of the First International Conference on Bioethics in Human Reproduction Research in the Muslim World*, 10–13 December 1991. Cairo: IICPSR.
79. Marshall, P. A. 1992. Development of ethical guidelines for research in human reproduction. Pp. 269–281, *in* Serour, G. A. (Ed.) *Proceedings of the First International Conference on Bioethics in Human Reproduction Research in the Muslim World*, 10–13 December 1991. Cairo, IICSPR.
80. Mcnaughton, M. (Sir) 1992. Medically assisted conception, dilemma of practice and research, global view. Pp. 229–233, *in* Serour, G. I. (Ed.) *Proceedings of the First International Conference on Bioethics in Human Reproduction Research in the Muslim World*, 10–13 December 1991. Cairo, IICPSR.
81. Gad, El Hak A. G. H. (His Eminence) 1992. Organ donation and Islamic Sharia. Pp. 143–160, *in Gynecological problems in the legacy of Islam* IICPSR.
82. Holy Qur'an, Sura Al-Israa 17:23-24.
83. Gad El Hak, A. G. H. (His Eminence) 1992. Islam—a religion of ethics, (the opening speech). Pp. 13–19, *in* Serour, G. I. (Ed.) *Proceedings of the First International Conference on Bioethics in Human Reproduction Research in the Muslim World*, 10–13 December 1991. Cairo, IICPSR.
84. Hadith Shareef, reported by Abou Dawood. Agreed upon.*

---

* 'Agreed upon' means that all authorities of Hadith agree that the attributed saying was said by the Prophet.

9

Islam and the Four Principles: a Pakistani View

DR K. ZAKI HASAN, MB, FRCP, FCPS(PAK)

Dean and Professor of Behavioural Sciences, Baqai Medical College, Karachi, Pakistan

The first problem that a discussion such as this encounters is the wide gulf that exists in most Islamic—indeed all Third World—countries between the clerical and the professional groups. In the traditional systems of medicine there was considerable interaction between religious scholars and those who practised the healing arts. One reason was that the ecclesiastical courses included elements of the healing arts. In the colonial era the traditional systems of medicine were replaced by the western system which received official patronage, at the expense of traditional systems. The emerging and more dynamic western systems were adopted by the elite who became more and more westernized. The two systems (and their practitioners) began to differ in content and in form. In form, the economic levels, the modes of living and the social circles of the traditionalists differed from the emerging west-oriented elite groups. The practitioners of traditional systems of medicine continued to have more in common with religious and clerical groups than professionals practising modern systems of medicine, essentially because of a common spiritual content. When the colonial era was replaced by nationalist trends, attempts were made to bridge this gap. This process is best exemplified in the subcontinent of India. The last of the Moghul kings was replaced by British rule in the early part of the nineteenth century. During the Moghul period the system of medicine called 'Unani' or 'Greek', which indicated its origin which lay in the teaching of eminent Greek physicians, was rendered accessible to the Muslim world. 'It was in fact an eclectic synthesis of more ancient systems, chiefly Greek, but in a lesser degree Indian and old Persian, with a tincture of other exotic systems less easily to be identified' (1).

The practitioners of that system were drawn from the same stratum of society as the clerical group. The teacher, cleric and healer had a common role in society and they shared a common culture. The social nexus was status, not a monetary

Principles of Health Care Ethics. Edited by Raanan Gillon.
© 1994 John Wiley & Sons Ltd

contract. Also, within the prevalent extended family system there were more points of intellectual contact and social intercourse. The gradual introduction of the modern medical system without concomitant social change and technological advance created conflicts in society. The result was that the modern-educated section of the population found itself at one end of the social scale while at the other end were the traditional medical groups and religious scholars. An epistemological reason for the absence of dialogue between these groups lies in the fact that, unlike the Christian clergy, Muslim clerics did not have state authority directly or indirectly. Nor was there a transfer of power from the feudal groups to the mercantile. Instead, society changed into groups of hierarchical families, not guilds or fraternities with their own codes of honour. This left little room for intellectual dialogue. The same is true for all dialogue between clerics and the scientific professions.

In most Third World countries medical ethics is not a discourse that forms part of the mainstream thought process in those societies, or even within the medical profession. It is alluded to briefly whenever an event concerning negligence or medical malpractice makes newspaper headlines. The result is that the dialogue which is ferocious in the west is virtually absent in the Third World. One would have expected that where religious scholars also form a political power this dialogue would be more frequent and more intense. Iran represents one such example, but even there, dialogue on medical ethics does not form a major concern. This lack of dialogue is because the thought of theocrats is divorced from modern advances in science and philosophy and therefore no mechanisms exist for establishing a dialogue. This may also explain why no desire for social equity, altruism, and idealism lingers in the young medical person for very long, even when it is ardently professed in the early years of medical school.

THE NATURE OF ETHICS IN ISLAM

Islam has a very wide spread. There are 1.2 billion Muslims who form 18.3% of the total world population, spread over 20% of the land mass. Islam is the religion of certitude and equilibrium as Christianity is the religion of love and sacrifice. It is founded on the total character of human intelligence in free will and in the gift of speech and is represented by *Iman–Islam–Ihsan* (Faith–Law–Way) (2).

It is embraced by peoples from a large number of ethnic and linguistic groups. Over the years these cultures have modified some of the basic principles to suit political and cultural expediencies. Islam's original address was to humanity as a whole; 'Insan' or Man was the prime objective. The main source of guidance is the *Qur'an* followed by *Hadith/Sunnah*, *Ijmma* and *Qiyas*. Since the contents of the *Qur'an* did not cover all possible religious and ethical circumstances, devout Muslims patterned their life after the words and actions of the Prophet. This took the form of the *Hadith/Sunnah*. *Ijmma* is the interpretation of law by a consensus of scholars. Although this has considerable potential for a progressive interpretation in the light of new knowledge it is no longer in vogue. *Qiyas* is analogy where a previous example is used for a decision on the present problem, except that it is more objective and more free of personal philosophy. *Ijtehad* or 'enterprise', accepted by certain schools and denied by others, depends on reasoning on the basic principles and its application to the present situation.

The concept of Unity in Islam implies a single source of divine knowledge, and this source allows evolution of laws as society develops, and its problems become more complex. Commenting on the social mores in Islam, Wilfred Cantwell Smith says: 'While Christianity in recent years has moved towards a social gospel, Islam has been a social gospel from the very start' (3). Islam's social gospel is based on religion and morality, as opposed to secular social philosophies.

Moral acts in Islam may be divided into five categories: (a) acts which are obligatory, (b) acts recommended by law, (c) acts which are permitted, (d) acts disapproved by the law, (e) acts forbidden by law. Thus the entire spectrum is covered in such a way as to make Islamic law an important arbiter (4).

In the light of its religious basis, it is apparent that the core of Muslim ethics, in contrast to that later known mainly from Greek philosophy, is to be found in the *Qur'an* and *Hadith*. The ethics of Mohamed and the traditions, in the ninth century, ran head on into the struggle between the Mu'tazilah school and the reaction to it in the form of exegesis known as *Kalam*. The former reserved some moral decision and responsibility for the individual while the latter remained orthodox, opposing any free will. During this contention, Greek ethics entered the intellectual scene, gradually to make itself more and more influential (5).

Ethical values are universal but are deeply embedded in cultural contexts. They are adaptations which have roots in local circumstances. The interpretation of ethical values is also determined by the resources that are available to individuals, families and communities. They are also heavily influenced by the prevailing economic and political systems. Over the years there has been much local interpretation of Islam, sometimes determined by political necessity, but often as a social imperative to suit the needs of technological advance and cultural developments.

There are instances where original concepts are superseded by pragmatic considerations. Some interpretations appear to distort original concepts, others represent adaptations which remain true to the meaning but the adaptation becomes a distortion.

The discourse that forms the basis of this book can be considered as a discussion of medical ethics on a micro level which is mostly valid for those societies where ethical problems at a macro level have been addressed through a prevailing system of justice that has provided equity and access to health services as part of social progress. In the Third World, social development has yet to reach a level of development where these concerns can assume a central position. The other point that must be made in this context is the need for new research to become part of beneficence. We can now turn to the responses that Islam offers to the four principles.

The four principles can be either considered separately, as has been done for the purposes of discussion in this book, or justice can be considered as a cluster complex which would include these four principles.

AUTONOMY

There is considerable room for personal autonomy in Islam. The rapid and all-round progress and spread of Islam, and its assumption of world leadership in civilization and culture, was due to the definiteness of its healthy outlook on society and its embodiment in a progressive system. It spread rapidly because it offered equality before law, and social justice, to large groups of humanity who had suffered under all types of tyranny. A relative liberty was encouraged by some of the social conditions of the mid-arid zone itself where the tribes lived. Individual liberty often went to great lengths. The sense of personal liberty that this allowed contributed to the strength of the social system. The progressive era lasted several centuries. Later, the momentum weakened and it became fossilized in various forms of orthodoxy and the universal and eternal character of Islam was eroded.

Islam recognizes many Prophets of God and their injunctions; this implies that it accepts that laws have to evolve to suit the needs of society as it changes. The teaching of the *Qur'an* is that life is a process of progressive creation which necessitates that each generation, guided but unhampered by the work of its predecessors, should be permitted to solve its own problems.

According to the *Qur'an*, the first and foremost attribute of God is Rabb, which means provider, sustainer, and cherisher. This makes God immanent in the universe as a creative and evolutionary purpose. The *Qur'an* says that the spirit of man is the divine spirit itself; if God is free, His essential attribute of freedom is shared by man, being God's viceregent on earth; hence he too possesses delegated freedom. Adam's first exercise of liberty was in disobedience. Liberty itself may not be an intrinsic value but it is an indispensable condition for the realization of all the intrinsic values of life (6). It is in this context that *Qur'an* constantly exhorts people to use reason, and to reflect. Wisdom is called 'a great good'.

Diversity in Islamic thought started to appear very early in the history of Islam. This has had its positive aspects. Since Islam rejected any priesthood, there was no authoritative interpretation of the divine message. There were no ecclesiastical courts and no central authority to enforce any of their verdicts. The progress that Protestant protest achieved for the Christian faith became available to Islam earlier, since no immutable ideology was ever established. Sometimes dissent became so strong and established as to change what could be the very basis of the faith. The Shi'ite faith has designated justice as the second major principle of religion. Later, Mu'tazili thinkers who were deeply influenced by Greek thought used the method of rational discourse to refine further the concept of justice as part of their emphasis on temperance along with wisdom and courage; and the corresponding vices are designated as ignorance, incontinence, cowardice and injustice (7).

Islam believes that its finality is not in the immutability of legislation but in the fact that there will be no more divine revelation; and the legal system is left to be determined by the people in the light of their own reasoning. This concept is specially applicable to individual autonomy.

A study of the social history of societies in the west indicates that the achievement of individual autonomy has been a gradual process, the rate of which varied from one culture to another. In the US and the Scandinavian countries, which did not have traditional societies, individual autonomy was easily achieved. In France, Germany, and the USSR the process was accelerated by revolutionary changes in the political systems assisted by the transfer of social and political power from the landed gentry to the commercial and industrial groups. The movement towards individual autonomy has been slower in the UK and Japan. Islamic countries are a part of the Third World where these social and political changes have not taken place. Here progress towards political autonomy has been extremely slow.

Any discussion of autonomy will also include the question of paternalism, as the two are interdependent though sometimes contradictory. Unlike autonomy, paternalism is not a finite principle. It is dependent on many variables, especially socioeconomic systems. It can be considered as a mode of life where the individual is dependent on a wage-earner, a feudal or religious leader, or state power which controls the finances. In a hierarchical society one section is considered more dispensable than another, be they the poor or the elderly. Islam disapproves of this.

Societies in developing countries are essentially traditional and require for their existence a focus on the family rather than the individual. This has influenced all aspects of life. Paternalism thus becomes a mode of life. It is exercised within the family. The family also wants the physician to exercise paternalism.

Paternalism was originally an essential part of a tribal culture where collective decisions were needed. As tribal societies evolved into feudal societies, the collective decisions became family decisions. This was accepted more in feudal societies where paternalism by the head of the family is part of a hierarchical order, a protective mechanism which also supports and helps in maintaining the social system. It is exercised within the family and the family expects the doctor to exercise varying degrees of medical paternalism. Gillon puts it succinctly when he says

> Put in terms of various real life circumstances, however, with patients terrified by their diseases, perhaps suffering from pain and other highly unpleasant symptoms such as breathlessness, intractable itching, disordered sensation, misery and depression, and, often, utter bewilderment, it becomes far more plausible to think, especially if one is that patient's doctor relative or friend, that the last thing one should do is add to the misery and worry by passing on the results of biopsy, the risks of treatment, the unsatisfactory option, or whatever other nasty bits of information the doctor has up his sleeve. More plausible indeed, but how justifiable? (8).

Withholding information is not technically the same as lying. It is believed in Islam that sometimes truth can be harmful to some people if they are not 'spiritually' strong. The spectrum ranges from giving all the information (which may not be absorbed, accepted/handled properly), censoring, i.e. withholding some information, and fabrication/deception. Informed consent lies in this grey area produced by the philosophical clash between beneficence and autonomy as principles governing the consent doctrine (9).

Cultural attitudes in Pakistan towards informing patients about cancer or similar irreversible conditions tend towards caution, and relatives usually request that information be withheld not only from the patient but also from other near relatives who are believed to be specially vulnerable. Kauser very perceptively observes: 'Ethics is the expression of human values. Cultures are primordial sources of values, which have often been amended by religions' (S. K. Kauser, personal communication).

BENEFICENCE

Beneficence (*birr*) is one of the great pillars of the Message of Islam and a clear way to social righteousness.

The term appears with many meanings in the Qur'an, depending on the context. It may signify truthfulness, goodness and right-doing in the broadest sense as well as obedience to God.

> By beneficence is meant here acting rightly by offering comfort to the poor, to the less fortunate, and to those of our brethren in the community who have fallen on evil days ... owing to natural handicaps, orphanhood, illness, misfortune, or ignorance, among other causes (10).

Beneficence refers to the moral duty of doing good. Islam lays great stress on doing good, and there is a great and clear distinction between good and evil. The former will be rewarded and the latter punished.

There is also a violent debate within Islamic thought on the subject of goodness between the Ash'arite and the Mu'tazilah schools.

> For, whereas the latter held that man can determine rationally what is good and evil, prior to Revelation, the Ash'arites adhered to a strict voluntarist ethics. Good is what God has prescribed, evil what He has prohibited. In keeping with this voluntarist thesis, they were reluctant to admit that any merit attached to that type of rational knowledge which is attainable through unaided reason. God's power and sovereignty are such that the very meaning of justice and injustice is bound up with His arbitrary decrees. Apart from those decrees, justice and injustice, good and evil, have no meaning whatsoever. Thus God is not compelled, as the Mu'tazilah had argued, to take note of moral or religious interests, so to speak, but is entirely free to punish the innocent and remit the sins of the wicked. And had He so desired, He could have created a universe entirely different from the one which He has in fact created, or refrained from creating this universe or any part of it altogether (11).

In Islam there also exists the concept of Shifa, which means recovery from illness and is part of the rubric of beneficence in the particular context of the process of healing or recovery from illness. God is especially endowed with this capacity, very kin to a comparable Christian concept. He is depicted frequently as the source of healing and Reliever of distress. 'Then eat of all the fruits and walk in the ways of the Lord submissively. There comes forth from within it a beverage of many colours in which there is healing for men; surely there is a sign in this for a people who reflect' (16:69). Here He not only assumes responsibility for healing the sick but also exhorts search and reflection (in that pursuit). The Muslim medical practitioner traditionally superscribes his prescription with an invocation to God to grant His beneficence to the recipient.

Beneficence in the medical context is considered very important by Islam. It exhorts members of the medical profession to put the interest of patients above their own interests. This applies to the present-day controversies raised by the generally accepted right of the medical profession to go on strike in pursuit of its economic demands. Since a strike may place the life of some individuals in jeopardy this goes against the concept of beneficence and almost reaches the mischief of maleficence. Governments in Pakistan and in other Islamic countries have been known to invoke religious principles to dissuade members of the medical profession from going on strike. This is one example where beneficence may conflict with a principle of justice. On the same principle the physician is supposed to respond to every call for help, believing it to be a religious duty. The elderly are particular recipients of beneficence as enjoined by Islam. They are not only to be treated with reverence but are considered the special responsibility of the young. The concept of beneficence is also extended to include concern for animals. Unkind modes of killing animals are considered reprehensible; massacre is not tolerated. Animal research should not entail cruelty to, or torture of, animals.

One of the earliest known books on medical ethics in the Islamic world is attributed to Ishaq ibn 'Ali Al-Ruhawi who lived in the ninth century. All through Al-Ruhawi's treatise the author is deeply concerned with the standards of medicine and the dignity of the physician. He states that since the dearest possession of man is considered to be health, those who have adopted the profession of medicine are on the side of the virtuous and rational ones, 'the foremost of the people in station, highest in rank, greatest in worth, and most truthful in speech'. This, says the text, is because, when this art was bestowed upon mankind, God did not consider all persons fit to learn it and so He gave it to some virtuous ones 'whose hearts are pure, with a sharp intellect, and who love the good, have mercy, sympathy and chastity' (12).

As to the Hippocratic oath, this is not required of a physician by Al-Ruhawi. Since the profession is given only to those who are qualified, an oath would hardly be necessary. Thus, in this deontological text, the practice of the art of medicine, being God-centred, is bracketed together with ethics.

Magic (mind control) is certainly mentioned in the Qur'an, but is to be deprecated unless it is subordinated to the Will of God. The implication in this context is the avoidance of magical cures and the substitution of rationality for naive hopes of miracles. This indicates that a large place was allotted to reason not only in theological theory but also, and especially, in the actual intellectual activity of education for Muslims.

NON-MALEFICENCE

It is possible to accept non-maleficence as the exact opposite of beneficence, but that would be making it a negative quality. In a just system of moral philosophy it is imperative that non-maleficence should be a positive and determined attitude. In fact avoidance of doing harm should take priority over beneficence (see ref. 8, p. 31). The most obvious relevance of this element to the Islamic thought process would be in the area of therapeutic nihilism. In the practice of modern medicine there are occasions when practitioners resort to nihilism, or minimalism. This cannot be accepted as an absolute principle. As mentioned earlier, in a Muslim society there is a prevailing belief that God has a remedy for every illness. Taking a rational view of this means that withholding from a patient what he therapeutically needs can never be justified. The guiding rule in matters falling under no extant text or law, is the Islamic dictum: 'Wherever welfare is found, there exists the statute of God' (13).

Organ donation has also been a subject of debate in Muslim society, and the consensus is that while it is not prohibited, 'Organ donation shall never be the outcome of compulsion, family embarrassment, social or other pressure or exploitation of financial need' (see ref. 8, p. 81). There are many other tracts which support the concept of organ donation positively.

There exists a debate initiated by Jonsen and quoted by Gillon (see ref. 8, p. 84), which suggests that sometimes non-maleficence can be used as a justification for termination of life. From an Islamic point of view symptomatic treatment such as replacement of fluids, maintenance of airways and attention to rigors and shivering, even for the irretrievably comatose, can never be denied. Beneficence of God can be expected to save the patient until the last moment. Discontinuation of life support systems is always a difficult decision in a society where not only the immediate, but also the extended, family is intimately involved in the final moments of the life of the member of the family. This is often a dilemma which faces modern tertiary care institutions patterned on the western model but located in a Third World milieu.

JUSTICE

Justice may be defined as 'giving to everyone his due on the basis of equity'. In its widest sense *the pursuit of Justice* relates to two levels, individualistic and collective. The individualistic level has two dimensions, *viz.* justice to one's self and justice to other individuals. Then, there are two aspects of the pursuit in each case, *viz.* positive and negative. Thus, at the individualistic level, four basic rules of justice emerge in Qur'anic ethics: (a) establish positive devotion to the harmonious development of personality; (b) remain constantly on guard against all negative factors in respect of every aspect of personality; (c) give unstintedly to others what is due to them; (d) refrain absolutely from defrauding others in what belongs to them.

At the collective level, justice takes the following four forms, which have been projected by the Qur'an: (a) justice in social relations; (b) justice in respect of the process and enforcement of Law; (c) economic justice; and (d) political justice. The healthy growth of society, which greatly influences the growth of the individual, demands the enforcement of all these forms of justice.

There is a metaphysical concept of ultimate justice and then there is the application of justice in practical matters. To combine justice with goodness is perhaps a primitive concept. The latter, equated with righteousness—comprising faithfulness, loftiness of character and sincerity towards onself—cannot become a useful ingredient in medical ethics.

Social justice which borders on political philosophy is certainly relevant, as it deals with equity and access to health services. Islam lays great stress on justice and equity and vehemently supports the cause of the oppressed and the disadvantaged. It holds the oppressor in contempt, strikes terror in the hearts of the oppressor, vows to punish the culprit, and cites instances where this has been done.

The first conflict that becomes apparent in the medical context is that between the concept of cost-effectiveness and justice. Justice demands that service to an individual must continue even if the service is not cost-effective. A health system based on cost-effectiveness using modern equipment as part of a service industry in a society too poor to allow access to the great majority cannot be considered just. A duty-first doctor is to be preferred to a fee-first doctor. Beneficence is *im#tatio dei*. This Islam shares with Judaeo Christian concepts (14). By the same inference, illnesses produced by the society should also be its responsibility.

Justice is not measurable; therefore the decision in a given situation must appear to the people concerned to be just in its totality. This will include the private life and lifestyle of the person concerned; in this case a physician. His lifestyle should be ruled by the three tenets of Galen which Al-Ruhawi applied to medical deontology. These are from the former's *On the Passions of the Soul*: (a) stress on the Aristotelian mean, i.e. moderation and temperance; (b) liberation from passions by training and practice; and (c) nature, or the temperament of the body, as an ethic forming factor (see ref. 12, p. 17). The medical practitioner thus schooled will do justice, not only in outward appearance, but also in his behaviour.

Distributive justice is also an important concern of Islam. This principle, which is most relevant to our discussion, was discussed by a group of medical students in Karachi. They were told:

> Assume two proposals are before the Government, both of which are involved in health care in Karachi. Proposal A calls for heavy investment in the major hospitals including that required to back up a community-based primary health care (PHC) programme. Proposal B calls for immediate launching of a new approach to community-based PHC over the next three years, which may be followed by increased support to the hospitals, including emphasis on hospital back-up for the PHC programmes.

For the young students this case raised questions about equity, principles of social justice and who shall receive care when all cannot be served. It illustrates the dilemmas involved in resource allocation when cogent arguments can be put forward in support for either of two important choices. It also calls attention to the social obligations of physicians and institutions. Relevant here, too, is that Islam is perhaps the religion most suited from the perspective of its fundamental principles to the support of primary health care (J. H. Bryant, personal communication).

CONCLUSION

A large number of moral dilemmas can be associated with the practice of medicine, complex and highly technological as it has become. This book has confined itself to dilemmas involving four moral principles. These principles are respect for a person's autonomy, beneficence, non-maleficence, and justice. These principles provide a useful analytical framework for practitioners of medicine anywhere. The issues are particularly germane to problems in those societies that are in transition towards modernity. The term modernity is being used to describe a societal process towards a higher level of socioeconomic development. The discussion in this chapter has confined itself to the responses that Islam, as a metaphysical system based on faith, offers to these four principles. Islamic society has a vast storehouse of revealed and deductive logic, as well as solutions to problems as they existed in the days of its ascendancy. Intellectual and technological progress raised the level of civilization of the time to unprecedented heights. Medical science also flourished at the time, and appropriate ethical principles were enunciated.

Absence of major transitions in relation to economic changes in most Islamic societies has resulted in their now being included in what is called the Third World. In the process of decline historical interpretation of basic Islamic thought was distorted particularly because there were no imperatives to progress. In the present day, with expansion of science and technology across national barriers and the ever-rising expectations of people, there is an urgent need to rethink some of the questions that were not relevant, or never asked. This chapter has attempted to do that.

ACKNOWLEDGEMENTS

Acknowledgements are due to John Bryant, Manzoor Ahmed, Mubashir Hasan, Karrar Hussain and Kausar Khan for useful discussion and advice; and to Sabiah Askari who valiantly edited the text.

REFERENCES

1. Browne, E. G. 1921. *Arabian medicine*. Cambridge University Press, Cambridge.
2. Schuon, F. 1986. *Understanding Islam*, pp. 15–16. Unwin, London, Boston, Sydney.
3. Smith, W. C. 1946. *Modern Islam in India*. London.
4. de Boer, T. J. 1961. *The history of philosophy in Islam*, pp. 39–40. London.
5. Walzer, R. and Gibb, H. A. R. 1960. *Encyclopaedia of Islam*, new edition, vol. 1, pp. 325ff.
6. Hakim, K. A. 1974. *Islamic ideology*. Institute of Islamic Culture, Lahore.
7. Miskawayh, A. 1966. *Tahdhib al-Akhlaq*, pp. 16ff. Beirut.
8. Gillon, R. 1986. *Philosophical medical ethics*. John Wiley & Sons, Chichester.
9. Veatch, R. M. 1991. Accomplishments in bioethics, quoted by J. H. Bryant in *Ethics and epidemiology: international guidelines*. CIOMS, Geneva.
10. Azzam, A. R. 1965. *The eternal message of Muhammad*, p. 89. New American Library, New York, Toronto.
11. Fakhry, M. 1970. *A history of Islamic philosophy*. Columbia University Press, New York and London.

12. Al-Ruhawi, 1967. *Adab-al-tabib*, translated by Martin Levey. Transaction of American Philosophical Society, New Series, vol. 57, Part 3, fols 70b to 71a.
13. *Islamic code of medical ethics*, IOIM, Kuwait, 1981.
14. Glick, S. 1990. *A view from Sinai*. National Academy of Sciences, Washington, DC.

10

Buddhism and the Four Principles

R. E. FLORIDA, PhD

Associate Professor, Brandon University, Manitoba, Canada; Visiting Professor, Mahidol University, Bangkok, Thailand

INTRODUCTION

Before considering to what extent the four principles, autonomy, beneficence, non-maleficence and justice, can be applied to Buddhist medical ethics, there are three preliminary observations to be made. First, Buddhism is a tremendously diverse tradition with some 2500 years of development in Asia behind it, and it would be incorrect to think that there is only one normative view on biomedical issues. Buddhism in Asia can be classified into two major schools, which have much more in common than they have differences. The older tradition, now centred in Sri Lanka, Thailand, Burma, and Indo-China, is called Theravāda, the way of the elders, and is somewhat more conservative in many ways than the other major school, the Mahāyāna. The large vehicle, or Mahāyāna, is the Buddhism of North Asia, predominating in China, Korea, Japan, and the Himalayas. Mahāyāna Buddhists have a much larger canon of scriptures than the Theravādins and tend to be a bit less literal in their interpretations and a bit more liberal in practices. Through immigration, missionaries, and scholarship both schools have recently established beachheads in the western world.

Buddhist ethical teachings and medical practices vary enormously from country to country. Buddhism has a tradition of tolerance and generally adapts itself readily to local customs, allowing its adherents much freedom in matters of belief, worship and religious practice. Thus, in a country such as Japan, individuals freely consult modern technical specialists, traditional doctors and religious healers all for the same illness. To make things even more complicated, without any sense of contradiction or conflict in a Japanese patient, Buddhist, Shinto, Confucianist and Taoist religious cures may all be routinely resorted to (1,2). Thus, it is often not easy to sort out what is Buddhist in the thought and actions of a given person, and Buddhist theories and practices differ quite a bit

Principles of Health Care Ethics. Edited by Raanan Gillon.
© 1994 John Wiley & Sons Ltd

from place to place. It is not to be expected, necessarily, that exactly the same Buddhist health care ethical principles will be held by Thai, Chinese and Tibetan Buddhists, for example.

Second, it would be dangerous to assume that the four principles of autonomy, beneficence, non-maleficence and justice are foundational in Buddhist ethical theory and practice. Indeed, all or some of them may be absent altogether. There is no reason, on the face of it, to think that ethical principles developed in the west from a Christian background and from the Hippocratic tradition in medicine will be important or even present in non-western cultures.

Finally, it is only recently that Buddhists have begun to try to work out systematic medical ethics, and there is still much to do. So far none of the works are comprehensive, and Dr Pinit Ratnakul and Shoyu Taniguchi, the authors of the two most extensive studies, both stress that Buddhists have only begun to contribute to biomedical ethical thought. As Taniguchi puts it, 'it is very difficult, if not impossible, to find any contribution towards solving ... biomedical problems from the Buddhists' (3).* Taniguchi's thesis, *A study of biomedical ethics from a Buddhist perspective*, is a major Buddhist contribution to the field. Dr Ratnakul, a Thai Buddhist who received his doctorate from Yale, also notes, in his excellent book, *Bioethics: an introduction to the ethics of medicine and life sciences*, that Asian cultures have lagged behind the west in developing biomedical theory and applications to practical problems, and thinks, 'It is time that discussion of a more systematic and intensive nature ... be developed in Asian societies' (see ref. 6, p. 18). Indeed, the Faculty of Social Sciences and Humanities of Mahidol University in Bangkok, Dr Ratnakul's home institution, has taken a leading role in this task in Thailand, as detailed in a recent article (7).†

Taniguchi's methodology is to apply models drawn from Pali texts, the scriptures of the Theravādin Buddhists, to current biomedical issues. Ratnakul, in *Bioethics*, writes from a primarily western philosophical standpoint but is also often guided by his Thai Theravādin tradition. His more recent article, which will be considered later in detail, is a very interesting attempt to specify a set of basic Buddhist principles for bioethics (7). To my knowledge there are no large-scale studies in a western language to look systematically at health care ethics from a Mahāyāna perspective.

In the remainder of this chapter these three problems should be kept in mind: the difficulty of generalizing from such a diverse tradition as the Buddhist; that it should not be assumed that autonomy, beneficence, non-maleficence and justice are central to Buddhist ethical thought; and, finally, that Buddhist bioethical thinking is just beginning to be systematically developed. I will

---

* Neither the most recent nor the earliest major publications in the field of Buddhist ethics directly mentions medical applications: see refs 4 and 5.
† In two articles, which reached me too late to consider fully in this chapter, Ratnakul has discussed ethical issues, including medical ones, in the Thai context with much less reliance on western models than in his earlier work. The articles are 'The dynamics of tradition and change in Theravada Buddhism' and 'Reflections on development and tradition in Thailand', both in Ratnakul, P. and Than, U. K. 1990. *Development, modernization, and tradition in southeast Asia: lessons from Thailand*, pp. 115–152 and 259–278. Mahidol University, Bangkok.

attempt to advance the discussion somewhat in all three of these areas, but first, for the benefit of those readers who are not familiar with Buddhist thought, some exposition of basic Buddhist principles will be necessary.

BASIC BUDDHIST ETHICS*

Ethics, in Buddhism, are part of a religious path and are based on religious insight rather than coming from philosophical argumentation. Ultimately, the fundamental principles derive from the enlightenment experience of Buddha, the founder of the faith, but Buddhists would insist that they are confirmed by the continuing experience of Buddhist practitioners over the centuries. The test of Buddhist morality is pre-eminently practical. If something conduces to the alleviation of suffering and the elimination of delusion, then it is proper to be done. The point of such good action is to help one along the path that Buddha discovered, and which leads to a state of enlightened wisdom.

The wise person realizes that anything at all that exists in our world exists only in relation with everything else that exists. Nothing at all has independent self-being. I am here and you are there only as the result of temporary, contingent causal relationships with similar beings. All of us are in constant flux, unsubstantial, and prone to suffering. Thus Buddhist ethics is essentially global, holistic and contextual. Ethical questions are to be rationally analysed as problems in co-conditioned causality (*pratītyasamutpāda*). This great insight, that all phenomena are interrelated (co-conditioned causality), which has been taken as Buddhism's first principle (10,11), can be understood from the ultimate or the relative viewpoint.

Since all things are radically contingent and co-dependent, everything, including all living beings and of course our selves, is fundamentally empty. To the extent that one sees this directly, one tastes wisdom, and recognizes that we are all caught up in foolish selfish patterns of grasping that can never lead to peace. Insight into the absolute truth of emptiness leads directly to the relative truth of compassion. Compassion, or *karuṇā*, is the practical expression of wisdom, or *prajñā*, and together wisdom and compassion are the essence of the Buddhist way. Compassion involves living in the world in such a way as to reverse habitual patterns of selfishness because wisdom has shown the pointlessness and painfulness of ignorant grasping; and *upāya*, skilful means or the ability to serve others on the path, is a fundamental Buddhist practical virtue, necessary to function properly in the relative, conditioned world.

Thus moral behaviour in the Buddhist way is not an ends unto itself. It is a

---

* The following section I believe generally applies to both the Theravāda and Mahāyāna traditions. I am deeply indebted to the generosity of Buddhist teachers over the last decade for whatever understanding I have. In particular, I gratefully acknowledge the patience and kindness of the people of the Naropa Institute (Boulder, Colorado), Rissho Kosei Kai (Tokyo), the Diamond Sangha (Honolulu), the Faculty of Social Sciences and Humanities of Mahidol University (Bangkok), and the Chung Hwa Buddhist Institute (Taiwan). Perhaps the best concise and easily accessible introduction to Buddhist ethics is Reynolds and Campany (8). Taniguchi (3), chapter 4 and Ratnakul (6) chapter 1 and appendix III are also useful. Dharmasiri's *Fundamentals* (5), although rather long for a quick grounding, is a very good introduction to the subject. Finally, see my earlier article (9).

way to advance towards an ultimate religious' goal, the transcendence of those cravings which bind us to the dreary round of selfish existence. So acts are judged by their effectiveness to help one along the religious path. Those which are helpful are called *kuśala karma*, or skilful deeds; those which impede progress are *akuśala karma*, or unskilful deeds. Basically anything which harms oneself or others or both is unskilful while all acts which are non-harmful are skilful. This means that there is no absolute judgement of a person in terms of good and evil. What you do, and what you are, are matters of skill. If you are wise, then you will be able to apply your insights skilfully to the path.

Therefore Buddhist moral precepts are not understood to be absolute. Even the five basic moral precepts of Buddhism are explicitly understood to be 'rules of training' which the practitioner undertakes as vows for specific, temporary periods. For example, a lay person might undertake to abstain from the taking of alcohol for the duration of a certain holy festival. The relativity of the basic precepts is illustrated by the fact that they vary from five for the ordinary lay person, to eight for the advanced laity, and more than 200 for monks and nuns. Also the severity of interpretation of the precepts and of the social penalty, exacted within the religious community, for breaking vows varies according to the status of the person concerned, with monks and nuns being judged the most severely.

To a large extent, in Buddhist thought, a person's place in the world, one's destiny, and even one's character are predetermined by one's previous acts or *karma*. Unskilful acts (*akuśala karma*) lead to unfortunate states, and skilful acts (*kuśala karma*) have the opposite effect. But the Buddhist law of karma is far from a fatalistic determinist system. Each person has considerable opportunity to improve his or her fate by living according to *dharma* (law or the Buddha's teachings). Such skill in living (*upāya*) comes about through volition (*cetanā*). All acts start by an act of will when the mind undertakes to do something. Ignorant, unskilful acts are the product of an untamed will, dominated by the poisons of greed, hatred, and delusion. Any act so motivated will be unskilful, bringing harm to the actor and generally to others as well. On the other hand, acts which come from positive motivation will be skilful and will bear good *karma* for all involved. Ideally body, speech and mind all work harmoniously in accord with both ultimate and relative truth (*prajñā* and *karuṇā*).

The point of the Buddhist religious path is to transform the practitioner's mind so that it is no longer driven by the poisons but functions in a positive way. Precepts are useful tools in training the mind, but should not be reified into something absolute. This would be the extreme of eternalism and would surely lead to dogmatic inflexibility, the opposite of *upāya* or skilful means. Buddhist morality as part of the middle way avoids extremes, the other of which would be the antinomian or nihilist view that there are no moral or karmic consequences to one's actions. Both extreme views are errors to be avoided. Finally, it should be emphasized that morality, while an essential part of the discipline, cannot by itself lead to enlightenment or ultimate truth. It is an important step on the path, but for all of that, the path is not the goal.

DO THE FOUR PRINCIPLES APPLY IN BUDDHISM?

Now, having reviewed some of the background, we can move to consider whether or not the principles of autonomy, beneficence, non-maleficence and justice would be foundational in a Buddhist formulation of health care ethics. As a first step it would be good to see what Buddhist writers have done in this regard. The two who have written the most in the field are P. Ratnakul and S. Taniguchi. In Ratnakul's 1986 book (6) he takes fidelity to the medical profession, autonomy, beneficence, non-maleficence and justice as the *'prima facie* duties' that underlie bioethics (p. 86). While these cohere very well with the four premises of the current study, Ratnakul does not develop them from Buddhist texts, traditions, or arguments. Rather they come from the western philosophical and medical traditions.

Taniguchi, on the other hand, works practically exclusively from within a Buddhist context but does not attempt to isolate a limited number of essential Buddhist principles on which to develop a system. The study develops Buddhist models and processes and then proceeds rather discursively. Therefore, *A study of biomedical ethics from a Buddhist perspective* (3), although extremely valuable, does not immediately apply to the question at hand.

Interestingly enough, Ratnakul in his recent 1988 article, 'Bioethics in Thailand' (7), turns to his Thai Theravādin tradition as the source for fundamental bioethical principles and comes up with four. They are veracity, non-injury to life, justice and compassion. Non-injury to life (*ahiṁsā*) applies to all sentient life, but otherwise is the same as non-maleficence, which in the past in the western world has usually referred only to human life, although this seems to be changing now. Thus two of the Ratnakul's principles coincide with the four which make up the major themes of this book. In the spirit of his comment, 'There is much work to be done both in clarifying these and other principles and in applying them' (ref. 7, p. 312), let us turn our attention to his 1986 and 1988 formulations, starting with autonomy.

AUTONOMY

Dr Ratnakul describes autonomy as the ability of an individual 'to order, plan, and choose among the diverse human potentialities, the pattern of their own lives, as long as it is consistent with meeting the rightful claims of others upon them and the fulfilment of their responsibilities as moral agents' (ref. 6, pp. 83–84). In traditional Buddhist ethics, autonomy is not featured as a major category. However, the Buddhist emphasis on the responsibility of each person for his or her own *karma* or moral character implies autonomy. As outlined above, each person is responsible to order his or her own will, speech, and actions to achieve progress along the path to religious deliverance.

However, there is something in this modern notion of autonomy that goes against the Buddhist grain. While Dr Ratnakul is careful not to fall into this extreme, autonomy of the individual could be understood in a way contrary to the central Buddhist insight of co-conditioned causality, which insists on the co-dependency of all beings in opposition to radical autonomy. At any rate, we note that in his later formulation, autonomy has dropped from Dr Ratnakul's list of fundamental principles.

NON-MALEFICENCE OR AHIMSA

Non-injury to living beings must, I think be central to any Buddhist medical ethical system. As Dr Ratnakul puts it, 'In a Buddhist society it is well known and accepted that a primary obligation is non-injury *ahiṁsā* to others' (ref. 6, p. 54). It is after all closely related to the first of the 'rules of training' that guide all Buddhists on the path. In Buddhaghosa's formulation of this rule, the importance of will is very clear, as is the interaction of body, speech and mind:

> 'Taking life' is then the will to kill anything that one perceives as having life . . . in so far as the will finds expression in bodily action or in speech . . . In the case of humans the killing is the more blameworthy the more virtuous they are. Apart from that the extent of the offence is proportionate to the intensity of the wish to kill (12).

Although the precept is worded 'I undertake to observe the rule to abstain from taking life', it is interpreted to apply to all harm to fellow creatures. Obviously it is very powerful as a general principle in health care ethics, and is continuously applied by both Ratnakul and Taniguchi.

JUSTICE

In his 1988 article (7) Dr Ratnakul identifies justice as a basic Buddhist teaching, and singles it out as one of the fundamental principles on which to base a Buddhist bioethical system for Thailand. He explains his concept of justice to be:

> understood in terms of impartiality and equal treatment, giving to each one what is his due. People may be different from us either by their economic condition or by their social status, but as moral potentialities they are equal to us and therefore deserve equal treatment (p. 311).

This concept of justice is, it seems to me, a modern western one, and is indeed very like the ideas developed in his earlier book, from western sources. In checking traditional Buddhist sources I find very little about justice. Buddhaghosa, a Theravādin scholar of the fourth or fifth century AD, who may be the greatest exegete that Buddhism has produced, for example, does not seem to mention justice at all in his masterpiece, the *Visuddhimagga** (13).

Tachibana, in his still valuable 1926 path-breaking book, *The ethics of Buddhism* (4), attempts to formulate a comprehensive ethical system from the texts of Theravāda Buddhism. In the early parts of his book he stays very close to the

---

* Lamotte (11), and several other basic source books yielded nothing on justice as an early Buddhist concern. Similarly, Punyanubhab (14) and other contemporary popular treatments of Buddhism fail to include justice as a fundamental tenet.

traditional terminology and formulations, and does not mention justice at all. Then he changes his tack and decides to reformulate Buddhist ethics according to modern categories. 'This is firstly to make the moral ideas of the Buddha clearer, and secondly to see how far a moral system designed twenty-four centuries ago can appeal to the modern mind' (p. 95). Justice appears as a major category in his modern reformulation, but he notes that it is not at all easy to find precise equivalents from Buddha's time to our own twentieth century for such basic terms as justice, righteousness and impartiality (pp. 264–265).* In effect, he seems to admit that he was unable to show that justice is a fundamental ancient Buddhist principle of social ethics. Nonetheless, recognizing that justice is a keystone for any ethical system which is to appeal to people shaped by modern western thought, he goes ahead in a very appealing but not quite convincing way to use justice in his scheme of Buddhist ethics.

I also have not found much evidence that justice in an egalitarian sense is a major theme in Buddhist tradition. Recall, for example, the way that Buddhaghosa interpreted the precept against taking life as quoted above. The severity of the offence is a function of the amount of virtue that the victim has; hardly an egalitarian concept of justice. Dharmasiri points out that the Buddha taught that class society is inevitable, and that classes do not have equal rights and duties, but rather that 'classes should have reciprocal moral relationships with each other' (see ref. 5, p. 61). Indeed, this seems to be the major Buddhist philosophy behind social relationships in Thailand and other Theravādin countries.

Phra Dhammadhajamuni, Secretary General of Mahamakut Buddhist University in Bangkok, has written a useful practical book to explain the fundamentals of how Buddhism is practised in Thailand today. He expounds the social teachings of Buddha found in the Theravāda scriptures and applies them to everyday life. The basic principles that govern the relationship between people are not egalitarian but are determined by the age, gender, or class of the persons involved. For example, the categories that he treats are the following: parents and children, husband and wife, master and servant, teachers and pupils, leader and subordinate, king and official, and friends (16). Within these categories, only amongst friends is there equality. Otherwise there are reciprocal duties and obligations between relatively high and relatively low individuals.

Teachers, for instance, are to be knowledgeable, helpful, protective, fair, and generous to their students, who in turn are expected to be grateful, to show their gratitude, to obey, respect and wait upon their teacher (ref. 16, pp. 45–46). Leaders are to be compassionate, fair, and helpful to their subordinates, who in turn first must obey orders and then should work hard and responsibly with the master's interests as their own (ref. 16, pp. 46–48). The basic model is paternalistic as is very explicit in the case of the king, who, the Buddha taught, should rule according to *dharma*, 'treating his subjects as parents treat their own children' (17). My sources do not mention medical matters, but likely the doctor–patient model relationship would be hierarchical, with the doctor taking a paternal role and the patient a subservient one. Perhaps the relatively inferior

---

* See Basham (15), pp. 114–117 and *passim* for an indication of how different the ancient Indian concept of justice is from the current western notion.

quantity and quality of heath care that the poor masses of Thailand are given is partially due to traditional hierarchical social practices.

Yet part of these ancient, traditional social teachings strongly supports the provision of adequate health care for all people, even all living creatures, in society. The higher individuals in the reciprocal relationships have a duty to be concerned for the welfare of those in their care, and this most definitely includes health matters. For example, masters are taught to give their servants help in times of sickness (ref. 16, p. 43); and at the highest level, the king's first duty to his subjects is to give the 'help when and where it is needed, i.e. a material or verbal or manual help' (ref. 16, p. 53). Secondary royal duties include the development of human resources and philanthropic activities to provide a benign infrastructure in the kingdom (ref. 16, p. 55).

In Buddhist political thought the *dharmarāja* (the king who rules by righteousness or by Buddhist principles) or *cakravartin* (literally, the wheel turner, or the king who turns the wheel of righteousness) is the ideal ruler (18). The royal precepts and virtues that Phra Dhammadhajamuni enumerates are drawn from that tradition and still very much apply to the monarch in Thailand. Aśoka, an emperor in India who reigned in the third century BC, is the king revered today as the one who most nearly embodied the *dharmarāja* ideal, and he was very vigorous in promoting non-harm as a principle of governance and as a way of life for his subjects. He also took a great interest in the physical welfare of his subjects and provided health care medical herbs to be distributed free of charge to the people of his kingdom and also to the animals (ref. 16, pp. 53–57, 500). The royal family of Thailand today live up to these same Buddhist ideals by sponsoring and financing many public health and other health-related projects (19).

On the practical side, Dr Ratnakul (7) notes that the poor of Thailand, who make up most of the people, have very little access to health care as compared to the wealthy, and what care they do get is all too often 'degrading, humiliating, and dehumanizing'. Arguing from the 'Buddhist principle of justice', he concludes that the state, since it is the major source of medical care in Thailand, has a duty to provide adequate services for anyone who needs them (p. 311). While, in my opinion, his conclusion is certainly correct, it seems that egalitarian justice does not have a firm base in Buddhist traditional thought. Perhaps a sounder Buddhist case for an equitable distribution of health services could be built on the foundations of *karuṇā* (compassion), a fundamental virtue for all Buddhists, and on the *noblesse oblige* expected of the ideal Buddhist monarch. Both of these would entail helping the poor: *karuṇā* should motivate individuals whether commoners or royal; and the state should manifest the ideals of the *dharmarāja*, the king who rules according to the teachings of the Buddha.

COMPASSION (*KARUṆĀ*) AND BENEFICENCE

Compassion is one of the four principles that Dr Ratnakul identifies as central to Buddhist medical ethics, and it is clear from my discussion of justice, and from the section on 'basic Buddhist ethics' above, that I agree with him. Compassion is one of the most fundamental Buddhist categories, so fundamental that the entirety of the tradition can be described as compassion (*karuṇā*) and wisdom (*prajñā*) working together. It is important to keep in mind that the two are linked, and one without the other is dangerous. For example, a person who is not wise may cause enormous problems by witlessly attempting to be compassionate, and a person who has penetrating insight without compassion is very dangerous indeed.

In order to help one attain this balance, to make sure that the practitioner develops skilful means (*upāya*), certain sublime states of mind are cultivated in Buddhism. There are four of these taught by all schools of Buddhists and recognized as essential if a person is to live a moral life, generating *kuśala karma*, skilful deeds, rather than the opposite. The four are loving kindness for all sentient beings, compassion for the unhappiness of others, sympathetic joy for the happiness and good fortune of others, and equanimity (3,20). Were a nation and its people to be governed according to these impulses, then the health care system would be a most excellent manifestation of Buddhist beneficence. Dr Ratnakul agrees that this religious ideal of compassion, which goes far beyond what is called for in natural reason, is at the deepest level the Buddhist foundation for medical ethics (ref. 7, p. 312 and ref. 6, introduction and *passim*).

VERACITY

The fourth principle which Dr Ratnakul sees as essential in Buddhist biomedical ethics is veracity, which he firmly bases on another of the five basic moral precepts: 'I undertake to observe the rule to abstain from false speech'. In applying this to medical ethics he concludes that one must always tell the complete truth to the patient. Failure to disclose the truth is generally, he argues, due to denial and fear on the part of the medical personnel. If the patient does not know all the facts of his or her condition, then his or her 'strength, will power, and endurance' (ref. 7, p. 308) will be compromised. Buddhists know that life is hard and full of suffering, and have always taught that these truths must be dealt with frankly and openly. Hiding from the unpleasant sides of things is not part of the Buddhist way.

This insistence on veracity fits in very well with the current doctrine in western medicine that the patient as an autonomous moral agent has a responsibility for his or her own health and care. However, in the Mahāyāna tradition there is a rather different approach to the issue of veracity. In chapter 16 of the *Lotus Sutra*, one of the most influential Mahāyāna scriptures in East Asia, there is a parable, where Buddha describes himself as a skilful doctor.* All his sons have foolishly taken some powerful, poisonous medicine. Those who are deranged by the poison refuse to take the antidote which he has quickly prepared. Therefore, he deceives them by feigning his death, thereby shocking them back into their right minds so that they will take the remedy.

---

* In early Buddhist literature the skilful doctor occurs quite often as a metaphor for the Buddha and in the descriptions of bodhisattvas. See Birnbaum (21) for a review of the literature. Although this is not the place for it, I believe that these sorts of parables could be useful in producing models for contemporary Buddhist health care ethics, and I am currently working on this topic.

Buddha rhetorically asks: 'Is there any man who can say that this good doctor is guilty of the sin of wilfully false speech, or is there not?' (22).

This parable is taught as an example of *upāya*, or skilful means. In the Mahāyāna tradition, deception on the level of relative truth is quite justified as long as it advances the cause of absolute truth and, as in this case, is beneficent. Of course, if a deception led to harm of sentient beings, it would be unskilful rather than skilful. Thus, in Mahāyāna thought at least, a case could be made for the health care team withholding the truth, or even deceiving a patient if it was thought to be therapeutic.

This sort of paternalism is no longer stylish in the west, and many current health care ethicists reject it, including Dr Ratnakul, who writes, 'The practice of paternalism in regard to truth-telling is therefore unacceptable to Buddhism' (ref. 7, p. 308). Although his argument for veracity on medical, general ethical, and Buddhist grounds is very appealing, it nonetheless seems to me that his conclusion is perhaps overstated. Medical paternalism may be justifiable in traditional Buddhist societies, where society is governed by ancient hierarchical principles. It certainly is the current practice in Japan in regard to cancer diagnosis, where doctors practically never reveal the truth to their patients. While Mahāyāna teachings on skilful means provide a theoretical justification for this, Japanese pre-Buddhist attitudes towards bodily disintegration are also important (ref. 2, pp. 62–65, 207–208).

This issue of veracity illustrates some of the difficulties alluded to in the introduction to this paper. With the Buddhist tradition being diversified in theory and localized in practice, it is often very difficult to give a definitive or universal Buddhist answer to a specific health care ethical question. However, surely this is to be expected in a non-dogmatic, practical, and relativistic religious tradition.

CONCLUSION

In the study of ethics in the west there is widespread agreement, perhaps an emerging consensus, that certain principles, autonomy, beneficence, non-maleficence, and justice apply *prima facie* to health care issues. Buddhist health care ethics is very much in a preliminary stage of development, but it would seem that these four principles do not all fit into a Buddhist framework. Two of them, however, do fit well. Non-maleficence and the Buddhist principle of *ahimsā* (non-harm) appear to be practically identical. Furthermore, *karuṇā* (compassion), which perhaps is the central ethical principle of the Buddhist tradition, is very similar indeed to beneficence. Autonomy is also important in Buddhist practice but, as argued above, is not central and has some important differences both in theory and in its application to health care from the way it is understood in the west.

Justice seems to be the sticking point. Egalitarian justice is not part of traditional Buddhism, although using other Buddhist categories and principles, the aims of justice in health care are included. However, as noted in the introduction, Buddhism has a wonderful flexibility, enabling it to adapt to and to learn from new situations. It is noteworthy, I think, that converts to Buddhism in the western world, eastern Buddhists who have settled in the west, and those like Dr Ratnakul who have been influenced by western thought, are tending to make justice a Buddhist value (ref. 23 is a good introduction to this phenomenon).

'Cease to do evil, learn to do good, cleanse your own heart', the catchphrase which is popularly used to sum up the essence of Buddhism, suggests how important non-maleficence, beneficence, and self-reliance or moral autonomy are in Buddhist thought. All three are aspects of *karuṇā* (compassion) and *upāya* (skilful means), the qualities necessary to function well in the world as a Buddhist. These relative qualities must, of course, work in conjunction with *prajñā* (wisdom), insight into absolute truth. To be true to the Buddhist tradition, any theoretical system of health care ethics must be based on wisdom and compassion, and all applications should manifest skilful means. At the present, with the tremendous changes and challenges taking place in the heath care field, Buddhist thought, by applying wisdom, compassion, and skilful means to both theory and practice can make a tremendous contribution to bioethics.

REFERENCES

1. Ohnuki-Tierney, E. 1989. Health care in contemporary Japanese religions. Pp. 59–87, in Sanderson, L. E. (Ed.) *Healing and restoring: health and medicine in the world's religious traditions*. Macmillan, New York.
2. Ohnuki-Tierney, E. 1984. *Illness and culture in contemporary Japan: an anthropological view*. Cambridge University Press, Cambridge.
3. Taniguchi, S. 1987. *A study of biomedical ethics from a Buddhist perspective*. Berkeley: Graduate Theological Union and Institute of Buddhist Studies, MA thesis, p. 2.
4. Tachibana, S. 1975. *The ethics of Buddhism*. Curzon, London (reprint of the 1926 Oxford University Press edition).
5. Dharmasiri, G. 1989. *Fundamentals of Buddhist ethics*. Golden Leaves Publishing, Antioch, California.
6. Ratnakul, P. 1986. *Bioethics: an introduction to the ethics of medicine and life sciences*. Mahidol University, Bangkok.
7. Ratnakul, P. 1988. Bioethics in Thailand: the struggle for Buddhist solutions. *Journal of Medicine and Philosophy* **13**: 301–312.
8. Reynolds, F. E. and Campany, R. 1987. Pp. 498–504, in Eliade, M. (Ed.) *The encyclopaedia of religion*, vol. 2. Macmillan, New York.
9. Florida, R. 1991. Buddhist approaches to abortion. *Asian Philosophy,* 39–40.
10. Kalupahana, D. 1975. *Causality: the central philosophy of Buddhism*. University of Hawaii Press, Honolulu.
11. Lamotte, E. 1976. *Histoire du Bouddhisme Indien*, vol. 1, pp. 25ff. Université de Louvain, Louvain-la-neuve.
12. Conze, E. (trans.) 1959. *Buddhist scriptures*, pp. 70–71. Penguin, Harmondsworth.
13. Buddhaghosa. 1976. *The path of purification (Visuddhimagga)*, 2 vols. Shambhala Berkeley and London.
14. Punyanubhab, S. 1981. An outline of Buddhist tenets. Pp. 19–28, in National Identity Board (Eds) *Buddhism in Thai life*. Funny Publishing Ltd Partnership, Bangkok.
15. Basham, A. L. 1959. *The wonder that was India*. Grove Press, New York.
16. Phra Dhammadhajamuni, BE 2530. *Outline of Buddhism*, 2nd edn, pp. 37–61. Mahamakut Buddhist University, Bangkok.
17. Indr, S. B. 1981. The king in Buddhist tradition. P. 61, in National Identity Board (Eds) *Buddhism in Thai life*. Funny Publishing Limited Partnership, Bangkok.
18. Tambiah, S. J. 1976. *World conqueror and world renouncer: a study of Buddhism and polity in Thailand against a historical background*. Cambridge University Press, Cambridge.

19. Kraivixien, T. 1982. *His majesty King Bhumibol Adulyadej: compassionate monarch of Thailand.* Kathavethin Foundation, Bangkok.
20. Conze, E. 1972. *Buddhist meditation*, pp. 118–132. Unwin, London.
21. Birnbaum, R. 1979. *The healing Buddha*. Part One, Shambala, Boulder.
22. Hurvitz, L. (trans.) 1976. *Scripture of the lotus blossom of the fine dharma*, p. 240. Columbia University Press, New York.
23. Eppsteiner, F. and Maloney, D. (Eds) 1985. *The path of compassion: contemporary writings on engaged Buddhism.* Buddhist Peace Fellowship and White Pine Press, Berkeley, California and Buffalo, New York.

11

Principles and Life Stances: a Humanist View

DR HARRY STOPES-ROE

Moseley, Birmingham, UK

Humanists accept that the moral constraints that a society imposes on its members should be fair to each, and impartial between all. This principle, if valid, limits the claims that any life stance should make concerning these constraints. In this sense, the Humanist view of health care ethics should be the same as that of any other life stance; for a Humanist will seek to be impartial between Humanism and the other life stances.

INTRODUCTION

The value of morality lies in its capacity to bring out the best in individuals and society, so that people may have the best in life. But 'society' is not a single, monolithic, will. It is constituted by a multiplicity of individuals, and they have different ideas on what 'the best' means; and some of these differences represent fundamental divisions in morality. What then are the moral constraints that society can, and should, place on the health worker in her* relationship with her patient?

I do not mean that we, the members of society, disagree totally on morals—that would be impossible, for some degree of agreement on right and wrong is essential if a society is to exist. In fact, in our society, there is good agreement on a wide range of very important moral principles. But at the same time there is profound *dis*agreement on certain other moral principles which are of the greatest importance; and it so happens (not surprisingly, if one thinks about it) that the matters of disagreement are particularly significant for health care ethics. Further, this disagreement in practice is in part founded on disagreement on the deepest theory: we do not agree where to look to settle our moral

---

* With two personal pronouns available, 'he' and 'she', one can simplify expression and avoid ambiguity. I will use 'she' for the health worker and for anyone in authority, 'he' for the patient, except where the gender is relevant.

Principles of Health Care Ethics. Edited by Raanan Gillon.
© 1994 John Wiley & Sons Ltd

disagreements. Some of us hold that morality is rooted in human nature alone; others hold it to be rooted in God. How do we resolve such disagreements as this?

My purpose in this chapter is to discuss the implications of these deep assumptions, and (more particularly) of their diversity, for health care ethics. These issues may be unfamiliar because they are seldom explicitly recognized as such in this area. Often debate is conducted between protagonists (say Roman Catholic and Humanist) who seek to prove that each is right. I will argue that this is (largely) to misconstrue the role and nature of health care ethics. So I will start, in the next two sections, by setting out some basic concepts; and in the remainder of this chapter I will focus on examples which illustrate these issues. I will look in particular at the first of the 'principles of health care ethics', autonomy. This and the fourth, the principle of justice, seem to me fundamental. I will argue that the second and third, beneficence and non-maleficence, are not of primary value in health care ethics.

MORAL THEORY AND LIFE STANCE

I will accept, as did Mill and Kant, that right and wrong and moral duty do not depend on the knowing mind; that is to say they are *objective*. Objectivity does *not* mean that, in any particular circumstance, there is only one act which is right, the rest being wrong; this is a common misunderstanding. In most circumstances there are many alternative right acts, and it is eminently appropriate for the agent to apply his or her own personal values within the framework of morality. But the force of morality is no less objective because it leaves a range of options.

The first point I wish to make, however, comes not from the freedom within morality, but from the divergence of claims about what the constraints of morality are; and the absence of any secure way of settling these disputes. On the one hand there is the objective framework of right and wrong; on the other hand we do not *know* exactly what it requires. In other words, the moralist in general, and in particular the moralist in health care ethics, can deal only in *moral theories*. I use the word 'theory' to bring out two points: that moral judgements claim objective validity; and that we have no secure way of finding out whether they are valid.

My use of the word 'theory', however, does not imply that moral judgements are factual, nor even like factual judgements. They are profoundly different. Moral judgements are not intellectual beliefs merely, but express human duties and commitments. They reflect the ultimate questions of life and death—the facts and values that define, limit and empower human life, and give it meaning and direction. All this has traditionally been looked upon as the province of *religion*. But this word can be a source of prejudice, because it means different things to different people. For some 'religion' implies God. For others the word refers to the response to ultimate questions, whatever it may be, whether it involves God or not.

It is of the very essence of the project I am engaged upon in this chapter that it shall be fair and impartial between the ultimate beliefs of all members of our society. So the first thing I need is a vocabulary that does not prejudice the commitments of individuals. I need two words: a genus-word, an umbrella concept which all can share, from which each can set out his or her own distinctive commitment; and a specific word, which implies acceptance of God or some 'supernatural' state, element or power. (The technicalities of defining this interpretation of 'religion' are not here relevant.) The term *life stance* is now widely used for the former. I will use the word *religion* in the latter sense.* The concept of a 'life stance' differs from that of a 'religion' *only* in that 'life stance' does not carry the implication that ultimate questions *can only* be answered by reference to God. Thus 'religion' precisely equals 'life stance which involves a "supernatural"'. Therefore 'life stance' can no more be given a truly adequate definition than can 'religion'; but one can give a dictionary-type definition:

> *Life stance* The style and content of an individual's or a community's relationship with what is ultimately important; the commitments and presuppositions of this, and the theory and practice of working this out in living.†

A moral theory is set in the context of a life stance, and this provides the roots which support it. The essence of the term is that it must be an umbrella which can be used without prejudice by all.

No life stance is monolithic: even the leaders disagree (to a greater or lesser extent) on its beliefs and values. It is notable, however, that beliefs and values do fall into broad groups, with the *religious* (in the above sense) and the *naturalistic* being particularly significant. The former find God to be ultimately important, most of them tending to accept that morality is rooted in God; the latter find the natural world to be ultimately important, and accept that morality is rooted in this and in the human sense of responsibility.

HEALTH CARE ETHICS: THE ETHICS OF A SOCIETY

If there is a multiplicity of contradictory life stances and moral theories in society, and no secure way of settling which is right, how can society, the collectivity of individuals, find any moral principles? This leads me to the distinction between *collective morality*, which embodies the moral principles which should govern the rules set up by a society, and the actions it takes collectively; and *individual morality*, which sets the moral limits on what an individual may and may not do.

Health care ethics is that part of collective morality which requires society to construct codes and regulations which limit what a patient may ask for and a health worker may give. We form a theory of it as best we can.

What are the principles of collective morality, from which one may derive health care ethics? Three points are basic:

---

* In British law the word 'religion' is firmly established in this sense, so a naturalistic life stance such as Humanism is not a religion. The legal usage is more ambiguous in the USA, so in some contexts there Humanism is a religion. The common use in both countries is totally confused.
† Adapted from *A dictionary of religious education*, edited by John Sutcliffe, London: SCM Press, 1984.

A. The principles of morality are not absolutely clear and straightforward, so it is not possible to achieve security in our moral judgements; any formulation anyone attempts may be in error.
B. Morality requires a degree of respect for the autonomy of the moral agent. (This is one thing that does seem clear.)
C. Different individuals want things which mutually conflict. Thus a basic requirement of collective morality is to adjudicate between individuals, according to some principle of justice.

The first two points come together to mean that collective morality cannot be the same as any individual morality; it is looser. When presented with a concrete situation an individual cannot avoid acting one way or another, and should make up his or her own mind and conscience to guide the decision. A collectivity is not called upon to make rules governing every situation. It should not make a rule where it has no secure basis for a decision. Respect for autonomy, particularly in the absence of certainty, means that society should give a wide range of discretion to individuals. Morality tells an individual that he or she should not act outside the range of what is morally acceptable; but morality does not require that society should act or make regulations which require its individual members never to act immorally. For example, society does not intervene to force a Jehovah's Witness to receive the blood transfusion which would save his life, even if he has a wife and young children, despite the general recognition that a father should not thus ignore his responsibilities.

But collective morality does exert constraints. Some acts are so clearly wrong that society must do what it can to stop them. For example, society prohibits murder, even by a woman who sees no other way of escape from her husband's violence.

Thus the central question of health care ethics is: When does morality allow, or require, society to infringe an individual's conscience, and even to contradict his or her life stance? How does one draw the lines? This will be my leading question.

RESPECT FOR AUTONOMY

The question of autonomy well illustrates both the agreement and the disagreement between life stances. All agree that autonomy is important, and also that it must be restricted; but they differ on where to draw the border-lines. I will look at the agreements first. I think the following formulation of patient autonomy could be generally agreed. I will look at the health worker's autonomy in a later section (see p. 128).

Principle I below might seem to give excessive rights, even powers, to the patient. But the qualifications are of the essence. In particular, it in itself gives the patient no right to any particular treatment, or indeed to any treatment at all. I will not in this chapter consider the patient's right to treatment.

Principle I
Respect for the patient's autonomy. The health worker who is treating a patient

must not flout or ignore the patient's view of what outcome is best for him, where the outcome and necessary treatment are morally acceptable in themselves and the patient is not misguided in preferring the outcome, and giving the treatment to the patient does not have morally unacceptable wider implications. However, a health worker may decline to treat, or to continue treating, a particular patient.

But the health worker *must not* accede to the patient's wishes when the above conditions are not satisfied to a degree which is morally important.

However, this principle can be generally accepted only because it contains value-words, namely 'morally (un)acceptable', 'misguided' and 'morally important', which each reader interprets according to her or his own moral theory. All readers can agree with the formulation because it means something different to each.

The qualifications look in two directions. The two concepts, the 'moral acceptability in itself' of the course of action desired by the patient, and 'misguided', look to the state of the patient and those immediately involved with him, and I take them up in this section. The 'wider implications' of what the patient desires raise questions of justice: the balance between the patient on the one hand; and other individuals, and society in general, on the other. The border-line is not sharp, however. The question of justice includes the rights of the health worker (see p. 128). I take up the broader question in the section entitled 'Justice'.

The Failure of the Patient's Autonomy

Central to the health worker's responsibility, which she accepts in accepting the patient, is the commitment to act in the patient's 'best interests'. There are two problems in this: the interpretation of 'best interests' where the possible treatments considered do not have implications beyond the patient; and where the treatments do have wider implications. I now look at the interpretation of 'best interests' in the former situations.

The concept of 'best interests' is essentially ambiguous: how, then, is it to be defined—by the health worker, the patient, or the principles of morality? Personal feelings enter, and also deep moral convictions. I claim that central to the patient's autonomy is his right to determine the outcome which is best for him, from amongst those of the available treatments—subject to the limitations stipulated in the Principle. This is the point of Principle I.

The limitations are essential. One may wish to reject the patient's view of what treatment is best for him for many different reasons. I list below six situations in which one might say that the patient's wishes fail to be morally acceptable in themselves, or because they are misguided. The first four situations turn on either the validity, or the effectiveness, of the patient's sense of right and wrong, his conscience. I think one would say the patient was 'misguided' in the first, and second, and the less extreme examples of the fifth and sixth situations. Which of the following give morally valid grounds for rejecting the patient's *prima facie* right to determine the desired outcome of his treatment?

1. The patient may have a good conscience in the sense that his conscience

knows what is right and wrong, and he tries to follow it; but sometimes it is *not effective*. We each of us can provide examples of this situation: I suppose we all believe we have at least a reasonable understanding of right and wrong, and we try hard to do what is right; but sometimes we fail, for our personal reasons. In such a situation as this the health worker is able to counsel the patient using his (the patient's) own moral understanding. Selfishness by the patient leads to the question of justice.

2. His conscience may be effective in the sense that he is sincere and acts according to it; and it may be founded in a coherent life stance—but it and the life stance are *wrong*. I will make my example for this second situation hypothetical, because I do not wish at this point to enter into controversy: if abortion really is murder, a Humanist patient who asks for abortion is an example. This situation presents the deepest problems for health care ethics, for it turns on conflicts of life stance.

3. His 'conscience' may be *perverted*, in that he is fully aware of the consequences of his actions but does not recognize the wrongness of certain of them. In extreme cases he may have no concern for anything that can be accepted as 'right' and 'wrong'. I will turn to forensic psychiatry for an extreme example: the patient who is liable to knock people down if they look at him, because he does not like people looking at him.

4. He may have a *limited* conscience, or no meaningful conscience at all. This may be because he has a limited capacity to understand. The patient suffering severe Alzheimer's disease is an example here: he is simply not responsible for his wishes and actions. One will not let him dance in the snow in his night-dress. A child provides another, very different, example.

5. His judgement may be based on a false or otherwise *inadequate understanding* of the facts of his situation, and of the possible consequences of alternative courses of action. This type of situation covers a wide range: the failure may be because he suffers the misinformation of common prejudice; or he may never have recognized the problem *as* a problem; or he may be unable to understand because of mental defect; or he may suffer a functional psychosis. In the simpler cases the patient may be brought to a more correct understanding if he is given an explanation. This introduces the consideration of autonomy as 'informed consent'. The more extreme examples may raise psychiatric problems.

6. He may be subject to *undue pressure*, which may prevent his acceptance of information, or make him forget his conscience. This pressure may be imposed by those who seek to advise him; or it may be the emotional pressure inherent in a fatal, or painful, medical condition.

The scope for controversy is obvious. But I think one can state two *sufficient* conditions for the *rejection* of autonomy, which do have some meaning to them:

Principle II
A: *First condition for the rejection of autonomy.* Autonomy should *not* be respected if the individual's conscience is deeply perverted (situation 3) or absent (situation 4), or his perceptions are deeply disturbed (extreme examples of situations 5 or 6)—if there is consensus in society on this and on the underlying moral issues;

and there is no other way of achieving the desired end, which is agreed to be important.

B: *Second condition for the rejection of autonomy.*   Autonomy should *not* be respected if his expectations do not take due account of the welfare of others.

Consensus, I think, is here sufficient; that is to say, the overwhelming majority of the people can accept the decision, even if they do not really agree.

Principle IIA would, I think, be generally acceptable. I return to IIB, which is a form of the principle of justice, later.

The health worker's role is relatively clear in so far as her intrusions are restricted to situations which satisfy the first condition above, and in particular if the patient is a danger to himself or others. (The 'desired end' in these applications of Principle IIA is then the avoidance of the danger.) For example, psychopathic (situation 3) or psychotic (situations 5 or 6) individuals must sometimes be restrained, and in some cases the worker in mental health should explicitly seek to change the moral sensibility of the psychopathic patient (situation 3). The wishes of the patient who has 'lost his mind' will often legitimately be overruled (situation 4). I have given examples above. In these situations all would agree that the patient's wishes cannot be acted upon—though there is, of course, ambiguity over the border-line. I say that these judgements are clear and agreed, but nothing in morality is *universally* agreed: some people find difficulty in the idea of psychiatry seeking to mend the patient's moral sensibility (situation 3); and there are some who find difficulty in psychiatric constraint as such. I would urge the acceptance of Principle II into any theory of health care ethics.

The young child also is an example in situation 4, for by definition his moral sensibility is unformed. Thus the educator has a role in moral education: she seeks to help the child to establish moral understanding and sensibility. She will avoid deep controversy in so far as she guides her pupils towards moral principles that are clearly right and also subject to consensus. Likewise an education about life stances would not infringe the autonomy of either child or parent if it treats religious and naturalistic life stances in a way which is objective, fair and balanced. If these principles are followed, it is possible to give all children moral and life stance education in schools together, in a way which would be of value to all, and pressurize none. Principle IIA would be satisfied, and this example illustrates its significance in the general theory of collective morality. Principle IIB also is, of course, satisfied.

I will not pursue further the particular problems of psychiatry. I have referred to situations 3 and 4, and extreme examples of 5 and 6, where the patient (or pupil) may not be voluntary. More typically, psychiatry is conducted with a voluntary patient, so one can suppose that the treatment does not conflict with his wishes. The problems then are different—and include the question whether this supposition is legitimate. Situation 6 raises particular questions of principle for mental health workers.

In most circumstances society does not lightly reject the patient's conscience, as with the Jehovah's Witness refusal of blood. The attitude to a minor, however, is different: the doctor will give a transfusion to a Jehovah's Witness child even if the child objects to it. Here the child's autonomy is overridden because his conscience is unformed (situation 4); and perhaps one may say the child is under undue pressure (situation 6). These examples also exemplify Principle IIA. But further, the *parent's* autonomy also is rejected in this second case. This is a clear example of situation 2, his conscience being deemed unacceptable. The parent is not the patient; but normally society accepts the parent as speaking for a patient who is a minor. The rejection of the parent's authority here is an application of a very general principle of collective morality, that society assumes responsibility for a minor (or any other individual in situation 4) if his interests are seriously at risk. The definition of damage to the child extends widely, and includes failure of physical or moral nurture, or education, and is based on an interpretation of consensus which sometimes excludes those who share the contrary view. Thus the consensus on blood transfusion excludes Jehovah's Witnesses, and the consensus rejecting corporal punishment excludes those who accept it.

The 'Normal' Patient

Situation 2 raises really the most profound question: can society refuse the autonomy of the patient when he is neither deeply perverted nor deluded? My main concern in this chapter is situations where the patient is, as one might say, 'normal'; and yet there is conflict between his conscience or his view of his interests, and the conscience or values held by the health worker, or between either and significant sections of society. I cannot in this chapter look at the question of 'informed consent', which arises in situation 5, though it also involves autonomy. In situation 2 we meet disagreements between life stances, with the Jehovah's Witness as a simple example; more difficult ones will come later. Can society impose moral values on the patient, or authorize the health worker to impose moral values, where Principle II is *not* satisfied?

Here we have a major division between life stances. Some claim that their beliefs and values are, in their essential core, certain and secure: 'Others may be confused; God has given us the truth' or 'False consciousness is induced by capitalism; dialectical materialism gives the truth.' Or they may say simply 'Our claim is *obviously* right.' In either case it follows that, as they have the truth, therefore where the application is important their views should be imposed. What happens is all too often a matter of power. The Jehovah's Witnesses are not in a position of power; so they have only limited scope for maintaining their own autonomy in the health care situation, and none for imposing their moral theories on others.

Many religions, and also Marxism, when in a position of power often seek to enforce their moral theory. The Humanist position is very different. It fully accepts the reality of right and wrong, but it claims *as a matter of fundamental principle* that no-one has certain and secure knowledge on the fundamental questions of fact and value that determine moral issues. This follows from their rejection of revelation. It follows that Humanism accepts Principle I more fully than these other life stances; and it accepts the two parts of Principle II together as the only conditions under which intrusion is justified. Religious people may claim the right to go further, on the basis of their revelation (see the section entitled 'Beneficence and non-maleficence', p. 129).

It may be useful to introduce this discussion with a clear example from outside health care ethics, which illustrates the contrasting positions of different life stances: the life stance education of children (situation 4). Certain groups of Christians have sufficient power in Britain to have secured the enactment of legislation (the 1988 Education Reform Act) which those involved intended should not only establish the primacy of Christianity in 'religious education' but also exclude the recognition of the non-theistic life stances. As RE is normally the only place in the school where education about life stances is practised systematically, this exclusion from RE of the non-theistic gives authority to the religious life stances, and in effect indoctrinates with religion. Such a treatment of life stances does not satisfy Principle II, and Humanists reject it. They endorse one which does satisfy this Principle, as indicated above.

Metaphysical Questions

All moral theories are built on basic claims of value and of fact. Some of the factual claims, however, have a 'metaphysical' quality. I am here using the word *metaphysical* somewhat loosely, to refer to such claims as the reality of the soul, of God* and of the after-life; the rejection of a metaphysical claim is also metaphysical. The theory of health care ethics must come to terms with the range of contradictory metaphysical claims that are made by the different life stances.

It is a question of fact whether the soul, God and the after-life are real or not. Christianity claims they are; Humanism says no. No proofs on these matters are available in this life, but if Christianity is right then Humanism is wrong, and a Humanist will know this after he or she dies. On the other hand, of course, if the Humanist is right the Pope will never know he is wrong. We do not, now, *know* which is right; but the hypothetical statements which I have just made are *certainly* true. The different life stances stand or fall according to the truth or falsity of the claims they make: thus one or the other of Christianity and Humanism *may* be true; *one* is certainly false in its assumptions concerning the soul, God and the after-life. Where can we look to find understanding of the metaphysical assumptions, and the values, which should guide health care?

Science gives a context for the consideration of the metaphysical questions, and may help us towards an answer, but answers are beyond its power.

Questions of value are quite beyond the scope of science, by its definition. By definition it offers statements on questions of fact only; and it is widely accepted by philosophers that one cannot derive value judgements from factual statements—facts do not imply values. But certain facts do 'drive' evaluations,

---

* Like the word 'religion', 'God' is interpreted in many ways. Though it may be said that some ideas are meaningless, many are not, and these latter are the ones that matter. To claim a 'mythical' view of God (as for example Don Cupitt: *Taking leave of God*, London: SCM Press, 1980) is, for the purpose of health care ethics, a form of atheism; for it does not allow the strong conclusions which can be reached if a 'real' God is real.

for (on the one hand) if the facts go one way people feel driven intuitively to accept that they reveal something which is important; and (on the other) if the facts go other ways, these value judgements become incredible or absurd. For example: if God created us for his purposes, to be finally discharged in the after-life, then the shift from the present life to the next is both momentous and beyond our understanding; should we not submit to God in it? If the factual claims are true, then these value judgements would seem unavoidable. Or again: if the soul 'enters' the human body at conception, then one can hardly deny that the embryo is a human person from that time, and to kill it may indeed be murder. But if the factual claims are not true in each case, then the value judgements do not follow: if there is no God one cannot owe a duty to 'him'; and if there is no soul 'it' does not endow the embryo with personhood.

Abortion and voluntary euthanasia well illustrate these issues. They raise different questions, and I will consider one typical argument from each. I will first take the fundamental Roman Catholic argument against abortion. This is based on metaphysical premises which give a uniquely strong conclusion: there is an innocent third person whom we are threatening to kill, so such an act would be murder. Clearly this would justify overruling the autonomy of the patient. But if the embryo does not constitute a third person, it cannot be murder. What can society do in such a dispute as this? Is it ethically acceptable, or ethically obligatory, for society to prohibit abortion?

On the basis of one metaphysical theory the Roman Catholic sees abortion as murder. Against this, the Humanist considers that this metaphysical theory is absurd, on the basis of the known facts. Further, both the Humanist doctor and her patient may consider that the prohibition of abortion leads to consequences which are morally wrong: for example they may have the deepest conviction that it is profoundly wrong to bring a seriously deformed child into being. Is it right for society to impose a particular metaphysical theory, when the two individuals concerned consider the theory to be absurd, and to lead to immoral conclusions?

How can we develop our theory of health care ethics further? The religious believer may put forward the following principle:

Principle III
The absolute wrongness of murder. In a situation of uncertainty the wrongness of murder is such that society cannot authorize acts which risk it, whatever the alternative, unless the only alternative also involves death.

On this basis an impartial moralist may argue against the Humanist doctor and patient as follows. 'The Roman Catholic moral theory may be right; if it is, the act of abortion would be murder. Therefore, however much you protest, and reject the religious claim, and however much the patient suffers (short of death), the above principle requires society to impose the religious view upon you.' I consider here only those cases where the patient's life is not at risk.

But does Principle III extend to interpretations of 'murder' which rely on a metaphysical premise? Can a metaphysical claim have the *prima facie* plausibility which is necessary for it to be part of an acceptable theory of health care ethics?

I will argue that the answer to the latter question must be 'no'. Then Principle III must exclude metaphysical claims, and it cannot support the argument.

If one is trying to develop a theory of collective morality, one must test any general principles that may be proposed against a *range* of moral theories. Would the principle be acceptable if our society included a large contingent of people of the corresponding life stances, with their metaphysical presuppositions? The Roman Catholic claim that the embryo carries a soul must be set alongside, for example, the Jain claim that every living thing carries a soul. Jains claim that this soul should progress to humanity and finally to liberation or *nirvana*. Corresponding to their metaphysics, Jains make every effort to avoid killing any living thing. Should we, then, prohibit all killing? Why discriminate between Jains and Roman Catholics?

The point I am here considering is not objective right and wrong, but what morality allows a collectivity to impose on individuals. To kill an innocent person is certainly wrong; but the moralist developing a theory of collective morality can no more accept the Humanist theory that '[the Roman Catholic] theory is absurd, on the basis of the known facts' (as I put the claim above) than she can accept the Roman Catholic theory—or the Jain theory. I am arguing that *none* of these metaphyiscal theories is such as may be imposed on individual patients or health workers. By the same token, health care ethics cannot require a Roman Catholic doctor to perform an abortion at the request of a Humanist patient.

This conclusion, that metaphysical theories cannot be accepted into a theory of collective morality, like health care ethics, is reinforced by a legal maxim:

> 'The faithful must embrace their faith believing where they cannot prove; the court can act only on proof.'* The reference was to the efficacy of intercessionary prayer. The court concluded that it could not accept that the prayers of an enclosed order of nuns gave public benefit.

Another example which tells against the acceptability of Principle III, if it were interpreted to encompass metaphysical theories, is the currently accepted response to the claim that war is murder; collective morality as practised, and most Christians, pay no attention to the possibility that the pacifists are right. Principle III is ignored. Society goes no further than to allow the individual pacifist his conscience, by exempting him from military service; it does not even exempt him from military taxation.

Though (I have argued) metaphysical claims cannot play a part in health care ethics, other arguments may legitimate constraints on later abortions. For example, where the patient could have requested an abortion earlier one may argue that she should have done so: she has a duty to take reasonable responsibility for her actions. Or again, present scientific evidence allows that a fetus might have some degree of consciousness some time after about 24 weeks, and hence might feel pain: this is another example of a factual statement

---

* *Gilmour v. Coates* [1949] AC 426 *per* Lord Simmonds, at p. 446.

that may call for an evaluative response. I give these examples but cannot discuss them.

Voluntary euthanasia also is the object of both naturalistic and metaphysical arguments. Its moral quality is simpler because no-one claims that a third *natural* person is intimately involved. The metaphysical claims which would support its rejection are that the patient owes a duty to his God; and that his eternal life depends on it. It really does seem clear that collective morality *cannot* impose a duty to God on an unbeliever, health worker or patient; and it must allow each individual to look after his own soul. It is the province of particular life stances to include, or not, their own metaphysical arguments against voluntary euthanasia; but these are not relevant to collective morality. Collective morality can only take account of naturalistic–social arguments.

The Health Worker's Autonomy

The health worker has a general right to just consideration, and also a specific right to the protection of her autonomy, guaranteed by the qualification in Principle I: 'However, a health worker may decline to treat, or to continue treating, a particular patient.' In particular, she may decline to treat a patient when the treatment requested conflicts with her conscience. In fact, no responsible proponent of voluntary euthanasia or abortion, or any other medical procedure, claims for the patient the right to demand action from any particular health worker. They ask only for the *willing* doctor's *right* to observe the patient's autonomous desire. Thus the legality of these treatments makes no problem for the health worker's autonomy. It is the *prohibition* of voluntary euthanasia and abortion that is an infringement of her autonomy.

The immunity of a health worker is limited, however, in so far as a proposed treatment has consequences of great importance (for example to secure the life of the patient), and no other qualified person is available: she may be required to perform the treatment, even against her conscience. Thus a health worker who is a Jehovah's Witness will be expected to administer a life-saving blood transfusion if no-one else is available.

A health worker cannot be required to act against her conscience except in extreme circumstances. She may be required rather more frequently to provide information. If a medical procedure is forbidden then of course the health worker is not expected to provide information on 'back-street' opportunities. But if the procedure is permitted by the principles of health care ethics as they are generally accepted, then the health worker must give the information necessary for the patient to find a suitable practitioner. For example, if a patient comes to a Roman Catholic general practitioner asking for an abortion, the doctor may quite properly refuse. But if the patient then asks 'What can I do?' the doctor must give a full and fair answer—as she would if the patient asked for any other help beyond her professional competence. In both cases the health worker must pass the patient on to an appropriate specialist, with all due speed. It cannot be morally acceptable for the health worker to set herself up above the community so far as to refuse legitimate information. Unfortunately this rule is by no means universally respected in the matter of abortion in Britain.

A fitting coda to this section may be to note the difficulty of the health worker who is subjected to legal or professional constraints which conflict with her understanding of health care ethics. Many health workers have shown great courage in defence of the rights of patients, and been vindicated over the years by the reform of law and practice; others have defended false principles to the harm of their patients. It may be that some have done harm to their patient, as the patient defined it, but been morally right in so doing. It is not for me to adjudicate which historical cases fall under which description.

BENEFICENCE AND NON-MALEFICENCE

Everyone should sometimes seek to do good, and always try to avoid doing bad. This *is* morality; but such a statement as this is a 'platitude' not a 'principle'. Working out the demands of morality in real cases requires the two principles: respect for autonomy (with its restrictions), and justice. These do not give specific guidance, but they do point one in the directions where one should be looking. Each is necessary for health care ethics, and together they are sufficient.

In so far as a treatment affects only the patient, the principle of respect for autonomy gives the patient the right to decide what is best, subject to the restrictions the principle imposes. In so far as a treatment affects others, the treatment is governed by justice. There is no room for any other independent principle governing the choice of treatment. (Principles II and III above are subsidiary.) I wonder if the call for the two further principles 'do good' and 'do no harm' arises from the inner forces of a theory of morality which derives from metaphysical sources? On such a basis one can claim:

Claim X
The best interests of the patient. There are certain, critical, 'best interests', such that one should always act for the 'best interests' of an individual in this sense, regardless of what the individual himself sees as his 'best interests', and however otherwise 'normal' the individual may be, and however otherwise moral his request.

Anything that is against the patient's 'best interests' in this sense may be called an 'absolute harm'. If there were such 'best interests' and 'absolute harms', then the principles of respect for autonomy and justice would not be sufficient, and the principles of benevolence and non-malevolence would be required also. Accepting a patient's request to be helped painlessly to die might be an example of an 'absolute harm'.

Such a system of principles cannot stand by itself. A theory of morals which includes 'absolute harms' which the health worker must not commit is tenable only if it is restricted by the addition of criteria which allow exemptions, because sometimes in health care one cannot avoid choosing between two 'absolute harms'. For example, both mother and child may die in a difficult labour, unless the health worker intervenes to save the mother in such a way that the child will die. It would be unconscionable to forbid causing a death in such circumstances. The theory of double effect resolves this problem. It allows the health worker to act in such a way that will involve the 'absolute harm' of the fetus being killed, on condition that *her intention* is to preserve the life of the mother, not to kill the fetus. She is, of course, aware that both consequences will follow.

Real cases often require agonizing decisions, and no-one should try to pretend otherwise. But the supposed principles 'do good' and 'do no harm' have no *specific* consequences unless conjoined with the absolute claims of a metaphysically based morality. Their relevance evaporates when one accepts that metaphysical claims are not within the province of collective morality. I, of course, do not deny that such principles may hold in the true theory of individual morality. My claim is that such Absolute Goods and Absolute Harms cannot feature in health care ethics, because they come from metaphysical premises.

If one does not seek to impose absolute prohibitions and duties, one should simply exhort the health worker to do her best. Health care ethics does require one further principle, to govern the health worker:

Principle IV
The health worker's professionalism. The health worker should commit herself to her patient, with skill and with fairness.
(a) Her skill means that the treatment she adopts will minimize the harm and maximize the good; while her fairness means she will properly balance the patient's decisions and the needs of others, rejecting the former only if justice demands it, or the conditions of Principle II are satisfied.
(b) Her skill also means that she will give the patient all possible support, and in particular support in making his decision; while her fairness means that she will avoid improper intrusion on the patient's proper choices.

This statement also does not give the answer, but it points one where to look. Nothing more is required at this level of generality.

JUSTICE

'Justice' in health care ethics means 'distributive justice': that is to say, the distribution of benefits and harms between two or more people, or between an individual and the generalized good of society; and it becomes important in those situations where one cannot do all one would wish, for all the parties. The possibility of distributing benefits is usually limited. The reason for the limitation need not be a single resource in short supply, such as money; it may be an inherent contradiction between two quite different things, both of which one would wish to do. The mother and fetus of the last section illustrates this, and I make it the first example of this section.

As a second example, suppose a patient tests HIV positive and then makes it clear that he will carry on as before and not reveal his condition to his partner, who is a patient of the same doctor. Suppose he further instructs the doctor not to inform his partner, despite the doctor's moral arguments. The doctor will wish to preserve both confidentiality, and the life of the partner. But if she accepts the patient's demand she will be an element in the cause of the (probable) death of the partner; if she rejects it she will break confidentiality.

Morality is, of its essence, impartial between individuals; but it does not require that each action shall distribute 'good' equally to all. This would quite stultify action. In the end, most 'good' is done person-to-person, and cannot be spread out over many persons. Consider a third example: the provision of family planning facilities in developing countries. The health worker in the clinic is very partial in her attention to her client; I am impartial between many individuals in the developing world when I give my few pence to Marie Stopes International. We are both acting morally, but the impartial good I do is realized by the personal good done by another. There are different jobs to be done, at different 'levels': world, community, friends, family; and a person of good will may focus his or her effort on any of these levels, and act on more than one at different times.

Morality requires, however, that one shall at all times take account of the impact of one's current action both on wider groups, and on smaller groups and individuals. This does not mean that an act can never be moral if it benefits some individuals at the expense of causing injury to 'innocent others'. In some situations it is unavoidable that the best thing one can do involves as a consequence that some individual or individuals suffer harm—as in the first two examples of this section, and the fourth.

The requirement of impartiality operates differently in individual and in collective morality. The individual who is deliberating and acting has a unique role in individual morality, for individual morality applies to each individual separately. Collective morality, however, does not pick out a particular individual as its concern. All theories of individual morality that have any credibility put quite a stress on one's duties to others—much more than most individuals choose to admit! On the other hand, all also accept *in practice* that radical altruism is sometimes beyond the call of duty: the individual may be excused if he is somewhat selfish. But collective morality may have to take a more stringent view, because its reference is of necessity all the members of the collectivity.

A central problem in collective morality is the extent to which an individual with power and responsibility should condone, or enforce, selfishness; and to what extent she should disregard the wishes of the selfish individual and do the right thing. What does 'justice' require? The problem is an open one; in fact it seems to me that *all* life stances are in confusion on how to draw the line. However, I can see nothing in the essence of either religious or naturalistic life stances that drives the balance towards the limit where the selfish person is immune from restraint.

In the section entitled 'Respect for autonomy' I stressed the right of the patient himself to determine which outcome is in his best interests. But his decision may not be acted upon if it impinges seriously on other people. This restriction is essential, and it was set out explicitly in Principle I. I am now pursuing this situation, where the patient has the opportunity to call for action which could seriously prejudice the welfare of others. Where questions of justice are relevant, I argue for the duties of the health worker, and against the rights of the patient, because the health workers must also protect the autonomy of others.

The principle of respect for autonomy applies to all persons affected by a treatment, whether directly or indirectly, by commission or by omission. When it is impossible to secure the best interests of all those whose interests will be affected, the health worker is not oppressing one individual, but balancing the oppression of one individual against the oppression of another. She must be just between them. A collectivity should exercise restraint in the rules it imposes, based on recognition of the *prima facie* right to autonomy; but where the moral balance is clear, then collective morality demands action.

Where the consequences of giving treatment A to patient P can be traced to individuals, each should be allowed to make his own assessment of his 'best interests', so far as this is possible; and where the consequences cannot be traced to individuals, a generalized assessment must be made. The requirements of justice then adjudicate between the resultant contradictory demands.

The range of consequences to be taken into account is extensive, complex and subtle. My fourth example is a continuation of the second. One can argue that the two patients, the one with HIV and his partner, are not a sufficient basis for the ethical consideration of this case. For suppose the doctor tells the partner: by this act she would have undermined the rule of confidentiality. This rule is fundamental to the freedom which the patient feels in consulting the health worker, so that if it is lost some people might decline to seek medical aid, sometimes with killing effect. In other words, the alternatives before the doctor are not 'patient's confidence' and 'partner's (possible) death' but 'patient's confidence and the lives of many unknown patients of unknown doctors' and 'partner's (possible) death'. This example illustrates the important possibility that unless certain rules are maintained *without exceptions*, greater suffering may be feared. Here the beneficiary would be society in a very generalized sense.

How far should this go? What kinds of rule should be maintained so absolutely that identifiable individuals may be required to suffer for the preservation of the rule, and how much suffering should society expect? Conversely, how much selfishness should be condoned by the health worker? The principle of confidentiality is already broken for some notifiable diseases.

Is it necessary for the medical profession to pander to the selfishness of the patient when he demands that the health worker consider *only his* 'best interests'? Should it, perhaps, make clear that the individual's right to health care is conditional on his accepting his duty to recognize the rights of others to health care? Would such a recognition really make the public lose its trust in doctors?

Consider a fifth example: a society which offers free health care, and consider it at a point in its history when the rising scope of health care has led to demand for it which has become insupportable. I suggest that it is legitimate for the society to limit the resources made available for health care. But if so, it must also take the responsibility of defining the basis on which these resources are to be made available to individual patients. These collective decisions must, of course, be taken within the constraints of collective morality—whatever they may here be. Doctors must then apply these definitions; they cannot, morally, respond to the situation by the claim that their responsibility is to their current patient and him alone. They have, of course, the right of all citizens, and also the responsibility of specially informed citizens, to use proper democratic means to influence the community to give more money, or to spread the benefits differently.

The health worker has a unique commitment to the patient before her, in two respects. First, in the professional context she is committed to action, whereas in general she could choose to do something else. Second, as the health worker treating this patient, she is directing her attention to him. These requirements are stated in the two clauses in the first sentence of Principle IV. The moral necessity of such personalized action was illustrated in the third example above. But the necessity of person-to-person action does not imply that the health worker should consider only the best interests of the patient before her. If she claims that she acts as advocate for that individual, and therefore she cannot also act as judge, then she must accept that someone else must intervene in the clinical consultation to act as judge—which clearly is absurd.

The failure of many proponents of health care ethics to recognize that their subject is a particular development in collective morality, not an extension of individual morality, has led to a quite inadequate response by doctors to their social responsibilities, as these have recently become pressing. Everyone, doctors and the public alike, should recognize that the doctor is not acting solely as the agent of her particular patient, but also as the judge who balances the interests of all. Health care ethics cannot accept that a health worker should act as would her patient, if he applies a rather lenient and selfish individual morality.

ACKNOWLEDGEMENTS

I would like to express my enjoyment of Raanan Gillon's stimulating and perceptive book *Philosophical medical ethics* (Wiley, 1986), and my appreciation of the understanding I gained from it; and I would like also to record my indebtedness to Tom Beauchamp and James Childress's book *Principles of biomedical ethics* (Oxford University Press, 2nd edn, 1989).

12

The Four Principles of Health Care Ethics and Post-modernity: why a libertarian interpretation is unavoidable

H. Tristram Engelhardt Jr, PhD, MD

Professor, Department of Medicine, Baylor College of Medicine; Professor, Department of Philosophy, Rice University; Adjunct Research Fellow, the Institute of Religion; Member of the Center for Ethics, Medicine and Public Issues; Texas, USA

Kevin William Wildes SJ, MA, MDiv

Managing Editor of the Journal of Medicine and Philosophy, Texas, USA

INTRODUCTION: THE FOUR PRINCIPLES RECAST

Over the past 20 years health care ethics has become an established field of scholarship and an area of public debate. Interest has been spurred by developments in the biomedical sciences, the costs of health care, the difficulty of making moral decisions regarding novel issues, and the weakening of traditional moralities. The hope has been that health care ethics could provide, through philosophical reflection, content-full guidance to direct health care policy and give moral authority to health care choices. A prominent way of justifying moral judgements and recommendations in health care ethics has been by an appeal to the 'middle-level principles' of autonomy, beneficence, non-maleficence, and justice. This approach has been articulated most prominently in the work of Beauchamp and Childress (1) and has been widely deployed in many areas of controversy in biomedical ethics (2). The appeal to middle-level principles, at least in the Beauchamp and Childress model, attempts to circumvent the difficulties of deep theoretical disagreements. By invoking the principles the

Principles of Health Care Ethics. Edited by Raanan Gillon.
© 1994 John Wiley & Sons Ltd

expectation on the part of many is that normative moral judgements can be authoritatively justified and controversies resolved. The appeal to principles is in the service of a *modus vivendi*, a way of framing public policy in a morally pluralistic society. While the appeal to middle-level principles in order to justify rationally moral choices in health care ethics has become *au courant*, it has also been subjected to criticism (3).

This chapter provides a radical criticism of the four principles. It leads to their being recast in light of (a) the failure of philosophy to justify a particular content-full ethics, and (b) the persistence of a theoretically intractable secular moral pluralism. The criticism is from the perspective of the post-modern condition. The post-modern condition is, on the one hand, a sociological and cultural fact. 'The grand narrative has lost its credibility, regardless of what mode of unification it uses, regardless of whether it is a speculative narrative or a narrative of emancipation' (ref. 4, p. 32). On the other hand, the post-modern condition is the recognition of the fundamental limits of the modern moral philosophical project: there is no way to discover either a canonical content-full secular morality or the correct morally content-full solutions to secular moral controversies. As a consequence, individuals meet as moral strangers when they are not bound by the communality of a shared moral vision that binds moral friends. Moral strangers do not see the world in the same way. They do not possess common content-full moral premises so as to resolve concrete moral controversies or agree regarding the nature of true human flourishing. A consequence of this predicament is that a variety of libertarianism is morally unavoidable for peaceable secular pluralist societies. The moral pluralism of post-modernity leads both to recasting the meaning of libertarianism under such circumstances, as well as the significance of the four principles of health care ethics.

In the course of this chapter, a number of theoretical terms are introduced. One is the notion of a moral stranger. Moral strangers are individuals who do not share sufficient content-full moral premises in order to resolve content-full moral controversies by sound rational argument. Moral friends, on the other hand, are individuals who do share such premises in common. The same individuals can in different contexts be both moral friends and moral strangers. In this chapter a distinction is also drawn between the various content-full secular moral visions on the one hand and the canonical secular moral vision towards which modern moral philosophy has striven on the other. The second would be a moral vision that should be shared by all persons. This chapter concludes that there is a moral vision, or at least a moral perspective, that can be shared by moral strangers. However, that moral perspective is without content. Finally, a special sense of privacy emerges. A domain of activity is within a moral sphere of privacy if others cannot show in general secular terms that they have the moral authority to enter. In this regard both the moralities of Christians and secular egalitarians are privatized. The definition of these terms and the development of the arguments within which they are advanced have been undertaken at greater length in ref. 5.

This chapter provides by default a libertarian approach to health care policy and a libertarian understanding of the four principles of health care ethics. Its libertarian character is grounded in the failure of health care ethics to provide what it has promised. A libertarian understanding must be accepted because of the failure of the modern philosophical project to discover by rational reflection a content-full, canonical morality that can bind individuals outside of commitments to particular religious faiths or particular ideological understandings. This chapter will not argue for the virtues or usefulness of a libertarian health care policy. Instead, it will show why a libertarian public policy in the sense of one that acknowledges the fundamental limitations of the moral authority of secular governments is morally inescapable.

An examination of the failure of the modern moral philosophical project leads to recasting the four principles because of the inability to justify the content usually ascribed to, derived from, or presupposed to be in them. The principle of autonomy becomes the cardinal principle, now best understood as the principle of acting with the right and authority derived from permission. Authority must be derived from the consent of actual individuals, when all do not hear God in the same way and if reason cannot disclose a canonical, content-full morality. Against the failure of the modern philosophical project, the four principles are evacuated of content, not because this is desirable, but because of what is left in principle for men and women to share as a common fabric of secular morality. This chapter will in part be a criticism of the unwarranted over-optimism of contemporary health care ethics. There is no canonical, content-full, secular ethics for applied ethics to apply. It is not possible to employ middle-level principles as means of discovering content-full solutions to public policy controversies without covertly presupposing a canonical content-full secular ethics.

In anticipation of the arguments in the sections that follow, we offer here the four principles as they must be recast.

The Principle of Autonomy as the Principle of Permission

If one cannot discover content-fully what one ought to do, one can at least derive moral authority from the consent of those who collaborate in a project, whether this is as citizens of a secular state or as doctors and patients meeting in secular health care institutions. If one rejects the principle of autonomy so construed, and if all do not hear God in the same way, and if secular reason cannot deliver a content-full canonical moral guidance, then one cannot complain in generally defensible secular terms when visited with defensive or punitive force. On the other hand, those who accept the principle find a basis that can bind moral strangers, which basis does not presuppose a particular content-full moral vision, a prior ranking of liberty, or require that a special value be assigned to individuals or individualism. One has a straightforward answer to the question, by whose authority are you doing this? If one acts with permission, one acts with the authority of those who collaborate.

The Principle of Beneficence

Morality focuses not just on acting with moral authority, but on doing the good. Morality involves willing the good of others. But since there is no canonical, content-full account of the good outside of particular moral narratives, there must be an agreement on what will count as the good and regarding the correct ordering of goods. In particular, one will need to take account of how such goods as individual liberty and freedom must be weighed against other goods, so as to set limits on moral obligations to be beneficent to others. One will need to know how one ought to balance concerns of general altruism with concerns to have one's own good and the good of one's intimates flourish. It is within particular visions of human flourishing that one learns how to balance duties of beneficence to one's self and intimates with duties to others. Such concrete guidance can only be given within a particular moral vision. If a canonical, content-full secular moral vision cannot be discovered, it must be fashioned by mutual agreement, by permission of those who act together. In any concrete situation, when moral strangers meet, the principle of beneficence will depend on the principle of autonomy. The principle also highlights the difference between the best interests of others (and what will count as harms to others) as understood by them, and their best interests (and harms) as understood by third parties.

The Principle of Non-Maleficence

This principle stresses that one should not act in ways one understands on balance to be harmful, even if those involved consent to be harmed. This principle stresses that permission is necessary but not sufficient in order to show the moral appropriateness of an act.

The Principle of Justice

In his *Institutes*, Justinian (6) understands justice as 'the constant and perpetual wish to render every one his due' (5,I.1). But this understanding reveals a fundamental ambiguity. On the one hand, it requires giving each person that to which the person is entitled, in the sense that persons or their property should not be used without their permission, and that they should be made whole if they have been so used. The principle of justice is here dependent on a fundamental notion of acting rightly, which in secular contexts will in the end be reducible to considerations best understood in terms of the principle of autonomy. In this context the focus is primarily on retributive and restorative justice. On the other hand, the principle may identify the good of giving persons that to which they are entitled in virtue of a particular vision of the good or human flourishing. In this context issues can be reduced to concerns that fall under the principle of beneficence, and the problems that beset beneficence show themselves here in full embarrassment. There are as many theories of fairness and content-full understanding of distributive justice as there are major world religions.

THE BOND BETWEEN A SECULAR PLURALIST STATE AND LIBERALISM: LIBERTARIANISM REDEFINED

The liberal state of the modern era developed against the background of religious wars and persecutions. In many respects the liberal state is a response to the plurality of moral visions that emerged after the Renaissance through the Reformation. The hope was to bind together moral strangers, persons who possessed radically different views of what was of ultimate importance. The modern liberal state is largely neutral towards religious and moral commitments, out of a consideration of the usefulness of that policy, as well as due to diverse views regarding the policy's intrinsic desirability. This chapter leads to a justification of the state and a public morality in many respects similar to that which characterizes the moral neutrality of the liberal state. The justification, however, is not in terms of the usefulness or the intrinsic desirability of such an account of the state or view of public morality. It is instead derived from considering the only remaining possibility for justifying a moral vision that can compass moral strangers.

Within particular moral communities, within particular moral visions, individuals usually possess sufficient moral premises and commonly acknowledged moral authority such that moral disputes can be resolved by sound rational argument. The hope of the liberal state was that individuals separated by confessional and moral difference would find that they share enough as humans or persons so that sound moral arguments could lead to a common morality independent of, and transcending, the moralities of particular religious and moral communities. If sound rational argument could deliver content-full moral conclusions and establish the moral authority of particular political and social structures, then those who disagreed could be dismissed as irrational. Moreover, the conclusions would bind all persons, insofar as they were derived from premises reflecting moral rationality itself. The particularity of individual communities could be overcome and the liberal state would represent the morality of moral rationality. Individuals who seemed to be moral strangers would find that in fundamental philosophical terms they shared content-full moral premises and could resolve moral controversies by sound rational argument. In addition, when the state coercively constrained individuals to conform to morally rational policies, such coercion would not be alien to the true nature of the individuals subjected to its force, for they would be constrained to act in conformity with their rational selves.

Because this hope to establish rationally a content-full morality fails, there is no canonical content-full morality for the state to impose. The moral authority of the state is brought into question. The libertarianism endorsed by this chapter is thus the result of a moral catastrophe that marks the failure of the modern moral project to establish a content-full, canonical morality. On the other hand, the proposal in this chapter represents at least the partial success of the liberal modern moral project of providing justification for a state compassing moral strangers. It is just that the justification is limited, leading the state to have only limited moral authority.

The libertarianism that must be endorsed is thus not one embraced because of its consequences or because of its desirability. Because a canonical understanding of content-full moral activity cannot be justified in general secular terms, the state loses authority to forbid what individuals agree peaceably to do with themselves and consenting others. In addition, the limited authority conveyed to the state limits its capacity exhaustively to claim the energies, resources, and possessions of its citizens. For example, there is no canonical view of appropriate distributions of resources that can provide a secular substitute for a divine right of majorities or of overwhelming consensus. As a consequence, moral rights to privacy loom large and private resources and energy set limits to redistributional goals. In these circumstances the state may appropriately use force to protect the unconsenting from being used without their permission. It may record contracts and then enforce them. It may also, through established procedures, determine how to use commonly owned resources (bearing in mind that all resources will not be commonly owned). This may include the creation of refusable welfare rights, including rights to health care. But the state will lack the authority to limit the use of private resources so that the rich may purchase more food or health care than is provided through basic welfare entitlements.

There will still be grey areas. Where answers to unavoidable questions cannot be discovered they will need to be created with as much moral authority as possible; that is, with as much democratic participation as is feasible. But democratic authority will always be limited because consent, especially the consent to be governed, is limited. The right of individuals to act with consenting others and to use their private resources peaceably is not justified in terms of the consequences of this policy or in some particular view of human flourishing. Rights here mark the limit of the moral authority of large-scale states.

THE POST-MODERN CONDITION: WHY THE MODERN MORAL PHILOSOPHICAL PROJECT MUST FAIL, AND ITS IMPLICATIONS FOR HEALTH CARE ETHICS

A concrete moral vision allows one to judge what ought to be done in particular circumstances. It provides principles for moral guidance and for resolving moral controversies. It may even provide explicit principles such as the four principles. Within a concrete moral vision moral controversies can be resolved by sound rational argument because the disputants share sufficient common moral premises. These premises may include claims regarding the morally authoritative judgement of particular individuals. Roman Catholics, for example, hold that papal definitions *ex cathedra* on matters of faith and morals are infallible. A moral theological dispute can then in principle be resolved for Roman Catholics by the Pope of Rome speaking to a particular issue. Within the moral domain of Roman Catholic disputants the papal pronouncement is morally authoritative, just as finding a particular bacterium can be a clincher in a dispute among doctors as to the cause of a particular disease. A concrete moral vision can provide authoritative moral axioms. Within a concrete moral community defined by a moral vision, there tend to be moral authorities, who know the basic moral premises that frame the moral vision and how to apply that knowledge in particular disputes. There may as well be individuals who are recognized as having the moral authority to close debates by deciding what ought to be done.

Philosophical moral accounts advance claims regarding the overriding character of particular goods, interests, duties, or rights. Such accounts or theories have implications regarding the propriety of different trade-offs between concerns about freedom, equality, prosperity, and security. As with Roman Catholic moral reflection, secular moral reflections seek to establish particular individuals or groups as having moral authority. In particular, secular moral reflections attempt to provide accounts of the circumstances under which public policy and governmental action have moral authority. They attempt to account for the moral authority of constitutional conventions and democratic processes. The philosophical difficulty is to identify one among the many rival moral accounts as authoritative. The post-modern context is defined by the realization that this difficulty is insuperable. A particular, canonical, content-full, philosophical account of morality cannot be identified.

One cannot derive canonical, secular moral guidance or authority by turning to reason in the hope of discovering moral content. At the most, one finds particular logical constraints tied to different systems of preserving truth in reasoning. One cannot find an authoritative way to rank or compare competing human claims regarding human goods, obligations, or rights. To derive content-full conclusions, particular content-full premises must already be presumed. This, of course, is the difficulty. One is not able to find an uncontroversial starting-point. The elaboration of a particular theory or account of morality, justice, or political authority appears to be nothing more than the elaboration of one among many particular clusters of moral sentiments without the possibility of showing it to be the correct cluster. Nor can one turn outward to the world and discover moral facts in order to choose among different moral theories. One must already know the correct way of interpreting states of affairs morally in order to draw the correct conclusions from them. One must already know the answer one is seeking before one can find it.

This presupposition of a particular moral vision prior to the elaboration of a secular philosophical account of proper moral actions can be illustrated by reviewing the usual ways in which moral controversies are alleged to be soluble. Consider, for example, hypothetical choice theories. For the hypothetical choosers or contractors to choose in one way rather than another, the choosers or contractors must already be fitted with a particular moral sense, thin theory of the good, moral sensibility, or set of moral interests. If the hypothetical choosers or contractors are truly disinterested, they will not be able to make a choice between different rankings, for instance, of the goods of liberty, equality, prosperity, and security. If they are not truly disinterested, it is because one has already begged the question by fitting them with a particular thin theory of the good, moral sense, or moral vision. The same will be the case in terms of any appeal to moral rationality. In order for moral rationality to have concrete implications it must be a sense of moral rationality with a particular moral content.

The same difficulty besets consequentialist accounts. In order to compare the different consequences of different public policies one must be able, for example, to compare liberty, equality, security, and prosperity consequences. One must already know the proper relative moral weight of liberty considerations, equality considerations, prosperity considerations, and security considerations; which is to say that one must already have a concrete background moral vision in order to calculate the moral significance of different public policy choices. To compare pleasures and pains, or to hold that all pleasures and pains are equal, already presupposes a particular interpretative account of pleasures and pains. Moreover, an appeal to preferences will not solve the difficulty. One must already know how to compare present and future preferences, rationally considered versus impassioned preferences. One must know how one ought to discount time.

One might seek to avoid the problem of choosing the correct lexical ordering of goods or values by appealing to intuition, so as to balance the principles in different conflict situations. It is this method of intuitive balancing to which Beauchamp and Childress appeal. However, this approach again begs the central question: what intuitions or moral sense one ought to use in the process of balancing. An appeal to intuitive balancing will not resolve a conflict of moral principles unless those involved in the controversy share the same intuitions. In an attempt to remedy this difficulty, Henry Richardson has recently argued for an alternative to lexical ordering or intuitive balancing as a model of specification (7). Proponents of specification argue that, when norms are in conflict, the norms embraced by interlocutors can be specified and re-specified in debate so that the norms can come to cohere with one another, leading to the resolution of the controversy. The process of specification, so they contend, allows a flexibility not found in lexical ordering in that the way the norms are specified will change from case to case. It is also argued that specification has the advantage of being public and discursive, thus avoiding the privacy of intuitions. The insurmountable difficulty for this model is that the process of specification and re-specification will depend on a particular set of moral senses or of understandings of values and rights. Such a process will succeed only when moral strangers meet, insofar as there is a sufficient prior coincidence of moral senses. That is, the process will succeed only if the individuals are not really moral strangers. In particular, people may be unwilling to 'specify' or qualify the principles they hold, since they believe them to be absolute. One can easily imagine individuals absolutely committed to particular value hierarchies or understandings of rights, so that the resolution of moral controversies will not just be practically impossible, but impossible in principle.

Nor will it help to appeal to human nature, which as a biological phenomenon is the outcome of random mutations, varying selective pressures, genetic drift, the constraints of physical, chemical, and biological laws, as well as various catastrophes. Human nature is a biological fact, which must be placed within a moral vision in order to derive moral consequences from it. Moreover, a contemporary understanding of human nature suggests that it is pleomorphic and that people very likely have different diatheses towards being egoistic or altruistic, aggressive or pacific. Nor is it possible, outside of a value framework and other choices, to distinguish between successful versus unsuccessful adaptations. To be well adapted is, after all, to be well adapted within a particular environment with respect to particular goals. To determine which human traits should be favoured requires seeing human nature within a particular moral, metaphysical, or religious vision. The difficulty is to choose the correct vision. This, though, was the initial question at issue.

Secular moral philosophy is thus unable to select the canonical moral vision. Moral visions require and involve the choice of particular moral premises and particular moral commitments. This has profound implications for the use of the four principles of health care ethics. On the one hand, they can provide a general reminder about the kinds of considerations to which one ought to attend. On the other hand, they cannot disclose content-full solutions to content-full moral controversies. They may help sort out mistaken assumptions. They may lead individuals to convert to the moral vision of their interlocutor; but they will not help resolve real moral controversies that turn on real differences in views regarding the proper ranking of moral goods or the priority of competing moral duties and obligations. The principles are useful if they are placed within a context where they can actually provide guidance. They are, however, misguiding if they suggest that they can bridge the gulf between individuals separated by real differences in moral vision. The principles are likely to be misunderstood by those who do not recognize the full force of the post-modern predicament.

WHY THE FOUR PRINCIPLES MUST BE RECAST: MIDDLE-LEVEL PRINCIPLES PRESUPPOSE A CONTENT-FULL MORAL VISION

What appear to be the same words often identify quite different circumstances or things. Thus, the term 'mass' is substantially different in meaning, depending on whether it is understood within a Newtonian or Einsteinian framework. So, too, the term 'oxygen' means something different to us than it meant to Lavoisier. Terms are embedded in theoretical and value frameworks, which give to them their meaning. The same is the case for the elements of actions in the moral world. Thus, though the same term 'priest' can be used to identify a 'hiereus' in classical Athens (8), a 'kohen' in Orthodox Judaism, and a 'presbyter' in Orthodox Catholicism, the terms identify individuals performing profoundly different functions with radically different significance. One must be very careful to understand the context and significance of the request, 'please call a priest', or one will both disappoint and cause confusion.

So, too, there are ambiguities regarding the meaning of autonomy, beneficence, maleficence, and justice. Some, following Kant, may argue that the principle of autonomy requires one to choose as rational agents would choose, undetermined by heteronomous inclinations. Others will argue that one should respect an uncoerced choice made by a self-conscious rational agent, even if the choice is heteronomous in Kantian terms. The same difficulty besets appeals to beneficence. Is doing the good to be regarded as constrained by definitions of what is right? Or ought one to achieve the good whenever there is a general balance of benefits over harms. Here one must determine whether they are intrinsic evils which cannot be outbalanced by good outcomes. Similar questions will beset the principle of non-maleficence.

Similarly, the profound differences that underlie the various competing accounts of justice and fairness make impossible an appeal to the principle of justice in order to discover a content-full resolution of a moral controversy regarding fair action. Consider the different notions of justice that separate disputants, if one is a Rawlsian, and the other a Nozickian. On the one hand,

John Rawls (9) indicates that there are the following principles of justice for institutions.

> *First Principle*: each person is to have an equal right to the most extensive total system of equal basic liberties compatible with a similar system of liberty for all. *Second Principle*: social and economic inequalities are to be arranged so that they are both: (a) to the greatest benefit of the least advantaged, consistent with the just savings principle; and (b) attached to offices and positions open to all under conditions of fair equality of opportunity (p. 302).

Rawls provides an account of justice crucially driven by a particular thin theory of the good (p. 396). In contrast, Robert Nozick (10) provides an account of the justice of institutions that depends on using individuals, their energies, and their possessions only with their consent. 'From each as they choose, to each as they are chosen' (p. 160). Nozick's account does not incorporate or presuppose a theory of the good. As a consequence, when a Nozickian and a Rawlsian appeal to a principle of justice to resolve a controversy in health care ethics, they appeal to quite different principles. One has an ambiguity as deep as that involved in a contextless request, 'Call a priest'.

The point is that one cannot know in a content-full fashion what it is to appeal to a principle of justice or to call a priest unless one knows the moral context in which the appeal or call is made. Granted, each of these appeals is useful in the very general sense of calling attention to the need for certain moral considerations or some variety of religious help. There are certain family resemblances among considerations and theories of justice, as well as among notions of priesthood, even if they do not all share certain essential features. But if what is sought is someone to provide absolution and remission of sins at the point of death, it is very important that the correct priest is called. So, too, in order to have substantial help from an appeal to the principle of justice, the disputants must already share a common understanding of what it is to act justly.

The gulfs that loom between different meanings of justice and priesthood can be papered over by various forms of ecumenism, which identify certain social similarities and common historical influences. But for those who are serious believers the differences are decisive. Only the priest of the right kind blesses in the synagogue. It would be a profanation were a pagan priest to bless from the bema. So, too, partisans of a Rawlsian view of justice will not find a Nozickian answer acceptable, and a Nozickian will find a Rawlsian answer to be equally morally outrageous.

These difficulties can be illustrated by two examples drawn from health care ethics. First, consider the issue of whether patients should be allowed to purchase kidneys from individuals in the Third World. Opponents of such a policy will argue that these practices exploit the vulnerability of inhabitants in the developing world, taking advantage of their poverty. The purchase of organs can then be opposed by appeals to both the principles of beneficence and justice, if not in addition the principle of non-maleficence. On the other hand, proponents of the practice of purchasing organs will argue that those who forbid the sales are in fact exploiting the poor of the Third World to satisfy their own moral sentiments, which are not shared by many inhabitants of the developing world. One charge of exploitation will thus be met by a contrary charge. This contrary charge will be buttressed by appeals to the principles of beneficence, non-maleficence, and justice. There will be arguments that the transfer of funds from the developed world to the developing world will redound to the greatest good for the greatest number and will on balance be good, and that such a policy is in the long run most beneficent and just. The calculations of benefits will depend on different views of human dignity, responsibility, and freedom. Controversies will be irresolvable unless individuals come to share a common moral vision. The appeal to the principles of health care ethics may help define and sharpen the character of the conflict. But if the individuals possess different rankings of values and different understandings of exploitation, the appeal to principles cannot lead to resolving such controversies by disclosing hidden grounds for their resolution.

This point can be underscored by changing the case slightly to consider the issue of commercial surrogacy. Here, the controversy is often sharper, given the special moral values that traditionally cluster around sexuality. The sale of reproductive services will be considered by many to be analogous to the sale of sexual services, which in many secular, not to mention religious, contexts is considered an undignified and demeaning activity. In addition, within a number of secular as well as religious moral visions, the intrusion of a third individual into the process of child-bearing may be viewed on analogy with adultery. Such controversies will not be resolvable when the participants share divergent moral visions of human dignity or of the purposes of reproduction and sexuality.

In that there is no possibility in general secular terms of resolving the disputes regarding the moral probity of the sale of human organs or of commercial surrogacy, choices in this area fall by default beyond general secular moral authority. They become issues to be decided within the domain of moral privacy, not because this is good, but because no-one can in general secular terms show what the good choice is, or who has moral authority to intervene and why. By default, then, the appropriate secular moral position should be one of toleration: one of allowing the sale of organs and of commercial surrogacy, while also allowing partisans of various religious and particular secular moral visions to condemn such practices openly and vociferously.

Similar conclusions are equally unavoidable in the case of health care social welfare. Because there is no canonical secular content-full understanding of the good, and because there is no canonical secular understanding of distributive justice, health care welfare rights will need to be created out of common resources by democratic procedure. The correct pattern and character of health care welfare rights will not be discoverable by secular philosophical reflection. They must instead be created by democratic processes. But since the authority of democratic social institutions is limited, governments will consequently not own all the energies and resources of citizens. After a government has created a web of health care welfare rights, it will not have the moral authority to forbid the creation of private insurance systems through which individuals will be able to purchase health care not available through the governmental systems. That the rich may purchase more health care than the poor, that the rich in this circumstance will not be equal to the poor will be fortunate for the rich, unfortunate for the poor, but not unfair. That is, it will not be possible to show that such a circumstance violates a canonical secular understanding of distributive justice because such does not exist.

Appeals to the principles of health care ethics will not be able to resolve the content-full moral controversies. Depending on whether one ranks more highly liberty of choice or equality, one will morally endorse one policy over the other. Depending on which content-full principle of distributive justice one invokes, one will see different patterns of possession as constituting an unjust social institution or unjust social distribution of resources. It is because the principles of health care ethics cannot disclose the correct content-full moral vision that they cannot bring such real controversies to closure. Again, they can help sharpen the character of debates by revealing the stark divergence of actual views regarding autonomy, beneficence, non-maleficence, and justice. But since a correct vision cannot be disclosed, one is left with the need of tolerating that which one does not have the moral authority to change.

These cases underscore not just the limits of secular moral authority, but the ambiguities of autonomy, beneficence, non-maleficence, and justice. There is no canonical, content-full sense of autonomy. Autonomy can be understood as a choice that a self-conscious person affirms in the absence of external coercion, or autonomy can be understood as a choice that expresses the authentic nature or character of that agent. Beneficence and non-maleficence will be defined differently, given different understandings of benefits and harms. The differences will spring from different rankings of goods, which will include different rankings of liberty and free choice. Finally, as has already been noted, there is not one content-full understanding of distributive justice. Therefore, appeals to the principle of justice, if undertaken honestly, disclose the moral diversity and separation of interlocutors in real moral controversies. Beauchamp and Childress (1) in part recognize the difficulty by underscoring the historical embeddedness of content-full principles (p. 24). The difficulty is that there is not one content-full history of ethics. There are histories of ethics. In content-full debates, disputants stand within different moral visions, each with its own canonical history.

The principles of health care ethics do not escape the difficulties disclosed by post-modernity. It is not as if middle-level principles could disclose something shared by partisans of diverse moral visions. As a consequence of the deep differences in the ways in which the principles will be understood, depending on the moral vision and theory of those who use them, one must conclude that the four principles of health care ethics function not as (a) principles in the sense of sources of justification for particular actions or for grounds for resolving substantial moral controversies, but rather as (b) chapter headings under which one clusters together theoretically different philosophical considerations which, because of certain family resemblances, can usefully be placed under a particular rubric. Understood in this fashion, middle-level principles are middle-level not in a chain of justification or reflection between theories and actual judgements or choices. They are rather middle-level as mediating middlemen who bring together diverse philosophical considerations in a way that can help organize the analysis of health care controversies.

LIBERTARIAN DESPITE OURSELVES

The principles of health care ethics, properly understood, disclose the limits of secular moral reasoning, secular morality, and the secular moral authority of common endeavours. Because there is no canonical content-full secular moral vision that can be established in general secular rational terms, and because in such circumstances the secular moral authority of communal undertakings derives from actual individuals, secular morality has a libertarian cast. The failure of the modern philosophical project defines the post-modern condition, and conditions the moral authority of public policy in general and health care policy in particular. For general secular moral considerations the accent is unavoidably on free and informed consent, rights to privacy, private property, and limited democratic decision-making. In terms of the morality that can be justified in secular contexts to moral strangers, we must be libertarians in our public lives, despite our private moral convictions. Or to put the matter more precisely, insofar as one wishes to act in terms of a morality that can be justified in general secular terms, that morality will have an unavoidably libertarian character. Individuals will be at liberty to do with themselves what many, if not most, find to be morally improper. One fails to be able to justify the secular moral authority to set aside inequalities in health care distribution. Private tiers of health care become morally unavoidable. In all of this, appeal to the principles of health care ethics can be heuristic. Such appeals can help make differences clearer, and in so doing help disclose the limits of the secular morality that moral strangers can share. But such principles cannot set those differences aside. They cannot lead to discovering content-full resolutions of content-full moral disputes between moral strangers.

REFERENCES

1. Beauchamp, T. L. and Childress, J. F. 1989. *Principles of biomedical ethics*, 3rd edn. Oxford University Press, New York.
2. National Commission for the Protection of Human Subjects of Biomedical and Behavioral Research. 1978. *The Belmont Report: ethical principles and guidelines for the protection of human subjects of research*. US Government Printing Office, Washington, DC.
3. Clouser, K. D. and Gert, B. 1990. A critique of principlism. *Journal of Medicine and Philosophy* **15**: 219–236.
4. Lyotard, J.-F. 1984. *The postmodern condition* (trans. Bennington, G. and Massumi, B.). Manchester University Press, Manchester.
5. Engelhardt, H. T. Jr. 1990. *Bioethics and secular humanism: the search for a common morality*. Trinity Press International, Philadelphia, PA.
6. Justinianus, F. P. S. 1970. *The institutes of Justinian* (trans. Sandars, T. C.). Greenwood Press, Westport, CT.
7. Richardson, H. S. 1990. Specifying norms as a way to resolve concrete ethical problems. *Philosophy and Public Affairs* **14**: 279–310.
8. Beard, M. and North, J. (Eds). 1972. *Pagan priests*. Cornell University Press, Ithaca, NY, especially pp. 73–91.
9. Rawls, J. 1972. *A theory of justice*. Belknap Press, Cambridge, MA.
10. Nozick, R. 1974. *Anarchy, state, and utopia*. Basic Books, New York.

13

Utilitarianism and Deontological Principles

RICHARD M. HARE, FBA

Graduate Research Professor of Philosophy, University of Florida, USA;
White's Professor of Moral Philosophy Emeritus, University of Oxford, UK

As well as being a general introduction to medical ethics this volume as a whole is dedicated to the exposition, defence and application of the four principles of medical ethics of which Dr Gillon, following Professors Beauchamp and Childress, has been an advocate. These have been given names, but need to be spelt out as clear prescriptions, in universal terms, for action—that is, in the form of universal imperative or moral sentences. Their names are: 'autonomy', 'benefi-cence', 'non-maleficence' and 'justice'. It is appropriate that the book should contain a chapter relating the four principles to utilitarianism, which is one of the chief traditions in ethics, often contrasted with deontology. But this presents a difficulty for anyone like me who, even if he recognizes (as I do) that deontological principles have a part to play in moral thinking, does not think that the four principles are necessarily the only ones to be considered, nor that they can, without reducing them to vacuity, be so stretched that they cover everything that a doctor ought to consider his duty. I therefore asked to be allowed to change my title from the original one given me, which was 'Utilitarianism and the Four Principles'. This however is not a big difficulty, because what I have to say about deontological principles in general will cover the four principles in particular, which is what I was asked to do.

There is another difficulty to be got over at the start. Many people think that utilitarianism is in some way *opposed* to deontological principles. This is not so. A properly formulated utilitarianism can find a place for such principles in our thinking. The name 'utilitarianism' covers a wide spectrum of theories, some of them fairly easily demolished, and philosophers who claim to have demolished one or two of them often think that they can throw out the lot as not worth further consideration. I shall therefore confine myself to the utilitarian theory which I have myself advocated (1) and which, I hope, survives such attempts at demolition. A utilitarian of my sort can speak with confidence about rights and

---

duties, which are what deontological principles lay down. I could probably agree with nearly all that deontologists say about rights and duties, if they were able to satisfy three conditions for thinking rationally about them. I do not think that deontologists are able in fact to satisfy these conditions; but a carefully formulated utilitarianism can satisfy them. So it is not a question of me trying to stop people talking about rights and duties. It is a question, rather, of showing how we can talk about them in a way that we can defend in argument.

The three conditions are these:

1. We have to have a way of deciding rationally *what* rights we ought to respect and *what* duties we ought to observe (that is, *what are* people's rights and duties).
2. We have to have a way, when two or more of these duties or rights are in conflict in a particular case, as they often are, of deciding rationally which of them ought to prevail (that is, to determine what we ought to do in that case).
3. We are owed an account of how moral thinking of both these kinds fits into a coherent logical structure of moral thinking, such that we are able to tell whether the thinking has been well or ill done. It must not be the case that, in moral thinking, anything goes.

It does not seem to me that typical modern deontologists have satisfied in a convincing way any of these conditions. All they do is to appeal to our intuitions, which is the term philosophers of this stamp use for opinions about moral questions about which we are very sure. We might call them 'our moral convictions'. Sometimes we meet somebody who does not share these convictions, and *he* will call them 'prejudices'. The trouble with deontologists is that they leave us defenceless against this attack. To defend our convictions, we should have to produce arguments for them. It will not do just to go on insisting that we, and others of our way of thinking, feel very strongly that they are right. But arguments are just what deontologists are usually unable to provide. They rely on an appeal to convictions; but if it is the convictions themselves that are being questioned, of what use is that?

On the other hand, I think that someone like me, a utilitarian of a sort, and therefore not in the ordinary sense a deontologist, *can* provide arguments to show why we ought to have the convictions that most of us have, and how to tell whether we ought to abandon any of them, and what to do when they conflict. I cannot here do very much to explain how my account of moral thinking works (see ref. 1). I can give only a very rough sketch, and shall not have room to answer all the objections that have been raised to my account, though they can be answered.

I can best explain the account of moral thinking that I am advocating by taking a particular example of a real moral dilemma. I have chosen one which has actually occurred, and which shares features with many other real-life examples. This is the case of Dr Arthur, whose trial and acquittal in Leicester Crown Court on the charge of murder (later changed to attempted murder) of a neonate in July 1980 was extensively reported in the press. Briefly, the facts were these. The baby was born with Down's syndrome and the parents were very distressed and rejected the baby. Dr Arthur then made a note: 'Parents do not wish it to survive. Nursing care only'. He prescribed dihydrocodeine (DF 118), a morphine-type drug, to be given orally in 5 mg doses, to alleviate distress as and when it arose, not more than every four hours. Sixty-nine hours later the baby died. The cause of death was given as 'bronchopneumonia due to consequences of Down's syndrome' (2). The baby's weight at death was similar to that at birth. It was established in the trial that the baby had other defects which could have led to pneumonia, although when he made his note Dr Arthur did not know this. This was why the charge was altered to attempted murder. It seems that his intention was that the baby should die from lack of either food or drugs, water only being given, but that distress should be avoided by means of the dihydrocodeine and the other nursing care.

There has been much discussion of this case in the literature (3–6). A number of senior and distinguished medical colleagues testified in court on Dr Arthur's behalf, and it appears from their evidence that his treatment of the baby did not deviate from standard practice in the profession. But considerable doubt has been cast on whether this standard practice is in accordance with the law; and the result of the case did almost nothing to determine this legal question. The reason was that the facts of the case made available to Dr Arthur a number of different defences, and it is impossible to know which of them convinced the jury. Nor did the judge do enough to clarify the law.

I shall therefore not go any further into the details of this particular case, but discuss in general terms what we ought to say about such cases, what deontological principles can be applied, and how to resolve conflicts between them. The main problem concerns *who* are to be the parties whose interests, etc., are to be taken into account in applying the principles. Whose autonomy has to be respected? To whom should a doctor be beneficent and non-maleficent? And between whom has he to do justice? The narrowest answer to this question limits the parties, to whom these duties are owed, to the doctor's patients. Wider answers extend them to cover the patient's parents or next of kin, and the immediate family. But wider extensions still of the principles will allow the interests and preferences of the doctors and nurses concerned to be considered, and, even wider, those of the whole of society. All these parties do have preferences which a principle of autonomy could respect, and interests which a doctor could handle beneficently, non-maleficently and justly. Unless the four principles tell us how to limit the scope of their application, they will not settle many questions in medical ethics.

One possible view is that a doctor's prime duty is to his patient, and that others, if considered at all, should have a much lower priority. This is a principle which many would add to the four principles in order to get determinate answers. It too needs justification, and can be given one by utilitarians, but not easily, so far as I can see, by deontologists. The utilitarian justification for this principle is that unless doctors follow it, their practice of their profession will not be very successful. Unless patients can rely on the almost whole-hearted devotion of their own doctors, they will not be looked after as they should be. But we might wish to make qualifications to this principle. There are cases where the interests of some other party than the patient are so strong that they should be served even at some cost to the patient. For example, if an airline pilot has epilepsy, it might be the doctor's duty to reveal this to his airline. The patient might suffer, but fewer people might die in crashes.

On the case under discussion, are there any such interests outside those of the patient? Obviously there are. The parents, as was evident, did not want to have to bring up a child with Down's syndrome. If they rejected the child, then, in default of adoption, which was unlikely, the child would have had to be looked after in an institution, probably at cost to the taxpayer. The health service would probably have incurred additional costs, which would have resulted in other patients getting less care. We do not take these costs into account when thinking about normal babies; but they are considerable, and in the case of severely defective neonates it needs at least to be asked whether *their* interest in survival is so great as to outweigh the other costs. In the extreme case it may not even be in the interest of the neonate to survive, if the quality of his life would be very low. Though this was probably not true of the baby in Dr Arthur's case, there are many in which it is.

A helpful way of looking at this question is to ask about the interests of a class of people that we have not yet considered. This is the class of the people who will be born if, but only if, this baby is allowed to die. These include, obviously, any further children that these parents will have if they do not have to look after this one. I have always found it surprising that in discussions of the treatment of defective neonates the interests of these possible future children are usually ignored. This may be because of a mistaken idea that people who do not yet exist cannot have interests. This mistaken idea might be dispelled if we considered the situation which would obtain if these future children *were* born. We could then ask one of them, 'Was it in your interest that the earlier defective neonate was allowed to die, this being a necessary condition for your being born?' He (or she) would surely, if leading a normal and happy life, answer 'Yes', and we should accept this answer. So if he can truly say that it *was* in his interest, then at the time when the decision had to be taken whether to preserve the life of the defective neonate, they could truly have said 'It is in his interest.'

A full consideration of the duties of the doctor and parents in cases like Dr Arthur's would therefore demand that we take into account the interests of these possible future children, at least those that could be born to these parents. My argument does not imply that the parents have a duty to have more and more children indefinitely. If they did that, the time would come when they could not support any further children, and those that were born would not have happy lives, and might even think that it was *not* in their interest to have been born. The argument only implies that parents should have children up to the limits of a proper family planning or, on the larger scale, population policy, a policy that has to be argued for on other grounds.

Reverting then to the four principles: we cannot fully understand their status until we have done justice to the complexity of the activity that we call moral (or ethical) reasoning. It is not a simple matter. In particular, we have to distinguish between the thinking that we do when we are confronted with a particular case (often in difficult and stressful circumstances, and without as much information as we need about the medical and other facts and possibilities) and the thinking that we can and ought to do when we are not under stress, about the general principles which ought to guide us in such situations. To questions about the second of these kinds of thinking a Kantian and a utilitarian, if they are true to their theories, will give substantially the same answer. The general principles that ought to guide us are those whose general adoption will be likely to do the best to serve the interests, or promote the ends, of all those affected by our actions. At this level of thinking we are not confronting particular cases, but seeking general guidance.

Because the principles we adopt will have to be to some degree simple and general, there will arise particular cases where they come into conflict; and then we shall have to think again about the particular case. But it would be wrong to say, as advocates of situation ethics do, that therefore we ought not to have any general principles. Edmund Burke ironically called these general principles 'prejudices', and of these he said, 'Prejudice is of ready application in the emergency; it previously engages the mind in a steady course of wisdom and virtue, and does not leave the man hesitating in the moment of decision, sceptical, puzzled and unresolved. Prejudice renders a man's virtue his habit, and not a series of unconnected acts. Through just prejudice, his duty becomes a part of his nature' (7).

Doctors therefore should seek to develop in themselves what Burke calls 'just prejudices'. And that means that they have to have a way of deciding what prejudices *are* just. It would not do if what had become part of their nature were not their duty, but only what they wrongly thought to be their duty. That, I am convinced, is the situation of doctors who think that their absolute duty is at all costs to preserve life, even when life is not in the interests of their patient. And it became evident in the Arthur case that many distinguished medical people, no doubt after careful thought, had abandoned the simple absolute principle that life should be preserved at all costs. Rather, it seems to have become accepted in the profession that there are exceptions to this principle, and that they include cases like Dr Arthur's. But the thought which went to the abandonment of the simple absolute principle, and the substitution of a more qualified one, had not been made articulate. It needs to be, so that in future doctors may have clearer guidance. And no doubt the law will follow suit, as it usually does in the end.

The four principles to which this book is devoted are best thought of as, in Burke's (7) sense, prejudices (I think just ones). We have to ask, then, first of all what makes them just; secondly, whether these four are the only prejudices that doctors ought to have; and thirdly, what to do when they give conflicting answers. Let us begin with autonomy. Why is it a good principle to respect the autonomy of patients? There are two good reasons, both of them available to a utilitarian. The first is that on the whole people prefer to make decisions affecting their own future. In the great majority of cases, patients do not like doctors to decide on their treatment without keeping them in the picture and respecting their wishes. We may call this the *direct* value of autonomy. It must be admitted, though, that there are exceptions. Sometimes patients *want* their doctors to do the deciding—whether because they trust the wisdom of the doctor more than their own, or because the whole process of decision-making is too anxious and stressful. This preference too should be respected.

The other reason is that on the whole people are the best judges of what will be best for them in the future. They are likely to predict more correctly than any doctor what will be best for *themselves*. For people's ideas of what is a good life vary enormously, and doctors are, these days, seldom in a position to know a patient well enough to predict them. The doctor can usually predict better than the patient what the consequences of a particular treatment will be; but he is no expert on how the patient will like these consequences. Therefore, in deciding on a treatment, the doctor should be guided by the patient's idea of the best life, and not impose his own. There are exceptions to this too. In some cases patients may be quite unable to form clear preferences about their own future. They may prefer to hand over to the doctor, if they think him wise, the decision as to what is best for them. As before, this preference also should be respected. And of course the fact that the doctor is better able than the patient to predict the consequences of alternative treatments may add to the patient's confidence in the doctor's choice of treatment. If the relationship between doctor and patient is good, they will make the decision together, each contributing the knowledge that he has, and the question of autonomy will not arise.

We see, then, that the principle of autonomy can be given a utilitarian justification, and so can the exceptions to it. Spelt out, it will run something like this: a doctor ought always, having informed the patient as fully as he can of the consequences of alternative treatments, to respect the preferences of the patient in choosing between them; but if the patient prefers that the doctor decide, this preference too should be respected. Additional exceptions will have to be made to deal with cases of incompetent patients, such as children, the mentally disturbed, and the unconscious. In such cases a doctor may have no option but to decide what will be for the best for the patient, sharing this decision with the patient's family as proxies. The adoption of this principle has, as we have seen, an obvious utilitarian justification.

The second and third principles, beneficence and non-maleficence, can be taken together. Indeed, both in theory and in their application, it is rather hard to draw the line between them. To deprive someone of a benefit is, at least in the most natural senses of the words, a harm. But although we shall be able easily to give these principles a utilitarian justification, we must be careful not to confuse them with the principle of utility itself, which is a feature of many utilitarian theories, though not of my own. My own theory contains, not a principle of utility, such as that we ought always to maximize preference-satisfaction, but rather a method for either choosing particular principles, or dealing with individual cases. It says that in making these choices one should imagine oneself in the places of all those affected, and treat them on a par with oneself, as if one were going to be in their situations. This method will give results similar to a principle of utility, and the difference between it and commoner forms of utilitarianism is not important for our present purposes.

If, when choosing general principles for the guidance of doctors, we are trying to adopt those whose general adoption will be for the best for all, treated as if we were they, it is obvious that we shall include in the list principles of beneficence and non-maleficence. For obedience to those principles is likely on the whole to be for the best for all. But only on the whole, and not in every case. As we have seen, there is at least one other principle, the principle of autonomy, which can seem to conflict sometimes with beneficence or non-maleficence, but whose general adoption would be recommended by a clear-headed utilitarian. The same applies, as we shall see, to the fourth principle, that of justice. There are cases in which a direct application of the principle of beneficence might lead a doctor to try to do good to a patient against the patient's will, thus infringing the principle of autonomy. He (or she) will be restrained from this, not by the principle of beneficence, but by a much more general consideration, reaching right back into the roots of morality itself. He will reflect, if he is wise, that if autonomy comes to be disregarded, much harm will ensue both for the profession as a whole and for individual patients. This is a principle to be held to tenaciously for fear of impairing the whole relationship between doctors and the public.

So, paradoxically, he may think that the bad consequences of being beneficent on a particular occasion outweigh the good aimed at for the individual patient. The four principles, being general guidelines which can conflict with one another, have in such cases of conflict to be balanced against one another, and beneficence may lose out and be overridden. But the correct method of moral thinking, relying on putting oneself in other people's places and acting for the best for them, is not overridden; indeed, it is just this method which leads us to override the principle of beneficence, because if we thought only of beneficence we should end up doing more harm than good. Beneficence and non-maleficence are principles which have always to be considered, but which can on occasion conflict with other principles which we ought not to disregard; and then there is a problem of deciding between the principles. This problem has to be solved by ascending to a higher level of thinking than that of the four principles, and using the method I have outlined.

If we try to spell out these two principles, we shall see that there are more difficulties, already hinted at. Does the principle of beneficence say that a doctor ought to aim at the good of *his patient*? Or of his patient and the patient's family? Or of all those affected, extending to society as a whole? And similar problems arise for non-maleficence. It is necessary for doctors to find for themselves guidelines which tell them whose interests should be considered in what kinds of cases. Those who have homicidal maniacs or airline pilots as patients may think that beneficence to *them* ought to be tempered by non-maleficence to the public. And even in more humdrum cases a doctor might think he was offending against the principle of justice, to which we shall come in a moment, if he wangled a supply of a scarce drug for his mildly ill patient, so depriving other doctors' patients, who were more seriously ill, of the drug. Such conflicts between the four principles make it imperative to have a method of deciding between them in particular cases, and this the utilitarian, unlike most deontologists, can provide. He does this by seeking to do the best, all in all, for all those affected.

Lastly, justice. The utilitarian reason for giving great weight to a principle of justice is that enormous good comes of observing such a principle, and enormous harm from disregarding it. No society can be happy unless there is justice between its members. In the context of the health service this is obvious. A society in which everybody can get a decent level of health care is almost bound to be happier than one in which an underclass is deprived of it. Justice has enormous utility, and that is the justification of the fourth principle.

But the principle of justice needs, even more than the others, to be spelt out; and there are a great many different ways of spelling it out. In its simplest, formal expression it operates at a higher level than that of the distribution of health care. The utilitarian method for choosing guiding principles is itself an embodiment of justice in this formal sense of the word. Jeremy Bentham, the great utilitarian (1748–1832), had a maxim 'Everybody to count for one, nobody for more than one'. This is to be formally just between all the parties affected. It enjoins a moral thinker to love his neighbour as himself, and to do to others what he wishes to be done to himself if he were in their situations. The Golden Rule is, properly understood, the foundation of morality.

But when we come to more substantial principles of justice, especially justice in distribution, which are what most concern doctors, there is a bewildering variety to choose from. It is possible, even, that different principles of justice are appropriate for different societies. This is not to advocate relativism in any but a harmless sense; for even the most objectivist of moral philosophers must agree that the best principles of justice may vary with the circumstances in which they are to be applied. Some principles will be more egalitarian than others. The benefits of just arrangements in society depend in large measure on their acceptance as just by the members of the society; so if the members of one society think their arrangements unjust, the benefits will not be realized, as they might be in another society that accepted them as just. This is too large a question to be dealt with in a short article (see ref. 1, Chapter 9 and References).

So then we have these four principles. I have shown that they are not by themselves enough to determine the duties of doctors. We need at least to have a principle which tells us *whose* autonomy we have to respect, to *whom* we have to be beneficent and non-maleficent, and between *whom* we have to be just. And we need a level of thinking at which we can formulate and select principles for the guidance of doctors—not only these principles but possibly others. For example, it is not clear that a duty to tell the truth to patients (a duty about which there has been a great deal of dispute) can be subsumed under any of the four principles. So, although all of the four principles are important and can be justified, they are only general guidelines. In deciding on them and on their precise formulation, as well as in adjudicating between them when they conflict, doctors and medical authorities will have to do more and higher-level thinking than the mere unquestioning and mechanical application of the principles.

REFERENCES

1. Hare, R. M. 1981. *Moral thinking*. Oxford University Press, Oxford.
2. Brahams, D. 1981. Medicine and the Law. *Lancet*, 14 November.
3. Brahams, D., Brahams, M., Ferguson, P. and Havard, J. 1983. 'Symposium' on the Arthur case. *Journal of Medical Ethics* 9: 12–20.

4. Kuhse, H. 1984. A modern myth: that letting die is not the intentional causation of death. *Journal of Applied Philosophy* **1**: 21–38.

5. Gormally, J. 1982. Note: Regina v. Arthur. Pp. 85–88, *in Euthanasia and clinical practice.* Linacre Centre, London.

6. Gillon, R. 1985. *Philosophical medical ethics.* Wiley, Chichester, pp. 2–7, 174–183.

7. Burke, E. 1815. *Reflections on the revolution in France,* Vol. 5, p. 168: as cited in ref. 1, p. 45.

14

Medical Ethics, Kant and Mortality

S. H. FURNESS, BA, PHD

The Former Vicarage, Whissendine, Oakham, Rutland, UK

INTRODUCTION

A frequent picture of Kantian ethics is of empty and formal rules (1) which are of little use in making decisions. If reference is made to the Kantian theory of knowledge then Kantian ethics may look even more unpromising, with unknowable agents performing atemporal acts (2). I offer an alternative which avoids these problems. It is based upon Kantian insights and connects Kantian ethics to the theory of knowing. My aim has been to see how useful Kantian ethics can be to medicine if Kant's professed intentions of providing a Copernican revolution in thinking are taken very seriously and applied to ethics. The result is 'Kantian' in inspiration but is not a detailed textual Kantian exegesis.

Uncontroversially, I take respect for autonomy as central for any account of Kantian ethics. This may not appear a fortuitous starting point for medical ethics because patients' autonomy is often impaired, but thinking in terms of an ideal autonomy is mistaken. If Kant is understood in a non-Cartesian way, through the Copernican revolution, and finite mortal human autonomy is taken into account, then respect for autonomy has much to offer medical practice.

Respect for autonomy can be shown to generate the other principles of health care ethics. From this Kantian horizon ethical principles should guide all that is done, whether by individuals or collectives, committees or governments.

AUTONOMY AND ETHICAL OBLIGATION

Explanation of why we *should* act in certain ways is not provided by observation that we do. If moral principles are to have obligatory power they must be more than cultural or context-related norms. Just as a doctor will achieve little progress in treating a disease if she deals with the disparate symptoms without understanding the pathogenesis, so we must understand *why* we should hold moral principles.

Principles of Health Care Ethics. Edited by Raanan Gillon.

The 'pathogenesis' of the four principles in this Kantian-inspired paper is our capacity for self-conscious activity, which is the basis of all knowing and therefore must be respected. There is no reason why this respect should be limited to one's self; respect must be extended to all others. From respect for autonomy we can generate the other principles of health care ethics.

Kantian ethics centre upon autonomy. For the Kantian humankind's capacities to form intentions and act upon them, rather than unreflectively reacting to circumstances, is what distinguishes us fundamentally from machines and some (perhaps all) animals. For example a doctor's job is considered of ethical importance, unlike a garage mechanic's. While a vet may have ethical duties to avoid unnecessary pain she may also behave in ways which are quite unacceptable in human medicine. ('Putting down' animals which are no longer wanted, or that behave aggressively, is acceptable practice in veterinary medicine, for example.) Neither a garage mechanic nor a vet can seek the consent of their 'patients'. Why should the practice of human medicine be so different—or should it?

Much medical ethical thinking does not account for what makes human welfare of particular ethical importance; it simply assumes that it is. Justification in terms of 'humanity' may miss the point and fall foul of a type of 'speciesism'. It is not humanity as such which makes our welfare of importance—we can imagine other species and types of being who are not human, yet require ethical consideration and respect. It is humanity's self-conscious capacities to act, which could be shared by other types of being, which can account for the difference. Human beings are fundamentally self-conscious beings that can make and act upon decisions, and direct and reflect upon their lives.

RESPECT FOR AUTONOMY IN MEDICAL EXPERIENCE

If Kant's emphasis upon autonomy allows us to make a fundamental distinction between the practice of medicine, and the practice of veterinary medicine or the 'art' of car maintenance, it may at the same time appear to undercut the distinction through its apparent incongruence with medical experience. The central place given to autonomy in Kantian ethics makes it apparently unsuited for, or possibly antagonistic to, medical situations in which patients often, indeed more usually, have impaired autonomy. Patients routinely do not know as much about their medical condition as their doctors do. If patients are to exercise autonomy when making decisions about treatment they will require sympathetic explanations which they can understand. More seriously for the Kantian position, many patients will have impaired autonomy. The dementing, the frightened and confused and the very young do not have full autonomy. To treat them as if they do may at best fail to respect what autonomy they have, and at worst may be life-threatening. To treat a very young child or a demented adult as if they were fully autonomous may be to leave them to suffer and starve. For example, to say to a dementing elderly patient 'Go home take this medication three times a day, keep warm and well fed and come back in three days if you don't feel better' could be life-threatening to someone with variable capacities for independence and whose grasp of time and number is insecure.

Yet it may be perfectly appropriate to a young adult with the very same condition; a throat infection, for example.

If Kantian autonomy is taken seriously it might seem that it can only be applicable to the most knowledgeable, fittest and least worried or intimidated of patients. Kantian ethics would then seem incapable of addressing many— perhaps most—medical situations. When we are ill we are usually frightened and we are often intimidated by the greater knowledge and perhaps the social position of the doctor dealing with us. We are not usually in a position to make confident and reflective decisions without help. If respect for autonomy is taken as respect for an ideally autonomous agent, we may well fail to respect the actual autonomy of actual agents (3).

This would be a serious blow for a Kantian position if it were not for the fact that Kant repeatedly stresses that his ethical theories are not for 'holy wills', but are for finite human beings. Kantian knowing is perspectival and limited. We do not even necessarily have insight into a full picture of our own motivations, let alone know what is best for others. The applications for medical situations open when autonomy is put in the context of finitude; that forms, at least, the necessary limits of any human knowing. Kantian ethics may be more successful and have more to offer the practice of medicine if related to the fundamental Kantian move which informs the whole Kantian philosophy—the Copernican revolution.

THE COPERNICAN REVOLUTION

Kant presents the Copernican revolution in the context of his exploration into a new way of thinking about knowing. Explanation of what we know, the objects of the world, apart from our knowing of them, has been a traditional problem for philosophers. How is it that we know the world? This is particularly difficult if we carry assumptions about the self as an indivisible spirit essentially distinct from matter. Descartes put forward just such a theory, and painted a picture in which what we know first and most easily is the self. Knowledge of the world, which is essentially different from self, is problematic and has to be 'guaranteed' through the goodness of God. This image of the self not only leads to problems with knowledge of the world, it also leads to problems of knowing any other selves. Kant rejects this problematic (4) and suggests rather that we do not know objects apart from our capacities to know them, we do not know them as they are in themselves. He writes:

> Failing of satisfactory progress in explaining the movements of the heavenly bodies on the supposition that they all revolved around the spectator, he [Copernicus] tried whether he might not have better success if he made the spectator to revolve and the stars to remain at rest. A similar experiment can be tried in metaphysics, as regards the *intuition* of objects. If intuition must conform to the constitution of objects, I do not see how we could know anything of the latter *a priori*; but if the object (as object of the senses) must conform to the constitution of our faculty of intuition, I have no difficulty in conceiving of such a possibility (*Critique of pure reason*, Bxvii).

This passage has resonance for all that will follow. The metaphor works by placing the 'spectator' within the same realm as the planets. The spectator has position in relation to the planets and is not in some Olympian role with no position but able to see all. Further, it is only because Copernicus thinks himself into the position of the spectator and knows that he moves that he can explain the position of the planets.

THE COPERNICAN REVOLUTION: KNOWING FINITE AGENTS

This metaphor provides us with a route map for the Kantian theory of knowledge. From the Kantian viewpoint, knowledge is gained by beings placed within a world, not outside it, who construct their concepts through synthetic activity. We cannot know things as they exist in themselves, thus knowledge is perspectival; we have it because of our activity and capacities, but these also provide the limits of it. All knowing by finite beings is limited. It is not such a large or unKantian step to add to this that the capacities for knowing can develop and degenerate, as studies of child development (5) and dementia (ref: 4, p. 164) would suggest. Such studies (6,7) illuminate Kant's philosophical insight that the distinction between self and world is not something miraculously given. It is a distinction built up through use of synthetic and embodied capacities. It is made when we are able to distinguish between sequences of experience over which we have control, and which we know could have been otherwise, and sequences which we could not order in any other way and perceive as objective events. (This is the point of the Second Analogy in Kant's *Critique of Pure Reason*.) Knowledge of ourselves as *actors* is necessary for any distinction to be made between self and world, subjectivity and objectivity (ref. 4, pp. 278–283). Our activity is at the heart of all knowing. It is no coincidence that Kant sees autonomy as fundamental to ethics. However, this picture of knowing as activity leaves room for recognition that there are degrees of consciousness and self-consciousness, as study of child development and senility would also suggest. This provides a pointer to what respect for autonomy might amount to, for if we recognize that there can be degrees of consciousness and self-consciousness, we may recognize that respect for autonomy is not so simple as assuming that all others are ideally autonomous agents. It may place us under obligations to empathize with others and respect what self-determination they actually have, rather than what might be ideal.

THE COPERNICAN REVOLUTION: AN ANSWER TO PATERNALISM

I suggest that the Copernican metaphor can also provide a useful signpost for our route through Kantian ethical thinking. If the assumption of an Olympian position leads to problems with accounting for all knowing—and a long philosophical tradition recognizes the problem, if not its cause—then this must include problems with ethical knowing as well. Here is a Kantian line against paternalism. Kant argues that we have no Olympian position from which we can know anything, let alone what is best for what happens in a world construed as far below and distinct from us. It is a mistake to assume a transcendent viewpoint—as the paternalist must—and behave as if it were possible to leave our own subjectivity out of the picture. This may be a particularly important line of thought for medical ethics.

Doctors particularly must be tempted to think of themselves as in such a position, for they, when dealing with others who are patients, will usually be in a position of having greater medical knowledge and they must, as a requirement of their profession, keep a distance from their patients. However, greater medical knowledge and professional distance does not necessarily equate to knowing what is best for the patient. For example, a woman who at 38 has just lost a child after a second difficult Caesarean section may be in an ideal position to have a time-saving, money-saving, and possibly in the long term, life-saving, sterilization. It might seem obvious that at her age and with her past history she would not wish to take the risks of a further pregnancy. Sterilization from a purely medical viewpoint would seem to be wholly advantageous, but if performed without consultation, or with consultation only while the woman was upset at the news of her lost baby, is a kind of arrogance, and she may feel this as a violation for the rest of her life.

Paternalism may be necessary in specific instances. Accident victims who arrive unconscious and in need of urgent medical attention clearly require such an approach until such time as they are able to exercise some autonomy. The fundamental problem with paternalism as an approach to conscious patients is that it assumes that it is possible to know what is best. In medicine the paternalist may assume that knowing what is best from the mechanical viewpoint of knowing what is best for the working of the body, amounts to knowing what is best for the patient; and that the medical viewpoint is the only viewpoint, or is superior to that of the patient's. The Kantian Copernican perspective suggests that we not only need to recognize the limitations of others but that our own viewpoint is limited too.

The Kantian Copernican revolution places us firmly within the orbit of what we know. We are not ideal, rational, all-knowing agents, but sensible, feeling and rational beings who live embodied lives alongside others (8,9). We have knowledge because of our embodied capacities, our situatedness, because of our place alongside other beings. Knowledge is perspectival; it may be limited, but it does exist. If we are to see beyond our immediate perspective we must take that perspective into account. If all knowing is limited and dependent upon our synthetic capacities, it is clear that we will not know what is ethically right immediately or without guidance. Indeed it is only when we accept that knowing what is right may not be immediate or easy that we have need for ethics at all. The Kantian acceptance of our finitude and our spontaneity, our activity, requires the provision of the categorical imperative.

THE CATEGORICAL IMPERATIVE

The categorical imperative is a means by which—without assuming an Olympian standpoint—we can glimpse beyond the boundaries of our own position and context and see a wider horizon. The categorical imperative is the Kantian replacement for the transcendent viewpoint or Olympian standpoint assumed by paternalists. Yet it is not derived from any account of human nature as it actually exists. It is a thought experiment, an abstract test which can be applied to different particular situations and, when so applied, will provide principles which may guide our lives. These are supposed to be universal, that is, applicable at all times and in all situations.

I do not wish to dwell upon the question of the equivalence or non-equivalence of the various formulations of the categorical imperative. What is of importance here is to provide a working model and show how it works and what results from its working.

The central thrust of Kantian ethics is to respect our capacity to act rather than to react. It is this which differentiates us from machines, and in Kant's view animals, which are determined and can be used by us as tools or means. This capacity for self-conscious action we must respect in ourselves; it marks us out as an end. Kant writes:

> Act so that you treat humanity, whether in your own person or in that of any other, always as an end and never as a means only (10).

However, in so far as we are rational, we do not and should not make an exception of our own case, because it is our very rational capacity to see beyond our own position sufficiently to realize that we have one (that is, we are self-conscious) that allows us to act rather than react. If we do choose to make an exception of our own case, we choose to act irrationally (Kant calls this the freedom of the turnspit). We must therefore ask whether a maxim could be acted upon by others, that is, whether or not it is universalizable. (Universalizability is not by itself a sufficient ground for a moral rule. Clearly, everyone can stretch at six o'clock in the evening, but this has no moral significance.) Thus the most famous formulation of the categorical imperative is:

> 'Act only on that maxim which you can at the same time will to become universal law.'

Kant claims that by seeing whether our maxim, the basis upon which we act, is universalizable, we will see if we could will it were we in the position of some other being. By asking ourselves whether a maxim could be applied to all other agents we can achieve a degree of self-consciousness; we can think for ourselves and beyond our immediate position, rather than simply base our thinking upon the prevalent assumptions of the society around us. This supreme principle of morality is claimed to be a means by which we need not be passive in relation to our assumptions. We may start with ourselves, our needs, wants and assumptions, but we need not end up with a purely personal or context-related viewpoint. The categorical imperative is supposed to allow us to think from the standpoint of everyone else, to detach ourselves from a purely personal viewpoint. It also allows us to think consistently. If it works, then its use is the supreme manifestation of our autonomy, because through it we can be self-conscious and choose by what our actions are to be determined.

WHAT IS A MAXIM?

What is a maxim (11,12)? If a maxim is understood as an individual intention then it is unlikely that these could be universally acted upon. Individual intentions will include reference to an individual's particular situation and context. Further, there are many specific intentions involved in an action, but, according to Kant, only one maxim. Moreover, if maxims are understood as conscious intentions, agents are most likely to be self-conscious about them. Kant insists that we are not always conscious of our maxims; the thought experiment of the categorical imperative may reveal aspects of a maxim about which we were unaware. O'Neill (11) has argued persuasively for understanding maxims as fundamental intentions rather than specific ones. She gives as an example making a visitor welcome by making her a cup of tea, and writes:

> —there are numerous specific intentions: the warming of the pot, the offer of sugar and the like. But what guides and makes sense of these ancillary intentions is the underlying one. Had that underlying intention differed, then I would not have done just those acts or not just in those ways.... In a different social setting— for example among the Athenians, who had no tea—the same underlying intention would have had to be expressed by way of a different set of specific intentions: wine or conversation, perhaps (p. 394).

Understanding maxims as fundamental intentions is fruitful, for it allows maxims to be universalizable. O'Neill makes it clear that making welcome—the maxim— can remain the same while taking different forms in different ages or social contexts. It takes these different forms because it will be supplemented by different specific intentions according to context. It is these specific intentions with which we would have difficulty if we were to try to universalize them. Another advantage of this understanding of maxims for medical ethics is that it does not commit Kant to any kind of individualism. If maxims are understood as an agent's future intentions, then it seems that institutions, governments and administrations cannot act upon them. However, when they are understood as fundamental intentions there is no reason why collective agents cannot hold maxims or use the categorical imperative. In medicine ethics are often thought to be only useful for individual doctors or nurses in dealing with patients, and not for collective administrative decisions. This understanding of maxims means that Kantian ethical examination need not be left at the finance committee room door just because decisions made there are non-individual.

GENERATING THE PRINCIPLES

The Principles of Justice, Non-coercion and Non-deception

What maxims cannot be universally shared by other rational beings? Coercion, deception and the control or enslavement of others cannot be universally shared. These forms of behaviour require agents *and* victims. They are not universalizable because not everyone can be agent, nor can everyone be a victim. To coerce, deceive, control or enslave is to use others as tools and not to respect them as agents or as ends. If we are coerced, we are made to act in ways not of our choosing, but chosen by others. If we are controlled or enslaved we have no possibility of determining our own behaviour; we are some other agent's tool. Deception cannot be universalized because it is parasitic upon trust. If deception were universal there would arise mistrust and the whole notion of deception would fail. It too uses others as tools, for it does not allow for the possibility of consent being given to the deception by the deceived. Non-coercion and non-deception are the duties of justice for Kantian ethics; they are perfect duties and must apply to all and any rational beings.

What does non-deception amount to in a medical context? If our image is of an ideal rational being, non-deception will amount to something very different than if we face actual finite agents. For example, thalidomide is being given to fertile women to treat certain conditions provided that they are on the contraceptive pill. It has been suggested that although these women have been told a trade name, told it will help their condition, that they must not have babies, and have been asked for their consent, the generic name 'thalidomide' with all its connotations has not been used. If this were so, and if these women were ideal rational agents, did not have limited knowledge and were not likely to be frightened by their illness, if they were not in awe of the medical profession and system and were instead all-knowing ideal rational beings this treatment would not be deceptive. (They would know that the two names of the drug were equivalent, and would in addition not be afraid to ask for the further information that only a finite agent would need.) However, for finite agents such treatment is deceptive, and the consent given to it by them is spurious. Deception may take place even when a description of an action can be given which not only makes no mention of deception, but can point to efforts that have been made to gain consent—thus apparently showing respect for autonomy. Deception takes place when it has not been made possible for patients to consent to fundamental aspects of the treatment, but when patients have been allowed to think that they have done so. Those whose business it is to gain a patient's consent can question their own motives, by asking why the name 'thalidomide' was not used, even though this would have been familiar to the patient? What was the fundamental principle guiding the description of the proposed treatment that they gave? Kantian duties of justice are guiding principles which are to be actively pursued. Efforts have to be made at all times not to deceive, and ways in which deception might take place have to be anticipated and avoided.

Coercion can also take place when a description of treatment need make no mention of it and when, were the same treatment to be given to an ideal rational agent, it would not be coercive. For example, a very thorough, completely technical account of a proposed treatment and its effects could be given in a brisk business-like manner, followed by the remark: 'and if you allow this to take place you have a chance of getting better, and if you do not you won't'. This would be totally non-coercive to an ideal rational agent. To a finite human being it may be the opposite. What happens if this approach is taken with someone who has just been diagnosed as having cancer. She is frightened, she may be intimidated by the presence of someone better educated, of a higher social class, who is behaving in a way which makes it clear they have little time. She will consent and walk out of the room with little or no idea of what she has consented to. She certainly could not have given consent to the fundamental aspects of her treatment, because care has not been taken to make sure that she had any grasp of them. Coercion takes place when there is no real chance of someone saying 'no', or 'can I think about it?'

The duty not to coerce in medicine requires a degree of imagination from the practitioner and a positive effort to gain informed consent rather than an effort to gain a signature on a consent form. The Kantian distinction between acting in accordance with duty and acting out of duty (10) has much to offer in illuminating this type of medical situation. To act in accordance with duty is to gain the signature on the consent form, but to act out of duty is to make sure that the patient has understood at least the fundamental aspects of the treatment for which consent is being sought, and knows that he or she can say 'no' as well as 'yes', or can ask for more time.

The medical system can itself be coercive. The hours worked by junior doctors are often twice the hours of an average worker, and those hours which are 'extra' are paid at a much lower rate. Those hours are compulsory, but it is possible to describe this treatment without any mention of coercion and to make it look as if respect for autonomy is present. A line such as this is familiar: 'Those training to be doctors know the system, and in training and qualifying they tacitly consent to it. Patients know that junior doctors are working long hours but if they choose not to question every doctor as to how long they have been on duty they too give tacit consent.' Ideal rational agents may not suffer from sleep deprivation, but finite embodied doctors do. Ideal rational agents may have the courage to ask awkward questions, but ill finite patients do not. For both finite doctor and finite patient there is no real possibility of doing other than accepting the *status quo*. The finite doctor will have little idea how lack of sleep will affect her, so when she begins her training she will not be in a position to give informed consent to the system, nor is any provision then or later made to make sure that she can do so. Once she qualifies there is no possibility of her refusing to do the required hours, including the on-call hours, without losing her job; even if this makes her ill or makes her lose her professional judgement. Indeed, if that happens she is likely to find herself unemployed once her short-term 'houseman's' contract has run out. For finite patients—ill, frightened, vulnerable, in their pyjamas (a very private form of attire for a public place), possibly feeling that the profession around them manifests a higher social status, certainly knowing that these professionals are more knowledgeable than they are about their medical condition—it would be a very difficult thing to ask a doctor how long she has been on duty. However, given that this is how the health service is run, and that the health service is the only option for most patients, it may appear to patients that they have to accept the system unless they can afford to be treated privately.

To avoid coercion and deception, non-coercion and non-deception have to be fundamental guiding principles for all actions and systems, whether set up by individuals or collectives. It is not sufficient to be able to describe actions or systems in ways which do not mention either term. Finite beings must have their finitude taken into consideration if they are not to be deceived or coerced;

that is, if they are to be given a real possibility of consenting to or dissenting from treatment. This is the point of the Kantian emphasis upon acting out of duty rather than merely in accordance with duty. To act merely in accordance with duty is sufficient for some ideal rational being, but we are not; acting out of duty requires positive efforts.

These duties of justice are not the only obligations for finite beings. Respect for the autonomy of ideal rational beings might amount to not coercing or deceiving them. However, finite embodied beings live in a world surrounded by other finite and embodied beings, to whom they are vulnerable and upon some of whom they depend, in a variety of ways. Finite embodied beings are mortal; they develop and (usually) degenerate, before dying. Respect for them will amount to more than not coercing or deceiving them. The principle of beneficence is important when we recognize our finitude, of which mortality is an all-important part. This recognition places us under obligations to respect others in ways which make allowances for that finitude. Obligations to finite beings are to help and to cooperate, and to develop talents.

Beneficence and Non-maleficence

Beneficence is the positive side of non-maleficence. It is an active duty which includes making sure that no harm is done. Not to be beneficent, and to be maleficent, is non-universalizable—if we take our finitude seriously. We all start life as babies, we are creatures who develop. If we universalize non-cooperation and non-development of talents, non-support and non-help of others, then we will not survive babyhood and there will be no autonomous finite beings to respect. Dependence upon others does not end at babyhood; we are dependent in a variety of ways throughout our lives. We have at the very least some emotional or psychological needs for others during adult life, as is witnessed by the damaging effects of long-term solitary confinement. Towards the end of a life that has not been cut short, our dependence upon others increases. We cannot universalize maleficence for adults because we must all recognize that we will at some point be in need.

The forms that beneficence (respect, cooperation and the development of talents) take will vary according to context. How can this obligation manifest itself in medical situations?

Clearly respect for others requires provision of help in response to needs, and this must include medical help. If we take our finitude (of which mortality is an essential part) seriously then medicine is of major ethical importance and medical help to prolong, increase or maintain autonomous finite life should not be dependent upon an individual patient's capacity to pay for it. It is a moral obligation and as such is to be met not just by individual members of the medical profession but by society as a whole—that is, government (13).

Full acceptance of our finitude, our needs and our mortality (that we develop and degenerate) is difficult even, ironically, within medical practice. If we accept that we are developmental and degenerative beings with variable capacities for autonomy, and with needs for specific others such as mothers, fathers, husbands, wives, etc., then we must accept that the expressed wish of a child (a developing autonomy) for its mother or family is one that is 'reasonable', and grant it. As little as 20 years ago babies and young children who needed to stay in hospital were cut off from their families, visiting was limited during the day and not allowed at night. Nurses were expected to step into the mothering role—and of course step out of it when they changed shift and when the child went home. This situation has largely changed. That it once existed shows the difficulty of thinking in terms of an ideal rational being whose full autonomy is not dependent upon others. If we think in those terms, then clearly children are not such beings, and so need not be treated with respect. If we recognize the nature of our finitude then children should be treated with respect about fundamental wishes, such as their emotional ties with those upon whom they are dependent for survival. Likewise the child's need for stimulation through play has to be met; beneficence and the obligation to develop talents require this. Respect for a child's limited autonomy is not the same as respect for an adult's less limited autonomy. For example, the child may wish to leave hospital; but to grant that wish when the child is in need of medical help would be a failure of beneficence and a failure to recognize that while they have some autonomy, it is a lot less than that of an adult.

If the situation has changed for children it has certainly not changed significantly for the elderly, and with an increasing ageing population this is an area in which ethical examination is urgently needed. It is ironic that within the National Health Service the elderly and dying will often be given privacy to discuss their condition with a doctor or senior nurse, but may be given no privacy in which to see, chat to, hug or love their spouse or other loved ones, at least within the hospital. If you are on a ward you are usually in the presence of other patients and their relatives and visitors. Clearly, privacy to discuss a medical condition with medical staff is part of dealing or being dealt with respectfully. However, the presence, comfort and conversation of a life's companion must be much more important to most patients when facing the possibility of the end of their life. Drawing the curtain around the bed is a pathetically inadequate means of privacy, and the curtain is of course liable to be whisked back at any moment by a nurse or doctor busy about their business. Even in a separate room, staff may burst in unannounced. To respond to this situation by saying that provision could be made for any patient who expressed the wish for private time with their spouse or loved ones, to say in effect that there is no demand for it, is again to treat patients as if they were ideally autonomous. Whereas a child will have no inhibitions about demanding 'Mummy', an adult may well be embarrassed to demand private time with their loved one. In Britain many old people remember the days before the National Health Service when ill health could mean large bills and financial ruin. Often they are pathetically grateful for their treatment and feel they must not 'cause trouble'. They may also readily perceive the pressure under which medical staff work, and do not wish to add to their burden or cause offence. For these sorts of reasons, people will not make demands which are perfectly reasonable.

Many 'homes' for the elderly are single-sex, and very few indeed make any provision for married couples. This can lead to marriages of 50 years being ended. For example, take an old man looking after his dementing wife at home.

She is unable to look after herself but still knows her husband and loves him. He falls down and breaks his hip and will not be capable of looking after her. They may both wish to be together, but without the money to provide private nursing care they are split up and sent to separate homes—a 50-year marriage finished. If we really took our mortality seriously could we allow such situations to happen? If our lives are not cut short we too will be old one day.

Respect for finite beings must include respect for their relationships too. These are positive obligations which must guide all aspects of practice and planning within a health service. This must include work practices; thus it should be possible for employees within the health service to meet their family commitments. The provision of creches, allowance of maternity and paternity leave and job-sharing schemes might all be means through which collectives such as health authorities and government could meet obligations of beneficence.

CONCLUSION

We have travelled a *broadly* Kantian path. My aim has not been to provide detailed Kantian exegesis, but to explore Kantian insights through practical reasoning on medical issues in a way which, I hope, is open to non-philosophers. We have seen that respect for finite human mortal autonomy can and should be important within a medical context. I hope to have shown through use of commonplace examples that if we move away from a Cartesian picture of a self, cut off and distinct from the world, to one in which our subjectivity is situated within it, then we perceive differently. The Kantian picture of a limited self, set within and as a part of the world, means that we should take finitude in its variety (limited knowledge, emotional and physical needs and mortality) seriously. When we do this, we move from thinking of ideal rational autonomies to finite human mortal autonomies, and our obligations change too. My examples have been chosen because they are commonplace, and can illustrate all the more clearly the power of the Cartesian picture of the self even upon a discipline so concerned with the body as medicine. We have seen that what might be respectful and just to an ideal autonomy can be coercive or deceitful to a finite human mortal one. Behaviour which to an ideal rational autonomy with no emotional or familial ties can be acceptable, or even beneficent, can be maleficent to a finite human mortal autonomy with such ties. Through use of commonplace examples I hope to have illustrated that, even if medics and medical administrators know nothing of Descartes, they feel the power of that picture of the self. In doing this I hope not only to have offered an alternative picture, but to have illustrated the Kantian point that we are not always or easily self-aware. Commonplace examples are important; it is too easy to think that moral principles only have power when we are faced with powerful examples of dilemmas, such as 'is euthanasia appropriate in this case?' or 'should I treat the child of this Jehovah's Witness in spite of the family's objections?' Difficult though resolution of such cases is, they do seem to arrive almost 'ready labelled', 'this needs ethical examination'. The Kantian point is that respect for autonomy, and from this, justice and beneficence, are positive guides for the conduct of everything. They are not just to be got out of the cupboard and dusted off when a 'dilemma' arises. We will not always be aware that we have failed to respect others if we think that moral principles are only for certain difficult cases. Commonplace and apparently trivial occurrences, such as saying to the spouse of a patient who is being discharged 'you can have her back now' (as if the spouse had no right to their relationship while in hospital), are failures of respect, too: My object in using commonplace examples has been to show this, and to demonstrate the Kantian insight that we are not always aware of our presuppositions, and so we have need of the categorical imperative. Examples of medical ethical 'dilemmas' may be misleading in a further way; they may make it appear as if ethical life were only the province of the relationships between individuals. I hope to have shown that, from a Kantian horizon, it is possible to see ethical life extended to collectives, committees and governments.

REFERENCES

1. Macintyre, A. 1981 *After virtue: a study in moral theory*. Duckworth, London.
2. Broad, C. D. 1978. *Kant, an introduction*, pp. 290–291. Cambridge University Press, Cambridge.
3. O'Neill, O. 1984. Paternalism and partial autonomy. *Journal of Medical Ethics*, 173–178.
4. Furness, S. H. 1986. A reasonable geography. PhD thesis, University of Essex.
5. O'Neill, O. 1984. Transcendental syntheses and developmental psychology. *Kant Studien* **75**, Heft 4: 145–167.
6. Piaget, J. 1975. *The development of thought*. Viking Press, New York.
7. Issacs, A. D. 1977. *Studies in geriatric psychiatry*. John Wiley & Sons, Chichester.
8. Kant, I. 1781. *The critique of pure reason*, 1781, (trans. Kemp Smith, N.) St Martin's Press, New York 1965; A359–60, 363, 379–8, 385. B409, 415, 428.
9. Kant, I. 1798. *Anthropology from a pragmatic point of view*, p. 323.
10. Kant, I. 1785. *Groundwork of the metaphysics of morals* (trans. Paton, H. J.) Harper Torch Books, 1964, second section 9IV 286–287; and 397.
11. O'Neill, O. 1984. Kant after virtue. *Inquiry* **26**: 387–405.
12. O'Neill, O. 1986. *Faces of hunger; studies in applied philosophy*, pp. 131–140. Allen & Unwin, London.
13. H. M. Government, 1991. *The patient's charter*. HMSO, London.

15

Marxism, Health Care Ethics and the Four Principles

PROFESSOR DR ERNST LUTHER AND DR VIOLA SCHUBERT-LEHNHARDT

Martin-Luther-Universitat, Halle, Germany

WHY A CHAPTER ABOUR MARXISM IN THIS BOOK?

It could be asked after the failure of 'real socialism' what health care workers could possibly learn from Marxism? We believe there are things to be learned from Marxism because:

1. Marxism, like Christianity, is one of the philosophical and intellectual streams of thought running through history. Founded in the middle of the nineteenth century, it captured the minds of millions of people in all parts of the world who felt repressed by capitalism and who hoped for a more just world.
2. Some special principles and experiences in health care existed in countries that were formerly socialist and these continue in those countries which remain socialist today. These must be considered and evaluated.
3. A lot of the global problems arising from the lack of the basic prerequisites of health such as peace, shelter, education, food, income, social justice, equity and a stable ecosystem with sustainable resources, are not provided by the free market system. Which means that to say 'Marx is dead' makes just as little sense as to say—like Nietzsche—'God is dead' (1).

For followers of Marx, which we regard ourselves as being, it is necessary to be self-critical and ask why the ideas of Marx became so rigid, how they came to be used to harm the people, and what must be done to make them open to a pluralist world without their making any claim to the right to dominate this discussion. The term 'Marxist' was already under discussion in the lifetime of Karl Marx (1818–1883). Friedrich Engels mentioned in letters to Eduard Bernstein and Paul Lafargue that Marx said, in order to dissociate himself from intellectuals who called themselves Marxists: 'All I know is that I am not a Marxist' (2).

Principles of Health Care Ethics. Edited by Raanan Gillon.
© 1994 John Wiley & Sons Ltd

Engels accepted the term after the death of Marx; he said that the theory correctly had his name (3). Nowadays the philosophical and political spectrum of people who called themselves Marxists is very heterogeneous. However, this is not peculiar to Marxism: the same could also be said of many other ideologies and religions.

THE PATERNALISTIC AND DEONTOLOGICAL TRADITION

In the first place medical ethics arise independent of ideology and politics from the need to react to the new opportunities and dangers presented by scientific and technical progress. This progress also took place in countries in which Marxism had become the 'ruling ideology'. From the tradition of socialist development, which has always conceived of itself as diametrically opposed to liberalism, it followed that the principle of autonomy would be subordinated to the principle of beneficence.

Where Marxism was, or is, the ruling ideology, the traditional principle 'Salus aegroti suprema lex' ('the patient's interests always come first' (4)) is understood to be the fundamental principle of health care. The doctor is immediately responsible for the well-being of the patient. Only the doctor has the competence, the knowledge, the ability, to help. It is not his place to judge or to apportion blame (for instance in the case of alcohol abuse). One particular code for doctors obliges them 'to engage fully all my knowledge and all my strength for the good physical and mental health of man, as well as for the cure and prevention of sickness' (5). E. Seidler asserts that a paternal health care system which was conscious of its authority was dominant in both West and East Germany (6). The principle of paternalism was also supported by governmental decisions in Eastern Europe and in other socialist countries. The Social Democratic Party (SPD) of Germany had already resolved in 1891 at a party rally, to demand 'free medical care including obstetrics and remedies, and free burial' (7). This demand for free health care was included in the constitution, and relieved doctors of having to ask for payment for the treatment. In the very beginning this paternalism had a beneficial effect (8). However, the principle of paternalism in health care proved disadvantageous in two respects as the costs of treatment increased: (a) doctors could not fulfil their obligations to treat patients because of a permanent shortage of medicine and outdated techniques; and (b) because treatment was free patients were not motivated to safeguard their own health in order to save the money incurred by treatment.

Sanctity of Life, Quality of Life and Autonomy

Since the 1970s medical ethics has been examining the claim of the concept of the principle of the sanctity of life to be the unique, overriding, fundamental principle of medical ethics. The discussion has been broadened to include the concept of the quality of life and the principle of autonomy. How can a Marxist perspective accommodate the principle of autonomy, we must ask. Two points must be emphasized: Marx's image of man and the political ideals which he stood for. As a critical follower of Ludwig Feuerbach, Marx was of the opinion that the human being is what the human being values most. Here we see a clear exclusion of religion and the affirmation of the idea of self-determination. In Marxist thinking life is not sacred in the sense that life is given to human beings by God and so should not therefore be touched or interfered with by human beings. Life is held to be sacred because each human being's life is unique and irreplaceable; each human being has responsibility for shaping his or her own life.

That is why from a Marxist viewpoint suicide is not something to be morally condemned but a misfortune, a crisis, a dilemma to be avoided. Respect for life, especially because of the experiences of eugenics in the nineteenth and up to the Nazi period in the twentieth century, must exclude any notion of someone other than the person concerned evaluating whether her or his life is worth living. The Marxist understanding of euthanasia and of the care of the most sick and dying, is not very different from that of other humanistic positions. Its aim is the respect for autonomy of the person, consistent with a belief in a 'soft' or 'weak' paternalism. In 1989 the Marxist position concerning this problem was made public: The terms 'euthanasia' and 'mercy killing', as used in a number of countries, were inappropriate. Careful analysis of the socioeconomic, political, and ideological roots of Nazism led to the conclusion that a term which is so tremendously tainted by the murder action 'Tiergartenstrasse 4' (the secret action was named for the street Tiergartenstrasse 4 because in this street Adolf Hitler placed an administration building) of the Nazis, is thereby utterly unsuitable for reference to well-intentioned action. Furthermore, the distinction between 'active' and 'passive' euthanasia rather than helping to clarify matters only serves to confuse them. The term 'Sterbehilfe' (letting die), as it is used in Switzerland, Austria and in Germany, has to be excluded from philosophical and ethical discourse because it leads to confusion. The supporters of the use of this term have, of course, emphasized that 'Sterbehilfe' is understood and used by them to mean 'Lebenshilfe' (help for life), i.e. as assistance throughout the dying process, and assistance to bring about death. The possibility of misinterpretation of the term as assistance in bringing about death results, however, from the distinction between 'active' and 'passive' 'Sterbehilfe'. Since 'active' obviously connotes killing, passivity is the only alternative meaning left to 'Lebenshilfe', and this is exactly what we do not want.

In the eastern part of Germany the term 'Betreuung Sterbender' (care of the dying) became generally accepted in the first half of the 1980s. This term implies two main ideas: first, an active devotion to the patient based upon the respect for life as a fundamental value, and second, the acceptance of death as that which determines the nature of the devotion to the dying patient. This was the background for discussion in the literature about many recommendations and criteria for basic attitudes and partial decisions, and it indicated there was an emerging consensus with respect to a system of standards. Basic to that system is the principle that the care of dying patients is to be regarded as a task for society as a whole, and that this task should promote security and confidence in society, as well as a high valuation of life. The provision of care for the dying is a humane task of all health care and social care workers, and one which has to be fulfilled in a careful and devoted way. The following constitutes a challenge to the providers of care to think about their readiness to devote themselves to the dying:

1. the care of dying persons requires that the provider of care thinks about his own attitude to dying and death;
2. the provider has to accept the dying person as he or she is;
3. the provider has to be sincere.

The care of dying persons therefore requires that their basic social needs are met. Among them are:

1. the need for adequate physical care and hygienic living conditions;
2. the need to avoid suffering and pain;
3. the need for communication with relatives and friends or caring people;
4. the need to be informed about one's own prospects for life;
5. the need to be respected, even at this last stage of life, as a personality, and to be given the opportunity to exercise their personalities—to be themselves (9).

Agreement exists between Marxist and religious thinkers in Eastern Germany on this problem. This was especially emphasized at the main session of the houses of deacons (Diakonisches Werk) of the Protestant churches of the GDR in June 1988 (10). The Christian thinker K. Nowak mentions that this agreement between Marxist and religious thinkers has historical antecedents in Germany. In 1931/32, he said, Marxists and Christians acted together in the Prussian Privy Council against the position that the so-called 'unworthy-life' (lebensunwertes Leben) would simply be excluded from funding when funds being made available for medical institutions were in the process of being reduced (11).

However, in practice the policy in the socialist countries was characterized not by a soft, but a very strong, paternalism which not only interfered considerably with the work of doctors (with serious effects, for example in psychiatry) but which also hindered and obstructed the development of important forms of help for lay-people, for example self-help groups. A weighty two-fold point of Marxist theory itself was: (a) its pretension to define politics scientifically and (b) the principle of organization within the party that such 'scientifically' defined politics must be accomplished through the power of the working class. Thus was Marx's understanding of autonomy turned on its head, a process which has been described by Stefan Hermlin in his book *Abendlicht* (*Evening light*) (12). He underlined that in 1848 in the Manifesto of the Communist Party Marx and Engels wrote the sentence 'In place of the old bourgeois society, with its classes and class antagonisms, we shall have an association, in which the free development of each is the condition for the free development of all' (13). However, in practice, in practical politics the opposite was understood. In other words that sentence was understood to mean that the free development of all— realized through the abolition of exploitation—is the condition for a free development of each individual. This interpretation was obviously aimed at limiting anarchy, liberalism and individualism; obviously towards this end,

Marx was read, was 'understood' in this way. The book *Abendlicht* was published in 1979 and gives a literary expression to the fact that the idea of autonomy was slowly beginning to catch on.

As far as the care of patients was concerned, this meant a more critical way of looking at the risk in medicine and increasing demand from patients for better information. While it has been generally acknowledged that the principle of informed consent must be respected it is held to be wrong recklessly to impart information as to diagnosis, for instance in the case of cancer. This problem was discussed in the book *Ethics in Medicine* (14). The book also explored the idea of 'soft' paternalism; it maintained that two meanings of autonomy should be accepted: if the patient did not want information it should not be forced upon her; however, if information was wanted it should be given with the aim of helping the patient to live with his illness and of explaining to him his chances of survival.

The idea of autonomy is directly connected with the Marxist understanding of freedom and responsibility and it has an important consequence concerning lifestyle. Freedom is not seen as the state of being able to do everything one wants without any thought being given to preconditions and consequences. The Marxist position concerning freedom was described in Engels' book against Dühring (the *Anti-Dühring* (15)), a book written by Engels during his continuous exchange of ideas with Marx. Firstly Engels warned of the illusion of a dreamed-of independence from natural laws, and, secondly of ignorance. The result of this illusion and this ignorance would be uncertainty (for example in the case of addiction to drugs), 'it is controlled by the very object it should itself control'. Engels concludes from this: 'Freedom therefore consists in the control over ourselves and over external nature, a control founded on knowledge of natural necessity; it is therefore necessarily a product of historical development.' (ref. 15, p. 106).

It is remarkable that the right for a woman to make up her own mind about continuing her pregnancy was achieved in most eastern countries many years ago, yet now that these countries are gaining political freedom, this right is in danger (compare developments in Poland and Germany).

From a Marxist viewpoint the necessity that women make their own autonomous decisions is pre-eminent, because the dignity of women is seriously affected by making such decisions. At the same time we demand that in this interpretation of the right the newest scientific knowledge be included. We understand abortion as the destruction of developing life. We recognize this as a dilemma which includes an ethical conflict for women as well as for doctors, a dilemma which cannot be solved by legal sanction. In applying the principles of beneficence and autonomy it is impossible not to allow for individual decisions being different. However, the Marxist orientation in ethics is to connect analytical and normative moments, and so the actual situation is always included in the theory governing the decision-making. The idea of decision-making case by case is rejected.

The Utopia of Justice

Marx's understanding of justice is always a point of discussion among Marxist thinkers (16–19). It was the concern of Marx and Engels to distinguish and to bring some order to ideas of moral, legal, social and historical justice. They distinguished what is just by law (legal justice) from what is just by history (by this they understood the objective results of the historical process). They have distanced themselves from any appeal to an 'eternal justice' many times, and underlined the need for a neutral analysis of economic relations as the basis of all politics and ideology. Engels wrote in *Anti-Dühring*: 'From a scientific standpoint, this appeal to morality and justice does not help us an inch further; moral indignation, however justifiable, cannot serve economic science as an argument, but only as a symptom' (ref. 19, p. 138).

This opinion was what Allan Wood was referring to when he asked if it would be possible to speak about Marx's thought being amoral; he answered this question with only a qualified 'yes' (20). It is indeed legitimate to say that Marx refused any moral critique of injustice within his economic theory. But this did not stop him from interceding for justice in politics and in the evaluation of human relationships.

Within this framework the following designation of justice is emphasized:

1. Justice always exists in direct or indirect relation to equality.
2. Both terms must be seen in an 'historically concrete' context. This means that there cannot exist any 'eternal justice' or any 'general equality'.
3. Social justice, as a criterion for the evaluation of social relations from the viewpoint of justice, means above all that people are equal in relation to the means of production and that they have equal political and legal rights and duties.

The realization of these principles should guarantee equal (just) possibilities for a free and all-round development of a person's skills and abilities. Bearing in mind the historical character of these terms, it has been pointed out that in socialism, as the first phase in social development, it is impossible to create full justice. This would be possible only through communism. This was expressed in the well-known principles of distribution—in socialism distribution should be carried out according to the achievement principle; in communism distribution should be carried out according to the principle 'from each according to his ability, to each according to his needs' (21).

With this common understanding as a basis, justice in health care in Marxist thought is understood as:

1. constitutional guarantee of the right to health protection and to health and social care (constitutional guarantee means here the same rights for all citizens);
2. the principle of free health care and cure as an inalienable part of the ideal of social equality;
3. social equality with the accessibility of medical institutions and a free choice of doctor.

At this point it must be mentioned that the principles named here could only be realized to a certain extent in the socialist countries. For example, there has always existed a 'hierarchy' for the care of the person according to his or her social status (special programmes for high-level 'party workers', special hospitals for members of government). Access to some drugs and medicines also depended on this status and the geographical location of the chemist's (drugs in short supply were often only available in the capital). The objectives mentioned above were the historical aim. The fact that they could not be realized is a result of the real problems in these countries after World War II and of the increasingly subjective and distorted interpretation of Marx's ideal.

If the trend of historical development is seen as geared to the further development of human skills and abilities (development of the species *Homo sapiens*, self-development of every one), then such an understanding has a good chance of making distribution possible according to actual existing needs (and not, for example, on the basis of financial considerations or by thoughts about the utility of the patients). But before this a decision must have been taken about the relationship between general welfare and individual welfare. In socialism this decision was made to the effect that when resources were running low, the needs (groups of illness) of these people were attended to and cured where possible, where there was an interest on the part of the whole community in this being done. In practice this led to a good working system of inoculation (and so *de facto* such illnesses as poliomyelitis, smallpox, and so on, were eradicated), and a good system of health care in factories and for mothers and children.

At the same time this system has had the disadvantage that needs which where not seen to be in the interest of the whole community to meet were difficult to satisfy. For example, in a paper about the situation of women in the German Democratic Republic it was estimated that women had been disadvantaged because they usually were not so often in positions of work or at places of work where regular check-ups took place (22) (furthermore, in the same paper the situation of women pensioners and invalids is assessed and it is described as shameful) (pp. 171ff).

Just as limited was the development of fixed medical techniques and the accessibility of these techniques if such accessibility was not directly in the interest of the whole community (for example, relatively late development of *in vitro* fertilization (IVF), difficult or complete lack of access to IVF for unmarried women or lesbians, and so on).

In some degree these difficulties were neutralized (or tolerated) by a feeling of social security and welfare, which should not be undervalued. In other words everybody was sure that in situations of vital importance he would be cared for and hopefully cured, even if this was very expensive and the person in question was poor. Also everybody was also sure of receiving many health check-ups, aimed at preventing ill-health. Prophylactic measures for mother and child were guaranteed by law, regardless of social and financial status. The lack of any kind of financial link or contract between patients and doctors has led to the development of a relationship of confidentiality and trust that could serve as a model for the doctor–patient relationship today. It must be mentioned here that such a relationship could run the risk of favouring paternalism, but altogether we regard the absence of any kind of financial relationship between patients and doctors as a positive factor (this understanding is supportd by the results of investigations) (23, 24).

NON-MALEFICENCE—A PRINCIPLE FOR CONFIDENTIALITY AND QUALITY

Arthur Schopenhauer wrote, in his paper 'Über die Grundlagen der Moral' (The foundation of morality), that between all ethical systems there exists a consensus about the principle 'Neminem laede, imo omnes, quantum potes, iuva' ('do no harm, and help all persons as well as you can') (25). Of course everyone in the medical profession knows that damage cannot be excluded from medical practice; for example, amputations are sometimes necessary to save lives.

To be precise, the principle of non-maleficence is a principle of quality and confidentiality which primarily focuses on the confidence of the patient in the doctor. The doctor's specialist knowledge is what enables him to do his work, and he does it with the benefit of the patient as his foremost aim. The doctor thinks about any risks involved and discusses them with the patient before proceeding. Also included in, or covered by, this principle is the promise of the doctor to do exactly what he has said to the patient that he will do. The principle of non-maleficence implies the principle of informed consent. In the German (and European) tradition the principle of non-maleficence has always been linked with the care-principle 'beneficence'.

In countries which aspire to Marxist and socialist aims special efforts were made to reduce the harm done by doctors. One way of doing this was through a well-established system of continuous professional training aimed at maintaining and improving the quality of doctors' work and at motivating health care workers to be exact and precise in their work (*Sorgfaltspflicht*). Reference was made in this training to the harm that doctors could cause (26). Another method of attempting to reduce the effects of the harm that might be done by doctors was the establishing of a special insurance system, for patients as well as for doctors and other health care workers. In the governmental health care system primary liability for damage caused to patients was placed on the hospital or clinic. The duty of evidence did not lie on the side of the patient: the duty of evidence lay with the institution (27). In other words it was not up to patients to prove that what they said was true it was up to the institution accused of harming a patient, accused of negligence, to prove that it was not responsible for damaging that patient. A special positive ruling was drawn up in the GDR in 1974 which established that patients would receive financial support (*erweiterte materielle Unterstützung*) if the duty of being precise and exact in their work (*Sorgfaltspflicht*) was not to be violated, resulting in harm to the patient either through surgery or radiotherapy. The extent of the harm caused was estimated and evaluated by the doctors concerned. In contrast with the USA or western European countries such conflicts have been rare and of a fairly trivial nature. These legal rules also encouraged in doctors a moral readiness to examine any damage caused in a self-critical manner.

Under the new conditions after the failure of socialism the process of trust-building is increasing in importance. However, demands that the sanctity or, on the other hand, the quality of life, be regarded as absolute principles, are not generally accepted. In detailed cases there will be preferences, but in general there must be independence, interaction. The contradiction, the necessary tension between general welfare and individual welfare, must be accepted.

From the Marxist perspective medical ethics cannot exist without values and principles. But if they are understood as something external to the way we live our lives they must fail.

REFERENCES

1. Nietzsche F. 1986. *Die fröhliche Wissenschaft.* 125. *Stück,* p. 14. A. Kronenverlag, Stuttgart.
2. 'Alles was ich weiß, ist, daß ich kein Marxist bin': Engels an Paul Lafargue 27 August 1890. *Marx Engels werke,* Bd. 37, p. 450. Dietz Verlag, Berlin. Engels to Eduard Bernstein 2/3 November 1882. *Marx Engels werke,* Bd. 35, p. 388. Dietz Verlag, Berlin, 1967.
3. Engels F. Ludwig Feuerbach und der Ausgang der klassischen deutschen Philosophie. *Marx Engels werke,* Bd. 21, p. 292. Dietz Verlag, Berlin, 1962.
4. Gillon, R. 1986 *Philosophical medical ethics,* p. 73. John Wiley & Sons, Chichester, New York, Brisbane, Toronto, Singapore.
5. Physicians' solemn vow (German Democratic Republic, 1976). *Journal of medicine and philosophy* **14**: 351 (1989).
6. Seidler, E. 1971. Grundformen ärztlichen Selbstverständnisses. P. 70, in Engelmeier, M. P. and Popkes, B. (Eds) *Leitbilder des modernen Arztes.* Thieme Verlag, Stuttgart.
7. Berthold, L. and Diehl, E. (Eds). 1964 *Revolutionäre deutsche parteiprogramme,* p. 85. Dietz-Verlag, Berlin.
8. Helbing, K. and Hermann, S. 1989. *Vergleich des gesundheitswesens in der BRD und DDR während der Jahre 1950–1989.* Institut für medizinische statistik und datenverarbeitung, Berlin: Information No. 5.
9. Luther, E. 1989. Medical ethics in the German Democratic Republic. *Journal of medicine and philosophy* **14**: 295–299.
10. Luther, E. 1989. 'Gemeinsame humanistische ziele?' Gedanken zum thema aus der sicht marxistischer ethick. and Krusche G. "Gemeinsame humanistische ziele?"— Das besondere des Christlichen in unserem Dienst, in: *Diakonie. Information 1 Handreichung des Diakonischen Werkes—Innere Mission und Hilfswerk—der Evangelischen Kirchen in der DDR.* Evangelische Verlagsanstalt GmbH, Berlin.
11. Nowak, K. 1977. *'Euthanasie' und sterilisierung im 'Dritten Reich'.* Niemeyer Verlag, Hale.
12. Hermlin, St. 1979. *Abendlicht.* Verlag Ph. Reclam, Leipzig.
13. Marx, K. and Engels, F. 1976. Manifesto of the Communist Party. *Karl Marx–Frederick Engels collected works,* Vol. 6, p. 506. Progress Publishers, Moscow.
14. Luther, E. 1986. *Ethik in der Medizin.* VEB Verlag Volk und Gesundheit, Berlin.
15. Engels, F. 1976. *Anti-dühring.* Herrn Eugen Dühring's revolution in science, *in Karl Marx–Frederick Engels collected works,* vol. 25. Progress Publishers, Moscow.
16. Cohen, M., Nagel, Th. and Scanlon, Th. 1980. *Marx, justice, and history.* Princeton University Press, Princeton, NJ.
17. Haney, G. 1967. *Sozialistisches recht und persönlichkeit.* Berlin.
18. Klenner, H. 1979. Gerechtigkeit—eine rechtsphilosophische kategorie. *Deutsche zeitschrift für philosophie,* 7.
19. Leist, A. 1985. Mit Marx von gerechtigeit zu freiheit und zurück. *Philosophische Rundschau,* 32, J. C. B. Mohr (Paul Siebeck), Tübingen.
20. Wood, A. W. 1986. Marx' immoralismus, in: Angehrn, E. and Lohmann, G. (Eds)

Ethik und Marx. Moralkritik und normative Grundlagen der Marxschen Theorie. Hain Verlag bei athänäum, Königstein/Ts.

21. Marx, K. 1969. Kritik des Gothaer Programms. *Marx Engels Werke*, Bd. 19, p. 21. Dietz Verlag, Berlin.

22. Winkler, G. 1990. *Frauenreport 90'*, p. 161. Verlag Die Wirtschaft, Berlin.

23. Winter, K. (Ed.) 1974. *Das Gesundheitswesen in der DDR*, chapters 1–8. Verlag Volk und Gesundheit, Berlin.

24. Helbrug, K. H. 1990. *Vergleich des Gesundheitswesens in der BRD und der DDR während der Jahre 1950–1989.* Institut für medizinische Statistik und Datenbearbeitung. Berlin; Information No. 5.

25. Schopenhauer, A. 1979. *Sämtliche Werke*, Bd. III, p. 9. Insel-Verlag, Leipzig.

26. Lignitz, E. and Mattig, W. 1989. *Der iatrogene Schaden.* Akademie Verlag, Berlin.

27. Mandel, J. and Lange, H. 1985. *Ärztliche Rechtspraxis.* Verlag Volk und Gesundheit, Berlin.

16

African Ethical Theory and the Four Principles

PETER KASENENE, BA, DipEd, MA, PhD

Senior Lecturer and Head, Department of Theology and Religious Studies, University of Swaziland, Kwaluseni, Swaziland

INTRODUCTION

The African world-view, in which people's ethics is rooted, is life-affirming, and societal activity centres on the promotion of vitality and fertility of human beings, livestock and the land on which their livelihood depends. Sickness and disease, which disrupt people's well-being, have always been unwelcome, and when they are experienced, attempts are made to restore a state of wholesomeness using both natural and supernatural means.

What is African?

It should be noted that writing about an aspect of life from an African perspective creates a number of problems. One of them, for example, is that Africans are not a monolithic society, Africa being home to a variety of between 800 and 1200 peoples, with different cultures (1). It means, therefore, that generalization in this chapter is inevitable. This comment should not give an impression that one cannot speak of an African view or an African perspective. Despite variety, there is a common Africanness about the culture and world-view of Africans.

The second problem arises from the changes that are taking place in Africa. In recent years Africa has experienced profound and radical changes as a result of colonialism, foreign religions, western education and technology, contact with both the west and the east and the inevitable changes arising from within. The process of acculturation and general adaptation has undermined or even disrupted, to some degree, the traditional ethos. Thus there are remarkable differences in values among Africans; urban and rural, educated and illiterate, Christian or Muslim and traditionalist.

This does not, nevertheless, mean that the African traditional values, attitudes,

---

Principles of Health Care Ethics. Edited by Raanan Gillon.
© 1994 John Wiley & Sons Ltd

ideas and norms have been completely abandoned. The traditional ethos still dominates and it is this ethos we shall discuss in relation to health care.

Ethics in Traditional Societies

In traditional societies moral authority is enshrined in custom, the basis of which is the belief in ancestors who, after their death, retain their authority over the living. Right actions are defined as those forms of conduct which are approved by the traditional standards or customary modes of behaviour of a society to which an individual belongs. Everyone is expected to conform to established norms and standards. An aspect of custom, however, is a people's philosophy of life. At this point it is pertinent to discuss briefly the basic philosophical principles underlying African ethics.

TWO BASIC ETHICAL PRINCIPLES

In 1945 Placied Tempels, a Belgian missionary in the Congo (Zaire), published his celebrated work *Bantu philosophy*, based on his experience and knowledge of the Baluba people (2). In this book Tempels discusses African ontology and ethics. Although the volume aroused great controversy, it was gradually endorsed by many African philosophers and theologians, though reservations were expressed regarding certain details. According to Tempels, 'life' or 'vital force' is central to African philosophy (ref. 2, p. 44).

The Vital Force Principle

According to Tempels, vital force is the meaning of 'to be'. The ultimate goal of anyone is to acquire life, strength or vital force; to live strongly. Everyone strives to make life stronger and to be protected from misfortune or from a diminution of life or of being (ref. 2, pp. 44–45). Supreme happiness is to possess the greatest vital force, and the worst misfortune is the diminution of this force which is brought about by illness, suffering, depression, fatigue, injustice, oppression and any other social or physical evil. This vital force is hierarchical, descending from God through ancestors and elders to the individual. Whatever increases life or vital force is good; whatever decreases it is bad. Human society is organized on the basis of vital force; life growth, life influence and life rank. This structure must be respected, and the individual is good in so far as he or she fulfils his or her duties to promote, support and protect the vital force within the community, according to his or her rank.

The Communalism Principle

J. Mbiti discusses another aspect of African traditional ethics. According to him the key value in African societies is community (ref. 1, p. 205). This is influenced by the African understanding of being.

In African societies to be is to belong, and an individual exists corporately in terms of the family, clan and whole ethnic group. As Mbiti observes:

Only in terms of other people does the individual become conscious of his own being, his own duties, his privileges and responsibilities towards himself and towards other people. When he suffers, he does not suffer alone but with his corporate group: when he rejoices, he rejoices not alone but with his kinsmen, his neighbours and his relatives whether dead or living. . . . Whatever happens to the individual happens to the whole group, and whatever happens to the whole group happens to the individual. The individual can only say 'I am, because we are; and since we are, therefore, I am' (ref. 1, pp. 108–109).

This is the key to understanding the African view of a person, in relation to the community. A person's identity and indeed his or her very life are through a group. Thus the Venda saying *'Muthu ndi muthu nga numwe'*, meaning 'A person is person through another person'. The deeper meaning is that an individual by himself or herself is helpless and has little value. Another proverb of the same people expresses this idea clearly: *'Muthu u bebelwa nunwe'*, meaning 'A person is born for the other'. This shows that, according to the Venda philosophy, which is similar to the philosophy of other African peoples, one cannot regard even one's own life as purely personal property or concern. It is the group which is the owner of life, a person being just a link in the chain uniting the present and future generations. For that reason one's health is a concern of the community, and a person is expected to preserve this life for the good of the group.

IMPLICATIONS FOR HEALTH CARE

African ethics based on the preservation and promotion of life or vital force and communitarian living present no problems in the application of the principles of beneficence and non-maleficence in health care. Respect for autonomy and justice and their applications, however, seem to create problems. It is upon these principles we shall focus in our discussion, but first let us examine health care in a traditional African setting.

Traditional Health Care

Health and disease are not universal concepts; they are shaped by a people's philosophy and culture. Health care, too, is determined by a people's view of a person and his or her relation to the environment. Health care attitudes and methods, therefore, have to take into account a people's philosophical and cultural concepts of health and disease.

Health, in traditional African societies, is all-inclusive, taking into account a whole person and his or her social environment. Briefly stated, health means personal integration, environmental equilibrium, and harmony between the integrated person and the environment. If any of those three factors is missing a person is not regarded as being healthy. Personal integration is achieved when all the major aspects of a person, namely the physical, mental and social, are sound and operating normally and successfully. On the other hand, environmental equilibrium means a harmonious natural and social surrounding. Health, therefore, does not mean only the faultless mechanical functioning of the body, but also prosperity and mutal coexistence and contentment. Even when one is physically well, for example, in an environment of war, famine, drought, envy, hatred, poverty and similar social or natural calamities, there is no state of health. Health means wholesomeness in a harmonious environment.

This is similar to the World Health Organization (WHO) understanding of health as 'a state of complete physical, mental, and social well-being and not merely the absence of disease or infirmity' (3). Following from the above understanding, health care touches a very broad range of personal experience. Over and above the malfunctioning of the biological mechanism, the whole person and his or her social environment call for health care.

In a modern setting it may not be possible to regard health care in such an all-encompassing way. Nevertheless, this African holistic approach provides a challenge we cannot ignore completely. In health care it is not adequate to concentrate exclusively on the body. The psychological, social and environmental aspects of the person also need to be attended to.

The introduction into Africa of western medical institutions, medicines and technology has complicated and introduced ethical problems in health care. One case will be related to show some of the issues that are raised by medical care in an African setting.

The Maze Case

This is a real case the names having been altered to preserve confidentiality and a few additions having been made to make the issues clearer.

Mrs Maze, five months pregnant, went to hospital with swollen legs and hands. She also complained of severe headache, drowsiness and vomiting. On examination the doctor diagnosed her problem to be pre-eclampsia. He admitted her for constant and expert care and ordered complete bed rest for her. Mrs Maze asked the doctor not to reveal the nature of her sickness to her husband because if he knew he would think of marrying another wife. In fact she told the doctor to tell her husband a lie about her condition. In the evening Mr Maze came to visit his wife and wanted to know what she was suffering from. The doctor did not want to tell a lie; at the same time he did not want to violate the rule of confidentiality and so he told Mr Maze that he could not disclose the nature of Mrs Maze's sickness.

Three days later, Mr Maze and his relatives went to the hospital to collect Mrs Maze, arguing that an *inyanga* (traditional healer) would heal her faster. The doctor who had admitted her was called in by the medical staff and he pleaded with them to leave her in the hospital. According to the doctor, what Mrs Maze needed was sleep and rest. Mrs Maze's husband and in-laws insisted on taking her. The doctor explained to Mrs Maze the seriousness of her condition and advised her to stay in the hospital, but Mrs Maze said that she wanted to go. The doctor tried to persuade her to stay, but she refused. In the end the doctor gave her a form to sign confirming that she was leaving against medical orders. She did, and her in-laws took her to the traditional healer.

Two weeks later Mrs Maze was returned to the hospital in a coma and having continuous convulsions. At the hospital the medical staff were divided as to whether she should be attended to or not, having brought herself to that condition. The doctor who had admitted her was called and immediately started giving her treatment, which annoyed those hospital staff members who had wanted her to be sent away. She died three hours later.

The four ethical principles are called into play in this case.

Autonomy

In African traditional ethics, autonomy, the ability to think and act independently and freely, is limited by the emphasis put on communalism. African societies emphasize interdependence and an individual's obligations to the community. An individual who disregards the family or the community and does what he or she thinks to be right, is regarded as anti-social. Thus, excessive individual autonomy is regarded as being a denial of one's corporate existence.

This should not be misunderstood to mean that a person does not have an individual existence, personality and a certain degree of autonomy. Communalism permits a degree of personal independence. In fact a person, in African ethical thinking, has to think and act independently. This is what distinguishes one person from another. A person who becomes famous and respected in the community as a hero or heroine, or as a virtuous person, is one who has proved to be superior to the ordinary person in some way, and has evolved a life plan of his or her own, achieving through his or her own efforts and ingenuity what is admired by the community. This life plan, however, is moulded in agreement with the traditional norms of the community. An individual has to strike a balance between creativity, originality and independence on the one hand, and conformity on the other.

Some members, however, must remain under the control, guidance and protection of the community, especially the mentally deformed, the insane, the senile, children and those who are temporarily unable to depend on themselves. Traditionally, women too were expected to be dependent on their husbands or fathers. This, however, has changed and women, especially those living in urban areas and working in the professions, have regained their independence and can act autonomously in many respects. The problem which remains, apart from male attitudes, seems to lie in the basic differentiation of male and female biological and social roles, and how to respect these without subordination. Mrs Maze was from a rural community where a woman still has to listen to and obey her husband and in-laws.

Quite apart from the dependent members of the community, African societies practise a high degree of paternalism. Although we have stated that African societies respect individual autonomy, and that a person is free to think and act independently, as long as his or her actions do not harm others or restrict their rights, this autonomy is not respected when the community believes that the person is acting against himself or herself. The community will restrict the free action of that individual for his or her own good. The good of the individual and of the group is more important than personal freedom or autonomy.

We need to keep in mind that, in the African concept of corporate existence, what harms an individual is considered harmful to the community. Thus it is accepted that it is right to interfere with a person's actions to prevent harm to others. Paternalistic intervention is justified on the grounds that the experience and knowledge of the elders should benefit the younger or less wise members of the community who might not understand the implications of their decisions or actions. Thus the communalistic value of mutual responsibility and caring often leads to paternalism.

One of the issues raised by the Mrs Maze case is confidentiality. A person's autonomy includes the right to privacy. In the hospital the health care worker has an obligation of confidentiality with regard to information about the diagnosis, treatment and prognosis of the patient's illness unless the patient has given permission to him or her to disclose them. Yet, because of the communal nature of African societies, relatives often want the doctor or nurse to let them know what the patient is suffering from, what treatment he or she is receiving and what the possible outcome of the treatment will be. Failure of the doctor or nurse to cooperate and reveal information sought by relatives can lead to the patient being 'stolen' from the ward by the relatives. This is perhaps the reason why Mr Maze and his relatives decided to take Mrs Maze out of the hospital to a traditional healer.

The second problem raised by this case is the freedom of the patient to choose the nature of medical care to be received. It was clear to the medical staff in the hospital that the traditional healers were not able to treat this case of pre-eclampsia. Many cases of this nature were known which, in the past, had been handled by traditional healers, leading to the death of the patient. All the patients with this disease who had been taken to traditional healers had either died or been returned to the hospital in a worse condition.

On the basis of respect for the autonomy of a patient to decide what treatment to receive, and from whom to receive it, Mrs Maze was allowed to go to a traditional healer and was accepted back by her doctor when she was returned. The cultural factor in respect for autonomy, however, is the group or communal influence on the patient. It may be argued, in relation to respect for autonomy as understood in western culture that insofar as an autonomous agent's actions do not infringe upon the autonomous actions of others, that person should be free to perform whatever action he or she wishes, even if it involves serious risk for the agent and even if others consider it to be foolish (4). This is not the case in African thinking. In African societies which emphasize corporate existence, a person is expected to conform to communal decisions.

It is debatable whether the decision of a patient should be respected when he or she 'decides' under the pressure of the family. Many people would say that a patient who decides or acts under the influence or pressure of his or her family is not acting autonomously. In Africa, however, autonomy, as we have noted, is both individual and communal.

In traditional health care usually it is the person providing the care, not the patient, who makes decisions on what action is to be taken. In this case Mrs Maze was given a chance to decide; a decision which cost her her life. The question is who should decide on the course of action in health care? Should it be the patient, the relatives or the doctor or nurse giving the care? The obvious answer is that there should be cooperation, and when possible agreement, among all the parties involved. The problem which still remains is, what happens when there is no agreement among them? This introduces the issue of competence in decision-making during health care.

In traditional health care it is common for the traditional healer or the family to decide for the patient. They may do something against his or her wishes or for his or her care without consulting him or her, if it is believed that what they are doing is for his or her good. Beneficence is a higher value than autonomy. However, health care is now complicated, especially when modern technology is involved. In many cases the patient and even the family do not have a minimal required knowledge of the problem and how to deal with it. Should the doctor, in such cases, not act without consulting the patient or the family or ignore their views for the good of the patient?

Beneficence

Following from the vital force principle, everyone has a duty to do good to his or her neighbour, especially to friends, relatives and clansmen, in order to promote the vital force. Generosity, kindness, hospitality, sharing and charity, all of which promote vital force, are basic values. In African ethics these beneficent qualities are not mere virtues, but duties. When one is in a position to do so, for example, one is duty-bound to give food to a stranger, unless doing so will mean someone else in the family going hungry. Not to do so is regarded as immoral. This is based on the conception of community as one family, with mutual obligations. It is done in order to preserve and enhance vital force, or to restore it when it has been disrupted.

One also has an obligation to prevent harm from happening, when one can. Members of the community must oppose any action which diminishes vital force or must apply remedies if the event has already occurred. Thus, in terms of health care, mutual obligation extends to preventive and curative medicine.

In order to promote or restore vital force, health care is highly valued. It should be emphasized, however, that when care is being administered the interests and needs of the patient are weighed against the good of the whole community. It is for this reason that people suffering from contagious diseases are traditionally isolated, or even helped to die, if they threaten the health of the community. The good of the patient is considered in the context of the good of all parties concerned, especially the good of the patient's immediate family.

As noted above, the concept of a person's wholeness underlies the African understanding of health and health care. The challenge to modern health care is that beneficence should not be directed only to the elimination of the disease, but rather it should be concerned with the patient's whole person and his or her social involvement in the community, in order to promote and enhance his or her ability to play his or her social role.

Non-maleficence

The vital force principle establishes the duty not to cause harm, injure or do anything that reduces the vital force of the individual members of the community or threatens its collective existence. One should not even refrain from doing what would stop harm being done to others. However, the vital force philosophy also recognizes the existence of abnormal and yet potentially powerful influences from minerals, plants, and animals, which can be manipulated as forces for evil or good. There are also human beings who are believed to harm others although unaware of their own power and unable to stop themselves. These are witches who, according to the traditional ethos, must be neutralized by rituals or even eliminated. Other people are harmful voluntarily; these include sorcerers and murderers, who are regarded as anti-social because they are anti-life and are therefore hated. In the past such people could openly be killed by the community in order to save the rest. These days, because of modern laws, their power is either 'neutralized' with Christian rituals or, when this fails, they are secretly killed. All anti-life forces, substances and people must be neutralized or even be eliminated in order to preserve and promote the vital force in the community.

In terms of health care the traditional healer and the community are required never to do harm to the patient unless it is in his or her best interests or for the good of the community. In modern health care this is a principle worth following; never to do harm to a patient unless the nurse or doctor, after serious consideration, believes that it is in the interests of the patient or it is necessary for the protection of other patients. According to African ethics, harm should be allowed only as a lesser evil or when all means to stop it have failed. In doing so justice, if possible, must be done.

Justice

Justice is highly valued in communal existence in order to maintain social order, peace and solidarity and to avoid disintegration of the community. Because of the communal nature of African societies, justice is first and foremost a social affair. An offence against an individual is an offence against the community, and for the good of the community everyone's needs must be attended to without discrimination. Health care is, consequently, made available to everyone according to his or her needs. Since health care, in a traditional setting, is simple and inexpensive this is easy to do.

African societies, however, emphasize a social hierarchy, consisting of, in descending order of prestige, kings, chiefs, religious specialists, grandparents and parents, older brothers and sisters down to the youngest member of the family and community. Justice, like any other aspect of society, is understood in hierarchical terms. It is giving or receiving what one deserves according to one's status in the community. No-one has rights other than those given him by membership in the community. Justice in African societies is based on each according to his or her needs and status in society.

In medical care, faced with patients whose interests or needs conflict, the doctor or nurse is faced with the dilemma of whose needs or interests should be attended to first. In the case of Mrs Maze, she was readmitted to the hospital in a critical condition requiring immediate attention, yet humanly speaking she was responsible for her own state, having refused to follow the doctor's advice. Was it fair for the doctor to leave the other patients in order to attend to her?

Was it fair that more expensive and intensive care, at the expense of *bona fide* patients, should have been afforded her, whereas if she had listened to the doctor probably all she would have needed was bed rest and probably occasional mild sedatives? However, the principle of justice had to be weighed against beneficence.

Availability of health care services is another moral challenge. The state has an obligation to provide at least a minimum standard of health care available to those in need of it. According to African ethical principles, once health care facilities are provided, accessibility should not be based on need alone, but also on status. Since ethical rules and principles often change with time and circumstances, this view is changing and emphasis is put on need more than on status. This, it is believed, is a more just and objective approach.

CONCLUSION

From the above discussion it is apparent that cultural and individual ethics influence people's understanding of health and health care activities. In providing health care these factors have to be taken into account so that the care given is adequate and relevant to the situations in which people live. In the African context, and in accordance with the traditional ethical values, health care should extend to the whole person, seriously taking into account the interdependence of the various aspects of a person. A patient should be helped, for example, to heal his fears, misunderstandings, quarrels, jealousies, hatreds and other factors which militate against health. Secondly, both the patient and the whole family should be involved in health care. This approach is extremely important in the application of the four principles if we are to avoid health care turning into a mechanical exercise, but instead want it to be a personal relationship with its part to play in the attempt to bring about wholesomeness for the person.

On the subject of autonomy, it is important that the patient's independence is respected in deciding the nature of health care to be provided, especially if he or she is competent to take a rational decision in the matter. However, unless the patient objects, his or her relatives, especially the close ones, should be regarded as part of the team which is involved in the patient's care; therefore they deserve to know about the patient's sickness and treatment, and should have a say in the whole healing process.

In some societies autonomy may be regarded as of higher value than beneficence, non-maleficence and justice. In general this should be respected. In African culture, however, beneficence has a higher value, which justifies paternalistic interventions either by the doctor, who is supposedly more knowledgeable than the patient in the matter, or by the family, who may be in better condition or position than the patient to judge wisely what is best for him or her.

In health care it is important to help those in need in order to enhance their vital force. In doing so, however, it is important to consider the social nature of a person and to balance the patient's needs, rights and interests with those of other patients, the family and the community as a whole.

It is also important to avoid any action or non-action which weakens the vital force and harms the patient. In African ethical thinking, however, harm may be done to avoid greater harm either to the patient or to the community as a whole.

In doing all this justice must prevail. Those in need of health care should receive it according to their respective needs. There are situations when social status, which is an important consideration in Africa, is not a relevant factor, i.e. when people's lives are threatened. In such cases it should not be a determining factor in the provision of health care. As elsewhere, in the matter of healing, those with equal needs should be treated equally and those with unequal needs should be treated unequally (4). Again this should be balanced with the general good of the community.

It should be emphasized, finally, that in African ethical thinking, of supreme and simultaneous importance is the good of the patient and the welfare of the community. Principles are secondary, and only a means to an end.

REFERENCES

1. Mbiti, J. 1969. *African religions and philosophy*, p. 101. Heinemann, Oxford.
2. Tempels, P. 1959. *Bantu philosophy*. Presence Africaine, Paris.
3. Gillon, R. 1985. (quoted). *Philosophical medical ethics*, p. 148. John Wiley & Sons, Chichester.
4. Beauchamp, T. L. and Childress, F. J. 1979. *Principles of biomedical ethics*, pp. 59, 174. Oxford University Press, New York.

17

Feminism and the Four Principles

REBECCA J. COOK, JD, LLM

Member of the Washington, D.C. Bar; Member, Ethics Committee of the International Federation of Gynecology and Obstetrics; Associate Professor (Research), Faculty of Law, Faculty of Medicine and Centre for Bioethics, University of Toronto, Canada

INTRODUCTION

What characterizes a feminist approach, whether to ethics, bioethics, health care, law or society, is an acceptance of a perspective that women have been and are oppressed, and that such oppression is morally and politically unacceptable. The challenge that feminists accept is to demonstrate the fact of women's subordination within the social systems in which they exist, to convince others that women are afforded less than just access to their fair entitlements, and to achieve reforms through recognition of the legitimacy of women's experiences in shaping a society to which women contribute equitably. In short, the feminist commitment is to the relief of women's oppression through the introduction of social fairness.

Readers unfamiliar with feminist analysis tend to react with shock, denial and outrage. Conscientious professionals who have made efforts to advance their prestige do not easily come to identify themselves as oppressors, and find feminist explanations of injustices, in which they might have been complicit, to be radical, extremist and 'shrill'. Equally, those who have become absorbed in feminist analysis and advocacy may lose vision of the virtues that health professionals have long manifested. Their demands for justice should not be made through unjust criticism.

The special obstacle to the feminist agenda is that the marginalization of women has been so pervasive that it has been traditionally accepted by both leaders and followers of social movements to constitute the natural order. That is, the subordinate and servile role of women has been invisible because it has been an essential feature of society itself. Women are defined as people who alone are responsible for rearing children, nurturing, supporting and comforting spouses and maintaining the welfare of the elderly, including their and sometimes their spouses' parents.

The disadvantage of women in many societies is perceived as a condition of the societies themselves, so that those who function within society cannot isolate themselves sufficiently to recognize women's systemic disadvantages, or conceive of how their societies could be structured differently. In this sense the challenge of feminism is a political challenge. Susan Sherwin has observed that

> Ours is a world permeated by sexism. In virtually every sphere of life, women's interests are systematically subordinated to those of men; and yet, these arrangements are so extensive, so familiar, and so entrenched in our habits of thought that it is possible not to notice them at all. Such all-encompassing exploitation is harmful to women. It is unjust and unacceptable (1).

The feminist perspective is critical of the fact, for instance, that religious institutions that make definitive statements on such matters as family life, contraception and abortion, which critically affect the control that women can exercise over not just their bodies but their very lives, frequently exclude women. For example, the Roman Catholic Church interprets its teachings to preclude the ordination of women, and speaks authoritatively from within the ranks of the ordained. Small, elite groups of men interpret the divine will to authorize the power of small, elite groups of men (2). Orthodox Judaism and Islamic sects are similarly exclusive of women, and attempts to accommodate women's equality within Judaism and some Islamic sects have met with resistance similar to the resistance within the Roman Catholic Church. Feminists question whether religions that exclude the full participation of women are credible in formulating ethics of human conduct and look to religious reconstructions that accommodate women's spiritual needs (3).

Similarly, the world of medicine has historically been dominated by a male standard of normality. Women's failure to share male satisfactions in life has disproportionately been analysed as psychopathological, and the research that has established standard physical responses has centred on men. Women's experiences with heart disease, cancers of the non-reproductive organs and, for instance, diabetes have tended to be inadequately researched (4,5) (see also Sherwin (1), pp. 158–175). It has been noted, for instance, that leading US legal cases in which patients' preferences regarding terminal care have been doubted or questioned have predominantly concerned women (6). Physical and psychological injuries caused by violence against women, including assaults by husbands, have been inadequately recognized, diagnosed and treated, in part because of the social stigma attached to the causes of such injuries* (7).

Some feminists, such as Karen Lebacqz, charge that

> medicine, like other social institutions, does not take women's moral agency seriously, and that traditional bioethics is deficient because it fails to recognize and address this gender gap. Traditional bioethics is often conducted as though

---

* See also Rosenberg *et al.* (8), explaining that assaults by husbands, ex-husbands and lovers cause more injuries to women than do motor vehicle accidents, rape, and mugging combined.

we all 'know' that medicine has a benign purpose: to heal disease. Such assumptions are challenged by feminists. Feminists charge that 'disease' itself is a social construction, that medicine has functioned not simply to heal disease but also to reinforce sex, class, and race stereotyping, and that the real question, therefore, is whether the institution and practice of medicine is good for women (9).

'Feminism' is the name given to the different theories that help to reveal the many gender-specific patterns of disadvantage of women that constitute their oppression, and is also the term that generally characterizes the movement to eliminate such forms of oppression. A feminist approach to ethics, and to such keys to an understanding of modern bioethics as the four principles, is not necessarily one that all women share. Similarly, the approach is not available exclusively to women. Not all women are feminists, and not all feminists are women.

Feminist commentators face the dilemma of seeking credibility among prevailing schools of philosophers and ethicists while some of their number demand and work for the overthrow of prevailing doctrines and institutions and their replacement by agencies sensitive to the impacts of policies and practices on women. The moderate middle ground that seeks reform towards necessary sensitization and the evolution of the *status quo* to the recognition of women as equal partners in their societies is unsatisfactory to those who favour radicalism, and to those who are distrustful or impatient of progressive reform.

FEMINIST THEORIES

Feminism is no more monolithic than are the philosophies and politics from which feminist analysts draw inspiration in explaining sexist structures of society and proposing reforms, compelled by justice. Distinctions may be drawn by using such labels as liberal, socialist, radical, cultural, lesbian, post-modern and, for instance, ecological feminism. Distinguishable and in some details mutually exclusive though such approaches are, most forms of feminism share many principal values; labels often exaggerate contrasts in order to establish boundaries or to link approaches with broader philosophical or political movements. Feminists of different persuasion frequently identify women's oppression with that experienced by people disadvantaged on such grounds as their race, colour or poverty.

Liberal feminism is derived from the general political theory of liberalism, and is committed to the legal and political reforms necessary to ensure that women enjoy rights and opportunities equal to those of men. Feminism is committed to emancipation through the destruction of oppressive patterns of social structure and functioning. Liberal feminists' commitment to a rights-based analysis and reform is opposed by more radical feminists who believe that rights are by definition claims staked within a given social order, and fail sufficiently to challenge prevailing social structures and relations (see, generally, Kingdom (10)). Rights that individuals can invoke to oblige others to observe duties can too easily become instruments of oppression of those others. Feminists are guarded, for instance, about movements to accord rights to fetuses, since those rights are frequently invoked by those whose purpose is to regulate how women may behave when they are, or are liable to be, pregnant.

Socialist feminists frequently draw on socialist or Marxian analysis that shows how dominant groups in society use economic, legal and related power to protect their privilege and sustain subordination of the oppressed. Replacing capitalist institutions as oppressors are male-dominated institutions, although capitalist, bourgeois and patriarchal institutions themselves can be shown to have been repressive of the distinctive influences of women, and to accommodate only women who are obedient to male authority. Socialist feminists tend to be suspicious and critical of pharmaceutical entrepreneurship, for example, especially through promoting therapeutic and cosmetic drug use among women, and internationally question the promotion in developing countries of pharmaceutical products and, for instance, infant formula, to enrich corporations of the industrialized world.

Cultural feminists embrace the view that there is an essential female nature distinguishable from the male nature. They challenge feminists who urge sex-neutrality and political asexualism by asserting that women speak and hear 'in a different voice' (see, generally, Gilligan (11)). They claim that, in contrast to a rights-based ethics, female and male feminists are motivated by an ethics of caring for individuals who are affected by decisions. Rather than 'let justice be done though the heavens may fall', they would risk inconsistency among objectively similar cases by resolving them according to the different needs, desires and aspirations of the different actors within such cases, which, because of those differences, are considered not to be similar to each other. Caring resolutions may be different in their outcomes, but are linked through the personal regard and respect given to individuals (12).

FEMINIST APPROACHES TO THE FOUR PRINCIPLES

Feminist orientations to bioethics do not necessarily reject the four principles, but address them through their potential to promote women's interests in self-determination and in injecting their experiences in life and insights into the reconstruction of their societies. The significance of the four principles to women can be approached by what has been described in feminist jurisprudence as 'asking the woman question'. What Katherine Bartlett says of law is equally applicable to health care and bioethics. She states that:

> asking the woman question means examining how the law fails to take into account the experiences and values that seem more typical of women than of men, for whatever reason, or how existing legal standards and concepts might disadvantage women. The question assumes that some features of the law may be not only non-neutral in a general sense, but also 'male' in a specific sense. The purpose of the woman question is to expose those features and how they operate, and to suggest how they might be corrected (13).

Similarly, the application of the four principles bears analysis in light of impacts on women and the potential for correction.

Respect for Persons

Feminists endorse the principle of respect for persons, but conditionally on 'person' being recognized to include all human beings. Both law and culture disclose understandings of the word or status 'person' that did not include women.* Too often, women have been considered to be less than full persons, and to lack the capacity of persons because they make decisions conditioned by their own experiences and perceptions, which differ from those of persons who are accustomed to the role of authoritative decision-maker, particularly in hospital and medical clinic settings. Practices remain of health facilities seeking husbands' authorizations for health care requested by women, for instance concerning family planning, when wives are not similarly approached regarding procedures requested by husbands (14).

Women find it incongruous that the same agencies that have failed to consider women fully fledged persons sometimes deliberate about whether fetuses are persons. The emergence of the 'fetal patient' is positive and protective in anticipating the health circumstances that will affect children to be born. However, health professionals have been seen to subordinate the interests of women patients who seek their help to the interests of such women's fetuses, of which the health professionals appoint themselves protectors. That is, fetal rights are invoked to diminish the respect that is paid to decisions that women make regarding the health and welfare of their families (15).

Autonomy

The principle of autonomy may promise women true self-determination, but feminist approaches distinguish circumstances to which it is appropriate. Autonomy is appropriate to relationships between strangers and to purely professional relationships, in contrast to relationships based on what feminists describe as connectedness. Women find connectedness to characterize the lives and experiences of women, symbolized initially in the umbilical cord through which all human beings survive, and projected through bonding of mother and child and women's discharge of the caring, nursing and nurturing role, including care of sick relatives and dependent parents.

Feminists consider the independence and isolation implicit in autonomy to be based on male-derived values, reflected in such idealized abstractions as 'the reasonable man'. Susan Sherwin (1) expresses scepticism about the priority that is accorded to autonomy, since it is alien to women's experience. She observes that:

> Ethical models based on the image of ahistorical, self-sufficient, atom-like individuals are simply not credible to most women. Because women are usually charged with

---

* *In the matter of a reference as to the meaning of the word 'Persons' in section 24 of the British North American Act, 1867* [1928] S. C. R. 276: Supreme Court of Canada ruled that women are not among the 'qualified persons' who may be called to the Senate under the terms of the B. N. A. Act, since that Act was passed in 1867 when women had no legal capacity. Reversed by the Privy Council in *Henrietta Muir Edwards v. A. G. for Canada* [1930] A. C. 124.

the responsibility of caring for children, the elderly, and the ill as well as the responsibility of physically and emotionally nurturing men both at work and at home, most women experience the world as a complex web of interdependent relationships, where responsible caring for others is implicit in their moral lives. The abstract reasoning of morality on the rights of independent agents is inadequate for the moral reality in which they live (p. 47).

Reinforcing this feminist scepticism in health care is a perception that autonomy is inappropriately emphasized when people are sick and critically dependent on others for comfort, sustenance and the means of life itself. Nevertheless, the right to respect for autonomy is seen to afford women a potential for the same respect that men enjoy to protect their physical integrity and resist patriarchal control exercised under claims of protecting people incapable of autonomy, and of protecting fetuses that fall under the allegedly unreliable judgement of the women who bear them. Autonomy fails not necessarily in principle, but in practice; historically, health professions have disregarded or distrusted women's right to or capacity for autonomy.

Jennifer Nedelsky urges a view of autonomy that is conducive to the reality of women's lives, not as atomistic individuals, but as related to family, friends and community. She explains that '[w]e see that relatedness is not, as our tradition teaches, the antithesis of autonomy, but a literal precondition of autonomy, and interdependence a constant component of autonomy' (16). This is a sense in which feminists may support and apply the ethical principle of autonomy in health care decision making, and women's status as ethical agents.

Recognition of women as ethical agents in their own health care arises when women can volunteer to accept the risks of being subjects of medical research. Misdirected paternalism has caused both investigators and research ethics review committees to exclude from pharmaceutical and other research protocols women who were or who might become pregnant, for fear that they would experience fetal damage through participation. The result has been the approval and marketing of products that were never tested on adult women, so that their safety, efficacy and interaction with women's physiology were unknown, although they are prescribed for women, frequently more often than for men. In the United States since 1986, the National Institutes of Health and the Alcohol, Drug Abuse, and Mental Health Administration have required that clinical research findings should be of benefit to all persons at risk, regardless of sex (17).

The ethical right of women to volunteer to be subjects in health research of concern to them, based on their informed choice and judgement of the effect of participation on their pregnancies, will be respected under the principle of autonomy. That is, women's informed autonomy and beneficence aimed at other women will be given priority over investigators' and review committees' beneficence aimed at potential fetuses and protectiveness or paternalism aimed at women. Further, justice will be served in that women, as intended beneficiaries of research, will accept the burden of deciding on its risks. This remains subject to the general principle that some risks of injury may be so great that no investigator or review committee may conscientiously invite even an informed potential subject to take them.

Protection of the Vulnerable

Feminists are not of one mind concerning women's entitlement to protection because of their vulnerability. Some take the normative approach that women should not be considered incapable of autonomy, and therefore vulnerable, but should be treated as capable of informed self-determination. Others take an approach based on the experience of women's long subjection to patriarchy. They point, for instance, to women's lower rates of literacy and education than men, their lack of experience in operating political and legislative systems in their self-interest, and their absence, silence or under-representation among leaders of traditional religious institutions. They therefore consider women vulnerable to exploitation by professional and quack health service entrepreneurs who promote diets, fitness programmes, cosmetic enhancements such as breast implants, and techniques of assisted reproduction. Some, indeed, claim that women have been brainwashed into believing that they are unfulfilled unless they have children, and that they owe it to themselves and their partners to explore every medical means of achieving parenthood, particularly through recourse to the new reproductive technologies (18). In contrast, however, some feminists reject a Luddite approach to reproductive technologies, and trust women to exercise judgement without the need for paternalistic protection, and to acquire the information they find that they need for this purpose (19).

Where feminists of different persuasion find common ground is on the need to focus on the causes of women's vulnerability in order to enable vulnerable women to exercise autonomy. The conditions and policies that facilitate autonomy will vary according to the degree and kind of exploitation that women have experienced, and cannot be exclusively dependent on a signed informed consent sheet.

Beneficence

The ethical duty of beneficence poses the question for feminist analysts of determination of the 'good' that it is mandatory to pursue. Answers will be found according to the inspiration of different schools of feminist theory. Liberal feminists define good according to liberal values, and, for instance, socialist feminists identify good through socialist principles. The different approaches have in common their commitment to asking the woman question (11).

A frequent dilemma in beneficence is that health policies and practices that are beneficial for some are non-beneficial or even harmful to the interests of others. A modern expression of this incompatibility of interests arises in so-called 'maternal–fetal' conflict. This is characterized by mothers who resist pre-natal care or Caesarean deliveries that health professionals consider essential for the welfare of their fetuses. It also appears in instances in which women intend to pursue use of alcohol, tobacco or prescription or illicit drugs during pregnancy, or intend to pursue employments in work environments that pose a danger to the children they are gestating. Respect for women's autonomy may prejudice the children to which they will give birth, but to constrain them in order to compel protection of their fetuses would require oppressive and perhaps physically invasive non-consensual treatment, which itself may pose risks to such women and compromise the welfare of others who depend on them, for instance for economic support.

A beneficent perspective on this dilemma is one in which the maternal–fetal relationship is viewed not as adversarial in nature but as an interaction in which the needs of one define the needs of both (20). The adversarial view of pregnancy is a regrettable but persisting legacy of the abortion debate, which pits a woman against her fetus and interprets her quest for self-determination as contrary to the best interests of the fetus. The woman's behaviour or intentions may be considered deviant, and by legal or other means of intervention she may be compelled to observe a discipline that will give effect to intervenors' views of her responsibility. In reality, a balance must often be struck regarding choice of abortion between the interests not only of the woman and her fetus but also between those of other children for whom she is responsible and of other children as yet unconceived whose future would be better assured by therapeutic birth spacing.* Further interests may have to be balanced of a spouse and of elderly parents or other relatives of the woman or her husband.

Beneficence requires a reformed understanding of pregnancy as affecting an interconnected and interactive unit (see King (20), p. 614) and affecting the functioning of a family unit. Fetus and woman are vulnerable to forces that have an impact on the woman's body, and when the woman is treated well the fetus shares the advantage. For instance, policies of fetal protection should at least include adequate prenatal and nutritional care for the woman, whose collaboration should be invited and encouraged rather than coerced. Law may play a role by requiring that women working to support families be assured of paid maternity leave, and no job discrimination on return to work. More enlightened schemes may require public or employment-related day care services for dependent children of working parents. Any policies aimed at fetal protection cannot be developed in isolation from women and should respect the role of women as mothers.

Similarly, the resolution of conflicting interests within a family triggered or aggravated by pregnancy should be resolved in ways that respect and reinforce the integrity and cohesion of the family unit, and not risk these values by the coercive interventions of strangers and their ideological agendas. Pressures to risk the welfare of unborn children, like pressures to abort pregnancies, are frequently related to economic necessity and the taint of social stigma associated with pregnancy out of marriage. Agencies anxious to coerce pregnant women to observe behavioural discipline are sometimes conservatively resistant to women in the workforce, and critical of sex and pregnancy out of wedlock. Beneficent obligations require at least a non-judgemental approach, and reconsideration of attitudes and characterizations that seek to promote benefits to one interest while ignoring or suppressing measurement of the costs imposed on others.

---

* In general, one in five infant deaths could be averted if children were spaced more than two years apart (21).

Non-maleficence

The ethical duty of non-maleficence is the principle to which physicians claim that they are most responsive, because of their historical acceptance of the mandate to do no harm. The Hippocratic oath that established and reinforces this mandate also illuminates, however, areas in which physicians may be liable to violate it. The oath is explicit concerning the obligations of physicians not to abuse access to their patients' bodies to satisfy their sexual appetites or curiosity. Modern reports indicate, however, physicians taking sexual advantage of patients, sometimes by female physicians of male patients, sometimes homosexually, but in the overwhelming preponderance of cases by male physicians taking advantage of female patients (22). Medical associations and licensing authorities have until recently not been sensitive to the incidence of sexual abuse of patients, and have appeared sceptical or hostile to complaints, rationalizing them as expressions of women's emotionalism, spite over doctors' rejection of their affection (ref. 22, p. 166) or hysteria.* Abuse of female patients ranges from indifference to their embarrassment or compelled immodesty through to cynical and exploitative sexual intercourse repeated over long durations.

Sensitivities to how men treat women are particularly acute in feminist analysis, and may at times approach extremes. In observing the traditional imbalance of power and authority between the sexes that favours men, feminist commentators accurately identify the capacity for exploitation that has been associated with the historically male institution of medicine, demonstrated in the refusal of medical schools until quite recent times to consider women suitable for admission. The more extreme feminist critics may perceive as exploitation, however, or as sexual harassment, familiar courtship patterns between doctors and nurses, junior instructors and graduate students and office personnel and secretarial staff. However, authentic courtship is usually distinguishable from professional misconduct by physicians with those in dependent patient relationships with them. Professional licensing authorities and medical associations have tended to pay lip-service to duties of sexual non-exploitation, occasionally satisfying themselves with severe punishments of blatant cases, but have not been proactive in monitoring physicians' conduct, or facilitating complainants to come forward and be heard in an environment that finds them credible.

It is a general complaint that, while men are seen as individuals and their failings as personal traits, women tend to be seen as representatives of their sex, and their failings to be typical of women. In health care, women similarly tend to be seen less as individuals than as representatives. Further, women tend to be stereotyped by the extreme ends of a spectrum. Their complaints have often been dismissed or trivialized, including by attributing complaints of physiological conditions to emotional causes, or dissatisfactions (see Carter (23), pp. 179–180). Another extreme stereotype views women as sources of infection of men, particularly women who have sex with more than one man, and are therefore 'promiscuous' or prostitutes. This stereotype, and health policies based

---

* Historically related to disorders of the womb, see Carter (23). Freud based much of his work on cases of sexual neurosis associated with hysteria.

upon the stereotype, have evolved regardless of the epidemiological data of sexually transmitted diseases in a given subpopulation of men or women. For example, between 1918 and 1920 more than 18 000 women suspected of prostitution were detained in the United States by governmental initiative for fear that they would spread venereal disease especially to returning soldiers and sailors conscripted to fight in World War I (24). A response to modern concerns with AIDS and HIV infection has recycled the image of women 'not as individuals, but merely as vectors of virus transmission' (25).

HIV infection also confirms the way in which women are harmed by being considered through stereotypes (26). AIDS is seen pre-eminently as an infection of men (27), and women's need for protection and treatment is a low priority. Indeed, protection of women through the promotion of condom use has been actively resisted by church and other conservative agencies that consider publicizing means of safer sex to endanger public morality (28). Condom availability is of little avail, however, where men consider their use unmanly or unpleasurable, and women cannot deny them unprotected sex for fear of violence or abandonment of them and their dependent children (29). Ignorance and denial by health professionals of women's vulnerability to coerced sex, particularly in jurisdictions that continue to accept husbands' criminal immunity for rape of their wives, aggravates women's hardship. Women using female-dependent barrier methods have been shown to be significantly more effective in preventing sexually transmitted diseases than those relying on condoms (30). In ideal circumstances where women have equal negotiating powers with their sexual partners, the condom could protect much more.

Only recently has attention been given to the very small amount of information available from clinical studies on HIV infection regarding the effects of disease processes or medical interventions on women (31). It has further been observed that:

> the original interest in HIV-infected women centered on their relation to paediatric AIDS through perinatal transmission. A search of the medical literature yields only a handful of papers focusing on the consequences of the infection in nonpregnant women (32).

In some communities where health professionals discriminate in services to HIV-infected patients, women's liability to HIV infection has been recognized by health professionals to women's detriment. Gynaecological examinations, prenatal care, abortions and services in childbirth may become unavailable to women who are HIV positive, or who are suspected of being HIV positive, perhaps because of the status or lifestyle of their partners. Health professionals have been seen to react judgementally to patients who engage in high-risk behaviour for suffering or transmitting HIV infection, without being subject to discipline for professional misconduct or violation of their employing institutions' bylaws or regulations (33,34).

Justice

An obligation of justice to treat like case alike and different cases with acknowledgement of the differences raises the question for feminist analysis of whether men and women are to be treated essentially as alike notwithstanding genetic, hormonal and reproductive differences, or whether women are so unlike men, for instance in the way they conceive of reality, experience life and relate to others, that they should be treated as different from men. The risk to women of finding men and women essentially like each other is that the model for their treatment will be the male model. It is already observable that women who do not meet male standards of performance and reaction will be considered pathological or paternalistically regarded as 'the weaker sex'. There is equal danger, however, that treating women differently from men will take effect not on a horizontal plane of equality but on a vertical plane of superiority and inferiority, women occupying the lower, subordinate and passive position.

A branch of feminist analysis has been seen that claims that women experience, perceive and express relationships 'in a different voice' (11). This leads to the ethical conclusion that it is proper that women should be treated differently from men but with equal respect taking due account of differences. Instances abound, however, of women being offered and receiving health services differently from men in a tradition of medical paternalism. Feminist sensitization to the obligation to apply health services justly compels acceptance of the challenge to render health care to women that is different but equal, recognizing how claims to provide services by this standard have failed in US treatment of its black population, and in *apartheid*. These instances illustrate through race the oppression that women have suffered through sex, and the comparable challenge, constituting political revolution, of just reform.

The ethical principle of distributive justice has greater significance for feminist analysis. In nurturing their children, husbands and elderly family members, women are health care workers. Their status as such is rarely recognized, valued or paid. Women are expected to understand and apply the advice (commonly described as 'orders') of doctors and other health professionals, but are considered their inferiors in awareness and status. Further, having devoted their lives as 'non-working' homemakers to rearing and nurturing others, the present generation of elderly people constituting the geriatric population in western countries, among whom women are the overwhelming majority, are being told that health services for them will be the first to be limited (35). That is, the last generation of women who rendered unpaid care to others will be the first to be denied medical services under the impact of financial economy in health care.

Bioethicists addressing rationing by age have paid little attention to the differential impact of their proposals on women. The argument in favour of inter-generational justice is that distinctions drawn by age are unlike distinctions drawn on race, sex or culture in that individuals progress in life through different ages, whereas other distinctions are constant. Accordingly, a health policy favouring expenditures on the young in order to enhance their prospects to survive to middle years and advanced age may be just, in that all individuals would receive comparable lifetime benefits, distribution being allocated more at the earlier than the later ages of life. The policy would nevertheless have a differential impact on women where demographic evidence shows a significantly greater proportion of women who reach advanced age. Implementation of such a programme of inter-generational justice would require a concurrent affirmative action component to redress the disproportionate impact that would be felt by a generation of women who did not receive health benefits when they were young, and who may be the first generation to be denied them because they are old.

An injustice already visited disproportionately upon women has resulted from policies of de-institutionalization of mental health patients, community care of long-term patients and those undergoing rehabilitation, and growing preferences that hospital care be delivered on an out-patient rather than an in-patient basis. Each of these policies has burdened women who serve as the unpaid and frequently unacknowledged care-givers in their families. The care they give is often given lovingly, but at a cost to them and their future well-being, including their physical and emotional well-being and their economic well-being when they give up pensionable employment, that goes unrecognized. This is not to argue that such policies are misguided or driven only by a governmental incentive to save expenditures, but to argue that the interests of women should be more justly represented in advisory and decision-making tribunals. A response that decision-making tribunals are democratically composed and accountable is not sufficient while women lack political opportunities to influence decisions proportionately to the impact that decisions make on them. Oppression by a democratic majority remains oppression, and violates the ethical duty to act with justice and not merely by exercise of political and legal power.

CONCLUSION

The purpose of feminist analysis in health care to achieve just recognition of women's concerns can be implemented and advanced through recourse to the four principles. They are not the only means to this end, but they serve helpfully to demonstrate proper goals of health care ethics, and means of analysis by which feminist bioethics can be advanced; that is, they may serve both as destination and vehicle. The four principles have emerged from a comparatively limited environment in which women were under-represented, but they have the potential to grow instrumentally in feminist hands. Health professionals and others who claim the inspiration of the four principles can be required to show that they apply them to achieve the vision of ethical conduct held within the different schools of feminist theory.

The four principles can have a widening and liberating effect in that they can permit feminist analysts to explain their criticisms of and ambitions for health care through concepts and language with which non-feminists are familiar, and can make clear to feminists the concepts and orientations that others apply to reach the conclusions they hold. The four principles can thereby serve as a *lingua franca* or common language through which differently directed analysts of the ethics of health care can explain themselves and comprehend each other. They can offer a universal ethical language in which to 'ask the woman question'.

They may serve to resolve misunderstandings and even antagonisms, and expose the goodwill that different and even opposing analysts bring to their tasks, and thereby encourage dialogue and wider discussion conducted in good faith.

ACKNOWLEDGEMENT

The author is grateful to Sir Malcolm Macnaughton, Vice-Chair of the Ethics Committee of the International Federation of Gynecology and Obstetrics, for comments on an earlier draft of this chapter. The author is solely responsible for the views expressed in this chapter.

REFERENCES

1. Sherwin, S. 1992. *No longer patient: feminist ethics and health care*, p. 13. Temple University Press, Philadelphia, PA.
2. Ranke-Heinemann, U. 1990. *Eunuchs for the Kingdom of Heaven: women, sexuality and the Catholic Church.* (Peter Heinegg translation). Doubleday, New York.
3. Ruether, R. R. 1983. Sexism, religion, and the social and spiritual liberation of women today. Pp. 107–122, *in* Gould, C. C. (Ed.) *Beyond domination: new perspectives on women and philosophy*, at p. 117. Rowman & Allanheld, Totowa, NJ.
4. Council on Ethical and Judicial Affairs, American Medical Association. 1990. Gender disparities in clinical decision making. *Journal of the American Medical Association* **266**: 559–562.
5. Society for the Advancement of Women's Health Research. 1991. Towards a women's health research agenda: findings of the Scientific Advisory Meeting. Society for the Advancement of Women's Health Research, Washington, DC.
6. Miles, S. H. and August, A. 1990. Courts, gender and the right to die. *Law, Medicine and Health Care* **18**: 85–95.
7. White, D. G. 1991. Wearing a wife-assault button: impact on family practice. *Canadian Medical Association Journal* **145**: 1005–1012.
8. Rosenberg, M. L., Stark, E. and Zahn, M. A. 1986. Interpersonal violence: homicide and spouse abuse. Pp. 1399–1426, *in* Last, J. M. (Ed.) *Public health and preventive medicine*, 12th edn. Appleton-Century-Crofts, Norwalk, CT.
9. Lebacqz, K. 1991. Feminism and bioethics: an overview. *Second Opinion* **17**(2): 11–25 at p. 16.
10. Kingdom, E. 1991: *What's wrong with rights? Problems for feminist politics of law.* Edinburgh University Press, Edinburgh.
11. Gilligan, C. 1982. *In a different voice: psychological theory and women's moral development.* Harvard University Press, Cambridge, MA.
12. Noddings, N. 1984. *Caring: a feminine approach to ethics and moral education*, p. 5. University of California Press, Berkeley, CA.
13. Bartlett, K. T. 1990. Feminist legal methods. *Harvard Law Review* **103**: 829–888 at p. 837.
14. Cook, R. J. and Maine, D. 1987 Spousal veto over family planning services. *American Journal of Public Health* **77**: 339–344.
15. Field, M. A. 1989. Controlling the woman to protect the fetus. *Law, Medicine and Health Care* **17**: 114–129.
16. Nedelsky, J. 1989. Reconceiving autonomy: sources, thoughts and possibilities. *Yale Journal of Law and Feminism* **1**: 7–36 at p. 12.
17. *National Institutes of Health Guide*, Vol. 19 (31), 24 August 1990, p. 18.
18. Corea, G. 1985. *The mother machine: reproductive technologies from artificial insemination to artificial wombs.* Harper & Row, New York.
19. Andrews, L. 1989. *Between strangers: surrogate mothers, expectant fathers and brave new babies.* Harper & Row, New York.

20. King, P. A. 1991. Helping women helping children: drug policy and future generations. *Milbank Quarterly* **69**: 595–621.
21. Maine, D. and McNamara, R. 1985. *Birth spacing and child survival*. Centre for Population and Family Health, Columbia University, New York.
22. Task Forces on Sexual Abuse of Patients: Final Report, 1991. An Independent Task Force Commissioned by The College of Physicians and Surgeons of Ontario (Chair: Marilou McPhedran).
23. Carter, R. B. 1853. *On the pathology and treatment of hysteria*. Churchill, London.
24. Brandt, A. M. 1985. *No magic bullet: a social history of venereal disease*. Oxford University Press, New York.
25. Mitchell, J. L. 1988. Women, AIDS, and Public Policy. *AIDS and Public Policy Journal* **3**(2): 50.
26. Overall, C. 1991. AIDS and women: the (hetero)sexual politics of HIV infection. Pp. 27–42, *in* Zion, W. P. (Ed.) *Perspectives on AIDS: ethical and social issues*. Oxford University Press, Oxford.
27. Murphy, J. S. 1988. Women with AIDS: sexual ethics in an epidemic. Pp. 65–66, *in* Corless, I. B. and Pittman-Lindeman, M. (Eds) *AIDS: principles, practices, and politics*. Hemisphere, New York.
28. Aiken, J. H. 1987. Education as prevention. Pp. 90–105, *in* Dalton, H. L., Burris, S. and the Yale AIDS Law Project (Eds) *AIDS and the law*. Yale University Press, New Haven, CT.
29. Stein, Z. A. 1990. HIV prevention: the need for methods women can use. *American Journal of Public Health* **80**: 460–462.
30. Rosenberg, M. J., Davidson, A. J., Chen, J. H., Judson, F. N. and Douglas, J. M. 1992. Barrier contraceptives and sexually transmitted diseases in women: a comparison of female-dependent methods and condoms. *American Journal of Public Health* **82**: 669–674.
31. Minkoff, M. L. and DeHovitz, J. A. 1991. Care of women infected with the human immunodeficiency virus. *Journal of the American Medical Association* **266**: 2253–2258.
32. Mitchell, J. L., Tucker, J., Loftman, P. O. and Williams, S. B. 1992. HIV and women: current controversies and clinical relevance. *Journal of Women's Health* **1**: 35–39 at pp. 35–36.
33. Gillon, R. 1987. Refusal to treat AIDS and HIV positive patients. *British Medical Journal* **294**: 1332–1333.
34. Melica, F. 1992. Fear of contracting HIV infection and ethical behaviour in medical care. Pp. 178–182, *in* Melica, F. (Ed.) *AIDS and human reproduction*. Karger, Basel.
35. Bell, N. K. 1989. What setting limits may mean: a feminist critique of Daniel Callahan's Setting Limits. *Hypatia* **4**(2): 167–178.

18

The Four Principles and Narrative Ethics

HOWARD BRODY, MD, PhD

Director, Center for Ethics and Humanities in the Life Sciences; Professor, Family Practice and Philosophy, Michigan State University, USA

INTRODUCTION

I have spent nearly 20 years seriously thinking about medical ethics. During the first portion of that time I assumed that any approach to ethics, if it were to be philosophically rigorous and if it were to appeal to the scientific sensibilities of doctors, would include some framework of formal reasoning, of which the four principles constitute one example. Indeed I prepared a textbook of medical ethics which began with a diagram of a sequential method, roughly a preference–consequentialist approach (1).

More recently I have become convinced that formal frameworks, for all their value, need to be supplemented with other ethical approaches, based more on interpretation and judgement than on formal deduction or algorithm. My shift in viewpoint derives from two sources. First, my own work as an ethics consultant and as a member of a hospital ethics committee has caused me to join similarly placed colleagues in finding that formal methods of ethical reasoning describe very poorly our actual day-to-day practices. Second, I have been influenced by theoretical movements in ethics in the USA, of the sort that have been somewhat harshly labeled as 'anti-theory' (2).

The alternative description of what ought to happen in ethical reasoning in health care settings could go by various names. Elsewhere I have suggested a 'conversation model' (3,4). For this chapter I will adopt the term 'narrative ethics'. I will address three questions:

1. What is narrative ethics?
2. How does narrative ethics fit in with contemporary criticisms of the four principles and other formal approaches?
3. What role would the four principles play within a narrative-ethics approach?

Principles of Health Care Ethics. Edited by Raanan Gillon.
© 1994 John Wiley & Sons Ltd

WHAT IS NARRATIVE ETHICS?

The meaning of narrative ethics will become clear by contrast with what I have been calling 'formal approaches', which have the following characteristics:

1. A small number of very general principles or concepts promise to provide an ethical resolution to the entire range of cases one will encounter.
2. Rational manipulation of the principles or concepts is the philosophically interesting task, on which most energy is focused in typical ethics courses. Fitting the particular facts of any case into the formal framework is a fairly mechanical exercise requiring much less philosophical insight.
3. The unit of ethical analysis is the single case or the single moral decision.
4. The key facts of the case can usually be summarized in a paragraph or two. Details regarding the life histories and prior experiences of the participants, or the social and cultural setting in which the case occurs, are seldom critical in applying the general principles.
5. Ethical analysis is an intellectual, dispassionate exercise. Emotion is to be avoided as it is likely to cloud objectivity.

Narrative ethics, by contrast, may be characterized as follows:

1. Decisions require a detailed inquiry into the case and into its historical and cultural context and antecedents. No single formal framework can be predicted to yield a sound resolution, *in advance of* knowing the specific facts of the case.
2. Ethical case analysis can be rational and rigorous, but not according to a deductive or mathematical model. Skills include:
   (a) *interpretation* of what the particular facts of the case mean, within the specific context and history;
   (b) *reasoning by analogy* with other cases, to catalogue the similarities and dissimilarities and ultimately to draw insights into the resolution of this case.
3. Combining the above two points reveals that, after all the facts of the case are known, one can arrive at a sound resolution and give good reasons in defense of that resolution. However, before one heard the facts one could not have predicted exactly which aspects of the case would be morally weighty in reaching a conclusion and which morally trivial.
4. Ethical reasoning cannot focus solely upon a single case or decision. Issues of moral character are also critical; and these involve questions of what it means to live a complete life in such a way that one's actions embody one's core moral values and commitments.
5. When one knows the detailed story of a situation, one is likely to find oneself identifying emotionally with the participants. This is an aid to ethical insight, not a threat to objectivity, since it is often through such empathy that one first glimpses a morally critical factor in the case.

This approach to ethics is *narrative* in the sense that one tries to decide what to do in a given case by telling a very detailed story about that case; and one tries to decide on issues of moral character and integrity by telling a detailed story of a person's life. Facts acquire moral significance not because they fit into a particular slot in a general moral framework, but rather because they hang together with other facts in the story, and the 'plot' of the story reveals the critical interconnections. While this analogy should not be overdrawn, it may be illustrative to compare this mode of ethical analysis to literary criticism. The good critic, presented with a story or a novel, can tell whether it is complete or incomplete, and whether it is well constructed or whether it is full of loose ends. Moreover, the critic can give fairly rigorous and scholarly reasons to support these judgements. But the critic cannot describe any formal framework of reasoning that will unerringly provide a thorough analysis of a piece of writing that has not yet been seen; and still less can the critic produce an algorithm that will generate a 'good' story from scratch.

A CASE EXAMPLE

The difference between the two ethical modes may be illustrated further by a case study:

> Mrs L.W. is a 58-year-old woman who has been treated for the past two years for lymphoma. Initially she did well, but recently the malignancy has recurred and spread. The doctor presented the options for treatment, including a new course of aggressive chemotherapy, but indicated that the likelihood of success was limited and that the treatment was quite toxic. Mrs L.W. stated that she did not want another course of chemotherapy, and instead would like to go home, be with her family, and receive palliative treatment for any symptoms that might develop. But after three days, following discussions with her husband, her sister, and her three children, Mrs L.W. announces that she has changed her mind and wishes to receive chemotherapy, to the surprise (and chagrin) of the doctor.

A formal approach to this case would focus upon respect for autonomy, beneficence, and non-maleficence. (This assumes that the chemotherapy is not a scarce medical resource; else considerations of justice might also enter the picture.) To apply these principles to the case, the following facts seem pertinent:

1. Mrs L.W.'s prognosis with and without chemotherapy.
2. Mrs L.W.'s personal preference for treatment.
3. Mrs L.W.'s mental capacities and ability to choose rationally.
4. The nature of the discussion with family members, including the possibility of manipulation or coercion being applied to Mrs L.W. by others.

If these facts are 'fed into' the formal reasoning method, some conclusions emerge. The doctor, motivated by beneficence and non-maleficence, would have preferred that Mrs L.W. avoid chemotherapy as he feels that the toxicity will probably outweigh any positive effect upon the course of the disease. However, the doctor feels obligated to honor Mrs L.W.'s request so long as he is convinced that her choice was truly autonomous. To judge this he has to consider two possibilities. First, perhaps Mrs L.W. really wanted not to have the treatment, but the family members, motivated by guilt or fear, wished her to have it and succeeded in putting enough pressure on her to make her change her mind. Second, perhaps Mrs L.W.'s initial refusal of treatment was not fully consistent with her own well-established values; by discussing matters with her family she was reminded of her true value commitments and came to see that they would best be furthered by accepting chemotherapy. The case description does not provide the precise facts needed to resolve this question; but further discussion with Mrs L.W. with and without her family present will probably bring these additional facts to light. At any rate, if the doctor thinks Mrs L.W. was manipulated by her family members, he would appear obligated not to begin administering treatment until this issue is clarified.

Narrative ethics would probably, in the end, come to some of the same conclusions, but it would look very differently upon at least one aspect of the case—the role of the family in the decision. How would I approach a momentous decision in my own life? First, I am conscious at some level of wanting my life to unfold in a coherent narrative. I want my actions to appear reasonable and responsible, as the sorts of things that the principal character in my life story would do, given what we know of his past history, his value commitments, and his relationships with others. I do not want my actions to appear as whimsical or aberrant. Moreover, I want my life story to be the story of a person who cares what his close associates think of him. If the only action I could take with a good conscience would be one that all my family and friends would condemn, then perhaps I would follow my moral integrity rather than their opinions of me; but in the more usual case, how my associates would react to my choices would be a serious factor in the decision I eventually make.

Now, how will I know what decision seems best to fit with the history and the character of the principal figure in my life story; and how will I know how my associates will respond to my decision? Typically this requires fairly extended conversation. I may have to 'try on' different choices, both to see how my family and friends react to them, and also to see how well I can envision myself following out that course of action. Perhaps my family will initially be opposed to a choice, but will come around to support it after they can better see me living out the remainder of my life in accordance with that choice. Or perhaps it will only be after I have spent a couple of days 'trying on' a choice, thinking what life would be like and what would change for me in my activities and relationships, that I will be able to conclude, 'That just wouldn't be me.' And it might be the objections that I receive from my friends and family that help me to see that this is so.

Thus a change of mind in the case of Mrs L.W., following extended conversation with her family, need not signal manipulation, coercion, or threats to her autonomous choice. According to the formal approach, Mrs L.W.'s 'true' preference, the preferences and interests of other family members, and Mrs L.W.'s mental capacities are all facts that are known in advance, and which need to be processed in accordance with the general principle of respect for autonomy. According to a narrative approach, Mrs L.W.'s preference *emerged from the process of conversation*. What might to an outsider seem to be 'manipulation' might have been instead a necessary component of a conversation, without which Mrs L.W. would never have discovered her preferences and values. The doctor could assess what happened over the past several days only by hearing the detailed story of Mrs L.W.'s conversations with her family and her own deliberations.

This is not to suggest that families never put undue pressure on their members because of selfish interests. But the difference between coercive, selfish relatives and concerned, involved relatives will emerge from a careful analysis of the detailed narrative of the case. It will not simply pop out of a mechanical application of the four principles.

In its worst form a formal approach will view Mrs L.W. as an autonomous individual and ask whether there are conflicts of interest between her and other autonomous individuals. This would effectively portray her and her family as adversaries. But that would grossly distort the process of reasoning by which Mrs L.W. seeks to arrive at her decision. For her, the choice of treatment must make sense *within* her family network of roles and relationships; whereas the ethical analysis would try to solve the problem by abstracting her out of this network and pretending that it was of no moral consequence.

CURRENT CRITIQUES OF FORMAL APPROACHES

The discussion so far has hinted at several ways in which formal approaches have come under fire in recent years. Critics of formal approaches have come from at least three alternative vantage points: casuistry, virtue ethics, and some versions of feminist theory. Each of these three alternative approaches contains important narrative elements.

Casuists (5–7) argue that there will always be too much space between general, abstract ethical principles and the concrete facts of particular cases for a formal approach to generate realistic action guides—unless a variety of concrete assumptions are smuggled in along with the general principles. For example, consider a general ethical principle that prohibits stealing. This principle gets us nowhere in judging a concrete case unless we have a sense of what counts as the ownership of property. And there is no general, abstract theory of ownership; instead there are many traditions, all of which are bound up in the history and the culture of different societies. Thus no purely general (i.e. culturally and historically neutral) ethical principle can give us the guidance we seek in such cases (2). Casuists seek instead an understanding that ethical insight can come from case and context, and not only from abstract theories (8).

Virtue ethics (9–11) points out that many qualities of the moral life simply defy analysis in terms of formal principles. For instance, it would seem to be a very shallow and truncated view of medical ethics that would be unable to provide any account of the qualities of kindness and compassion. But understanding these qualities requires at least two factors that are missing from formal approaches. First is a broader perspective that embraces the whole of a life and not simply the one decision that is at hand. Virtues are excellences in how one lives one's life (9); the way one internalizes these excellences into one's character cannot necessarily be determined by how one behaves in any given case. The virtuous person asks not, 'What do I do now?' but rather 'How can I go about becoming a certain sort of person?' The second factor is a type of judgement or discernment which is itself a developing trait of character. To know what it means to act kindly or compassionately *in this situation* requires a very delicate appreciation of the situation, of a sort for which no automatic formula can be given. (Indeed, if one engages in *too much* intellectual analysis, one is no longer acting kindly or compassionately.)

Some feminist critics of formal approaches have called instead for an ethic of caring and relationships (12,13). They argue that formal approaches invariably rely on the sorts of rules that appropriately govern contacts among strangers. While a stranger ethic may be unavoidable and even desirable for many aspects of our lives, it cannot do justice to many of our most important relationships and responsibilities. This seems especially important for medicine, if our profession thinks that doctors and patients ought to be something more than strangers to each other. This is particularly true of primary care medicine, where it could be argued that maintaining a positive helping relationship over time is as important as making any particular decision correctly (4,14).

In the past, women have sometimes been degraded as reasoners because they are supposed to be 'emotional' rather than 'objective'. The ethic of caring, by contrast, insists upon the importance of emotion in ethical reasoning, particularly in two ways. First, empathic identification with the other parties to a case is essential in order to discern what truly counts as a caring response to their predicament. Second, relative to virtue ethics, emotion plays a role in the manner in which one carries out an action, and often that determines the sort of action that it is—a kind or compassionate act is an act which is carried out in a certain emotional state (13).

Defenders of formal approaches will object that these alternatives all fail to provide the level of rigor and certainty that one ought to expect of ethical methodology. According to this objection, approaches such as the four principles represent a 'hard' method for applying well-grounded ethical truths to particular factual situations. By contrast, casuistic, virtues, and caring analyses seem intolerably 'soft', relying far too much on intuition and on *ad hoc* opinions. It would appear that much more agreement will be possible around the application of the four principles than around what is virtuous or what is caring.

The rejoinder to this objection is that we are the heirs to a philosophical tradition beginning with the Enlightenment, which has confused rationality and method with one particular form of abstract, universalizable reasoning. It is wrong to dismiss (say) Aristotle and the American pragmatists as lacking rigor or method in ethical reasoning, simply because they do not fit into the mold of Descartes and Kant (15).

Another rejoinder points out that formal approaches will always appear to be superior in medical ethics so long as the 'cases' are presented as is now most typical in textbooks and journals—one- or two-paragraph synopses, like the case of Mrs L.W. above. These brief descriptions have room only for a few very general facts, and necessarily omit almost all of the narrative details about the social or institutional context in which the case occurs, and about the uniqueness of the people involved. (To mention just one example: the case of Mrs L.W. omits all mention of the previous career of the doctor, what happened to the last several patients of his who underwent chemotherapy, and how those experiences may have shaped his advice to Mrs L.W.) When cases provide no grist for the narrative mill, the formal approach will always appear to provide the 'right answer'. By contrast, when a single case is discussed in sufficient depth to allow a full understanding of its history and context (16), then the weaknesses of a formal approach and the need for a narrative approach will become apparent.

NARRATIVE AND THE FOUR PRINCIPLES

Some have been sufficiently swayed by recent criticisms of formal approaches to suggest that abstract principles and ethical theory be dispensed with entirely. My argument is that the moral life is rich and complex, so that no single approach is likely to do justice to all its aspects. It is clear from the contents of this book that the four principles are capable of adding considerable illumination to many topic areas in medical ethics. The question, then, is how the four principles can be accommodated in an overall approach which also includes a central role for narrative ethics.

The psychologist Jerome Bruner has suggested that the most basic way human beings have of coming to understand or to assign meaning to the world that they live in is by telling stories about it. Bruner claims that all other ways of knowing—including the scientific—are in some way derivative from the more basic narrative mode (17). That is, science is not the rejection of narrative, but rather a particularly sophisticated way of constructing special types of narratives for special purposes. It is only a small extension of this idea to see, in the four principles, a compressed form of narrative about human behavior and human reasoning.

Our culture has a long history of reasoning about what people ought to do in difficult life situations. While much of what we draw from our culture as we grow up consists of common-sense folk beliefs and various religious dogmas, the culture also includes important elements of the work of previous philosophers. For instance, in any extended, searching conversation about a moral issue conducted among a group of typical persons without special training in ethics, it is very likely that there will eventually emerge some discussion of respect for others' basic rights; some mention of what it means to respect another's dignity as a person; and some attempt to calculate good or bad consequences. This means that the ideas of past philosophers such as John Locke, Immanuel Kant, and John Stuart Mill are alive and well within our culture.

The narrative approach to ethics focuses upon the uniqueness of human problems. And yet the reason that we have sciences of human biology and human behavior is that there are also important patterns of similarity among human experiences. If we temporarily put to one side the unique features in a large set of cases, and consider only those features that many or most of the cases have in common, then we are likely to discover that those common features can be described with fair accuracy by a small number of general and abstract concepts.

Thus, the four principles can serve as a tightly compressed synopsis of a very large body of case experience during a good portion of the history of our culture. If the casuist is correct, and moral judgements often proceed by comparing a new case with a set of known and carefully analyzed past cases, then it follows that those who are most conversant with the four principles and all their implications will be very richly supplied when it comes to reasoning about a new case. They will be able very efficiently to pick out features of the new case which are likely to be morally relevant. The only danger will come if they fall into the trap of thinking that the features that this case has in common with all previous cases *exhausts* the moral content of the case at hand.

There are some circumstances in which the four principles legitimately take precedence over a narrative approach. We have to make many ethical decisions about people who basically are and will remain strangers to us, and about whom we will never know very much of their life histories and contexts. For us, these people are like the standard cases printed in the ethics textbooks. The four principles give us a firm ground upon which to base our moral decisions.

Moreover, there will be people for whom we are in the process of learning more about the uniqueness of their circumstances, to allow us eventually to reach a moral conclusion that is fully informed by narrative and contextual insights. However, while we are in the process of learning, we need to know how to approach these people. If the principle of respect for autonomy causes us to do two things—first, not to subject the person to interventions that she does not wish; and second, to listen carefully to what she says about her preferences and values—then it serves the purposes of the narrative approach. By contrast, if we had no notion of respect for autonomy, it is quite possible that we would already have committed irrevocable ethical blunders by the time we had enough information to construct a narrative understanding of our choices.

But the debt is not all on one side. Whenever we try to apply the four principles to a particular case, we need somehow to find a way to link up very general and abstract ideas to concrete circumstances and actions. Often, we would be lost in doing this, if we did not have a narrative account of the case to aid us in interpreting the significance of its various features. In the case of Mrs L.W., does the principle of respect for autonomy require that we accept her refusal of chemotherapy on day 1, or her request for chemotherapy on day 4? Unless we can tell a coherent story about how Mrs L.W. got from the first point to the latter, it is very likely that no formal principle of ethics will conclusively guide us. (Indeed, if we relied only on purely formal principles, we might see the decisions on day 1 and day 4 as essentially *unlinked*—which hardly seems to do justice to Mrs L.W.'s needs or circumstances.)

SUMMARY

Narrative ethics in medicine suggests that we supplement the four principles with an appreciation of the following factors:

1. The choice that the patient is now making, or the way the doctor now behaves toward the patient, is going to become one episode in the unfolding

narrative of the patient's life, and will acquire meaning within the context of that narrative.

2. The action the doctor is now about to take will also become an episode in the doctor's life narrative, and will reflect upon the doctor's core commitments and values.

3. The action that doctor and patient are about to take is embedded in a context that consists of their life histories, the lives of other involved parties, and the customs and practices of the community and the institution (such as the hospital). A full understanding of the action requires that it be interpreted within that context. The 'right course of action' to resolve a problem is not necessarily the action that conforms to an abstract principle; rather, it may be the action which, without violating any moral principles, most successfully navigates all the contextual factors to move the situation in a direction that best serves the major interests of all involved parties.

REFERENCES

1. Brody, H. 1981. *Ethical decisions in medicine*, 2nd edn. Little, Brown & Co., Boston, MA.
2. Clarke, S. G. and Simpson, E. (Eds) 1989. *Anti-theory in ethics and moral conservatism*. State University of New York Press, Albany, NY.
3. Brody, H. 1989. Applied ethics: don't change the subject. Pp. 183–200, in Hoffmaster, B., Freedman, B. and Fraser, G. (Eds) *Clinical ethics: the nature of applied ethics in medicine*. Humana, Clifton, NJ.
4. Brody, H. 1991. *The healer's power*. Yale University Press, New Haven, CT.
5. Jonsen, A. R. and Toulmin, S. 1988. *The abuse of casuistry: a history of moral rasoning*. University of California Press, Berkeley, CA.
6. Murray, T. H. 1987. Medical ethics, moral philosophy, and moral tradition. *Social Science in Medicine* 25: 637–644.
7. Arras, J. D. 1991. Getting down to cases: the revival of casuistry in bioethics. *Journal of Medicine and Philosophy* 16: 29–51.
8. Zaner, R. M. 1988. *Ethics and the clinical encounter*. Prentice-Hall, Englewood Cliffs, NJ.
9. MacIntyre, A. 1981. *After virtue*. University of Notre Dame Press, South Bend, IN.
10. Shelp, E. E. (Ed.) 1985. *Virtue and medicine*. D. Reidel, Boston, MA.
11. Drane, J. F. 1988. *Becoming a good doctor: the place of virtue and character in medical ethics*. Sheed & Ward, Kansas City, MO.
12. Gilligan, C. 1982. *In a different voice: psychological theory and women's development*. Harvard University Press, Cambridge, MA.
13. Carse, A. L. 1991. The 'voice of care': implications for bioethical education. *Journal of Medicine and Philosophy* 16: 5–28.
14. Brody, H. *Stories of sickness*. Yale University Press, New Haven, CT.
15. Rorty, R. 1979. *Philosophy and the mirror of nature*. Princeton University Press, Princeton, NJ.
16. Campbell, A. V. and Higgs, R. 1982. *In that case: medical ethics in everyday practice*. Darton, Longman, & Todd, London.
17. Bruner, J. 1986. *Actual minds, possible worlds*. Harvard University Press, Cambridge, MA.

19

Needs, Rights and the Moral Duties of Clinicians

LEN DOYAL

Senior Lecturer in Medical Ethics, Department of Human Science and Medical Ethics, The London and St Bartholomew's Medical Colleges, London, UK

Beauchamp and Childress's *Principles of Bioethics* has been enormously influential (1). Reference to and discussion of their four principles—autonomy, non-maleficence, beneficence and justice—have been endemic in debates among moral philosophers specializing in medical ethics. There can be no doubt that the moral imperatives to which they allude dominate the national and international moral codes of the medical profession, as well as much current argument about medical law.

This said, the philosophical justification which Beauchamp and Childress offer to explain the importance of these principles is, at times, shallow and eclectic. On the one hand they stress the compatibility of the four principles with competing utilitarian and deontological moral theories, and to this extent place argumentative priority on the intuitive clarity of the principles themselves. On the other hand, they also demonstrate how these different theories can lead to inconsistent interpretations of each principle in the face of specific clinical dilemmas and describe a consequent moral indeterminacy from which their intuitionism provides no escape.

What is required to account for the undoubted importance of the four principles (or their equivalent formulation) for the practice and teaching of medical ethics is a moral theory from which their substance logically follows. Such a theory must coherently account for their intuitive appeal while at the same time specifying how whatever moral determinacy they do possess can be made compatible with the accepted indeterminacy of many specific clinical dilemmas.

In this chapter I will attempt such a derivation based directly on the second part of my book with Ian Gough, *A Theory of Human Need* (2). In so doing I will argue—as we do in our book—that human needs are the preconditions for participation in moral life, that for this reason the two most basic needs are

Principles of Health Care Ethics. Edited by Raanan Gillon.
© 1994 John Wiley & Sons Ltd

physical health and autonomy, that the serious imputation of moral duties to others entails their right to optimal need satisfaction and that the recognition of this entails the adoption of procedural rules for rationally debating what follows from this right in practice. It will then be demonstrated how a deontological interpretation of Beauchamp and Childress's four principles derives from these arguments and does so in a way that demarcates morally determinant clinical reasoning from that which remains open to further debate.

THE CONCEPT OF HUMAN NEED

The word 'need' is used explicitly or implicitly to refer to a particular category of *goals* which are believed to be *universalizable*. Examples would be: 'This person needs (and should have the goal of) more protein' or 'These families need (and should have the goal of) proper shelter this winter'. Needs in this sense are commonly contrasted with 'wants' which are also described as goals but which derive from an individual's particular preference and cultural environment. Unlike needs, wants are believed to vary from person to person. The difference between goals thought of in these distinct ways is explicitly recognized by such an uncontentious statement as: 'I want a cigarette but I need to stop smoking'.

Referring to needs as universalizable goals risks obscuring the reason why universality is imputed to some aims and not others. The imputation rests upon the belief that if needs are not satisfied by an appropriate 'satisfier' then serious *harm* of some specified and objective kind will result (3) (cf. Wiggins (4)). Not to try to satisfy needs will thus be seen to be against the objective interests of the individuals involved, and viewed as abnormal and unnatural. When goals are described as 'wants' rather than needs, it is precisely because they are not believed to be linked to human interests in this sense.

But what counts as serious harm? Unless we can identify some universalizable characteristics, any conception of need which is linked to its avoidance must be hopelessly relative. Our approach equates serious harm with fundamental disablement in the pursuit of one's vision of the good. Thought of in these terms, the objectivity of harm is ensured through its not being reducible to contingent subjective feelings like anxiety or sadness. For one can experience both and still successfully achieve aims to which importance is attached by oneself or others (5).

Another way of describing such harm concerns the impact of poor need satisfaction on the success of social participation. Unless individuals are capable of *participating* in some form of life without arbitrary serious limitations being placed on what they attempt to accomplish, their potential for private and public success will remain unfulfilled—whatever the detail of their actual choices. Whatever our private and public goals, they must always be achieved on the basis of past, present or future successful interaction with others. We build a self-conception of our own personal capacities through learning from others— how they assess what we think we have learned and how they respond to changes in our actions on the basis of such assessment.

It follows from the preceding arguments that the search for objective basic needs becomes that for universalizable preconditions which enable non-impaired participation both in the form of life in which individuals find themselves as well as any other form of life which they might subsequently choose if they get the chance. Without the discovery of such conditions, we will be unable to account for the special moral significance which we wish to impute to basic need satisfaction (6).

PHYSICAL SURVIVAL/HEALTH AND AUTONOMY AS BASIC HUMAN NEEDS

Against the background of the body conceived as a deterministic process, Kant searched for the conditions to which persons must conform if they are to be capable of initiating actions and assuming responsibility for them. Although he was not directly concerned with the character of human need, he did articulate many concepts and arguments relevant to its theorization. Kant showed that for individuals to act and to be responsible they must have both the physical and mental capacity to do so: at the very least a *body which is alive* and which is governed by all of the relevant causal processes and the *mental competence to deliberate and to choose*. Let us identify this latter competence and capacity for choice with the existence of the most basic level of personal 'autonomy' (7).

To be autonomous in this minimal sense is *to have the ability to make informed choices about what should be done and how to go about doing it*. This entails being able to formulate aims, and beliefs about how to achieve them, along with the ability to evaluate the success of beliefs in the light of empirical evidence. Aims and beliefs—'our own' reasons—are what connect us logically with 'our own' actions. The capacity to make 'our own' mistakes performs the same role as regards the successes and failures of our actions. In these minimal terms, autonomy is tantamount to 'agency' and is a clear precondition for regarding oneself or being regarded by anyone else as being able to do, and to be held responsible for doing, anything. Its existence is expressed in the unique repertoire of successful and unsuccessful manual and mental activities which constitutes the story of how we became who we are (8).

A person with impaired autonomy is thus someone who temporarily lacks the full capacity for action through his or her agency being in some way constrained. Examples would include a person who is physically forced to do something against her will or who has been duped into thinking that she has done one thing when, in fact, she has done another. Someone would fall into the first category, for example, if she were raped. The second category would be illustrated if you were deceived into doing something which you did not intend, such as committing a crime. It makes sense, therefore, to claim that since physical survival and personal autonomy are the conditions for any individual action in any culture, they constitute the most basic human needs— those which must be satisfied to some degree before actors can participate in their form of life to achieve any other valued goals.

Let us now look at each of these basic needs in further detail. Beginning with survival, it is clear that the need for physical survival on its own cannot do justice to what it means to be a person. The victim of a motor accident who survives in deep coma on a life-support system, incapable of independent action, demonstrates why. This is not an idle philosophical point. Whether or not such victims regain the capacity to act will eventually determine their fate. Despite physical survival, if the best clinical advice continues to be that the chances of regaining consciousness are non-existent, or even extremely remote, then the ventilator may eventually be turned off.

So it is *physical health* rather than just mere survival which is a basic human need, one which it will be in the interest of individuals to try to satisfy before they address any others. To do well in their everyday lives—whatever they do and in whatever cultural context—people have to do much more than survive. They must possess a modicum of good physical health. To complete a range of practical tasks in daily life requires manual, mental and emotional abilities with which poor physical health usually interferes.

On this view the physical health needs of individuals have been met if they do not suffer in a sustained and serious way from one or more particular diseases (9). For our purposes the usefulness of such a perspective should be clear. Serious diseases ordinarily keep sufferers from participating as well as they might—and as might be expected of them—in the particular form of life in which they find themselves.

In short, physical health can be thought of transculturally in a negative way. If you wish to lead an active and successful life in your own terms, it is in your objective interest to satisfy your basic need to optimize your life expectancy and to avoid serious physical disease and illness conceptualized in biomedical terms. The same applies to everyone, everywhere (10).

Yet clear and potentially useful as the negative definition of physical health is, it is rightly regarded by many as problematic. For much more is involved in the preconditions for sustained successful human action than the absence of serious biological disease (11). Individual autonomy must also be sustained and improved. One can easily imagine a situation where an actor has met her primary need for physical health but is still capable of initiating very little.

Three key variables affect levels of individual autonomy: the level of *understanding* a person has about herself, her culture and what is expected of her as an individual within it; the *psychological capacity* she has to formulate options for herself; and the objective *opportunities* enabling or impeding her to act accordingly (12).

The degree of understanding of self and culture depends on the availability and quality of *teachers*. People do not teach themselves to act—they have to learn from others. Which skills are learned will differ from culture to culture, but they are not totally variable. All children must learn, for example, to interact socially in minimally acceptable ways, irrespective of the specific cultural rules they follow in the process. Similarly, in all cultures, language skills are necessary as the medium through which actors learn conceptually to order their world and to deliberate about what to do in it. In this sense, individual consciousness is essentially social—the by-product of interaction with others.

Some forms of learning and teaching will be more conducive to high levels of autonomy than others. Much will depend on what is taught. There are some activities which are common to all cultures and for which everyone must be prepared if they are to be able to participate successfully and to understand what goes on within those cultures. Braybrooke correctly classifies these social roles as those of parent, householder, worker and citizen (13). The strength of our autonomy when negotiating with experts will also be related to our understanding. In medical relationships, for example, patients who know more about medicine and health can and do demand more from their doctors and from themselves—they have more choices than they would otherwise have (14).

The second key determinant of autonomy is the individual's *cognitive capacity and emotionality*—ultimately his or her *mental health*. Rationality is an important component in all the definitions of autonomy which we have considered. But what does it mean in relation to mental health?

Since all actions have to embody a modicum of reason to be classed as actions at all, it is difficult to give a precise definition of the minimum levels of rationality and responsibility present in the autonomous individual. Generally speaking, the existence of even minimal levels of autonomy will entail the following sustained characteristics:

1. that actors have the intellectual capacity for the formulation of aims and beliefs common to their form of life;
2. that actors have enough confidence to want to act and thus to participate in some form of social life;
3. that actors sometimes actually do so through consistently formulating aims and beliefs and communicating with others about them;
4. that actors perceive their actions as having been done by them and not by someone else;
5. that actors are able to understand the empirical constraints on the success of their actions;
6. that actors are capable of taking moral responsibility for what they do.

Therefore, again like physical health, autonomy at its most basic level should be understood negatively—with reference to the serious objective disablement to which the absence of one or more of these characteristics will lead (15).

When the preceding characteristics are absent in individuals, they may be deemed either emotionally or mentally disabled. Leaving aside specific symptomatology, the main difference for our purposes is that, for some reason, those who are seriously and permanently ill in this sense have either lost or never possessed a level of autonomy sufficient for more than minimally successful levels of intentional social interaction—if that.

The third variable which affects the degree to which autonomy can be increased is the range of *opportunities* for new and significant action open to the actor. By 'significant' we mean activities which are deemed of social significance in any of Braybrooke's preceding categories, or which the actors deem of significance for the rational improvement of their participation in their form of life. This means that when we link improvements in autonomy to increased choices, we do not mean any old choices (16). Significant choices require social opportunities. Those who are denied them have their freedom and their autonomy artificially constrained and are unable to explore some of their capacities as a person (17). More than anything else, it is this that makes tyranny so abhorrent.

In further exploring the links between autonomy and freedom, many writers within the liberal tradition argue that both should be seen as the absence of constraints on actions which have not been chosen by actors themselves. Yet if 'constraint' is taken to mean 'self-sufficiency' then we must take great care. For the opportunity to express individual autonomy requires much more than simply being left alone—more than *negative* freedom. If we really were ignored by others, we would never learn the rules of our way of life and thereby acquire the capacity to make choices within it.

In other words, to be autonomous and to be healthy, we also require *positive freedom*—material, educational and emotional need satisfaction of the kind already described (18). Against the background of the general socialization on which their cognitive and emotional capacity for action depends, autonomous individuals (who are not slaves) must understand *why* they should not physically constrain the actions of others and must possess the emotional competence to act accordingly. But again, they can only learn to follow the rules embodied in such constraint with positive assistance.

Further, to wish to act in an unconstrained fashion still entails participating in a form of life to which the positive actions of others give substance. For example, for an individual to deliver a successful lecture involves much more than her listeners not intervening to stop it! They must also have the physical, intellectual and emotional competence to give serious consideration to her arguments. Otherwise, why should the lecturer bother? This is why the concept of serious harm is so intimately linked with that of impaired social participation.

DUTIES, RIGHTS AND MORAL RECIPROCITY

To be a person rather than just a living body or animal entails more than consciousness and an ability to communicate and to formulate aims and beliefs. The individual must also be the bearer of responsibilities. Whatever their specific content, the normative structures of particular cultures would be unintelligible were it not for the assumption that their members could accept responsibilities toward, as well as recognizing them in, others.

Not only does social life require moral responsibility; the same can be said for the success of our own individual participation within it. Unless we just happen fortuitously to have the power to inflict our will on others, social success will depend on our capacity to understand what our moral responsibilities are and our willingness to act accordingly. The duties which moral responsibilities entail are just as *real* for us in our social lives as is our physical environment. For example, a statement to the effect that someone is acting in accordance with a specific duty has empirical conditions under which it will be true in the same sense as are descriptive statements about the natural world (19) (cf. Arrington (20)).

The reality of duties apparently entails the reality of *rights*—the entitlement of one group of individuals to what is required for them to carry out obligations which they and others believe they possess. However, the logical relationship between rights and duties is highly complex. For this reason we shall argue that duties only entail rights against the background of an already existing network of moral beliefs which clearly specify the conditions of entailment (21) (cf. Doyal and Gough (2), chap. 6, footnotes 1 and 2).

Let us begin with an individual A who believes that she has a duty of some kind toward others in group B who expect her to act accordingly. Also assume that she is aware of and accepts the legitimacy of their expectation. The group in question could be a small face-to-face community or a large anonymous collectivity. But whatever its size, and however well its members know each other, for her and them to believe that she should do her duty, presupposes that they also believe that she is in fact able so to do. In other words, 'ought' implies 'can'.

The Right to Minimal Levels of Need Satisfaction

Therefore, the ascription of a duty—for it to be intelligible as a duty to those who accept it and to those who ascribe it—must carry with it the belief that the bearer of the duty is entitled to the level of need satisfaction necessary for her to act accordingly. Thus A must believe that she has the right to such satisfaction if, say, she suddenly becomes impoverished but is still expected by the members of B to execute the duties she did before this occurred. For *without at least minimal levels of need satisfaction, A will be able to do nothing at all, including those acts that are specifically expected of her.* And the same applies to those who believe that they have a right to A's actions. They also must accept that, unless her basic needs are minimally satisfied, she will be unable to do what they think she should. Therefore, she has a right to such satisfaction in proportion to the seriousness with which they take her duty and expect her to comply with it. And the converse also holds.

Of course, the acceptance of such a right does not specify exactly how it should be respected in particular circumstances. The members of B, for example, may accept that A has a right to a minimal level of need satisfaction without accepting that they have a corresponding duty *directly* to provide it. This will be likely if, say, welfare agencies exist which have the institutional responsibility for meeting needs. But remember, someone or some group must accept the duty to act for A if her right is to have substance. Therefore, the members of B cannot escape from the responsibility at least to *contribute toward* A's minimal need satisfaction—provided that an *agency* exists for this purpose (22).

The same argument concerning the right to minimal need satisfaction applies to those from alien cultures. To take a topical example, if we think that individuals should not be killed for their beliefs or for what they write and publish about them, then we identify this position as one aspect of what we accept to be the moral good. It is the categorical status of this principle which leads us to condemn anyone who violates it, whether they are a member of our own culture or of another which embodies opposing moral views. To say of those in another culture that they should do otherwise presupposes that they can, and that they have the right to minimal need satisfaction to the degree that we are capable of providing it.

The Right to Optimal Need Satisfaction

The argument so far has justified the rights of all peoples to the *minimal* satisfaction of their basic needs. It has not, however, provided a justification for anything more than the avoidance of gross suffering, or enabling people just to 'get by'. Let us now extend the argument to higher levels of need satisfaction, up to and including 'optimal' levels.

Fulfilling one's perceived obligations in public and private life usually involves much more than the minimal amount of action made possible by a minimal level of need satisfaction. There will always be some goals which individuals take very seriously and which they believe that they have a duty to achieve *to the best of their ability*. These will usually be aims which they perceive as central to the conduct of their lives, the successful achievement of which will determine whether or not they will regard themselves and be regarded by others as of high moral character. Personal goals of this kind are informed by cultural values—the types and levels of performance expected by those toward whom one experiences moral obligations.

Thus attempts at excellence are symbolic of the commitment to a specific way of life and thereby to a particular vision of the good. The degree of this commitment will ultimately be judged by others who share the same values. In these situations, for us to expect *less* of ourselves than our best, or to believe that less would be acceptable to those to whom we are obligated, calls into question our and their commitment to the shared good which informs our action. It would mean that the good was not really believed to be *that* good after all.

If, however, we agree that those who are committed to the same morality have the duty to do their best—to be good in its terms—then this commits us to a further belief: the *right* of those concerned to the goods and services necessary for their best effort to be a realistic possibility. It is inconsistent for us to expect that others should do their best and also to think that they should not have the wherewithal to do so—the *optimal* as opposed to the minimal satisfaction of their basic needs. And, of course, the same applies to ourselves. The only way in which this conclusion does not follow is for us to believe that, all things being equal, less than the best effort is compatible with the pursuit of the good.

But again, what would 'the good' mean in this context? If we really take our moral beliefs seriously, then we have no option but to take equally seriously the entitlement of other members of our community to those things which will optimize their capacity for moral action. As was the case with minimal need satisfaction, this entails two things: negatively, not inhibiting persons from trying to do their best, and positively, doing what we can to provide access to the same levels of need satisfaction that we claim in our own pursuit of moral virtue. All other members of our own culture who take their morality seriously incur the same duties toward us, and for the same reasons (23).

Of course, what is regarded as 'best' and 'optimal' in the above terms will vary between cultures, depending on their particular moral codes and the resources which are available for need satisfaction. Therefore, when we use the term 'optimal' we are obviously not maintaining that those who share moral values have a right to *everything* that might conceivably reinforce their pursuit of moral excellence. Since the scope of such satisfiers is potentially infinite, no individual or group within the culture could assume the corresponding duty of providing them, and without such a duty there can be no identifiable right.

The point is rather that the members of specific cultures will already have reasonably clear ideas of what doing one's best amounts to *in practice*. These will be linked to exemplars of what ordinary individuals can hope to achieve if they apply themselves to the best of their ability, along with theories about the levels of health, learning and emotional confidence which are usually associated with such application. To be consistent, therefore, a commitment to a vision of the good must be linked to that culture's best available understanding of what is required for optimal individual effort. Consistency also dictates that everyone who is expected to do their best to be good in our terms—and is encouraged to try to do so—is given a fair share of the resources available for this to be a real possibility.

SUBSTANTIVE AND PROCEDURAL NEEDS

The discussion thus far has focused on our substantive theory of human need. Equally as important is our procedural theory of the necessary conditions for discovering more about and prioritizing basic need satisfaction. There is no space to discuss this at length. Suffice it to say that, even if we are clear about the substance of need and need satisfaction, there will still be disagreements about which areas of satisfaction and which specific satisfiers should be prioritized in conditions of scarcity—for example, educational v. medical provision v. housing v. employment. The list is long.

Here, answers which are in some sense correct may well be elusive. However, it does not follow that in many instances, some answers will not be much better than others. Therefore, to optimize their rationality and collective acceptability, public policies should be formulated on the basis of the best technical information available and through democratic and representative debate which precludes the arbitrary influence of vested interests (see chapter 7 in ref. 2). If compromise is inevitable, the most acceptable result will be the one which has won the widest consensus.

Further, it is the rationality of related debate which fuels progress in need satisfaction, which in turn increases the ability of individuals to participate in such debate. The fact that the likelihood of rational discourse about needs is limited by the defence of privilege and power within the political process in no way detracts from the importance of struggling to achieve it. One of the most important dimensions of such struggle is the attempt constitutionally to guarantee the right to basic need satisfaction, including the right of participation within all stages of public policy formation.

BACK TO BEAUCHAMP AND CHILDRESS

The right to optimal need satisfaction—or more precisely to access to those goods and services which are preconditions for it—has been shown to carry with it corresponding duties. Translated into a clinical environment, these become precisely those which Beauchamp and Childress outline. Leaving aside justice for the moment, let us assume that their other three principles can be reduced to two. First, clinicians have a duty to provide good medical care—to use their expertise to protect the life and health of patients to an acceptable standard. Second, they have a duty to provide good moral care—to respect the right of patients to informed consent, to correct information about their illness and treatment (and enough of it to make informed consent a practical proposition) and to confidentiality.

If our more general arguments are correct about the rights and duties associated with the universal basic needs of health and autonomy, both sets of associated duties of good clinical care obviously follow from the existence of such rights. These arguments are based on reason and not moral intuition. From the perspective of their own moral commitments, all clinicians believe that both they and their patients have certain duties. One of these is to be a good patient—once the choice has been made to have medical treatment, to act responsibly through doing one's best to follow whatever plan of medical management that has been prescribed. Yet for such beliefs to be consistent—for good citizenship and compliance to be a practical proposition—patients must have the competence physically, emotionally, intellectually and socially to choose to act accordingly.

This in turn implies that clinicians must strive to do what they can to optimize this competence or, which is just another way of saying the same thing, to act to optimize the physical health and autonomy of their patients. Of course, it is not being suggested that most clinicians primarily see patients as good or bad compliers. No doubt they also perceive them as good or bad citizens in a much wider sense. But this only strengthens the argument that patients will not be able to do their best, either as citizens or patients, to lead the sort of life the clinician deems morally acceptable unless appropriate clinical help is provided.

To be sure, such a derivation of Beauchamp and Childress's principles places a distinctly deontological interpretation on what beneficence, non-maleficence and respect for autonomy should mean in practice. If, to be consistent, clinicians have a duty to facilitate in their patients the capacity for being good, they cannot do so with crude utilitarian arguments associated with questionable medical paternalism. Deliberate deception is not acceptable, for example, either for reasons of beneficence or non-maleficence. For as a result of the deceit, the patient would not be able actually to *do* the very things which probably prompted the deceit in the first place—to take charge of his or her life or what is left of it in a way that conforms to the clinician's own vision of the good. For reasons of this sort, deriving the moral importance of clinically protecting health and respecting autonomy from our theory of need leads to a moral determinacy which is missing from Beauchamp and Childress's initial formulation.

This said, the deontological emphasis which we have stressed should not be taken to suggest that consequential modes of reasoning are not also crucial to the application of our theory of need to the medical encounter or even, with this in mind, that the moral consequences of more sophisticated versions of rule utilitarianism might not overlap with our own. Now placing their fourth principle of justice on the agenda, it is clear that we ourselves have been employing consequential reasoning through stressing what has to be done if optimizing health and autonomy is going to be achieved in whatever professional context (24). Compare ref. 25.

However, to argue that social programmes can be evaluated in these terms—with respect to the related degrees of social justice-through-need-satisfaction which they achieve—does not let crude utilitarianism in through the back door. Rather, it demonstrates that consequential reasoning should not be confused with it, provided that one of the consequences is the optimization of individual autonomy. For to the degree that this is so, it is just another way of saying that the individual clinician has no right to dictate or manipulate the choices of competent patients, no matter how much doing so is argued to be in their best interests.

Of course, the rule utilitarian might retort that a similar emphasis on rights can equally be justified through arguing that if everyone acted as if they possessed such rights—even though they really don't—then collective welfare would be increased (26). The problem here is what is meant by 'welfare'. If it is a subjective conception then the basis for moral decision-making collapses back into a collective form of act utilitarianism with the majority literally being able to dictate any moral terms it likes to the minority.

Conversely, if welfare is thought of more objectively along the lines outlined by our theory of need then, again, the majority must respect the right of members of the minority to choose, even if their choices are not perceived to be in their interests.* Not to conceive of welfare in these terms throws us into the inconsistency of expecting patients to conform to one's vision of the good—whatever that is—while undermining their human capacity to do so.

Therefore, a deontological interpretation of Beauchamp and Childress's principles follows from the preceding theory of need—one which takes rights seriously in Dworkin's terms (27). This has a clear cutting edge both as regards the morality of the clinical relationship and the just distribution of scarce medical resources.

As regards the former, little more needs to be said other than to direct the reader to some of the most forceful attacks on paternalism in medicine. The denial of the right of patients to be the autonomous gatekeepers of their own bodies—either through straightforward deception or even more devious manipulation—simply cannot consistently be justified and should always be morally condemned. Of course, sustaining this right in the heat of the clinical encounter can be difficult either because of the patient's lack of competence to understand, possibly compromised by illness itself, or the clinician's poor communication skills ... or both.

Where moral dilemmas seem indeterminate for these sorts of reasons, the most that can be expected is that clinicians do the best they can to resolve them

---

* This, of course, assumes that the physical health and autonomy of others are not impaired in the process. When such a threat is present then individual rights must be modified accordingly. Yet note that the moral and legal force of such a threat is only sustained when the harm that is threatened is objective in our terms.

in ways which respect the rights of those involved. The question of whether or not they are doing their best should not be obscured by the fact that, in some instances, clinicians may disagree about the most appropriate course of action to take. It simply underlines the importance stated in our general theory of need for the institutionalization of procedural guidelines which ensure that the final decision is as rational and as fair as possible given the particular circumstances surrounding it (28).

Finally, returning to Beauchamp and Childress's principle of justice, the interpretation which follows from our theory of need continues to remain strongly deontological in the face of the problem of the distribution of scarce medical resources. One way or another—and there are many different ways in which this might be administratively envisaged—a morally just health service must, as a matter of individual right, incorporate the mandatory provision of a broad spectrum of basic medical services with equal access to everyone on the basis of need.

Remember, our theory sharply distinguishes between need and preference. No injustice is done through ignoring the latter in situations of scarcity. However, as regards the need for appropriate medical care to optimize the basic need for physical health, an injustice will occur if some illnesses are generally viewed as warranting no or very little provision. For then sufferers will be treated unequally—their right of equal access to the particular need satisfiers they require will be violated. This will be so, however others might rank their preferences for treatment in different clinical circumstances. Thus the argument from equality draws attention to the central moral problems confronting utilitarian approaches to health care rationing which maintain the general public is entitled—just because they are the general public—to decide which medical treatments should and should not be on offer (cf. the articles in Bell and Mendus (29)).

It follows that when rationing becomes inevitable, as will always be the case for some treatments and for some patients, it can only justly take place *within* the provision of treatments but not *between* them. But how should just rationing occur within the provision of types of treatment? Again, the answer harks back to the assessment of need and entails two principles.

On the one hand, patients who possess morally similar prognoses and ages should be randomized (30). If properly administered within a national health service like the one in the UK, waiting lists provide a rational and effective way for this to occur. Here, the randomization is created, so to speak, by the lottery of life. On the other hand, there will obviously come a point when prognosis and age are so different that randomization through the administration of fair waiting lists will itself be seen by almost everyone as unfair. Treatment—as opposed to palliative care—may well be given to one patient and denied to another.

Of course—and returning to the notion of moral indeterminacy—where to draw the line for rationing between morally relevant and irrelevant age and prognosis remains unclear. There may be general agreement that a 95-year-old does not have the same right of access to scarce medical resources as a 35-year-old. Yet what about 35 v. 50? Similar dilemmas confront us with respect to prognosis. It may be fair to randomize patients for a particular treatment with, say, roughly the same life expectancy and/or probability of pain or mobility. However, this will not be so for those who differ greatly on any of these counts.

In both cases, the most just decision will require very detailed information on the comparative benefit of the treatment, along with a forum of discussion where views reflecting the capacities and interests of those who stand to lose and gain are rationally debated. Given our preceding argument about the relationship between rights and duties, such decisions will inevitably lead to a suspension of moral obligation on the part of those who have been declared moral unequals. In practice this should be because they are no longer capable of anything resembling moral reciprocity due to the impact of their age and illness on their human agency. Interestingly, much clinical intuition about rationing reflects this judgement, even when it is not articulated precisely in these terms. In any case, the results of such discussions of comparative need— assuming that they are truly democratic and representative—should then be incorporated in rationing policy.

Suffice it to say, that attempts to devise just methods of rationing do not preclude political struggles to diminish the scarcity which gives rise to their necessity. Indeed, it follows from the preceding theory of need that justice demands no less. Yet, as we have also seen, since 'ought implies can', we must sometimes make decisions which are as just and as rational as possible. Rough justice is better than no justice at all.

CONCLUSION

This chapter has argued that a consistent deontological interpretation of Beauchamp and Childress's four principles follows from Doyal and Gough's theory of human need. This provides a meta-ethical justification of the general moral importance of such an interpretation. The relevance of this justification for the theory and practice of medical ethics has also been outlined. Good and just practice of medicine has been shown not to be based on moral intuition, nor the greatest utility (of some subjective sort) of the greatest number. Rather medicine at its moral best derives from an understanding of the objective preconditions of human flourishing and a commitment to the consistency of whatever vision of the good which we accept. It is the failure of such understanding and commitment which leads to immoral medicine and to immorality generally.

REFERENCES

1. Beauchamp, T. and Childress, J. 1989. *Principles of bioethics.* Oxford University Press, New York.
2. Doyal, L. and Gough, I. 1991. *A theory of human need.* Macmillan, London.
3. Feinberg, J. 1973. *Social philosophy*, p. 111. Prentice Hall, Englewood Cliffs.
4. Wiggins, D. 1985. Claims of need. Pp. 153–159, *in* Honderich, T. (Ed.) *Morality and objectivity.* Routledge, London.
5. Thompson, G. 1986. *Needs*, pp. 35–54. Routledge, London.
6. Goodwin, R. 1988. *Reasons for welfare*, pp. 32–35. Princeton University Press, Princeton.

7. Lindley, R. 1986. *Autonomy*, chap. 2. Macmillan, London.
8. Parfitt, D. 1984. *Reasons and persons*, Pt. III. Clarendon Press, Oxford.
9. Stacey, M. 1988. *The sociology of health and healing*, pp. 169–172. Unwin Hyman, London.
10. Doyal, L. 1987. Health, underdevelopment and traditional medicine. *Holistic Medicine* **2**(1): 27–40.
11. Salmon, J. (Ed.) 1984. *Alternative medicines*, pp. 254–260. Tavistock, London.
12. Beauchamp, T. and Faden, R. 1986. *A theory and history of informed consent*, pp. 241–256. Oxford University Press, New York.
13. Braybrooke, D. 1987. *Meeting needs*, p. 48. Princeton University Press, Princeton.
14. Gorovitz, S. 1982. *Doctors' dilemmas*, chap. 4. Oxford University Press, New York.
15. Fulford, K. 1989. *Moral theory and medical practice*, chs. 8 and 9. Cambridge University Press, Cambridge.
16. Dworkin, G. 1988. *The theory and practice of autonomy*, chap. 5. Cambridge University Press, Cambridge.
17. Haworth, L. 1986. *Autonomy*, chap. 6. Yale University Press, New Haven.
18. Berlin, I. 1969. Two concepts of liberty. Pp. 118–172, in Berlin, I. (Ed.) *Four essays on liberty*. Oxford University Press, New York.
19. Platts, M. 1979. *Ways of meaning*, p. 243. Routledge, London.
20. Arrington, R. 1989. *Rationalism, realism and relativism*, chap. 4. Cornell University Press, Ithaca.
21. White, A. 1984. *Rights*, p. 70. Oxford University Press, Oxford.
22. Goodin, R. 1985. *Protecting the vulnerable*, pp. 151–153. University of Chicago Press, Chicago.
23. Gewirth, A. 1978. *Reason and morality*, pp. 240–248. University of Chicago Press, Chicago.
24. Hare, R. 1983. Ethical theory and utilitarianism. Pp. 23–38, in Sen, A. and Williams, B. (Eds) *Utilitarianism and beyond*. Cambridge University Press, New York.
25. Sen, A. 1982. Rights and agency. *Philosophy and public affairs*, **11**(1): 18–19.
26. Sen, A. and Williams, B. 1983. Introduction: Utilitarianism and beyond. Pp. 1–22, in Sen, A. and Williams, B. (Eds) *Utilitarianism and beyond*. Cambridge University Press, New York.
27. Dworkin, R. 1978. *Taking rights seriously*. Duckworth, London.
28. Doyal, L. 1990. Medical ethics and moral indeterminacy. *Journal of Law and Society*, **17**: 1.
29. Bell, J. and Mendus, S. 1988. *Philosophy and medical welfare*. Cambridge University Press, Cambridge.
30. Harris, J. 1985. *The value of life*, chap. 5. Routledge, London.

20

Rights and the Four Principles

Sophie Botros

*Lecturer in Medical Ethics, Centre of Medical Law and Ethics, King's College,
London, UK*

Puzzling ambiguities surround the claims made by Raanan Gillon for the four
principles* in his *Philosophical medical ethics* (1) (hereafter *PME*, with figures in
parentheses being page numbers in that book). They are said to be 'acceptable
within a wide range of very different moral theories' (quoted from a talk given
by Raanan Gillon, personal communication) and 'defensible from a variety of
theoretical perspectives' (*PME*, viii). Does this just mean that apparently conflicting
moral theories, such as Kantian deontology† and utilitarianism, recognize to a
greater or lesser extent the importance of all four principles for the guidance of
conduct in general? Or is a stronger claim being made, that deontologists and
utilitarians can agree in a wide range of medico-moral situations, where there is
an apparent conflict in application of the principles, which one should be given
priority, and hence what action to recommend? In addition, are these claims
concerning the principles to be substantiated simply by the neutral way in which
they are formulated, or by modifications of one of the theories?

In the following I confine my comments to just two of the four principles,
those of autonomy and beneficence, and argue that Gillon wishes to make the
stronger claim that deontologists and utilitarians could generally agree, at least
as regards these two principles, as to which principle should be given priority
in medico-moral disputes. This in turn seems to rest upon the contention that
the 'deontological'‡ principle of autonomy can be accommodated within a

---

* These are principles of autonomy, beneficence, non-maleficence and justice. In this chapter I shall
be concerned only with those of autonomy and beneficence. Moreover my references are all to
competent patients.
† Gillon appears to use the terms 'Kantian' and 'deontologist' almost interchangeably. Indeed he
describes Kant as a deontologist and stresses Kant's concern with autonomy as the overriding moral
principle. I follow this usage, although I would prefer a further distinction to be drawn between
duty-based and right-based deontologists. See Ronald Dworkin's interesting discussion (5) of the
relation between (what he calls) duty-based and right-based moralities and deontology.
‡ I follow Gillon in using quotation marks here, see *PME*, 22.

Principles of Health Care Ethics. Edited by Raanan Gillon.

utilitarian framework. But this contention, I suggest, receives perhaps insufficient support in *PME*, raising questions about how far it might be necessary or appropriate to acquaint health care workers with the philosophical underpinning of the moral import of their decisions.

I finally suggest that medical ethics should be more than just the judicious balancing of principles in order to reach practical moral decisions, and should involve a close scrutiny of the highly equivocal and theory-loaded language of current medico-moral debate, which centres largely upon rights.

NEUTRALITY AND THE FOUR PRINCIPLES

Near the beginning of *PME*, Gillon praises the American medical ethicists, Beauchamp and Childress, whom he describes as 'one a utilitarian, the other a deontologist' for 'showing how in practice both sides of this philosophical divide can agree on what might be termed working moral principles to be used in consideration of medico-moral issues' (26). At this point, Gillon might seem to be merely maintaining that it is possible to formulate moral principles, so detached from any justification in terms of moral theories as to obviate any need, at least in the limited context of health care, for an inquiry into how fundamentally irreconcilable these theories are.

Now of course it would be absurd to deny that in some sense or other all of the four principles could be acceptable to widely divergent moral theorists. Kant (2), for instance, though primarily concerned to insist that we should respect people's autonomy, treat them justly and never deliberately harm them, is hardly likely to deny that we should also treat people benevolently where we can. Indeed he makes helping others a moral duty, albeit an 'imperfect' one. Likewise it would be a brash utilitarian who would countenance our violating someone's autonomy when we could see no clear utility in doing so either for an individual or for people generally. Indeed as Gillon points out 'in practice everyone accepts [the] principle [of autonomy] to some extent' (63). If, of course, the principle stated that we should respect a person's autonomy *even if doing so would have deleterious consequences* it would evidently entail a rejection of utilitarianism. Nevertheless, provided that the principle of autonomy is so formulated as to be free of any tell-tale marks of its moral provenance, it can hardly offend even utilitarians.

According to Gillon, one advantage of showing that both deontologists and utilitarians have all of the four principles within their moral repertoire is that it would encourage people 'to consider the possible relevance of each of these principles to the particular circumstances' (viii). This, however, would seem of no help at all in settling the important question as to *just which* of these principles are to take priority in situations of apparent conflict in their application, and indeed practical decision-making is in danger of running aground. For a doctor to know how to settle a medico-moral conflict between, say, the principles of autonomy and beneficence, he must surely know whether to respect autonomy for its own sake, or only for the sake of any beneficial consequences it might have. But to recommend that a doctor respect a patient's autonomy for its own sake, rather than for its consequences, is already, it might seem, to favour one moral theory over the other.

It is, however, doubtful whether Gillon's obvious desire to remain neutral between these theories (23) would allow him to make such a biased judgement. In fact he deals with the problem of how neutrality could be maintained, yet specific moral recommendations made (118)*, by arguing that both utilitarians and deontologists would generally resolve medico-moral conflicts between the principles of autonomy and beneficence, such as whether to deceive a patient in order to spare him anguish, by giving priority to the principle of autonomy (102). Of course utilitarians and deontologists would have very different reasons for recommending that a doctor should not deceive her patient about his prognosis, and hence should respect his autonomy, even though the knowledge might 'cause [him] some immediate distress' (105). For utilitarians, the principle of respect for autonomy is a crucial moral principle only to the extent that it maximizes welfare and minimizes harm 'while (for deontologists) respect for people and their autonomy is itself the overriding moral principle' (102). But it can apparently be left up to the doctor herself to choose (8) whether to refrain from deceiving her patient on the deontological ground that the patient's autonomy must be respected *for its own sake* or on the utilitarian ground that the long-term benefits of respecting autonomy are likely to outweigh the short-term disadvantages.

But how is the ambitious claim that both utilitarians and deontologists could agree as to which principle should have priority, in a wide range of situations where autonomy and beneficence are in conflict, to be supported? Attempts, or partial attempts, at reconciling utilitarianism and deontology are typically made by utilitarians themselves,† and it is hardly surprising that Gillon, in his own attempt to effect some kind of reconciliation between these theories, reveals strong utilitarian proclivities. Although in his introduction (8), he states that 'the purpose of [his] book is not to promulgate a particular theory', he concedes (23) that utilitarianism, given its promise of 'a reliable decision procedure' and the absence of troublesome internal conflicts, would be, provided 'criticisms could be countered . . . an extremely attractive moral theory, offering considerable advantages over pluralist deontological theories'. Moreover his remark (26) that 'in practice at least it seems to me that there need be no unbridgeable incompatibility between non-absolutist pluralist deontological theories and utilitarianism' would seem, given its context, to be an endorsement of the utilitarians' claim to be able 'to encompass the ordinary deontological principles used in everyday moral and medico-moral decision-making' (22). Indeed

---

* The moral recommendation that Gillon makes in regard to conflicts between the principles of autonomy and beneficence is as follows: 'in normal cases respect for patients' autonomy takes moral priority over medical beneficence and generally precludes lying to or otherwise deceiving patients even in their own interests, breaking their confidences even in their own interests, and failing to obtain their adequately informed consent to medical intervention even in their own interests' (*PME*, 118).

† Gillon himself acknowledges this: 'contemporary utilitarianism in several of its variants purports to encompass the ordinary *prima facie* "deontological" moral principles used in everyday moral and medico-moral decision-making' (*PME*, 22).

utilitarians, we are told, 'have developed complicated ways of accommodating the standard deontological counterarguments to utilitarianism based on the counterintuitive results of a gross or simplified version of utilitarian thinking' (26). It might seem already therefore that one of the most damaging criticisms of utilitarianism—that it runs counter to our ordinary decent moral intuitions—can possibly be overcome. Nor is it simply a matter of a utilitarian *toleration* of deontological values, such as autonomy; respecting people's autonomy, it is claimed (65), must be a major *obligation* for utilitarians if their objective of maximizing welfare is to be achieved. For this very reason, Mill, 'a founding father of utilitarianism' (63), would have argued hardly less strongly for autonomy than Kant (65). Several chapters of *PME* are accordingly given over to showing that, for a very wide range of cases where the principles of autonomy and beneficence appear to be in conflict, a utilitarian backing can be found for allowing the 'deontological' principle of autonomy to predominate.

Now representing the four principles as effectively ungrounded in moral theory tends to encourage the conception of medical ethics as just the refining of a professional code of conduct. However, to advance the four principles on the basis of sophisticated philosophical claims, such as those mentioned above, far from representing a severing of decision-making from moral theory, appears, quite contrarily, to be part of an attempt to bring moral theory to bear on medical practice, and would have both important theoretical and practical implications.

Nevertheless a discrepancy now becomes apparent between Gillon's theoretical aim of showing how deontological concerns, such as respect for autonomy, can be accommodated within a utilitarian framework, which would involve lengthy and contentious philosophical argument, and his practical aim of helping health care workers make better medico-moral decisions. This dual aim compels the following question: how far is it necessary, possible, appropriate or even advisable to reveal the philosophical foundations of their moral practice to the busy doctors and other health care workers at which *PME* is primarily directed? Gillon evidently recognizes that health care professionals cannot be expected to become proficient in a style and intricacy of philosophical argument more suited to professional philosophy journals than to a medico-moral case presentation. His solution, as I show in the next section, is to endeavour to strike a balance between argument, on the one hand, and appeal to philosophical authority, on the other. However, as we shall see, he tends to appeal to authorities (e.g. J.S. Mill and R. M. Hare) just where the standard utilitarian arguments that they can accommodate 'conventional' (26) deontological principles, such as respect for autonomy, seem to be in danger of breaking down. Thus the perplexed reader may well find that it is just when she most requires it to resolve her medico-moral dilemmas, that further philosophical help is lacking.

UTILITARIAN DOCTORS AND THE PRINCIPLE OF AUTONOMY

With some apparent medico-moral conflicts a utilitarian backing can be found for respecting a patient's autonomy, rather than for being beneficent, just by pointing to the long-term cost of sparing the patient immediate distress. Thus Gillon (68–69) writes of the effects of deceiving a patient about a dire prognosis:

The assumption, however, that this generally makes such patients happier is highly suspect ... what is more, it is often only the patient who is deceived and treated thus, while a relative or relatives are told the truth; the deceit that this imposes on the family (and also on other medical and nursing staff) may itself provoke considerable distress, not to mention the breaking of normal medical confidentiality and the effects of doing so. Then there is the suffering of the patient who suspects that something nasty is afoot but cannot discover what. Finally, there is the suffering of a fatally ill patient on discovering that he or she has been deceived by his or her doctor and family. What a way to go.

But even an act-utilitarian, assessing the rightness or wrongness of an action by calculating the amount of good in its consequences, and defining good in terms of overall welfare, would give priority here to respecting the patient's autonomy. Hence there is really no disagreement in the first place between utilitarians and deontologists as to what should be done. Indeed, it is only if the principle of beneficence is interpreted so narrowly as to require the doctor merely to spare her patient immediate pain, rather than being (what Gillon sometimes calls) a principle of 'real beneficence' (74), that being beneficent could ever have seemed to be in conflict with the principle of autonomy.

Suppose, however, that a doctor is quite certain that, even considering the possible long-term repercussions, to conceal from this particular patient his prognosis will best promote the welfare of everyone concerned. Gillon seeks to show that, even here, utilitarians can agree with deontologists that the doctor should not deceive her patient. He appeals to the traditional utilitarian strategy of asserting that no-one is more qualified to determine which course of action will promote the most welfare than those whose welfare is at stake. A long list of factors is cited (70–71), including the psychological make-up of the people concerned, which would have to be taken into account if someone else was to make this decision for them. The upshot is that it would quite probably be disastrous for a doctor to assume the role of the 'happiness' predictor for the patient and his family. Hence utilitarians, as well as deontologists, have reason to recommend that the doctor tells the truth and lets her patient deal with the facts himself.

This application to the medical context of the somewhat overworked utilitarian strategy for accommodating the deontological concern with respect for autonomy is genuinely illuminating here because it brings out (71) the important distinction between a technical medical decision, which only doctors are competent to make, and a medico-moral decision, which they are arguably no more competent to make than their patients. Nevertheless, as we have seen, once the doctor discriminates between these two types of decision, she will have good reason, even as a utilitarian, not to pre-empt the decisions of her patients. It is therefore doubtful whether Gillon's manoeuvre amounts to a demonstration that the two apparently divergent moral theories can after all be reconciled. Rather, it shows that utilitarians ought to be properly sensitive to the limits of a doctor's special expertise, and so recommend that doctors tell the truth here, just as the deontologist insists.

Similar qualifications apply to several other useful reminders that Gillon provides for doctors. A doctor who neglects to discover a patient's own wishes regarding treatment, not only fails to respect her autonomy but may therefore be unable 'to do [her] good', as the principle of beneficence requires. Thus Gillon writes (75):

> If one wants to do good for a patient one generally needs to find out what he or she actually wants one to do. In even the simplest of interactions patients in similar circumstances want different things from their doctors. One patient with a sore throat wants antibiotics, another wants a pain killer, another wants information about what it is, whether it is likely to go to his chest . . . and a fourth wants a sick note for his employer but refuses treatment, preferring to let nature take its course. The doctor who 'knows' what his patient wants without asking him is quite likely to get it wrong.

It is also pointed out (75) that respecting a patient's autonomy in the sense of fully and frankly explaining to her a proposed treatment is probably the most effective way of achieving the compliance necessary if she is to get better. There is thus not only 'an independent presumption' (75) in favour of respecting the patient's autonomy in such cases, but doing so is also a means to promoting a medically beneficial outcome. The reader may at this point be wondering why it was ever supposed in the first place that there was a 'divide' between deontologists and utilitarians, since it may now seem to be a relatively simple matter to show how they can be brought to agree in most of their moral recommendations, at least where the principles of autonomy and beneficence are in apparent conflict.

But consider the following situation. A woman, A, has breast cancer. There are two possible treatments: mastectomy and lumpectomy. Her doctor believes that mastectomy will give her a better chance of avoiding serious medical complications later, and hence is the better treatment for her. Knowing how fearful she is of major surgery, he is convinced that if he were to tell her of the less aggressive option, she would demand it. He also believes that if he then refused her demand, she would consult another less responsible but more obliging doctor, with potentially disastrous consequences. He decides that the best thing to do is not to inform her of what he believes to be the inferior treatment option. Now obviously deontologists will condemn any deliberate manipulation for her own good of a competent patient's decision. Can it be shown that utilitarians also have a good reason for challenging the doctor's decision?

The reference in *PME* to the views of J. S. Mill (3) are relevant here. Mill claimed that the utilitarian goal of happiness or welfare is 'constituted to a large extent in the exercise of people's autonomy' (65, also 26). He believed that it is destructive of their happiness for people to be treated as mere passive beneficiaries of others' good offices, even if this could save them from making terrible mistakes and spare them much anguish. It might plausibly be denied, then, by a utilitarian of Mill's complexion that manipulating her decision would contribute to A's welfare, despite the possibly damaging consequences of letting her make her own choice.

But suppose A's doctor is willing to concede *some* moral weight to respecting his patient's autonomy in determining how best to promote her welfare. Nevertheless he urges that being respected as an autonomous person is only *one* of the things in which the patient has an interest, and so only one of the values that should guide a doctor's choice of whether to inform her of certain treatment options. He also believes that she has an interest in getting better. But there is a limit, which any good utilitarian would recognize, as to how much a patient may be allowed to damage herself by choosing a medically inferior treatment, and by revealing both treatment options here he would step over that limit.

But the deontologist is unlikely to accept this modest role for respect for autonomy in the hierarchy of values. Indeed he will claim that it defeats the whole purpose of insisting on autonomy as a *right*. For if respecting autonomy is only one of the values that the doctor must feed into his computation of how best to promote his patient's overall welfare, it is potentially overridable, just like any other consideration. But the existence of a right to autonomy is a guarantee that the decision of an autonomous person may never be manipulated, even though others judge that it will be for her own good.

Here then is a situation of conflict between the principles of autonomy and beneficence where utilitarians and deontologists appear not to be able to agree, even in practice, as to which principle should be given priority. Unless some further strategy can be found for reconciling the two types of theorist, one of the central claims of *PME* may seem to be threatened. A further strategy, however, is implicit in the discussion (71) of the Christian Scientist 'whose decision to turn to orthodox treatment for her thyrotoxicosis [comes] too late to save her life'. Here Gillon writes that 'those for whom the principle of respect for autonomy is morally important' would respect her right to refuse medical treatment 'even though this was highly likely to be fatal and thus cause her family and medical attendants great anguish and even though paternalistic intervention would have saved her life'.

But the principle of respect for autonomy is, Gillon claims, important for both Kantian deontologists and many utilitarians. Hence many utilitarians would argue that the patient's autonomy should be respected, even though it will 'result in an obviously worse decision in terms of the patient's, the family's or even, a particular society's happiness'. But what could possibly be the utilitarian justification for respecting autonomy in such a case? Such respect is required, Gillon claims, 'if human welfare *really is to be maximized*' (my italics). The reference in the notes (72) to R. M. Hare's *Moral Thinking: Its Levels, Method and Point*, suggests that this apparently paradoxical position is being maintained by appeal to an *extra* or *meta-consequentialist* rule to be followed on the basis of the promotion of welfare. Hare's position here is more fully expounded by John Mackie (4) thus:

> At the level of ordinary practical day-to-day thinking, actions and choices are to be guided by rules, principles [and] dispositions . . . rights will be recognized at this level. But at a higher level of critical or philosophical thinking these various provisions are to be called in question, tested, explained, justified, amended, or rejected by considering how well practical thinking that is guided by them is likely to promote the general happiness. Such intermediate devices, interposed between practical choices and the utilitarian goal, may for various reasons do more for that goal than the direct application of utility calculations to everyday choices.

It seems then that, once more, Gillon is offering two reasons for respecting a patient's autonomy. It is, of course, in accord with ordinary deontological principles to respect autonomy. Also, however, and quite independently, respecting autonomy is more likely to further the utilitarian goal of maximizing welfare, even though it may not seem to. It must hence be required both by deontologists and many utilitarians. But why should the utilitarian doctor accept this bare assertion that respecting a patient's autonomy, though it so patently leads to a disastrous outcome, will really maximize welfare? Is the doctor just to accept it on authority, and if so, on whose? Is the cryptic reference to Hare enough to establish such an authority? Moreover, if the doctor is at all inquiring, she may well already have doubts (shared by many of Hare's opponents) about the viability of this 'split-level' thinking. Mackie, for instance, asks how a person is to maintain the two levels of thinking whilst keeping them insulated from each other: can a person, who is 'for part of the time a critical moral philosopher in the utilitarian style' (ref. 4, p. 173) prevent this method of thought from 'infecting his everyday moral thought and conduct'? Mackie concludes that such a person would not be able to take seriously, e.g., rights when he knows that these are just 'devices to compensate for the inability of everyone, himself included, to calculate reliably . . . in terms of aggregate utility'.

One solution, Mackie suggests, would be for these two different types of thinking to be done by 'two different classes of *people* . . . those who follow a practical morality devised for them by others, and those who devise this, but themselves follow a different, more directly utilitarian morality' (my italics). But it would surely be odd if, having been encouraged critically to appraise their medico-moral practice, doctors were finally told that there were things here that only the experts, namely philosophers, could properly understand and hence make decisions about.

At the very heart of Gillon's treatment in *PME* of at least two of the four principles (namely the principles of autonomy and beneficence), I thus detect misgivings about the whole enterprise of opening up the critical resources of philosophy to health care workers in order that they can examine for themselves the foundations of their medico-moral practice. Sometimes such critical thought seems to be encouraged; at other times it almost seems as if doctors are being shielded from possibly unsettling reappraisals on grounds that these are better left to philosophers.

Gillon, the key British exponent of the four principles, has undoubtedly made a notable contribution to the difficult problem of how to make moral theory bear on medico-moral practice. It is a pity therefore that the four principles seem nevertheless to relegate medical ethics to a shadowy hinterland between applying pre-established criteria to practical decision-making and doing philosophy.

MEDICAL ETHICS AND THE LANGUAGE OF RIGHTS

Putting to one side Gillon's own position, I want now briefly to argue that the idea that a checklist of principles, effectively detached from any grounds in moral theory, and encouraging a false sense of security about the extent to which moral conflicts may be resolvable, *could* be of help to health care workers involves a mistake. It is that of failing to realize that the language of current public moral debate, centring largely around rights—those of fetuses, of the senile and of autonomous persons—is grievously ambiguous and theory-laden. A major service that philosophers could render to health care workers, faced with acute moral dilemmas, is to make them aware of the confusing way in which the rhetoric of rights is used both to advance different moral theories and to express conflicting moral claims.

Two examples will help to illustrate this. An anti-abortionist will typically support his position by pointing to the fetus's right to life. A proponent of voluntary euthanasia will typically support his position by claiming that autonomous persons have a right to self-determination. But have the rights mentioned here anything in common morally? It would hardly seem so. For the anti-abortionist appeals to the rights of the fetus precisely in order to emphasize the absolutely binding nature of the prohibition against intentionally killing innocent human beings. The proponent of voluntary euthanasia, by contrast, appeals to the rights of autonomous persons in order to *deny* the binding quality of the prohibition on intentional killing. For him, an autonomous person may exercise her rights just in order to cancel another person's duty not to kill her. The ambiguities are clear.

A second illustration of the highly ambiguous and theory-loaded nature of the language of rights concerns the frequently heard contention that patients have a right to information (about their illness and about any proposed treatments or alternatives). But why, one may well ask, is this claim formulated in terms of *rights*? Does it really make a moral, as opposed to a rhetorical, difference whether it is formulated thus or in terms of duties? If a patient has a right that her autonomy be respected by being given information about a proposed treatment, then doesn't her doctor have a duty to respect her autonomy and, if so, is not this duty properly part of his ethical code? But if respect for patient autonomy can so comfortably be accommodated within the confines of the medical ethical code, why should doctors often so hotly contest this claim? What consideration is it being pressed against that makes it so controversial and so likely to be rejected by doctors?

To answer these questions it is necessary to recall the position of the American informed consent theorists who first* advanced the claim that patients have this right to information. For them, this claim had a special moral force. It entailed that a patient's autonomy must be respected for its own sake and not merely because doing so was in the long run in the patients', or in society's, best interests. Moreover even if the doctor were prepared to respect a patient's autonomy for its own sake, it must not be thus respected only so long as it did not conflict with the duty of care. Thus a show-down is forced between those who regard autonomy as the pre-eminent value and their moral opponents.

But against this background, interpreting the claim that patients 'have a right to information' as merely part of the doctor's duty of care (since they are more

---

* See reference to Justice Schroeder in *Natanson v Kline,* in Veatch (7), p. 45.

likely to get better if they feel that they are being respected as people) can be seen as itself a counter-move, favoured by conservative doctors, to accommodate such a right, whilst not fully yielding to the patient's autonomy. Thus a doctor may continue to deny important information to a patient because he thinks it will be damaging to her health, and yet concede that patients have a right to important information concerning their prognosis, etc. For him, however, such a right cannot override his duty of care; it merely arises out of, and is complementary to, one of the duties that comprise his duty of care—namely the duty to give information so long as it is not damaging to his patient. We might therefore perhaps coin the term *'duty-based* right' to describe it, in contrast to the *'right-based* rights' which informed consent theorists are evidently concerned to assert.

It is difficult to see how the confusing and complex relationship between rights and duties that I have sketched here, their varying significance within different claims and contexts, the ongoing debate between different types of moralist, and the major collisions of values that are involved in the above examples, could possibly be articulated within the conceptual resources of the four principles. This is especially true if their own putative grounds have been deliberately disregarded, and where it is immaterial to their proponents whether, say, the principle of autonomy is taken as an ultimate principle or grounded in the promotion of welfare.

My own suggestion would be that the framework of the four principles be replaced by one in which three types of moral approach, namely 'duty-based', 'right-based' and 'goal-based', are contrasted. This would involve applying to the moral domain a terminology originally introduced by the legal theorist Ronald Dworkin (5) to differentiate between types of political theory. This framework alone, I believe, is flexible enough to allow us to take account of the different types of moral right mentioned above, and hence to accommodate the huge shifts in moral perspective that they entail. I have pursued these suggestions in more detail elsewhere (6).

ACKNOWLEDGEMENT

I owe a debt of gratitude in writing this paper to Dr A. R. Jonckheere, who has constantly forced me to clarify my points and produce better arguments.

REFERENCES

1. Gillon, R. 1986. *Philosophical medical ethics.* John Wiley & Sons, Chichester.
2. Kant, I. 1964. Groundwork of the metaphysics of morals. *In* Paton, H. J. (Ed.) *The moral law.* Hutchinson University Library, London.
3. Mill, J. S. 1974. On liberty. *In* Warnock, M. (Ed.) *Utilitarianism.* Collins/Fontana, Glasgow.
4. Mackie, J. 1990. Can there be a right-based moral theory. Pp. 172–173, *in* Waldron, J. (Ed.) *Theories of rights,* Oxford University Press, Oxford.
5. Dworkin, R. 1977. *Taking rights seriously,* pp. 171–172. Duckworth, London.
6. Botros, S. 1992. Duty-based, right-based and goal-based approaches: sketch of a new framework for medical ethics. (Unpublished manuscript.)
7. Veatch, R. 1981. *Theory of medical ethics.* Basic Books, New York.

21

Ideals, the Four Principles and Practical Ethics

ALASTAIR V. CAMPBELL

Professor of Biomedical Ethics and Director of the Bioethics Research Centre, University of Otago, New Zealand

INTRODUCTION

Is there a place in health care ethics for actions beyond the call of duty? It very much depends how we phrase the relevant ethical questions. If we start from the assumption that professional ethics is best understood in terms of general principles which delineate the scope of moral obligation, then we shall find no place for moral ideals in the general scheme of things. Of course, acts in excess of what the principles require may be seen as admirable, exemplary even, but (in this moral scheme) they cannot form part of that general morality which is to be expected of every practitioner. Ideals are for the exceptional few: but for the many the observance of the numerous interlocking (at times conflicting) requirements of the principles is all that should be demanded.

But what if this is the wrong place from which to start the discussion of health care ethics? What if the provision of helping relationships to people in times of a crisis in their health cannot be properly understood without appeal to ideals which transcend the boundaries set by principles? What if the virtuous practitioner is a better model for health care ethics than the conscientious one? Moreover, what if ideals are equally needed by those who seek professional help, and by those who help or support others in a non-professional capacity? Perhaps the stress on principles guiding health care practice is caught in both an over-rationalistic and an over-professionalized mould.

In this chapter I shall be considering these questions, first by exploring the implications of three case examples, each of which illustrates how ideals enter into the substance of health care practice. I shall discuss whether these cases could have been dealt with simply by recourse to the relevant principles of ethics. My conclusion will be that the principles become devoid of useful moral content unless they are made to intersect with a set of ideals which are beyond

Principles of Health Care Ethics. Edited by Raanan Gillon.
© 1994 John Wiley & Sons Ltd

the call of duty. I shall try to formulate this conclusion without falling into the trap of portraying the health care provider as some kind of saint, angel or heroic figure. The emphasis in my conclusion will be on the *practicality* of ideals, and their applicability to all parties in health care relationships, and an example of a 'virtuous' patient will serve to reinforce this point.

THE CASE OF THE FOOLISH DOCTOR

Once upon a time a doctor who specialized in intensive care within a high-tech hospital setting was confronted with a request he would rather not have ever heard, yet in his field the request is not an uncommon one. His patient wanted nothing more than to die, and to die in a way that was not too prolonged and not too frightening. We do not need to dwell on the patient's medical condition, for, although no-one would deny that it was severe, unpleasant and incurable, she alone could judge whether it was unbearable, and she did so judge. She expressed her desire to die in such a consistent and reasoned manner that no psychiatrist could diagnose depression as a let-out for his clinical colleagues.

So the foolish doctor began to rehearse his ethical principles. His patient's choice appeared to be an autonomous one—should it not be honoured? His patient's life was miserable—would it not be a beneficent act to help it to an end? He need not do active harm, just switch off the life-support and increase the medication to avoid anxiety and respiratory distress. And would it not be just to make his expensive equipment available for other patients who had greater use for it? With such a battery of green lights on a principled ethic, the foolish doctor worked out a plan with the patient and with other staff that resulted in her peaceful death, in the presence of family and friends, a few hours after the respirator was switched off. The patient's last words to the doctor were 'Please tell others about this, so they know they have a choice.'

And so the foolish doctor wrote a brief report on the case for a professional journal, and wrote a plain-language version for a popular magazine, and offered to present his case at a conference for his fellow-specialists. His colleagues were horrified! Did he really want to publicize how his patient gained a peaceful death from his ministrations? Did he want to make himself, and all his fellow-specialists, vulnerable to the attacks of the 'pro-lifers'? Why had he acted without covering his tracks more carefully under advice from his medical protection society? Why draw attention to himself now, when it would be easy to keep the whole incident under wraps?

But all the foolish doctor would answer was, 'I owe it to her, and I cannot let her down.' Thus he risked more than was reasonable, more than was a duty, out of loyalty to the dead, or perhaps out of concern for those in the future who would not know to ask for such an easy death.

So was our 'foolish doctor' an idealist, going beyond the requirements of ordinary medical duty? In their very clear and useful analysis of moral ideals in *Principles of biomedical ethics* Beauchamp and Childress (1) suggest that ideals 'transcend ordinary universal duties without violating them' (p. 255). Following an account by Urmson, they describe the features of saints and heroes, who consistently do their duty when others normally do not or who go beyond duty at some risk to the self. Such categories, however, obscure the real issue, which is whether at the level of ordinary non-saintly, non-heroic morality there is a need for moral ideals, in order to give a proper expression to the nature of the moral life. Our 'foolish doctor' was neither a saint nor a hero, but many would regard him as an example of a good or virtuous doctor, because he was committed to acting against his own self-interest for the benefit of patients.

Thus we need to consider a goodness or virtue which does not 'transcend' moral obligation, but which rather gives it its specifically moral character. (This is expressed in accounts of religious ethics by speaking of the *spirit*, not merely the *letter* of the Law.) This requirement to blend virtue and obligation is acknowledged by Beauchamp and Childress later in the same chapter (p. 265), when they state 'character and virtues are indispensable in the moral life and cannot be ignored in ethical theory' (1). This leads them on to a brief discussion of the nature of goodness or virtue in professional health care. My argument in this chapter is that such an account needs to be greatly expanded and to be given a more central place in health care ethics.

Let us return, then, to our foolish doctor. I have suggested that his actions exemplify a moral ideal which is central to the ethical treatment of patients or clients. Yet, paradoxically, his actions may not have been morally right. It could be argued with some force that removing artificial ventilation (even at the patient's request) and (more seriously) using medication to ensure that the patient did not survive this removal was tantamount to killing the patient. Some requests, it could be argued, must never be granted, since to do so would be to act immorally and (probably) illegally. The only right course of action for the doctor—so this argument goes—would be to help the patient change her mind about wanting to die. Colluding in her plans is failing in one's duty to her.

We do not need to resolve this argument about whether the doctor acted rightly in order to establish whether he followed a moral ideal. The possibility of being wrong is part of that ideal, for this possibility is present in every moral decision made by ordinary mortals. It is the acting in good faith *for* the patient and *against* the dictates of prudence that embodies the moral ideal. We may describe that ideal as the risk of self for others, or more simply as loyalty. (The nature of that loyalty was very fully discussed in one of the first works in modern medical ethics—Paul Ramsey's *The patient as a person* (2).) Thus the folly of the doctor is like the folly of the fool in *King Lear*:

> That sir which serves and seeks for gain
> And follows but for form
> Will pack when it begins to rain
> And leave thee in the storm.
> But I will tarry; the fool will stay,
> And let the wise man fly. (3)

Like Lear's fool, the foolish doctor stays loyal when there is no possible advantage to be gained, no contract to require him to stay on the side of the vulnerable person when the storm rages.

THE CASE OF THE ERRANT PATIENT

I turn now to a second case, one which tests in a different way the character of the helping relationship. In this case more than loyalty is required. Rather, the moral ideal is that of perseverance, or of a hope beyond hope.

One day in a medical ward the truth was vindicated by means of deceit, but lying was closer to the truth. In this unhappy scenario it was of no help to anyone that a professional judgement triumphed, since this victory was really just a form of therapeutic defeat.

These strange contradictions arise from a fairly familiar problem in health care: self-induced illness. A young woman re-appeared constantly on a medical ward for tests to establish the cause of her very severe gastric problems. With all other diagnoses eliminated, the staff became convinced that she was inducing her symptoms with frequent heavy use of purgative drugs. Yet this she strenuously denied. A way to circumvent this denial was planned by all and executed by the charge nurse, who searched her locker after having her leave the ward on a false pretext. Professional judgement 'triumphed' when a large container of the relevant medicine was found in her handbag. When confronted with the 'evidence' the patient agreed that the pills belonged to her, but was unable to admit even then that she ever took them. She also adamantly refused any form of psychiatric help, and bitterly accused the hospital of invading her privacy and of failing to give her the treatment she required. The outcome was a therapeutic defeat, with every prospect that after a rapid discharge from hospital (which seemed inevitable) she would find another group of professionals to treat her once again as a 'real' patient, at least for a time.

This case illustrates the poverty of an approach to health care ethics which tries to 'fix' an interpersonal dilemma by working with just one half of the relationship. When the providers and user of health care have such totally different perceptions of the 'truth' of the situation, the only viable ethic is a mutual ethic, in which provider and user sink or swim together. The health care provider cannot create hope where none exists, and cannot force upon the recipient of care answers to questions which are not being asked or solutions to problems which the recipient cannot perceive.

We could, of course, try some application of the four principles to the case of the 'errant' patient, in an effort to guide the decisions of the professionals involved. We could consider whether the deceit and intrusion of privacy were justified by their beneficent intent. We could ask whether the patient's autonomy must be wholly respected when it is so obviously impaired by a driving need to be ill. We could justify the confrontation with the 'evidence' and the subsequent discharge from hospital on the principle of non-maleficence, since continued investigations would clearly be futile, if not dangerous. The principle of justice would certainly suggest that resources of potential use to others were being wasted by this patient, and that she should be flushed out of the health delivery system as quickly and effectively as possible. ('Bad' patients who waste professional time and resources are a familiar problem in every system.) But all this would be to miss the moral point. We would be trying to apply the rules of rugby, while the patient is really immersed in a game of cricket! We may be utterly right according to our rules, but for the patient our 'right' actions are both meaningless and useless. We are not in any sense a co-player in her potentially lethal game, and so, however 'right' we are, we are total failures as helpers. It is like a rehearsal of the old medical joke: 'The operation was a success; regrettably the patient died.'

So what is the ideal which must guide us in this situation? It has to do with the rejection of a 'fix-it' approach to health care and with a willingness to share in the ordeal of the person's illness, as she perceives it.* I have described it above as 'hope beyond hope', because the perseverance required entails for the professional a profound sense of defeat as the first step towards a mutual hope. The required idealism is a two-stage affair—recognizing failure, and being willing to start again in a way which will try to meet the patient where she is. An ethic of simple duty makes no such requirement. It allows the professional to say, after honest attempts to help, that the patient has only herself to blame for her condition. It does not require the helper to question his or her part in the failure.

LOVE'S LABOUR LOST

In a third case we shall see that the moral ideals required in confronting illness are as relevant to the relatives of sufferers as they are to the sufferers themselves or to their professional helpers. The moral ideal highlighted by this case is that of acting with courage.

> Harry had always tried to be a kind and considerate husband to his wife, Susie, but somehow he had always failed her; fallen short of what she expected. His sense of inadequacy was compounded by their long and futile efforts to have children, eventually traced to his infertility. His wife had been becoming increasingly demanding and aggressive as she neared the end of her childbearing years, and eventually (after much hesitation on her part, but on urging from her husband) a donor insemination was carried out. The resultant pregnancy caused a puzzling reaction in Susie—she was at first overjoyed, but then began to have violent mood swings and incidents of somewhat bizarre behaviour, rather like a caricature of her usual quite assertive personality. In a lull between these violent outbursts she agreed that they should consult their general practitioner together to see if he could help them understand what was happening. At the consultation the practitioner pointed out to her that (as she already knew) there was a history of Huntington's disease in her family. He said that one possible explanation for her sudden changes in mood was that she was experiencing the early symptoms of the disease which begins to manifest itself in middle age and results in increasingly disabling mental changes. These suggestions provoked an outburst of rage in Susie. She swore that she would have nothing more to do with that doctor, that there was nothing the matter with her (apart from the usual moodiness of early pregnancy) and that she would refuse to have any of the tests suggested by the GP to seek to establish a diagnosis and to predict an outcome for her baby. Switching from anger to pleading, she clung to her husband and tearfully demanded, 'Harry, don't let them take my baby away from me!' Harry—who had always tried so hard to please her—found himself desperately looking for a way to be a loving husband, as he had always been. Where was he to turn to do the right thing by her and the baby?

Had Harry known about the four principles of biomedical ethics it would not have helped him much with his dilemma. True, he might have considered the balance of his obligations to his wife and to the child as yet unborn, each deserving of his beneficent attention—but to what degree? He might have contemplated the harms entailed in trying to overrule Susie's determination to

---

* For a powerful exposition of the theme of the patient's experience of illness see May (4).

avoid a definitive diagnosis, and the harms to himself and especially to the child to be born in letting her will prevail. He might have sought professional advice about the extent to which his wife's capacity for autonomous choice was already affected by her developing illness. But none of this would be of any use to Harry so long as he continued to perceive love as appeasement, and so long as he saw himself as always the one in the wrong—the failed lover. To deal with the morality of the choices facing him and his wife Harry needed courage, a capacity to face up to his wife's anger and to take the steps necessary to minimize the harm in their tragic situation. He needed courage not as some admirable extra which would put him into the category of romantic hero, but as a simple and totally necessary component of his moral responsibility as the spouse of an increasingly mentally disturbed pregnant woman. Thus the ideal of courageous decision-making was integral to his moral choices.

ANGELS, HEROES AND PRACTICAL IDEALISM

The three case examples I have chosen have a common thread running through them. They illustrate the testing nature of moral choice in health crisis situations. Much of our day-to-day experience of health care is really of little interest to a theoretical approach to health care ethics, since it consists of formed habits of attitude and action, which we follow without reflection upon what we are doing. The fact that such habits are of minimal theoretical interest does not mean that they are unimportant to morality. On the contrary, without such habits our daily interactions—in health care and in life more generally—would be fraught with danger and uncertainty. We rightly assume that most health care providers most of the time will act (without having to think about it) in a way which respects their clients' or patients' wishes; we assume that most patients most of the time will give accurate information about their thoughts, feelings and actions; we regard relatives, most of the time, as the advocates and supporters of the patient, enabling the patient to have her wishes fulfilled. But habitual approaches to choices break down when the assumptions upon which they are based no longer hold. Harry had to find a different kind of care for his wife; the errant patient was seeking someone who would accept the importance of her 'lying'; the foolish doctor had a risky choice to make—in both a moral and a professional sense—and so found himself at odds with the ethos of his own profession.

In such testing situations there is more than a rational task to be performed in order to make effective and informed choices. The test is not simply one of reasoning ability (though clear thinking about principles is always important): it is a test of character. Beauchamp and Childress perceive this point (at least in part), and put forward the following description of the place of virtue and strength of character in health care ethics:

> Our willingness to *trust* a health care professional will depend on what we think about that person's character. To trust others is to have confidence in and to rely upon them to act in certain ways ... A person is worthy of such trust only if he or she has displayed a character that includes several virtues (ref. 1, p. 263).

But although this is a clear expression of the importance of character for the *habitual* practice of morality in health care, it lacks direct application to the critical choices which must be taken. Moreover, it also fails to perceive the qualities of character required also of patients and of relatives in such critical situations. Indeed, there is a grave danger that too much emphasis on the required virtues in the professional character will perpetuate that inequality between provider and user in health care, which has been the mainstay of paternalism in the past.

What is required, then, is an entirely practical form of idealism; one which aids the choices of all parties and which avoids the error of making the health care professional into an angelic or heroic figure. Until relatively recent times the irrational, frightening aspects of our confrontation with illness have been dealt with by investing nurses and doctors with powerful images of care and healing, based upon stereotypes of femininity and masculinity. The nurse becomes an angel of mercy, floating ethereally above the pain, fear and mess of illness. Nowhere is this more powerfully portrayed than in Longfellow's poem, *Sancta Filomena* (Holy Florence), a poem in praise of Florence Nightingale:

> Lo! in that house of misery
> A lady with a lamp I see
> Pass through the glimmering gloom,
> And flit from room to room.
>
> And slow, as in a dream of bliss,
> The speechless sufferer turns to kiss
> Her shadow, as it falls
> Upon the darkening walls. (5)

This soft image of the nurse was complemented by a hard image of the doctor, the heroic fighter against the forces of illness and death. The superior knowledge of the doctor and the skill in overcoming disease gave god-like properties, creating a hero of semi-divine potency. So an ancient fragment portrays the doctor as both god and brother to the sick: 'He would be like God, saviour equally of slaves, of paupers, of rich men, of princes, and to all a brother' (6). These images linger on in contemporary health care, despite the changes in gender balance in both professions stereotyped in this manner. But the total passivity of the patient in both scenarios (Miss Nightingale's patient does not even speak!) and the unrealistic sentimentality of the imagery must surely force us to find alternative ways of conveying the necessary confrontation with illness. We need an idealism which provides a shared framework of resolve for all those caught up in the crisis of illness. Such a framework will be found by discovering a shared imagery of heroism and hope.

But where are we to turn for such a shared imagery? The traditional approach to virtues and vices has a quaintly outmoded ring. Most people have heard of the 'seven deadly sins'—though they probably would find difficulty in naming them all.* But how many people would even have heard of their counterparts:

---

* For those who failed this test the answer is: pride, avarice, lust, gluttony, envy, anger and sloth.

the four cardinal virtues (prudence, temperance, justice and courage) and the three theological virtues (faith, hope and charity)?* Such shopping lists of vices and virtues, which derive from the writings of Plato and Aristotle and their Christianization by the Church Fathers, seem to embody both psychological and religious assumptions which our era has outgrown. The Freudian dissection of motives has left temperance and courage suspect, and we tend to perceive a conflict rather than a complementarity between prudence and justice. As for faith, hope and charity, what more are these to our secular age than preacher's rhetoric, appealing only to the religiously devout?

Yet something is required to fill the gap left by the rejection of a simplified moralism and an unquestioned religious world-view. Perhaps the answer lies in seeking to delineate *virtue* rather than *virtues*.† In so doing we would be trying to describe actions not merely by their external form, but by their origins in the character of the agent. Here we shall find the need of descriptions like 'wise' (as opposed to merely clever), 'brave', 'tolerant', 'persevering', 'dependable, 'sincere', 'loyal', 'humorous', 'humble', 'open', 'warm'. These are all ways of describing not just what a person does but how he or she does it. We will seek different aspects of moral character for different situations. To some extent we can connect these to social roles. For example, we might want the police to be courageous and dependable, but not feel it essential that they were warm and humorous! We will look for loyalty and perseverance in a parent, but might settle for dependability and sincerity in a salesperson. A witty magistrate may help pass a tedious day in court, but we would prefer that she were both tolerant and wise.

It must be accepted that all such attempts to describe character as opposed to a specified set of actions which conform to moral principles will have an arbitrary and imprecise feel about them. The words we use are attempts to convey perceptions of the actions of others which are largely intuitive and may be far from the truth. (Think of the millions of Americans who perceived some notoriously dishonest tele-evangelists as 'sincere'!) The creation of the right personal image has become a major industry in itself, and, of course, if virtue is no more than appearance it ceases to be virtue. It is hardly surprising, then, that we are often prepared to settle for an assessment of the rightness or wrongness of a person's actions as a more reliable yardstick than subjective perceptions of a person's character. (In many a medical disciplinary case there has been no shortage of witnesses to describe what a wonderful doctor Doctor X was.)

But in the situations which face people during illness the need to go beyond the externalities of actions is very great. The reason for this is obvious. All serious illness or injury presents a threat to the individual (and the individual's family) of such a magnitude that the ordinary ways of coping with life's problems are rarely sufficient. The possibility of death or of permanent disablement creates special demands on the relationships available to a person in such a crisis. A

---

* For an admirable account of the virtues as traditionally understood, see the relevant entries in Ref. 7.
† See Stanley Hauerwas's helpful discussion of this distinction in ref. 7, p. 649.

search for 'virtue' from those involved can be seen as a search for relationships of the appropriate quality to enable the person to come through the crisis in his or her unique way, and in a way which is also fulfilling for those who offer assistance and support. Illness is first and foremost a test of the character of the ill person, before any question arises about the character of that person's helpers, and in this respect most health care ethics is sadly deficient in its stress on the duties or the virtues of helpers only.* My concluding case example is an attempt to remedy this deficiency by portraying a not-uncommon example of heroism in the face of incurable illness, and then to specify why this exemplifies an ideal which could both enrich and correct any approach to health care ethics which talks merely of principles.

ON REFUSING TO SACRIFICE ONESELF

To many people the news that they have a fatal illness which has a short-term survival rate represents a kind of altar of a baleful deity upon which they must sacrifice themselves in the hope of some rescue from the inevitable. They diminish themselves, seeking to atone for they know not what; they become depressed and over-cautious, fearful and less than themselves; they begin to die already in the hope that they will miraculously live after all. Such self-sacrificial behaviour is often expected of them by those around the terminally ill. Dying people are supposed to be quiet, humble, and not too assertive. Of course they are permitted to be angry, but only for a while, and only for a therapeutic end, the acceptance of the inevitable. Society seeks to put a veil of comely gloom over the features of those who have the shocking attribute of dying before their time—and many people meekly accept the assigned role.

> Tim, a student in his early twenties, would have none of this correct behaviour for the dying. He knew that he must soon die of an incurable cancer before he was fully into his third decade of life. All that seemed so important to him was to be swept away within months, perhaps weeks, and the prelude to this would be some deterioration and loss of dignity that would take away even that which he now held onto so fiercely. He knew that his career was ended, that his intimacy with several friends and the warmth of his relationship with his partner were now very transient things, to be measured only qualitatively, without any knowledge of how much longer they would be part of him. But Tim simply was not interested in being the tragic hero bemoaning the losses he faced. All that mattered to him was to be allowed to have the whole range of feelings that were his of right—to be angry, depressed, elated, hopeful and hopeless, to be as wild and devil-may-care as young men of his age, to be not the person about to die, but the person still now alive and allowed to live that life like any other young person. In other words, Tim asked for nothing else than just to be himself, nothing special, nothing different. He did not want to sacrifice on the altar of death. Being a 'terminal case' was something he would fight off to the end, not because he denied his situation, but because he did not see any usefulness in such a category. So he sought the company of friends who would just let him be what he had always been to them. The more unctious of his helpers soon had to correct their professional bad habits, or find someone else to 'care for'.

---

* William F. May (4) provides a very notable exception to this generalization.

Tim's determination presents a very simple ideal to which all in the health care arena (in whatever role) might aspire. One can translate it into 'respect for autonomy' if one so wishes. But I would prefer to describe it as the virtue of being oneself. This may sound so simple and so obvious that it is mere platitude. Yet simplicity of this kind seems to be one of the hardest lessons to learn in health care ethics.

REFERENCES

1. Beauchamp, T. L. and Childress, J. 1983. *Principles of biomedical ethics*, 2nd edn. Oxford University Press, New York.
2. Ramsey, P. 1970. *The patient as a person*. Yale University Press, Newhaven.
3. Shakespeare, W. 1606. *King Lear*, Act 2, scene 4.
4. May, W. F. 1991. *The patient's ordeal*. Indiana University Press, Bloomington, IN.
5. *The writings of Henry Wordsworth Longfellow*, vol. 5 (Routledge, London, 1886), p. 53.
6. Oliver, J. H. 1939. Hymn of Serapion: an ancient poem on the duties of a physician. *Bulletin of the history of medicine* 7: 315–323.
7. Macquarrie, J. and Childress, J. (Eds) 1986. *A new dictionary of Christian ethics*. SCM Press, London.

22

Morality vs. Principlism

K. Danner Clouser

University Professor of Humanities, Pennsylvania State University College of
Medicine, Pennsylvania, USA

Bernard Gert

Eunice and Julian Cohen Professor for the Study of Ethics and Human Values,
Dartmouth College, New Hampshire, USA

INTRODUCTION

It has become *de rigueur* to cite 'the four principles of bioethics' in dealing with problems in biomedical ethics. Throughout most of the bioethical literature writers seem to believe that they have brought theory to bear insofar as they have mentioned 'the four principles'. Indeed the prevalence of the 'principles' extends to framing the problems as well as to solving them. That is, commentators frequently organize the various ethical problems of medicine according to which principle is 'needed' to 'solve' the problem at hand.

It is our contention that invoking the 'principles' is only and necessarily ceremonial. That is, we argue that the 'principles' are not action guides at all, but that at most they represent a category of concerns, a listing of issues, that should be considered in dealing with the problem in question. Traditionally principles have been action guides; that is, they summarized a whole theory and thus, as shorthand for the theory, assisted the agent in making a moral decision. For example, Rawls's two principles of justice are meaningful directives for action because they not only are based on his theory of justice, but they also have a priority ranking.

However, the 'principles' as dealt with by principlism are not systematically related to each other by any underlying unified theory. Of course each 'principle' is an expression of one or another important and traditional concern of morality. But there is no priority ranking; in fact, there is not even any specified procedure to be used in resolving particular cases of conflicts between the principles. This

Principles of Health Care Ethics. Edited by Raanan Gillon.

is not surprising, inasmuch as the 'principles' are not action guides but only checklists of moral concerns. Furthermore since they have neither foundations nor clear interrelationships, we believe they are useful primarily as a means of consciousness-raising, but not as a means of clarifying the moral issues involved in any particular moral problem nor in providing guidance toward a solution. We argue these points more extensively elsewhere (1).

The point of this chapter is to explain in what way we find the 'principles' to be inadequate, and to describe what we would put in their place. Both aspects of this charge require extensive arguments well beyond the space allocations of this chapter. However, we will articulate our objections and our own position with as much supporting argument as space allows.

Our plan is to discuss very briefly the principles of non-maleficence and justice in order to set the context for our argument. Then we will discuss in some detail the principles of autonomy and beneficence in order to demonstrate the force of our arguments against principlism. These latter two were chosen not only because they are the ones most often employed in bioethical discussion, but also because they best illustrate the most problematic aspects of principlism. In particular, we will show that principlism embodies the inadequacies of most previous accounts of morality by failing to appreciate the significance of the distinction between moral rules and moral ideals, and by misrepresenting the ordinary concept of duty. Finally we will show how a systematic account of morality provides a useful guide to action that can prevent much of the confusion that results from trying to use the four principles as action guides.

THE FOUR PRINCIPLES

Non-maleficence

We have very little quarrel with the principle of non-maleficence. It is the only one of the four principles that does not blur the distinction between moral rules and moral ideals. Indeed, this principle would most reasonably be interpreted as merely summarizing some of the moral rules. The moral rules 'don't kill', 'don't cause pain', and 'don't disable' are clearly included in this principle, and probably the rule 'don't deprive of pleasure' is as well. Even the rule 'don't deprive of freedom' could be included in the principle of non-maleficence, but perhaps principlism would prefer to have it included under the principle of autonomy. We see no reason for distinguishing the rule concerning the deprivation of freedom from the other four rules, for all five of these rules prohibit causing what are universally recognized as evils, i.e. death, pain, disability, loss of freedom, and loss of pleasure.

The principle of non-maleficence *does no more than* simply collapse four or five moral rules into one more general rule—'do not cause harm' (see ref. 2, p. 109). That general rule—*'primum non nocere'*—is often taken as the first principle of medicine. It is primarily a matter of purpose and style whether one prefers to list five distinct moral rules or to have one general rule which includes them all. We prefer the former because it makes more salient the fact that there are different kinds of harms (or 'evils', as we call them) and that rational persons can and do rank them differently. Neglecting the fact that there are different rational rankings is one of the primary causes of unjustified paternalism. Thus, specifying the different harms that one must avoid causing must be explicitly and carefully done in any event, so that the gain in simplicity of one general rule is minimal at best. Nonetheless, this principle, even as it stands, has no major problems. That fact is not surprising, since it is the only one of the principles that is not an invention of philosophers, but is a long-standing principle of medicine.

Justice

Our discussion of justice will be equally brief, but not for the same reasons. Far from finding this principle closely related to some specific moral rules, we find this principle does not even pretend to provide a specific guide to action. We doubt that even the proponents of principlism put much stock in it as an action guide. It is the prime example of a principle functioning simply as a checklist of moral concerns. It amounts to no more than saying that one should be concerned with matters of distribution; it recommends just or fair distribution without endorsing any particular account of justice or fairness. In the texts of principlism the principle of justice seems, in effect, not to be an action guide at all, but rather a chapter heading under which one might find sophisticated discussions of various theories of justice. After reading such a chapter one might be better informed and sensitive to the differing theories of justice, but when dealing with an actual problem of distribution, one would be baffled by the injunction to 'apply the principle of justice' (see also ref. 1, pp. 225–227).

The principle of justice has an additional problem that it shares with the two remaining principles—it blurs the distinction between what is morally *required* (obeying the moral rules) and what is morally *encouraged* (following the moral ideals). Since the principle of justice can hardly be taken seriously as an action guide, this blurring is not as obvious as in the two remaining principles. In this, as in other matters, principlism simply takes over errors of those theories which suggested their principles in the first place. For example, the most prominent contemporary discussion of justice is by John Rawls (3). Rawls describes what he calls the duty of justice as follows:

> This duty requires us to support and to comply with just institutions that exist and apply to us. It also constrains us to further just arrangements not yet established, at least when this can be done without too much cost to ourselves (p. 115; see also p. 334).

Thus Rawls includes in what he regards as a single duty (a) the moral rule requiring one to obey (just) laws and (b) the moral ideal encouraging one to help make just laws, without even realizing how different these two guides to action are.* As we shall see, this failure to distinguish between what is morally required (the moral rules) and what is morally encouraged (the moral ideals)

---

* For further discussion of Rawls on this point, see chapter 13 of ref. 4.

creates significant confusion in both the principle of autonomy and the principle of beneficence.

Autonomy

This principle seems to be the centerpiece of principlism. It is cited more frequently than the others and has really taken on a life of its own. The concept of autonomy has come to dominate discussions of medical ethics—to the point that there is a growing and focused opposition to its predominance. Attention is being drawn to concerns that outweigh autonomy; its claim of trumping every conflict of interests is being questioned. (It is to the credit of Beauchamp and Childress that they make it clear that other considerations can outweigh autonomy; for example pp. 101–102 of ref. 2). But these developments are only symptomatic of deeper theoretical problems with autonomy as a principle. As close as Beauchamp and Childress get to stating the principle of autonomy is this:

> Hence, we shall here understand the principle of autonomy as follows: *Autonomous actions and choices should not be constrained by others.* . . . It asserts a right of noninterference and correlatively an obligation not to constrain autonomous actions—nothing more but also nothing less (p. 62, their emphasis).

As stated here it is surprisingly akin to the principle of non-maleficence, and as such we would of course have little disagreement with it. In fact it simply seems to pick out one evil, the loss of freedom, and gives it a principle all to itself. Interpreted simply as an alternative formulation of 'do not deprive of freedom' we obviously have no objection to this principle. However, this principle does not say merely that one should not constrain anyone's actions and choices; rather it says that we should not constrain their *autonomous* actions and choices. The addition of 'autonomous' is what causes most of the problems with the principle of autonomy. The principle does not prohibit constraining non-autonomous choices and actions, thus making what counts as an autonomous choice or action a matter of fundamental moral concern. As we shall see later, the principle is also often taken as requiring one to promote autonomous actions and choices, not merely to avoid constraining them.

Autonomous Actions and Choices

In practice the basic difficulty with autonomy, dogging it throughout all its uses, is knowing whether or not the actions and choices one is concerned with are autonomous. Is the choice to give up drinking the autonomous choice or is the autonomous choice the choice to continue? Is the choice to withdraw from expensive life-prolonging treatment to save his family money and anguish the autonomous choice or is the autonomous one the choice to go on living a while longer? Which choice is it that we are being admonished not to constrain? This ambiguity invites a conflict between people who differ on which choice of the patient is the autonomous one. One side may favor overruling a patient refusal on the ground that the refusal is irrational, claiming that therefore the choice is not autonomous; whereas the other side may favor going along with the patient's explicitly stated refusal on the ground that, though the refusal is irrational, the patient is competent and therefore the refusal is an autonomous choice. Both sides can claim that they are respecting the autonomous choice and, hence, acting on the principle of autonomy. A principle which can be used to support two completely opposing ways of acting even when there is no disagreement on the observable facts of the case is obviously not a very useful guide to action.

There may be times when it is appropriate to question whether what the patient chooses is an autonomous choice, e.g. when he is delirious, or intoxicated, or under the influence of drugs, and the views he expresses significantly differ from those he expresses when he is in a normal state. But when the significant departure from previously expressed views is not temporary and not explained by medical reasons, then it is inappropriate to be deciding what to do by focusing on the question of whether the patient's choices are autonomous. To do this is to substitute a metaphysical question for a moral one. Following the principle of autonomy may encourage one to act with unjustified paternalism; that is, to overrule the patient's explicit refusal, simply because one views that choice as not being autonomous. Thus the principle of autonomy may lead one to deprive a person of freedom without an adequate justification for doing so.

Moral Rules and Moral Ideals: a Fundamental Distinction

At the core of many problems with the principle of autonomy is its failure in practice (and the failure of principlism generally) to recognize the significance of the distinction between what is morally encouraged (following the moral ideals) and what is morally required (obeying the moral rules). This distinction, or rather one that seems closely related to it, has traditionally been made by distinguishing between duties of perfect obligation and duties of imperfect obligation ('perfect' and 'imperfect' duties). However, this indiscriminate use of the term 'duty' (a matter we will discuss later in connection with beneficence) has made it almost impossible to make this distinction in the correct way. The first five moral rules listed in our earlier discussion of non-maleficence would be examples of perfect duties, as would be the moral rules requiring one not to deceive, not to cheat, and not to break promises. 'Perfect duties' are those which one *is required to obey impartially all of the time.* One is morally allowed not to obey a perfect duty only when one has an adequate justification for the disobedience.

On the other hand, the moral ideals would be 'imperfect duties', that is, those duties that it is impossible to obey either impartially or all of the time, such as working to help the down-trodden. One may pick and choose not only which of the down-and-out one will help, but also when and where one will help them. Furthermore, one may even choose not to act on that imperfect duty at all, but rather to act on some other imperfect duty such as preventing the deprivation of freedom of someone, somewhere. It seems as if an imperfect duty is a duty that one is not required to act on at all; morality certainly does not *require* one to work for either Oxfam or for Amnesty International, let alone both. It is not morally required to give to or work for any charity, although morality certainly encourages such behavior. Doing so is following an imperfect duty (moral ideal), not a perfect duty (moral rule).

Because this traditional distinction between perfect and imperfect duties embodies a confusion about the notion of *duty*, we would make the distinction in a different and less misleading fashion. *Moral rules* prohibit causing evil— and that is what morality requires. *Moral ideals*, on the other hand, encourage the prevention of evil—but morality does not require following them. The moral rules must be followed all the time, toward everyone, equally (except, of course, in cases of justified exceptions). But that is impossible in the case of the moral ideals since those involve positive action. Doing what morality requires (i.e. obeying the moral rules) is not usually praiseworthy; rather it is normally expected, and failing to do it makes one liable to punishment. Doing what morality encourages (i.e. following the moral ideals) is usually praiseworthy and failing to follow them is not punishable. Therefore it is not surprising that appreciating the distinction between the moral rules and moral ideals within the moral system is basic and crucial.

Eliminating the misleading use of 'perfect and imperfect duties' makes clear that the distinction between moral rules and moral ideals is quite significant. The ordinary use of 'duty' suggests that punishment is deserved when one fails to do one's duty, perfect or imperfect. We are morally required to obey the moral rules impartially all of the time. All instances of killing, deceiving, cheating, etc. are immoral unless one has an adequate justification for doing so. For example, whenever one deprives persons of freedom (principlism might call this violating their autonomy), one needs an adequate justification for doing so. But one does not need a justification for failing to help them to *increase* their freedom (principlism might call this promoting their autonomy), unless one has a duty to do so, e.g. because of one's profession. In the absence of such a duty it is following a moral ideal to help someone to increase her freedom—it is something that morality certainly encourages us to do, but not something that it requires us to do.

Autonomy As Rule and *Ideal*

The principle of autonomy requires respect for autonomy, but it fails to distinguish between 'respecting (not violating) autonomy' and 'promoting autonomy'. Since that crucial distinction is not made explicitly, the important differences between 'promoting autonomy' and 'respecting autonomy' are often neglected. Indeed, Beauchamp and Childress, after emphasizing and developing the intimate connection between autonomy and informed consent, state that they 'accept the view that the primary function of informed consent is the protection *and promotion* of individual autonomy' (ref. 2, p. 67; our emphasis). If these are not distinguished then we lose sight of the greater stringency of the former; not protecting (i.e. violating) autonomy is breaking a moral rule and thus requires adequate justification. Not promoting autonomy is not following a moral ideal and hence does not require justification. This is not to deny that promoting autonomy may sometimes provide adequate justification for violating autonomy, but not distinguishing clearly between 'protecting autonomy' and 'promoting autonomy' inevitably leads to confusion.

Principlism's coalescence of respecting autonomy and promoting autonomy compounded by its need to search for the 'genuinely' autonomous actions and choices invites a kind of activism wherein an agent promotes those choices and actions of another that the agent regards as the latter's autonomous choices and actions, even though that involves depriving the person of freedom. Such manipulation seems to conflict with morality itself insofar as it leads one to deprive people of freedom simply in order to promote what one decides would (or should) be their autonomous choice. Thus, principlism's centerpiece, 'the principle of autonomy', embodies a deep and dangerous level of confusion. That confusion is created by unclarity as to what counts as autonomous actions and choices and the consequent blurring of a basic moral distinction between moral rules and moral ideals. The unnecessary introduction of the metaphysical concept of autonomy inevitably results in making it more difficult to think clearly about moral problems. The goal of moral philosophy is to clarify our moral thinking, not to introduce new and unnecessary complications (see also refs 5 and 6).

As an aside it is worth observing that the principle of autonomy probably caught on so tenaciously for two reasons. One is that Kantian ethics was experiencing a renaissance, and that his notion of autonomy was central to his account of morality. The other is that the medical profession had become so markedly paternalistic that patient self-determination had all but vanished. So the emphasis on autonomy became the banner under which forces rallied to regain lost territory. Allowing the patient to decide what treatment he would receive became the main issue, and thus momentum and conviction—rather than conceptual clarity or theoretical soundness—perpetuated the emphasis on autonomy. Even the fact that the principle of autonomy did not really embody Kant's notion of autonomy did not detract from the overwhelming political appeal of invoking the principle.

An example of how confused the general understanding of autonomy is comes from examining Kant's view of autonomy. On Kant's view one is not acting autonomously if one kills oneself or allows onself to die because of intractable pain. That would be allowing pleasure and pain—which according to Kant are not part of the rational self—to determine one's actions. Thus it is not an autonomous action of the rational self. To act autonomously one must always act in accord with the Categorical Imperative. In *Groundwork of the metaphysics of morals* (7), Kant explicitly states that the Categorical Imperative requires one not to commit suicide because of pain. By way of contrast, note that one of the major arguments in favor of allowing people to die when they are suffering from intractable pain is the principle of autonomy. The seeds of confusion were present in the initial planting of the concept of autonomy. This explains, in part, why we prefer the simple rule 'don't deprive of freedom' to the fancy principle of autonomy as the preferred method of protecting patient self-determination.

Beneficence

More Blurring of Distinctions

As used by principlism, this principle suffers similar shortcomings as the previous principle. As popularly used in the biomedical ethics literature this principle is cited simply to give 'validation' both to preventing or relieving evil and to doing good or conferring benefits. Beauchamp and Childress, who are the major messengers of principlism to medicine, though much more cautious in their discussion of the principle of beneficence than many, do not avoid the errors. For them the principle of beneficence 'asserts the duty to help others further their important and legitimate interests' (see ref. 2, p. 148). In the biomedical context the principle becomes the duty to confer benefits and actively to prevent and remove harms, in addition to balancing the possible goods against the possible harms of an action (see ref. 2, pp. 148–149). Even though Beauchamp and Childress are well aware that many philosophers treat beneficent acts as 'morally *ideal*', they still regard beneficence as morally required.

Thus the principle of beneficence not only succumbs to the same criticisms that we earlier leveled at the principle of autonomy for ignoring the distinction between the moral ideals (preventing harms) and the moral rules (avoid causing harms) but it falls victim to a new criticism—namely, failing to distinguish between the preventing (or relieving) of evil and the conferring (or promoting) of goods. This distinction is especially important for medicine, inasmuch as preventing or relieving harm often justifies violating moral rules when conferring benefits would not.

Beneficence and the Concept of Duty

Furthermore there is another major confusion perpetuated by the principle of beneficence. Though it arises from the mistake of turning moral ideals into duties, the problem itself has nothing to do with the rules/ideals distinction. Rather it concerns the concept of duty. Principlism regards the following of the principles to be a duty. This especially comes clear in the frequent references to 'the duty of beneficence'. It is not that it is incorrect to call beneficence a duty simply because it is a moral ideal. (It would be equally incorrect to call 'do not kill' a duty, even though it is a moral rule.) Rather it is incorrect because such usage distorts and obscures the primary meaning of 'duty' which basically refers to the specific duties that come with one's role, occupation, or profession. Though it is correct to say 'we ought not to kill' or 'we ought to help the down-trodden', it is cultivating significant confusion to label these 'duties'. For some philosophers 'do your duty' has come to mean no more than 'do what you morally ought to do'. But using the term 'duty' in this way makes it very difficult to talk about *real* duties, those that are associated with one's profession and whose content is not determined by philosophers but by the members of that profession and the society in which they live.* However, morality does put

---

* For more on using the concept of duty in medical ethical considerations, see ref. 5, p. 387, and refs 8–11.

a limit on what counts as a duty: there can be no duty to violate unjustifiably any of the other moral rules (ref. 4, p. 156). Thus it is not only misleading to talk of the moral *ideals* as imperfect duties, it is also misleading to talk of the moral *rules* as perfect duties. For reasons of conceptual soundness and clarity we think it best to use the term 'duty' only in its ordinary sense—that is, for what is required by one's role in society, particularly by one's profession. Thus 'do your duty' is a distinct moral rule, on a par with the other moral rules; it is not a meta-rule telling one to obey the other rules. It is justified as such because of the harm that would be caused by one's failure to do that which others are justifiably counting on being done. We are morally required to do our duty, but it is misleading to say that we have a duty to do our duty (11). (see also 'Rejoinder' in ref. 11, Shelp, pp. 115–116).

In medicine it is especially misleading to use the principle of beneficence as if it created a general duty for all health care professionals. This obscures the role of real duties; that is, the specific duties that come with one's role or profession. Beauchamp and Childress (2) seem to recognize the significant difference between what they call the general duty of beneficence and the specific duties of beneficence. They state:

> Even if our general duty of beneficence derives in part from reciprocity and fair play, our specific duties of beneficence often derive from special moral relationships with persons, frequently through institutional roles (p. 156).

They are clear that doctors, nurses, and others in the health care field have specific duties to their patients that are determined by their profession and by the practices of their specific institution. But to lump these widely varied and richly detailed duties to the well-being of their patients together with the misconceived 'general duty of beneficence' under one principle of beneficence is to substitute a slogan for substance. Indeed, the principle of beneficence, like the other three principles, is more of a slogan than anything else. It provides no useful or practical guide to behavior.

Principles, Slogans, and Morality

The popularity of the principles rests in large part on the fact that the principles serve as slogans that are used to support conclusions that one has reached without really using the principles at all. Use of these slogans undercuts the much more sophisticated knowledge of morality that all of us in fact have.* This knowledge of morality (or 'the moral system') is used by most people when they think seriously about making a moral judgement or deciding how to act when confronting a moral problem. We do not claim that everyone *explicitly* holds the moral system that we will espouse and briefly describe in this chapter. A useful analogy is the knowledge of the grammatical system used by all competent speakers of a language. Even though almost no such speaker can explicitly describe this system, they all know it in the sense that they use it

---

* For an elaboration of this point see ref. 12, pp. 165–171.

when speaking and in interpreting the speech of others. If presented with an explicit account of the grammatical system, competent speakers have the final word on its accuracy.

In a similar fashion a moral theory that provides a description of a moral system for acting in a way that conflicts with one's own considered moral judgements normally should not be accepted. However, recognition of the systematic character of morality may make apparent some inconsistencies in one's moral judgements. Morality is a system and the acceptability of the answers that this system gives to any particular problem is affected by the acceptability of the answers that it gives to all other problems. Moral problems cannot be adequately discussed as if they were isolated problems whose solution did not have implications for all other moral problems. Making one's moral views explicit may reveal that some few moral judgements are inconsistent with the vast majority of one's judgements. Thus one may come to see that what was accepted by oneself as a correct moral judgement is in fact mistaken.

Principlism oversimplifies our moral reasoning. In this it follows in the great tradition of moral slogans that are recited but not used, such as the Golden Rule, 'Do unto others as you would have them do unto you.' Do we really want judges and policemen to follow the Golden Rule with respect to criminals? Furthermore, in many cases doing to others what you would like them to do to you could result in some very unacceptable behavior! No doubt there are many times that the Golden Rule has great rhetorical value, but by itself it has no value in determining what is the morally right way to act. In a similar fashion, the four principles often have great rhetorical value, but they play no useful role in determining how one morally ought to behave. Morality is a complex matter, and any attempt to reduce it to slogans is bound to distort it. But because morality is complex, that does not mean it is difficult. Grammar is complex, but even high-school students are able to speak grammatically and to use their knowledge of grammar to understand extremely difficult sentences.

What we shall attempt to do in the next section is to make explicit a very brief outline of the moral system that we all actually use when making a moral judgement or when deciding how to act in confronting a moral problem. Though this system will be complex, all of its parts should be completely familiar. This is as it should be, for we are not presenting some new morality, but simply making explicit our common morality. We are aware that the test of the accuracy of our account is the degree to which every clear moral judgement follows from our account. Our account will also explain why there is disagreement on some moral judgements. In any event, we are prepared to submit our account of morality to this test.

MORALITY AS A PUBLIC SYSTEM

The Moral Rules

Morality is what all impartial rational persons would choose as a public system that applies to all rational persons. It includes rules prohibiting causing each of the five evils (or harms, if you prefer) that all rational persons (by virtue of their rationality) want to avoid. Thus it includes the following five rules (see ref. 4, chapter 6).

Don't kill (don't cause permanent loss of consciousness).
Don't cause pain (including mental suffering).
Don't disable (don't cause loss of ability).
Don't deprive of freedom (including opportunities).
Don't deprive of pleasure.

Morality also includes rules which when not followed usually cause harm; whenever they generally are not obeyed, the result is always an increase in the amount of harm being suffered. Thus morality also includes the following five rules (see ref. 4, chapter 7).

Don't deceive.
Don't break your promise.
Don't cheat.
Don't break the law.
Don't neglect your duty. (The term 'duty' is being used in its everyday sense to refer to what is required by one's role in society, primarily one's job, and not as philosophers customarily use it, namely, simply as a synonym for 'what one morally ought to do'.)

There should be nothing surprising in this list of moral rules. All that is being claimed is that there are certain simple kinds of actions that everyone counts as immoral, e.g. killing, causing pain, deceiving, and breaking promises, unless one can justify doing that kind of act. Although moral or religious philosophers differ on the theoretical justification for these rules, they, like everyone else, accept the rules.

Although it is usually clear what counts as a violation of any of these rules, there are sometimes slightly different interpretations of the rules. It is clear that withholding some idle unsupported thought about the prognosis of a patient is not deceiving, but that withholding facts about significant side-effects of a drug being prescribed is deceiving. Various professions often determine slightly differently what counts as deceiving or keeping a promise of confidentiality. Doctors do not regard themselves as having violated confidentiality when they consult with other doctors about a case.* This is another reason, in addition to the importance of the specific duties of the profession, why one cannot do professional ethics, including medical ethics, without a full knowledge and understanding of the profession and its practices.†

Justifying Violations of the Moral Rules

Almost everyone agrees that these rules are not absolute; that is, all of these rules can have justified exceptions. The attitude that all impartial rational persons

---

* For more on interpreting the rules in different contexts, see ref. 8, pp. 116–120; ref. 9, pp. 657–658; ref. 12, pp. 170–172.
† For a fuller discussion of these matters, see ref. 4, pp. 111–116; see also refs 8–11.

would take toward these rules when considering them as moral rules (i.e. as rules in a public system applying to all rational persons) is the following: everyone is always to obey the rule unless an impartial rational person can advocate that violating it be publicly allowed. Anyone who violates the rule when an impartial rational person cannot advocate that such a violation be publicly allowed may be punished. (The *unless* clause only means that when an impartial rational person can advocate that such a violation be publicly allowed, impartial rational persons may disagree on whether one should obey the rule, not that they agree one should not obey.)

In determining whether or not to advocate that a violation of a moral rule be publicly allowed, a person should use only the morally relevant features in describing the proposed violation. What constitutes morally relevant features of an action are contained in the answers to the following questions:

1. What moral rules are being violated?
2. What evils or harms are being (a) avoided, (b) prevented, (c) caused?
3. What are the relevant desires of the people toward whom the rule is being violated?
4. What are the relevant rational beliefs of the people toward whom the rule is being violated?
5. Does one have a duty to violate moral rules with regard to the person(s), and is one in a unique or almost unique position in this regard?
6. What goods are being promoted?
7. Is an unjustified or weakly justified violation of a moral rule being prevented?
8. Is an unjustified or weakly justified violation of a moral rule being punished?
9. Is the situation sufficiently rare that no one would ever plan or prepare for being in it?*

When considering the evils being avoided, prevented or caused, and the goods being promoted, one must consider not only their intensity, duration, and probability; one must also consider the kind of good or evil involved. If more than one person is affected, one must consider not only how many people will be affected, but also the distribution of the harms and benefits. If two violations are the same in all of their morally relevant features then they count as the same kind of violation, and any impartial rational person who advocates that one of them be publicly allowed must advocate that the other also be publicly allowed. However, this does not mean that two impartial rational persons, who agree that two actions count as the same kind of violation, must always agree on whether or not to advocate that that kind of violation be publicly allowed, for they may differ in their estimate of the consequences of publicly allowing that kind of violation, or they may rank the goods and evils involved differently.

Once one has determined what kind of violation is involved by using the morally relevant features (that is, described the violation using only the morally

---

* See ref. 4, pp. 141–145 for a more complete account of these morally relevant features. Feature no. 9 is a newly discovered feature not listed in that book.

relevant aspects), an impartial rational person decides whether or not to advocate that a violation be publicly allowed by estimating what effect this kind of violation, if publicly allowed, would have.* (A rational person would be one who would avoid harm unless he had an adequate reason not to.† Impartiality requires considering that everyone knows that the violation is allowed in these specified morally relevant circumstances.‡) If all impartial rational persons would estimate that less evil would be suffered if that kind of violation were publicly allowed, then all impartial rational persons would advocate that that kind of violation be publicly allowed and the violation is strongly justified; if all rational persons would estimate that more evil would be suffered, then no rational person would advocate that that kind of violation be publicly allowed and the violation is unjustified. However, impartial rational persons, even if equally informed, may disagree in their estimate of whether more or less evil will result from that kind of violation being publicly allowed. When this happens they will disagree on whether or not to advocate that that kind of violation be publicly allowed and such a violation counts as weakly justified.

Moral Disagreements

Disagreements in the estimates of whether a given kind of violation being publicly allowed will result in more or less evil may stem from two distinct sources. The first is a difference in the rankings of the various kinds of evils. If someone ranks a specified amount of pain and suffering as worse than a specified amount of loss of freedom, and someone else ranks them in the opposite way, then although they agree that a given action is the same kind of violation, they may disagree on whether or not to advocate that that kind of violation be publicly allowed. The second is a difference in estimates of how much evil would result from publicly allowing a given kind of violation, even when there seems to be no difference in the rankings of the different kinds of evils (see also ref. 5, pp. 385–386). These differences may stem from differences in beliefs about human nature or about the nature of human societies. Insofar as these differences cannot be settled by any universally agreed upon empirical method, such differences are best regarded as ideological. However, it is quite likely that most ideological differences also involve differences in the rankings of different kinds of evils.§ On the other hand, of course, there often seems at first to be an unresolvable difference, but careful examination of the issue shows that there is actually a correct answer.

The Moral Ideals¶

The moral rules, together with the procedure for determining when it is justified to violate the rules, including the list of morally relevant features, make up the

---

* This is the morally decisive question. See ref. 4, pp. 145–146.
† For a fuller account of rationality, see ref. 4, chapter 5.
‡ For a fuller acount of impartiality, see ref. 4, chapter 2.
§ For a fuller account of evil, see ref. 4, chapter 3.
¶ For a fuller account of moral ideals, see ref. 4, chapter 8; for an early employment of this concept to describe some puzzles of bioethics, see ref. 13, pp. 50–56.

core of morality, as is recognized even by the utilitarians (see J. S. Mill (14)). However, even from the above it should be clear that that is not all of morality. For morality not only requires us to act in certain ways—namely, obey the moral rules—but it encourages us to act in certain other ways, *viz.* follow the moral ideals. These ideals tell us to prevent and relieve the evils that the first five moral rules tell us to avoid causing, *viz.* death, pain, disability, loss of freedom and loss of pleasure. Since unjustified violations of the moral rules almost always result in more evils being suffered than if the violations did not occur, one is also following moral ideals when one acts so as to prevent unjustified violations of the moral rules.

It is relatively unimportant how many moral ideals one specifies. We could have a specific moral ideal related to each of the first five moral rules, encouraging us to prevent or relieve the evil or harm that the related rule tells us to avoid causing. We could then have a specific moral ideal telling us to prevent the unjustified violation of each moral rule. Or we could have only one moral ideal which encourages us to do that which lessens the amount of evil suffered. As long as no moral rule is broken, any action which lessens the amount of evil suffered is morally encouraged. If a moral rule is being violated, then we follow the procedure for determining if the violation is justified, and that includes noting what kind of evil is being avoided, prevented, and caused, as well as how much.

The importance of distinguishing between the moral rules and the moral ideals lies not in our motivation for following them. In both cases the primary motivation may be our concern for others, i.e. our desire to avoid causing evil to others and our desire to alleviate the evil suffered by others. Rather, the importance stems from the fact that it is only for a violation of a moral rule, not for failing to follow a moral ideal, that we may be punished. Only the moral rules can be enforced; the moral ideals can only be encouraged. This is because only the moral rules, not the moral ideals, can and must be impartially obeyed all of the time with regard to everyone. When the facts are known, it is usually quite clear when a moral rule has been violated, and if that violation is justified. Thus punishment can be effectively used to deter unjustified violations.

Moral ideals cannot be impartially obeyed all of the time with regard to everyone. It is humanly impossible to do so. Thus it must be left up to all persons to determine for themselves when they will follow the moral ideals. This makes enforcement of the moral ideals and punishment for not following them more than pointless. Everyone knows that even with regard to people who do not act immorally, some people are morally better than others. This is possible only if there is more to morality than doing what is morally required (i.e. obeying the moral rules). After all, there is also doing what is morally good (i.e. following the moral ideals). Making the distinction between moral rules and moral ideals explains why not every doctor who is, morally speaking, not the best that he or she can be, is not thereby subject to moral censure.

Doctors, like everyone else, are not allowed unjustifiably to violate moral rules, which includes the rule 'do your duty'. Thus, for example, a doctor must provide sufficient information for valid consent and to provide the patient with at least a minimum standard of quality medical care. If doctors do not do so, they are properly open to censure; but some go far beyond what they are morally required to do. That is, they act on the moral ideals with regard to their patients, and often with regard to the wider community, in a way that deserves moral praise. They are not merely doing their duty, as the principle of beneficence would suggest. Rather they are setting a standard of behavior for other doctors to emulate—though not, of course, for the profession to enforce.

We know that it is impossible to do away with slogans in one's moral thinking; they are not necessarily bad or misleading, and they can be helpful. But they must be based on a unified moral system and be reminders of the complex moral system rather than being replacements for it. Given that the moral virtues and vices are intimately related to the moral rules and ideals, one might use the virtues and vices in appropriate slogans, e.g. 'don't be cruel' (don't unjustifiably violate the first five moral rules); 'be kind' (follow the moral ideals); 'be truthful, trustworthy, fair, law-abiding, and dependable'.* (These obviously relate to each of the second five moral rules.) These slogans seem to us quite respectable, even though seven or eight of them are needed to summarize the whole system.

If slogans somehow are needed, we would recommend a single slogan that is both engaging and incisive, yet when unpacked, summarizes the whole moral system: 'care without arrogance'. We would define 'caring' as being motivated to act by the belief that one's action will lessen the suffering of others.† We define 'arrogance' as acting as if one is not subject to the moral requirements that apply to all rational persons.‡ Using these definitions, the elements of which are grounded in a unified moral system, we can provide a slogan that has general appeal as well as a special application to medicine. 'Care without arrogance' means acting according to the moral ideals without unjustifiably violating the moral rules. Of course, for any practical work to be done, one must apply the whole moral system, but at least this slogan should not mislead one into thinking that it can be applied in place of the moral system.

REFERENCES

1. Clouser, K. D. and Gert, B. 1990. A critique of principlism. *Journal of Medicine and Philosophy* 15: 219–236.
2. Beauchamp, T. L. and Childress, J. 1983. *Principles of biomedical ethics*, 2nd edn. Oxford University Press, New York.
3. Rawls, J. 1971. *A theory of justice*. Harvard University Press, Cambridge, MA.
4. Gert, B. 1988. *Morality: a new justification of the moral rules*. Oxford University Press, New York.
5. Clouser, K. D. 1975. Medical ethics: some uses, abuses and limitations. *New England Journal of Medicine* 293: 384–387.
6. Clouser, K. D. 1973. Some things medical ethics is not. *Journal of the American Medical Association* 223: 787–789.
7. Kant, I. 1785. *Groundwork of the metaphysics of morals* (trans. Paton, H. J.). Harper Torch Books, 1964.

---

* For a fuller account of virtues and vices, see ref. 4, chapter 9.
† For a fuller account of caring, see ref. 4, pp. 176–177.
‡ For a fuller account of arrogance, see ref. 4, pp. 256–258.

8. Clouser, K. D. 1978. Bioethics. Pp. 115–127. *In* Reich, W. T. (Ed.) *The encyclopedia of bioethics*, vol. 1. Macmillan, London, and Free Press, Glencoe, IL.

9. Clouser, K. D. 1974. What is medical ethics? *Annals of Internal Medicine* **80**: 657–670.

10. Clouser, K. D. 1977. Allowing or causing: another look. *Annals of Internal Medicine* **87**: 622–624.

11. Clouser, K. D. 1983. Veatch, May, and models: a critical view and a new view. Pp. 89–103. *In* Shelp, E. E. (Ed.) *The clinical encounter: the moral fabric of the patient–physician relationship*. Reidel, Boston, MA. (Reprinted in Veatch, R. M. (Ed.) 1989. *Cross-cultural perspectives in medical ethics: readings*, 174–186, Jones and Bartlett, Boston.)

12. Clouser, K. D. 1989. Ethical theory and applied ethics: reflections on connections. Pp. 161–181. *In* Hoffmaster, Freedman, and Fraser, (Eds) *Clinical ethics: theory and practice*. Humana Press, Clifton, NJ.

13. Clouser, K. D. 1977. Biomedical ethics; some reflections and exhortations: *Monist* **60**: 47–61.

14. Mill, J. S. 1863. *Utilitarianism*, chapter 5, paragraph 31.

23

Limitations of the Four Principles

R. H. NICHOLSON, MA, BM, BCH, DCH

Editor, Bulletin of Medical Ethics, London, UK

It was Hamish Macarthur who first made me aware of the practical limitations of the four principles. Hamish was a ghillie—a gamekeeper—who lived by himself in an isolated bothy miles from the nearest village in the northern Highlands of Scotland. He was good at his job and well-respected in his scattered community, but he had a problem. He was a binge drinker.

I first heard of him late on a spring evening in 1978. I was duty doctor at Craig Dunain, the psychiatric hospital for the Highlands in Inverness, when Hamish's general practitioner rang me. Hamish, he said, was on his annual binge, drinking two or three bottles of whisky each day. Because he lived by himself, and it was a busy time of year, he had not been missed until 10 days after the start of the binge. By now he was well-poisoned and in urgent need of supervised drying-out. But Hamish was large and very fit, and he was adamantly refusing to go into hospital.

What his GP, Dr Logie, wanted was for me to accept him as a compulsory admission under the 1959 Mental Health (Scotland) Act. That Act permitted people suffering from mental disorder to be compulsorily admitted to hospital, and detained for seven days, at the request of a general practitioner acting on his own without any supporting professional opinion. Seven days was long enough to dry out an alcoholic. The only problem was that alcoholism was not a mental disorder under the Act, and Hamish had no other mental problem. So I refused to accept him on those terms.

This surprised Dr Logie. He explained that Hamish's binges were a regular annual occurrence and that, for years, they had been terminated in the same way, by compulsory admission to Craig Dunain. I reiterated that he was asking me to break the law. Moreover, since Hamish did not want to come into hospital, I should have to send out two nurses with a large supply of intramuscular sedatives, which they would have to give him in order that he could be safely

Principles of Health Care Ethics. Edited by Raanan Gillon.
© 1994 John Wiley & Sons Ltd

and quietly transported 100 miles to the hospital. So I should be asking them also to break the law.

AUTONOMY OR BENEFICENCE?

In other words, I was all in favour of promoting Hamish's autonomy. Not only was he saying that he did not want to come into hospital, but there was no legal basis for his compulsory admission, which would in effect be kidnapping. Dr Logie, however, produced the beneficence argument. If Hamish was not admitted to hospital he would continue to drink, and would probably kill himself in another day or two. There was no way that Dr Logie could be certain to remove all his supplies of whisky. Nor was there anyone who could stay with Hamish waiting for him to become unconscious, at which point he could legally be admitted as an emergency without consent. Moreover, Dr Logie pointed out that Hamish had never previously complained about being carried off to hospital illegally. (It was, of course, highly unlikely that anyone had ever told him about the limits on compulsory orders under the Mental Health (Scotland) Act.)

So we were at an impasse. We could respect Hamish's autonomy, with the likelihood that he would drink himself to death within a couple of days, or we could follow the dictates of beneficence and dry him out, but that would require two doctors, two nurses and two ambulance drivers to conspire to kidnap him. Although I had read widely about medical ethics as a student, and had worked for a few months for the Society for the Study of Medical Ethics, I had read nothing about the four principles that would suggest a way out of the impasse. So we chose instead to muddle through, in the way that Barry Hoffmaster (1) suggests nearly all moral decisions are in practice made. I gave Dr Logie the home number of the duty consultant; the latter decided to follow the previous routine and instructed me to admit Hamish. That I could do happily, knowing that the legal responsibility was the consultant's, but aware also that the ethical problem remained unresolved and admitted of no easy route to a solution.

THE MANTRA IS PROVISIONAL

Hamish provided my first indication that the four principles might not after all be the last word in medical ethics. Since then many more problems have become apparent to me, in addition to the absence of any coherent mechanism for resolving conflict between the principles. Some problems are inherent, some lie in the application of the principles. A philosopher could no doubt write at great length analysing these problems, but that is not what seems to be needed here. I propose to discuss the problems polemically, rather than analytically, to show the limitations of the 'Georgetown mantra', as the four principles are now colloquially known. That name arose from the promotion—indeed, the 'devotional incantation'—of the four principles by scholars at the Kennedy Institute of Ethics at Georgetown University in Washington, DC. At times, however, the constant repetition of the four principles by some scholars has seemed less mantra-like, and more reminiscent of a line in Lewis Carroll's 'The Hunting of the Snark': 'What I tell you three times is true.'

Perhaps the most basic limitation of the four principles is their aridity. They are reminiscent of the stony ground on which seed fell in the Parable of the Sower (2). At first the corn sprang up, and then it withered because there was nothing to sustain it. The four principles are rationalist and derived from theory, with little to say to the complexity and joyful variety of real life. Yet some scholars believe that they provide a complete and potentially permanent framework within which to analyse bioethical problems, not acknowledging that even much more comprehensive principles should only be regarded as provisional. Stephen Toulmin (3) quotes Goldsworthy Lowes Dickinson's summary of the place of reason in ethics:

> It is the part of Reason ... to tabulate and compare results. She does not determine directly what is good, but works, as in all the sciences, upon given data ... noticing what kinds of activity satisfy, and to what degree, the expanding nature of this soul that seeks Good, and deducing therefrom, so far as may be, temporary rules of conduct. ... Temporary rules, I say, because, by the nature of the case, they can have in them nothing absolute and final, in as much as they are mere deductions from a process which is always developing and transforming itself. Systems of morals, maxims of conduct are so many landmarks left to show the route by which the soul is marching; casts, as it were, of her features at various stages of her growth, but never the final record of her perfect countenance ... in a sense, they are only to be understood in order to be superseded. (4)

Advocates of the Georgetown mantra tend not to acknowledge that it might be—indeed, should be—only of temporary value. Valuable it certainly has been, in providing a simple framework comprehensible to non-philosophers. But one of the great dangers of the mantra is precisely that it has become ossified and formulaic, and is no longer viewed as just a step to further development. It is of course immensely attractive to doctors, brought up in medical school on a diet of anatomical mnemonics. What could be more attractive than being reminded of all your ethical obligations by swiftly chanting 'autonomy, justice, beneficence, non-maleficence' as you come to each patient on a ward round or in the clinic? It certainly requires no more effort than the crude and unconsidered sort of utilitarianism—'How can we get the most benefit out of this situation?'— most often used by health care workers in earlier decades.

WHY BENEFICENCE AND NON-MALEFICENCE?

Problems with the mantra are much greater, however, than just the ease with which it may be misused. One of the more curious inherent problems lies in the apparent need to have separate principles of beneficence and non-maleficence. It would seem, at first sight, that the duties to be beneficent or non-maleficent were two sides of the same coin. How could one duty exist effectively without the other? Gillon, however, explains that one is a perfect duty, the other is not: 'we do not have a duty to benefit all other people; apart from everything else it is incoherent to talk of a duty which is impossible to fulfil. Thus at most we can have a duty only to benefit some other people (an imperfect duty), while we have a perfect duty to everybody not to harm them' (5). In other words, it is possible, in his view, to fulfil a duty not to harm all other people. For those living in small, isolated, primitive societies this may just be a possibility; for anyone living in developed countries it is nonsense.

In the west we all use a disproportionate share of most of the world's resources. We acquiesce in social and political structures that ensure the poverty of a substantial proportion of the world's population—poverty not only in material terms, but in education, health care, personal development and the absence of leisure. In our own countries we have seen this century a move away from the social group to the paramountcy of the individual. Concentration on the importance of the individual leads inevitably to greater competition between individuals; as we each strive to improve our standing in various ways other than the spiritual, we are likely to do so at the expense of others.

Just by living in western society and accepting some—and by no means necessarily, all—of its standards of behaviour, one is harming others. Most of those harmed may not be people one knows. But just as that was a contributory factor to the impossibility of benefiting all other people, so it ensures that one cannot avoid harming some others. Thus the idea that non-maleficence could be a perfect duty is folly. To attempt to distinguish between beneficence and non-maleficence on such grounds just demonstrates a weakness at the heart of the principles.

XENOPHOBIC JUSTICE

Another weakness was hinted at above, when mentioning use of the world's resources. The health care systems of Western Europe, North America, and Japan and Australasia account for approximately 9% of the world's total economic activity. Those systems make a significant contribution to the net outflow of resources from the least developed parts of the world. They have helped to ensure that in some countries in Africa in the last decade, health expenditure per capita has dropped from about $2 per annum to $1 per annum. In other words, demands for ever more to be spent on health care in the west contribute to the failure to increase, and in some cases the reduction of, health care services in the 40 or 50 poorest countries of the world.

Yet where in the thousands of books and papers about allocation of health care resources does one find this inequity considered? Who is the bioethicist who has argued that the principle of justice in the Georgetown mantra must apply equally to all men if it is to retain any value? One may find plenty of papers advocating more equal resource allocation within a particular developed country, but where is the man, or woman, who argues that human life is as valuable in the least developed country as in the most, and that the principle of justice therefore demands that as many resources be used in the least developed country as in the most? What appears all too obvious is that those who rely on the Georgetown mantra as the means to solution of practical problems can only apply it to people like themselves.

This is not to say, of course, that the principle of justice, as expressed in the mantra, is wrong. It is to suggest that, as a practical tool, it gives its practitioners enough help or strength only to enable them to tackle minor problems, not the major ones. This may perhaps be inevitable, in that the mantra had to be developed in a particular sort of society. As Vaclav Havel, when President of Czechoslovakia, said:

> ... modern thought—based on the premise that the world is objectively knowable, and that the knowledge so obtained can be absolutely generalised—has come to a final crisis ... the era of arrogant, absolutive reason is drawing to a close. ... It was an era in which there was a cult of depersonalised objectivity, an era in which objective knowledge was amassed and technologically exploited, an era of belief in automatic progress brokered by the scientific method. ...

How does one find a way forward out of this crisis? Not, Havel suggests, by more of the same:

> We are trying to deal with what we have unleashed by employing the same means we used to unleash it in the first place. We are looking for new scientific recipes, new ideologies, new control systems, new institutions, new instruments to eliminate the dreadful consequences of our previous recipes, ideologies, control systems, institutions and instruments. We are looking for an objective way out of the crisis of objectivism. (6)

ARE THE PRINCIPLES PRACTISED?

If it seems unfair to suggest that practitioners of the four principles deal only with minor, not major, problems, it is perhaps worth asking what any approach to bioethics, and its practitioners, have achieved. Can one suggest any medical or biological development that has been prevented, or significantly slowed down, because of the intervention of bioethicists? Occasionally, as in the early days of DNA recombinant experiments, there was a voluntary moratorium by scientists themselves on further work. If anything, however, the intervention of bioethicists has tended to make it easier for doctors and scientists to go ahead with whatever technological innovation they have developed.

Alderson has made the latter point elegantly in a paper looking at the protection given to children in guidelines on the conduct of research produced in the last half-century. She comments:

> Successive bioethics guidelines are like a series of doors, opening to involve children increasingly in research. Restrictive labels on the doors—'danger', 'adults only', 'in the child's best interests'—change to permissive ones—'therapeutic research', 'allow children to be included', 'not against the child's interests', 'preferably in early childhood'. (7)

The last label above is taken from the Clothier report on gene therapy (8), which reverses the previous injunction that research should always be conducted first on voluntarily consenting adults before being tried on children. It is now suggested that young children be the first experimental subjects of gene therapy.

An equally elegant example of how bioethicists have failed to influence routine practice was contained in a 1988 paper in the *British Medical Journal* (9). One hundred consecutive patients in the professorial surgical unit of a Scottish teaching hospital were asked, two to five days postoperatively, what had been done to which organ. Twenty-seven did not know which organ had been operated on, and 44 did not know what procedure had been performed. Those who did not know were older on average than those who did (63 years old v. 50 years).

The unit's procedure involved a ward round the day before operation 'when the consultant tells the patient of the nature of the intended operation'. Later that day a junior doctor repeated the details of the intended operation and obtained the patient's signature on a standard consent form. The authors acknowledged that the information given 'was possibly inadequate', but concluded that this was 'unlikely to be the major factor' in the poor results. They preferred an explanation of an unexpectedly high level of cerebral atrophy, aggravated by anaesthesia and analgesia!

More recently a paper examining the ethics of clinical trials concluded that multi-centre trials should be reviewed by a national ethics committee, rather than local ones. The (medical) authors continued:

> In certain cases the committee may take the decision that for a particular trial, in consideration of all the issues, the principle of non-maleficence should override that of autonomy. In such cases informed consent need not be sought since . . . the best medical care is randomisation into a trial. (10)

Medical paternalism is alive and well. That it is reflects the failure of the four principles to be powerful enough in themselves to tackle the issues of where power lies, and how it is used, in health care. Obviously the issue of doctors' power over patients or research subjects is frequently examined, but any amount of preaching of the principle of autonomy has brought us no closer to power-sharing in the doctor–patient relationship. Other power relationships are examined less often. The power of politicians over health care users, for instance, and of developed countries over developing, are rarely considered. Most importantly, it is only in the last decade that issues of men's power over women, and the relationship of that power to ways of dealing with moral problems, have been discussed, but not in terms of the contribution of the mantra. Almost invariably, examples used to discuss the application of the four principles focus attention on a male doctor; rather than questioning the power structure, such examples tend to promote a white, male, western power centre.

GENDER DIFFERENCES ARE IMPORTANT

It is the work of Carol Gilligan in particular that has recently drawn attention to the need to focus on gender differences in approaches to moral issues. She re-examined Piaget's and Kohlberg's work on moral development, showing how it was based entirely on their observations of males. Those observations fitted the theories they as males had developed; when girls were found to approach moral issues differently from boys, it was automatically assumed that their moral development was less. She postulated an alternative theory to explain their findings and supported it with her own work. Women construct moral dilemmas as issues of the duty to care and of responsibility in relationships:

> The moral imperative that emerges repeatedly in interviews with women is an injunction to care, a responsibility to discern and alleviate the 'real and recognisable trouble' of this world. For men, the moral imperative appears rather as an injunction to respect the rights of others and thus to protect from interference the rights to life and self-fulfillment. Women's insistence on care is at first self-critical rather than self-protective, while men initially conceive obligation to others negatively in terms of noninterference. Development for both sexes would therefore seem to entail an integration of rights and responsibilities through the discovery of the complementarity of these disparate views. (11)

Gilligan herself acknowledges that she has drawn the distinction between the sexes too sharply in order to make her point. But her work has a self-evident ring of truth about it. The mantra and the rights it entails are largely built on non-interference. Autonomy is almost invariably presented as a right to non-interference. The spurious claim of a 'perfect' duty to non-maleficence, with beneficence as an imperfect duty, again reflects a need not to interfere.

The contrast between Gilligan's observations of how at least half of the population deals with moral issues and the artifice of the mantra approach is not new. It closely reflects the distinction between situation ethics and rule ethics that Joseph Fletcher described:

> ... rule ethics eliminates what we call conscience—that is, the responsible exercise of moral decision making. If you follow a rule your choice is dictated by the rule. If certain forms or kinds of acts are forbidden in advance of the variables or circumstances of the actual situation, then all decision making has been preempted by the rule. Conscience is irrelevant. The rule decides, and you, the moral agent, have no part to play. (Yours not to reason why, yours but to do and die.)
>
> Situation ethics is the other approach. ... In situation ethics the moral agent, the decision maker, judges what is best in the circumstances and in view of foreseeable consequences. (12)

ON BEING A MORAL AGENT

Fletcher reminds us of the importance of the moral agent, someone absent from the four principles. This perhaps is the root cause of the aridity that was not fully explained earlier. They are an abstraction, plucked from one knows not where, and there is a presumption that they can always be applied objectively, dispassionately, by rational people. But life ain't like that; I am reminded of Robert Louis Stevenson: 'Books are good enough in their own way, but they are a mighty bloodless substitute for life.' Real moral agents do not always work in the abstract; they exhibit emotions which get mixed up in decisions that are not always rational. Hoffmaster, for example, quotes the example of one of Abby Lippman's early studies on decision-making in genetic counselling:

> The first step [prospective parents] take is to discard the probabilities the counsellors

have given them. They reduce the alternatives to two equally likely outcomes—either we will have a defective child or we won't. Then they imagine what it would be like to care for and raise a defective child. If they feel they can cope with these scenarios, they try to conceive; if not, they seek permanent contraception. And if they cannot make up their minds, they play 'reproductive roulette', that is, they engage in unprotected intercourse, thereby abandoning the decision to fate. (1)

The ways in which moral agents do make moral decisions and the wide range of influences on an individual conscience have been examined most effectively in a recent book by Sidney Callahan, an American psychologist married to a bioethicist. Amongst her conclusions are:

Reasoning, human intuition, emotions, and social communications are integral to the scientific and moral quest for personal conviction. Knowing this, we should also beware of overanalytic rationalist methods of moral decision making, which fail to take into account the subjective person's moral resources of nonconscious mental and emotional signals. Emotional commitment, care, and desire are never irrelevant in morality. (13)

Some of the limitations of the four principles discussed above seem to arise from a basic contradiction in the approach of some philosophers to bioethics. Bioethics is, *par excellence*, an example of applied ethics, ethics at work in the world, yet philosophers who promote the mantra seem to eschew the techniques of observing the real world used by social scientists, and to stick with their need for abstraction. Gilligan is a professor of education, Callahan a professor of psychology, and it is a professor of the history of medicine, George Weisz, who provides the most succinct summary of the Georgetown mantra's problems:

No one disputes the significance and often the painfulness of the issues and choices being addressed. But there is something about the way these issues are usually handled which seems somehow inappropriate if not wrong-headed to one trained in a discipline like sociology or history. In their analyses of complex situations, ethicists often appear grandly oblivious to the social and cultural context in which these occur, and indeed to empirical referents of any sort. Nor do they seem very conscious of the cultural specificity of many of the values and procedures they utilize when making ethical judgments. (14)

IS DUTY THE WAY FORWARD?

Cultural, psychological, gender and geographical limitations to the four principles have been discussed. Are they fatal to any worthwhile continued use of the principles? The answer has to be yes to their use as a self-sufficient basis of bioethical analysis. As an observer of the bioethics scene I cannot say with authority in what direction bioethics should now go. It seems most likely, however, that development of duty-based ethics will be of value (15). This approaches moral problems by seeking an answer to the question: 'What ought I to do?' Thus it includes consideration of the moral agent, taking on board many of the strengths of virtue ethics but avoiding the latter's tendency to exclusion of other pertinent interests. And duty-based ethics avoids the limitation of deontological approaches, such as the Georgetown mantra, that regard duties only as responses to the rights that have been claimed.

An answer to the question 'What ought I to do?' also depends on detailed information about the particular situation, so that such an approach encourages the development of casuistry. Good casuistry depends on thorough case descriptions, rather than the very brief outlines often used in teaching, and one volume (16) of such detailed case-histories has already appeared. If bioethics turns to duty-based ethics as its way forward, then there will be a place for the four principles, but only as one consideration among several, reflecting the complexity of real life.

REFERENCES

1. Hoffmaster, B. 1991. Morality and the social sciences. Pp. 241–260, *in* Weisz, G. (Ed.) *Social science perspectives on medical ethics*. University of Pennsylvania Press, Philadelphia, PA.
2. *The Holy Bible* (King James version). *Gospel according to St Luke*, **8**: 4–15.
3. Toulmin, S. 1950. *An examination of the place of reason in ethics*. Cambridge University Press, Cambridge.
4. Lowes Dickinson, G. 1901. *The meaning of good*. George Allen & Unwin, London.
5. Gillon, R. 1986. *Philosophical medical ethics*. John Wiley, Chichester.
6. Havel, V. 1992. Address to meeting of World Economic Forum. Davos, Switzerland; 4 February.
7. Alderson, P. 1992. Did children change, or the guidelines? *Bulletin of Medical Ethics*, No. 80: 21–28.
8. *Report of the committee on the ethics of gene therapy (Cmnd 1788)*. 1992. HMSO, London.
9. Byrne, D. J., Napier, A. and Cuschieri, A. 1988. How informed is signed consent? *British Medical Journal* **296**: 839–840.
10. Baum, M., Zilkha, K. and Houghton, J. 1989. Ethics of clinical research: lessons for the future. *British Medical Journal* **299**: 251–253.
11. Gilligan, C. 1982. *In a different voice: psychological theory and women's development*. Harvard University Press, Cambridge, MA.
12. Fletcher, J. 1979. *Humanhood: essays in biomedical ethics*. Prometheus Books, Buffalo, NY.
13. Callahan, S. 1991. *In good conscience: reason and emotion in moral decision making*. Harper Collins, New York.
14. Weisz, G. 1991. Introduction. Pp. 3–15, *in* Weisz, G. (Ed.) *Social science perspectives on medical ethics*. University of Pennsylvania Press, Philadelphia, PA.
15. O'Neill, O. 1991. Introducing ethics: some current positions. *Bulletin of Medical Ethics*, No. 73: 18–21.
16. Ackerman, T. F. and Strong, C. 1989. *A casebook of medical ethics*. Oxford University Press, New York.

24

Against the Four Principles: a Nordic View

HENRIK R. WULFF, MD

Professor of Clinical Theory and Ethics, Consultant Physician, Herlev University Hospital, Denmark

HOW CAN ANYBODY BE AGAINST 'THE FOUR PRINCIPLES'?

The idea of human autonomy constitutes the very basis of western ethical thinking, and everybody must agree that it is evil deliberately to harm others, and that it is commendable to do good deeds and to seek justice. In other words, the principles of respect for autonomy, non-maleficence, beneficence and justice are so fundamental that they cannot be contested.

I appreciate that the distinction between the four principles may be useful when authors of textbooks of medical ethics wish to explain the complexities of their subject to the uninitiated reader (1,2), but the four-principles approach has no guiding force in real life, unless the principles are interpreted and ranked.

The four-principles approach to medical ethics originated in the United States, and in this chapter I shall argue that the interpretation and the order of priority of the four principles within the American moral tradition do not accord with the prevailing moral tradition in other parts of the western world, e.g. the Nordic countries.

First, it is necessary to discuss briefly the derivation of moral principles and their role in ethical reasoning. According to the conventional point of view, fundamental moral principles are primary and moral practice is secondary. The allegedly universally valid principles are regarded as the starting-point of a deductive reasoning process which leads to the solution of the ethical problem. This point of view, however, is hardly tenable today when most people have abandoned fundamentalist religious beliefs, and philosophers have given up the hope that universal moral principles can be derived by reasoning alone. Moral principles are always extracted from a particular moral tradition—moral practice is primary and moral rules secondary—and the guiding force of a set of principles depends on their accordance with current practice. This view takes into account

Principles of Health Care Ethics. Edited by Raanan Gillon.

the importance of cultural differences, but, as pointed out by Kekes (3), it need not lead to extreme cultural relativism, as some moral traditions guarantee better than others that the members of a society can pursue what they regard as good lives.

Ethical reasoning cannot be described in simple terms, but anybody who has seriously tried to analyse an ethical dilemma will know that it is an elaborate process. It is necessary to reason backwards and forwards, seeking and weighing all the relevant moral aspects of the case, in order to reach a balanced conclusion. The initial moral judgement may have to be revised when it is confronted with a careful evaluation of the consequences of different decisions and with accepted moral principles, and all these deliberations take place within the framework of those theories of man and society which are ingrained in the culture to which the persons belong. The end-result of such a process, which may vary considerably from one case to another, has been called a *wide reflective equilibrium* (4).

With these considerations in mind I shall briefly sketch some of the main trends of the moral traditions in the United States and the Nordic countries, and I shall try to illustrate how the *four-principles approach* and the alternative *Golden-Rule approach* are embedded in these traditions. Then, I shall consider the problems of health care, both on the individual and the societal level, in the light of the two traditions.

THE AMERICAN MORAL TRADITION AND THE FOUR PRINCIPLES

The moral tradition of any society to a large extent reflects its historical development. The immigrants who came to the United States had very different cultural backgrounds, and many of them had fled from religious, racial and political oppression. It is easy to understand that the resulting pluralistic society would cherish the right to self-determination as the supreme moral principle. Paramount importance is attached to the right of individuals to shape their own lives and to pursue their happiness with a minimum of interference from other individuals and from society. All over the world this love for freedom has served as an inspiration to those who are politically oppressed, and due respect must be paid to its moral significance. It is this aspect of American culture that is reflected by *the principle of respect for autonomy*, which in the context of this tradition may be defined as respect for *the right to self-determination*. However, it goes without saying that individual freedom of action must have its limits and that everybody has an obligation not to harm others. All civilized societies, including the American one, recognize *the principle of non-maleficence*.

These two principles do not suffice. In any society there will be those who cannot manage their lives without the help of others, and a *principle of beneficence* is needed. The important role played by organized charity shows that this principle is a very active component of the American moral tradition, but nonetheless the outside observer can hardly fail to notice that American society in spite of its immense wealth tolerates great social inequalities. This state of affairs suggests that the principle of beneficence has only a limited scope and a lower priority than the others. It follows that the *principle of justice* (in the sense of distributive justice), although it may be seen as a moral ideal, also has a fairly low status when it comes to moral practice.

This brief presentation of the chief characteristics of the prevailing American moral tradition serves to show that the four-principles approach fits this tradition when the principles are interpreted in certain ways and when they are ranked in a certain order of priority.

I shall now illustrate that this particular interpretation of the four-principles approach has influenced medical ethics, and for that purpose I shall quote the published proceedings of the Appleton Consensus Conference which took place in 1988 (5). At that conference a group of ethicists from the United States and other western countries met to formulate a set of 'guidelines for decisions to forgo medical treatment', and the introduction to the proceedings contained the following brief formulations of the four principles:

1. *Autonomy.* All persons have a *prima facie* moral obligation to respect each other's autonomy insofar as such respect is compatible with the respect for the autonomy of all affected . . .
2. *Non-maleficence.* All persons have a *prima facie* moral obligation not to harm each other . . .
3. *Beneficence.* All persons have some moral obligation to benefit others, to some degree, including, perhaps even especially, those in need . . .
4. *Justice.* All persons have a *prima facie* moral obligation to act justly or fairly to others in the context of the distribution of scarce resources, in the context of respecting each other's rights, and in the context of obeying morally acceptable laws . . .

It is obvious that these formulations differ markedly from the brief incontestable ones which I included at the very beginning of this chapter. The four-principles approach originated in the United States, and this interpretation illustrates that the principles can be extracted from the American moral tradition. The formulation of the principle of beneficence is loaded with qualifications, and the authors of the document do their very best to stress that the principle of justice must not interfere with any other moral consideration. One may even interpret the formulation to mean that the principle of justice is not 'a morally acceptable law' in its own right.

One may, of course, argue that this presentation is much too simplistic, as American society is highly pluralistic and there is no single moral tradition. It is, for instance, well known that there is a strong liberal opposition, including philosophers and medical ethicists, who oppose the libertarian tradition which I have described. However, I believe that it is true to say that it is that tradition which has determined the social structure of contemporary American society or, in other words, that it is the libertarian tradition which has determined moral practice on the societal level.

According to the libertarian tradition, individual freedom is interpreted as *negative freedom,* i.e. the idea that a person is free if he or she is not restrained from seeking the realization of his or her wishes in life, and it is this idea which justifies the ranking of the four principles. As I shall explain below, others favour the concept of *positive freedom*, i.e. the idea that the members of a society are not really free, unless they also have the opportunity to realize their wishes.

THE NORDIC MORAL TRADITION AND THE GOLDEN RULE

In contrast to the United States, the populations of the Nordic countries (Denmark, Finland, Iceland, Norway and Sweden) are very homogeneous. There has been some immigration during the past few decades, but the vast majority of the inhabitants have the same cultural and religious background. The number of active members of the Lutheran churches may be relatively small, but very few people have joined other religious communities.

I shall confine myself to describing very briefly some aspects of the development of Danish society. In the nineteenth century Denmark was a poor agricultural country. It went bankrupt in 1813 at the end of the Napoleonic wars, became a democratic constitutional monarchy in 1849 and had to cede to Germany one-third of its population after the war in 1864. Against this background an economic, educational and spiritual revival took place. The farmers, most of whom were smallholders, formed the cooperative movement and gathered round the so-called folk high schools, i.e. institutions for adult education inspired by the ideas of the Lutheran theologian and educationalist N.F. S. Grundtvig. Towards the end of the century, when industrialization gathered speed, workers joined forces in the social-democratic movement with its egalitarian concept of social justice, and in this century emerged the ideal of a democratic welfare state based on mutual obligations. That ideal has left its mark on many of our social institutions: the Danish school system is mainly public and the few private schools receive large grants from the state; higher education, including university education, is practically free; the hospital system is almost exclusively public and everybody is entitled to free hospital treatment; the income taxes are among the highest in the world.

The history of the other Nordic countries differs from that of Denmark in many important respects, but they, too, have cherished the ideal of the welfare state, and the prevailing moral traditions in the Nordic region are very similar.

The moral codex to be extracted from this tradition is not the four principles in a particular ranking order, but the Golden Rule as it is formulated in the Sermon on the Mount: 'And as ye would that men should do to you, do ye also to them likewise' (Luke iv. 31). This principle must not be taken to mean that we should attribute to others our own wishes and preferences, but rather that we should help others to pursue their happiness as we wish to pursue ours. The Golden Rule interpreted in this manner entails the idea of positive freedom. It is extremely difficult to define in exact terms what is meant by justice, but the closest that we shall ever get to the idea of a just society is probably the society where everybody lives according to the Golden Rule, and in this sense the Golden Rule also entails the principle of justice.

It follows from the Golden Rule that individual man must not regard himself in a privileged position, and in this respect there is considerable similarity between traditional Christian ethics and Kantian moral theory. In one of the formulations of the categorical imperative, Kant stresses that a moral agent must always act as if the maxim of his action (i.e. the principle guiding the action) were to become a universal law, and, just like the Golden Rule, this principle of universalizability serves as a protection against ethical egoism.

The Nordic moral tradition is, of course, not uniform, and there have always been those who favoured the libertarian approach, but it can hardly be denied that the idea of mutual obligations has been an important guiding force in the development of the Nordic societies. It is a fact that no political party in any of the Nordic countries advocates the dismantling of the national health services, and I have yet to meet somebody who does not take it for granted that two people suffering from the same disease should have the same medical or surgical treatment, regardless of their social status and economic means. However, it is also true that in recent years the very ideal of the welfare state has come under attack, and that the libertarian way of thinking is gaining ground also in this part of the world. In Denmark the first private 'for-profit' hospital has been established, and it is quite possible that the American and Nordic norms will converge in the years to come.

THE FOURFOLD TABLE OF HEALTH CARE ETHICS

So far the two moral traditions and the principles to be extracted from these traditions have been discussed from a general non-medical point of view, and it remains to apply the ideas to the problems of health care. For that purpose I shall introduce 'the fourfold table of health care ethics', which may provide the necessary common ground for the discussion.

As explained in the introduction to this chapter, the reasoning process which leads to the 'solution' of an ethical dilemma is extremely complex, but nonetheless, everybody facing an ethical dilemma, either in their daily or in their professional lives, must take into account the consequences of the possible actions; this is the *consequentialist* component of ethical thinking. It is also a common characteristic of all cultures that obedience to certain rules of behaviour poses a constraint to the consequentialist considerations. Truth-telling, for instance, is a generally accepted *prima facie* obligation (which perhaps ought to have been added to the 'four principles'). This is the *deontological* component of ethical thinking. Utilitarians will, of course, object to this expression, but they may rephrase the argument to mean that in all cultures some 'goods' are considered so important that their attainment overrules other consequentialist considerations. Mill's emphasis on the importance of the liberty of man is the classical example.

It is also uncontroversial to state that deliberations about health care ethics usually take place on one of two levels: the *individual* level and the *community* level. Typically, dilemmas on the individual level arise in everyday clinical practice when the individual doctor faces an individual patient, whereas dilemmas on the community level occur when, for instance, administrators and politicians concern themselves with the distribution of limited resources. The distinction is, of course, not clear-cut, as the doctor treating the individual patient must also consider the general interests of the community which he serves.

TABLE 24.1 The fourfold table of health care ethics

	Reasoning	
Level	Deontological	Consequentialist
Individual	**A** Respect for right to self-determination	**B** Consequences for patient
Community	**C** Justice	**D** Universal consequences

These considerations may serve as a rough framework for a discussion of the fundamental problems of health care ethics, most of which take the form of tensions between the rows and the columns of the resulting fourfold table (Table 24.1).

The prevailing American and the Nordic traditions resemble each other to such an extent that we are on common ground not only when we construct this table, but also when we consider the contents of the four fields which have been labelled A, B, C, and D. The clinician will in each individual case consider which decision has the best consequences for that particular patient, but he is also well aware of the fact that he acts under a deontological constraint. According to both traditions he must consider the patient's right to self-determination.

Ethical reasoning on the community level presents a similar tension. Administrators, health economists or policy-makers tend to reason much like the utilitarians of the eighteenth and nineteenth centuries as they seek those decisions which have the best general consequences. However, they, too, are acting under a deontological constraint as they must at the same time seek a just distribution of the limited resources. As discussed above, the status of the principle of justice may differ, but it is recognized by both traditions.

Ethical dilemmas, however, do not only arise out of tensions within the two levels. It is also necessary to consider the tension between the two levels, i.e. one must also balance the interests of the individual patient against the interests of the community.

THE FOURFOLD TABLE AND THE FOUR-PRINCIPLES APPROACH

The European reader of American reports of ethical problem cases is often astonished by the legalistic nature of the discussions. Who has the right to decide what in that particular case? Does the patient have the right to refuse further treatment? Does the doctor have the right to turn off the respirator against the wishes of the relatives, or do the relatives have the right to demand cessation of treatment against the doctor's best judgement? Frequently, the case is brought to court and the verdict is presented as the 'solution' to the ethical dilemma. Thus, the important distinction between legal and moral norms is completely obliterated. This legalistic approach to medical ethics accords well with the Appleton formulation of the four principles where the right to self-determination receives such high priority that the other principles are practically forgotten.

Of course, I do not wish to imply that American doctors do not to the same extent as their European colleagues try to do the best for their patients, and that they do not seek to provide compassionate care, but one gets the impression that the moral norms on the societal level and the resulting structure of the health care system have had an effect on the patient–doctor relationship which has forced them to focus on the legal aspects of clinical practice to such an extent that the discussion is limited to field A in the fourfold table.

The tension between the two levels, especially the tension between respect for individual autonomy (field A) and the duty to ensure justice (field C), is also resolved in favour of the former consideration; the members of a society favouring the idea of negative freedom will feel no strong moral obligation to provide equal health care, but at most an obligation to provide that minimum of care which is justified by the low-priority principles of beneficence and justice. The authors of the Appleton guidelines also draw this conclusion. They write:

> The principle of justice requires universal access to an acceptable, decent minimum of basic health care.

The ideal, according to this point of view, is a two-tiered system of health care. As stated by Engelhardt: 'It provides at least some amount of health care for all, while on the other hand allowing those with resources to purchase additional health care' (6).

THE FOURFOLD TABLE AND THE GOLDEN-RULE APPROACH

The Golden Rule provides less specific guidance in the concrete case; the secondary principles to be derived from that rule are not ranked, and the tensions in the fourfold table remain. On the individual level the clinician must subject each case to a careful analysis. He must seek a reflective equilibrium which takes into account the right to self-determination (field A) but does not exclude paternalistic action grounded on compassion (field B). Individual rights are not belittled, but it is recognized that ethics is much more than the mutual respect of rights. Most people would agree that the author of a book on the ethics of marriage ought to discuss not only the rights of husbands and wives, but also such concepts as love and mutual trust, and in much the same way the primary concern of medical ethics ought to be the positive aspects of the patient–doctor relationship. Patients' and doctors' rights are important, but controversies about rights are always the result of the breakdown of a human relationship, and it is the cause of that breakdown which ought to interest medical ethicists.

Contractual relationships between two persons based only on the mutual respect of individual rights can be subjected to a legalistic analysis, but relationships based on the Golden Rule require empathic understanding. Therefore, in the case of conflicts between doctors and patients, one ought to ask questions like these: Did the doctor sincerely try to understand the patient's experience of the illness in the context of the patient's own life? Did he explain the diagnostic and therapeutic options so well that the patient did not feel estranged and ignored in the unfamiliar hospital environment? Did he spend sufficient time with the relatives to be able to alleviate their worries? Those who adopt the legalistic approach rarely try to answer such questions when they publish their reports of ethical problem cases.

In other words, the Golden-Rule approach invites a distinction between moral and legal norms, and it becomes possible to discuss even the delicate topic of patients' duties without denying their legal (or quasi-legal) rights. One may, for instance, argue that patients who benefit from the results of clinical trials in which earlier patients took part have a *prima facie* moral obligation to participate in new trials in order to benefit future patients. There may, of course, be good moral reasons why individual patients should not wish to fulfil this obligation, and the only ones who can decide this are the patients themselves. Therefore, informed consent is still indispensable. Patients' duties are rarely discussed in the American literature on medical ethics, but it remains a fact that the prime motive of many patients for participating in clinical trials is to benefit future patients (7).

On the societal level the Golden Rule invites the establishment of an egalitarian public health system based on national insurance. However, the resources available for such systems are never unlimited, and the distribution presents considerable difficulties. Health economists often aim at maximizing the expected utility of the resources, and for that purpose they may recommend the calculation of QALYs, i.e. the resulting number of 'quality of life'-adjusted life-years. This mode of thinking is clearly utilitarian and the calculations are reminiscent of the 'felicific calculus' suggested by Jeremy Bentham 200 years ago. Here I shall not discuss the methodological problems, but only point out that decisions based on such calculations may seem highly unjust (8). They do not, for instance take into account that proportionally more money must be spent in sparsely populated than in densely populated areas in order to ensure equality of access. The administrators of a public health care system must always consider the constraint posed by the ill-defined principle of justice; they experience the tension between field C and field D in the fourfold table, and once again there is no easy solution.

The tension between the two levels is equally important. Doctors employed in a public health service, like those found in the Nordic countries, will want to do their best for each of their patients, but they must also ensure that everybody gets a fair share of the limited resources.

THE IMPORTANCE OF CULTURAL TRADITION

For the sake of simplicity I have used the expressions the *four-principles approach* and the *Golden-Rule approach*, and I have discussed the relationship between these approaches: the Golden Rule encompasses the four principles while the four principles, when ranked, seem incompatible with the Golden Rule.

However, as already explained, the use of the word 'approach' does not imply that decision-makers simply deduce the solution to an ethical problem from one or more fundamental principles or rules. The principles must always be seen as part of a moral tradition, and all the components of that tradition, including the accepted background theories of man and society, enter the reflective equilibrium. Moral principles cannot be interpreted in isolation.

The two traditions which I have described are in agreement in one very important respect: the belief in the autonomy of man—the belief that man is capable of moral deliberations and of acting freely on the basis of such deliberations—but the moral consequences which are derived from that belief differ. Those who favour *the Golden-Rule approach* will argue: man is autonomous, therefore man has duties towards others. It is this aspect of Christian ethics (and of Kantian moral theory) which entails the idea of positive freedom and ensures the symmetry in human relationships which is the basis of the concept of justice. Human rights are seen as secondary to human duties, which means that the violation of rights can always be blamed on those who did not fulfil their duties.

In contrast, those who accept the conventional *four-principles approach* seem to argue in this manner: man is autonomous, therefore man has certain natural rights which must be respected. This is the basis of the concept of negative freedom which pervades that approach. Human duties have a lower priority than human rights, and the resulting asymmetry in human relationships will by necessity entail social injustice.

The main conclusion of this chapter is not, however, that one approach ought to be preferred to another (although I have not tried to conceal my own preference), but only that cultural traditions differ and that, consequently, the problems of medical ethics must always be viewed in the perspective of a particular culture. International cooperation is extremely important as the introduction of new medical technology creates similar ethical problems all over the world, but the answers to those problems are bound to differ. Those who read the international literature on medical ethics must always be conscious of their own cultural background, so that they do not unwittingly import professional norms which do not fit the society which they serve.

REFERENCES

1. Beauchamp, T. L. and Childress, J. F. 1989. *Principles of biomedical ethics*, 2nd edn. Oxford University Press, Oxford and New York.
2. Gillon, R. 1985. *Philosophical medical ethics*. John Wiley & Sons, Chichester and New York.
3. Kekes, J. 1985. Moral tradition. *Philosophical Investigations*, 252–268.
4. Daniels, N. 1980. Reflective equilibrium and archimedean points. *Canadian Journal of Philosophy* **10**: 83–103.
5. Stanley, J. M. (Ed.). 1989. The Appleton consensus: suggested international guidelines for decisions to forgo medical treatment. *Journal of Medical Ethics* **15**: 129–136.
6. Engelhardt, H. T. 1986. *The foundations of bioethics*, p. 361. Oxford University Press, New York and Oxford.

7. Lynöe, N., Sandlund, M., Dahlqvist, G. and Jacobsson, L. 1991. Informed consent: study of quality of information given to participants in clinical trial. *British Medical Journal* **303**: 610–613.
8. Harris, J. 1987. QALYfying the value of life. *Journal of Medical Ethics* **13**: 117–123.

25

The Four Principles in Practice

POVL RIIS, MD (UNIVERSITY OF COPENHAGEN), FRCP

Professor, physician-in-chief, Herlev University Hospital (University of Copenhagen), Herlev, Denmark

The interactions between ethical principles and practice, at least outside the religious spheres, inevitably raise a chicken-and-egg-which-comes-first problem.

The principles (PRI) most probably are secondary to established practice (PRA), introduced in clinical practice as implicit projections of attitudes and norms in society as a whole. At least this has been the case until the last decade, when ethical analyses have been introduced in the health research sector, in hospital departments, primary health services and in the education of health professionals. In other words, the egg seems to have been first on the scene, giving a sequence of PRA → PRI, and not PRI → PRA. But already now there is a growing tendency to introduce the ethical principles earlier in daily decision-making, that is to apply a sequence of PRI → PRA, with an ever-ongoing adjustment to new ethical problems, necessitating further ethical analyses leading to supplementary principles (PRI$_2$) or maybe even exchange of established ones (PRI$_1$). The sequence of events in the future will consequently by PRA$_1$ → PRI$_1$ → PRA$_2$ → PRI$_2$ → PRA$_3$. At this stage the bird reproduction analogy seems no longer applicable.

WHAT IS PRACTICE?

A multitude of health care workers meet ethical aspects and problems in their daily work: nurses, midwives, technicians, doctors, etc. Most of these groups confront ethics and the four principles during their *implementation* of clinical or scientific decisions, taken by others, mainly doctors. In contrast, doctors, responsible scientists and other direct decision-makers will meet the ethical aspects in a stronger form, linked as they sometimes are to their personal involvement in decision-making of paramount importance to patients and research subjects. Furthermore, such decisions are often part of several activities by the same doctors.

Decisions on clinical interventions, diagnosis, treatment and prevention, are

Principles of Health Care Ethics. Edited by Raanan Gillon.
© 1994 John Wiley & Sons Ltd

integrated in every *clinician's* daily work, thus representing a never-ceasing component of the patient–doctor relationship (1).

If the clinician is an active *researcher*, involved in projects on human subjects, he will be confronted with a new set of ethical problems, and consequently will meet again the four principles (2). Linked to the research activities is the clinician's function as a *scientific author*. This activity further introduces publication ethics, with another reappearance of the fundamental ethical principles.

Even without inventing a medical Jack of All Trades the clinician may be a *clinical teacher* too, involving patients in bedside or lecture room demonstrations; and some of the clinicians will even be *participants in the public debate* on health policies, ethics, etc. Again, such activities cannot be performed in an ethical vacuum, and the principles applied will have to be in accordance with the person's ethical conduct within the other areas of his or her professional life, in order to accord with personal integrity.

IMPLICIT AND EXPLICIT ETHICAL PRINCIPLES

Health personnel as a group have never worked in an ethical vacuum. Historically they have long been educated in, and controlled by, comprehensive ethical systems, for instance the Hippocratic system, Christianity structured in a strong church system, etc. However, in the twentieth century an ethical reference system has been much less visible, until the last two or three decades. In other words, explicit ethical norms for doctors and other health personnel have been declining, leaving for a time only implicit residues in the minds of doctors and others, until now they are being re-invented, or re-discovered, sometimes with a strength similar to a religious revival.

Tracing the four principles will consequently be a way of looking for both implicit and explicit markers.

The implicit principles are still far the most common, and lie behind all routine work with patients and research subjects. When for instance a nurse or a doctor meets a mentally handicapped patient, after having noticed the mental retardation, he or she does not start by analysing the situation, asking which principle is needed? 'Number four of course, that one expressing the necessity of justice—I'd better behave as if I was confronted with a person with equal rights.' If they have or have had prejudices against the mentally retarded, or if they need repeated *ad hoc* analyses in such situations, they would probably not have stayed within the health sector for very long.

The explicit principles are unmasked or encircled during the analyses of unusual professional situations. If an 82-year-old demented man with severe chronic obstructive lung disease is admitted to a hospital department in a bad condition, selecting the level of active therapy will probably evoke a brief discussion of the ethical aspects, in the light of principles such as the right to autonomy, the expected ratio between benefits and costs, and that of equity and justice, in order not to let age and related factors weigh too much without a thorough analysis.

THE DREAM OF A COMMON CURRENCY

Complex ethical weighing of the four principles is usually not difficult, when the principles are applied one by one, as if they were isolated determinators for the resulting decision-making. Further, such single-factor analyses give rise to much less intra- and inter-individual differences. Problems arise when benevolence, non-maleficence, right to autonomy and justice, as different starting points, must converge on one single decision, for instance not to operate versus to operate, or to include patients in a planned controlled trial versus not to allow such a trial for ethical reasons, etc. Clinical and scientific decision-making cannot survive with answers like 'It is a very complex and difficult problem that has no easy solution—or no solution at all.' The health sector has to be operational, to make decisions, even when it is saying clearly no to individual interventions.

It would be easier if doing good, not doing harm and acting fairly could all be measured in one unit, an Ethic, like an ECU, etc., and if the measures could be added, subtracted etc. It is, I believe, without sense—yet still the dream of making ethical characteristics numerical recurs, for instance in many clinical indices and in the concept of Quality Adjusted Life Years, QALYs.

THE ACCEPTANCE OF THE FOUR PRINCIPLES IN DAILY WORK

In contemporary democratic societies it is probably unlikely that any major groups would *publicly* reject the four principles, and even more unthinkable that groups of health personnel would express such views. On the contrary, the explicit acceptance of the principles varies from an attitude of wearily accepting truisms to one of considering the principles as valuable parts of the national culture and legal philosophy and not just a question for the health sector, the scientific community, university teachers and medical journal editors. Consequently, the visibility of, and the need to introduce, the four principles varies from country to country.

In a democratic welfare society, with a national health service accessible to all citizens, the justice principle will seem to be an inborn part of the national health system, leaving equity and justice to be a question of counterbalancing personal prejudices, etc., but not of questioning equal access even to scarce resources.

Along the same lines, doing good is a part of the initial, and later continued, motivation for health workers, in other words a built-in constituent, whether from a personal, professional or societal perspective in a welfare state.

Not harming people within the health system of stable societies similarly seems to be an integrated part of a long tradition, and to be explicitly expressed in national laws on nurses' and doctors' work, besides being a fundamental part of the criminal law.

The fourth principle, citizens' right to autonomy, is the most paradigm-influencing of the four in the modern development of ethical concepts. Its appearance is mainly due to the 1968 movement, or at least this historical turning point brought the principles from philosophers' and political ideologists' minds out into the open. This principle is linked primarily to human integrity, dignity and the concrete signs of equity in person-to-person-relationships and person-to-society relationships that are so common in the health sector and the scientific community.

APPLYING THE FOUR PRINCIPLES IN PRACTICE

The interaction between ethical principles and daily situations is often exemplified by testing the application of fundamental principles on constructed and often very overloaded examples. Questions related to the ethics of artificial insemination, for instance, can be exemplified by a synopsis, describing two lesbian women, wishing to have a child, without sexual or other contact with heterosexual men, planning artificial insemination with semen from a coloured, homosexual man, paying for the 'delivery' without full security against HIV contamination, and so on (the additional layers can be added almost indefinitely). Such cases can ease the teacher's mastering of the educational situation, but they create a feeling among health workers that medical ethics taught in this way is a kind of intellectual hobby and has nothing to do with their professional life. Fiction has a tendency to exaggerate, whereas real life contains all the variation we need (and good art, consequently, lets us feel that its fiction reflects the real world).

In the following a small number of synopses from contemporary life will serve as test-targets for the four principles.

> A 79-year-old rather demented man, whose wife is mentally well preserved and the only close relative, is admitted to hospital with a gastric bleeding. After three transfusions gastroscopy is performed, disclosing a 5 × 5 cm polypoid tumour in the fundus. Biopsies show adenocarcinoma. Ultrasound does not show metastases of the abdomen. The wife makes a plea for not intervening surgically. The patient gives no clear-cut answer. Technically the patient is operable, yet with an increased per- and postoperative mortality risk.

Applying the four principles will lead to the following reasoning. 'Doing good' by operating is not an obvious outcome due to the major intervention (probably a total gastrectomy) and the increased risk of dying postoperatively. Life after a gastrectomy might easily be considered socially harmful, even if it is still linked with life and not with death. Beside these potential harms the anaesthesia and the postoperative days might well worsen the patient's dementia. His right to autonomy presupposes a competent person that sufficiently understands the situation, and these conditions are certainly not fulfilled in the present case. This means that his old wife and the department will have to exercise a 'kind paternalism', at least partially, and help him to take or accept a decision. The final conclusion in this case was to abstain from surgery, and instead arrange for extensive home support, pain treatment, and the patient's easy re-admittance to hospital via a standing admittance paper given to him. To include the fourth principle: was justice fulfilled? Probably. He was not rejected for surgery because of some unjust criterion such as income, social grouping, etc. Rather, the decision not to operate was the result of a fair balancing of all pros and cons.

> A 45-year-old man with an advanced amyotrophic lateral sclerosis (a severe

neurological degenerative disease), had tried unsuccessfully to commit suicide on an earlier occasion before his present admission. He is now admitted acutely half a year later due to a new attempt to commit suicide. His farewell letter expresses clearly that his situation is hopeless, that he is tired of suffering, and is not depressed in any psychiatric sense. He wishes the department to respect his wish not to be resuscitated this time. He is deeply comatose on arrival, with signs of ischaemic brain damage, yet with all the prognostic doubt related to a severe case of poisoning. His only relative is a sister living in another part of the country. She confirms that the patient has often expressed a wish to 'end this tragedy soon'.

Here 'doing good' by supporting life would be considered by the patient as doing him harm. Further harm might result from an attempted resuscitation, because brain damage might well be the end-result, leaving the patient still more helpless. The patient's autonomous wish was clearly expressed both in a written form and through a spokesman or 'proxy', his sister. Was the decision to respect the patient's will just? Yes, probably. He was not unjustly deprived of any health resources, because the decision not to intervene solely stemmed from his personal wish.

A 64-year-old woman, a heavy smoker through 35–40 years, and still a smoker, is admitted for the eighth time during the last year. She has severe respiratory insufficiency, with breathlessness and asthmatic wheezing. She is afebrile. All kinds of treatments have been unsuccessfully tried during the earlier admissions, including those aiming at the 'asthmatic' element. The department has tried to persuade the patient to stop smoking on several occasions, but has failed. 'I cannot stop.' During the present admission the patient does not improve, but is constantly bedridden.

Here 'doing good' with therapy for her respiratory failure is not possible. 'Not doing harm' has complex relevance as a principal analytic approach. Certainly one could harm the patient's respiration by prescribing morphine or morphine-like drugs, yet these might be considered as doing her good in the terminal stage by relieving her severe breathlessness and anxiety. Autonomy presupposes a set of options, but here there were almost none, except the one rejecting any kind of resuscitation in case of an acute exacerbation. The only autonomous action of importance would have been an earlier decision to stop smoking. Justice comes in through the question: is it fair to shunt so many resources to one group of patients, while others are excluded because of finitely restricted health resources?

A large national collection of post-mortem brains and brain specimens was established over a number of years, obtained from a large series of patients with psychoses and other severe psychiatric states. A comprehensive study is planned, applying modern genetic techniques to the specimens and to blood from their living first- and second-order relatives in three generations. The purpose is to try to determine genetic factors underlying manic-depressive states, schizophrenia, etc. The protocol is sent to the regional and the central research–ethical committee for consideration and possible approval.

Once more applying the four principles, 'doing good' to the deceased persons has no real meaning. Nor can exploiting a unique possibility to advance psychiatric research, with the hope of alleviating the kind of suffering that filled the probands' lives, harm them. The brain tissues were collected at autopsies at a time when national legislation did not demand informed consent to autopsy from patients (through an advanced directive) or from relatives. Would they have said yes, had they known? Maybe, maybe not. Is it fair or just to preserve such a collection of brains, 'the centre of the soul and the personality'? The psychiatric patients' supportive society finds it unjust, but is it not unjust to deprive future patients and their families of a possible prevention or therapy resulting from such research? Do we not have a duty to be just in a historical perspective, considering the benefits that we have gained from autopsies and patients' participation in research in previous generations? And have we no obligation to hand knowledge from one generation to future generations? Seen from such perspectives respect for autonomy, or even only presumed autonomy, can result in a very restricted and selfish outcome of ethical analyses (3).

> A large controlled trial of a new anti-rheumatic drug is planned and carried through, based on cooperation between a university hospital and a drug firm. After completion of the trial the drug company makes preliminary calculations of the data, showing that the drug effect is a little less good than that of the existing non-steroidal anti-rheumatic drugs, and it decides not to publish the results. Their reasons are 'deficiencies in the design and the compliance of patients and researchers'. The clinical scientists cannot accept these criticisms and the decision to abstain from publication: 'The trial followed a protocol that we all agreed upon before embarking'. Both sides have their copies of the raw data, but the firm claims that 'they own the data' because they delivered the drugs, etc. Negotiations between the firm and the scientists do not lead to a solution. Finally the disagreement is presented to the national scientific–ethical committee for the health services, in order to reach a solution.

How would the four principles fit in when the committee tries to analyse this conflict of interests? Both parties point to a solution that benefits them and does not harm them. Instead, two groups of patients are to be placed in the centre of the ethical analysis: the trial patients have done a serious job to help medicine to deal better with rheumatic complaints. If the design and compliance were in order, then they are harmed in case of no publication, because their efforts have been in vain. If the design was invalid, they have again worked in vain. They are, however, not asked their views about publication or not, i.e. their right to collective autonomy is not respected. Can one introduce justice in this context? In a way, yes. Judging all accessible documents from the planning phase, the protocol, etc., might enable an independent body to judge between the two parties. The members of the appeal body will probably introduce a fifth principle, the right to scientific freedom, and decide to favour the publication of research results as the responsibility of the individual scientists. This was actually the result that the central scientific–ethical committee reached. If the individual scientists, or groups of scientists or the firm representatives disagree, and if they cannot solve the matter themselves, they are free to publish their own versions after three months (3).

> Two relatives of a hospital patient publish a long letter to the editor of a national newspaper, accusing the responsible doctor and the department of misconduct,

malpractice, inadequate standards, etc., with many technical references to what has happened during the patient's stay for more than one month in hospital. Neither the newspaper nor the family have informed the accused department and its leaders about the appearance of a critical article.

Normally doctors, social workers, etc., and their institutions find that they are obliged *not* to comment on such articles publicly, at least not by commenting and correcting factual parts of the patient's social and medical record. The reason is the legal protection of patients' and social clients' right to privacy. In this way medical and social personnel stick vigorously to the principle 'do not harm', even if they are strongly attacked with doubtful and sometimes false accusations. If the accusations are false or wildly exaggerated, with reference to the facts of the case, then not accepting harm caused by the accusations might justify an answer in the media, including facts of the case, as seen from the department's point of view. In this way the right to autonomy can result in a right of defence, after the patient himself has waived, in effect, the fundamental principle underlying the Data Protection Act and legislation on professional duties, requiring non-disclosure of any information from case records, etc. In this way justice as the fourth principle steps in. Justice is not only about distributional problems *among* patients, it also concerns the acceptance of duties and rights as complementary, not only in a linguistic universe, but also in a social one. No patient has only rights, and no health worker only duties.

CONCLUSION

The four principles can act as philosophical catalysts for development of an individual's personal network of ethical concepts and norms, especially in the analytic part of a professional life. They can, however, also act as daily tools, applied whenever their user meets an ethical problem during his or her daily work.

In countries with a tradition of accepting and applying ethical obligations within a health care system, the four principles probably have their biggest influence on the individual health employee's analytic and conceptual ability, helping his or her overall competence to deal with ethical dilemmas (4).

However, on the contrary, where health personnel are educated within a weaker tradition of ethical reasoning and decision-making, an early introduction of the four—or more—principles might help them deal with the ethical dilemmas they encounter in their everyday work. But, this is probably only feasible if the principles are tested against a number of realistic problems during their training in medical ethics.

A serious problem is the still-existing, and in places increasing, gap between ethical principles and the reality of everyday life in many countries. The right to respect for one's autonomy, for instance, has little meaning in a country where patients and other citizens alike are subjected to a totalitarian regime. Further, the principle of justice in a health service context has little or no meaning if the country's citizens are forced to accept heavy social imbalances, because some patients can pay, others have health insurance, and a large residual group can only expect health care through charity. Poverty in itself, even in the context of a reasonable and democratic constitution, can overrule the ethical principles, because the daily fight for 'food, fibre and shelter' absorbs all physical and mental resources.

There is a danger that if fundamental ethical principles are published and given weight by philosophers, ethicists, doctors and health authorities, and if citizens increasingly expect and look out for benevolence, non-maleficence, the right to autonomy and justice in their daily life, the result may be a paradoxical and undeserved distrust, not only of the principles, but of ethics as such. An analogy is easily found in the targets of the World Health Organization's adopting the programme Health for All by the Year 2000 (5). This programme was established with a clear, long-needed and highly desirable objective, and has been worded accordingly. But due to recession, poverty, and political movements in an antidemocratic direction, the concepts of justice, etc., in health care seem to be situated beyond the horizon for many citizens of the Third World.

In other words, life continuously tests the reliability of words, irrespective of the speaker's or writer's good will.

Judged against a background of clinical work, clinical science, teaching, writing and debating, one can try to answer the question: Do the four principles applied in practice represent a step forward? The answer is 'To some extent, but not as much as is often thought.'

The main problems are their lack of mutual exclusiveness and their failure to incorporate exhaustively the ethical universe of health care.

Doing good must sometimes be effected when at the same time one also does harm. One person's right to autonomy may well reduce another person's similar right. Doing much good for one patient may reduce the resources available to other patients. The case-histories above illustrate that ethical analyses often need the inclusion of other basic principles, freedom for instance, even in societies accepting a similar commitment to justice.

If ethical principles are presented in a very dogmatic style, which is often the case in ethical writings, clinicians with their main role as daily, practical decision-makers are often discouraged from bringing such principles into their daily work.

However, expressed in plain language, the four principles can act as important eye-openers, especially when they are supplemented by further principles, and if they are presented in relation to what is called 'the jungle of experience'.

REFERENCES

1. Andersen, D, Mabeck, C. E. and Riis, P. 1987. *Medicinsk etik* [*Medical ethics*]. FADL, Copenhagen (in Danish).
2. Andersen, D., Havsteen, B., Juhl, E. and Riis, P. 1988. *Lægevidenskabelig forskning—en introduktion* [*Medical research—an introduction*]. FADL, Copenhagen (in Danish).
3. Central Scientific-Ethical Committee of Denmark. 1991. *Annual Report for 1990*. Ministry of Education and Science, Copenhagen.
4. Ministry of Health. 1989. *Research involving human subjects—ethics and law*. Ministry of Health, Copenhagen.
5. World Health Organization. 1985. *Targets for health for all: targets in support of the European regional strategy for health for all*. Regional Office for Europe, Copenhagen.

26

The Four Principles in Practice: Facilitating International Medical Ethics

JOHN M. STANLEY, PhD

Edward F. Mielke Professor of Ethics in Medicine, Science and Society, Lawrence University, Wisconsin, USA

This chapter is about principles, about decisions that will determine whether a patient lives or dies, and about attempts to understand differences and agreements regarding such decisions across national boundaries and medical cultures.

PRINCIPLES

By 'principles' I shall understand any principle-based approach to provide guidance in medical decisions. There are four problems that any such approach should consider:

1. *The problem of justification or legitimization*: Why these principles rather than some others? What is the source and scope of their authority? How are they derived? How justified?
2. *The problem of selection*: Which principles are to be considered relevant to a particular case or set of cases—however they are derived or justified?
3. *The problem of context*: In what way do the particular conditions of the individual case affect the application of a particular set of principles to it—whatever the principles are and however any conflict amongst them has been resolved?
4. *The problem of conflict*: How are conflicting principles to be weighed and balanced? How are particularly difficult conflicts among principles to be sorted out? What procedures and mechanisms should be in place to adjudicate irresolvable conflicts?

Principles of Health Care Ethics. Edited by Raanan Gillon.
© 1994 John Wiley & Sons Ltd

These four 'problems' constitute a kind of a test maze for any principle-based approach to decision-making. Later in this chapter I will use these four problems as just such a test maze to examine one particular attempt to stimulate international discussion of principle-based guidelines for medical decisions near the end of life.

MEDICAL DECISIONS CONCERNING THE END OF LIFE

I am throughout using the category 'medical decisions concerning the end of life' (MDEL) as identified by van der Maas, van Delden and others (1) in their report on life-terminating decisions in The Netherlands. Their very useful taxonomy distinguishes between three kinds of MDEL: (1) decisions 'to provide alleviation of pain and symptoms with such high dosages of opioids that the patient's life might be shortened'; (2) decisions to withhold or withdraw life-sustaining treatment, including decisions not to resuscitate, decisions to withdraw from dialysis, to discontinue antibiotics, or to disconnect respirators and feeding tubes; (3) decisions to provide euthanasia, doctor-assisted suicide or other life-terminating acts.

There are a number of reasons for focusing particularly on the applicability of a principle-based approach to MDELs. MDELs heighten and intensify all of the problems a principle-based approach must address, and are therefore instructive regarding the problems of a principle-based approach to any medical decision.

Both the usefulness of a principle-based approach to decisions of this sort and its risks and limitations will have been discussed elsewhere in this volume. There are, however, two particular contexts where the usefulness of principles is particularly noteworthy: in contexts of pluralized MDELs and in attempts at building international and cross-cultural understandings of what is at stake and what needs to be protected in MDELs.

PRINCIPLES AND PLURAL DECISIONS

Increasingly over the past several years end-of-life decisions have become pluralized. Ten years ago solo clinical decisions in MDELs were still commonplace. Today nearly all MDELs in hospitals are plural decisions, many employing formal structures for pluralizing decisions, such as ethics committees or critical-care review boards. Even MDELs made in a home context are often pluralized to some extent. Plural decision-making requires a framework from which to understand what is at stake in a particular case in terms that can be efficiently communicated across significant differences in clinical and personal perspectives. In many cases a principle-based approach has been helpful as a framework for such communication across different perspectives of medical specializations, as well as across different individual values.

Of course, some caveats are in order. Any structure that is imposed on any problem to help understand the problem and communicate that understanding to others runs the risk of concealing potentially important dimensions of the particular case being examined, and it well may be that a principle-based structure, depending on its rigidity and the solution it works out to the four problems mentioned above, may be in more danger of this tyranny of perspective than some other approaches. Howard Brody's chapter (Chapter 18) on narrative approaches to clinical decisions is an interesting and challenging corrective of some possible excesses in principle-based approaches.

If principles are helpful, in spite of their risks, in plural decision-making within the same medical culture, they are all the more helpful in attempts to achieve degrees of understanding across different medical cultures and across the different philosophical and religious cultures that support them, which brings us to the third thing that this chapter is about.

INTERNATIONAL UNDERSTANDINGS

It is, of course, quite possible for clinicians with far different value and belief systems to agree that a principle or a set of principles speaks, indeed often in a rather precise sense, to an ethical dimension of clinical decision-making that they all hold important even though each of them would justify their selection of the principles in different ways, weight them differently when they came into conflict and, quite possibly, disagree somewhat in the scope of their application. This is surely a less than profound insight, yet it is one for which, until recently, the possibilities have been insufficiently tested.

In the spring of 1988, intrigued by the possibilities that serious attention to this insight promised, 33 delegates from 10 different countries set out to create a set of guidelines for discussion in medical and medical ethics communities internationally that would address both decisions to forgo medical treatment, including life-prolonging treatment, precipitated by autonomous requests by patients or their surrogates, and decisions to forgo medical treatment as a result of pressure due to scarcity.

Most of that group of 33 had met a year earlier at a specially invited conference where each had presented a case from his or her own practice in which a decision whether or not to initiate or continue a treatment or procedure had caused particular ethical anguish. The cases had been discussed openly and candidly both in small groups and in plenary sessions; participants probed for underlying agreements, sometimes across some very different perpectives, on which they could make some basic distinctions and work towards a common basis of understanding of what is at stake in these decisions. We appealed to several different conceptualizations of authority: the Hippocratic tradition, notions of human rights, the art of medicine, respect for human life. I remember Grant Gillett, especially, speaking eloquently about the integrity of the practice of medicine and the norms and standards that such integrity both required and made possible.

And I remember well the crucial point at that first working conference when, to the astonishment of the moderator, the group agreed that for the purpose of discussing the cases before us we could accept that the four principles articulated by Beauchamp and Childress (2) provided a useful starting point for considering what is at stake in such decisions. By the end of the second conference, a year later, we were ready to refer to the four principles as 'summarizing the norms of integrity', and we had produced for international discussion a set of model guidelines for decisions to forgo treatment based on those principles.

That set of guidelines was published as 'The Appleton Consensus: Suggested International Guidelines for Decisions to Forgo Medical Treatment' in the *Journal of the Danish Medical Association* (3). In the winter and spring of 1990 an annotated study edition (4) of this set of guidelines was produced and distributed to 152 discussion groups that met in 15 different countries for systematic study and comment. Those discussion groups included hospital ethics committees, hospice teams, two groups of health care economists, several groups of health care professionals (nurses, social workers, hospital chaplains, administrators and doctors), and a strong representation of groups of interested people from the 'grass roots' of several societies. A total of 1450 persons were involved in the 152 discussion groups. The 94 groups from the US met in 23 different states, and the 58 foreign groups met in 14 countries (Denmark, Scotland, Israel, Sweden, Australia, Malaysia, Guinea, the Netherlands, England, Norway, Canada, India, Colombia and New Zealand). The groups spent a total of 731 hours discussing the study edition, with average length of discussion per group equalling 4.9 hours. The average size of the discussion groups was nine members. Thirty per cent of the participants were doctors; the other 70 per cent were from a variety of professions and vocations.

Each discussion group sent a report documenting its reactions to, and its suggestions for, the guidelines. A total of 749 participants returned individual participant evaluation forms. These results were tabulated and summarized for the delegates to a third working conference: 'The Appleton International Conference: Developing Guidelines for Decisions to Forgo Life-Prolonging Medical Treatment', which met once again in Appleton in May, 1991, to respond to the suggestions, comments and challenges from the 152 discussion groups and to revise and refine the guidelines in light of those discussions.

This project as a whole, from the first working conference in 1987 through study group meetings and responses to the final revisions at the 1991 conference, will be referred to as the Appleton Project. It is that project which I now want to examine in light of each of the test problems I enumerated at the beginning of this essay.

The Problem of Justification and Legitimization

In the Appleton Project we recognized in the first few hours of discussion at the first conference that we faced, just within the scope of those present (not to mention the perspectives we were already talking about adding), both personal and cultural value differences of immense proportions. While some felt that we did not yet have enough diversity for the global nature of the task we had identified, most felt we should see what agreements we could find within the diversity we already had on board, before attempting to broaden the base of participation. Could we, for example, find a basis for thinking about the difficult issues raised in the cases we had presented and discussed in the previous working conference? Could we agree that we were in possession of a significantly similar understanding of the demands or requirements implicit in an individual principle or a set of principles, however differently we might derive the principles or whatever authority or authorities might be appealed to for legitimization?

It was, as I recall, about halfway through the first conference in the spring of 1987 that one of the delegates asked, 'Can't we agree that, however they are derived or justified, the four principles articulated by Beauchamp and Childress offer a helpful starting point for this kind of discussion?' We all agreed that, in fact, those four principles had already been providing a framework from which we had been discussing and analysing many of the most troublesome and anguishing of the cases we were sharing with one another, that indeed the four principles seemed to constitute a kind of summary of the values and standards we had been appealing to, however we might, individually, regard their authority. We also agreed they might provide a basis on which a second working conference aimed at producing a set of suggested guidelines for decisions to forgo treatment might legitimately be based.

So in the Appleton Project we did not acquire our four principles the way principles are usually acquired. We did not discover them or derive them or find them revealed. We simply 'agreed' to accept them. We assumed them, at first as a heuristic strategy, then as a working assumption and finally as a summary of all the values and norms we had found ourselves appealing to for guidance from the perspectives of our various medical cultures.

We also at this point noted two caveats about the use of these principles. First, principle-based approaches, however helpful they might be in getting started, can screen out details that could be very important in a decision. Howard Brody's excellent note in the study edition of the Appleton Guidelines (1990) carried this warning:

> One suggestion holds that only by turning attention from the isolated individual to the community can medical ethics make progress. Another is that we must replace rules-language with virtue-language and return to the task of addressing questions of character and integrity, which a rules-approach tends to ignore. A third suggestion is that we must ask, not how each of us as individuals can know that our ethical position is correct, but instead how groups or teams can reach workable compromises in the face of continued deep disagreements about moral principles.

Second, while there may be considerable agreement across medical cultures that a given principle is important, either in an individual case or in the process of guideline building, there may remain significant disagreement on how heavily to weight that principle when it comes into conflict with other principles. One who regards a principle that informs his or her guidelines as derived or revealed may weight principles differently from one who regards them as something in the order of an heuristic assumption. Thus the problem of the authority of the principles, agreed upon at one level, may well reappear at another level. Even so, the initial agreement that the principle was important, and the communication established by that agreement, may provide possibilities for resolution of many of these second-order conflicts of weighting and, in any case, will provide a better foundation than previously existed, and perhaps the only one available, for the analysis and understanding of the different degrees of authority assigned to the principles.

The Problem of Selection

Once we had accepted the four principles, the problem of selection for the Appleton Project essentially amounted to whether not to admit any other principles—most notably the principle of respect for human life. At the first conference when this possibility was first discussed, it was suggested that respect for human life is not really a separate principle at all, but that it is rather 'understood' as what the four principles were expressing and, as such, did not need to be listed as a principle. Thus, although it was considered early in our deliberations, the respect for human life was not added as a separate principle in the first published version of the guidelines. In fact, it was not even mentioned. Its omission stimulated, in the second phase of the project, the second-largest number of challenges that we received from the study groups around the world. More than half of the study groups charged us to either add it as a fifth principle or explain why we did not. In the revisions and reconsiderations at the third working conference the delegates decided that reference to respect for human life should be explicitly mentioned, but it would not be listed as a fifth principle. Rather, it would be mentioned as a basic value which all four principles, taken as a whole and properly balanced, express. Further, because of the perceived need to guard against overemphasis on this value to the extent of endorsing an unexamined vitalism, a strong note was included explicitly rejecting vitalism. Our final statement in our revised guidelines on the issue of respect for human life.

> All of the principles in the preamble reflect respect for the dignity of human life. The extent and scope of this respect is expressed in the application of the four principles. In applying respect for human life to specific cases it is important to remember that the prolongation of life, without consideration of the quality of life, may not always be preferred by a patient, may not be evaluated as being in a patient's best interest, and may not in some cases be compatible with respect for the dignity of human life.

The Problem of Context

Principles must be applied in a context. There are three basic patterns of solution of the problem of context: (a) use no principles because of the danger that principles will be misleading when applied to an individual, unique case; (b) use principles seriously, even rigidly, and trust that a principle-based approach will always, on balance, do more good than harm; (c) use principles cautiously and flexibly, more as ideals to be approximated than rigid patterns to be imposed on unique cases.

Avoid Principles

According to this solution, the context of each case is unique. Any sorting of cases into categories suitable for a principle-based approach will necessarily filter out from the individual cases assigned to that category some of their unique particularity, and any consideration of a particular case in the light of other cases in the category runs the risk of overlooking ethically relevant differences in the case under consideration from ones for which the principle may be appropriate. There are, of course, many times when this is not a problem at all. In such cases nothing is lost and, quite possibly, a great deal gained by the use of both the category and the principle. But there are other times when the use of guidelines based on principles appropriate to other cases in a given category would obscure enough ethically relevant particulars of an individual case to be misleading. Since MDELs are usually irreversible, some have argued that even the remote possibility of a principle-based approach obscuring relevant ethical dimensions of a decision is enough to dictate against its use.

Apply Principles Rigidly

According to this solution, principles are to be taken very seriously. They may very well reflect the structure of reality itself from which they have been discovered, or the mind of God from which they have been revealed. When in doubt, one should trust the structure and the pattern visible in the principles. One should not fear to fit the individual cases into the pattern of the principles, maybe even force them a bit, if necessary. The instruction gained from the pattern that the case almost fits will justify the force-fit. Indeed, all possibility to make the individual case fit the pattern should be exhausted before sensing that it could possibly be an exception. Of course, a mechanism must be in place to cope with genuine exceptions, but genuine exceptions are rare, and though one should be open to their possibility, a high standard of evidence should be required to justify an exception.

Context-sensitive Application of Principles

According to this solution to the problem of context, principles are better understood as ideals rather than binding laws. They 'exist' or have their 'being' at the metaphysical level of ideals and can only be imperfectly reflected in the practical realities of 'real life'. These ideals become reified in social life: (1) in society as laws, policies, directives, funding decisions; (2) in medical institutions and professional organizations as guidelines and professional standards, and (3) at the individual level as 'middle axioms', or 'rules of thumb'. The purpose of the reification of the principles at all levels is to create conditions in the real world that will, as closely as possible, approximate the ideal embodied in the principle. According to this understanding principles are not kept or broken as much as they are 'approximated' or 'almost realized' or 'fallen far short of'.

I am sure it is fair to say that all three of these basic patterns of solution to the context problem were represented in the Appleton Project working groups. A few delegates were consistently worried over the shift from cases to principles. A few had started with a principle-based orientation and could be comfortable with the rigid application pattern of addressing the context problem. Most of us were quite comfortably firm in the middle pattern. We had started, it must be remembered, with cases. We had discussed, analysed and probed for reasons behind decisions in cases before we began looking for summaries of the norms of professional integrity. In the last conference we reminded ourselves several times that we did not want to lose the sensitivity to the cases with which we had started. Certainly the predominant pattern in all our discussions and deliberations was that of a context-sensitive application of agreed-on principles to cases, to be accomplished always with great respect for the particularity of the case.

The Problem of Conflict

Principles conflict with one another. Any approach based on principles should realize that, and have both some notion of a theoretical solution to the problem of conflict among principles and a set of practical procedures for sorting out conflicts in specific clinical cases. Several things should be considered. Are, for instance, some principles more important than others? More troublesome, is one principle to be paramount? If paramountcy and all its attendant troubles is avoided, is there a systematic understanding of the weights given to conflicting principles? Is there an agreed-on procedure to formally resolve conflicts that require formal resolution?

The Appleton Project avoided the problem of paramountcy. While some delegates complained that in every conflict between the principle of autonomy and that of professional beneficence we had sided with autonomy, and that we thus were *de facto* making autonomy paramount, others argued that we had not made autonomy paramount, but that in a conflict with effectively deliberated autonomy professional beneficence would most often lose out, largely because beneficence itself entailed an obligation to respect well-informed patient autonomy.

When we addressed the issue of scarcity it became clear that we had not made autonomy paramount. Autonomy may nearly always trump beneficence, but it did not so obviously trump justice and efficiency.

Although it took us some time to understand some of the implications of our discovery, we very quickly noticed that most of our cases involved two different kinds of conflict: (1) those where the central conflicts are between patient autonomy and professional beneficence, and (2) those where, usually after scarcity is introduced as an element in decision-making, the central conflicts are between the concerns of justice and efficiency on the one side and patient autonomy, often now in allegiance with professional beneficence, on the other.

As we addressed the first set of conflicts, we were in territory that was not altogether unfamiliar or uncomfortable. Conflicts between what a patient wants and what a representative of the medical profession, either as an individual doctor or as an institution, thinks is good for the patient could be serious, but resolution did not test the limits of the thinkable. Since professional beneficence respects fully informed and responsible autonomy, guidelines are needed to make sure the autonomy is fully informed, that the patient really wants what he or she says she wants. Then we can respect autonomy. If we create conditions to maximally inform autonomy and create safeguards against errors of inauthentic or impaired autonomy, while keeping those safeguards free from abuse, the conflict is resolved. There is no reason for the doctor's beneficence to override the patient's autonomy. On the contrary, respecting the patient's autonomy is now consistent with the professional beneficence. There are, of course, some caveats: be very careful, but also be open-minded, on the edges of the allowable, and be willing to employ what John Arras (5) has called an 'ethics of ambiguity' which has room in it for moral praise and support for those who make difficult dilemma-filled decisions whatever the outcome of the decision.

It was, of course, the second group of conflicts that was especially difficult for us. First of all, the conflicts were more complex. A conflict between professional beneficence and autonomy was still, for the most part, a face-to-face conflict. The players were visible and identifiable and the rules, on the whole, comprehensible. But the conflicts generated by scarcity that pit justice and efficiency on one side against autonomy and beneficence on the other are much more difficult to resolve. They are necessarily played out on several different levels of decision-making. Decisions made at one level both affect and are affected by decisions being made at several different levels; communication between the levels may be poor, players not always visible and rules often hard to discover. Such decisions involve new kinds of uncertainties about both risks and benefits, uncertainties often very difficult to measure or understand. And, most troublesome of all, assessment of the conflicts almost invariably requires weighing the well-being of an aggregate of individuals (society, community or members of the same health care plan) against the well-being of an individual patient and the integrity of the medical profession.

CONCLUSION

The Appleton Project did not begin as a project to apply a system of principles to clinical decisions to forgo treatment. We started with cases, real cases of our own, difficult cases that had required decisions that had caused us anguish. We started by talking about those cases and those decisions. We were really just beginning to look for some kind of structure to organize the almost surprising agreements we had discovered in our discussions of our cases when we asked ourselves if Beauchamp and Childress's four principles could help. We tentatively tested them, embraced them as summarizing the norms and standards that we had found when probing our cases, and enshrined them in the preamble of the guidelines statement. The responses from the 152 study groups indicated that the principles in the preamble significantly enhanced their discussions of what was at stake in the guidelines.

We maintained for the most part a context-sensitive pattern of applying principles to cases, though we did not formally address the problem of a principle-based approach to MDELs. We did address the problem of conflicting principles and indeed probably accomplished some of our best work on this topic.

The adoption of the four principles by the Appleton Project was enormously enabling. In spite of individual and cultural differences among the delegates, a level of consensus was reached about the content of guidelines for a variety of MDELs that none of us would have thought possible at the outset. It is important to remember, as Howard Brody reminds us, that a principle-based approach cannot exhaust the moral content of medicine any more than ethics can be reduced to a set of rules to govern individual behaviour, but it is also the case that the kind of search for common understandings and the kind of reaching across differences for agreements and consistency that became characteristic of the Appleton Project could not have happened without the acceptance of the four principles by the delegates at the first working conference.

REFERENCES

1. van der Maas, P. J., van Delden, J. M. M., Pijnenborg, L. and Looman, C. W. N. 1991. Euthanasia and other medical decisions concerning the end of life. *Lancet* **338**: 669–674.
2. Beauchamp, T. L. and Childress, J. F. 1979. *Principles of biomedical ethics*. Oxford University Press, New York.
3. Stanley, J. M., Abrams, F. R., Admiraal, P. V. *et al.* 1989. The Appleton consensus: suggested international guidelines for decisions to forgo medical treatment. *Journal of the Danish Medical Association [Ugeskr Laeger]* **151**(11): 700–706.
4. Stanley, J. M., Abrams, F. R., Admiraal, P. V. *et al.* 1990. The Appleton consensus: suggested international guidelines for decisions to forgo medical treatment, study edition (Proceedings of Guidelines for Non-treatment Decisions: an international working conference, Lawrence University Program in Biomedical Ethics).
5. Arras, J. 1989. The ethics of ambiguity. Pp. 231–240, *in* Arras, J. and Rhoden, N. (Eds) *Ethical issues in modern medicine*. Mayfield Publishing Co., Mountain View, California.

27

Legal Approaches to Health Care Ethics and the Four Principles

Bernard M. Dickens, PhD, LlD

Barrister (England), Barrister and Solicitor (Ontario), Professor of Law, University of Toronto, Canada

RELATIONS BETWEEN LAW AND ETHICS

Both law and ethics provide rules or norms by which individuals are expected to regulate their conduct, meaning their advancement of their wishes, including pursuit of both their selfish and their altruistic interests. Law is expressed, interpreted, applied and enforced more systematically than are ethical norms, through the legal system. This includes a policing service to monitor how the law is respected, lawyers who give advice about the law and represent clients by advocating the interests clients instruct them to advance, courts and judges, and appeal tribunals. Laws are made by legislatures that, in democracies, are elected by popular vote, and by courts. In the Common Law tradition, based on English historical experience, courts both interpret legislation and identify the principles of customary law into which legislation may fit. In the Civil Law tradition, in which the laws are contained in comprehensive codes modelled on that established in France by Napoleon, customary laws have been superseded and legal rights are derived from the code, as interpreted by judges.

Ethical decision-making is not undertaken by equally accessible and authoritative institutions. Ethics derived from religious principles may be explained by ministers of religion, and in societies where a distinction between secular laws and religious principles is not recognized, such as Islamic societies, they are as authoritative as legislatures and courts. Where secular ethics prevail, however, decision-making involves personal perception and conscience, peer review and various institutional ethical review processes, and outcomes of reasoning from principles of which the four principles are the best articulated.

The relationship between law and ethics is a common topic of discussion and

Principles of Health Care Ethics. Edited by Raanan Gillon.
© 1994 John Wiley & Sons Ltd

disagreement. Law is often described as a minimal ethic, meaning that there is an ethical obligation to keep the law but that many decisions, such as whether or not to invoke a legal power, are based on ethics and not simply on law. For instance, courts have ruled that prison authorities have no legal duty to force-feed hunger-striking prisoners, but that they have a legal capacity to do so (1). Whether authorities and individual doctors will use this capacity is a matter of ethical judgement. Similarly, regulations often provide that hospital staff members may legally consult patients' identifiable records for purposes of research, but whether they may use this power without seeking patients' prior consent is an ethical decision. Neither force-feeding nor record consultation without consent is ethical simply because it is lawful.

Law often invokes ethical justifications for its provisions. Both political legislatures and judges in courts tend to explain their shaping of the law by reference to ethical values, or to claim that, while pragmatically inspired, the law is in harmony with ethical principles. The law usually tries not to obstruct the exercise of ethical judgement, to accommodate ethical choice, and not to compel unethical behaviour. At times, however, laws may be criticized from an ethical standpoint because they deny ethical choice. Legislatures and courts may invoke ethical principles in order to reform the law, and many jurisdictions have law reform commissions that keep the law under review and recommend change such as when ethically justified.

Whether ethical outcomes of socially contentious issues should be embodied in law and enforced by legal systems has been the subject of classical debates (2). Ethical behaviour may be regarded in terms of right conduct, and law can to an extent compel compliance with behavioural ideals and prohibit forms of unethical conduct. Behaviour that merely conforms to the law, however, is not necessarily ethically inspired. A woman's decision not to have an abortion because it is legally prohibited provides her with no opportunity for ethical reflection, for instance on the competing claims of the sanctity of human life on the one hand and her capacity to discharge moral duties to others such as her dependent children and, for instance, her dependent parents or parents-in-law, on the other. Laws enacted to advance an ethical value may compel obedience, but risk impoverishment of experience of ethical judgement. Laws may compete against ethics for popular allegiance. When ethical behaviour is regarded as that which results from ethically inspired choice among options, the law's denial of options will decrease the exercise of ethical judgement.

How far civil disobedience to law can be ethically justified depends on the ethical character of the law disobeyed. Resistance to oppressive laws has a distinguished and liberating political history such as in anti-slavery and anti-colonial movements, but, for instance in the United States, obstruction of access to legally operated abortion clinics by protesters against abortion has been held lawfully indefensible (3). An issue that has arisen, initially in The Netherlands but now far beyond where attempted suicide is not an offence, is the role that doctors should ethically be allowed to play in assisting or inducing patients' voluntary deaths (4). Assisting suicide is usually illegal, and deliberately inducing death, including accelerating natural death, is usually liable to prosecution for murder.

The law will usually accommodate ethical choices, but whether a society's ethical preferences should be compelled by mandatory legislation, such as through prohibition of less ethical or unethical alternatives, or be directed by courts of law, remains a matter of contention and of personal and political judgement. Laws tend not to address the peculiarities of particular circumstances as sensitively as ethical assessments and judgements may. In medical settings, furthermore, a danger exists that law may consume ethics, so that the dominant medical ethic becomes reduced simply to obeying the law. Accommodation of ethically inspired choice may, however, require legal tolerance of ethical errors.

LEGAL RESPONSES TO THE FOUR PRINCIPLES

Respect for Persons

The ethical principle of respect for persons is conventionally considered to include at least two elements, namely respect for autonomy of competent persons, and due protection of persons incapable of exercising autonomy.

Autonomy of Competent Persons

The law has historically been a conservative influence protective of paternalism. This has been true both of judgements and of legislation. Adults with capacity to be assertive of their rights have frequently been able to employ laws to prevail, but in borderline cases involving such persons as married women, minors and mentally impaired individuals, the law has tended to favour health protection over autonomy. Autonomy has been legally respected when invoked for protective purposes. The modern tendency, however, particularly in westernized legal systems, has been for courts and legislation to promote the individual autonomy of competent people. The 1914 judicial statement has been frequently invoked by subsequent courts of law that:

> Every human being of adult years and sound mind has a right to determine what shall be done with his own body (5).

This principle is now being applied to justify patients' refusals of life-sustaining care. In the 1990 Ontario case of *Malette* v. *Shulman* (6), for instance, a Jehovah's Witness was awarded $20 000 in damages for battery when a doctor aware of her religious convictions gave her a blood transfusion while she was unconscious. The doctor considered the transfusion necessary to save her life when she suffered loss of blood on being injured in a vehicle accident. It was held, however, that there was no legal power to disobey her competently exercised autonomous choice, even under the inspiration of saving her life. The court noted that there would have been no risk of legal liability for her death resulting from respecting her wishes.

Courts and legislatures are also recognizing that individuals are legally entitled to be treated according to their competently formed wishes, even when they are no longer able to express them. Legislatures are recognizing this in enactment of so-called durable power of attorney laws. Historically, anything people could do for themselves they could authorize to be done through attorneys, who were frequently but by no means necessarily lawyers. Powers of attorney lapse, however, when those who created them lose competence to act by themselves. Legislation increasingly now provides, however, that people can anticipate incompetency, such as when they undergo general anaesthesia or suffer neurodegenerative diseases, and make arrangements while competent that legally will endure their loss of competency.

Courts of law are also being respectful of advance medical directives. In a sense, the court was so respectful in the case above concerning the unconscious Jehovah's Witness (6). When individuals have not clearly expressed their wishes, however, such as to forgo invasive artificial or mechanical life-support once they are in a terminal stage, or to forgo artificially supplied nutrition and hydration if they fall into a persistent vegetative state, it is difficult to know what standard of proof must be established to discover what their competently formed wishes were. Information may be found in statements they made to family members, friends, and work colleagues. The US Supreme Court has upheld a finding that proof of their wishes must be established by 'clear and convincing' evidence, and not just a mere balance of probabilities of what a person's wishes were prior to loss of competency (7).

The right of autonomous medical decision-making is often expressed as the right to give 'informed consent' before being subjected to medical treatment. Health professions are required to disclose information that is material to the choice a reasonable or prudent person in a patient's circumstances has to make. 'Informed consent' is an unfortunate misnomer, because it incorrectly suggests that:

1. the purpose of giving information is to gain consent;
2. patients who do not consent are not adequately informed;
3. patients who refuse proposed treatment need not be informed, or need not be as well informed as those who consent; and
4. health professionals simply give information, and patients respond by giving or denying consent.

A better expression than 'informed consent' is 'informed decision-making' or 'informed choice'. The legal duty to give information serves the goal not of inducing consent, but of facilitating autonomy. Similarly, a decision not to have treatment must be as well informed as a decision to accept it. Historically, consent was legally relevant to prevent touching from constituting a compensable civil battery or a punishable criminal assault, and doctors' decisions not to touch patients, for instance because patients would not allow it, did not require doctors to make disclosures or obtain further consent. Now, however, the duty to disclose is considered relevant to negligence law, so that a doctor must ensure that patients' choices are adequately informed, whether the choices are to accept or to reject proposed treatments, lest the doctors be held liable for professional negligence.

Courts are finding that decisions whether to have medical treatment are not themselves medical decisions, but personal decisions to be made by patients. Doctors' duties are not to make decisions, but to ensure that patients' decisions are adequately informed about medical and related matters, such as the implications of having and of not having treatment options. In order to discharge their duty of giving adequate and appropriate information, doctors may have to ask patients questions, concerning not only their symptoms and care preferences but also their hopes for their future opportunities and security in life. Accordingly, doctors may have to ask questions in order that their patients will give them information. Based on that information, doctors will give advice on appropriate treatment options and their implications.

Legal systems approach the duty of disclosure rather differently in principle. In the United Kingdom, for instance, the highest court, the House of Lords, has claimed that the doctrine of 'informed consent', as developed in the US and Canada, is not accepted (8). According to legal precedent, doctors satisfy their duty of disclosure if they give such information to patients as their medical professional peers would give. This professionally based standard of disclosure is to be contrasted with the patient-based standard associated with the doctrine of 'informed consent', and reflects an historic paternalism that the professional knows best, rather than the autonomy of entrusting patients with responsibility for decisions that affect them. The House of Lords rejected informed consent as a 'transatlantic' doctrine, apparently unaware that it had long been the law in such countries as France, Germany, Switzerland and Austria (9). A leading US judgement observed that 'Respect for the patient's right of self-determination ... demands a standard [of disclosure] set by law for physicians rather than one which physicians may or may not impose upon themselves' (10).

Protection of Persons Incapable of Autonomy

Paternalism is inappropriate and demeaning when applied to adults, but provides the quality of care that parents should apply to their dependent children, and that others should apply to protect the interests of similarly dependent people who cannot protect their own interests. Childhood itself in health-related law is a quality of immaturity rather than simply an age. Those below a given age set by legislation to achieve, for instance, majority status, or medical autonomy, may individually be capable of exercising autonomous rights when they are found to display the maturity to make, and to bear responsibility for, their own decisions (11). They may accordingly be legally capable of making autonomous decisions about even contentious matters such as contraception and abortion.

In historical law, mentally impaired adults were considered to be 'Nature's children', and were subject to paternalistic protection. Capacity was once considered 'global', in the sense that those who possessed it had it for all purposes, and those found to lack legal capacity were incapacitated to discharge any legal function. Modern law is influenced, however, by the principle of accommodating only the least invasive inroads into autonomy. One expression of this is the autonomy in health matters that mature legal minors may be found to possess. Another is that adults whose intellectual capacities are compromised, whether chronically, temporarily or transiently, may have legal capacity for some functions but not others.

An example of this from law is that a person may have capacity to enter into a simple contract, such as of employment, but not be able to make a will. Similarly, legal standards of capacity are higher to make a will than to revoke one. To make a will, a person must have a sense of what and where the person's assets are, or of how their extent and location can be determined, of at least close family structure, and of financial and moral obligations. To revoke a will, a person need know little more than that the arrangements in an existing will are no longer acceptable. The law acknowledges these differences by requiring evidence, usually from a lawyer, accountant or doctor, that a person making a will possessed testamentary capacity at the time, and a witness to say that the will was signed freely and with apparent comprehension. To revoke a will, however, a testator may strike a line through it, tear it, burn it, or throw it into a waste container.

The law similarly recognizes different capacities to consent to and to decline recommended medical care. A low threshold is set for a person to consent to medically recommended routine treatment. A higher level exists for more speculative and less established forms of treatment, and a higher level still of competence to consent to invasive procedures proposed as non-beneficial medical research. A higher standard is set for refusal of recommended routine care than for its acceptance. It may appear self-serving and manipulative for a doctor to find a person of uncertain or borderline competence fit when giving consent to advised treatment, but to question the person's mental competence when such treatment is refused, but that approach may be legally sound. The law affords more protection against a poorly considered decision to forgo advised routine care than a similar decision to consent to it.

The law may protect all weaker partners in unequal relationships by a presumption that when any disproportionate advantage passes from the less powerful to the more powerful party, it has been induced by the exercise of undue influence, and is voidable. The presumption arises from a number of predetermined relationships, and applies without regard to the more powerful party's good reputation. Such relationships include those between lawyer and client, minister of religion and congregant, and doctor and patient. The lawyer, minister and doctor all have the power of superior knowledge, and if they acquire more than a regular professional fee or bequest in the relationship, the courts will set it aside.

Accordingly, the law respects the ethical obligation of protecting vulnerable persons incapable of autonomy by determining individuals' capacities to consent by reference to their comprehension, and their relative bargaining power. Vulnerable and dependent persons will be under the legal care of others. Children are legally protected by their parents or other legally appointed guardians, and, for instance, disabled parents may be the legal responsibility of their children. When the law recognizes one person's responsibility for the welfare of another who is dependent, it charges the guardian to supply or arrange for necessary care, which includes reasonably recommended health care.

The law may enforce this protective responsibility through punitive sanctions against a guardian who is neglectful.

More legally challenging are cases of guardians, such as parents, who may care dearly for their dependants but whose medical decisions are influenced by religious, philosophical or other convictions that cause them to reject routine medical advice, such as to approve an indicated blood transfusion. The law usually holds guardians to objective standards of medical care. They may martyr themselves for their convictions, but not those who depend on them for protection. Courts will either order Jehovah's Witness parents to consent to medically necessary blood transfusions for their children, give consent themselves or place the children in the medical care of other guardians who will make appropriate decisions. Courts may even order pregnant adults at risk of death to submit to transfusions for the sake of unborn children or so order parents with very young dependent children (12), although they will be very reluctant to do so and in the latter case will review whether such children may retain adequate protection if the parent dies (13). In the event of peril to a dependent child, however, the law may discount the guardian's autonomy by reliance on the ethical principles of beneficence to the vulnerable, and non-maleficence.

Beneficence

There is no general legal duty to do good to strangers, so that health professionals may decline to accept people as patients, although when they are accepted they cannot be abandoned. It has been seen that in special relationships, however, such as between parent and child, enforceable legal duties arise to supply or consent to indicated health care. Some jurisdictions impose duties of reasonable rescue of those in demonstrable peril that may bind neighbours and those who are aware and able to give help, but the usual legal encouragement of rescuers is that they will incur no legal liability to those they try to help if they act negligently. Only acts of gross or extraordinary negligence may expose them to legal liability. Doctors may accordingly give assistance at traffic accidents, and like cases of need of medical care, with little fear of incurring liability.

It is a general principle of tort law in the English Common Law tradition and perhaps beyond that, in special relationships, a duty arises to take care for the well-being of those one foresees or reasonably should foresee being injured as a consequence of one's act or omission to act. It has been legally recognized that the relationship between a psychotherapist or psychiatrist and a patient is special in this sense, and that it creates a legal duty to warn or otherwise protect a third party the health professional identifies as being at risk of injury by the patient's conduct. This duty to warn, given expression in the US in the *Tarasoff* case (14), transcends the ordinary obligation to preserve confidentiality. The California Supreme Court in *Tarasoff* observed that 'The protective privilege [of confidentiality] ends where the public peril begins' (see ref. 14, at p. 347), indicating that the beneficent duty to warn potential victims, in order that they may take due precautions, supersedes a patient's autonomous right to control information about the patient's condition and prognosis.

The AIDS epidemic has given the law additional occasions to apply this principle. A doctor aware of a patient's infected condition and liability to spread the infection through sexual or drug-taking conduct may have a duty to consider a third party's beneficial care. A patient's spouse may be notified, for instance, if the patient fails to respond to a doctor's request to notify the spouse of the risk of transmission of the infection (15). Courts are being increasingly invited to consider holding liable people who wilfully or negligently risk spreading the infection through sexual or other conduct, but no clear jurisprudence has yet emerged, in the absence of infected persons' deceptive assurances that they are not infected.

Even when no duty to warn of a health danger is recognized, courts may recognize a power to warn where this is beneficial to the interests of individuals, or indeed to those of the public at large. Courts will protect the power to give information to police, child protection, public health and comparable authorities of a perceived risk, by ensuring non-disclosure of informant's identities, even at the cost of occasionally protecting malicious and false reports (16). Patients' general legal rights of confidentiality, which may yield to the public benefit of disclosure of hazards to health, protect revelations of truths. Communications of falsehoods fall under the law of defamation, but here again disclosures made in good faith, non-maliciously and non-negligently, that are beneficial in the public interest, will not attract liability. For instance, a doctor who acts to give warning to a spouse apparently at risk because a patient has tested positive for the AIDS virus will be protected if the test result proves to be a false-positive.

An instance of how a judge can act against the ethical principle of beneficence occurred in 1980, when the Royal College of Nursing sought an interpretation of whether the British Abortion Act 1967 protected nurses from criminal liability for undertaking abortion by the more recently developed method of administering prostaglandin drugs. The method, which consisted of a doctor installing the means of administering the drug but a nurse doing the actual application of the drug and managing the consequent abortion, was considered more beneficial to many patients than surgical methods that existed when the legislation was enacted in 1967. In the English Court of Appeal, however, Lord Denning concluded that the superior technique was not protected by the 1967 law, observing that 'the doctor will have to use the surgical method with its extra hazards' (17) or the patient would have to forgo therapeutic abortion. On higher appeal, the House of Lords reversed this decision and found that nurses performing the more beneficial method were legally protected, because they were acting under doctors' orders. The higher decision illustrates the ethical principles both of beneficence and non-maleficence.

Non-maleficence

Courts will seek to prevent harm by such means as limiting the scope of parental power over children's medical treatment, so that parents can use their legal authority only for a child's benefit (18). The same limit applies to others who act *in loco parentis*, and to courts that exercise the state's *parens patriae* power to protect mentally impaired persons. There may be legal uncertainty and disagreement, however, regarding what treatment is harmful and what may be beneficial.

A procedure on which the highest courts of the UK and Canada have differed is sterilization proposed only for contraceptive reasons, as opposed to on therapeutic grounds. In the *Eve* case (19), the Supreme Court of Canada held that contraceptive sterilization of a mentally impaired adult woman suffering from extreme expressive aphasia, which doctors proposed to achieve through hysterectomy, was not in her interests, and would be a harmful invasion of her physical integrity. In a following case in England, however, the House of Lords held that a suitable sterilization procedure could be beneficial for a mentally impaired adult and could be approved (20). The facts of the two cases are not necessarily incompatible, but the Canadian court approached the issue in an absolute manner, whereas the House of Lords was more open. Both agreed, however, that parent-like powers could not be employed in non-beneficial ways, and differed only on the classification of contraceptive sterilization performed on a non-consenting person. The English decision may accommodate social advantages that a sterilized person may enjoy, such as more private time with members of the opposite sex.

The House of Lords had already been willing to take account of psychological and comparable factors in the assessment of benefit of a non-therapeutic medical procedure. Lord Reid had found, for instance, that a parent can lawfully require that a young child be compelled to submit to a blood test, with the use of reasonable constraints if necessary, for determination of paternity, because of the 'financial advantage' of legitimacy (21). It is instructive that the court found such blood testing not to be harmful, because medical literature records such anecdotal consequences as haematoma, dermatitis, cellulitis, abscess, osteomyelitis, septicaemia, endocarditis, thrombophlebitis, pulmonary embolism and death (22). Further, the 'financial advantage' would be absent if the test was to result in a finding of illegitimacy and the consequent forfeiture of inheritances. Nevertheless, Lord Reid found that a court 'is not really protecting the child to ban a blood test on some vague and shadowy conjecture that it may turn out to be to its disadvantage' (see ref. 21 at p. 43). This reflects a general view that it is not harmful or unlawful for dependent persons to be exposed by their legal guardians to the risks of everyday life. It is questioned in Canada, however, under the *Eve* decision, whether incompetent persons may be exposed to venepuncture for the purpose only of non-beneficial medical research (23).

Laws frequently recognize that some medical procedures that may be undertaken for financial advantage are sufficiently liable to prove maleficent to justify prohibition. A person who is willing to donate a kidney or other solid organ to another in exchange for payment will violate the legislation of many jurisdictions, and contracts for such commerce will judicially be held void as contrary to public policy, public order or public morality. Legislation may not be as rigid concerning tissues, which are usually understood to be body materials that are replaceable by natural processes of repair. Blood, bone marrow, and sperm are tissues most often concerned in transfers between living donors and recipients. Some legislation that prohibits sales of any body materials, including tissues, makes an exception for blood and blood constituents. Where no exception exists, however, such as for sperm donation, payments may be made to compensate donors for their out-of-pocket expenses and inconvenience in submitting to human immunodeficiency virus (HIV) testing on donation, and having a repeat test six or more months later for determination of whether the previously donated sample may be unfrozen for use. Donation is viewed as a service rather than a commodity transaction, and legislation prohibiting commerce does not bar payment or recovery of costs actually incurred.

Legislation that prohibits organ donation by legal minors may not address donations of tissues. Blood and similar tissue banks may decline minors' donation on ethical and legal grounds, but a dilemma may arise within a family. If one child suffers from such a condition as leukaemia, and requires a bone marrow transplant, the only genetically compatible donor may be a sibling. A parent of both a potential recipient and a donor child faces a conflict of interest, in that a legal responsibility exists to protect the interests of both children. It has been seen that a parent cannot use legal authority over a child in a manner that is not in that child's interests, and that legislation confirms this in prohibiting donation of a solid organ. Bone marrow donation is uncomfortable, presents risks such as infection, and cannot be considered beneficial to undergo unless benefit can be assessed in psychological terms.

If a potential donor child has no personal relationship with a potential recipient, such benefit will usually be absent or illusory. If a genuine affection or affinity exists, however, donation may constitute a sufficient benefit to the donor to justify the donation in law. More speculative benefits, such as avoiding fear of remorse and self-recrimination if a sibling dies without the donation, or avoiding persistent parental grief or resentment following such death, may be more difficult legal justifications for allowing donation. The potential donor's age and maturity are also factors to consider, since it has been seen that mature minors may be accorded the same autonomy as competent adults. As against this, if donation appears sufficiently beneficial to be justified but the potential donor resists or otherwise denies assent to the procedure, it cannot be pursued.

Research procedures that are non-beneficial and that pose risks may be accepted by competent altruistic subjects when there is a favourable risk-to-benefit ratio, determined to the satisfaction of an independent ethics review committee. The acceptance of risk without benefit may at first appear to violate the principle of non-maleficence, but it may be acceptable, within reasonable limits of likelihood and extent of injury, as serving the ethical values of autonomy and beneficence.

Justice

The ethical principle of justice is the principle that the law claims primarily to serve. Law respects precedents, for instance, because of the rule of justice that like cases should be treated alike. Similarly, in the context of health care, general medical practitioners' standards of proficiency are measured against the standards of other general practitioners in like circumstances, and specialists are measured against the standards of other practitioners within the same specialty.

It was once an additional feature that medical practitioners were measured against others in their locality, but the 'locality rule' is in decline for reasons both of pragmatism and principle. Now that, in most developed countries, ease of transport gives patients access to services throughout expanded geographical areas, and one practitioner can refer a patient to another, usually a specialist, in another locality, the proposition that patients are entitled to no higher performance than can be achieved by practitioners in their locality has lost much of its force. Other reasons for the decline in the locality rule are that, in confined localities, medical practitioners may be reluctant to testify as expert witnesses to the effect that a colleague's practice was below standard, so that courts may be impaired in establishing what the standard is in the locality (24), and that, where tax-funded health services exist, those equally liable to taxation are entitled to equal standards of service.

Classical concepts of justice traceable to the time of Aristotle distinguish distributive justice from corrective justice. Distributive justice is concerned with the allocation of rights, duties and burdens among community members. Corrective justice redresses imbalances of rights and duties among community members by restoring the position that existed, or that justly should have existed, before a wrong or injustice was done. This is the basis of awards of financial compensation, although these aim to achieve the position that would now have existed had a wrong not been done, rather than simply the position that preceded it.

Both corrective and distributive justice include a concern with relations between individuals, but the latter is more concerned in addition with collective or group rights, and with relations between communities and individuals. Ethical relations between one person and another are sometimes described as microethics, whereas ethical relations between groups and between a group and an individual may be described as macroethics. The law is often engaged in issues of macroethics through, for instance, criminal law, constitutional law and administrative law.

Human rights law, derived in modern times from the international legal instruments that give effect to the Universal Declaration of Human Rights, which was adopted by the United Nations Organization General Assembly in 1948, concerns in particular how states and their governments treat individuals. Implementing legal instruments include such regional treaties as the European Convention on Human Rights, the American Convention on Human Rights and the African Charter on Human and Peoples' Rights. Judicial institutions created under these conventions, particularly the European Commission and the European Court of Human Rights, may compel member-states to reform the content or effect of their national laws. In 1981, for instance, the European Court of Human Rights condemned certain English legislation that was found to operate unjustly regarding mental health detention (25), although a year earlier the European Commission rejected a challenge that the British Abortion Act 1967 was unjust to the unborn (26). European tribunals have more recently been hearing challenges to abortion law provisions in Ireland, and the Commission upheld Germany's abortion law in 1977 (27).

The international level of legal decision-making has a potential to affect macroethical concerns in health care that transcend medical care. The levels of health that major populations of the world achieve are influenced less by advances in medical technology and, for instance, legal reforms regarding patients' rights, than by their access to clean water for drinking and sanitation, and by the quality of the air they breathe. Environmental law, concerned with pollution control and preservation of natural resources, seeks justice in communities' health standards not only among developed countries, underdeveloped countries and countries in the process of becoming newly industrialized, but also between existing and future human generations. The quality of the world one generation passes to following generations, and the environment's capacity to sustain people in health and nutrition, are perhaps the most profound issues of justice that national and international legal systems face.

REFERENCES

1. *Re Attorney-General of British Columbia and Astaforoff* (1983), 6 C.C.C. (3d) 498 (B.C.C.A.).
2. Lord Lloyd and Freeman, M.B.A. (Eds) *Lloyd's introduction to jurisprudence*, 5th edn, pp. 61–64. Stevens, London.
3. Cadigan, L. T. 1991. Balancing the interests: a practical approach to restrictions on expressive conduct in the anti-abortion protest context. *Boston College Law Review* **32**: 835–897.
4. de Wachter, M. A. M. 1989. Active euthanasia in the Netherlands. *Journal of the American Medical Association* **262**: 3316–3319.
5. Justice Cardozo. In *Schloendorf* v. *Society of New York Hospital* (1914), 105 N.E. 92 (N.Y.C.A.).
6. *Malette* v. *Shulman* (1990), 67 D.L.R. (4th) 321 (Ont.C.A.).
7. *Cruzan* v. *Director, Missouri Dept. of Health* (1990), 110 S.Ct. 2841 (U.S.S.C.).
8. *Sidaway* v. *Bethlem Royal Hospital Governors*, [1985] 1 All E.R.643 (H.L.).
9. Giesen, D. 1988. *International medical malpractice law*, p. x. J.C.B. Mohr (Paul Siebeck), Tübingen.
10. *Canterbury* v. *Spence* (1972), 464 F.2d 772 at p. 784 (Dist. Columbia Circuit Ct.).
11. *Gillick* v. *West Norfolk and Wisbech Area Health Authority*, [1986] A.C. 150 (H.L.).
12. *Raleigh Fitkin-Paul Morgan Memorial Hospital* v. *Anderson* (1964), 201 A.2d 537 (N.J.S.C.) (8 month fetus) and *State* v. *Perricone* (1962), 181 A.2d 751 (N.J.S.C.) (dependent infant).
13. *Fosmire* v. *Nicoleau* (1990), 551 N.E.2d 77 (N.Y.C.A.).
14. *Tarasoff* v. *Regents of the University of California* (1976), 551 P.2d 334 (Cal. Sup. Ct.).
15. Dickens, B. M. 1988. Legal limits of AIDS confidentiality. *Journal of the American Medical Association* **259**: 3349–3351.
16. *D.* v. *National Society for the Prevention of Cruelty to Children*, [1978] A.C. 171 (H.L.).
17. *Royal College of Nursing* v. *Department of Health and Social Security*, [1981] 1 All E.R. 545 (Q.B.D., C.A. and H.L.) at p. 556.
18. Dickens, B. M. 1981. The modern function and limits of parental rights. *Law Quarterly Review* **97**: 462–485.
19. *Re Eve* (1986), 31 D.L.R. (4th) 1 (S.C.C.).
20. *Re F (Mental Patient: Sterilization)*, [1989] 2 W.L.R. 1025 (C.A.) 1063 (H.L.).
21. *S.* v. *McC., W.* v. *W.*, [1972] A.C. 24 (H.L.) at p. 42.
22. *Cobbs* v. *Grant* (1972), 501 P.2d 1 (Cal. S.C.) at p. 11, n. 2, citing Harrison, *Principles of internal medicine* (5th edn, 1966) p. 726, 1492, 1510–1514.
23. Medical Research Council of Canada. 1987. *Guidelines on research involving human subjects*. Ministry of Supply and Services, Ottawa.
24. Furrow, B. R., Johnson, S. H., Jost, T. S. and Schwartz, R. L. (Eds) 1991. *Health law: cases, materials and problems*, pp. 132–138. West Publishing Co., St Paul, MN.

25. *X* v. *United Kingdom (Re Detention of a Mental Patient)* (1981), 4 E.H.R.R. 188 (Eur. Ct. H.R.).
26. *Paton* v. *United Kingdom* (1980), 3 E.H.R.R. 408 (Eur. Comm. H.R.).
27. *Bruggeman and Scheuten* v. *Federal Republic of Germany* (1977), 3 E.H.R.R. 244 (Eur. Comm. H.R.).

28

The Four Principles Revisited—a Reappraisal

RAANAN GILLON

When I first read Beauchamp and Childress I recognized what I thought was a very important framework for medical ethics—a common basis of moral commitment (admittedly only *prima facie*, but nonetheless common to all) a common basis for moral analysis and the elements of a common moral language—that would overcome a major and common problem that I encountered in medical ethics. This was the problem of ethical relativism ('well we can't really talk about medical ethics because we have such very different ethical/religious/secular/philosophical/political/cultural/professional/personal backgrounds and perspectives—we'll simply have to beg to differ'). As I began to teach using this framework I was impressed by the readiness with which doctors could agree that the four principles were indeed consistent with their own perspective on medico-moral issues. When I lectured more widely I found similar reactions from nurses, other health care workers, medical students and more recently members of the general public. I began to think that the four-principles-plus-scope approach was not only helpful in health care but seemed equally relevant to other ethical issues.

Then a philosophical backlash emerged with a small but very vocal minority of philosophers vigorously attacking the 'Georgetown mantra', and a variety of others finding fault with it. It seemed worth while extending the discussion by asking writers from a very wide range of viewpoints to consider not only substantive issues in health care ethics but also the relevance of the four-principles approach within their own perspectives. I must confess to being very reassured by the remarkably positive response manifested in this first section of the book. Time and time again the basic relevance of these four principles plus consideration of their scope of application is acknowledged, whether in law or religion, whether in Marxism or Roman Catholicism, whether the latter

Principles of Health Care Ethics. Edited by Raanan Gillon.

is liberal or more orthodox, whether in Judaism or in Islam, whether in utilitarian philosophy or Kantian, in international consensus building or in clinical ethics. Almost every writer, even the most critical, acknowledges that the Beauchamp and Childress four *prima facie* principles plus concern for their scope of application express important and common moral concerns, relevant to health care ethics.

And of course every writer also argues, at the very least, that the four slogans— autonomy, beneficence, non-maleficence and justice—are not and could not possibly be the whole of health care ethics, let alone ethics more generally. Anyone who has actually read Beauchamp and Childress's substantial book on the subject (1) could hardly accuse them of suggesting that those four slogans were the whole of health care ethics, and even my own far shorter book (2) indicates the very wide range of issues and problems encompassed by those slogans. Nonetheless just as the term 'solar energy' can be seen to encompass a wide range of issues relevant to light and heat on the earth, so the names of the four principles can be seen—and in the preceding chapters are seen—to be accepted as encompassing a wide range of moral issues relevant to health care ethics (and indeed to ethics generally). Of course they are interpreted very differently from different perspectives—see for example some of the religious chapters, all of them finding the four principles of moral importance but providing widely differing critiques of their inadequacy when shorn of the specific underlying religious understanding adhered to by the particular writer. Yet all indicate clearly that in contemporary contexts the four principles are acceptable and relevant within their religious perspective. And in so far as the term 'slogan' indicates some commitment, each of the four principles functions, or could properly function, not merely as a name of a moral concern but also indeed as a slogan, by virtue of naming a *prima facie* moral concern to which there is a moral commitment.

Even the most vigorous of the critics of the four principles—and I was keen to invite the strongest and most coherent of these critics, notably Clouser and Gert, as well as several others, to do their best to undermine the acceptability of the four principles—either provide alternative accounts of morality that include moral concerns easily encompassable within the general framework of the four principles (Clouser and Gert), or explicitly accept that the four principles 'are so fundamental they cannot be contested' (Wulff) or that 'it would be absurd to deny' that the four principles 'in some sense or another' would be acceptable to widely divergent moral theorists (Botros) but worry about their relative priority (Wulff), or wish to reduce the number of principles, e.g. by collapsing beneficence and non-maleficence (Nicholson), or are concerned about their lack of a decision procedure when the principles conflict in particular contexts (many of the contributors).

Perhaps the latter criticism is the one worth starting with substantively. The four-principles approach has never purported to provide a decision mechanism or procedure for application when the principles conflict in a particular set of circumstances. All they provide are a set of four *prima facie* moral principles, plus a concern for the scope of application of each, which anyone can accept as potentially relevant to his or her particular moral decisions. This may be dismissed with disdain as a 'mere checklist' of moral concerns (Clouser and Gert) but I prefer a positive approach to acceptance of such a checklist. Just like any other 'checklist' this one too points to a prior *commitment*; but rather more importantly than most 'checklists' this one points to the existence of four substantive, though admittedly only *prima facie*, moral concerns that *everyone can accept as of common and mutual moral relevance*. It seems to me to be of outstanding moral significance if a common commitment to a 'checklist' of certain specific moral principles can be agreed which transcends barriers of religion, culture, politics, nationality, philosophical stance, even gender (see Cook's contribution). The importance of this commitment is increased when it is made in common terminology—for now we have not only a *prima facie* international moral commitment to certain principles or values, but also elements of a common moral language. Thus the criticism that the four principles are a 'mere checklist' of potentially relevant moral concerns fails dismally.

The criticism that they fail to provide a decision procedure in particular circumstances when the principles conflict is entirely accurate but, as stated above, misdirected since they were never claimed to povide such a decision procedure. Undoubtedly there is a need for such a decision procedure or procedures, and a variety are explicitly or implicitly offered by the various contributors to this book; but whatever procedure is chosen it will require decision between competing moral concerns of the types encompassed by the four principles.

A third criticism (for example Clouser and Gert, Botros) is that the four principles do not provide a coherent moral theory. Once again the criticism is perfectly accurate, but misdirected, for the four principles were never claimed to provide a moral theory, coherent or otherwise; it was only claimed for them that they are *compatible* with many (I believe most) different moral theories, themselves often mutually incompatible. The fact that the four principles do *not* comprise a moral theory but are compatible with most if not all moral theories is one of their most valuable features, for they offer a way of bypassing the deep and probably unresolvable conflicts between competing moral theories. We can agree to differ about our basic moral theories and still agree about our acceptance of the four *prima facie* principles. One of the philosophical misunderstandings of the four-principles approach, manifested in this volume by Botros, is to assume that if the four principles are claimed to be compatible with several different moral theories then there must be an underlying philosophical claim that those theories are after all, must after all be, compatible with each other. Well of course at a trivially true level there is such a claim— notably that to the extent that mutually incompatible theories agree about the relevance of four *prima facie* moral principles they manifest compatibility. But that in no way entails any claims about the overall compatibility of the conflicting theories—such claims would be as silly as claiming that, because two political parties of mutually incompatible political beliefs find policies on which they can agree and cooperate in a coalition government, therefore they must have sunk all their political–theoretical differences and their political beliefs are no longer mutually incompatible. Needless to say, agreement on *a* and *b* and *c* and *d* neither entails agreement on *e* or *f*, nor entails agreement about the justification for such agreement as has been achieved.

In this context a further set of criticisms of the four principles certainly requires attention—notably the fact that there is *some* lack of agreement on their precise meaning. There are two sorts of task here, one philosophical (what do we *mean* by 'respect for autonomy', etc.) and the other partly philosophical, partly stipulative (are we to call positive action to enhance people's autonomy respect for autonomy or beneficence; are we to incorporate prevention and removal of harms under beneficence or non-maleficence?). While there is undoubtedly philosophical work to be done here, for both sorts of task, the lack of precision about the meaning of the principles need not undermine acceptance of the four-principles approach. I have several reasons for this assertion. The first is that there is already a considerable measure of agreement about the meaning of the principles. The second is that the ambiguities and disagreements that have emerged concern, or can be interpreted to concern, either how to classify certain sorts of moral obligation within the four-principle structure (is it non-maleficence or is it beneficence?—it's clearly one or the other); or disagreements about the boundaries of the particular concepts (is that child to be regarded as autonomous at all?); or of the scope of application of the principle (if the child is autonomous, is he adequately autonomous to fall within the scope of our *prima facie* obligation to respect his autonomy when to do so conflicts with our perception of his best interests?); or disagreements about the *substantive* theory of, for example, justice that should be accepted in a particular context (yes, we may accept the Aristotelian formal theory of justice, whereby equals must be treated equally, unequals unequally in proportion to the morally relevant inequality—but we may disagree radically about which substantive theory of justice to accept, even though they all are consistent with the Aristotelian formal theory). None of these disagreements and ambiguities need undermine acceptance of the four *prima facie* principles themselves. They all point to the need for more philosophical work to be done in clarifying and making more precise their interpretation and application for particular cases or types of case.

We should not, however, over-indulge the philosophical desire for definitional precision. As Aristotle so importantly advised at the beginning of the Nichoma-chean Ethics, 'our discussion will be adequate if it has as much clearness as the subject matter admits of, for precision is not to be sought for alike in all discussions'. And in speaking about 'fine and just actions' and of 'goods' we must be content 'to indicate the truth roughly and in outline, and in speaking about things which are only for the most part true and with premises of the same kind, to reach conclusions that are no better . . . for it is the mark of an educated man to look for precision in each class of things just so far as the nature of the subject admits' (3). Thus while the *precise* meaning of the terms respect for autonomy, beneficence, non-maleficence, justice, and a concern for their scope of application is open to considerable philosophical argument and debate, they are easily understood and accepted 'roughly and in outline' by philosophers and others alike. By all means let philosophers continue to fill in the pictures and smooth down the rough edges so far as possible—but given the fact that they are already reasonably clear, and given the widespread philosophical support from different moral theories for the families of *prima facie* moral principles denoted by 'respect for autonomy', 'beneficence', 'non-maleficence' and 'justice', there is no need to allow the residual 'roughness' of agreement about their precise meaning to undermine their acceptance, even though it provides an important area for continuing philosophical investigation.

One particular area of ambiguity concerns the issue of whether or not the principle of respect for autonomy encompasses positive actions to benefit others, or only covers obligations to desist from interference with people's autonomous choices for themselves. My own view, along with Beauchamp and Childress, is that the latter is the correct account of the principle of respect for autonomy (respect for people's deliberated choices for themselves is my own currently preferred short definition—with the essential rider that such respect must be compatible with equal respect for the autonomy of all others potentially affected— a qualification derivable from both Kant's account of the principle and Mill's (4). This in no way is to deny that we sometimes and in some contexts also have duties of beneficence which require us to act positively to increase certain people's autonomy. The most obvious example is the health care requirement for informed consent. Respect for autonomy does not require us to go around giving all other people information, it *prima facie* simply requires us not to interfere with their deliberated choices for themselves. *However,* if we propose to do something to them, purportedly to help them (the fundamental justification for all health care interventions), then our combined moral obligations of respect for autonomy, beneficence and non-maleficence, and perhaps justice qua respect for rights too, require us to consult them adequately and give them sufficient information (a) to ensure that our proposed interference does not infringe their autonomy, (b) to ensure that it is indeed likely to provide net benefit-over-harm as seen from their perspective rather than (merely) from our own and (c) to ensure that we do not unjustly infringe their rights (for example by cutting them up without consent).

A further ambiguity, at least in some people's perceptions, concerns the meaning of beneficence and non-maleficence. Why distinguish between them when, as some would claim, they are essentially the same principle? My first response to this is that if one is certain about them being one principle one is not debarred by the four-principles approach from treating them as one. It is important, however, to understand that for most people there is a very great distinction to be made between a moral obligation not to harm and a moral obligation to benefit. The distinction is most evident in contexts where we do not acknowledge any obligation to benefit others. If we are honest with ourselves most of us do not acknowledge a moral obligation—even a merely *prima facie* moral obligation—to benefit everyone else in the world, let alone people who have not yet been born into the world; or even, for example, an obligation to benefit all the poor people in the world; or even, as health workers, an obligation to benefit all the sick people in the world. We tend to acknowledge a moral obligation to help only *some* others in the world, and one of the enduring moral debates concerns precisely the scope of our obligations of beneficence—whom do we all have moral obligations to benefit—whom do I have moral obligations to benefit? But even to those to whom we acknowledge no obligation of beneficence we do acknowledge a *prima facie* moral obligation not to harm them—we acknowledge an obligation of non-maleficence that encompasses all the groups just mentioned.

Or do we? Nicholson, in rejecting the distinction between the principles of beneficence and non-maleficence, seems to argue that we do not. By living in developed western societies, he argues, we manifest that we reject even a *prima facie* moral obligation to avoid harming all others—because western societies *do* harm Third World societies and so by living in western societies we harm Third World societies and thus manifest our rejection of even a *prima facie* moral obligation not to harm all others.

This is to misunderstand the point. First, even if it were true that developed western societies cause overall harm to developing societies—and it is a hotly debated claim—this would not demonstrate that people in those western societies reject a *prima facie* obligation not to harm all others. They may instead be failing to live up to their perceived moral obligations; or they may be unable to prevent their governments from failing to live up to such perceived moral obligations; or they may consider that the harm caused is a necessary corollary in providing overall benefit (in medical practice we regularly do harm in order that net benefit will result; and indeed more generally it is true that whenever one sets out to benefit others one risks harming them and therefore in such circumstances the obligations of beneficence and non-maleficence must be considered together, with the moral objective being to produce *net* benefit—but none of that entails rejection of the *prima facie* obligation not to harm); or they may consider that the harm caused is acceptable in the pursuit of some other moral objective (an example of this is the acceptance of the harm of road traffic accidents in most societies as a consequence of allowing people to use private motor cars—respect for individual autonomy over-riding non-maleficence). None of these putative counter-examples negates my claim that most people acknowledge a *prima facie* moral obligation not to harm all others, whereas they deny a *prima facie* moral obligation to benefit all others. A simple test for those who still doubt this claim is to ask themselves: 'is there anyone in the world whom I do not consider myself to have a *prima facie* moral obligation to benefit?'; if the answer is 'yes' (can it be otherwise?) then ask 'do I nonetheless consider myself to have a *prima facie* moral obligation not to harm that individual or those individuals?'. If the answer is yes in both cases, a difference in the scope of application of one's duties of beneficence (restricted scope) and non-maleficence (universal scope) has been acknowledged.

Nonetheless, Nicholson is not alone in regarding non-maleficence and beneficence to be parts of a single moral obligation (5), and the four-principles-plus-scope approach has no more difficulty in accommodating this theoretical claim than it does in accommodating theoretical claims that the four principles are all parts or aspects of a single moral obligation (for example that they are all parts or aspects of a single moral obligation to maximize welfare, or of a single moral obligation to obey the Kantian categorical imperative, or of a single moral obligation to accept a particular theory of justice). Combiners of beneficence and non-maleficence can simply stipulate that one is a subclass of the other, or that both are subclasses of the combined principle. It seems clear to me, however, that it is essential to distinguish between non-maleficence and beneficence, at least for the purpose of providing a 'backstop' moral principle of universal scope of application—and one that all or most reflective moral agents would acknowledge—for any and all cases in which a duty of beneficence is for any reason rejected. However whether non-maleficence is separate from, part of, or explained by one or more of the other principles is not a concern of the four-principles approach which is neutral in disputes between overarching ethical theories—and as usual is consistent with them all.

Thus it is that moral theoretical positions as far apart as utilitarianism (see Hare's chapter) and Kantianism (see Furness's chapter) can accept the relevance of the four principles but only because they see them as generated by, and secondary to, their overarching and monist moral theories (based on welfare maximization and respect for autonomy respectively). The elegance of the four-principles approach is that it need say nothing about the deep, and some claim untraversable, philosophical chasm separating these two types of philosophical theory—instead it offers each a meeting place in practical ethics. Similarly, it is neutral between the various religious moral theories and indeed between different versions of the same religious theory (the most startling example of which in this book is afforded by the two contributions from the Roman Catholic perspective, by Finnis and Fisher on the one hand giving a traditionalist account of Roman Catholicism and of its interpretation of the four principles; and by Hoose on the other, offering a more 'liberal' Roman Catholicism and its interpretation of the four principles). So too do we find in this book Marxist (Luther and Schubert) and libertarian (Engelhardt) support for the principles—though of course very much qualified by the requirements of their underlying (or overarching) theories—once again the four principles approach is neutral between them and compatible with both.

Of course this moral–theoretic neutrality is not to everyone's taste, and one of its most vigorous critics in this book is Botros. On first reading her chapter I could not understand why she was spending so much of it attacking my own work, rather than writing about rights as requested. But on re-reading it I think that at the heart of her attack is a two-pronged claim; that acceptance of a set of moral principles without a supporting moral theory and worse, in the belief that opposing moral theories could accept the same set of moral principles (as what Habgood calls 'middle axioms'), is unphilosophical and therefore unacceptable; and that writing about and teaching medical ethics in a way that promotes acceptance of these *prima facie* moral principles without providing a supporting moral theory, and without arguing against those moral theories which in her view are both unacceptable and which do *not* purport to accept the four principles (in her case utilitarianism seems to be the moral–theoretic stalking horse) is also unphilosophical and therefore unacceptable. For her (and indeed many other philosophers), philosophy seems to require an intellectual 'showdown' with intellectual winners and losers—see for example her rejection of the possibility that utilitarians could *really* accept that patients had a right to informed consent, as contrasted with 'those who regard autonomy as the pre-eminent value'.

My own philosophical reading and thinking, by contrast, has led me to believe that where either moral theories or moral values conflict there is little point in pursuing moral philosophical argument in the hope of 'an intellectual kill' or 'showdown'—and no hope whatsoever that philosophers will come up with a moral philosophical theory that will either be so effectively supported by argument that it will supersede all competing moral theories, or that will provide similarly uncontested decision mechanisms for choosing between competing moral values when these conflict in particular cases.

What there *is* hope of achieving is a better-reasoned, more critical approach to personal and collective moral decision making, better awareness of opposing moral positions and especially of moral positions opposed to one's own, and an awareness that there are *some* moral values that are subscribed to by all, or most, competing and opposed moral perspectives. It is in these arenas that philosophy is helpful to health care workers (and where it is not helpful it may as well be abandoned—unlike philosophy, the *work* of health care workers requires moral decisions in the real world, and the only real purpose of introducing philosophy to health care is to help health care workers individually and collectively to make their decisions better (a deliberately ambiguous phrasing)). Philosophy is singularly unhelpful if it tries to turn health care workers into philosophers (there will always be a few exceptions who will become fascinated by philosophy for its own sake—I was one such—but that is not the function of philosophy in health care ethics); and it is singularly unhelpful if it tries to persuade health care workers that there is only one correct moral philosophical theory. Thus my own work has sought arenas of common agreement amongst opposed moral theories, and the Beauchamp and Childress *prima facie* principles plus attention to their scope of application provide just such an arena. There seems little doubt that whatever philosophical or religious moral theory is considered it will include support (however grudging in some cases!) for the purposes of practical ethics of the Beauchamp and Childress four *prima facie* principles. Of course we should ever remain open to argument for the need to reject or supplement them (and I shall consider putatively needed additions below); but given evidence of such widespread support for the principles, until and unless conclusive arguments for rejection or supplementation are produced it seems sensible to accept them as substantive moral premises upon which to base reasoning in health care ethics.

Nor, I believe, do all health care workers themselves need to try to acquire sufficient philosophical skills to come to a soundly based, well-defended philosophical decision about which moral theory they accept as grounding those principles and why they reject all the others. If life-long philosophers cannot succeed in this enterprise to the satisfaction of their philosophical opponents it would surely be ludicrous even to suggest that it is appropriate for health care workers spending a small part of their student and professional lives on the study of health care ethics to attempt it. Instead let us accept those (relatively few) moral claims that these competing philosophical theorists *can* agree on and use them as mutually acceptable *premises* in our moral reasoning and argument. Instead of wasting much time in health care ethics on fruitless argument about the underlying moral theories underpinning those moral claims, let us concentrate on learning to use the important philosophical techniques of clear, unambiguous, logical reasoning and argument in the light of the strongest counter-arguments, so as to help us make our moral decisions better.

Perhaps the most pervasive criticism of the four-principles approach is, however, precisely that it does not provide a moral decision-making procedure for when the *prima facie* principles conflict in particular cases (and Botros is simply mistaken when claiming that in my book I purport to offer a system for deciding 'which principle should be given priority in medico-moral disputes'). The four-principles approach was never devised or offered as a decision mechanism, and the fact that the *prima facie* principles can and do conflict in particular cases has always been explicitly acknowledged. Some moral religious or political philosophers may be brave enough to offer a moral decision mechanism or process for particular cases (see for example the chapter by Clouser and Gert), but the four-principles approach does not. What it does propose is that in any such decision process the potential relevance of the four principles (and their scope of application) should be considered. One of the most important such decision mechanisms, in my own personal opinion, is that of casuistry, outlined by Jonsen in his chapter. But as he also points out casuistry is the application of general principles to particular cases. Under a different guise this is also the basis of the case law approach in English law. The four principles as a set of general *prima facie* moral principles are entirely compatible with a casuistry which seeks to apply them in particular cases.

One aspect of such 'application' that I personally am increasingly dissatisfied with is the notion of 'balancing' the principles in particular cases (a description which I have previously repeatedly used myself). I now think that this description misleadingly suggests that the principles *have* determinate 'weights' in particular contexts such that they can be set upon some neutral balance in order to discover the morally 'weightier' course of action. My own and doubtless idiosyncratic tendency now is to speak not of balancing but of 'harmonizing' the principles in particular cases (and I am indebted to the crime writer Tony Hillerman and his accounts of Navajo culture for this insight, if such it be!). The advantage of this usage is that it reflects the possibility that the four principles can be 'harmonized' differently in the same particular case, depending on the particular culture's norms of harmony. Thus one culture may give greater 'dominance' to beneficence at the expense of say autonomy (see for example the chapters by Wulff, Riis and Steinberg), another may prefer the cool harmonies provided by a predominance of justice, and yet another culture may prefer the perhaps more dissonant harmonies resulting from frequent predominance of respect for autonomy. Despite some assertions to the contrary the four-principles approach is neutral between these different cultural perspectives, provided only that they take account of all the principles. Thus in very similar sets of particular circumstances different cultures may 'apply' or 'harmonize' the same set of principles differently—consistently within the context of their own cultures but inconsistently with the approaches of other cultures. This again seems to me to be one of the pleasing features of the four-principles approach—that it is consistent with such variety of application. In this way it permits the degree of moral variation that recognizes and accepts the moral importance of cultural variety, while maintaining a degree of universalizable moral agreement between cultures (notably agreement about the four principles themselves) that obviates the dangers of moral relativism.

Just as some critiques of the four-principles approach claim that the principles can be subsumed under fewer, more fundamental principles—all can be derived from, say, respect for autonomy or welfare maximization or a theory of need fulfilment; or two of them are really one (beneficence and non-maleficence)—so others claim that they need supplementing. Of course there is nothing intrinsically unacceptable about adding principles, but it is interesting to advocates of the four-principles approach to assess whether or not proposed additional principles are actually needed, or whether they can be accommodated within the four-principles-plus-scope structure. Two commonly proposed additional principles are a principle of the sanctity of life (or 'respect for life') and a principle of honesty.

So far as sanctity of, or respect for, life is concerned there is very major moral debate about just what sort of moral obligations are owed to just what sort of life. From the perspective of the four principles the additional issue here is not one of additional moral principles but of the scope of application of the existing principles. That is to say, for any living entity does it fall within the scope of our moral obligations (and why); and if it does which moral obligations do we owe it (and why)? In so far as we do owe any such moral obligations these will be encompassable within the framework of the four principles; that is to say the notions of sanctity of, or respect for, life do not add additional moral obligations over and above some combination of respect for autonomy, beneficence, non-maleficence and justice. But which of these obligations we owe to which sorts of life is a matter of major moral debate that is, I argue, easily interpreted as being a moral debate about the scope of application of each of the four principles, rather than being an additional moral principle itself. Thus we can all agree that *prima facie* we ought not to kill each other, that we have a right not to be killed unless we're aggressors (a right to life)—but we will disagree radically about what we mean by 'we'; about who or what falls within the scope of our moral obligations not to kill each other, about who or what has a right to life; most notoriously about whether human embryos and fetuses have such a right. But this radical disagreement is not about our substantive moral obligations but rather about their scope of application. They turn on disagreements about what attributes an entity must have to fall within the scope of our various moral obligations, not on disagreements about the obligations themselves. Thus I would reject the need for an additional principle, sanctity or respect for life, and instead argue for this issue to be seen as a scope issue; what attributes in an entity ground a right not to be killed unless it is an aggressor (I am of course simply assuming that aggressors do not have such a right).

A further principle sometimes proposed as a necessary additional moral principle (for example in this volume by Hare and by Wulff) is a principle of honesty or non-deceit or truth telling. Although, once again, there is nothing in the four-principles approach to prevent such additions, honesty as a *prima facie* moral obligation is easily supportable on the basis of some combination of the four principles themselves (for example it may be justified on the basis of respect for people's autonomy and/or on the basis of welfare maximization). There is an additional type of argument—one that I have used myself—that says that without a principle of honesty the very possibility of language acquisition would be undermined, and thus the very possibility of moral discourse. However, on reflection one still needs an answer to the question—so what? Why should language acquisition and moral discourse morally matter? Any attempted answers to such questions are likely themselves to depend explicitly or implicitly on considerations of respect for autonomy and/or the promotion of welfare, and/or (just possibly) considerations of justice. Thus it seems clear to me that there is no need for an additional principle of honesty or non-deceit, for such a principle can be derived from the existing four principles.

Later in this book Nylenna and Riis also propose the need for an additional principle, that of liberty. But the morally important principle of liberty is easily subsumable under the principle of respect for autonomy (or is indeed equivalent to it, as in Mill's 'On Liberty').

Two other important omissions for which the four-principles approach is sometimes criticized (though not within this volume) are the absence of a principle requiring respect for law and of a principle requiring respect for rights. While the moral functions of both laws and rights can be well understood and justified in terms of their tendency to promote the values encompassed by the four principles (6), with particular laws and particular rights being justified in so far as they promote respect for one or more of these principles, for my own part it seems clear that the formal moral requirements both to respect people's rights and to respect morally acceptable laws can be properly seen as subclasses of the formal principle of justice. Thus not only does the Aristotelian formal principle that equals be treated equally, unequals unequally in proportion to the relevant inequality, apply to distribution of inadequate resources; it also applies to our obligation to respect people's rights and to our obligation to respect morally acceptable laws.

Some of the many insights about supplementation of the four-principles approach that contributors in this section offer are particularly worth highlighting (though it should be stated that from the outset advocates of the four-principles approach have been perfectly aware of the relevance of such supplemental concerns!). I have already mentioned the decision-making approach based on what I have previously called the 'much-maligned method of casuistry'—the application of general principles to particular cases, discussed so well in Jonsen's chapter of this book. Another and related insight is that provided by Brody in his chapter, on the importance of empathy, narrative, conversation, sufficiently thorough investigation of particular circumstances before coming to moral decisions about them. Like several other contributors he also points to the need for virtue or good character in the good moral life—and of course there is no conflict between concern for the development of the virtues and discouragement of the vices and acceptance of the four-principles approach—on the contrary.

But in deciding what should *count* as a virtue or a vice the relevance of the four principles can easily be demonstrated. Indeed how else could one decide if some character disposition was virtuous or vicious other than by reference to its tendency to promote or undermine the moral values expressed by the four principles?

The relationship between desirable but not obligatory ideals and (mere) moral obligations is explored by Campbell. While he helpfully points out the moral importance of idealism, I cannot agree with him when he argues that the four principles 'become devoid of useful moral content unless they are made to intersect with a set of ideals which are beyond the call of duty'—with those ideals and the means to their achievement incorporated into the very characters— 'the formed habits of attitude and action'—not only of health care workers but also of their patients and their patients' families. Here there seems to be a danger of both ambiguity and of a false dichotomy. Ideals are those morally desirable objectives that are nonetheless not morally obligatory to achieve—not required as part of a person's moral duty. But if one accepts the four principles then one accepts certain obligations—admittedly *prima facie*, but obligations nonetheless that impose a moral duty unless other moral concerns over-ride that duty. Thus it seems odd—and false—to claim that they are 'devoid of useful moral content' unless they intersect with ideals that are beyond the call of duty. Surely the behaviour of anyone who took seriously the *prima facie* obligations of the four principles could not—and indeed *should not*—be said to be 'devoid of useful moral content', even if he or she does not act in pursuit of ideals beyond the call of those duties.

Furthermore the relation of the ideals and the four principles will inevitably be an intimate one, for the very possibility of justifying certain aimed-for states as 'ideals' requires some moral description of those states; and in the end that moral description will appeal to some combination of the moral values summarized by the four principles—the promotion of welfare, the prevention of harm, respect for autonomy and the achievement of justice. Similar comments apply to consideration of the 'virtues' discussed by Campbell. Descriptions such as wise, brave, tolerant, persevering, dependable, sincere, loyal, humorous, humble, open, warm, are all character descriptions. But whether or not they are to be classified as virtuous will surely depend on the extent to which they tend to produce morally desirable attitudes and behaviour (including mental responses of one sort or another) in the agent manifesting such character traits. And the assessment of whether or not those attitudes and behaviour are morally desirable will surely depend on whether or not they tend to respect autonomy, be beneficial, avoid harming, and be just. Similarly character traits would be described as vices in so far as they tended to produce behaviour that infringed these four *prima facie* principles.

Now it may be that I am quite wrong about these claims, and that character traits could simply be *stipulated* to be virtues or vices, or else specified to be such on account of attributes totally unrelated to the four principles. But so far I have failed to find plausible examples. I found it a useful exercise to go through Campbell's list of character traits noted above and ask myself; why do we think them to be virtues, and in what circumstances if any would we regard them not as virtues, as either morally neutral or even as vices? Tolerance, for example, is widely agreed to be a virtue; but if it is tolerance of despotism or other oppression then it is not a virtue; why? because it fails to prevent harm, to be just, to benefit others. Sincerity is widely agreed to be a virtue; but if it is a sincere belief in evil then it is not a virtue but a vice (Eichmann is said to have been a sincere Nazi; his conscience is said to have disturbed him deeply when on one occasion he took pity on a Jew and failed to have her gassed); what is different about virtuous sincerity and vicious sincerity? Virtuous sincerity tends to promote the values expressed by the four principles; vicious sincerity tends to undermine them.

Nonetheless, two insights are particularly worth highlighting from Campbell's chapter, both of them entirely consistent with the four principles. The first is that duty does not exhaust morality—one can be good if one does one's moral duty, but that in no way stops one from being even better by living up to one's ideals (assuming, I take it entirely reasonably, that one is not morally *obliged* to behave in a morally ideal way); the second—a point made by several contributors—is that character traits which tend to promote good attitudes and behaviour and discourage bad attitudes and behaviour (including merely mental behaviour) are a crucially important aspect of morality. As indicated above, in order to decide what those good or virtuous character traits are, we need to assess them against some moral standards, and this I have argued does involve reference to the four principles. But inculcating or helping the development of good or virtuous character traits need not involve such reference—though whenever such inculcation involves *justification* ('well you ought to try and help others because . . . ') then reference to moral values expressible in terms of the four principles will not be far behind.

A set of similar criticisms is that the four principles approach fails to recognize the importance of both conscience and emotion in practical morality. Again the importance of both is in no way ignored by the four principles, but on the contrary their importance is supported by reference to those principles (7). The main point to be emphasized is that in order to decide what constitute morally desirable and morally undesirable emotions, in order to decide whether one's conscience is giving one morally acceptable or morally unacceptable advice, one needs to make reference to moral values. Those moral values will involve reference to—or be redescribable in terms of—the Beauchamp and Childress four principles and their scope of application.

A minor criticism concerns the latinate names of the four principles. Doctors in particular are inclined to complain about the archaic-sounding vocabulary of 'beneficence', 'non-maleficence' 'autonomy' and perhaps even 'justice'—(which is ironic if one recalls the pidgin-ancient-greco-latinate nature of so much of my profession's own vocabulary). Nonetheless there is no reason why the names of the principles should not be translated into more accessible terminology, provided that such translation is accurate. A travesty of such translation is offered in a critical aside by Wikler (8) when he translates respect for autonomy as 'let people do what they want' (as distinct from something like: 'respect people's deliberated choices for themselves in so far as such respect is compatible with equal such respect for all potentially affected'!). The point of Wikler's translations of the four principles into simple (over-simple) colloquial English is to show that they are not a theory. This, as stated above, is perfectly true, but hardly a criticism given that the principles are not offered as a theory but only as a set of *prima facie* moral principles compatible with a wide variety of moral theories; and Wikler does not argue that the four principles are incompatible with any moral theory.

One recurrent criticism of the four-principles approach is that it can be misunderstood and misused, sometimes crassly so. This undoubtedly is true— as true of some of those who support and try to use it as of some of those who oppose its use and seek to denigrate it. In more than a decade of marking British medical ethics examination scripts in various contexts I, like any other teacher, have come across plenty of examples of crass misunderstanding and/or misapplication of what I have taught—including the four-principles-plus-scope approach to health care ethics. But which tools of ethical analysis are not capable of being misunderstood and misused? Of course anything that can be used can also be misused, but to judge a tool—any tool—not by its use but only by its misuse is surely mistaken.

So what in summary are the uses of the four-principles-plus-scope approach as a tool of practical ethics? The preceding chapters show that it offers a transcultural, transnational, transreligious, transphilosophical framework for ethical analysis; that it offers elements of a common language for such ethical analysis; and that it offers a common moral commitment upon which to base such ethical analysis. Because it is not itself a theory, but instead draws on elements common to most if not all moral theories, it can function peaceably as a tool of practical ethics that may be shared by those whose theories are totally incompatible and antithetical. Perhaps one of the most startling examples of such use is provided in Stanley's chapter on the development of the multinational, multicultural 'Appleton Guidelines' document on withholding and withdrawing of life-prolonging treatment.

From my own perspective the single most important feature of the four-principles-plus-scope approach is its flexibility within an agreed moral commit-ment. The approach does not seek to adjudicate between competing moral theories, religions, or political stances, provided they share compatibility with the common elements of moral commitment implied by acceptance of the four *prima facie* principles. Moreover, since one of those principles is respect for autonomy, and since it seems empirically indisputable that people's autonomous decisions are at least significantly influenced by their cultural environment, to the norms of which they tend to be deeply committed, it will follow that people in different cultures are likely to interpret these four principles somewhat differently, to 'balance', 'harmonize' 'apply' or otherwise prioritize them differently, and to have different views about their scope of application. Thus can acceptance of the four principles allow those who so choose to steer between the Scylla of moral relativism on the one hand and the Charybdis of 'moral imperialism' on the other; while at the same time allowing firm believers in a wide variety of moral theories on either side to accept them both because these *prima facie* principles are implied by their own theories and as a way of sharing moral thinking with those who, for whatever reasons, reject those theories.

Finally, two challenges to the reader: which, if any, of the Beauchamp and Childress *prima facie* moral principles do you personally reject—and why? And which moral concerns in health care ethics do you personally believe are not encompassable within these four principles, and why? For my own part the answer to each question is none, and this view has gained strength from the contributions to this book, including those purporting to undermine the 'Georgetown mantra'. Secondly, unless you positively do find good arguments for rejecting the approach please think carefully before scorning it. It is, of course, a duty of the philosopher to criticize. But when he or she joins in the enterprise of health care it is arguably also his or her duty to help to promote its morally acceptable objectives. An analytic framework, elements of a common moral language and a basic moral commitment for health care ethics that is neutral between competing religious, political, cultural and philosophical theories and that can be shared by all regardless of background is surely too important a moral prize to be rejected carelessly, or for the fun of being a 'Socratic gadfly'.

REFERENCES

1. Beauchamp, T. and Childress, J. 1989. *Principles of biomedical ethics*, 3rd edn. Oxford University Press, New York, Oxford.
2. Gillon, R. 1985, and subsequent reprints. *Philosophical medical ethics*. Wiley, Chichester.
3. Aristotle, *Nichomachean Ethics*, Book 1, chapter 3 (1094b, 12–26).
4. I offer outlines of their arguments for this principle in Gillon, R. 1985, Autonomy and consent. Pp.111–125, *in* Lockwood, M. (Ed.) *Moral dilemmas in modern medicine*. Oxford University Press, Oxford. The original arguments are to be found in: Mill, J. S. *On liberty*. Variously reprinted, e.g. in: Warnock, M. (ed.) 1974. *Utilitarianism*. Collins/Fontana, Glasgow; and in Kant, I. *Groundwork of the metaphysics of morals*. English translation in: Paton, H. J. (Ed.) 1964. *The moral law*. Hutchinson University Library, London.
5. See for example Frankena, W. 1973, *Ethics*, 2nd edn, Englewood Cliffs, New Jersey: Prentice-Hall. Frankena argues that there are four types of beneficence; do not do evil or harm (non-maleficence on the Beauchamp and Childress analysis); prevent evil or harm; remove evil or harm; do or promote good.
6. See reference 1, especially pp. 55–62, and 256–270; and reference 2, pp. 54–59 and 86–92.
7. See for example reference 1, Chapter 8, pp. 366–399 on 'Ideals, virtues, and conscientiousness'; and reference 2, Chapter 5, pp. 28–33 on 'Conscience, good character, integrity, and to hell with philosophical medical ethics?'
8. Wikler, D., 1991. What has bioethics to offer health policy? *Milbank Quarterly*, **69** (2): 233–251.

PART II

RELATIONSHIPS AND HEALTH CARE ETHICS

29

Client–Health Care Worker Relationships and Health Care Ethics—Introduction

RAANAN GILLON

In this second section of the volume aspects of health care ethics arising in the context of relationships between health care workers and patients or clients are considered. Certain themes arise recurrently and are perhaps worth noting. The first is that there is a common commitment to benefit patients or clients. Regardless of whose perspective is being addressed benefit to the patient/client is at its centre. Even the relatively neutral perspective of the ethicist is seen by Evans as promoting the interests of patients, either by explicitly being involved, as in Research Ethics Committees, in protecting those interests, or more generally by philosophical reflection on the functions of health care that are acknowleged by health care workers—with concern for *patients as persons* being seen to be a necessary condition of clinical practice.

This latter point underlies a second theme running throughout this section, notably the need to respect patients and their autonomy, even if for no other moral reason than to benefit them. Here changes in approach to patients are recurrently acknowledged by the doctor contributors. Both Pellegrino and Higgs, for example, indicate that medical attitudes have very properly changed over the past few decades as a result of clearer recognition by doctors of the need to respect the autonomy of their patients—and both also point out that such respect is needed in the context of the traditional Hippocratic obligation to benefit patients.

A further theme is that conflict between beneficence and respect for autonomy is fairly rare—especially once it is recognized that it is no more paternalistic (paternalism being the over-riding or ignoring of a patient's autonomy in order to benefit him or her) to respect a patient's deliberate wish *not* to be burdened with unpleasant information, than it is to respect a patient's wish to be given such information. This point emerges recurrently, again particularly in the medical contributions.

On the other hand sometimes there is a clear conflict between benefit to the patient and respect for the patient's autonomy—for example if a patient does want to know a suspected diagnosis (say suspected multiple sclerosis or Huntington's chorea or cancer) at a very early stage, even though it is clear that the person will worry about it for the rest of what may very well be a very long life and even though the diagnosis is not conclusively established. Interestingly even Shinebourne and Bush, who ostensibly write in favour of medical paternalism, tend not to favour paternalism, as defined above, and favour honest dealing with patients who specifically ask for full information. 'Of course if the patient does ask specifically, it would be wrong not to give full information', they write. Conversely Veatch, a philosopher renowned for his support of respect for patient autonomy, and his vigorous rejection of medical paternalism, nonetheless accepts that there are rare examples of morally justified paternalism— but they are rare, a conclusion that seems to be shared by all the contributors who consider this issue. Wilson–Barnett, writing from a nursing perspective, is one such, opposing paternalism. She exemplifies her argument with the case of an elderly patient who was forced to go into a nursing home against her will, 'for her own good', and whose remaining life was significantly reduced in quality if not quantity as a result. Just as deliberate choices to live precariously are respected in young people so they should be when made by elderly people, she argues.

A DANGER OF MANAGERIAL PATERNALISM

An interesting slant on the conflict between respect for autonomy and beneficence is offered by Downie. Whereas he praises the contemporary tendency within medicine to recognize that respect for patients' autonomy is an essential aspect of medical ethics—and acknowledges that 'consumerism' may function as a means towards encouraging such respect, he warns of the danger, in Britain at least, that current health service reforms are replacing old-fashioned medical paternalism with new-fashioned managerial paternalism. Instead of choices being made by doctors in what they perceive to be patients' best interests, choices are now increasingly being made by managers in what *they* perceive to be patients' best interests (and within their ever more strictly limited budgets)— but the patients' views on their best interests are still being inadequately ascertained. Furthermore, contemporary British government moves to enhance the entrepreneurial spirit in medicine (as a way of improving financial efficiency) run the major risk of weakening the traditional special 'bond' between doctor and patient—a bond based on acknowledgement by both parties that the commitment of the doctor is to benefit the patient. Without this traditional commitment Downie warns of the danger that doctors will increasingly see themselves as businessmen and, for example, reject 'expensive' patients who will be a burden on their budgets, and meanwhile try to persuade those patients whose care they have taken on to accept whatever medical services are profitable to the doctor, rather than strictly necessary to benefit the patient.

The conflict between benefit for the patient or client and concern for others permeates many of the contributions. Once again the special importance of the relationship between patient and health care worker is acknowleged by all the writers, but equally, all acknowledge that concern for the individual can never take absolute priority over concern for others. The conflict arises especially acutely in the matter of confidentiality, and Black and Kottow, both doctors, give different accounts of how they personally would draw the line. Similarly Almond, in her discussion of rights, argues that patients' rights can never be absolute and respect for rights involves respect for everybody's rights. Taking as an example the currently proclaimed right of people to remain in ignorance about their HIV status she outlines the standard arguments in favour of acknowledging such a right, and then offers important counter-arguments to each, considering both the cases of patients with HIV and of health care workers, especially doctors and dentists, with HIV.

Another aspect of the conflict between beneficence to the individual patient and concern for others is the threat to the traditional doctor–patient relationship posed by medical research. This is discussed by Neuberger and by Baum and colleagues. Rabbi Neuberger, a previous chairperson of the Patients Association in Britain, warns that both financial inducements to incorporate patients in clinical trials and the increasingly scientific- and research-oriented ethos of medicine threaten the traditional medical concern for the welfare of the individual patient. Patients, she argues, ought to be informed of the financial arrangements underlying any trial in which it is proposed that they should be involved, including, and especially, any financial benefit to the doctor; and if a conflict arises between the traditional support for the individual patient and the needs of 'hard science', then 'it may be worth sacrificing some of the "hardness" of the science for the sake of the relationship with the patient'.

The dilemmas generated by the dual role of personal doctor and medical researcher are acknowledged by Baum and colleagues who, however, point out that without research current treatment cannot be improved, and doctors will not be able to provide the most effective—and the most safely effective— treatments for their patients. Houghton, one of Baum's collaborators, outlines a novel proposed approach, itself yet to be researched, in which a researching doctor explains to the patient that he or she simply does not know which of the various treatment options is the best, but is part of a national research structure trying to find out. If the patient is interested the doctor will write to the research body with the patient's details, who will then send the patient information and a simplified protocol of the trial. Alternatively the doctor will, from his or her perspective of 'equipoise' (or agnosticism) about the relative superiority of the various available alternatives, help the patient to decide which he or she would prefer. The attractiveness of such a proposal is that it combines both honesty about the doctor's knowledge, or rather lack of knowledge, about the best treatment, and the offer of participation in trials to try to remedy this, with the traditional readiness of a personal doctor to try to help the patient reach the best available decision if he or she does *not* wish to participate in a clinical trial.

THE MORAL—AND LEGAL—IMPORTANCE OF GOOD COMMUNICATION

Underlying all the contributions are two shared assumptions—first that health care is essentially beneficial in intent; but second that health care is an enterprise crucially dependent on explicit or implicit consent of the cared-for. Thus health care is not only essentially a beneficence-oriented enterprise but it is also an essentially autonomy-respecting enterprise. And many of the contributors to this section point out that in order to achieve those joint moral objectives, good communication with the patient is a *sine qua non*. Nowhere is this more important than in explaining adequately to patients the anticipated risks and benefits of proposed treatments—as Henderson explains in his chapter on risk, and Kirby does in his account of consent from the perspective of the law. It is, says the latter, an abiding complaint of patients otherwise quite satisfied with their relationship with their doctors, 'that they are not allowed to participate sufficiently in deciding about their treatment nor given enough information to enable them to do so'.

Seeing the law as constantly developing, Kirby mounts a vigorous attack on the English legal doctrine known as the 'Bolam principle', whereby the standard of what is to be regarded as medical negligence is determined by a body of responsible medical opinion (even if there is another body of responsible medical opinion that disagrees). As applied to the question of what information a patient ought to be given it is 'a relic of an earlier time' and 'turns the nature of the profession on its head. It is not there for the good of doctors. It is there for the benefit of patients. The only authority and legitimacy of the doctor to intervene in the life and body of the patient is, respectful of the patient's individuality, with that patient's informed consent.' And he quotes with approval another judge, the English law lord, Lord Kilbrandon, on the relationship between doctor and patient: 'it is not fundamentally the expert instructing the ignorant, even though those terms may accurately classify the respective parties. One free human being advises and helps another. The relevant law exists for the purpose of supporting that relationship.'

The relevance of the Beauchamp and Childress four-principles-plus-scope approach recurs throughout these chapters, with the relationship between patient and health care worker emerging clearly as one that is essentially beneficent in intent and essentially respectful of the patient's autonomy, whether because such respect is morally necessary in its own right or because it is a means of achieving the intended benefits. However it is also constrained by the principle of non-maleficence, with harm only morally permitted as part of the overall objective of attaining net benefit. And it is also constrained by justice, whether in the context of fair distribution of scarce resources, in the context of respect for everybody's rights, or in the context of respect for morally acceptable laws.

What also emerges in these chapters is the fact that the Beauchamp and Childress principles do not provide a decision procedure for choosing between the principles when these conflict (these principles were never, of course, claimed to offer any such decision procedure). Several alternative methods for doing so are advocated in different contexts, and usually in passing, among them

Aristotelian 'practical wisdom' (Jackson), 'judgement' (Almond), legal mechanisms (Kirby, Kottow), professional consideration of cases (Black) and, perhaps most challengingly of all, explicit decision mechanisms based on numerical weighting of competing values (Dowie—his chapter can be seen as almost entirely concerned with methods of decision-making in the case of conflicting moral values). Suffice it to say that whatever method of deciding between competing moral values the individual moral agent decides to adopt, those values themselves can be seen to be encompassable within the framework of the Beauchamp and Childress four principles plus consideration of their scope of application.

30

The Doctor–Patient Relationship

R. S. Downie, MA, BPhil, FRSE

Professor of Moral Philosophy, University of Glasgow, UK

The doctor–patient relationship is commonly seen as the central feature of medical practice; it is by means of this relationship that a doctor exercises professional skills and pursues the aims of medicine. The analysis of this relationship and a consideration of the current challenges to it are the main concerns of this chapter.

THE TRADITIONAL VIEW

We can use the word 'relationship' in two ways: to stand for the bond which links two or more people, or to stand for the attitudes which bonded people have to each other (this argument is further developed in ref. 1). As examples of the first kind of relationship we might mention kinship, marriage, business association, or teacher–pupil. As examples of the second kind we might mention fear, pride, respect, envy, contempt, etc. Thus someone seeing an adult with a child might ask 'What is the relationship between these two?', and receive an answer in terms of the first kind of relationship: 'teacher and pupil', 'father and son', etc. Or he might ask 'What sort of relationship do Jones and his son have?', and receive an answer in terms of the second kind of relationship: 'Jones loves his son but his son can't stand him'.

The two kinds of relationship are connected in various complex ways. For example, if the situation is a business transaction then the attitude of the parties would not characteristically be one, say, of affection or friendship. There are, of course, no logical impediments to such an attitude developing out of the business transaction; indeed it is material for romantic comedy when the attitude in the relationship is inappropriate for the bond. What, then, are the special characteristics of a doctor–patient relationship?

Let us begin by anatomizing the attitudinal aspect of the relationship. To understand an attitude we must consider its object. The object of the professional attitude is the patient or client conceived in terms of vulnerability; typically there is inequality of power. This is obviously the case in a doctor–patient or

Principles of Health Care Ethics. Edited by Raanan Gillon.

teacher–pupil relationship. It can be argued that, because of the dominant position which doctors occupy in the relationship with their patients, and because as doctors they must supply a service, and often also assess its success, they must be governed more than many other people by principles of ethics; in particular in this context they must be governed by a desire to be of assistance to their patients, often called 'beneficence'.

The inequality of the professional relationship requires not only a special attitude, it also requires a special 'bond' which usually takes the form of an institutional role relationship. The need for a formal bond in addition to an appropriate attitude is evident if we consider the significant interventions which doctors can make in the lives of their patients. We could approach this point in another way. We can characterize the doctor as someone who necessarily aims at health. It follows that the doctor's activities intimately bear on human good and harm, and therefore the state will take an interest in them. For example, the state will lay down broad conditions for the qualifications of doctors, or specify when a patient has a legal right to medical care, to hospitalization and so on. There may even be cases, perhaps of certain infectious or psychiatric disorders, where the doctor has a duty to commit the patient to care against his or her wishes. In the latter case the authority by which a person may be compulsorily detained in a hospital obtains legally in Britain from an Act of Parliament. The professional bond is constituted, secondly, by rather more vague sets of rules, or even expectations, which doctors and patients have of each other. Doctors often refer to this as the 'ethics' of their profession, and the medical profession is very strict about enforcing its own discipline on these matters.

It is important that the doctor–patient relationship should be constituted, at least partly, by these legal and quasi-legal institutional bonds, for at least the following reasons. Firstly, because doctors and all health and welfare workers, by the nature of their job, intervene in existentially crucial ways in the lives of others. This is a serious matter and its consequences for a patient can be enormous. It is therefore in the interests of patients that there should be some sort of professional entitlement to intervene. In other words, if they are not simply to be busybodies, doctors must have the *right to intervene*, and if they have the right to intervene they must have duties and responsibilities; the concept of an institution encapsulates these ideas of rights, duties and responsibilities.

A second reason is that doctors must ask about many intimate details of people's lives, for example, about their marriages; and they also may conduct examinations of people's bodies. Questioning of this sort, far less physical examination, can create situations in which people can be exploited, or which could be embarrassing even to doctors themselves. The fact that it is an institutional bond which brings doctors together with their patients provides *emotional insulation* for both parties in such situations. Moreover, there must be some assurance that no untoward use be made of the information, that it will not be passed on to neighbours, etc. But the idea of an institution entails that of rules, and the rules can, thirdly, impose *confidentiality* on the doctor and provide security for the patient.

Fourthly, doctors are given a measure of *security* by virtue of the fact that they work inside an institutional framework. There are various aspects to this. For instance, it is good for all professions to have ways and means whereby new skills and knowledge can be shared, and in general whereby members of a profession can support and encourage each other. Again, doctors require legal or similar professional protection from exploitation, unfair criticism or legal action against them by their patients. Reciprocally there must be some institutional mechanism whereby the professions can criticize themselves and look for ways of improving their services to the public. These then are some of the reasons for which a complex legal and institutional structure has grown up governing directly and indirectly the relationships between doctors and their patients.

There are various desirable and undesirable aspects to this, but the relevant point for present purposes is that when the doctor or other health worker appears to be acting as an individual he/she is also acting as a *representative* of his/her profession, and to a lesser extent also of the state. In other words, the individual action of a doctor or other health worker expresses also the collective values of his/her profession; individual responsibility becomes collective responsibility since it is through individuals that their professions are represented. We might say that individual doctors represent their professions in two senses. First, they are the ascriptive representatives, in that the profession authorizes their actions, having sanctioned their training. Second, they represent the values of the profession insofar as they act in terms of its ethics, and its ethics are all-pervasive in the actions and attitudes of the individual doctor.

The aspects of the professional relationship which I have been discussing can be expressed through the concept of a social role, understood for this purpose as being a set of rights and duties to be analysed in terms of institutional concepts. When individuals have accepted a role they are authorized to act in certain ways. Thus, the traditional view of the doctor–patient relationship depicts it as a role relationship with the features I have noted; it is through the role so described that doctors and patients are bonded.

I have so far used the concept of a role as a way of linking medicine as an institution with the interests of *specific* patients, but it also enables us to refer to a broader social function which involves the doctor's duty to speak out with authority on matters of social justice and social utility. For example, doctors have a duty to speak out on broad issues of health, as, for example, they might speak out against cigarette advertising. In this kind of way the professions can be seen to have the important social function of regulators in the interest of general utility and justice. This is another aspect of the doctor–patient relationship; one in which doctors are concerned with categories or broad classes of patients, rather than with specific patients.

In sum, then, the traditional view of the doctor–patient relationship depicts it in terms of the doctor's attitude of beneficence toward the vulnerability of patients, and in terms of a set of institutional bonds, legal and quasi-legal, which can be united in the concept of a social role.

CHALLENGES

Consider the Following Imaginary Cases

> Dr G. has been qualified for many years and is well-liked by his patients. One of his female patients in her 20s has had a problem which has not been responding well to treatment. She approaches him saying that she has read in a magazine about new treatments for her condition. Dr G. feels slightly irritated, partly because he has not himself heard of the treatments and partly because he feels that it is not the business of patients to be suggesting their own treatments. He wonders what to do, and decides to tell her that his own treatment is the best.

> Dr H. comes from a medical family. His father had been a dedicated GP and his mother had been a nurse and eventually his father's receptionist. His uncle, now retired, had been a surgeon. It was always assumed that Dr H. would become a doctor and he has just passed through medical school and is in training as a GP. He was very upset to find that some meetings of the partnership were concerned with how to get rid of elderly patients who were likely to become expensive and a drain on the practice budget, and how to take on young and healthy patients. When he questioned these policies he was told: 'You've got to enter the real world—we're all businessmen now.'

These cases really contain two challenges to the traditional doctor–patient relationship which are connected but separable. The first is the challenge from patient autonomy, or the desire of patients to have more information and in general to be more involved in decisions on their treatment; the second is the challenge from the market-place, or the need for medicine to be a cost-effective service with all that that entails. Both challenges are being encouraged by the British Government, and both can be discussed under the heading of 'consumerism', but there are important differences between the two challenges. The first represents a challenge to the attitudinal aspect of the traditional relationship, but the second represents a challenge to the *financial infrastructure* of medicine, and therefore to the 'bond' between doctor and patient. The second challenge is more violent and radical. Let us look first at what can be called the challenge from patient autonomy to the traditional medical attitude.

The traditional attitude of medicine which I have discussed in my account of the doctor–patient relationship can be summed up as follows:

> *The over-riding obligation of the doctor is to treat her/his own patients to the best of her/his ability.*

In other words, doctors have traditionally seen themselves as dedicated professionals providing round-the-clock service to their patients—but service in terms of the medical perception of patients' needs. This is the attitude of beneficence in the face of perceived vulnerability.

The traditional attitude can survive several important modifications. For example, the idea of good treatment can be enlarged to include improved doctor–patient communication, for which there is currently much demand. Again, the individualistic, possessive ring of 'his/her own patients' can be changed into a more harmonious chime by introducing the idea of teams. The treatment of patients can be, and is increasingly being, shared by teams. It is true that many doctors express irritation at being lumped together with others as 'health professionals', but there is no question that increasingly health care is being delivered by teams. None the less, the teams are led by doctors and the crucial decisions are made by doctors. In other words we have a modification, rather than a change, in the traditional attitude.

The same conclusion can be reached if we stress the role of the doctor in providing preventive services or in health education. In these spheres developments involve the enlargement, but not the radical alteration, of the traditional attitude of beneficence, which is respected by a large number of patients.

The attitude, however, has also been challenged over the past 20 years, and the challenge can be expressed as follows:

The provision of health care is pre-eminently a matter of patients' rights to medical services, and doctors' duties should reflect this.

The main idea behind this challenge is that of personal autonomy. It should be assumed, according to this approach, that patients, like anyone else, are self-determining, self-governing people who are able to make up their own minds on appropriate treatment for themselves, provided doctors supply enough information. Emphasis on this approach is on the informed consent of the patient to any treatment offered.

If I were looking in detail at this approach it would be necessary to devote a large amount of discussion to questions such as the standard of information disclosure which is appropriate. Is it, for example, what patients happen in variable ways to want? Is it the standard of disclosure which would be typical of professional peers? Is it what the abstract 'reasonable person' might want? Similar questions can be raised about the nature of the voluntariness involved in informed consent; and there are obviously difficult questions about the elderly, the mentally handicapped, young children, and so on. These and many other questions related to the full articulation of the new attitude have been discussed by many others. My question is not here one of detailed analysis of the new attitude but of main principle. Can the traditional attitude which has been, and to some extent still is, transmitted by medical education be modified by this new approach without radical distortion?

My view is that it can. Indeed, it is already happening, for many medical schools now require courses which discuss such matters as patient access to medical records, communication skills, breaking bad news, and so on. In other words, the challenge can be met if medical education stresses *partnership* rather than paternalism. This change can be assimilated into medical practice because patients remain patients, except that they have heightened awareness of their rights as consumers of health care, and doctors are able to have cognizance of this.

In terms of the second and more radical challenge to the traditional doctor–patient relationship the financial considerations of being a consumer and being a supplier or provider of medical services come into the foreground. This is a radical challenge because traditionally doctors saw themselves, first and foremost, as being members of a profession; but now they are being encouraged by the government to see themselves as businessmen. Patients are to become customers or users, and doctors to become suppliers. In discussing this important development we must consider whether the changes are simply terminology. Are the changes simply in political rhetoric, or are they likely to be in the 'bond' of the doctor–patient relationship? What's in a name?

There are two approaches to the question of 'What's in a name?' which do not lead to anywhere of interest, but since it is tempting to go down these roads it may be helpful to show why each is a *cul de sac*.

It is not uncommon to assume that it is possible to determine what something is by using a dictionary. Thus a dictionary may tell us that a patient means (among other things) someone who goes to a medical practitioner, and a customer or consumer is someone who goes to a retailer. It seems to follow that these are two different concepts with nothing in common, and indeed the same might be thought to follow even if we adopt more sophisticated sociological definitions of each. But it is not possible to stop social and economic change by using a dictionary. The important question is rather whether patients are nowadays adopting some of the characteristics of consumers, and whether they should be encouraged to do so. Equally, we can ask whether doctors should be encouraged to see themselves as suppliers of services in a market.

Before we leave the unfruitful question of definitions we should also note a danger of the new rhetoric of health care—that the term 'consumer' becomes like the abstraction of the economic textbook 'rational economic man'. The truth is that consumers come in all shapes and sizes and can be disabled, mentally handicapped, elderly, etc. In other words we are not comparing just two concepts—the patient and the consumer—but a host of related concepts. So while it might be possible for *some* patients to adopt the characteristics of some consumers, it may not be possible for other patients to be like any consumer.

The second unhelpful approach to consumerism is from the moral high ground. The professions generally, and the medical profession in particular, sometimes approach the idea of business from a position of moral superiority. This superiority can be articulated in detail through a series of contrasts:

The professions	*Businessmen (the 'market')*
(a) Promote the interests of patients, clients, etc.	Promote their own interests, not those of customers.
(b) Fees incidental to professional activity.	Profits central to business activity.
(c) Professions concerned with real 'needs' of the public or important aspects of human life, such as 'health', 'justice' or 'education'.	Business concerned with wants or preferences (often trivial).
(d) Professions have duty to comment on broad matters of public policy.	No such public or social function.
(e) Professions have political and commercial independence which makes their comments relevant to public policy.	Business lacks independence and its comments on public policy express vested interests or right-wing politics.

(f) Professions have knowledge base which requires a broad education.	Business has shallower, opportunistic knowledge base for which 'training' is a more appropriate term than education.

These contrasts create a sense of moral superiority in the professions, whereas businessmen respond aggressively with claims such as 'We live in the real world not in an ivory tower', or 'We earn the wealth of the country on which the professions depend'. But the validity of the contrasts can be questioned: some are based on conceptual confusions and others are outdated by changes in the knowledge base of business and a changed economic structure in society.

Take first the issues of self-interest and profits. The idea here is that, on the one hand, the patient is vulnerable as we have said, in that he/she lacks information and may be sick, so that the doctor is able to provide a service to the patient within a framework of professionalized beneficence; whereas, on the other hand, the trader and the consumer are on an equal footing and can then, directly or indirectly, establish the best deal which suits their mutual self-interests. But to be fair the contrasts must be drawn at the same points in the chain of service. The professional is described as beneficent at the point where the service is delivered—during actual patient care. But this is compatible with saying that medical contracts for services rendered are being negotiated at another point in the chain in a self-interested manner. Equally, a business may establish its prices in a self-interested way—the astute businessman will consider what price the market will stand—but that is compatible with saying that at the point of delivery of service a salesman may offer his advice to a customer in a beneficent manner by considering what it is that would best suit the requirements of the customer.

It is simply a muddle to contrast the benign service at which the doctor aims with the self-interested profit at which the businessman aims. The doctor supplies medical services to the patient in a benign way but doctors are also fee-earners, and it would be disingenuous to pretend that their professional associations do not attempt to maximize their fees. Equally, businessmen are also suppliers of the goods and services necessary for the well-being of social life, and it is unfair to suggest that at the point of delivery there is no attempt to provide a service fitting the needs of the consumer.

Consider, secondly, the contrast between the alleged ideals served by the professions and the 'trifles of frivolous utility' offered by the market. Sometimes this contrast is stated as one between important human *needs*—health, justice or education—and superficial human *wants* or *preferences*. But this is unfair too. There are trivial sides to the professions—the cosmetics of health care or the frivolities of litigation—whereas the market characteristically supplies the necessities without which we cannot exist.

A third difference sometimes stressed between business and the professions concerns the alleged social function of the professions. It is clear that the health professions will be concerned with the interests of *specific* patients but, as we have seen, they also have a broader social function. For example, doctors have a duty to speak out on broad issues of health, as for example they might speak out against cigarette advertising.

But businessmen too can have a wider social function outside the concerns of their specific industries. Bodies such as the Confederation of British Industry are widely recognized as having the function of commenting on broad matters of social utility, and industry is increasingly involved in such matters as the sponsorship of the arts.

Fourthly, take the matter of independence. There was a historical period when it might have been claimed that only the professions had the political and commercial independence which enabled their comments to be disinterested. But this is no longer true. All the professions are in varying ways dependent both on governments and/or commercial support. For example, in medicine there is a suspicion that drug companies in many ways, some crude and some subtle, control at least some of the activities of the medical profession. On the other hand, whereas the primary duty of individual companies is to their shareholders, there are national bodies which speak their mind on broad policy issues and are no more subservient to the government than the British Medical Association.

Finally, it is certainly important that members of the professions should be educated as distinct from merely trained men and women. But the professions no longer have a monopoly of educated men and women. Large numbers of graduates enter industry and business; indeed if we consider the complexities of the technology involved at all levels it is clear that business requires educated as well as trained men and women.

The conclusion of this section is that the traditional contrast between the professions and business is based on misunderstanding of the present position of each group. As we move into the next century it is plain that there is going to be much more overlap, and that the professions have much to learn from business. It is therefore important to clear away uninformed, confused or emotionally based prejudice. It is also important to consider just what and how much the medical profession can learn from business which can improve the doctor–patient relationship.

The government, in a White Paper entitled *Working for patients* (2), is encouraging doctors to see their profession as a business. The hope is that there will be conspicuous improvements from the establishment of an internal market in health care services. What are these hoped-for improvements, and are there signs that they are likely to be achieved as the decade progresses towards the year 2000? There are three connected aspects of medical care where we might expect to see improvements with the establishment of an internal market: patient choice, quality of services, expenditure.

If patients are to be encouraged to see themselves as consumers or as customers then one obvious benefit which should be expected is improved choice. A criticism of medical services of all kinds, which has grown in volume from the 1970s, is that they are essentially paternalistic. To be paternalistic is to decide for others what they have a right to decide for themselves. Medical paternalism is thought to exist at two levels: at the point of delivery of the service (in the doctor–patient relationship), and in the selection of priorities in what is to be delivered (whether emphasis in the provision of services is to be, for example, on acute services or on the care of the elderly or the mentally handicapped). Will the much-vaunted internal market improve patient choice in either of these respects?

There seems little sign that this is happening. In the first type of situation—the doctor–patient relationship—choice *cannot* be achieved by a market mechanism, but only by the education of the doctor and the patient through medical ethics or the like. The greater the patient's information the more meaningful the choice, and the nearer the doctor and the patient come to equality. I have dealt with this in the first part of this section where I argued that paternalism can be changed to partnership without destroying the traditional relationship. But it is not at all clear how such a change could be assisted through the introduction of a market mechanism. Markets simply cannot help here.

When we move to the question of priorities in the provision of services, however, it is possible that market mechanisms can do more to improve choice. They can do so if patients, or at least bodies such as local health councils, patients' groups, etc., are allowed to participate in decision-making in the establishment of these priorities. For example, do we, the consumers, want a heart-transplant unit or do we want improved services for the mentally handicapped? The answer at present is that we have no choice. Decisions are made for political reasons, or as the result of powerful medical lobbies; they are not made by consumers. But local health councils could do a lot here. It is worth noting that *Working for patients* speaks of giving patients 'greater choice of the services available' (p. 3). But we might also want greater choice in *what* services are available. It might of course be argued that this is a *citizenship* rather than a *consumer* issue. The point is a nice one, but the issue remains.

Where, then, is patient choice thought to exist? Patients can choose what breakfast cereal they want in hospital! More seriously, they can choose their GP. But the latter choice can cut both ways. GPs with an eye to their budgets will not be anxious to accept high-cost patients such as the elderly. It is not even logically possible, far less practically likely, to change patients into consumers without also changing their GPs into financially interested suppliers.

Moreover, there is a serious risk of creating what economists call 'supply-induced demand'. To the extent that GP fees are linked to the supply of certain services, such as screening programmes, there is a danger that people will be encouraged to think that participation in these programmes is essential for their health, when in reality it is essential for GP fees. There are examples of this in the US (3). In short, in terms of possible increase in patient choice the introduction of business terminology has achieved little.

In the second place, is the introduction of an internal market likely to improve the quality of the doctor–patient relationship? Answers to this question will vary relative to the nature of those who are monitoring the services. In many of the large service industries, such as British Telecom, the Post Office or British Gas, there are consumer councils which monitor service. Those bodies have many lay members. In smaller businesses quality control is provided by the discipline of the market—competition from rivals. What happens in medical services? How are standards of care monitored? The position of the British government is that 'the quality of medical work can be reviewed only by a doctor's peers' (4). This does not sound like consumerism gone mad! It sounds more like the expression of a paternalistic monopoly. And what is being measured? Medical audit tends to stress outcomes, but there remains the quality of service in treatment. It is much harder to establish quality assurance here. Moreover, the whole issue of outcomes and quality of care is especially difficult in areas such as terminal care. The users of medical services, or their relatives or representatives, require to be empowered not only in the choice of services they wish, but also in the matter of evaluating the quality of that service.

The third area which was expected to improve by the introduction of a market is expenditure. Will a business approach to medicine cut costs as the decade progresses towards the year 2000? Will it have utility?

In answering this question we must avoid an oversimplification. It is easy to have a simple version of the market relationship in which we consider two parties only—the trader and the customer. But traders obtain their goods from wholesalers and manufacturers, and the market relationship holds there as well. In health care the market is one between different sets of managers—the managers of purchasing health authorities and the managers of provider units. The government may benefit here from cost-cutting—a reasonable objective— but the direct benefits to the patients or the users are marginal. Will the benefits even be passed on?

Some conclusions have emerged from this section of the paper. First, both the professions and business are evolving in this last decade of the century, and, in particular, concepts from business, such as information, choice, quality control and cost-cutting can be used to improve medical services, and therefore the doctor–patient relationship. There is a danger, however, that we shall have a manager-driven consumerism rather than a patient-driven consumerism, and it is far from clear that the result will be a user-friendly service. A genuinely market-based medical service might free us from most sorts of paternalism, but the service must be modelled on the right areas of the market or we shall simply be substituting managerial bureaucracy for medical paternalism. The doctor–patient relationship, either as attitude or as bond, will not be the better for the change.

REFERENCES

1. Downie, R. S. and Charlton, B. G. 1992. *The making of a doctor*. Oxford University Press, Oxford.
2. Ministry of Health. 1989. *Working for patients*. CM 555: HMSO, London.
3. Persaud, R. D. 1991. What future for ethical medical practice in the new National Health Service? *Journal of Medical Ethics* **17**: 10–18.
4. Ministry of Health. 1989. *Working paper on medical audit*, p. 5. HMSO, London.

31

The Four Principles and the Doctor–Patient Relationship: the Need for a Better Linkage

EDMUND D. PELLEGRINO, MD

John Carroll Professor of Medicine and Medical Ethics and Director, Center for the Advanced Study of Ethics, Georgetown University, Washington, DC, USA

INTRODUCTION

A little more than a decade ago, Beauchamp and Childress published the first edition of what has since become the most influential guide to biomedical ethics (1). They adapted W. D. Ross's notion of *prima facie* principles to the emerging field of medical ethics (2). Today, non-maleficence, beneficence, autonomy, and justice have become the reference *tetrad par excellence* which doctors and ethicists use to resolve ethical dilemmas and define the right conduct of doctors and patients.

As experience in the use of the four-principle framework has widened, shortcomings in its application to the clinical realities of the doctor–patient relationship have begun to appear. As a result, some moral philosophers today have called for the abandonment of 'principlism' (3) or its replacement by alternative theories based in virtue, feminist psychology, casuistry, or experience (4, 5).

In this chapter I shall argue that the four principles should not be abandoned. Rather, they need to be redefined and grounded in the reality of the doctor–patient relationship. This grounding can provide a standard against which the fundamental conceptual problem of conflict among *prima facie* principles can be resolved. This approach is also more congenial than 'principlism' to enrichment by moral insights from a variety of non-principle-based ethical perspectives.

The first part of this chapter describes how the emergence of autonomy as a dominant principle has altered our construal of the doctor–patient relationship. The second part details the conflicts that can occur among the four *prima facie*

Principles of Health Care Ethics. Edited by Raanan Gillon.
© 1994 John Wiley & Sons Ltd

principles when they are applied in clinical ethical decision-making. The third part offers a teleological foundation for the four principles as obligations of the good doctor. The last section re-examines the way philosophy itself is used as a tool in critical reflections on medicine.

AUTONOMY AND MODELS OF THE DOCTOR–PATIENT RELATIONSHIP

Nothing in medical ethics has changed so dramatically and drastically in the last quarter-century as the standards of ethical conduct governing the relationship between doctors and patients. In that time the center of gravity of clinical decision-making has shifted almost completely from the doctor to the patient. The traditional benign and respected image of the doctor as both moral and technical authority has been replaced by the doctor as protector, facilitator, and advocate for, the self-determination of the patient. Now, every facet of care, from the choice among preferred treatments to requests not to be resuscitated, and even for active euthanasia and assisted suicide, are construed as moral and civil rights with which doctors in good conscience are expected to comply.

This metamorphosis has been most evident and most advanced in the United States. But the sociopolitical and cultural forces that have nurtured such a drastic change are effecting similar transformations in almost every country of the world. Among these forces are the actualization of participatory democracy, the increasing moral pluralism and moral heterogeneity of modern society, expansions in public education by the media, the weakening of religion as an ultimate source of morality, a general mistrust of the exercise of authority in all spheres of life, and, of course, the unprecedented expansion of medical power through technology.

Not the least of the forces effecting change was the entry of the professional philosopher into the study of medical ethics. Curiously, philosophers historically paid little formal attention to the ethics of medicine. To be sure, there were 'philosophical' reflections by doctors on the nature of medicine and medical ethics, but this was philosophy only in the loosest sense. Until the mid-sixties, professional philosophers paid little formal attention to medical ethics.

This changed when medical ethics first came under serious philosophical scrutiny. Surely the most influential thrust in this direction was Beauchamp and Childress's *Principles of biomedical ethics*, first published in 1978, in which the four-principle approach around which this whole book is organized was first introduced (1). This book added the reinforcement of formal analysis to the more inchoate stirrings of social change which had already weakened the pediments of the traditional Hippocratic model of the doctor–patient relationship. In its place a variety of autonomy-based models have gained pre-eminence.

Given the confluence of forces we mentioned above as characteristic of modern democratic, secular, morally heterogeneous societies, the principle of autonomy has had understandable worldwide appeal within and outside medicine. Autonomy, self-governance, and the right to privacy have become symbols of resistance to the misuse of authority by professionals, institutions and governments. Respect for autonomy seeks to balance the enormous power of expert knowledge which figures so prominently in private and public decisions in industrialized and technologically oriented societies. Autonomy calls for protection of the moral and personal values of each individual and, thus, of the integrity of the person.

Autonomy has had a particular appeal in medical relationships. It counters the historical dominance of benign authoritarianism or paternalism in the traditional ethics of medicine. It assures that patients may choose among treatment alternatives, and accept or reject any of them and, thus, retain control over some of the most intimate and personal decisions in their lives. Respect for autonomy also protects patients against submergence of their moral values and beliefs. In morally diverse societies where doctors and patients may come from markedly different cultural, ethnic, and religious origins, observance of this facet of autonomy is especially and justifiably cherished.

The assertion of autonomy in medical ethics has been salubrious on the whole. It has become a powerful and increasingly effective deterrent to abuses of doctor power. It has served particularly well in placing the ultimate control of decisions at the beginning and ending of life more fully in control of the patient. It is the driving force behind judicial opinion and legislation which confirm the legal rights of patients to make their own decisions and to make use of advance directives to assure control of decisions if competence to do so is lost in the course of an illness.

The emphasis on autonomy has also fostered the emergence of several models of the doctor–patient relationship sharply divergent from traditional models (6). Two examples are the consumer and the negotiated contract models.

In the consumer model, health care is viewed as a commodity or service, like any other commodity, to be purchased in the marketplace on the consumer's terms, i.e. in terms of his personal assessment of alternative modes of treatment, their cost, benefits and risks. The doctor is a provider whose task it is to provide reliable information, perhaps to advise, but not to interject her own values. The patient's values must predominate and the doctor's moral obligations are to inform, to perform with competence, and to protect and enhance the patient's capabilities for self-determination.

In the negotiated contract model, doctor and patient discuss their relative values in advance—those related to health and those related to moral values in general. As in the consumer model, the doctor and patient are both autonomous persons entering a contract, but in the negotiated model the details of the contract are more intensively examined before any medical relationship is entered. Moreover, the nature of the relationship is determinable only by the contracting parties. In essence, they alone must determine what conduct is expected so that the ethics of the relationship varies with the ethics of the contracting parties. On this view, the notion of a universally applicable set of ethical principles beyond autonomy is irrelevant: doctor and patient may pursue any course they wish, provided it is mutually agreed upon. That which is agreed upon is no concern of third parties. It might include active euthanasia, assisted suicide or an advance directive that calls for involuntary or non-voluntary euthanasia.

These two examples of autonomy-driven models of the doctor–patient relationship make the relationship largely instrumental and procedural. They are legalistic in spirit, and the ethic they engender is one of minimal personal commitment and trust. Indeed, they are more based in distrust than trust. They are also destructive of the idea of a common medical morality since the participants give medical ethics any meaning they choose. The only ethical failure is failure to abide by a prearranged contract.

While these autonomy-inspired models seem to protect the patient's right of self-determination, on closer inspection they are also, in considerable measure, illusory and even dangerous to both parties. First, one thing they neglect is the fact that doctor and patient are not Lockean free agents equal in bargaining power. The patient is vulnerable since she is the one in need of help, has not the power to heal herself, is in pain, anxious, frightened, perhaps distressed. It is hard to imagine a valid contract in which one of the parties is so dependent upon the other for the information necessary to a choice, and upon the competence of the other to carry out the choice once it is made.

Autonomy-based models thus seem oblivious to the incontestable fact of doctor power, a power that arises from several sources. There is the *de facto* power mentioned above, which derives from the fact of illness itself. But there is also the power of the doctor's personality or charisma which operates in subtle ways often inapparent to both doctor and patient but, nonetheless, a powerful force in shaping even the independently minded patient's decisions. Finally, there is the force of social sanction of medicine and its monopoly of medical knowledge which operate regardless of the details of a negotiated contract.

The realities of these forms of 'Aesculapian power' make it amply evident that the desire to limit trust in the doctor which lies behind the autonomy models is often deceptive. There is no way to circumvent the doctor's character or her construal of what autonomy means in actual practice. In fact, to execute a contract is to send a signal of distrust of the doctor and to put her on her guard. As a result she might restrain her inclinations to be beneficent when the clinical situation changes in ways that could not be anticipated. In any case, there is no evidence that a relationship based in mistrust is any more protective of patient autonomy than one based in trust, i.e. in a covenant rather than a contract (7).

The deficiences of autonomy-based models of the doctor–patient relationship do not, of course, vitiate the validity of autonomy as a moral principle. There is no question that the centuries-old neglect of the role of the patient in decisions that affect him is not, and was not, morally defensible, even if it was socially tolerable. Respect for the patient's self-determination and, thus, for the integrity of the person, is a moral requirement in all human relationships and especially in those like medicine in which there is a *de facto* imbalance of power. What the deficiencies of the models that try to optimize autonomy reveal is not that autonomy is to be abandoned, but that absolutization is morally perilous. If autonomy itself is to be safeguarded, its expression must be more closely related with the other major principles of beneficence and justice, as well as with theories of medical ethics which are not principle-based.

CONFLICTS OF AUTONOMY WITH BENEFICENCE

A second consequence of the autonomy movement is the degree to which patient self-determination is set in polar opposition to beneficence. This emerges very clearly in Beauchamp's book with L. B. McCullough (8). Here, beneficence is erroneously equated with paternalism. The case examples used to illustrate the conceptual content of the text choices are framed almost exclusively as conflicts between beneficence and autonomy. Several misconceptions arise as a result.

First of all, beneficence and paternalism are not synonymous. Paternalism (or maternalism) assumes that the doctor knows better than the patient what is in the patient's best interests, or that a mentally competent patient cannot possibly know enough about the choices to be able to make intelligent decisions. Or, less benignly, the doctor may assume that it is her prerogative as the privileged proprietor of medical knowledge and skill to dispense it as she sees fit without the patient's interference.

Paternalism, whether benignly intended or not, cannot be beneficent in any true sense of that word. Beneficence, and its corollary, non-maleficence, require acting to advance the patient's interests, or at least not harming them. It is difficult to see how violating the patient's own perception of his welfare can be a beneficent act. Paternalism is obviously in a polar relationship with autonomy, but it is also diametrically opposed to beneficence and non-maleficence as well.

True beneficence, on the other hand, seeks the good of the patient. That good is a compound idea consisting in an ascending hierarchical order starting with (a) what is medically good, i.e. restoration of physiological functioning and emotional balance; (b) what is defined as good by the patient in terms of his perception of his own good; (c) what is good for humans as humans and members of the human community; and (d) what is good for humans as spiritual beings (9).

In this hierarchical order, autonomy is a good of humans as humans. Without freedom and the capacity to make choices about our own lives, to be responsible for those choices and to carry out a life-plan, we cannot express our humanity fully. To violate or impede a patient's autonomy is a maleficent act. To facilitate, enhance and restore the capability for self-governance is a beneficent act. Beneficence and respect for persons, which is the moral foundation for autonomy, are, therefore, congruent, and it is a misconception to see them as antithetical as some interpreters of the four principles do. Later in this chapter I will suggest an alternative perspective on the four principles which may help to resolve potential conflicts between autonomy and beneficence as well as the potential conflict with justice.

CONFLICTS OF AUTONOMY AND JUSTICE

If the antinomy between respect for autonomy and beneficence is more apparent than real, this is not the case with autonomy and justice. It can happen that respecting the autonomy of the patient may inflict harm on third parties near to, or distant from, the patient. Here we face a fundamental dilemma of the idea of *prima facie* principles. When two such principles are in conflict with each other we must choose between them. To do so one principle must trump the other. But how do we decide which one?

Justice is the most complex of the four principles, and the only one that is simultaneously a virtue and a principle. As a virtue it is a character trait, a habitual disposition to render to each what is due him. As a principle it ordains that we act in such fashion that we render to each what is due her, and that we treat like cases alike. There is, thus, an element of justice in each of the other principles since we owe it to humans not to harm them, to respect their autonomy, and to do good when we can. Justice, therefore, has a certain prior status in determining the right and the good. In this sense it limits the exercise of our own autonomy and our obligation to respect the autonomy of others. Justice thus sets limits on the absolutization of autonomy to which the autonomy-based models of the doctor–patient relationship tend.

Some examples in which respect for the autonomy of one person may impose injustice on another are these: the patient, seropositive for HIV infection, who refuses to disclose the fact to her sexual partners or persists in unprotected sexual intercourse; the airline pilot or railroad engineer who refuses to disclose her substance abuse to her employer; the patient who demands marginally beneficial treatments that use up inordinate amounts of health care resources; the psychiatric patient who intends to harm others (10).

Respecting the patient's autonomy can also compromise the autonomy of the doctor—not his autonomy to treat as he sees fit without reference to the patient's best interests, but his autonomy as a human being with his own values and beliefs. An example of this type is the demands of some patients, on grounds of patient autonomy, that the doctor violate standards of good care to provide treatments that are scientifically dubious. Of like kind are demands that the doctor perform abortion, participate in euthanasia, or withdraw artificial feeding and hydration when these actions would violate his personal conscience.

Instances of this kind are increasing as the pressure to absolutize the individual's autonomy become more insistent. There is a growing sentiment in certain public and private quarters that the doctor is merely the instrument of the patient's will. Some have even argued that the doctor should leave personal morality behind in her professional life. On this view, not to provide what the patient wants, or what institutional policy or financial considerations dictate, is to violate not only the rule of autonomy but also beneficence and, indeed, justice. On this view, the doctor's monopoly of medical knowledge is taken as warrant to justify the patient's claim irrespective of the doctor's values.

Judgements about how best to resolve the conflict between *prima facie* principles, or, perhaps more accurately, individual interpretations of how those principles ought to be applied, are difficult. I have suggested justice has a trumping function. Under what circumstances should it take moral precedence over autonomy? These circumstances would obtain when there is an identifiable harm of serious nature to a third party or parties and all other measures to protect autonomy have been taken. These conditions would be met in the case of the patient with HIV infection or the operators of public conveyances where even the small possibility of grievous harm to others outweighs the claim to autonomy and preservation of confidentiality. The harm to others is more remote and less clearly identifiable in cases where patients demand dubious, marginal, or excessively costly treatments. Here the doctor might more readily balance the psychological benefits to the patient against possible indefinite harm to others.

When the patient or social policy dictates that the doctor submerge her own moral values to accommodate patient demands, even if what is demanded is accepted practice, then the conflict is between the patient's and the doctor's autonomy. Here we must argue that the doctor, no less than the patient, is a moral agent, that her autonomy is as deserving of respect as the patient's, and that justice would require that neither doctor nor patient impose her values on the other. If it is maleficent to violate the autonomy of the patient, it is equally maleficent to violate that of the doctor.

In practical terms this will mean that, institutionally and ethically, mechanisms must be devised to permit doctors as well as patients to withdraw from their relationship. This must be done amicably, respectfully, and only after another doctor has agreed to accept the transfer of responsibility for the care of the patient. The doctor cannot withdraw without first making provisions for transfer to another doctor, because to do so would constitute abandonment, in itself a serious breach of ethical obligation.

Proxy and Surrogate Decisions

The potential conflict between autonomy, justice and beneficence becomes more acute and more complex when the moral right of autonomy is exercised by a surrogate. This is the case with infants and with adults rendered incapable of self-governance by virtue of severe illness, mental retardation, or severe brain damage. Under these circumstances the moral right to autonomous decisions is transferred to a morally valid surrogate or to an advance directive (living will or durable power of attorney for health care). The surrogate or living will are intended to assess what the patient would have wanted were he able to understand and evaluate his clinical state as it is when the decision is actually about to be made.

Here, again, autonomy cannot be absolutized, although doing so would simplify decision-making for doctors and families. The doctor can be caught in a serious conflict of obligations. On the one hand, she is bound to respect the delegated moral authority of the surrogate or advance directive; on the other hand, she is also bound in beneficence and justice to safeguard the welfare of the patient against possible abuse by the surrogate. Doctors must daily resolve these conflicts in obligation. They cannot debate endlessly. They must make a decision. They must sign the order. They are moral accomplices unavoidably.

Many practical problems complicate the doctor's decision to agree with, modify, or refuse to comply with the surrogate decision. Application of the four principles is dependent on many factual questions with moral implications. First, is the surrogate morally empowered to act for the patient? To be so qualified, the surrogate should, in fact, know the patient's values and give some evidence of the same; she must be free of obvious conflicts of interest, such as having a large stake in the patient's will; she must not be in an emotionally pathological relationship with the patient which might lead to unconscious over- or under-treatment.

Even if the surrogate is free of impediments to act on behalf of the patient, there are many other possible sources of difficulty (11). We must know whether the surrogate actually discussed the patient's preferences with her, whether they were understood in the same way by surrogate and patient, and whether the surrogate is transmitting the patient's meanings faithfully. When the time lapse between execution and application of an advance directive is long, the diagnosis/prognosis may have changed substantially. One might then question whether it is a beneficent act to follow the patient's advance statement of preferences. What about psychological discontinuity? Is the patient now before us in a permanent vegetative state the same person who told us her preferences when she was well? When, in the interests of beneficence and justice, may the projected autonomy which a surrogate or advance directive represents be overridden? May there be times when a 'best interests' or 'reasonable person' standard is more in the patient's interests? (12).

My purpose in reciting some of these difficulties is not to suggest that the four principles should be abandoned—as others have suggested. It is rather to point to some important philosophical questions that arise from the experience of applying principles in the moment of truth, i.e. in the actualities of the doctor–patient relationship. These experiences indicate that the four principles cannot stand alone, that they need linkages with other sources of ethical insight, and that they need a closer grounding in the phenomena of the relationship, itself.

'TUNING' THE FOUR PRINCIPLES PHILOSOPHICALLY AND CLINICALLY

To bring the four-principles approach into closer congruence with some of the realities of clinical decision-making, we need to examine at least three questions: (a) How are conflicts between *prima facie* principles to be resolved? (b) How may other sources of ethical insight be incorporated? (c) What, finally, should the relationship be of formal philosophy to medical ethics?

The Conflict Between *Prima Facie* Principles

The framework of *prima facie* principles has unquestionably advanced the quality of ethical decision-making at the bedside. Its utility must not be lost in the current zeal for replacing it with alternative approaches which have their own inherent difficulties. The four principles have put the whole process of moral decision-making on a more orderly, less idiosyncratic and more explicit basis. They have raised sensitivities to ethical issues among all health workers, patients and their families. The general moral precepts of the Hippocratic ethics have been 'fleshed out' where they have been deficient, and provided with philosophical grounding where this has been lacking. Principle-based ethics has also provided a *lingua franca* for communication among doctors and ethicists whose moral presuppositions might otherwise have been incommensurable with one another.

It would be a retrogressive step, indeed, to drop the principles and return to some simplistic conviction of the sufficiency of the Hippocratic Oath to which many doctors subscribe. Equally unsatisfactory would be a too-ready acquiescence to the arguments of the anti-principlists who would substitute important but insufficient bases for medical ethics drawn from virtue, feminist, or experiential systems. These alternatives, valuable as they are, also lead to subjectivism, emotivism and egoism, the major dangers to which non-principle-based approaches are susceptible.

This is not to deny a central difficulty in the design of the system of *prima facie* principles. If these principles are to be honored, unless there is an overwhelming reason to do so, what constitutes an overwhelming reason? Is the justification for overriding made in terms of some other *prima facie* principle or some special circumstance? If it is another *prima facie* principle, then we face the problem of one principle having greater moral weight than another. There is no formal mechanism or convincing argument that would grant trumping privileges to one principle over another.

Clearly, *prima facie* principles cannot be used to resolve conflicts among *prima facie* principles unless some external ordering mechanism is adduced, as I have done above in my discussion of the autonomy–beneficence polarity. Could the trumping justification then simply be the circumstances? If this were the case the circumstances would, themselves, take on the moral force of a *prima facie* principle, or they would have to be justified by one of the *prima facie* principles— but which one?

Any and all of these attempts to resolve the conflict between *prima facie* principles must eventually put one *prima facie* principle against another. This leads to the logical errors of begging the question or circular reasoning. If this is so, then some resolution must be sought beyond *prima facie* principles, and this could come about in one of five ways: 1. abandon principlism altogether in favour of some alternative theory like virtue, experience, or feminist psychology; 2. retain principlism, but supplement it by insights from other ethical theories; 3. ground principlism more fully in the phenomena of the doctor–patient relationship; 4. some combination of options 2 and 3; 5. retain the four-principle approach without emendation.

From what I have already shown thus far, it is clear that options 1 and 5 are not adequate in the face of the practical and theoretical complexities described here. Option 4 seems the most promising, and this option will be examined briefly, leaving to another occasion its more extended development.

Principlism has sustained its most radical criticism in the work of Clouser and Gert and others (3,13). These authors point out what they take to be fundamental conceptual flaws in principlism as they are exemplified specifically in the work of Frankena (14) and Beauchamp and Childress. Clouser and Gert (3) (and also in this volume, Chapter 22) assert that principlism lacks systematic unity and thus creates both practical and theoretical problems.

Since there is no moral theory that ties 'principles' together, there is no unified guide to action which generates clear, coherent, comprehensive, and specific rules for action nor any justification of those rules (ref. 3, p. 227).

On Clouser and Gert's view these inadequacies lead to relativism, since principles seem to stand free of any grounding and since they may conflict with each other without offering a path to resolution. Similar criticisms can be found in the articles by Brody (15) and Green (13). Criticism of another kind comes from the protagonists of virtue theory, feminist psychology, casuistry or ethics as narrative, experiential or existential phenomena. Space limitations prohibit serious examination of these alternatives. However, they share certain perceptions that principle-based ethics is too abstract, too removed from the actual moral and psychological realities of actual people making actual choices and too male-oriented in its psychology and reasoning. They also aver that principlism ignores the character, gender, life-stories and cultural identity of moral agents. On this view ethics is more than a technical exercise drawing clear conclusions from clear premises. It is a personal act nuanced in a variety of subtle ways principles do not touch. As Oakshott puts it 'moral conduct is art not nature' (16).

One may agree that there is substance in each of these varied criticisms of principle-based ethics without also agreeing that they do away with principles, or are themselves fully adequate replacements. It is too soon to know how, and to what extent, they will modify the four-principle approach. The likelihood is that they will enrich and refine principle-based ethics but not replace it (17,18). It seems clear that a unifying theory of biomedical ethics will need to link principles with insights from these other sources. This is the most serious conceptual task biomedical ethics faces in the immediate future.

Principles, Philosophy and the Doctor–Patient Relationship

If principles do remain integral to biomedical ethics they will have to be more firmly grounded in the phenomena of the doctor–patient relationship. One may approach this linkage in two ways: one is externally, by the application of an already developed philosophical or ethical system to the medical relationship. This is the method used by the four principles, whether those principles are conceived consequentially or deontologically. The second way is to examine the doctor–patient relationship with the method of philosophy (critical reflection) but without the content of a specific philosophy in order to derive from the relationship what is required ethically and what principles best exemplify what is required. This is the approach via the internal morality of medicine. This is essentially a teleological approach in the classical, not the consequentialist, sense—that is, it is oriented to the ends and purposes of the relationship, and it is the degree to which decisions and actions of the moral agents—doctors and patient—approximate these ends that determines whether they are right and good.

Briefly, the ends of medicine are ultimately the restoration or improvement of health, and more proximately, to heal, i.e. to cure illness and disease or, when this is not possible, to care and help the patient to live with residual pain, discomfort or disability. There are many decisions along the way to these ends, but in each decision there is a fusion of technical and moral elements. If it were merely a matter of technical correctness, of medical good alone, the major moral principle would be competence. But the subjects of medical decisions are humans, and humans in special states of vulnerability—anxious, in pain, dependent upon the doctor's knowledge, skill, and trustworthiness, and responsible management of the power his professional status confers *de facto*. Moreover, the doctor offers to help and, thus, promises the vulnerable patient that she will help attain the ends for which the patient seeks medical help. This implies that the doctor will use her promised competence not for her own ends but for those of the patient and will, in ordinary circumstances, efface her own interests in respect for the patient, i.e. she promises to serve the patient's good. But this good is more than simple medical good, it includes the patient's perception of good, material, emotional or spiritual.

If these ends are to be achieved, the good of the patient provides the architectonic of the relationship. Beneficence becomes a requirement not of a system of philosophy applied to medicine, but of the nature of medical activity. Respect for autonomy is required to achieve the ends of medicine because to violate the patient's values is to violate his person and, therefore, a maleficent act which distorts the healing end of the relationship. Justice is a requisite duty because what we owe the patient is fidelity to the trust we elicited when we offered to help, when we invoked confidence in our willingness to act beneficently. In like fashion the derivative obligations are mandatory if we examine the nature of the relationship. We must keep the promise we made, implicitly or explicitly, to be beneficent, to protect the confidentiality (except as outlined earlier when harm to others is at stake), and to tell the truth, since to violate any of these trusts and obligations is to go counter to the nature of the relationship itself.

On the view I am taking, the four principles are derived from obligations owed by doctors. These obligations, in turn, derive from the promise to provide competent help which is at the heart of the medical relationship. The primary obligation which unifies the theory of medical ethics is beneficence—beneficence not mistakenly equated with paternalism, but beneficence-in-trust, beneficence which fuses respect for the person of the patient with the obligation not just to prevent or remove harm, but to do good. The primary obligation is not non-maleficence, which is a negative obligation required even by law. Beneficence requires preventing harm, removing harm and doing good even at some cost and risk to oneself. Thus, there is an implicit promise of some degree of self-effacement of the doctor's interests in favor of the patient's interests.

The obligations that arise from the nature of the relationship provide the theoretical grounding lacking in the approach through *prima facie* principles. Rather than principles, we can speak of obligations freely undertaken when we freely offer to help a sick person. Beneficence-in-trust—that is to say beneficence that encompasses the whole of the patient's well-being and not simply his medical well-being, becomes the ordering principle. This form of beneficence cannot obtain if we violate autonomy, justice, truth-telling, fidelity to trust or promise-keeping.

Beneficence thus becomes a principle that is also a guide to action. 'So act in your relationship with your patients that your actions are directed by the good of the patient, the primary telos of the healing relationship.' Beneficence as a principle is grounded in the humanity of the persons interacting in the medical relationship. That relationship is, as Oakshott says of all ethics, a relationship *inter homines* (16).

This approach has the advantage of deriving its obligations and its principles from real phenomena of the real world of clinical medicine. It reverses the usual way philosophy is used to determine medical ethics. Rather than taking principles already formulated in an ethical theory—consequentialist, utilitarian, or deontological—it begins with the phenomena peculiar to the activity in question and examines them philosophically—i.e., critically, formally, systematically, in terms of the human realities they exemplify. It may indeed happen, as in the present inquiry, that the results are similar to the four-principle approach. But the principles are grounded in a more systematic use of theory; its principles flow from obligations grounded in the special character of the medical relationship. They become more than a checklist of considerations for ethical discourse. They have a moral binding power grounded firmly in clinical realities.

Clearly, the teleological approach suggested here does not, by itself, constitute a complete system of medical ethics. To do so it would also have to link obligations and its primary principles to virtue ethics and incorporate insights from casuistry, moral psychology and experiential ethical systems.

The four-principle approach does have its theoretical and practical inadequacies. However, it should not be abandoned because it still has much to offer. Its shortcomings can be remedied. The one direction for refinement I have suggested is a closer and firmer grounding in the doctor–patient relationship. Another direction, which I do not examine here, is to incorporate insights from experience, moral psychology, casuistry and virtue theories. In the years ahead, such efforts could produce a more complete theory and practice of medical ethics provided that theory is firmly situated in the central pediment of all biomedical ethics, the doctor–patient relationship.

REFERENCES

1. Beauchamp, T. L. and Childress, J. F. 1978. *Principles of biomedical ethics.* Oxford University Press, Oxford.
2. Ross, W. D. 1939. *The foundations of ethics.* Clarendon Press, Oxford.
3. Clouser, K. D. and Gert, B. 1990. A critique of principlism. *Journal of medicine and philosophy* **15**(2): 219–236.
4. Gilligan, C. 1982. *In a different voice: psychological theory and women's development* Harvard University Press, Cambridge, MA.
5. Drane, J. F. 1988: *Becoming a good doctor: the place of virtue and character in medical ethics.* Sheed & Ward, Kansas City, MO.
6. Emanuel, E. J. and Emanuel, L. 1992. Four models of the physician–patient relationship. *Journal of the American Medical Association* **267**(16): 2221–2226.
7. May, W. F. 1983. *The physician's covenant.* Westminster Press, Philadelphia, PA.
8. Beauchamp, T. L. and McCullough, L. B. 1984. *Medical ethics: the moral responsibilities of physicians.* Prentice-Hall, Englewood Cliffs, NJ.
9. Pellegrino, E. D. and Thomasma, D. C. 1988. *For the patient's good.* Oxford University Press, New York.
10. Beck, J. C. (Ed.) 1990. *Confidentiality versus the duty to protect: foreseeable harm in the practice of psychiatry.* American Psychiatric Press, Washington, DC.
11. Buchanan, A. E. and Broc, D. W. 1989. *Deciding for others: the ethics of surrogate decision-making.* Cambridge University Press, New York.

12. Robertson, J. A. 1991. Cruzan and the constitutional status of non-treatment decisions for incompetent patients. *Georgia Law review* **25**(5): 1139–1202.
13. Green, R. M. 1990. Method in bioethics: a troubled assessment. *Journal of medicine and philosophy* **15**(2): 179–197.
14. Frankena, W. K. 1973. *Ethics*. Prentice-Hall, Englewood Cliffs, NJ.
15. Brody, B. A. 1990. Quality of scholarship in bioethics. *Journal of medicine and philosophy* **15**(2): 161–178.
16. Oakshott, M. J. 1991. *Rationalism in politics and other essays*, p. 296. Liberty Press, Indianapolis, MO.
17. Carse, A. L. 1991. The voice of care: implications for bioethical education. *Journal of medicine and philosophy* **16**(1): 5–28.
18. Jonsen, A. R. and Toulmin, S. 1988. *The abuse of casuistry: a history of moral reasoning*. University of California Press, Los Angeles, CA.

32

The Nurse–Patient Relationship

JENIFER WILSON-BARNETT

Professor of Nursing Studies, King's College, London, UK

INTRODUCTION

In essence the effects of nursing depend on the quality and meaningfulness of the relationship established between nurses and those they care for. The expression of caring and empathy denotes what is valued and identified by patients as the special contribution of nurses. Because of this close and often intimate presence it is particularly important to have guiding principles which protect recipients and providers. Through recognition of rights and duties related to moral imperatives, priorities and decisions in care can be more reasonable and justifiable. In nursing as in other health care professions the principles of preserving autonomy, doing good, avoiding harm and being fair or just should prevail. However, the nature of the relationship provides a particular perspective and context for their application.

In this chapter the nurse–patient relationship will be explored and future directions for practice discussed in the light of ethical considerations. Current views of nursing as partnership with patients and clients, of negotiated plans for care and health promotion which negate professional dominance are in contrast to some illustrations on nursing care of the elderly. Here, in particular, the autonomy and rights of the individual must be explicitly recognized to avoid harm, and questions of justice in providing care are very pertinent. In common with many of these aspects of care is the closeness and emotional caring involved in nursing which could be seen to endanger the independence of choice and invade the personal liberty and privacy of patients and others who receive the attention of nurses. Thus it is vital for nurses to apply and integrate the accepted tenets of ethical thinking outlined in Beauchamp and Childress (1).

'Individualized care' has become one of the most important concepts in nursing. This implies that nurses should understand the particular needs, views and preferences of each person and care for him/her in a way which reflects his/her unique perspective and situation (2). Caring is thus dependent on

Principles of Health Care Ethics. Edited by Raanan Gillon.
© 1994 John Wiley & Sons Ltd

understanding what is relevant and right for each person. However, ideas of what that care involves differ to the extent that a nurse should form a close relationship. Some would emphasize that caring implies how nurses deal with a patient, not how they feel about the patient (3). Through caring for someone it is thought one can do good and affect well-being or independence without a necessary emotional involvement.

Other writers such Tschudin (4) and Campbell (5) stress the presence and emotional generosity of a nurse as cardinal to the process of recovery and adjustment. It is the understanding, sensitivity and genuine concern felt by the caring nurse which builds the patient's trust and provides the added faith and confidence necessary for recovery or therapy. Yet ideas of 'companionship' and 'feeling for' are criticized as sentimental by Thompson *et al.* (3) and unsuitable for many in the present varied contexts of care. I would contend that this not only negates human feelings but attempts to distance professional carers and denies what patients and relatives really value about the 'magic' or essence of good nursing. Clearly there are variations in the degree to which this emotional caring is appropriate and the breadth of nursing from health promotion, to extensive care and long-term non-acute home care determines this. For many, however, it is the very warmth and sometimes loving contact afforded by nurses which helps them tolerate or overcome infirmity. Having said this, both carers and those cared for need to be protected from over-extravagant expectations or obligations. Principles which guide such relationships are not only useful but enduringly necessary to avoid infringement of rights for both parties.

Caring in nursing, Rogers (6) advises, involves individuals who are honest and dependable, who are clearly able to express their willingness to be helpful. Within such a caring relationship respect is necessary and the other person must be enabled to express his/her freedom. Empathy, the ability to perceive the feelings of another and the ability to communicate this is seen as central to the relationship and fundamental to making the caring process explicit and specific. Through this another person can reach his/her potential for recovery or health. Despite the lack of concept clarification here, this type of relationship seemingly pertains most to a long-term situation.

In other more acute settings, patients also identify the quality of friendship and open communication as a most important contribution from nurses. Oakley's (7) moving account of a student who helped her reflects this empathy and courage. In anguish through lack of information and frustrated by not being able to obtain the truth about her condition Oakley learnt to appreciate the most important feature of her relationship with a student nurse. This girl understood her distress and shared the information documented in the medical notes. Although this was probably not condoned by the authorities it satisfied and relieved the patient. Only through recognizing her needs and caring sufficiently did this student manage to alleviate anxiety, and by doing so convey how much she cared; enough to risk trouble for herself.

The willingness to recognize, share and attempt to resolve emotional distress epitomizes the caring nurse–patient relationship; although this is so important to patients it is apparently under-valued in many health care settings. An analysis of this in the hospice setting by James (8) may help others to recognize the emotional burden that nurses attempt to carry. Identified as 'emotional labour' James discusses vignettes and descriptions of the working relationships of nurses with dying patients and their relatives. Their aim to comfort and contain the distress in that situation is heart-rending, particularly when so many feel ill-prepared for this. Perhaps the main point of her paper was to demonstrate the importance of emotional caring as axiomatic for these nurses, and yet also to analyse why this is so under-valued in health services.

ETHICAL PRINCIPLES IN THIS CARING RELATIONSHIP

Nursing must certainly combine emotional care and rational scientific approaches to treatment. As members of a discipline which integrates and applies many subjects nurses are realizing the importance of moral issues in care. Nightingale (9) discussed the 'sanitary and moral' dimensions of nursing and, of late, ethical concerns have been highlighted in most educational programmes. Some (10) feel that the contribution of nurse ethicists has not been sufficiently represented, and point to the International Council of Nurses' Code for Nurses: *Ethical concepts applied to nursing* (11), adopted by all member-states in 1973. Despite wishing to establish an independent discipline of nursing ethics, reflecting the unique characteristics applying to nursing, most nurse ethicists employ the four moral principles referred to previously (1). It is the context of responsibilities, and thus the nature of dilemmas, which seem to denote a difference from mainstream medical ethics. Above all preserving the autonomy and dignity of the individual underpins the principles for modern nursing practice. Through this it is conceived that nurses will be helping and not harming. However, the extent to which this can be seen and applied intentionally for all in need is becoming more openly discussed in some situations.

Recent nursing texts and research studies emphasize the importance of reflecting the consumers' wishes and enabling them to make choices and feel they can influence the process of their treatment. These aims are concurrent with increasing pressure from consumerism in health care. Many of the claims sought and the nursing care recommended reflect the ideal of full and open information-giving, of full access to staff at times of need and the right to negotiate plans for medical and nursing care, in particular. Following the earlier *Patient's bill of rights* (12), drafted by the American Hospital Association in 1972, British hospitals here now increasingly reflected this declaration in their own booklets. Such rights are succinctly expressed by Thompson (13) as the right to know, to privacy and to treatment. This 'rights' movement was necessary to raise awareness that institutional care, in particular, was seen as depersonalized and routinized. Reports from the Health Service Ombudsman (14) indicate that the majority of complaints concern poor communication and inadequate explanations when plans are changed or adverse events occur. Staff are frequently also criticized for not apologizing when appropriate, and for lack of time spent with relatives, leading, it was suggested, to more litigation, which could be avoided.

Systematic information-giving has been encouraged as a consequence of much nursing and psychological research which has demonstrated positive advantages of this approach for patients and relatives. Reviews of this work (15) show that stressful episodes associated with hospitalization, such as admission, surgery or invasive investigations, can cause emotional distress with related physical complications, but these can be alleviated by supportive and accurate information on what will occur and how the individual can cope or 'control' this experience. This should be tailored to the needs of that person, provided in a relaxed and careful way, giving a clear account of anticipated events. Learning to listen to the wishes of that person and his/her relatives on what they want to know or discuss before providing such information is vital. Once more this reinforces the benefits of a good nurse–patient relationship. With open communication, and the right questions, exploring worries or preferences a nurse can form a sound rapport in quite a short time. This is becoming increasingly necessary when hospital stays are much shorter.

This type of role is shared by other staff, but nurses do perhaps have more opportunities to establish a relationship with patients whether in hospital or at home. It is perhaps more difficult to understand or become able to provide psychological care in hospital than in the community where the family and friends and home life add meaning to the situation. For this very reason it is quite essential to remind ourselves of the oppressive and powerful nature of institutionalization and realize that this can be harmful to a family's well-being, deprive a patient of liberty and easily cause additional distress.

PARTNERSHIP NOT MATERNALISM

Ideas for partnership in care, for negotiated care plans and family participation in care are foremost in most modern nursing curricula. Clearly the dangers of professional dominance associated with patients' passivity and dependence have been recognized. With increasing numbers of the very elderly and chronically ill in our society, and the recent emphasis on community care, health carers should attempt to promote self or family care and prevent further illness. Research on patient teaching (16) over the past 10 years demonstrates a substantial shift away from the unequal arrangement where the professional acted as teacher and the patient as pupil in a structured pre-planned programme, to a facilitative partnership. More recent studies employ interactive approaches to help a patient and family to cope with health problems together. They set the agenda through discussion, determine the means to solve various physical and psychological problems, and decide when the 'professional' is no longer necessary. The development of many self-help and patient-spouse groups also shows that, after ensuring adjustment needs are met, staff can often enhance autonomy and promote well-being by withdrawing rather than continuing to care.

In the past nurses have perhaps been too intent on patient care rather than family care. So often in hospital relatives are not supported or included sufficiently. However, much of the research mentioned earlier now gives clear evidence that giving information and support to significant others is equally important. By helping family members understand an illness and recommending ways of managing this a nurse may do much to enhance total recovery or adjustment. Conflicts between family members are probably less likely if concerns are expressed together. Such conversations seem to occur much more easily if open communication and care plans are conventional in practice. Importantly hospital-based nurses cannot fail to consider the future life and home situation of patients when they provide individualized and holistic care.

Related to the preservation of autonomy, the right to decide, choose and act according to one's volition is, of course, the right to know what is best for one's health. Nursing students and staff are being encouraged to consider the meaning of health and how to maintain or retain this highly valued state. Of interest here are the varied interpretations given to health promotion. Whereas Campbell (17) warns of the commercial and proselytizing approach, nursing authors (18) interpret health promotion as a facilitative and liberating process which enables people to become more informed and autonomous. Through a thorough understanding of a person's social and health situation it is considered possible to assess needs and clarify problems. Individuals and their relatives are given opportunities through open communication with a nurse (or other) to review their own lifestyle and opportunities. Imposition of professional views is seen to be inappropriate and less effective. In recent work by Macleod Clark (19), for instance, health visitors who listened more, reflecting on what the client said, only giving information relevant, were found to be more effective in helping young mothers to stop smoking for longer than others who tended to adopt the professional information-giver or teacher mode.

If the nurse–patient or health visitor–client relationship is to lead to positive outcomes the consumer's autonomy must be preserved, not only because this is ethically correct, but because it is also shown to be more successful or therapeutic. Contrasting pictures of health visitors as inspectors or surveillance officers need to serve as a warning. Bloor and McIntosh's (20) work comparing a therapeutic community with health visitors' practice highlights the real social gap between professionals and clients. The view that health visitors were not visiting to do good but to snoop and make sure the rules were followed led to subterfuge and resistance from mothers. Harmful consequences of mothers directly going against advice in child-rearing shows that there was an inappropriate relationship. Failure to establish open communication and reassure mothers that they, the health visitors, understood their needs and problems prevented any positive outcomes.

ADVOCACY OR AUTONOMY

Discussion of advocacy in health care has probably resulted from the need to reassert consumer autonomy. Unfortunately this is seemingly viewed with suspicion by different groups within the health service. For instance nurses' claim as advocates for clients who are unable or unwilling to express their wishes has met with hostility from the medical fraternity (see ref. 10, pp. 208–225). Even if nurses were considered appropriate advocates for some people it is probable that the principle of self-advocacy is more constructive and indeed more healthy. If all health professionals were mindful of the morality in protecting autonomy, ideas of advocacy would surely be irrelevant. Johnstone (see ref. 10, pp. 208–225) criticizes those who base the justifications for nurse–patient advocacy on a special relationship. In a masterful piece she refutes both the idea and the feasibility of this in practice. Advocacy should be aimed at achieving the wishes of a client, and therefore reassert the importance of autonomy, but it also emphasizes a professional model of practice which runs the risks of paternalism and assuming (rather than really questioning whether) one is acting in the best interests of an individual. However, the close integration and importance of these concerns are expressed in Curtin's words (21) quoted by Johnstone (ref. 10, p. 12):

> the end or purpose of nursing is the welfare of other human beings
>
> this end is not a scientific end, but rather a moral end, and the relationship is what creates the benefit of health

Ideas such as advocacy have also gained credibility because of the inability of some to become free-thinking or make choices. Old age and infirmity do not necessarily lessen this ability or desire; in contrast it is extreme youth and disturbed cognition which affect this. When acting on another's behalf all of us need to ask whether someone else should or could do this more appropriately or accurately. Responsibility to care and give respect to others, even if they have not asked or have been unable to ask for this, is more completely conveyed by the fiduciary principle. This implies that authority to care in such settings is derived from the trust that others, near to that person, or society, place upon him or her.

LIMITS AND CONFLICTS TO THE NURSE–PATIENT RELATIONSHIP

Fundamental to the close and supportive relationship that nurses can build with patients is their need to understand individuals' experiences and preferences. In order to gain this degree of insight, systematic and comprehensive assessment 'interviews' or conversations are necessary. Clearly this type of thorough assessment is not appropriate for minor problems or short periods of treatment. During this type of process much information is requested; usually based on a framework which aims to cover most aspects of living activity. With an easy communication pattern a nurse can manage this in an interactive and informal way, and may complete this in several natural stages. In contrast this procedure may become routinized, meaningless, without sensitivity or proper analysis on which to base care. Despite advice that this initial stage of the nursing process should not be seen as a task, this has become a great risk.

Unless such information is gathered considerately and pleasantly, and is used to tailor nursing care to the individual's needs, it is clearly an infringement of privacy and a laborious nuisance for both patient and staff. Patients could well object to this waste of time—often up to an hour. Intimate subjects are also sometimes included, such as normal bowel habits (a subject which seems to interest nurses exceedingly), and even sexual habits and preferences. It is debatable whether such information should be discussed and documented unless it really is pertinent to nursing and medical care. Yet the justification lies in the necessity to care for the whole person and understand them well as a unique individual, and thereby form a therapeutic relationship.

Preservation of personal autonomy and self-determination should govern assessment of individual and family needs. Given the ideal of negotiated care plans the first interview should really introduce the ground rules. In my opinion nurses should not invade areas of a person's private life unless these are first broached by the patient. If such records are seen as working documents, to be used to identify needs or problems together with the patient and his family, it is obvious that certain information is unsuitable. Added to this are the problems of keeping such information confidential, or rather sharing it only with those who have a professional responsibility for that person. It follows that anything divulged in confidence as part of this process should not be documented, and in any case permission should be sought before getting or recording all information.

Building a partnership in care is not always easy. This may not be related to organizational constraints but to the novelty of this or unwillingness of the patient and relatives. Despite the ideas emerging in primary nursing when responsibility for an individual's continued care rests with one nurse, based on a sound assessment, patients may not be 'ready' to choose either that nurse or to participate. Negotiating plans for care may be seen as beneficial to avoid dependency, but this should not be imposed by enthusiastic nurses. Brooking's (22) research within acute care areas demonstrated that many patients resist taking on responsibility for decisions, and relatives do not necessarily wish to be involved in care. Obviously the principle of autonomy must apply, and flexible approaches to care should be adopted. It is the assumption by nurses that people either do or do not wish to form such an open and shared planning process which should be avoided. Careful assessment might indeed indicate preferences, but this should be checked continuously. More common though, at present, is the omission by nurses to consider negotiation with the patient, and perhaps even to dominate decision-making, failing to offer choice. Current thinking on partnership and care may influence practice in the next few years, and if so perhaps autonomy would be safeguarded.

ELDER CARE: A REAL CHALLENGE TO AUTONOMY

By focussing on dilemmas in caring for elderly people, I hope to reflect on the principles expounded above, and demonstrate how they may conflict in practice.

Peggy was an 83-year-old spinster who lived alone in a large suburban house which was surrounded by a spacious and beautiful garden. As a young lady Peggy had attended horticultural college, and her abiding passion was now her garden. Since adulthood she had cared for her mother who had died 20 years ago. However, Peggy was fully adjusted to what she called her selfish life at home, entertaining many friends to tea and welcoming the rather infrequent visits from two elderly sisters and a handful of nephews and nieces. Her charming old-world humour, warmth and kindness made her a great favourite with all who knew her.

Unfortunately, for the last five years she had found walking extremely difficult and arthritis was making her life rather 'slow'. She was housebound and took half-an-hour to go up or down stairs. Her worst days, she would chuckle, were when she left her spectacles in her bedroom. (She refused to sleep downstairs—'that was for invalids'!).

The crisis occurred when she fell and was found after 12 hours lying on the floor. Her gardener alerted the GP, who insisted she be admitted to a nursing home 'to build her up and get her on her feet again'. Unfortunately, family concern was expressed in an over-protective way. As no-one was able to care for her at home they insisted she stayed in the nursing home. Gradually after a few months, when neither her mobility nor her resistance increased, she became disoriented and depressed. A painful mouth abscess required antibiotics and made her anorexic. She constantly expressed her desire to be in her garden and go home.

The doctors, nurses and relatives were distressed about the situation but felt unable to allow her to go home and risk another fall and a further deterioration in health. She died one year after her admission, never having seen her new trees flourish.

The conflict to do good, or in this case avoid harmful accidents, was felt to be stronger than abiding by the wishes of the patient. Insufficient community support obviously played a part in this decision process, as did the pressure from the rather distant relatives. However, this type of situation is becoming more common, and nurses and others must learn not to be over-protective as the primary concern for the elderly (as with other individuals) must surely be to maintain their quality of life, their dignity and enjoyment. If they choose to live a precarious existence surely it is not right to interfere. After all, others take risks with their health throughout their life.

More and more nurses will engage in caring for the frail elderly, and perhaps one of the greatest challenges is to preserve choice and respect. If for one reason or another institutional care is desired by that person, deemed necessary and appropriate, it is often nurses and those who help them who can really do most to make life good. Pitiful pictures of old people's homes or geriatric wards should motivate us sufficiently to do more to individualize and domesticate such facilities. Real differences in standards can be achieved through reallocation of resources, change in attitudes and continued education. Baker's (23) moving descriptive comparison between two wards for the elderly demonstrated how the senior nurse could determine the quality of life, the degree of freedom to choose which activities to undertake and when, and the type of relationships that some individuals were permitted to develop with particular nurses. On the other hand, priorities for orderliness among nurses, ideas of ward ownership and of staff leadership can spoil the life of old people.

The gentle, loving, chaotic sister who decides what to do with her friends (patients), brings in her dog, has ward gardening, beer evenings and no uniform surely helps the autonomy and dignity of patients within a loving atmosphere more than a nurse who provides excellent physical care, has a superb filing system and is admired rather than loved by all the staff and patients. Thus within this environment choices have to be made by staff too. Values and priorities obviously influence the care that is given. In Baker's positive example psychosocial aspects of care took precedence, but within some wards caring for the elderly, severe physical infirmity is prevalent. From my experience this determines the majority of nursing care, staff still talking about the 'work' to be done. Consciously reordering the balance between physical and psychological care is not easy in such situations, but so often is really necessary to fulfil the total needs of the patients and sustain individualism among them. Ethicists may see this as a question of justice. If some individuals in (non-acute) wards for the elderly require only a little physical care and others a great deal, this seems to control the times nurses spend with each person. Is this not unfair, given that needs for companionship and stimulation may be greater for the first group? A full range of criteria should be applied when distributing this precious resource.

Scarce resources, that is nurses' time and efforts, should be tailored to the needs and priorities of patients. But judgements about these are based on many factors, including the skills and attributes of the nursing staff. It is rare for ward staff to decide priorities together explicitly, but this may be necessary in order to decide what not to do. Community nurses are also making such decisions. One inner London health authority district nursing team have very unwillingly 'closed the books'. This occurred after much discussion with management and reduction of care to those 'on the books'. In the UK some patients are thus either being deprived of nursing care or kept in hospital longer than deemed necessary. Such constraint makes discussion of autonomy and patient choice rather tangential. Justice cannot seem to be done to those deprived of care by nurses. It is also difficult but necessary for nurses to distribute their time more explicitly according to principles of justice, even if these are based on rather complex theories at times seemingly impossible to institute (ref. 24, p. 91).

Expectations for better standards and more conscious grounds for decision-making in nursing are ever greater. Devotion to, and emotional involvement in, care is also being encouraged in this chapter. So what are the acceptable limits to giving within the nurse–patient relationship? Certainly ethicists recommend that where a nurse may be exploited there should be an explicit contract, or as May (25) suggests, a covenant, in which terms for withholding or withdrawing from care, despite the vulnerability of the patient, are made explicit to both parties. Agreement for such a continued relationship should be updated with each changing situation. Certainly with private home nursing this is very appropriate to avoid feelings of failure or abuse. As Gillon (ref. 24, p. 85) says, the patient's interest cannot always come first. Rights and obligations should be finely balanced in any service-based relationship.

CONCLUSION

Opportunities for beneficial nurse–patient (or nurse–person) relationships can occur in acute or long-term situations. They can be rewarding or comforting to both parties when based on sound principles which aim to preserve the self-determination and well-being of those in receipt of nursing attention. Current ideas for nursing progress accord with such principles, and whether these were influenced by consumers or philosophers is certainly less important than their recognition.

ACKNOWLEDGEMENT

I acknowledge the helpful suggestions made by Alison Dines, Lecturer, Department of Nursing Studies, King's College.

REFERENCES

1. Beauchamp, T. L. and Childress, J. F. 1979. *Principles of biomedical ethics.* Oxford University Press, Oxford.
2. Wilson-Barnett, J. 1988. Nursing values: exploring the clichés. *Journal of Advanced Nursing* **13** (6): 790–793.
3. Thompson, I. E., Melia, K. M. and Boyd, K. M. 1988. *Nursing ethics,* p. 180. Churchill Livingstone, London.
4. Tschudin, V. 1956. *Ethics in nursing: the caring relationship,* p. 14. Heinemann Nursing, London.
5. Campbell, A. V. 1984. *Moderated love.* SPCK, London.
6. Rogers, C. 1961. *On becoming a person.* Constable, London.
7. Oakley, A. 1986. *On the Importance of being a nurse: nursing and health care division of labour, past, present and future.* WHO Symposium on Post-basic and Graduate Education for Nurses. Helsinki, Finland, 4–8 June 1984.
8. James, N. 1989. Emotional labour: skill and work in the social regulation of feelings. *Sociological review* **37** (1): 15–42.
9. Nightingale, F. (ed. C.Woodham-Smith) 1950. *Florence Nightingale 1820–1910.* Constable, London.
10. Johnstone, M.-J. 1989. *Bio-ethics: a nursing perspective.* W. B. Saunders/Baillière Tindall, Sydney.
11. International Council of Nurses. 1973. *Code for nurses: ethical concepts applied to nursing.* ICN, Geneva.
12. American Hospital Association. 1972. *A patient's bill of rights.* AHA, New York.
13. Thompson, I. E. *Dilemmas of dying: study in the ethics of care.* Edinburgh University Press, Edinburgh.
14. Ombudsman's Report. 1991. *Annual report.* HMSO, London.
15. Wilson-Barnett, J. 1984. Interventions to alleviate patients' stress: a review. *Journal of psychosomatic research* **28**: 63–72.
16. Wilson-Barnett, J. 1988. Patient teaching or patient counselling? *Journal of Advanced Nursing* **13** (2): 215–222.
17. Campbell, A.V. 1990. Education or indoctrination? The issue of autonomy in health education. Pp. 14–27, in Doxiadis, S. (Ed.) *Ethics in health education.* John Wiley & Sons, Chichester.
18. Macleod Clark, J. 1990. Health promotion: working together. *Nursing Times* **86** (46): 28–31.
19. Macleod Clark, J., Haverty, S. and Kendall, S. 1990. Helping people to stop smoking: a study of the nurse's role. *Journal of Advanced Nursing* **15** (3): 357–363.
20. Bloor, M. and McIntosh, J. 1990. Surveillance and concealment: a companion of techniques of client resistance in therapeutic communities and health visiting. Pp. 159–181, in Cunningham-Burley, S. and McKeganey, N. P. (Eds) *Readings in medical sociology. The professional–client interface.* Tavistock/Routledge, London.
21. Curtin, L. 1986. The nurse advocate: a philosophical foundation for nursing. Pp. 11–20, in Chinn, P. L. (Ed.) *Ethical issues in nursing.* Aspen Systems, Rockville, Maryland.
22. Brooking, I. J. 1985. Patient and family participation in care: the development of a nursing process measuring scale. Unpublished. PhD thesis, University of London.
23. Baker, D. 1983. 'Care' in the geriatric ward: an account of two styles of nursing. Pp. 101–118, in Wilson-Barnett, J. (Ed.) *Nursing research: ten studies in patient care.* John Wiley & Sons, Chichester.
24. Gillon, R. 1986. *Philosophical medical ethics,* p. 91. John Wiley, Chichester.
25. May, W. 1975. *Code, covenant.* Hastings Center Report no. 5.

33

The Patient's View of the Patient–Health Care Worker Relationship*

Rabbi Julia Neuberger

Chair, Camden and Islington Community Health Services NHS Trust; Vice-President, Patients Association, London, UK

PUBLIC PICTURES OF HEALTH CARE PROFESSIONALS

It used to be fashionable for fierce patient advocacy groups to criticize health care professionals, and particularly the doctors, as if doctors and patients were in direct competition with one another, as if there was no sense of idealism amongst doctors and no sense of trust amongst patients, as if the purpose of medicine was not to cure, nor to alleviate, human suffering. In that arena, George Bernard Shaw's quip about doctors was entirely in keeping with the prevailing mood (it was read to the Medico-Legal Society in 1909):

> If you are going to have doctors, you had better have doctors well off; just as if you are going to have a landlord, you had better have a rich landlord. Taking all the round of professions and occupations, you will find that every man is the worse for being poor; and the doctor is a specially dangerous man when poor . . .

In some ways his comments could be echoed by commentators on medical practitioners in the United States, and, in the face of a rapidly changing health care system, increasingly here in the UK. There are, of course, innumerable amusing, and sometimes less than amusing, quotations about doctors. Curiously, there are rather fewer about nurses, and about other health care professionals. Nurses have an image, even now, of the lady of the lamp, rather than that of Mrs Gamp, and the patients' and the public's perception of nurses is that they

---

* Part of this chapter was previously given as the Upjohn Lecture at the Royal Society, London, in 1992.

Principles of Health Care Ethics. Edited by Raanan Gillon.
© 1994 John Wiley & Sons Ltd

are sweet, overworked, underpaid and angelic. Hollywood's picture of 'The White Angel' dating back to 1936, has not really changed all that much (see Hudson-Jones (1), especially her contribution entitled 'The White Angel').

So much for the negative perceptions. There are positive ones as well. No-one who has read the doctor–nurse romances in plentiful supply in Mills and Boon covers, or watched TV series about hospitals, real of imaginary, could have failed to notice the way in which doctors are regarded as heroic and valiant, let alone the serious picture of heroic doctoring in Somerset Maugham's *Of human bondage*, whilst nurses are doughty troopers, as well as having their angelic quality.

But one might well ask whether these are the real perceptions of health care workers by the public and the patients. The answer has to be that of course they are not, though there are some elements of truth there.

At the same time as showing these different views it is essential to stress that patients do not have a single view of the relationship between themselves and health care professionals. The approaches vary in innumerable ways, but for the purpose of the present discussion it is worth making the point that patient preference will run the full gamut of preference for a paternalistic approach ('You, decide, doc!') to one where autonomy is stressed ('Tell me the alternatives, and I'll make the decisions').

Alongside this enormous variation there is a growing sense of unease amongst many professionals themselves, and members of the wider public, about the standards within the profession. The concern now is to keep within the law, and not get sued, rather than whether the highest professional standards of propriety and probity are being maintained. That unease has led to 'Values education' in medical schools all over the United States, where a key part of the course is a weekly session on 'patient–doctor' relationships.*

WHY THE UNEASE?

For what we have are health care professions which have their roots very largely in the medieval guild system. The idea of 'professionals' is modern—professing a calling or a skill. It has a variety of elements within it, but certainly for the health care professions there is expected to be an element of dedication in the profession, a sense of service to the public, a sense of wanting to do good, and a sense of idealism. That is one side of the modern picture of the doctor.

Both the medical and the nursing professions believe that they demonstrate these characteristics, though where they come from is unclear. Doctors have had academic training for the past century and more, and have a strongly hierarchical structure, as do nurses, as well as what can only be described as an apprenticeship system of entering the guild.

A medical student goes through her pre-clinical and clinical training, spending some of the time on the wards. That time is usually on the 'firm' of a senior

---

* See, for example, the patient–doctor course taught at Harvard Medical School under 'The new pathway', with materials available from the Division of Medical Ethics, Department of Social Medicine, Harvard Medical School, 641 Huntington Avenue, Boston, MA 02115, USA.

doctor, a consultant, who is often treated like God. On the impression that student makes on that consultant, her future reputation rests. If she wants to please, and it is clearly in her interests to do so, then she must imitate the behaviour of that consultant. She must act as the apprentice, learn from the man on the job, imitate, stay silent very often, and then practise in the same way. Now that in itself is not necessarily the recipe for a progressive profession. Indeed, it has all the makings of a very conservative one, with its emphasis on imitation, rather than independent thought. Junior doctors, housemen, spend up to 108 hours a week on the job and sometimes more. They are *expected* to do it. The explanations vary, but include: 'It's the only way of learning the job.' 'I did it, and it was the making of me . . .'. It has all the marks of a male initiation rite into a peculiarly male world. It appears to have nothing to do with those whom the profession is, after all, there to serve, the patients. Indeed, it can only be said to be harmful to the patients to have young doctors in charge who are exhausted, unable to think straight, and there not to learn (there's no-one there to learn from, except the patients and the nurses!), but to survive.

POSITIVE IMAGES

And this is what the patient sees. But she also sees the hospital doctors working unbelievably hard, with immense dedication, rushed off their feet. And so busy do they appear to be that she does not feel that they will have time to answer her apparently stupid questions; indeed, she would be wasting their time if she asked them. She rarely stops to ask herself whether all the work these doctors or nurses are doing is in fact necessary, or whether it is not a way of making it impossible for her to ask the questions, putting her at an instant disadvantage because she feels she is interrupting something really important, without recognizing that the most important person there is the patient. Without the patient, the medical profession and the nursing profession would have no function.

PRINCIPLES LYING BEHIND PROFESSIONAL BEHAVIOUR FOR HEALTH CARE WORKERS

In this area it is necessary to go beyond the simple breakdown into four discrete ethical principles of beneficence, non-maleficence, respect for autonomy, and justice, and ask about another principle, concerning primary purpose. Who is the system designed for? Is the health care system designed to provide employment for the hundreds and thousands of professionals working within it, or is its purpose first and foremost to help and enable patients? If the latter is true, then there are serious analyses to be made of patient–health care worker relationships, where what is done in the name of the patient or the public interest is in fact in the personal or professional interest of the doctor or nurse or other health care worker.

PUBLIC INTEREST, PATIENT INTEREST OR RESTRICTIVE PRACTICE?

What restrictive practices can we point to in medicine, which are clearly in the professional interest rather than the public interest? Does the battle over prescribing rights for nurses figure as a part of this, where the public, and the patients, might be well-served by nurses being able to prescribe a limited list of drugs, but the doctors have resisted? For simple, basic things, for repeat prescriptions which doctors will give over the phone in many cases, for the terminally ill being cared for at home by home-care hospice nurses, there can be no genuine argument against prescribing rights for nurses. But there has been considerable resistance from the medical profession, because it takes away a power they have had, and held dearly unto themselves. What message does that send out about the relationship between the health care professionals and patients? And about the relationship between one discipline amongst health care professionals and another?

Within medicine there has also been an uneasy hustling over powers for hospital doctors and powers for GPs. We have seen swings towards and away from general practice as the fashionable area into which to choose to go from medical school, as the GPs have been seen as having the most interesting work to do and the best remuneration, followed by rows over the GP contract and the insistence on the filling of quotas for a variety of procedures such as vaccinations, followed by a move back to general practice as the power is seen to lie with fund-holding, and the accusation from hospital doctors is that it will be in the financial interests of GPs not to refer their patients to specialists in the hospitals but to perform more and more procedures within the GP practice. This, they argue, will lead to it being done less well for patients (not in the patient's interest). The argument that has been used against many of the 1991 health service reforms, especially GP fund-holding, from the BMA, has been that most professional of all, that they lie against the patients' interests. But when the financial deals got better, the BMA seemed to mute its opposition, presenting a strange picture to the patients. That was the case despite the legitimate criticism that fund-holding, unless universal, may allow some GPs to get services more quickly for their patients, thus disadvantaging the patients of GPs who are not fund-holders, contrary to the principle of justice, or equity, usually listed amongst the four governing principles of health care ethics.

But though that may be a legitimate criticism, it is an extraordinary fact, pointed out by Professor Frances Miller of Boston University, that those who argue it is unethical to allow one group of patients to take precedence over another do not argue the same way over private patients, who are always seen first—for money. Nor is it a small percentage of doctors who see private patients. It is estimated to be some 50% of all doctors, which is perhaps why the BMA does not argue that private practice is unethical, although it gives some patients clear advantages over others—because so many of its members engage in it, and it may put the principle of justice in jeopardy (2). This use of the 'patients' interest' argument, or a statement that something is 'unethical', is a custom which requires close scrutiny, because of its tendency to muddy the waters over what is in fact in the profession's interest, or a section of it, what is in the patient's interest, what is in the public interest, and what is, in fact, genuinely unethical.

Where the system would be open to moral criticism is over the availability of expensive, or rare, services and treatments, which are not in the product range— yet where the assertion has been that everyone will be treated according to need, the principle of justice again. Where it is open to moral criticism is in treating some patient consumers better than others, but that is nothing new. These are questions which begin to muddy the waters in the relationship between the health care professional and the patient, and it is these questions which need clarifying for trust, and understanding, to be present.

THE REAL RELATIONSHIP

Downie and Calman, in their excellent volume, *Healthy respect* (3), suggest a wide-ranging list of roles which any health care professional might adopt, including healer, technician, counsellor, educator, scientist and friend. Yet the professional role, for example as a healer, may conflict with the role as a friend. The roles are confused in many cases, with conflicting values. The conflict between the role of friend and healer can be considerable, as can the conflict between the role of genuine scientist and friend. Scientific values are about finding out truths, investigating, experimenting in order to further human knowledge. A doctor, whether in general practice or in hospital medicine, may well be conducting some form of research. But it is remarkably difficult to include a friend in any randomized controlled trial. The whole point of such a trial is that neither the patient nor the doctor should know which arm of the trial the patient is in, so that for a friend to put a friend into such a blind study goes against the comforting and supportive values of friendship. All the theorizing in the world about how it may be therapeutic, because the patient may end up in the arm of the trial that has the most beneficial treatment, does not help in explaining to a friend that no-one knows the best treatment.

These are real conflicts, affecting crucially the relationship between the health care professional and the patient. But thinking has to go beyond the four principles of medical ethics which are normally cited—of beneficence, of non-maleficence, of justice and respect for autonomy—and look at what it is that is expected of health care professionals by patients, colleagues and superiors, and how these roles, and their underlying values, might conflict. And the friend–scientist or friend–healer conflicts are only two of many possible ones, such as the obvious conflict between trying to do the best for the individual patient, and looking at resources available for the totality of patients, when there is never enough to provide everything possible for all.

TRUTH-TELLING AND CONSENT

In all this, do patients get told the truth, about what treatments cost, about likely outcomes, and about how decisions are made? And are those decisions in the individual patient's interest, or in the public interest, or in the profession's interest, or merely the doctor's own?

Doctors do not, on the whole, want to take this on board. The Patient's Charter published by the British government in 1991 makes it clear that consent to treatment has to be requested. But that consent does not necessarily include details of cost and resource allocation, of public concern versus individual concern for the patient facing the health care professional at a particular time. The Patient's Charter merely requires that the patient 'be given a clear explanation of any treatment proposed, including any risks and any alternatives, before [you] decide whether you will agree to the treatment'. Informed consent, in the American sense of fully informed consent, with all the possible side-effects and risks explained, is not really known in the UK, let alone the added complications of cost and outcome analysis. Autonomy would appear to be limited in its application in Britain. But if there is no real informed consent, how is it possible to share with patients the difficult decisions about allocation of resources, or simply difficult decisions about which of a series of less than satisfactory treatments is the best?

But it also means that what has happened in the past—doctors making decisions that are, in effect, rationing decisions, for there has always been rationing of some kind in the NHS—by arguing that these are *clinical* decisions, can no longer continue. For there is going to be far more explicit decision-making, and gradually patients will come to realize that it is legitimate to ask about whether they are getting the best treatment available, or merely the best that the GP can afford. Alongside that will have to come explicit measures of outcomes of certain procedures, evidence that some standard procedures are of any benefit at all, and the realization that GPs will have to explain how they make their decisions on the basis of the individual patient's interests, the public interest, in terms of the public purse, and the GP's own personal financial interest, as a fund-holder with a clear interest in making the practice pay.

How does this fit with the professional–patient relationship? In order to make the system work, and to be true to the values of respecting autonomy, and acting both beneficently and non-maleficently, it is essential for decisions to be made explicit and for the patients, individually, and the public at large, to know the basis on which they are made. But that kind of explicitness has considerable difficulties for patients. The history of the relationship in Britain, at least, has been of a paternalistic one, with patients accepting large amounts of decision-making on their behalf. That is changing. There is resistance to paternalism from large numbers of patients, but there are also patients who find the openness and degree of decision-making expected from them very difficult indeed.

DOES EXPLICITNESS LEAD TO LOSS OF STATUS?

There is a fear amongst medical professionals and amongst patient groups that we might go down the US road, with doctors held in scant respect, being seen as driven wholly by the prospect of financial gain, with little in the way of real professional values. That does not need to be so. In these questions about allocation of resources, the fact that it will be wholly obvious, in the widest of possible public arenas, that doctors are having to give thought to the relative costs of treatments and procedures, terrifies doctors themselves. They do not want to have to say to patients that a particular treatment is too expensive. Nor do they want to talk about the financial implications of all sorts of other areas of practice, such as the fact that for most, but not all, clincial trials, particularly those sponsored by the pharmaceutical companies, doctors are paid for entering patients in a trial. To add to this, they are paid on a per capita basis, according to the numbers they recruit into the trial, a practice which is universal despite the Royal College of Physicians coming out strongly against it and arguing it is unethical (4). And whilst in hospital practice these monies tend to go into research funds for the department concerned, in the case of general practice, this money goes to the individual GP or the practice. Yet how many patients know this when they consent to enter a trial? And on what basis, if respecting the patients' interests is a key professional value, is it legitimate to keep this from them? In the case of GP trials, many of them never get vetted by a Research Ethics Committee at all (5).

HOW DOES RESEARCH AFFECT THE RELATIONSHIP? THE PATIENT'S VIEW

If patients have traditionally taken the view that the doctor and nurse are acting in their interests, the issue of clinical research throws up real problems. For in a randomized controlled trial, the one thing that can be certain is that the health care professional does not know whether she or he is acting in the patient's interest. The whole point of a trial is that it is being conducted in order to find out the answer to a problem. There might be a trial comparing two different forms of treatment, for instance. Or there might be a trial of a new drug for safety reasons, which could be very useful and beneficial to the patient, but which could also be damaging. There could be a question of surgery versus chemotherapy for various forms of cancer, or of high or low doses of the same drug. The problem is that if the answer is known, it is unethical to conduct the trial. Therefore it has to be the case that entering a patient into a trial cannot be said to be necessarily beneficent and, should the patient land up in the arm with the least good result, which happens to be the new treatment as opposed to the conventional one he would otherwise have had, it could be argued to be positively damaging. Add to that a question of whether it is possible ever to give the patient adequate information on which to make the decision, and the desire to get patients to enter the trial in order to get it going. Add into that the fact that doctors are often paid for entering patients into a trial, so that it is to the benefit of the health care professional, rather than the patient, for the patient to be in the trial, and one can see a complicated twist to the view a patient might otherwise hold of the health care professional! Consider the case below:

> A woman with ductal carcinoma *in situ* detected by mammography is asked, at the clinic appointment at which she is given her diagnosis, to enter a randomized controlled trial with four arms. They are: no further treatment, four weeks'

radiotherapy, tamoxifen in a small dose for five years, and tamoxifen plus radiotherapy. She is given two weeks to make up her mind, and told to telephone BACUP (the British Association for Cancer United Patients) for information on tamoxifen and radiotherapy. The information sheet describes the treatments, but does not give her any details of previous experience with the therapies under offer.

She is told she cannot ask the surgeon any more questions lest he influence her decision. She finds this difficult, in view of the fact that she would like further information about the exact nature of her carcinoma, the volume of tissue removed in the initial surgery, and oestrogen receptor status.

She decides to go and see her GP, who has a strong disinclination for radiotherapy; he quotes to her the Early Breast Cancer Trials collaborative groups' conclusion (6) that 'radiotherapy did not appear to produce any clear improvement in survival'. The GP did not comment, or feel it was fair to comment, on the tamoxifen option or on the no-treatment option. She continued to feel confused.

In analysing this question it is fair to ask several questions. First, what effect will it have on the relationship between patient and surgeon if the surgeon refuses to discuss it further because he does not want to influence the patient's decision? Is this a beneficent model of practice? Or has the interest of the entire patient population taken precedence over the individual patient, leading to a questionably disinterested air on the part of the surgeon, for the best of scientific motives?

Secondly, how can a patient give seriously informed consent when she cannot get any more information from those in charge of her treatment?

Thirdly, is it possible to ask a woman who has just been given the diagnosis of a form of breast cancer to take the kind of decision required at precisely the time when she is most in need of comfort and reassurance?

Fourthly, since the treatments vary so widely, should it not be possible for the patient to be given some choice in treatment, opting for an arm of the trial rather than randomization, when she might have clear preference?

Fifthly, what relationship can the patient have with her GP if the GP himself is not prepared to go into great detail about the trial, of which he has probably not been informed, or to go into the details of her condition? Should the GP express his preference for treatment?

It is clear that the relationship between the surgeon and the patient is critically damaged by asking her to take part in this trial. By that very request he has denied her the support, friendship and confidence in his ability she felt she ought to be able to rely on. He, however, has been honest in saying that the best treatment is unknown. He has been truthful and unsupportive. She has expected too much, and has been denied support. Her view of the relationship will be that it is not up to much. The doctor, on the other hand, might well feel he was respecting her autonomy, and that he was being honest in saying that it was not clear what the best treatment was. He is at fault in not being prepared to answer questions. But it would always be highly unethical to enter a patient into a trial without her consent, precisely because the interest of the individual is subsumed in that of the greater good of the masses.

Secondly, a lack of information is always the most keenly felt blow to a patient. Information is power. Information enables the individual to make choices. In this scenario the surgeon is denying information for what is an apparently good reason—he doesn't want to influence the patient's decision, but he is actually rendering her powerless to make her decision, because she does not have the information on which to make it, rendering the principle of informed consent meaningless.

Thirdly, asking patients who have just been given a diagnosis of a disease for their consent to enter a trial is always sensitive, and may have been done less than well. It is good practice to give the patient time to think about it. It would have been better practice to provide her with: more information about previous studies; more information about her own condition; and a nurse to whom she could put her questions, or another doctor, rather than tell her to contact an advisory service by telephone, however good that service might be.

Fourthly, the question remains open as to whether it is always necessary for these trials to be randomized, rather than the treatment arm being selected by the patient. The argument runs that patient preference skews the trial as much as doctor preference, making the scientific validity questionable. But it may be worth sacrificing some of the 'hardness' of the science for the sake of the relationship with the patient, particularly in an emotive area like breast cancer. The relationship with the patient is clearly damaged by her being unable to take control and make a choice in an area where she will have strong feelings about body image, and about mortality.

Fifthly, the role of the GP is complicated. The GP is often not informed about a trial taking place in a hospital setting. The GP then finds it difficult to comment, and may have views as strong as the surgeon's about hospital treatment. But the relationship with the GP is the most important one a patient has. It relies on a good working relationship, on trust, and to a large extent on the counselling and friendship roles of health care professionals cited by Downie and Calman (3). If a GP refuses to comment on these issues, it places that whole relationship in jeopardy. In thinking about this issue, GPs are particularly vulnerable to losing trust in the relationship, being seen by the patient to be acting either non-beneficently or, in the case of entering a patient into a study without knowledge or consent, maleficently, without respect for autonomy, because of inadequate information on which to make an autonomous decision, and arguably unethically. Indeed, in the research field, GPs are often the ones whose relationship with patients is most at risk.

(This is an altered version of a patient's account of a trial in 'Breast cancer trials: a patient's viewpoint', by H. M. Thornton. The alterations introduce the GP and ask the questions in accordance with the four principles used throughout this volume (7).)

This is an example of how the relationship can be thrown into jeopardy. Information is the key to the relationship. The patient who wants his autonomy needs to have as much information as possible, and not to feel that anything is being hidden. The most common complaint of patients is that they are given inadequate information, and at research ethics committees it is the information sheets which most frequently get criticized and are sent back for redrafting. The relationship rests on information and trust. That is how the patient's autonomy can be respected, and how the occasional 'You decide, doc' can be dealt with, because the trust is there. Without trust there can be neither support nor friendship. The counsellor role of the doctor or nurse is at stake here. Yet patients are rarely wholly satisfied with the information they are given.

If information is seen as empowering, as enabling patients to make choices, as allowing patients to behave like adults, it will change the way that practice is carried out. It will remove power from the health care professionals, but it will increase their influence, and will cast them in the light of genuine professional advisers. The relationship does not need to be paternalistic. It can be a relationship of equals, beneficent, non-maleficent, respecting autonomy, and encouraging the pursuit of justice. It will not be an easy relationship, and it requires a different approach from the standard Flexnerian scientific-based training of most medical schools. But medicine, now taught as what is effectively a technique, a series of skills, a discipline, *could* be taught with keen regard for the relationships, the human element, as Charles Odegaard put it (8). It would satisfy many patients whose power to choose is limited by lack of information and by being treated as idiots, and it would also sensitize both the patients and the health care professionals to the fact that health care is an art and not only a science, and that the relationship has to be worked on, by both sides.

REFERENCES

1. Hudson-Jones, A. (Ed.) 1988. *Images of Nurses: perspectives from history, art and literature.* University of Pennsylvania Press, Philadelphia PA.
2. Miller, F. H. 1991. Health policy, competition and professional behaviour, p. 142. *Healthcare UK.* King's Fund Institute, London.
3. Downie, R. S. and Calman, K. C. 1987. *Healthy respect—ethics in healthcare*, pp. 159–160. Faber and Faber, London.
4. RCP. 1990. *Research involving patients*, 7: 86. Royal College of Physicians, London.
5. Neuberger, J. 1992. *Ethics and healthcare: research ethics committees in the UK.* King's Fund Institute, London.
6. Early Breast Cancer Trials Collaborative Group. 1990. *Treatment of early breast cancer,* Vol. 1: *Worldwide evidence 1985-90.* Oxford University Press, New York.
7. Thornton, H. M. 1992. Breast cancer trials: a patient's viewpoint, *Lancet* **339**: 44–45.
8. Odegaard, C. 1988. *Dear doctor.* Henry Kaiser Foundation, Menlo Park, CA.

34

Ethicist and Patient: What is their Relationship?

DONALD EVANS, BA, PhD

Director, Centre for Philosophy and Health Care, University College, Swansea, UK

> The patient's essential being is very relevant in the higher reaches of neurology, and in psychology; for here the patient's personhood is essentially involved, and the study of disease and identity cannot be disjoined (ref. 1, p. x).

It is impossible to begin to determine the relationship between the ethicist and the patient without first identifying the two parties. Such identification is not straightforward.

For example, consider the identity of the patient. The label itself begs a number of questions in health care ethics. It denotes a passive recipient of treatments or services with a fairly well-marked-out place in the institutional hierarchy of health care provision. As such it embodies certain perspectives, attitudes and a *modus operandi* which have been subject to considerable criticism and change during relatively recent times. Should not the recipients of health care services be regarded as clients? Or are they better seen as customers? These are interesting and important questions. They will not be the focus of my concern in this chapter, though I shall have something to say of the significance of such labels. Suffice to say at this point that this side of the relationship shall be occupied by the persons receiving medical attention or health care provision of some kind.

The other side of the relationship is even more problematic, and it is necessary to be clearer about it before we can make progress on defining the relationship at all. There are numerous roles developing in health care which involve an explicit concern with ethics. Membership of Research Ethics Committees or Institutional Review Boards involves evaluation of the ethical dimensions of research protocols involving human subjects, whether healthy volunteers or patients. The terms of reference of members of these committees spell out a clear relationship with the subjects of research. For example the most recent

Principles of Health Care Ethics. Edited by Raanan Gillon.
© 1994 John Wiley & Sons Ltd

guidelines on the practice of such committees issued by the Royal College of Physicians define the objectives of Research Ethics Committees as follows:

> to maintain ethical standards of practice in research, to protect subjects of research from harm, to preserve the subjects' rights, and to provide reassurance to the public that this is being done (2).

The ethicist cast in this role is the advocate of the patients' interests. Given the power of veto which refusal to approve research protocols implies, the ethicist is in a position to act as protector of the patient.

The role of ethicists in ethics committees as opposed to Institutional Review Boards in the United States is not so clear. Practices vary considerably from state to state and even from hospital to hospital. What they have in common is a concern with the evaluation of clinical practice. They may be advisory, educational or even executive in the role they play in assessing the acceptability of therapeutic policies and particular clinical decisions. Here, however, the focus of concern may not be solely upon the interests of the individual patient. They may be concerned equally with the interests of the practitioner, the interests of the families of patients and the interests of other potential patients. It would, nevertheless, be very strange if the interests of particular patients dropped entirely out of the picture in their deliberations. Whilst membership of such committees, or even the activities of lone ethicists consulted on precisely the same issues, might involve advocacy on behalf of patients, they need not be responsible for protecting the welfare of patients exclusively.

Ethicists are to be found elsewhere than in such formal health care settings. The title is often given to those who are concerned to think, write and teach about health care ethics as a subject. Such persons may not have a formal relationship with patients set out in the terms of reference of their occupations. Some of them are unashamedly advocates of the interests of specific patient groups such as MIND, whilst others are explicitly advocates of the interests of patients as patients, irrespective of the conditions to be treated, such as spokespersons for consumer groups like the Patients Association.

My concern in this chapter is to say something about the relationship between those ethicists referred to above whose role does not carry with it any formal responsibility for advocating or protecting the interests of patients. They are engaged in the intellectual pursuit of examination and clarification of ethical issues in health care. In short they are those whose business is critical reflection. They will be made up of philosophers in the main, but may also include sociologists, lawyers, theologians and other interested parties. Can it be said of this group of ethicists that they too are related to the patient insofar as they are, amongst other things, advocates of the interests of patients? There is disagreement between philosophers about whether or not philosophical reflection is itself capable of providing answers to substantive ethical questions. Insofar as this is true it would not be possible to say that the critical reflector on health care issues should, or indeed could, speak with authority as the advocate of anyone's interests. Nevertheless it may still be that critical reflection will show that respect for the patient lies at the very centre of the clinical encounter. It follows that insofar as this is true the philosopher may dispassionately remind the practitioner that without taking due account of the subject matter of clinical practice, *viz.* patients as persons, clinical practice will be compromised. This is not to set one group of interests, the patient's, against another's, the practitioner's. Therefore it is not to advocate one set of interests against another. Rather it is to get clearer about the nature of clinical practice. The results of such clarification might well be to protect or improve the patient's welfare. This will, however, be a spin-off from the activity rather than constitute the motive force of the activity.

Such reflection does indeed place respect for the patient at the heart of clinical practice. Among the many values delineated in the literature as being integral to good health care provision—including the four values presented as principles by Beauchamp and Childress (3) (the authors present a case for regarding autonomy, beneficence, non-maleficence and justice as the four principles integral to biomedical ethics), the value which uniquely delineates the patient as person is autonomy. Respecting welfare, safety, dignity and even rights may be possible where the subject matter of concern happens to be non-human subjects. Animals can be harmed, threatened, treated unfairly and be subjected to indignities. In no circumstances, however, could we conceive of procuring the consent of a non-human subject for some veterinary procedure. By contrast, to proceed with a medical examination or with any clinical or nursing intervention without the consent of a patient, where such consent is possible, would constitute a battery. Thus the question of consent will always be chronologically prior to all other moral considerations in the treatment of patients. In this sense at least it may be said to lie at the very base of clinical and nursing practice.

However, the centrality of consent is more than a chronological matter. It is logically fundamental to the proper treatment of patients. If this thesis can be established in those clinical areas where the possibility of consent is a matter of dispute then we shall have no difficulty in accepting it elsewhere. It may be argued that clinical psychology, psychotherapy and psychiatry are such areas. We shall therefore concentrate on these for the remainder of this chapter. Here, it may be said, the very faculties necessary for the giving or refusing of informed consent are those which, in one way or another, call for treatment. If these faculties are at least a part of what makes up the personal individuality or identity of people, then treatment of them puts respect for that individuality at the very heart of clinical practice.

Such a case has been made eloquently by Tristram Engelhardt Jr (4). Great care needs to be taken in delineating the role of such respect, otherwise the case is overstated and the principle thereby compromised. I contend that this is true of Engelhardt's presentation.

His argument runs as follows: all medicine aims at liberating man from his afflictions, at increasing his freedom. The goal of all medical therapy is to increase autonomy. In the case of psychotherapy this may amount to liberating patients from unconscious drives and unacknowledged forces which hinder free action. Insofar as the therapist so acts he dedicates his energies to the autonomy of the individual. That is, he is concerned to get the patient to the place where he is able to act freely. The concern is not to get the patient to perform any particular act which is valued by the therapist, but rather to get the patient to act autonomously. In this sense psychotherapy may be said to be a form of meta-ethics. It does not advance particular ethical recommendations but rather, in its devotion to autonomy, enables the patient to engage in actions for which he may be morally commended or condemned because he will be enabled to act freely and thus be held responsible for his deeds. Engelhardt finds support in both Freud and Szasz for his account.

If we accept this account of clinical practice in psychology and psychotherapy, then the notion of respect for the patient is seen to lie at the very base of clinical practice, whether the client is able to give consent to a therapy or not. That is, not only in situations where consent properly can be sought but also in those cases where it cannot.

However, deciding between such cases is not a straightforward matter. This gives rise to suspicions that Engelhardt's thesis is flawed. It may tempt one to think that persons needing psychotherapy, people who in Engelhardt's terms do not value reality, need not be consulted about whether or not they should receive therapy, or what the nature of that therapy should be.

The danger arises from the indeterminate character of the notion of competence to consent. Think, for example, of the patchiness of the possession of this facility amongst those who present for treatment by psychotherapists. Autonomy may be something of which people may be capable at some times in their life, and not others, or in some areas of their life and not others. Correspondingly their competence to consent may vary. But competence to consent does not vary directly with the ability to act autonomously. This may appear to be plainly false when expressed in as many words, but some careful reflection will show it to be true.

Let us imagine that certain areas of my life are distorted by unacknowledged forces involving my relationship with my father. When such explanations begin to surface in the course of a therapy I might refuse to proceed. I may not wish, perhaps out of a profound moral regard for my father as my father, to uncover anything which would sully his memory in my eyes or the eyes of others. A whole set of regards bound up with the institution of the family may be central in my life, and may be valued above my desire for autonomy in those limited areas for which I am seeking help. In other respects people are constantly waiving their right to act with complete autonomy in order to realize things which are more highly valued. Such opting occurs when one becomes party to a contract, marries and so on. Why should not this freedom to act autonomously in certain areas of my life be waived in the course of a therapy? Why should I not be competent to decide to leave matters well alone? This may denote a willingness to continue to disvalue reality, as Engelhardt might express it, in that particular area, but it may also ensure that far more important and central concerns which give meaning to my life are preserved.

If the therapist insists that such a decision is unfree, that it cannot really be my decision because I have not yet been fully restored as an individual, then he is adopting an *a priori* position which dictates that no-one suffering from a neurosis is capable of giving or refusing a consent to therapy. Any request for consent would then be a charade, for refusal of therapy would simply be construed as a criterion of incompetence.

Now it is true that in any given case how far a disorder permeates a life will be a matter of judgement. More of this later. However, to determine before consideration of my particular circumstances that consent cannot be properly refused is to elevate one moral value to a position of supremacy over values which I, the client or patient, avow to be more significant. This constitutes a denial of the meta-ethical status of psychotherapy's pursuit of autonomy on behalf of the client. At certain points such a pursuit may well come up against other values. There it ceases to enjoy its meta-ethical status and has to fight for its life in the context of substantive moral disagreement.

Less problematic cases could be cited with ease. The alcoholic writer or artist whose creativity has been undermined by previous therapeutic interventions might refuse a further period of therapy. Surely it is conceivable for him both to be aware of the dire possibilities non-treatment will imply and yet, quite reasonably, decline therapy. His refusal will commit him to the hell of his addiction and the connected loss of control over large areas of his life. But it is still something which he may have good reason to enact.

Such criticism of Engelhardt's highly suggestive and promising thesis does not remove respect for the individual from centre stage. Indeed, it affords protection of such respect by warning against what could well become an *a priori* thesis about the competence of those suffering from mental disorders of varying kinds to give a proper consent to treatment.

Let us further explore the problem of consent in the treatment of mental disorder by comparing the alternative approaches to the sufferer marked out by the biological and behavioural models of such conditions. Each model may be thought to invoke a specific therapeutic relationship which has implications for the possibility of obtaining a consent.

The biological model suggests that the features of behaviour exhibited by those who are commonly described as being mentally disordered are symptoms of some disease or another. In physical diseases symptoms such as fever and weight loss are indicative of some underlying physiological condition, such as the presence of a tumour. The suggestion is that mental phenomena such as delusion and depression are also symptoms of some kind of lesion. There have been rival accounts of the character of the lesions in question, but much evidence has been gathered to support causal explanations in genetic, biochemical and cerebral damage terms. Psychiatry has commonly employed such a model.

There are well-established relations between certain genetic disorders and the kind of behavioural symptoms that interest therapists. Huntington's chorea springs readily to mind. Similarly the relation between disturbed behaviour and low blood sugar or intoxication has encouraged psychiatry to explore biochemical changes as the root of mental illness. The amelioration of symptoms by the use of drugs has offered further encouragement. Similarly the cerebral changes produced by syphilis in Cupid's disease are accompanied by startling changes in behaviour, suggesting causal explanations.

Such a working model of mental disorder invokes the therapeutic relation of doctor to patient. This relation is clearly unequal in a number of respects, thereby threatening the autonomy of the patient.

First the doctor is an authority in terms of being in possession of highly complex and specialized knowledge relating to the patient's condition, of which the patient is by force of circumstance generally ignorant. He thus presents to the patient as an expert, in contrast to which the patient is a layperson.

Second he enjoys a position in the institutions of health care which traditionally carries a fair degree of prestige. This further makes it difficult for the patient to relate on an equal footing.

Third the doctor is approached by the patient as a potential benefactor. He is in a position to confer something of great value upon the patient which the patient needs, sometimes urgently. What the patient needs is usually something important, such as life-saving intervention, pain relief, restoration of a feeling of well-being, the safe delivery of a child and so on. This tends to put the patient in the position of supplicant and at a disadvantage in negotiating any therapy.

Fourth the doctor is known to be in very great demand. His time is limited and the patient knows that others are queueing for his attention whether the doctor operates in the hospital setting or in the community. It is the doctor who allocates the time spent with the patient. It is the doctor who determines when the consultation terminates. This puts the doctor in the driving seat throughout.

What then are the dangers of this inequality? Can they be eliminated? If not, can they be ameliorated? The most worrying danger is the temptation to undermine regard for the patient as a person. In cases where the patient is not capable of giving or refusing an informed consent the doctor may well be justified in acting paternalistically. He might well know what is in the best interests of the patient and with beneficence act accordingly. The danger is in imagining that the doctor always knows what is best for the patient, and also that because he does then the patient's opinions or wishes are not sufficiently important to determine therapeutic policies.

As a safeguard of the autonomy of patients two qualifications have commonly been made to the consent to treatment which is sought by doctors. The first is that the consent is voluntary, the second that it is informed. These qualifications are designed to guard against coercion of any form and against judgements of ignorance on the part of the patient. Each of these threats is embodied in the inequality of the doctor–patient relationship.

The most difficult area in which to protect respect for the patient in treating mental disorder is that of determining the competence of the patient to give or refuse consent. Such competence involves both the ability of the patient freely to choose what shall or shall not be done to him or her, and the ability of that person to comprehend any information about his or her condition and alternative therapies which may be available. As we shall see, the therapists' values will inevitably colour the assessment of such abilities. However, may this difficulty not be confined to those practitioners employing the biological model of mental disorder? Might they not apply equally to the behavioural model? Before dealing with them let us identify that model and ask whether the same inequalities exist in the therapeutic relationship which it entails as in the doctor–patient relationship.

The behavioural model of mental disorder does not regard the various features of disturbed behaviour as symptoms of some disease which somehow underlies them. These features are simply regarded as behavioural reactions to life circumstances. They are themselves constitutive of a disorder and not symptomatic of it. Thus there is no need to reify such conditions in the form of this and that lesion or disease. On this view what is called for, if anything, in the way of help for the sufferer is some kind of assistance to modify the behaviour in question.

The contrast between the models can be illustrated by means of a simple example from the literature. A child not wanting to go to school is referred for behavioural therapy. Rather than diagnosing 'school phobia' or some other mysterious disease entity the behavioural model simply describes the child factually as being a low or zero school attender. The agreed goal of the therapy is to make her a 90–100% attender. On achieving the goal no claim need be made to have identified or cured any phobia. The behaviour of the child will simply have been modified (5).

This model of mental disorder invokes a quite different therapeutic relationship from that invoked by the biological model. There is no suggestion here that the therapist is party to complex and inaccessible information about the individual in question which is beyond the grasp of that individual. Thus it seems that the role of expert and the inequality of the therapeutic relationship which arises out of that have been eradicated. Furthermore it may be thought to be improper to call the child a patient, for she is certainly not being treated for any kind of disease or damage. She is simply seeking help to enable her to behave differently. She might thus more properly be called a client. As such she is using a service to achieve goals which she has by herself or with the advice of others freely chosen. The therapeutic relationship is therefore said to be egalitarian and enjoys something of a contractual character. The therapist and the client may be said to negotiate the therapy as equals.

If we adopt such a model of mental disorder have we automatically safeguarded the notion of respect for the individual? Have we avoided the pitfalls of the power relationship invoked by the biological model? Sadly we have not. Indeed to imagine that we have, as it will be tempting for the behavioural therapist to do, is to threaten that respect. An admission of the inevitable inequality in the therapeutic relationship is a necessary condition for safeguarding respect for the client. This becomes evident if we review the dangerous features of the biological model and consider whether they have disappeared in the new therapeutic relationship.

We need first to ask whether it is true that we have got rid of the expert–layperson relation. The answer seems to be that we have not. The behavioural therapist is highly trained and is party to a very sophisticated body of knowledge and techniques relating to human behaviour. Whilst he may not share the mystique of the doctor who knows much about incredibly small micro-organisms, sophisticated cerebral biochemical processes and so on, which baffle and impress the layman, he is still the subject of some awe in the client.

Indeed, the mystique may be all the more powerful in this case, being connected to a belief that the therapist knows much about the client and how he operates as opposed to knowing much about how his body functions. After all the client has come to the therapist precisely because he is impressed enough to believe that the therapist has the requisite knowledge and skill to be of help.

With respect to the position of prestige in the institutions of health care enjoyed by the doctor it is probably true that, in the eyes of patients or clients, if not in the ranks of the medical hierarchy, the behavioural therapist is indistinguishable from the doctor. This is an empirical matter. If it turned out to be false it does not follow that the therapist who practises with the *imprimatur* of the health authorities does not enjoy a certain prestige as a result.

There is no doubt at all that the therapist is approached as a benefactor. If the client did not think that he was going to derive help from the therapist then he would certainly not volunteer for therapy. Whilst this does not entail that the client adopts a cap-in-hand approach it certainly puts the therapist in the dominant position in the relationship. The therapist is in the position of offering or refusing something which the client wants and needs, often desperately.

The therapist is also the one who determines not only whether, but also when, the therapy shall begin and end. This may be negotiated with the client but the ultimate responsibility is the therapist's. This is well known to the client.

Thus whilst there may be differences of emphasis the therapeutic relationship invoked by the behavioural model embodies inequalities similar to those invoked by the biological model. To say as much is not to denigrate the relationship but to elucidate its character. For the therapist to proceed with the negotiation of therapeutic contracts unaware of this inequality is to run the serious risk of exploiting the inequality to the detriment of respect for the individual treated. And this in the firm conviction that he is profoundly preserving such respect as part of the ethos of an egalitarian methodology.

This brings us to the most difficult feature of the treatment of mental disorder with regard to preserving respect for the client or patient. It concerns the assessment of competence to consent. As we have seen, such competence involves both the ability to choose freely and the ability to comprehend on the part of the patient. Until such competence is accepted by the therapist the therapeutic relationship is inevitably unequal in a profound sense. The problems arise in assessing whether the patient is competent. It is the therapist who has to make such a determination. This is itself an important consideration in the power relationship with the client. The main question to be answered is whether such a determination can be made in a value-free manner. If the answer is no then the relation cannot be straightforwardly egalitarian, and special care will need to be exercised, otherwise respect for the client is undermined.

Can we find a set of objective criteria which will enable us to establish competence indifferently from the values of the therapist? Let us consider a valiant attempt to provide such a test (6). This test involves the application of five criteria:

1. There must be evidence of choice.
2. There must be a reasonable outcome of the choice.
3. The choice must be based on good reasons.
4. The patient must have the capacity to understand the issues in question.
5. The patient must actually have understood the issues when giving consent.

Can we call any of these criteria value-free? They might appear to be innocent of value commitment when spelled out in abstract, but the moment the therapist endeavours to apply them difficulties arise. Only the first on the list can claim with any degree of conviction to be objective. With respect to the rest it is impossible to divorce their application from the values of the therapist. Let us consider them separately.

The reasonable outcome criterion involves determining whether the choice made by the patient is that choice which would be made by reasonable persons in similar circumstances. The therapist will no doubt consider himself to be a reasonable person, and if the decision of the patient does not conform to the therapist's view of what ought to be done then the temptation will be to regard the patient as incompetent.

There are some safeguards which may be introduced to make such a test more reliable—that is, to insulate the assessment more securely from the values of the therapist. The first is to determine reasonable outcome in terms of the values which the patient holds fast when he is his authentic self. This relates to the restoration of autonomy as the central concern of psychotherapy discussed above. It is sometimes referred to as the 'thank you tomorrow' justification for treating without consent. There are unproblematic cases of this kind; for example, those undergoing manic episodes who engage in public behaviour which threatens their reputation (for a discussion of such cases, see ref. 7). On being restored to a normal state such patients may well be grateful for being treated against their will. Their autonomy is not overridden in such cases. Rather it is impaired while they are in the manic phase.

But not all cases will be as straightforward. Indeed the straightforward cases are likely to be those where the values of the patient when his authentic self accord more or less with those of the therapist. Determining what the authentic individual is is a matter of the therapist's judgement. It is not easy to insulate this determination from the therapist's values. There will be cases where the behavioural and attitudinal features of the patient's disorder are inseparable from the identify of the patient. The temptation here will be to produce a 'thank you tomorrow' from a patient, who might have become a very different person from his authentic self. Think of Witty Ticcy Ray, the patient of Oliver Sacks who suffered from Tourette's syndrome (ref. 1, pp. 87–96).

The syndrome, as Sacks describes it on p. 87, is characterized by 'an excess of nervous energy, and a great production and extravagance of strange motions and notions . . .. In its "highest" forms Tourette's syndrome involves every aspect of the affective, the instinctual and the imaginative life'.

Ray at 24 years old was severely incapacitated by violent tics which occurred every few seconds. This feature of his behaviour was clearly debilitating in the extreme and something from which he needed deliverance. But what of the other features of the case? What of the great nervous energy, the remarkable musicality? Were these features of the authentic Ray or of his disorder? Being a jazz drummer of rare virtuosity was largely due to his being a Touretter. When treated with Haldol he was delivered from the dreadful tics but he was also delivered from his remarkable creativity on the drums. He consequently chose to live on Haldol during working days and off it at weekends, when he would perform on the drums. Fortunately for Ray the outcome was something over which he could be said reasonably to have control. He was not grateful to be a dull person on Haldol, for that was not the real Ray. But what if he had been? Could we confidently say that he had been restored to his authentic self? Or should we have said that he was a different man? This problem of determining the degree to which a disorder permeates a patient's life is one which the therapist cannot avoid, and where his values will inevitably come into play.

The second useful safeguard when applying this criterion is to remember that people we regard as perfectly competent to make decisions about their lives are free to make foolish decisions.

The third test of competence to consent is also impossible to apply in a value-free manner. What may count as a good reason for adopting a particular therapy will vary from therapist to therapist. Consequently a patient judged to be competent by one may be judged incompetent by another. In setting the agenda of a therapy, even in consultation with a client, the therapist will face this difficulty. Take for example the treatment of homosexuals (8).

The case in point concerned a client who was sexually attracted to young boys. The behaviour therapist provided him with methods to transfer that attraction to men not women. The reason the therapist regarded this as a proper outcome was that the client wished to maximize the quality of his life as a homosexual. This seemed reasonable to this therapist but clearly it was not so regarded by others. Their view was that homosexuality was a 'sexual orientation disturbance', and that the reason the client had to proceed with such a therapy was a product of that disturbance.

What can we make of the test involving the client's ability to understand the information given about the possible benefits and risks of the therapy? It is easy to demand too much here. The client does not have to qualify as a doctor or psychologist to be able to make reasonable sense of the information proffered. To demand too much here threatens the autonomy of the client. But how much is too much? Therapists will not always agree about this. The following case illustrates how such disagreement can occur (6). A suicidal 49-year-old woman was offered electroconvulsive therapy. Her understanding of the treatment was otherwise intact, but when informed that there was a 1 in 3000 chance of dying from the treatment she replied 'I hope I am the one'. What does one say when what the therapist regards as a risk the patient construes as a benefit? That she had understood the meaning of his warning is quite clear.

The final test simply provides a reminder to the therapist to endeavour to inform the patient. The problems of its application are common with those of the test of the ability to understand.

So much for tests of competence to consent. They are fraught with difficulties yet they are not dispensible if respect for the client is to be preserved.

In this chapter I have endeavoured to show that respect for the patient is central to good therapeutic practice. I have tried to do so by emphasizing the importance of informed consent and its relation to the autonomy of patients. Even in the most problematic area of therapy where consent is not a straightforward matter it is not something that can be ignored. To ignore it in less problematic areas of health care would be necessarily to compromise that care. Philosophical analysis thus lays bare the nature of clinical practice and places respect for the patient at its heart. The ethicist, by means of critical reflection, can thus represent the interests of patients without prejudice to the interests of practitioners or providers of good health care.

REFERENCES

1. Sacks, O. 1985. *The man who mistook his wife for a hat.* Picador.
2. Royal College of Physicians. 1989. *Guidelines on the practice of ethics committees in research involving human subjects,* 2nd edn, p. 1. RCP, London.
3. Beauchamp, T. L. and Childress, J.F. 1983. *Principles of biomedical ethics.* Oxford University Press, Oxford.
4. Tristram Engelhardt, H. Jr. 1973. Psychotherapy as meta-ethics. *Psychiatry* **36**: 440–445.
5. Ayllon, Smith and Rogers. 1970. Behavioral management of school phobia. *Journal of Behavior Therapy and Experimental Psychiatry* **125**: 126.
6. Roth, L. H., Meisel, A. and Lidz, C. W. 1977. Tests of competency to consent to treatment. *American Journal of Psychiatry* **134**: 279–284.
7. Macklin, R. 1982. Refusal of psychiatric treatment: autonomy, competence, and paternalism. Pp. 331–340, *in* Edwards, R. B. (Ed.) *Psychiatry and Ethics.* Prometheus Books, Buffalo NY.
8. Karasu, T. B. 1980. The ethics of psychotherapy. *American Journal of Psychiatry* **137**: 1502–1512.

35

For Paternalism in the Doctor–Patient Relationship

ELLIOT A. SHINEBOURNE, MD, FRCP

Consultant Paediatric Cardiologist, Royal Brompton National Heart and Lung Hospital and National Heart and Lung Institute, University of London, UK

ANDREW BUSH, MD, MRCP

Senior Lecturer in Paediatric Respiratory Medicine, Royal Brompton National Heart and Lung Hospital and National Heart and Lung Institute, London, UK

Every adult, whether he is a follower or a leader, a member of a mass or an élite, was once a child. He was once small. A sense of smallness forms a substratum of his mind, ineradicably. His triumphs will be measured against this smallness, his defeats will substantiate it (Erik Erikson) (1).

Within every adult remains something of the child they once were.

For in every adult there lurks a child—an eternal child, something that is always becoming, is never completed, and calls for increasing care, attention and education (C. G. Jung) (2).

In times of illness or despair elements of the child remaining in our conscious or unconscious mind are more activated than at other times. This component of our personality, however mature, autonomous and self-reliant we are, may require care as well as information. In the same way as a child is in part dependent on the care, protection from harm and expertise of his parents, so is a sick patient *in part* dependent on the care, protection from harm and expertise of his doctor. Whether paternalism has any part in this relationship will be explored.

The title of this chapter—For paternalism in the doctor–patient relationship—was given by the editors. We note the next chapter to be entitled 'Against paternalism in the patient–physician relationship'. The juxtaposition of chapters

Principles of Health Care Ethics. Edited by Raanan Gillon.
© 1994 John Wiley & Sons Ltd

implies the need to defend paternalism—if it is defensible. We may not need to defend it, however; it may not be desirable, or even possible, to exclude paternalism from medicine. If a defence needs to be mounted it should take account of the stated *prima facie* ethical principles of respect for autonomy, beneficence, non-maleficence and justice. Is this possible? One essential question is to ask why most people (patients) go to see the doctor in the first place. Many will go primarily to seek information, but others will be in severe pain or distress, may be at risk of death or permanent damage, and their principal reason for seeking medical attention is to have their pain or condition relieved—any way that works.

FOR PATERNALISM

By 'for paternalism' is taken to mean on the side of, in support of, or perhaps in defence or paternalism. It could also be taken to mean in support of a measure of, or aspects of, paternalism and hence can imply support for some but not all aspects of paternalism. One can be 'for' sensuality, for religion, or for personal autonomy but not necessarily for all aspects of each, recognizing that unfettered expression or indulgence may cause more harm than good.

We have not, however, yet defined what is meant by 'paternalism'. 'The principle of acting in a way like that of a father towards his children' is the literal meaning (3), or 'behaving towards someone as a father would towards his children'. In *Moral dilemmas of modern medicine* (1985) Lockwood (4) defines paternalism as 'behaving towards someone in a way that does not respect his or her autonomy, for that person's own (supposed) good'. He continues 'Paternalism characteristically involves making people's decisions for them or keeping certain information from them on the grounds that it would be better for them not to know'. Medical condescension pervades this definition but is not implicit in the word paternalism.

What does acting like a father would to his children mean? On the positive side would be an absolute duty to safeguard the welfare and health of his child, to act always in the best interests of the child, to use his knowledge, skill and understanding to secure those interests, to take responsibility for decisions made and to be available to the best of his ability at all times when the child needed him. To act in this way imposes a tremendous duty on the father, a duty to act for the child's good. Why does this attitude imply not respecting the autonomy of the child? Surely the duty is to safeguard that autonomy or the potential for autonomy as much as possible. It may mean making judgements as to what or how much information is given, and indeed the manner in which information is given. To this we will return. Suffice it to say at this point that medical information, unlike packets of washing powder, depends very much on the way it is given. The manner of disclosure and a multitude of factors affecting comprehension are important. Both are infinitely variable and depend on the previous experience, knowledge and biases of those giving and receiving the information, as well as on the intelligence of doctor and patient and probably most importantly on the degree of anxiety or discomfort of the patient. Any doctor or patient who thinks it is even usually possible to give or receive unbiased, objective information is, in our view, unrealistic.

Even in the very simplest medical model, the prescribing of a drug by a doctor for a patient, paternalism is inevitable. The prescription of the drug will involve an assessment of risk versus benefit. The assessment of risk appears to be easy; the 'Data Sheet Compendium' contains a list of possible side-effects, and the patient can and should be allowed to read it. However, this list is itself a distillation of the published literature by one, or at best a few, people; and while usually representative is not exhaustive and is dependent on the views of others. The next step back would be for the patient to go to a computer and personally search the literature. Even here, editorial choice will influence what information is available, as much experience, particularly negative, remains unpublished. It is usual in practice that the patient will have to surrender some part of his/her control to others, or else risk failing to reap benefits. Paternalism becomes more inevitable as the medical situation becomes more urgent. When the heart has stopped beating, just as when the child runs in front of a car, the place for reasoned discussion is nil, the place for immediate, decisive action is central.

Autonomy also can never be absolute in a populated world. Originally autonomy meant living by one's own laws, a principle dear to the self-governing Greek city-states, but as Dunstan (5) commented, something of a hindrance when combination was required to meet a common foe or invader. We would argue that illness, including the need for medical or surgical treatment, can also erode absolute autonomy. While respect for this autonomy should be given, how much, by whom and whether under all circumstances, likewise, cannot be absolute. Paternalism does not have to imply disrespect for autonomy. It can, but it can also be used to protect someone whose autonomy or personal freedom has been eroded by illness until such time as he can regain control of his destiny.

PATERNALISM—AND THE FATHER

Why should acting like a father be construed as bad for the patient or in some way morally wrong? If one concentrates on the harmful effects of treating an adult like a child, this must be guarded against. On the other hand one might ask whether a sick patient would prefer the doctor not to care for him/her at all like a father. Perhaps it depends on the patient's (or reader's) view of the father. Particularly, if the doctor is considered to be in a way like a father to the patient then what will be the patient's response to this?

Every person has a father—a real father and an imagined archetypal father. The subjective experience of each may be transferred to the doctor. As an example of what might be termed projective identification some aspect of the personality which has been (unconsciously) split off is placed on the object (doctor or medical opinion) and is experienced as if it were an aspect or function of the object. If the aspect of the personality that is split off is regarded fundamentally with fear the doctor (medicine) will be seen as authoritarian, life-denying, not respecting autonomy, even castrating. If, on the other hand, it is perceived as devoted, wanting the best for, caring about the welfare of, nourishing, devoted to the service of, to the best interest of, and to promoting the autonomy of—then the 'paternal' component will be adjudged favourable. Personal experiences both of one's own father or of the father archetype will influence this.

WHY IS THERE A DOCTOR-PATIENT RELATIONSHIP?

In some books on medical ethics—particularly those written by philosophers, full-time medical ethicists, or even by doctors not looking after acutely sick people, one wonders whether the authors have ever been ill. There seems to be an assumption that the predominant reason a person consults a doctor is for information, not because that person feels terrible, is frightened, in pain, can't breathe, can't pass urine or feels life is not worth living. Such people want help, care, *therapos*. Do patients go to their doctor so that they can have a dose of information which allows them to make up their mind what treatment they want? Some, of course, do, but we would suggest that many don't—they 'just want to be made better'. The doctor has to make a judgement as to what the patient wants, or is in the patient's best interests. Sometimes it will be essential for full technical or medical information to be given in order for the patient fully to collaborate with the treatment—for instance if diabetes is diagnosed and control of blood sugar necessary—but sometimes not, and indeed sometimes full explanation is positively rejected. What the doctor *should* say to the patient is a matter of judgement. Indeed ethics is concerned with the taking of informed decisions in the light of values one holds to be good. For the doctor this has to be the welfare or best interests of the patient. To say that full information should be given—thus in some way protecting or respecting the full autonomy of the patient—is not necessarily either what the patient wants or what will produce the best result for the patient. Do people really want to know all the possibilities, even improbable ones? Can it seriously be argued that a middle-aged man with a cough should be told 'you probably only have a post-nasal drip, but you could have inoperable cancer, tuberculosis, or AIDS'? Certainly the actual diagnosis must be fully shared; but should every single possibility, even the remote and soon-to-be-eliminated? Of course, if the patient does ask specifically it would be wrong not to give full information—lying is extremely hard to justify under any (but not all) circumstances—but there is no absolute obligation for the doctor to say everything he knows (or to know everything). One pragmatic reason for this is that the doctor, for sure, will *not* know everything. What he does know will be limited, affected by his own emotional response to the information and his own previous experience of similar situations—which may well also be narrow, and possibly atypical. Some examples from clinical practice may illustrate these thoughts.

Information Given Before Performing Tests

Doctors are not permitted to carry out HIV testing without prior informed consent; the agony of people or parents contemplating AIDS in themselves or their children can hardly be imagined. If the tests are negative, does this anxiety serve any useful purpose?

One of us saw a child in whom the diagnosis of cystic fibrosis had to be ruled out; this could not be done without telling the mother, because of the nature of the test. The test was negative, all the child's symptoms disappeared without treatment, but the worry of the possible diagnosis caused the mother to go back to smoking. Would it have been better (though paternalistic) not to have told the mother about the possibility until it had been ruled out?

Informed Consent Before an Operation

The father of one of us required a prostatectomy; only after the operation did he realize that cancer was a possibility, a fact well known to his son. Happily he did not have cancer, and was glad that the stress of worrying about malignant disease had not been added to the stress of preparing for surgery; wrong paternalism by the surgeon (and the son)?

Lung Cancer

Patients with lung cancer are in general told their diagnosis. For planning their management an accurate diagnosis of the type of lung cancer is necessary. This may be made by looking at cells in the sputum but more commonly is obtained by taking a piece of tissue or biopsy via the fibreoptic bronchoscope passed into the lungs via the trachea under sedation and local anaesthesia. The average age of patients at diagnosis is around 65 years. The majority will have smoked cigarettes for many years and many will have associated conditions such as chronic bronchitis, emphysema, heart, kidney or cerebrovascular disease.

The outlook is not good, as many patients will already know, before their doctor discusses treatment options and prognosis. We argue here, as indeed does Spiro in *Doctors' decisions: ethical conflicts in medical practice* (6), that how much information is given, and the extent to which detailed description is given of the person's probable future or lack of it, is a matter of professional judgement. Not that the doctor should lie, but the information given should be adjusted to what the patient requests, and needs to know fully to participate in treatment. The way in which information is given in any case profoundly affects how it is received or perceived. Likewise, the extent to which a patient wants to be intimately involved in decisions about management, e.g. do nothing, surgery, radiotherapy, chemotherapy or a combination approach, is something to be determined overtly or tacitly by discussion between the people concerned. What is disclosed, required or requested by the patient may well change with time. It must also be appreciated that once certain pieces of information are given, such as (let us say) the probability of death within a few weeks whatever is done, the information cannot be withdrawn. It is true that the withholding of information—or economy with the truth—represents a form of medical paternalism. It is indeed the doctor acting in the best interests of the patient, as the doctor perceives them, but essentially because that is what the doctor believes or understands to be what the patient wants. If the patient requests more detail on his condition and asks questions directly then it would be wrong to lie.

Let's come back to the treatment options. First, what is the untreated survival time for different tumours? For squamous cell carcinoma a figure of 12 months is given. This accounts for about 50% of lung cancer. For adenocarcinoma 18 months (20% of tumours), small cell cancer two to three months, and large cell cancer, 10 months.

Surgery has a place for treating slower-growing tumours with a longer untreated expected survival time, providing the tumour has not already spread. Various tests can be used to confirm this, although none is completely reliable. In patients aged over 65 years surgery carries a mortality of 6–7%. Asking an older patient to decide whether or not to have this operation may be a means of respecting autonomy but most require guidance and in practice expect the doctor to guide or choose for them. In any case if the choice is put in terms such as—well I think there's a good chance of removing all the tumour (that we can see), you are pretty fit otherwise, and the success rate of the operation (i.e. not dying or having a major complication) is not much worse than 95%, most will, I suspect, agree to surgery. If, on the other hand, the surgical option is presented as—well there's almost a 10% risk of death from the procedure, and in any case we can't be sure that we'll remove all the tumour—then most will turn down surgery for something else. *Sotto voce* it might almost appear imprudent to suggest that who actually does the operation also makes a difference.

Since thoracotomy for lung cancer became established in the 1950s cure rate has not improved, but case selection and postoperative care has made surgery less harmful (safer), and immediate outcome more predictable. Some patients initially thought operable are then found to have too extensive disease within the chest shown either by computed tomography (CT) scanning or by mediastinoscopy (direct observation via a fibreoptic instrument inserted percutaneously). Many of such patients will have been told that they have lung cancer which may be able to be removed if the tests are satisfactory. The problem is then what to do, especially if the patients are asymptomatic. There is no evidence that five-year survival is helped by radical radiotherapy (i.e. therapy given with curative intent). Most surgeons or doctors, however, will feel it helpful to patients if they are offered a form of treatment other than surgery which *may* be curative, and in the case of radiotherapy not quite so restricted by anatomical boundaries as is surgery. The alternative, of no therapy until symptoms develop, can be a devasting blow for many—true some may choose it but others will not—and once the information has been given it cannot easily be retracted. Some patients, though, will not be told that radiotherapy is unlikely to be curative—an omission of information that could be deemed paternalistic. If the patient does ask outright if radiotherapy is going to be curative he should be given an honest answer, but if he does not, then this may be an instance when a paternalistic judgement to withhold information is justified. After all, autonomy or respect for autonomy also involves the right not to receive information if not wanted. Is not a doctor who has sensitively over a period of time sought to learn as much as possible about a patient's needs, vulnerabilities, family and social situation in as good a position as anyone to determine this, especially if the patient lives on his own with limited support? Even when there is a close family member such as spouse, son or daugher a judgement has to be made concerning what information is given (imposed) in the absence of direct questioning. Usually the doctor's conclusion will be that full prognosis, including the improbability of radiotherapy materially affecting life expectancy, be given to a family member, but perhaps not always. For instance in the absence of a son or daughter, and when the spouse is much older or already infirm, or when the prognosis of the spouse is considered shorter than that of the newly diagnosed patient with lung cancer it is not obligatory that information be given to the family member. Judgement is surely required, albeit with an element of paternalism.

CONSENT FOR MEDICAL TREATMENT FOR A CHILD

Parents have a duty to bring their child to autonomy free from avoidable harm— in a way they have a right to exercise that duty. This duty *is* paternalistic and hence can logically be described as an exercise in justifiable paternalism. Respect for that autonomy is one of the bedrock principles on which much of this book is based, but like all ethical principles is not absolute. There may be circumstances where the person's apparent autonomy can or should be overruled. A distinction is made between autonomy and respect for autonomy. Autonomy implies freedom of thought, of decision and of action, and includes freedom either to permit or not to permit something to be done to one's own person by a doctor. This should normally be respected provided that autonomy is not impaired by drugs, coercion, or, in the case of a child, by incomplete maturation or understanding. In an adult autonomy may be impaired by anxiety, depression, pain, toxaemia or severe illness, so that decisions about short- or long-term future health may be better decided by a doctor than by the patient. While there will be many occasions where this is not the case, to believe there are no circumstances where this is so is surely erroneous. If the doctor has as his principal concern the overall welfare of the patient, if there is reason to believe the patient's judgement may be affected by illness, then the doctor may well be ethically correct in adopting a strategy to produce what is in his professional opinion the best outcome or endpoint for the patient even if this involves an element of paternalism. Since Immanuel Kant's supreme moral law, ethicists have stressed the importance of treating people not merely as a means but also as an end in themselves. Here it would seem reasonable to treat a person so as to achieve the desired end rather than attaching greater importance to the means! An immediate objection to this view is that the end required by the patient may not be that of the doctor, and it is the patient's life, not the doctor's. True—but usually the shared aim is health and freedom from pain and disability, and the doctor may grasp the means to obtain this better than the patient.

When it comes to children and obtaining proxy consent for treatment from their parents, even more can there be occasion for a paternalistic element in management. This, of course, is enshrined in law. When parents of a child requiring surgery are Jehovah's Witnesses, the parents may request that no blood or blood products be given to their child. When the child requires open-heart surgery for congenital heart disease this may be difficult, but nonetheless responsible paediatric cardiologists and surgeons will do their utmost to avoid giving blood—until the child is bleeding to death. At that point, in the UK at least, if there is no conceivable alternative, blood will be given to the child. Normally the child will be made a ward of court, the parents will be spared the agony of a decision against their religious beliefs, and it is hoped that the child will be saved. Sadly, sometimes the decision is made too late. We have seen a child become so anaemic that although the circulating blood volume was adequate, blood loss having been replaced with non-blood plasma-expanding solutions, the oxygen-carrying capacity of the blood was so reduced that cerebral hypoxia resulted in brain damage. It would have helped had 'paternalistic' action been taken sooner. In the case of an adult similar circumstances can ensue. In most countries an adult patient has an absolute right to refuse blood, even if his life is in jeopardy from haemorrhage. Should such a patient become unconscious from inadequate delivery of oxygen to the brain—and then survive but with severe brain damage—it is again easy to argue that a more paternalistic attitude (the doctor believing he knows better than the patient!) would have a greater utility both for society and the patient. Against this view is a quote from an article commenting on blood transfusion, written under the auspices of the Watchtower Bible and Tract Society, Brooklyn, New York: 'Who would benefit if the patient's corporal malady is cured but the spiritual life with God, as he sees it, is compromised, which leads to a life that is meaningless and perhaps worse than death itself'. It is debatable whether the severely intellectually and neurologically impaired adult is still capable of a spiritual life with God similar to that of which he was capable before.

FOR—SOME ELEMENT OF—PATERNALISM IN THE DOCTOR–PATIENT RELATIONSHIP

In the majority of consultations between patients and doctors there is little place for paternalism. When the stakes are not high, when the decisions to be made are unlikely to have a long-lasting effect on quality of life—as adjudged by patient and doctor, there is no place for paternalism. The sicker the patient, the more vulnerable, the more regressed because of pain and anxiety, age, infirmity or debilitation, then in our view the more some patients will wish for an element of the sort of care a father may give his child. Some, of course, will not, but that has to be based on a judgement made by the doctor in consultation with close relatives or family members if available. In any case, is it really possible to eliminate paternalism when the medical stakes are high and the situation is acute—we have argued that it is not.

A doctor friend of ours in his late 40s, previously fit, played squash on Wednesday but on Thursday experienced severe chest pain sprinting up the third flight of stairs. Recognizing this may be angina, the following day an exercise test was organized, which proved to be positive. That is to say after 10 minutes exercise, chest pain recurred associated with ECG changes that confirmed the presence of myocardial ischaemia. Cardiac catheterization and angiography were arranged for the next week, but on the Sunday he developed chest pain at rest. Emergency hospital admission was arranged and catheterization the next day showed a localized area of narrowing in one coronary artery, the rest of the coronary arterial tree being normal and the function of the heart muscle otherwise unimpaired.

What to do? Medical treatment such as beta-blocking agents had not previously been tried, the area of narrowing could possibly be dilated with a small inflatable balloon on the end of a catheter (angioplasty), or the patient could have a very low-risk simple heart operation. Should the patient then leave the catheter laboratory to go back to the ward so that over the next few days informed discussion could take place over all the options? Should the patient, a doctor himself, review the literature, discuss mortality rates—not only for the different procedures but also—usually forgotten in the literature— discuss the mortality rates of the various operators who might undertake the angioplasty or the operation? Well, maybe that's what he should have done, but he chose to ask the cardiologists in the laboratory to make the decision. He trusted them and wanted an element of paternalism in his care. This was not demeaning; it didn't seem to him to threaten his autonomy or, for that matter, impair his or his cardiologists' respect for it. He wanted beneficence, hoped not to experience maleficence and as for some sense of overall justice, couldn't take that on board as well—at least at that moment. The justice, of course, related to resources. Maybe he should have declined further intervention in case there were others on the waiting list who needed treatment even more urgently. Nonetheless as virtually all hospitals work on a turnstile system—once through the door and in the bed, you usually get all the hospital resources can offer—he did not feel he was encroaching too much on the principle of justice by asking for his management to be carried out as soon as possible.

No, he did what many, but not all, patients will do: he left it to the doctors he trusted to make the decision for him. A choice for paternalism rather than its imposition maybe, but, we submit, a reflection of what many patients do wish for. That is to have medical care based on mutual trust between doctor and patient with the assumption that as a member of a profession the doctor will make choices in the best interests of the patient. The doctor must in turn realize that trust (of doctor by patient) has to be earned, gained, must not be abused and should not be assumed—indeed why should it be. Nonetheless, a doctor–patient relationship based on trust or covenant, albeit with an element of paternalism, seems better than a legal or commercial contract as seems so much to be the case in much of medicine in the USA. Doctors have a duty of care, and that includes a duty to recognize that this must include an element of the best of paternalism, without which care cannot be of the highest calibre. Failure to be paternalistic, in the proper sense of the word, deprives the patient and the family of real care in the time of their greatest need. Doctors have no need apologetically to defend paternalism.

REFERENCES

1. Erikson, E. 1977. *Childhood and society.* Paladin Books, London.
2. Jung, C. G. 1966. *The development of personality. Complete works,* 2nd edn, Vol. 17, pp. 284-323. Read, H., Forham, M. and Adler, G. (Eds). Routledge, London.
3. *Shorter Oxford dictionary.* 1983. Oxford University Press, Oxford.
4. Lockwood, M. 1985. *Moral dilemmas in modern medicine.* Oxford University Press, Oxford.
5. Dunstan, G. R. 1989. The doctor as the responsible moral agent. Pp. 1–9, *in* Dunstan, G. R. and Shinebourne, E. A. (Eds) *Doctors' decisions: ethical conflicts in medical practice.* Oxford University Press, Oxford.
6. Spiro, S. 1989. Clinical oncology: medical and surgical practice. Pp. 121–132, *in* Dunstan, G. R. and Shinebourne, E. A. (Eds) *Doctors' decisions: ethical conflicts in medical practice.* Oxford University Press, Oxford.

36

Against Paternalism in the Patient–Physician Relationship

ROBERT M. VEATCH, PhD

*Director and Professor of Medical Ethics, Kennedy Institute of Ethics;
Professor, Philosophy Department and Medical Center, Georgetown
University, USA*

CAROL MASON SPICER, MA

*Managing Editor, Kennedy Institute of Ethics Journal; Lecturer, Philosophy
Department, Georgetown University, USA*

Throughout history paternalism has characterized many elements of the patient–physician relationship. This chapter outlines what is meant by paternalism, the origins of physician paternalism, the moral arguments against paternalism, and, finally, some possible exceptional cases in which paternalism might be justified.

DEFINING PATERNALISM

Paternalism refers to behavior that attempts to interfere with the autonomy of an individual without his/her consent (explicit or presumed) for the express purpose of benefiting that individual. Thus the term is entirely descriptive. While this definition does not indicate whether paternalism is necessarily immoral, it does indicate that paternalism necessarily involves a conflict between two moral principles: autonomy and beneficence.

Philosophers have argued over the details of the definition. Gerald Dworkin, in an early discussion, defined paternalism as 'interference with a person's liberty of action justified by reasons referring exclusively to the welfare, good, happiness, needs, interests, or values of the person being coerced' (1). Culver and Gert have responded that defining paternalism in terms of coercively interfering with an individual's liberty of action is insufficient because numerous

Principles of Health Care Ethics. Edited by Raanan Gillon.
© 1994 John Wiley & Sons Ltd

cases of paternalism arise in which the recipient is neither coerced nor at liberty to take any sort of action (2). For example, one could act paternalistically toward a formerly autonomous unconscious individual who had a previously formulated life plan even though it would not interfere with that individual's liberty of action. What is at stake in the debate is whether the term paternalism should refer to actions against non-autonomous persons (for example, young children) or only to actions that violate autonomy. The term seems to include the way a father would act toward his child, but the morally interesting cases are those of actions directed toward autonomous or formerly autonomous persons against their will, but for their own good. Thus Dworkin in a later essay concludes, 'there must be a violation of autonomy . . . for one to treat another paternalistically' (3). If this is so, as we believe it is, then every act of paternalism will involve violating the principle of autonomy with regard to an individual without his/her consent and for the individual's benefit.

In order to play this crucial role in defining paternalism, the principle of autonomy must be distinguished from the 'liberty of action' initially referred to by Dworkin. Autonomy extends beyond freedom of action to encompass the idea of self-determination in accordance with a plan chosen by oneself. Anyone who deliberately chooses one course of action rather than another is, at least in some sense, autonomous regardless of whether the choice is considered rational. One problematic case is illustrated by the example of a clinician's transfusing a Jehovah's Witness against her formerly expressed wishes once she has become unconscious. Because she is no longer autonomous it may be argued that her autonomy cannot be violated. In such a case, however, it is reasonable to speak of extending the individual's previous autonomy into the period of incompetency just as we honor a person's will after death (4).

Paternalism, then, involves the attempted violation of an individual's autonomy, actual or extended, without explicit or presumed consent and for the express purpose of benefiting the individual.

We may further distinguish weak (soft) from strong (hard) paternalism. In strong paternalism the intervention takes place in spite of the fact that the one intervening knows the one acted upon is substantially autonomous and self-determining. By contrast weak paternalism takes place when one is unsure whether the individual is autonomous (5). We will refrain from referring to actions against clearly non-autonomous persons as paternalism of any kind (because there can be no violation of autonomy). We will, nevertheless, make clear that some interventions by physicians directed toward non-autonomous patients, while not technically paternalistic because they do not involve violations of autonomy, raise similar questions about the justification of the action.

The issue we must confront is whether paternalism, so defined, is ever justified morally and, if so, whether physicians are ever justified in acting paternalistically toward their patients. We will argue that clinicians not only generally must avoid all paternalism, but normally should avoid acting (without the consent of a surrogate) to benefit those whose plans cannot be known.

THE ORIGINS OF PHYSICIAN PATERNALISM

Before examining the morality of physician paternalism, it is important to be aware of the ancient and respected roots of paternalism in the practice of medicine.

The Hippocratic Oath

Medical paternalism dates back at least to the fourth century BC and the Hippocratic Oath. The Oath has the physician pledge that 'I will use dietetic measures for the benefit of the sick according to *my* ability and judgment' (emphasis added) (ref 6, p. 6). It is the physician, not the patient, who determines what counts as a benefit for the patient.

The Oath also has the physician pledge, 'I will keep them from harm and injustice' (ref. 6, p. 6). Ludwig Edelstein, a twentieth-century scholar who has studied the ancient oath in detail, rejected the possibility that the physician would protect the patient from the patient's enemies, from well-meaning friends, or from harm that the physician would himself do. Instead he concluded that the Hippocratic physician:

> promises to guard his patients against the evil which they may suffer through themselves. That men by nature are liable to inflict upon themselves injustice and mischief, and that this tendency becomes apparent in all matters concerned with their regimen, this is indeed an axiom of Pythagorean dietetics (ref. 6, p. 23).

Edelstein argued that the Hippocratic ethic in general is a manifestation of Pythagoreanism, the Greek philosophical–scientific school of thought that believed that knowledge was too potent and dangerous to be in the hands of ordinary lay people.

Modern Medical Ethics

This pattern of paternalism in professionally articulated medical ethics is reflected throughout the centuries. The most important modern Anglo-American discourse from within the health professions is Thomas Percival's medical ethics published in 1803 as a guide to the physicians, surgeons, and apothecaries at the Manchester Infirmary. Percival's ethics illustrates its general support of professional authority by counseling physicians 'to unite *tenderness* with *steadiness*, and *condescension* with *authority*, as to inspire the minds of their patients with gratitude, respect and confidence' (ref. 7, p. 71). The more specific notion that physicians know what is best for their patients and should promote that perception of patient welfare is illustrated by Percival's reluctance to disclose bad news to the patient, and his prohibition on 'quack medicines'.

The view that physicians generally ought not to make 'gloomy prognostications' although they 'should not fail, on proper occasions, to give the friends of the patient timely notice of danger, when it really occurs, and even to the patient himself, if absolutely necessary' (ref. 7, p. 91) reflects the belief that such disclosure would rob the patient of the benefits of hope and hence would not be in the patient's best interest. As in the Hippocratic tradition, the physician, not the patient, becomes the authority on what constitutes the patient's interests.

Similarly Percival says that a patient suffering from a 'lingering disorder' who insists on taking a 'quack medicine' should be given 'some indulgence' by the physician (p. 103). This passage implies that a physician should, at least to a certain extent, humor his/her patients when they persist in a course that the physician deems ill-advised much in the same way a parent might indulge a child in pursuing an ill-advised course of action. Like the parent, the physician should watch over the patient so that 'the consequent mischiefs, if any, can be obviated as timely as possible' (p. 104). There is no indication in Percival that the physician should respect a patient as an independent, autonomous agent who has the right to determine his/her own treatment however 'ill-advised' the choice might be.

Contemporary Medical Ethics

This tendency toward professionally articulated paternalism continued well into the twentieth century. For example, the 1957 *Principles of Medical Ethics* of the American Medical Association included a paternalistic exception to the duty not to reveal confidences. While it specified that the physician may generally not reveal confidences entrusted to him, a legitimate exception was the case in which breaking confidence was necessary in order to protect the welfare of the individual (8). (Other exceptions included breaking confidence when required by law, or when it was necessary to protect the welfare of the community, but neither of these is paternalistic since they would not be invoked to protect the welfare of the individual.)

Likewise, the British Medical Association's code of 1959 contained a similar paternalistic exception to the confidentiality rule. After spelling out the obligation to observe the rule of secrecy, the exception is added:

> The complications of modern life sometimes create difficulties for the doctor in the application of this principle, and on certain occasions it may be necessary to acquiesce in some modification. Always, however, the overriding consideration must be adoption of a line of conduct that will benefit the patient, or protect his interests (9).

In other words, a permissible exception to the confidentiality rule was the case in which the physician believed going against the wishes of the patient served the patient's interest.

Only in the 1970s was the paternalism of the professional associations tempered. In 1971 the British Medical Association changed its confidentiality rule to prohibit paternalistic breaking of confidence. 'If in the opinion of the doctor, disclosure of confidential information to a third party seems to be in the best medical interest of the patient, it is the doctor's duty to make every effort to allow the information to be given to the third party, but where the patient refuses, that refusal must be respected' (10). To be sure the rejection of paternalism was not complete, the British Medical Association reinstated the exception to confidentiality 'when it is undesirable on medical grounds to seek a patient's consent, but is in the patient's own interest that confidentiality should be broken' (11). Similary in 1985, the American Hospital Association, while strongly upholding the patient's right to confidentiality, allowed that 'subject to state law, confidentiality may be overridden when the life or safety of the patient is endangered' (12). The American Medical Association makes a similar exception to the rule of informed consent 'when risk-disclosure poses such a serious psychological threat of detriment to the patient as to be medically contraindicated' (13). Nevertheless, there was a dramatic shift away from paternalism in the direction of respect for the autonomy and self-determination of the patient *even in the case in which the physician believed such respect might harm the patient's interest.*

THE MORAL CHALLENGE TO PATERNALISM

The question is why did this dramatic change take place? What happened morally that accounts for the shift away from paternalism? We think that two major types of change, one social and the other moral, took place.

Social Changes Requiring Abandonment of Paternalism

First, the social setting in which health care was delivered changed dramatically in the 1960s and 1970s. As health care became increasingly complex technologically, more care was delivered in clinics, hospitals, nursing homes, and other sociologically complex settings (14). While the traditional model of the single, self-sufficient general practitioner providing long-term continuity of care was always somewhat of a myth, it cannot be denied that the setting of health care delivery changed during this period so that care was more institutionalized, bureaucratized, and sociologically complex. This made paternalism more difficult. Physicians would have a harder time withholding a terminal diagnosis from a patient even if they so desired, because there was less continuity of care and more people communicating with the patient.

Simultaneously the 1960s was a period of advocacy for the rights of minorities and other socially disadvantaged groups. Racial, gender, and social status rights all received much more prominent attention. Furthermore, in the United States, one effect of the Vietnam war was to teach lay people to be skeptical of the claims of military and political authorities. Similar doubts were expressed about the authority of educational leaders and other elites including medical professionals.

Moral Changes

These social changes were accompanied by shifts in the moral theory underlying professional medical ethics. Two major moral changes, we believe, rendered paternalism by physicians untenable and indefensible.

Changes in Consequentialist Theory

Medical ethics as articulated by physicians has traditionally been consequentialistic. Morally appropriate behavior is determined solely by examining the consequences of an action. In this regard Hippocratic ethics resembles utilitarian theory. Hippocratic ethics differs from classical utilitarianism, however, in the way it limits the consequences that are morally relevant. While classical utilitarianism considers every consequence for all affected parties to be morally relevant, Hippocratic consequentialism limits its calculations exclusively to the individual patient's interests. The morally right action is the one that most benefits the patient and protects the patient from harm. Sometimes Hippocratic consequentialism limits the consequences further by excluding all but the medical consequences to the patient. The goal, in that case, is the health and physical welfare of the patient and not the total good including economic, spiritual, and social well-being. These other areas are considered beyond the scope of the physician's expertise.

As the social setting of medicine became more complex, physicians began to realize that it was extremely difficult, if not impossible, for them to determine what served the welfare of the patient. Because of the more complex setting, they knew their patients less well. Especially in the United States there was less continuity of care. Because most patients were relatively healthy, and care got increasingly expensive, patients could go years without seeing their physician even if they had one. Increasing mobility meant that either physician or patient would relocate, further diminishing the continuity of care. When we realize that the total welfare of a patient covers many areas besides physical health, we see that it becomes almost impossible for a physician to guess accurately what would benefit the patient.

At this same time physicians were gaining the capacity to intervene in ways that led to more controversial outcomes. Ventilators made it possible to maintain for years patients bedridden without the ability to breathe spontaneously. Some of these patients were literally permanently vegetative (15). Chemotherapy, surgery, and radiation for cancers made aggressive, if painful, interventions possible, but physicians and patients increasingly realized that it was not obvious whether all of these interventions were in the patient's interest. Moreover, analysis in medical decision-making made increasingly clear that these questions were, in principle, not questions that could be answered on the basis of medical expertise. While clinicians could perhaps determine, at least to a first approximation, what the effect of an intervention would be, they could not tell whether that effect was good or bad and how good or bad it was.

Since Hippocratic consequentialism rests on these determinations of benefits and harms, medical professionals as well as lay persons increasingly concluded that, even if physicians wanted to be paternalistic, they would not be able to determine, based on their medical skills, what was good or bad for the patient. Hippocratic physicians had to involve patients more directly in determining whether the effect of treatment was good or bad *for the patient*.

Additional changes were taking place in ethical theory. The consequentialist theory manifesting itself thus far could be called a simple 'act consequentialism'.

Rightness or wrongness, according to this kind of consequentialism, is determined by assessing the benefits and harms envisioned for each individual action. The clinician by himself or herself standing at the bedside would estimate the consequences of alternative courses.

In the 1960s act consequentialism was challenged by much more sophisticated versions of consequentialism. Generally called 'rule consequentialism' (or 'rule utilitarianism'), these more sophisticated versions held that, for many reasons, it was not appropriate to determine the consequences of each individual instance of an action. Doing so was too time-consuming and too prone to error (especially in high-intensity, crisis situations involving complex actions among strangers such as those encountered in a hospital emergency room). Consequentialist theorists increasingly argued for a morality more oriented to a set of rules. The rules were chosen based on their consequences, but once the rules were chosen, moral action was, in most cases, simply a matter of following the rules. Only in special settings would the rules themselves be assessed based on their consequences (16–20).

A rule, for example one requiring that people acting strangely be committed for observation, might be paternalistic. However, individual clinicians, if they want to be good rule consequentialists, must follow the rule rather than make their own decision about what will benefit the patient. Some argue that the odds of benefiting the patient may be greater following the rule; others argue that it is just the nature of morality that it is a rule-governed enterprise, and hence the rule should be followed even if the clinician knows the patient's interest will not be served in the specific case. Either way contemporary consequentialists may be less inclined to be paternalistic in individual choices. Thus the physician at the bedside is not paternalistic even if the rule writers are.

Changes to Non-consequentialist Theory

While some consequentialist physicians have simply changed to the more sophisticated and defensible forms of the practice, many others have followed developments in moral theory that take them beyond consequentialism.

Some religious ethics (especially Jewish and Protestant) and many contemporary moral theories including liberal rights theory, Kantian theory, libertarianism, and contemporary theories of justice specifically reject all forms of pure consequentialism. The arguments are far too complex to trace here. They suggest that consequentialism misunderstands the nature of morality; mistakenly sees outcomes as the only morally relevant feature of actions; runs the risk of failing to respect individual persons; justifies gross injustices (such as slavery); and at the same time requires sacrifices well beyond what is morally plausible. These theories are collectively non-consequentialist or 'deontological'. They believe there are certain duties that people owe one another even if acting on those duties does not maximize the aggregate net good. Among the deontological principles characterizing morally right actions are veracity, fidelity to promises, not taking life (at least innocent, human life), and justice.

Another principle advocated as right-making by many is that of autonomy.

According to the principle of autonomy, an action tends to be morally right insofar as it respects the autonomy of another. Following this view, it is not automatically right to produce benefit for another without consent even if the consequentialists' terrible problem of determining what would really produce benefit could be solved.

The case of Karen Quinlan is the most famous American court case to establish legally that physicians no longer have the right to do what they think will benefit the patient in every case. Subsequent cases have recognized that the judgement of the patient while competent (21) takes precedence over the well-intentioned guess of the physician about what would benefit the patient. The autonomy of the patient generates a right of non-interference that remains even if the physician correctly believes that he/she could benefit the patient by violating the patient's autonomy.

No case in American law has recognized the legitimacy of a purely paternalistic intervention to provide treatment to a competent patient against his or her will. We know of no such case in British law either. Similarly, the *moral* right of non-intervention derived from the principle of autonomy is seen by most deontological theories to have absolute priority over paternalistic beneficence. Thus both sophisticated consequentialist theories and autonomy-based non-consequentialist theories reject paternalism at least as being justified by individual physicians.

POSSIBLE CASES OF JUSTIFIABLE PATERNALISM

Although both consequentialist and non-consequentialist theories have a very difficult time justifying physician paternalism, a paternalistic action is still not, by definition, immoral. Culver and Gert have suggested criteria that would tend to make paternalism more acceptable. For example, for a given instance of paternalism to be justified it would be necessary that the evil prevented or moderated by the violation of autonomy be so much greater than that inflicted by the violation that the individual would be irrational not to choose the violation (22, 23).

If paternalism is ever justifiable we believe two additional conditions would have to be met.

The Best Assessment of Interest

First, the one acting paternalistically would have to be able to make a legitimate claim that he or she was in a good position (perhaps the best position) to know what was in the interests of the patient. We believe that the physician is virtually never in the best position to make such an assessment. By contrast, the next of kin for incompetents who have never expressed their wishes while competent, as long as he or she is acting within reason, is more plausibly in such a position. Moreover, society gives families the authority to choose values for their incompetent members. Therefore, families should be given the presumption of authority to decide what is best for the patient in cases when the patient's wishes cannot be determined. This surrogate decision-making, however, is not paternalism. It is action on behalf of one whose wishes are not knowable and, hence, technically not paternalism at all in the sense of violating the patient's autonomy.

As we have seen, there are also cases in which we do not know if the one acted upon is a substantially autonomous agent. Interventions on their behalf would be what we call weak paternalism. Whenever possible such interventions are decisions for the courts, but private citizens may have limited authority to prevent persons from hurting themselves until the persons' mental state can be determined. The criteria we have summarized above would, however, still have to be met. This means that normally it should be the one who best knows the total, subjective interests of the patient—the next of kin rather than the physician—who would authorize such temporary weak paternalism.

Not all such interventions are justified, however. Only the person or people in the best position to know whether the patient is competent to act autonomously and know most reasonably what is in the patient's interest should have that authority.

Due Process

Second, maximum feasible due process should be provided. Normally, that will be within a court. Even then the minimal action necessary to stabilize the patient until mental status can be determined should be used.

It is striking that almost never will a physician be in a position to know best the full interests of a possibly non-autonomous agent. Almost never will the physician be in a position to offer due process.

David Jackson and Stuart Youngner report six cases of patient treatment refusal in which they believe that problematic questions about the patients' autonomy might justify physician intervention (24). However, none of those cases meets our criteria.

Arguably in all six cases there was sufficient time in which to seek due process in ascertaining whether the patients were substantially autonomous. In four cases it appears they were, and in the other two they had made choices before becoming incompetent. Furthermore in all cases family members were available who were arguably in a better position than the physicians to initially evaluate the patients' refusal.

As we have argued, those closest to the patient—family or friends—are usually in the best position to protect a formerly competent patient's extended autonomy by evaluating which actions best promote the patient's previously expressed desires. Health providers ought not to have the authority to determine the reasonableness of a surrogate's decision. If, however, a professional finds reason to question a surrogate's appropriateness as a decision-maker, the issue should be resolved by due process and not professional veto.

We believe there is only one type of case in which a limited professional paternalism might be justified. Such cases would rarely, if ever, arise. If they did, they would involve a patient in an acute and immediately threatening crisis who refuses treatment, and who the physician has good reason to believe is not fully autonomous. For example, a patient known by emergency room personnel to have a history of mental illness as well as asthma is brought to the emergency room in the midst of an asthma attack. She refuses treatment on the basis of quite evidently unjustified fears about the treatment.

This case is quite unique: unlike the blood transfusion or chemotherapy cases, the physician does not have even a few minutes to attempt to get a court order for the treatment. Unlike strangers in the emergency room, the physician has access to the mental history of the patient and good reason to believe she may not be acting autonomously (even though the physician has no legal authority to declare the patient incompetent). In this most unusual case no-one else can reasonably be expected to know better the patient's interests. Moreover, the patient will almost certainly be much better off with the intervention than without. In these very special circumstances one might argue that a very limited and temporary physician paternalism might, in theory, be justified, but only until those legitimated to act with due process, those in a better position to determine the patient's mental competence, can determine if she is, indeed, capable of acting autonomously.

However, because of the facts that weak paternalism by physicians is so rarely justified that terribly unusual conditions must be met, that both consequentialist and non-consequentialist ethical theories reject any more common physician paternalism, and that the data reveal that even experienced clinicians like Jackson and Youngner show high error rates in identifying cases of justifiable physician paternalism, we think it is reasonable to adopt a general rule of practice that prohibits physician paternalism as morally unacceptable.

REFERENCES

1. Dworkin, G. 1972. Paternalism. *The monist* **56** (January), 65.
2. Culver, C. M., and Gert, B. 1982. *Philosophy in medicine: conceptual and ethical issues in medicine and psychiatry*, p. 127. Oxford University Press, New York.
3. Dworkin, G. 1988. *The theory and practice of autonomy*, p. 123. Cambridge University Press, Cambridge.
4. Veatch, R. M. 1989. *Death, dying, and the biological revolution*, rev. edn, p. 112. Yale University Press, New Haven.
5. Feinberg, J. 1986. *Harm to self: the moral limits of the criminal law*, Vol. III, pp. 12–13. Oxford University Press, New York; Beauchamp, T. L. and Childress, J. F. 1989. *Principles of biomedical ethics*, 3rd edn, pp. 218–219. Oxford University Press, New York.
6. Edelstein, L. 1967. The Hippocratic oath: text, translation and interpretation. Pp. 3–64, in Temkin, O. and Temkin, C. L. (Eds) *Ancient medicine: selected papers of Ludwig Edelstein*. Johns Hopkins Press, Baltimore.
7. Percival, T. 1927. *Percival's medical ethics, 1803*, reprint, edited by Chauncey D. Leake. Williams & Wilkins, Baltimore.
8. American Medical Association. 1973. *Judicial council opinions and reports*, p. vii. American Medical Association, Chicago.
9. British Medical Association. 1963. *Member's handbook*, p. 58. British Medical Association, London.
10. Central Ethical Committee. 1971. *British Medical Journal Supplement* (1 May), p. 30.
11. British Medical Association. 1984. *The handbook of medical ethics*, p. 12. British Medical Association, London.
12. American Hospital Association, Special Committee on Biomedical Ethics. 1985. *Values in conflict: resolving ethical issues in hospital care*. American Hospital Association, p. 24.

13. Judicial Council, American Medical Association. 1989. *Current opinions of the Council on Ethical and Judicial Affairs of the American Medical Association—1986: including the principles of medical ethics and rules of the Council on Ethical and Judicial Affairs*, p. 32. American Medical Association, Chicago.

14. Rothman, D. J. 1991. *Strangers at the bedside: a history of how law and bioethics transformed medical decision making*. Basic Books, New York.

15. In re Quinlan, 70 NJ 10, 355 A.2d 647 (1976), *cert. denied* sub nom., Garger v. New Jersey, 429 U.S. 922 (1976), overruled in part, In re Conroy, 98 NJ 321, 486 A.2d 1209 (1985).

16. Rawls, J. 1955. Two concepts of rules. *Philosophical Review* **44**: 3–32.

17. Lyons, D. 1965. *Forms and limits of utilitarianism*. Oxford University Press, Oxford.

18. Ramsey, P. 1967. *Deeds and rules in Christian ethics*. Charles Scribner's Sons, New York.

19. Brandt, R. B. 1968. Toward a credible form of utilitarianism. Pp. 143–186, *in* Bayles, M. D. (Ed.) *Contemporary utilitarianism*. Doubleday & Co., Garden City, NY.

20. Veatch, R. M. 1981. *A theory of medical ethics*, pp. 291–305. Basic Books, New York.

21. Cruzan v. Director, Missouri Dept. of Health, 110 S.Ct. 2841 (1990).

22. Culver, C. M. and Gert, B. 1982. *Philosophy in medicine*, pp. 148–50. Oxford University Press, New York.

23. Gert, B. 1988. *Morality*, pp. 288–290. Oxford University Press, New York.

24. Jackson, D. L. and Youngner, S. J. 1979. Patient autonomy and 'death with dignity'. *New England Journal of Medicine* **301** (August 23): 404–408.

37

Decision Analysis: the Ethical Approach to Medical Decision-making

JACK DOWIE, MA (NZ), PHD (ANU)

Senior Lecturer in Social Sciences, The Open University, Milton Keynes, UK

INTRODUCTION

Medical practitioners should be able to engage in 'critical ethical thinking' so that they can go behind, rather than 'mindlessly' follow (or try to follow), the sort of exhortations and instructions embodied in professional codes (1). In this chapter I will be endorsing Gillon's argument, but only in a highly qualified way: along the lines of 'yes, provided it is part of the wider case that medical practitioners should be able to engage in critical thinking *in general* so that they can improve the quality of their judgements and decision-making'.

The goal of medical judgement and decision-making I take as being to *make the best decision in an individual case*, not to be 'ethically correct'—or 'technically correct' for that matter—in some abstract or general sense. An ability to engage in critical *ethical* thinking of the sort envisaged by Gillon is undoubtedly one of the *necessary* conditions for making the best decision in an individual case, but it is not a *sufficient* condition. Any critical ethical thinking must somehow be incorporated into the *general* thinking involved in the making of the decision, and failure to address the question of precisely how it is to be integrated is likely to leave it as a comforting (or disturbing) backdrop. Or as an appendage that has had an unknown, but possibly distorting, impact on the decision.

I suggest that the necessary integration of ethical into general thinking poses no problem *if* one employs the decision procedure that I believe is most likely to produce the best decision—'decision analysis' in its broadest sense. This procedure will involve drawing on ethical theory—not *medical ethics* (2)—in the same way as it will involve drawing on theory and knowledge of anatomy, physiology, biochemistry, statistics, etc. The quality of a practitioner's ethical thinking will impinge on the quality of the resulting decision in the same way

Principles of Health Care Ethics. Edited by Raanan Gillon.

as the quality of his or her knowledge of all the other disciplines that are necessary for good medical judgement and decision-making.

The ability to engage in 'critical ethical thinking' requires doctors to be familiar with the range of positions conventionally gathered under the 'absolutist–deontologist' and 'consequentialist–utilitarian' umbrellas. But Gillon goes on to argue that we can identify a set of four guiding principles—beneficence, non-maleficence, respect for autonomy and concern for justice—that are common to all of these approaches. Exploring the implications of these four principles in a case will ensure that no relevant moral concerns are overlooked.

Maybe so. But in relation to this aspect of Gillon's argument I suggest that, in the absence of any *well-specified* way of applying these principles to an individual case and, in particular, in the absence of any *well-specified* way of resolving the conflicts that are likely to arise from trying to respect all four simultaneously, they will also be set aside as interesting background, unhelpful in the precise decision-making task that the parties concerned face.

The answer is again to be found in decision analysis, broadly conceived, which provides the framework within which respect for autonomy can be given precise expression and within which the necessary 'filtering' of the other three principles into the inputs needed for actual decision-making—i.e. choice among actions in a specific case—can be undertaken. In a properly conducted decision analysis the importance of good ethical thinking is acknowledged at the same time as its particular, limited contribution to medical decision-making is demonstrated.

The reader will be aware by now that the present chapter is very much a personal statement. It is also a highly abbreviated one and what I regard as the supporting foundations and elaborations are to be found at greater length elsewhere (particularly in ref. 3).

ARE THERE 'ETHICAL DECISIONS'?

Listening to both everyday and professional conversations suggests many people believe there are some decisions in medicine that constitute 'ethical problems/dilemmas/decisions' and some that don't. This is a dangerous dichotomy, not because it is a dichotomy and dichotomies are usually dangerous (including the two implied in that statement!), but because it involves a serious distortion of the nature of medical decision-making.

All medical decisions—given that they are *genuine* decisions involving uncertainty on the one hand and outcomes of differing desirability on the other—involve value judgements of some sort and therefore raise 'ethical' issues in the widest sense. What seems to be implied in these overheard conversations is that because some medical decisions are 'easy' they are not to be thought of as 'ethical problems', whereas because others are 'tough' they are to be put into that box. But the term 'ethical' throws no particular light on these decisions *as decisions*, and it would be preferable to call them 'tough' decisions on the one hand (an extreme subset of these constituting 'tragic choices') and 'easy' decisions on the other. Better still, of course, get rid of the dichotomy and think simply of decisions varying in *degree* of 'toughness'.

Why decisions vary in 'toughness' will often be attributable to the sort of issues addressed in ethical discussions, such as the 'proper' trade-off between risks and benefits, or the case for or against providing the patient with 'therapeutic disinformation', and so on. But *how tough* a decision is is a judgement that logically should be made only at the end of, or well into, the decision process. It should not be decided on *ex ante*. Accordingly, even if one were to insist on retaining the 'ethical/non-ethical' dichotomy, there should be no question of deciding that a problem is an 'ethical' one or not before having undertaken a significant amount of systematic exploration of the case.

What will such 'systematic exploration' involve? In everyday terms it will involve meeting the criteria implied when people say that 'we really must think this thing through seriously'. More formally it means moving to a more *analytical* mode of decision-making.

MODES OF DECISION-MAKING

The appropriate *overall* framework for addressing the topic of medical judgement and decision-making is one that relates to judgement and decision-making as a human activity—and not to ethics, anatomy or any other contributory discipline. Cognitive continuum theory (developed by Kenneth Hammond) (4) provides such an overall framework.

Medical judgement and decision-making, like any other type of judgement and decision-making, can be tackled in one of six broad modes according to cognitive continuum theory. These modes are defined in relation to the two dimensions that make up the framework—the *cognitive* dimension (how we think about the task), running from 'highly intuitive' to 'highly analytical' and the *task structure* dimension (how the task presents itself), running from 'very ill-structured' to 'very well-structured' (Figure 37.1).

These six modes vary in their analytical rigour, their time and resource requirements and the degree to which they require manipulability of variables (i.e. ability to hold one constant while varying others).

Hammond's descriptive hypothesis is that the more structured the form in which the task presents itself the more analytically it will be tackled. For example, someone confronted by a *large* number of *non-numerical* cues *simultaneously* (e.g. a GP on a domiciliary visit to a previously unseen person) will be induced into adopting a much more intuitive/less analytical mode than someone presented with a *small* number of *numerical* cues *sequentially* (e.g. a hospital clinician reviewing the latest printout of results for a patient who has been well worked up over previous days).

As a *descriptive* theory, cognitive continuum theory will stand or fall by the results of its testing against real-world practice. As far as medical decision-making is concerned my hunch is that it will fall, because most current medical reasoning, judging and decision-making occurs at mode 6 or mode 5, *irrespective of the way the task presents itself and certainly irrespective of how it* **could** *present itself if it were so wished*. (I will ignore the reaction of some clinicians when I suggest this, which is that unnamed colleagues in other specialties operate at mode 7!) Whatever form the information comes in, the vast bulk of information

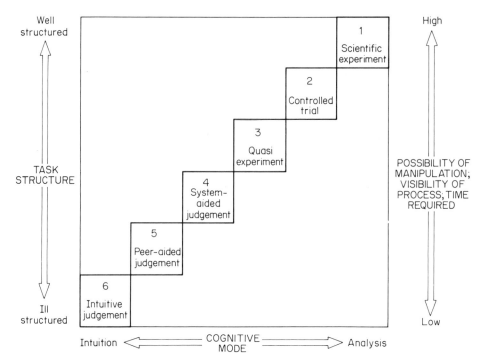

FIGURE 37.1 Cognitive continuum

processing for medical judgement and decision-making goes on inside the heads of individuals, either by themselves in their private rooms or with colleagues (and/or opponents) in group meetings. The key professional issue of our times is whether we stay at mode 6 and 5 or move along to mode 4, 'system-aided judgement and decision-making', with all its potential threats to professional autonomy and self-esteem.

System-aid is here defined very broadly to include almost any *formal* and *explicit* aid to reasoning. System aids range all the way from highly sophisticated systems accessed by computer (embracing both 'data-based scoring systems' and knowledge-based algorithms and 'expert systems') to drawing on simple analytical techniques such as, for example, listing *logical* possibilities on the back of an envelope.

One particular system aid which comes into use for the first time at mode 4 (in *my* experience of modes 5 and 6) is the number system. It has been around for a considerable time and been found to be of considerable help in many tasks where magnitudes of any sort are involved. All in the caring professions talk as if they're using numbers when they aren't. Here are some of the statements of intention that proliferate in mode 6 and particularly mode 5 decision-making, otherwise known as 'meetings' or 'case conferences'.

'We must take the home circumstances into *account*.'
'We must strike the right *balance* between risks and benefits here.'

'Clearly we need to give quality of life considerations proper *weight*.'
'We must keep the claims of autonomy and justice in *proportion*.'

At mode 4 we replace the metaphorical and rhetorical use of the concepts of 'weighing', 'balancing', 'taking things into account' and 'establishing a sense of proportion' with actual, *numerical*, weighing, balancing and—literally—taking into *a count* and establishing *proportions*. The decision analytic framework specifies the quantifications and calculations that are necessary for optimal choice.

Having acquainted ourselves with the cognitive continuum we are in a position to throw new light on an old complaint. As many who have consulted them complain, the problem with ethical philosophers—and even the ethical consultants/'ethicists' increasingly found in North American hospitals—is that they don't actually tell you *how* to 'take into account in the decision' all the things they introduce. (Of course no-one really expects or wants them to say what the decision itself should be.) They say that this isn't their job, which is to 'raise awareness' about various possibilities and factors and to increase the ability of those involved to 'think critically' in relation to the issues of the case. As I agreed at the outset, this can be an essential and extremely valuable contribution. But after the ethical consultation is finished the practitioner is effectively left back at mode 6 (or mode 5 if it is a team), where they started an hour—or several—earlier. They are left trying to 'weigh up the consequences and get the right balance between doing good and doing harm' (or something along these lines) if they have been listening to any sort of utilitarian, or trying to 'do what you think is right, taking everyone's interests and obligations into account' (or something along these lines) if they have been listening to any sort of deontologist. Or most likely a cuddly-sounding mixture of both!

The resolution of the inevitable conflicts between the claims of beneficence, non-maleficence, respect for autonomy and concern with justice that characterize most 'tough' medical decisions are therefore to be left to the unaided decision-maker(s). Even if all clinicians are 'brought up to speed' with their 'critical ethical thinking' as Raanan Gillon (and I) would hope, and even if they have access to 'clinical ethicists' (North America) or 'sensible chaps' (on this side of the Atlantic) at the end of the day the decision-maker(s) are to be left to their own cognitive resources and their unarticulated—probably unarticulable—'professional' or 'clinical judgements' as to what is 'reasonable' 'in the circumstances'.

Would mode 4 processes produce better medical decisions? This is an empirical question despite the obvious fact that value judgements and agreements are required before it can be answered. The odds, and the evidence, seem to me to be heavily in favour of an affirmative answer. Apart from the disturbing results from studies of clinical–pathological 'discrepancies', rapidly growing studies of 'small area variations' in medical practice, and numerous audit studies revealing significant proportions of 'inappropriate' or 'unnecessary' procedures, there is above all the vast literature on the 'clinical versus actuarial' controversy (5). The controversy relates to the comparative performance over a series of individual cases of unaided (but 'expert') human judges on the one hand and statistical models ('equations'), based on data drawn from similar cases, on the other. I have room for only my favourite quotation from this debate. It comes from the recent reflective paper by Paul Meehl (6), who set off controversy 35 years ago with what he refers to as his 'disturbing little book'.

> There is no controversy in social science that shows such a large body of qualitatively diverse studies coming out so uniformly in the same direction as this one. When you are pushing 90 investigations, predicting everything from the outcome of football games to the diagnosis of liver disease, and when you can hardly come up with a half dozen studies showing even a weak tendency in favour of the clinician, it is time to draw a practical conclusion (pp. 373–374).

> If I try to forecast something about a college student, or a criminal, or a depressed patient by inefficient rather than efficient means, meanwhile charging this person or the taxpayer 10 times as much money as I would need to achieve greater predictive accuracy, that is not a sound ethical practice. That it feels better, warmer, and cuddlier to me as predictor is a shabby excuse indeed (p. 374).

Predictably the clinicians' retort is, in one form or another, that the studies are all methodologically defective. One senses that unless the studies come up with a verdict in favour of the clinician this will always be their attitude.

Why could system-aided decisions be better? In brief, because at mode 4 we accept the well-established limits to human information processing (individual and/or group) and reduce the effects of these by raising the analytical level of discussion. Only an evaluation which regards a less analytical process as in itself a good thing (irrespective of the outcome results) seems likely to reach a contrary conclusion. And I insist that we judge processes (including decision analysis) by their results, not by their internal procedural characteristics or by their inputs.

It has to be accepted that the 'clinical versus actuarial' research relates mainly to *diagnostic and predictive judgements*, rather than to *decisions* involving outcomes that are value-laden. But on what basis could one assume that decisions made at mode 5/6 are superior to ones made at mode 4, when diagnostic or prognostic judgements are not? Is there any reason to believe that the processing of *information about values*, rather than about 'facts', will be less subject to the sort of biases and limitations that results in the superiority of mode 4 in diagnosis and prognosis? I think not, personally fear that the biases may be even greater, and as a patient certainly wouldn't want to bet that they aren't.

The implication is that we need help with the value aspects of decision-making just as much as with the more factual sides of the decision. And help also with the necessary integration of technical and value judgements—types of judgement that should have been made independently so as to avoid cross-contamination.

For a pioneering attempt to take decision-making up to mode 4 in a 'tough' case, I commend Candee and Puka's analysis of a case of a newborn baby with Down's syndrome and duodenal atresia (7). They undertake systematic and quantitative assessments within utilitarian and deontological frameworks (separately) and conclude that it is possible to reach either of the possible decisions within either approach. This is, of course, an important criterion for any decision-making procedure—it must be the *inputs* into the procedure rather than the procedure itself which determines the answer.

But it is not enough to show that one can move to mode 4 within two or more ethical frameworks. In order to *make a decision* all considerations relating both to rights/duties and consequences have to be filtered into the decision structure and into its detailed content in a well-specified way. Decision analysis provides the requisite (mode 4) procedure to achieve this. It enables the optimal choice to be determined, 'taking into a count' all the relevant clinical/technical and ethical/value issues. As a procedure it in no way determines the optimal choice. Nor, of course, does it guarantee that disagreements of any sort will be resolved. Parties may still disagree on what the best decision is, but the decision analysis will have established the set of elements on which agreement, or compromise, is logically necessary in order to make the decision.

DECISION ANALYSIS

Any systematic exploration of a decision problem will necessarily involve the framing of the problem as a choice among alternative actions (e.g. operate or not), with each action leading to a set of possible scenarios. Any one scenario will reflect particular uncertainty resolutions (e.g. the appendix was or wasn't the problem) and particular outcome states (e.g. good health or moderate disability).

Decision analysis is simply the formal modelling of these key components of a decision in the form of a 'tree' of which the simplest clinically relevant example is given in Figure 37.2. This simple tree suggests that there are only two available options, here labelled 'remove', the other 'leave' (for example, a possibly diseased appendix or a possibly abused child). It further suggests that there is uncertainty about whether or not the underlying condition (appendicitis, abuse) is present. Finally it suggests that there are four different outcome states, at least some of which will be regarded as more desirable than others. These four states are conceptually equivalent to the consequences that flow from making or not making the two sorts of error that are possible in this situation ('false positive' or 'false negative').

This tree has also been provided with the numerical 'fruit' necessary for establishing the optimal decision—*probabilities* on the chance branches to quantify the uncertainties and *utilities* on the outcome nodes to quantify the relative desirability/undesirability of the outcome states. Given the numbers inserted here, and given acceptance of the principle of maximizing expected utility, the optimal choice is to leave. Other numbers (and other principles) *could* change this (e.g. a probability of disease/abuse higher than 50% will make removal the optimal decision).

Fuller expositions of clinical decision analysis are to be found elsewhere (3,8, 9). No further details of the technique can be provided here, but it should be emphasized that there are few limits to the complexity of decision trees. While many (but not all!) real-life cases are more complex than the above illustrative one, the limitations of decision analysis lie not in the technique, nor in the computer software that is desirable for its implementation in anything but the

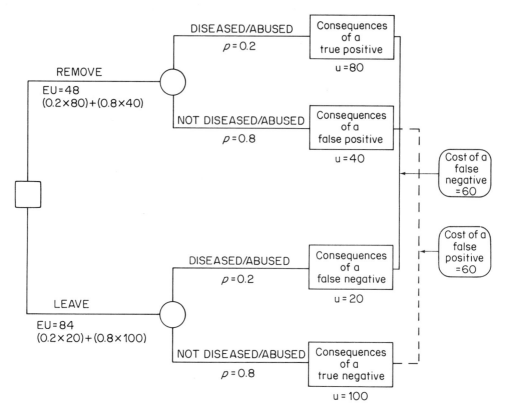

FIGURE 37.2 Example of a decision tree

simplest case, but in the ability of human beings to think clearly about great complexity and articulate it. It is simultaneously amazing and disturbing to find clinicians arguing that they cannot structure a problem as a tree (even with help) because of the complexity of the problem, nor provide the logically necessary chance and desirability assessments, while remaining utterly confident of their ability to make the decision successfully—or at least well.

We all *think* we can think immensely complex things. But for most of us this is a massive delusion insofar as *systematic analysis and modelling* is concerned. We *could* be much better at it if we were given lots of practice, lots of support and lots of reward, but at the moment we get none of these: professional (and ordinary) education is devoid of any attention to systematic analysis for judgement and decision-making, and the career rewards go to those who show disdain for such methods, claiming to be able to make good judgements and decisions by drawing on their intuitive powers of insight, based on 'my years of experience'.

In developing decision trees it is important to distinguish the *decision* from the *judgements* that need to be made within the decision structure in order to resolve it. A decision always involves choice among two or more options (e.g.

'remove' or 'leave'). Judgements do not involve choice. They involve assessment or valuation on some sort of scale.

In the case of most medical decisions, and hence in decision analyses of them, judgements of four broad types are needed.

1. Judgements as to the *'availability'* of various action options (what are the possible choices). What is judged as an 'available' option for a particular patient may be affected by clinical, religious, ethical, legal, economic or other considerations. For example, if the 'removal' concerned was of a fetus incapable of independent life, from the mother's womb, some people would argue that it is not an available option on the ground that abortion is simply wrong.

   This sort of judgement will determine whether an action option gets into the race. The three other sorts of judgements relate to the evaluation of the contenders.

2. Judgements as to the *chances* involved wherever there is uncertainty involved in an option scenario. The uncertainty may relate to whether an event will or will not occur in the future (e.g. the abuse will continue if the child is left) or whether something is or isn't the case (e.g. the appendix is or is not diseased).

3. Judgements as to the *desirability* of various possible outcome states (e.g. normal good health; confined to bed; unable to undertake self-care; dead). Making of this type of judgement may involve internal 'sub-judgements', for instance, of the relative importance of such health dimensions as mobility, mental function and pain.

4. Judgements as to the way *integration* of the foregoing judgements is to be achieved: how the uncertainty and desirability assessments pertaining to an option are to be integrated into some overall assessment for the option, so as to permit its comparison with the other available options. This will pre-eminently involve judgement as to 'risk preference' and as to whether or not 'maximizing expecting utility'—weighting utilities by their probabilities—is the appropriate way to integrate these sorts of judgements. While the present author does not find the arguments against MEU as a normative strategy convincing (10) the key point here is that the explicit specification of chance and desirability judgements in the tree enables the claims of any well-specified alternative integration strategy to be explored.

How does decision analysis relate to ethical debates? If we go along with a broad caricaturing of the alternative ethical schools as the absolutist–deontological and the consequentialist–utilitarian then in decision analytic practice their differences will usually be locatable in different judgements about (a) the 'availability' of a course of action and (b) the relative 'desirability' of certain outcome states.

In practice the deontological judgement that a course of action (e.g. abortion, euthanasia) is 'wrong' and should not therefore be included as a choice branch on the tree can equally well be achieved by giving any outcome node to which that choice branch leads a utility judgement of minus infinity.

Most ethical controversies therefore relate to the 'correct' utilities to be assigned to outcome states. The controversies are deepest when more than one party is involved in the decision (e.g. the mother and the fetus, the mentally ill patient and the family) and the question of resolving conflicting interpersonal interests arises. Alternative ways of systematically (numerically) rating and weighting the preferences of parties to a decision are available in 'multi-attribute utility theory'. Most of these procedures are instantly rejected by clinical practitioners on the grounds of their 'crudeness' or 'unacceptability' or 'impossibility', e.g. asking for the importance weights for the mother and fetus to be given as two numbers that add up to 100. To the decision analyst this is simply a signal that such logically necessary judgements are going to be made *implicitly* and *covertly* at mode 5 or 6.

Decision analysis therefore imposes two heavy psychological burdens on medical decision-makers. Firstly, it demands that all differences in beliefs and values that pertain to the decision be made explicit and resolved in the open. Secondly it demands that all verbal assertions of differences in magnitude be quantified. If the present chapter is based on any particular ethical presumptions, they relate to each of the foregoing. First, explicitness is to be taken as a moral imperative in medical decisions unless there is an *overwhelming* case against it on therapeutic grounds (or patient incompetence grounds). (This is apart from any legal imperatives to explicitness which are emerging from 'informed consent' requirements where the 'reasonable patient' standard is employed.) And secondly, there is no ethical implication in expressing magnitudes in numbers as opposed to words.

Decision analysis is particularly attractive in relation to the ethical issue of patient autonomy. Adopting a decision-analytic approach does not guarantee that claims for autonomy will be respected, but it does provide the framework within which the key issue in relation to autonomy—whose utilities are to count and for how much (patient, professional/s, family, community)—is made much more highly explicit. However it is resolved in the analysis, it cannot be resolved covertly or ambiguously.

It is important at this point to re-emphasize that the decision analyst has absolutely nothing to say about what the probability or utility numbers in an actual decision should be, only that it is necessary that the end-products of all searching of hearts, minds and literatures in the case are to be such numbers. While this requirement need not dominate every moment of discussion it is vital that that discussion be conducted under the assumption that these are what are needed at 'the moment of *decision*' (which it would conceptually be quite inappropriate to call the 'moment of *truth*').

HOW LONG SHOULD IT TAKE TO MAKE AN ETHICAL DECISION?

All decisions should be taken by the decision-analytic approach as modified in the light of the constraints of time pressure, resource scarcity, and the 'manipulability' limitations mentioned earlier. Clearly not all decisions require or justify decision analysis in its full quantitative rigour, although 'routine' decisions should in principle be based on a full-scale decision analysis of this type of case. One particular point to note, particularly relevant to *tough* 'ethical' decisions, is that it does not follow that decisions should have more resources and time devoted to them simply because the consequences to the patient and/or others are more serious.

Many decisions are tough decisions in the sense that the alternatives, even when thoroughly assessed (given the time judged to be available), are all highly unattractive, because of the consequences of 'errors' of both omission and commission. For example, the consequences of removing an unabused child and the consequences of leaving an abused child are both 'extremely serious'/'terrible to contemplate'/'very, very bad', etc. (In our earlier illustrative tree the costs of both errors are the same—60.) But unless there is reason to believe that further discussion will help *differentiate* the magnitude of these two error costs the fact that they are both absolutely highly negative is *not* a basis for postponing the decision and using up more time and resources. *Only the magnitude of the cost difference is relevant to the choice.* In other words, one should be seeking only to establish the *difference* between the 'cost of a false positive' and the 'cost of a false negative'.

For most people the *absolute* size of the consequences (either positive or negative) in these situations is thought to justify spending more time and resources on making the judgements necessary. It doesn't. One should devote extra time and resources to any process only because it will produce a better outcome, in this case a better decision. And one is on extremely dangerous ground if one argues that the amount of time and resources put into a decision process should, *per se*, be given any weight in evaluating the quality of that decision.

In many cases of so-called ethical decisions' the reason for the extra time and resources expended is actually to make the decision-makers happier (less anxious, etc.) rather than to produce a better decision, though of course they will not say or admit or perhaps even recognize this. I call this use of resources to increase the utility of the decision-makers, rather than that of the subjects of the decision (including the community), *process abuse* (cf. substance abuse).

There is even a peculiarly British form of *meta-process abuse* in which the community conspires. Vast and expensive public inquiries are held into cases where it is believed a process has gone badly wrong, based on a bad outcome. The series of inquiries into the distressing deaths of young children (Maria Colwell *et al.*) (14) and allegations of child abuse are classic examples. One thing these inquiries invariably avoid doing—the Butler-Sloss report (15) on Cleveland being just the most striking example—is actually to say what the decisions should have been or suggest, in any well-specified way, how they should have been taken!

THE ETHICAL DECISION PROCESS

Any decision process can be abused—which includes processes within any mode on the cognitive continuum, including 'scientific experiment', including any mode 4 process and therefore including decision analysis itself. But the difficulty and dangers of abuse are less the greater the openness and specificity (well-specifiedness) of the procedure. The argument that an innumerate population—and profession?—could be misled by numbers and equations deserves to be heeded and the appropriate therapy—remedial work—begun immediately.

There is, for instance, a fallacious argument concerning quantification to be disposed of. In the legendary TV series *The Prisoner*, the eponymous 'Number 6' sustains his morale by asserting 'I am not a number, I am a free man'. A fine sentiment, but one that, like many, is unhelpful in the real world if misinterpreted. The most prevalent misinterpretation in this case involves confusing being treated on the basis of statistical considerations with being treated as a statistic, i.e. as a dehumanized object in an experiment or trial. (Every medical encounter may conceptually be regarded as one or the other.) A truly free person is one who is able to benefit from being treated on the basis of his or her set membership when the limits of current knowledge mean that attempting to go beyond this will lead to inferior treatment. As a patient I say to doctors 'I am a free man—but please treat me as a number if it improves my odds'. And please 'accept error to make less error' (11), since I have no logical grounds for believing that I have any less chance than any other of your patients of being your needless error.

The ethical decision process is the one that produces the best decisions as judged by results over a large number of cases. Which process does this, whether intra- or inter-mode comparison is involved, can only be established by evaluation conducted at a mode 'higher' than the processes being evaluated. In medicine the controlled trial is accepted as the ideal mode for such evaluation. So, as with the evaluation of drugs or imaging technologies, decision technologies too need to be evaluated in controlled trials. (Familiarity means it is difficult to see 'clinical judgement' as a 'decision technology', but that is conceptually what it is.) The issue can then be clearly seen as not being whether decision analysis or any alternative mode is *perfect*, but which produces the *better* results.

What are the ethical implications of a commitment to mode 5 or 6 decision-making processes *not* based on any such systematic comparative evaluation? It involves acting on the assumption—or, more brutally, *faith*—that the results are better than those that could be produced by the alternative. It cannot (I argue) be ethical to refuse to carry out a controlled trial of one's judgement and decision-making and other alternatives simply on the ground that 'it's the way I/we as experienced practitioner/s do it' or 'it's the way things are done in this practice/hospital'. Nor can it be ethical to refuse a trial on the grounds that the alternatives are obviously 'defective' and 'unacceptable' *as processes*. There is a paradox here in that the alternatives to existing decision processes—such as decision analysis—are by definition more explicit and specific. Their potential limitations and weaknesses can be much more easily identified, even if we rule out, as we surely should, 'clinician acceptability' as a key criterion. (How can a fair evaluation of two things proceed when one is going to be the judge?)

A syndrome which I have labelled *quoplegic myopia* is rampant in the professional world. Quoplegic myopia is an acquired syndrome in which the sufferer, who can see weaknesses and deficiencies in the current or *status quo* way of doing things, including those identified in one's own processes by self-reflection, suddenly becomes blind to them as soon as any alternative to them is canvassed. The onset is particularly rapid when the alternative involves any change of behaviour on their own part (let alone income) and it is instant if it involves numbers or equations.

A truly free and truly ethical professional decision-maker is one who accepts his or her limitations as an information processor and decides whether or not to adopt a decision-support procedure on the basis of evidence, rather than *assuming* that he or she must be able to outperform it—as judged by results— because of its manifest internal defects. In other words he or she does not maintain that 'my clinical judgement must always take precedence', but adopts the reflective position that 'my clinical judgement will take precedence when I have good evidence to support the view that it will outperform the judgements and decisions produced with the help of a judgement and decision aid'.

> According to [the Hippocratic] tradition, only the physician who understands natural limits and uses this understanding to set wise boundaries, avoids the error of excessive confidence. The Greeks called this error *hubris* (ref. 12, p. 5).

Many of the judgements and decisions in health care effectively invite practitioners to play God, but that is no excuse for them confusing themselves with her. The awesome requirements of decision analysis quickly induce a sense of proportion.

REFERENCES

1. Gillon, R. 1986. *Philosophical medical ethics*. Wiley, Chichester.
2. Seedhouse, D. 1991. Against medical ethics: a philosopher's view. *Medical Education* **25**: 280–282.
3. Dowie, J. 1991. *Professional judgment and decision making: introductory texts*. (3 vols). Open University, Milton Keynes: [Course D300: first published in 1988 as D321.]
4. Hamm, R. M. 1988. Clinical intuition and clinical analysis: expertise and the cognitive continuum. Pp. 79–105, *in* Dowie, J. and Elstein, A. (Eds) *Professional judgment: a reader in clinical decision making*. Cambridge University Press, Cambridge.
5. Dawes, R. M., Faust, F. and Meehl, P. E. 1989. Clinical versus actuarial judgment. *Science* **243**: 1668–1674.
6. Meehl, P. E. 1986. Causes and effects of my disturbing little book. *Journal of Personality Assessment* **50**: 370–375.
7. Candee, D. and Puka, B. 1884. An analytic approach to resolving problems in medical ethics. *Journal of Medical Ethics* **2**: 61–70 (Reprinted in ref. 13).
8. Weinstein, M. C. and Fineberg, H. V. 1980. *Clinical decision analysis*. W. B. Saunders, Philadelphia.
9. Doubilet, P. and McNeil, B. J. 1985. Clinical decisionmaking. *Medical Care* **23**: 648–662 (reprinted in ref. 13).
10. Deber, R. B. and Goel, V. 1990. Using explicit decision rules to manage issues of justice, risk and ethics in decision analysis: when is it not rational to maximise expected utility? *Medical Decision Making* **10**: 181–194.
11. Einhorn, H. J. 1986. Accepting error to make less error. *Journal of Personality Assessment* **50**: 387–395 (reprinted in ref. 13).
12. Jecker, N. S. 1991. Knowing when to stop: the limits of medicine. *Hastings Center Report* **21**: 5–8.
13. Dowie, J. and Elstein, A. (Eds). 1988. *Professional judgment: a reader in clinical decision making*. Cambridge University Press, Cambridge.
14. DHSS 1974. Report of a committee of inquiry into the care and supervision provided in relation to Maria Colwell. HMSO, London.

15. Butler-Sloss, Lord Justice Elizabeth 1988. Report of the inquiry into child abuse in Cleveland, 1987. Cm. 412. HMSO, London.

38

Risk and the Doctor–Patient Relationship

MICHAEL HENDERSON

49 Bakers Road, Church Point, New South Wales 2105, Australia

THE EMERGENCE OF A PHILOSOPHY OF DISCLOSURE

A primary historical source for our understanding of the doctor's responsibility to the patient derives from the Hippocratic doctors of ancient Greece. The Hippocratic oath developed into a public pledge to uphold professional responsibilities, but it completely failed to address fundamental issues surrounding communication, disclosure and the giving of permission for treatment. Consent by patients, and the risks of treatment, go unmentioned.

The doctor is portrayed in Hippocratic writings as the one who commands and makes decisions, while patients must place themselves fully in doctors' hands and obey such commands. Indeed, the Corpus Hippocraticum commends 'concealing most things from the patient while you are attending to him ... turning his attention away from what is being done to him ... revealing nothing of the patient's future or present condition' (1). These attitudes hardly changed through medieval times, and it was not until well into the nineteenth century that medical writings record discussions between doctors and patients about the relative risks of treatment and the alternative of leaving well enough alone.

Even 100 years ago the doctor's relationship to the patient was very different from what it is now. Doctors still occupied a position of great authority. Suffering and death were part of our natural lot, and when things went wrong with medical treatment—and they often did—then that was a matter for the will of God. Most people, especially the poor, were grateful for any attention that the doctor would grant them, and accepted treatment willingly and uncritically. But today, people are more critical and they want to know more. In particular, they want to know more about the risks and benefits of medical treatment, topics they read about nearly every day of their lives.

Doctors are in a privileged position of trust, and this touches directly upon

Principles of Health Care Ethics. Edited by Raanan Gillon.
© 1994 John Wiley & Sons Ltd

the ways that they offer information and advice on risk. Doctors do traditionally adopt an authoritarian approach to their patients, and this has for many years been the style most expected by patients (2). In the end, however, and now to an increasing extent, it is the *patient's* perception and acceptance of risks which will help to determine whether to accept or reject any treatment that is offered.

Information leads to understanding, and understanding leads to consent (or rejection). Consent for medical intervention, therefore, is a subtle and complex outcome of the relationship of the doctor to the patient. The principles of respect for autonomy, beneficence and justice are directly relevant to whether consent is 'informed', and thus appertain to the assessment, perception and management of risk.

Until some 25 years ago the justifications for disclosure and consent-seeking were governed by beneficence rather than autonomy, centred on the idea that the primary obligation was to provide medical benefits for the patient. The welfare of the patient is the goal of health care, and thus the principle of beneficence is linked to the promotion of welfare: evil or harm should not be inflicted, they ought to be prevented or removed, and good should be promoted. The risks of harm caused by medical interventions must constantly be weighed against the possible benefits for patients, subjects or the public interest. The doctor who strives to 'do no harm' is not pledging never to cause harm, but rather to try to create a positive balance of benefit over imposed risk.

Today, however, beneficence is being replaced by autonomy as the most frequently mentioned moral principle in the literature on informed consent, rooted in the liberal western tradition that the individual's freedom and choice are important. Autonomy is loosely associated with ideas such as privacy, voluntary action, freedom of choice and acceptance of personal responsibility. Many issues about consent concern failures to respect autonomy, ranging from under-disclosure of relevant information on medical risks to non-recognition of a person's right to refuse medical treatment. To respect autonomy is to respect the right of the patient to hold certain views, make certain choices and take certain actions based on personal values, beliefs and perceptions of risk.

Respect for justice is the third of the moral principles that guide the doctor in discussing risk with patients. The principle of justice is upheld if a person has been treated according to what is fair, due or owed. Denial of information on risk to which a person has a right is an injustice.

THE PATIENT'S RIGHT TO KNOW ABOUT RISK

Part of the professional duty of care is the duty of a doctor to give information to the patient. A doctor may be held to be negligent if he breaches this duty in such a way that, by withholding information about a risk, the patient consents to a procedure which later causes harm, consent which would not have been given if the patient had been in possession of all the information beforehand. The essential premise is that the harm was caused by the non-disclosure of the risk.

The amount of information that must be disclosed about the risk and negative consequences associated with a medical procedure is still a controversial matter.

Two standards of disclosure have evolved in an attempt to resolve these problems, the 'professional practice' standard and the 'reasonable person' standard.

The professional practice standard holds that the scope of disclosure is determined by the customary practices of a professional community. Doctors commonly express concern that to give patients full information on risk would in fact be harmful. But the main objection to this standard is its assumption that doctors have sufficient expertise to know what information is in fact in the best interests of their patients. And a more fundamental objection is that this standard undermines individual autonomy, the protection of which is the primary function and moral justification of informed consent requirements.

The reasonable person standard has its basis in defining the information that the 'reasonable person' needs to know about risks, alternatives and consequences of medical procedures that are offered. The legal test is the significance of information on the process by which the patient makes decisions. Because the right to decide what information is reasonable is shifted from the doctor to the patient, the standard requires a doctor to divulge *any* fact that is material to a reasonable person's decision.

Despite its popularity with legal commentators and the courts in the United States, the reasonable person standard has been subjected to stern criticism. Critics have maintained that the standard is not in the best interests of either the patients or doctors, and is in any case impossible to satisfy (3).

Even more controversial is the 'therapeutic privilege' of a doctor to withhold information from a patient because of what are believed to be the risks of *disclosure*. Paternalism in this case may conflict with principles of respect both for autonomy and beneficence. The precise formulation of this privilege varies among the jurisdictions of the world. When framed broadly, it can permit doctors to withhold information if disclosure would cause any harm, however slight. If framed narrowly it can permit the doctor to withhold information only if the patient's knowledge would have serious consequences for health.

In the courts, the principles governing risk and the doctor–patient relationship have been argued in the stately manner so characteristic of the law.

The following example is one that is highly supportive of the principle of beneficence. In 1954 (4) a young freelance broadcaster developed a toxic goitre. A general practitioner asked a consultant physician at a London teaching hospital to see her, and he advised that a partial thyroidectomy as an alternative to medical treatment was the better course. The operation was performed by a surgeon who was asked by the patient whether there was any risk to her voice. He told her that there was none. Unfortunately, after the operation her voice was weak. There was paralysis of the left vocal chord from damage to the laryngeal nerve which passes behind the thyroid gland. Her complaint against the consultant physician was that he had, according to her, negligently advised that the operation involved no risk to her voice, and that had she known there was *any* risk she would have chosen medical treatment rather than the operation.

Lord Justice Denning held in his summing up of the case that it would be wrong and bad law to say that simply because a mishap occurred the hospital and doctors were liable, and it would be disastrous for the community. A doctor was only negligent when he had fallen short of the standard of reasonable medical care. The first question raised in the action was what should doctors tell patients. In this case the doctor had said that there was no risk to her voice, even though he knew there was in fact some slight risk. This, said Lord Justice Denning, he had done for her own good because of the vital importance to her that in her condition she should not worry. The doctor had told a lie which in the circumstances was justifiable. It was a matter in which the law was left to the conscience of the doctor himself, and the jury returned a verdict in favour of the doctor.

In the United States a series of important court cases in the late 1950s through the 1960s and into the 1970s firmly established a legal definition of 'informed' consent which substantially deviated from the attitudes expressed by Lord Denning and typified moves away from principles embracing beneficence towards those supporting autonomy. American courts found during this period that doctors had the duty to disclose any facts which are necessary to form the basis of an intelligent consent by the patient to proposed treatment. All pertinent topics of consent including the nature, consequences, harms, benefits, risks and alternatives of a proffered treatment were therefore perceived as information needed by patients in order for them to know what they are choosing. Self-determination—autonomy—was the central premise. People must be masters of their own bodies, and if of sound mind must be able expressly to prohibit the performance of even life-saving surgery or other medical treatment. The doctor's duty, therefore, becomes one of 'reasonable disclosure' of the risks or any alternatives to the proposed treatment, a duty based in the fiducial quality of the doctor–patient relationship.

An outburst of malpractice litigation in the 1970s saw the common-law basis of informed consent give way to statutes, and by the early 1980s 30 states in the USA had enacted informed consent legislation. In most cases the effect was to freeze the law where it already stood. This effectively wrote into a statutory legal framework the change from an exclusive preoccupation with a beneficence model for the doctor–patient relationship to an autonomy model of responsibility for the patient, including the full disclosure of the risks of treatment in a way that the patient could understand.

INFORMATION AND CONSENT

Consent in Britain has generally been held to be 'informed' if a doctor tells a patient the general nature of what is concerned in an operation or other treatment, but fails to disclose an improbable but serious risk. This has applied even if the patient could prove that, had information been given on the risk, consent would never have been granted. The method of judging the case has been the same as that for negligence; essentially whether comparable doctors would have done the same thing. It is the 'professional practice' standard of disclosure, founded upon the belief that describing all the risks would create harmful anxiety and might deter a patient from undergoing an operation.

The professional practice test took firm hold in England in 1957, based on the 'Bolam principle'. In this case, Mr Justice McNair instructed a jury that a doctor who administered electroconvulsive therapy to a mentally ill patient without informing him of the risk of fracture could not be criticized if he was acting in accordance with current medical practice.

A landmark case was that of *Sidaway* v. *the Board of Governors of Bethlem Royal Hospital and Maudsley Hospital* (5). This involved an elderly woman who claimed damages for negligence by a neurosurgeon, on the grounds of failure to explain to her the risks of the advised operation. The spinal cord was damaged during surgery, which was for a slipped disc in the neck, and she was left with some paralysis of the arm. Mr Justice Skinner dismissed the claim on the facts. However, he stated that the evidence of other neurosurgeons was that they would give such a patient some warning of the risks involved, although they differed about the nature and scope of the warning they would give, and each conceded that it might differ from patient to patient and from surgeon to surgeon. The doctor's duty was to take such action by way of giving or withholding information as is reasonable in all the circumstances, including the patient's true wishes. Too much information might hinder rather than help the patient in making a rational choice, and the mere fact that a patient asks to be told everything might not mean that he really wants to know the worst.

The judgement in favour of the defendant was upheld on appeal to the House of Lords. In a majority decision it was acknowledged that professional practice would usually determine what was reasonable for the doctor to say or refrain from saying to the patient.

The effect of this decision is to present some complications for the practitioner in the consulting room. Any doctor who declines to tell a patient about the risks of an operation might be in difficulty, the implication being that a patient has a legal right to know, and the doctor a legal duty to disclose, the risks inherent in any treatment recommended. Where there is a conflict over what should be disclosed, it then falls upon the courts to decide what is right, based on what is 'reasonable'. If a patient wished to know about a particular risk in order to decide whether to accept advice on treatment, a court in a subsequent hearing could rule that a doctor had neglected his duty if he did not disclose it. In other words, the issue is as much one of 'failure to warn' as it is of consent.

In the United States the matter is much clearer, although not less difficult to deal with in practice. The patient has an absolute right to know. He or she can determine whether or not to have an operation only after receiving full disclosure of all the risks. The basic elements of information needed in the United States were defined by the US Department of Health, Education and Welfare in 1978 (6). They include the following: an explanation of the procedures to be followed and their purposes; a description of any attendant discomforts and risks reasonably to be expected; a description of any benefits reasonably to be expected; a disclosure of alternatives that could be advantageous; an offer to answer queries; and an instruction that the person is free to withdraw consent at any time. The result is that surgeons present their patients with consent forms comprising several pages of complex information listing every conceivable complication.

It is easy to mock such efforts to inform, but studies of patients indicate that they do want to know. Alfidi (7) wrote to 100 patients before angiography, spelling out in reassuring language all complications including the 1-in-1625 risk of death. Most patients were found to want this information, and only an occasional one refused the investigation. It may be that people are more frightened of a little knowledge than of all the facts.

Whatever is indicated or compelled by law, just how much about risk a patient should be told by the doctor in the consulting room is not easy to decide. Among the factors will be the personality of the patient, age, temperament, clarity of mind, intelligence and the patient's desire to know everything there is to know about the treatment. In practice, often the circumstances will decide. When a patient is desperately ill and needs an urgent operation only a brief discussion will be either necessary or possible, whereas elective treatment with several options may require careful discussion of the alternatives and their resulting risks. No two patients are alike, but Hawkins (8) suggests that patients generally fall into two classes:

1. The patient who decides to place himself unreservedly in the hands of medical advisers and who signifies willingness to accept any decision that they may make as to treatment. Here the only question that arises is the extent of the doctor's duty to volunteer explanations of the treatment, its outcomes and risks.
2. The patient who makes it clear by questions about the nature of the treatment, and its consequences and risks, that the patient does not wish to surrender entirely to the hands of medical advisers, but wants to exercise personal judgement as to the type of treatment to be undergone. This patient should have questions answered fully and accurately and the doctor should explain fully the risks of any operation, investigation or medical treatment to be offered.

PRESENTING AND DISCUSSING RISKS

Sir William Osler wrote in 1906 that 'medicine is a science of uncertainty and an art of probability' (9). To a large extent it still is, and the array of different treatments now being offered by modern high-technology medicine presents a new array of risks. These lay a heavy burden on the doctor who tries to explain to the patient what the risks are, how big they are and what they mean. Patients are often particularly confused about drugs, reading on the one hand in the popular press about horrendous side-effects, and yet on the other hand being handed bottles of pills with no other information than that they should take one three times a day. Investigations, too, offering diagnostic but not necessarily therapeutic benefits, all carry risks that can be hard for a doctor to explain.

It is through the doctor–patient relationship that the patient will glean information on risk which will help to formulate a decision on what medical intervention to accept. The question then is not what doctors must disclose when discussing consent for a treatment or investigation, but rather, if patients are ignorant of risks, what can doctors do to facilitate an informed assessment of risks based on substantial understanding.

As a whole, patients are likely grossly to overestimate the doctor's capacity for accurately assessing risk. It is not an easy thing to do. At the individual level the doctor sees far too few patients to make a valid statistical calculation that the offered treatment carries, say, a 1-in-1000 risk of causing a given sort of harm. That kind of assessment can come only from large controlled studies, and while studies are mandatory before drugs are placed on the market that is not the case for most other medical interventions, including surgery. As it happens, the risk of surgery has been generally falling since analysts started measuring the outcomes of a selection of procedures (10), but nevertheless it will usually be the 'clinical judgement' of the doctor which is offered to the patient, not a summary of the statistical data.

The same difficulties with measurement apply to prescribed drugs, where a much lower level of risk than for surgery is generally considered acceptable. It may be years before a rare but severe side-effect is detected, and the publicity surrounding its detection is likely to raise the perception of risk so high that neither doctors nor patients will accept it, whatever its benefits.

The assessment of a risk will commonly differ between two parties to a discussion. Every therapeutic intervention—indeed, every human activity— carries some sort of risk. Therefore, the doctor may put to the patient that there is a 90% probability that the patient will survive the operation without significant harm. The patient may deal with this information in different ways. It may be seen as a 10% chance of a sentence of death. On the other hand it may be perceived as being no chance of dying at all: 'as safe as can be'. There are clearly grounds for substantial misunderstanding in presentation of risks unless all parties to the discussion clearly understand what the others are saying.

In an attempt to clarify explanations, probabilities are sometimes compared by doctors with probabilities in different contexts, equating the risks run by patients in accepting treatment to the risks they run in other walks of life, such as flying or driving a car. Pochin (11) has listed several such comparative examples. For example, vaccination and the taking of medicines prescribed by the doctor are comparatively minor risks compared with biopsy of the liver, having a child or scuba diving. And none of these pose as high a risk as hang-gliding or sport parachuting. Inman (12) has also compared risks, especially with those of drug therapy. But the doctor should be wary. For one thing, comparing the risk of bus travel to train travel is a very different matter from comparing bus travel to surgery. For another, the patient's assessment of the meaning of expressions such as 'likely' and 'possible' may be different from the doctor's. It is best that an attempt be made to give words such as 'small' or 'very unlikely' some numerical meaning, because it may be important for the patient to understand that 'very unlikely' does not mean that there is no chance at all.

Indeed, many problems of understanding and communication come together in the comprehension and assessment of information about risks and probabilities. People have problems processing information about risk, and these problems introduce errors, misunderstanding and exaggeration of risks in the making of choices. Even experts succumb to the influence of vivid and dramatic examples of events that are presented in ways that distort assessments of risk.

Examination of how various groups evaluate risk shows that while experts prefer to rely on statistics and fatality rates to assess and rank them, other people do not. They must, therefore, be using another set of concepts and beliefs to do so. Slovic has shown that three factors appear especially likely to affect the perception of risk: personal experience of the hazardous events; ability to control these hazards; and some concept of them which encompasses 'dread', a general feeling that the events are thoroughly nasty things (13). Clearly, then, perception of risk is a much more complicated matter than the use of statistics would indicate, and depends very much on personal biases and the context in which the risk is introduced into discussion between doctor and patient.

People's choices can be influenced by the way the risk information is presented or framed. These effects have been demonstrated in several studies involving assessment of information on medical risk. In a well-known study, different groups of people were asked to make a hypothetical choice between two alternative therapies for lung cancer: surgery and radiation (14). The preferences of all groups were affected by whether the information about outcomes was framed in terms of probability of survival or probability of dying. When the outcomes were framed in terms of probability of survival, only 25% chose radiation over surgery. However, when the outcomes were framed in terms of probability of death, 42% preferred radiation. The authors attributed the result to the fact that the risk of death at the time of operation, an outcome which would not happen at the time of radiation, became the pre-eminent factor in helping patients to come to a decision.

Individual perceptions, it is confirmed, are as influential as scientific variables. A patient's consideration of and response to information on risk will be more complex than a simple acceptance of 'facts'. Data should be placed in context by the doctor, and comparisons with other risks used carefully. Above all, uncertainty must be acknowledged, even if it is often hard for the doctor to say to the patient, 'I don't know'.

It is clearly undesirable for the doctor to present to the patient information on risk in a way which deliberately sets out to influence the patient's decision. Fear may be stimulated, for example, by the manner of presentation on the manifestations of a particular side-effect of a drug or unwanted outcome of surgery. This is not assisting understanding; it is coercion. The patient's choice of treatment should be an autonomous one, not under the doctor's control and based on as full an understanding of the risks and alternatives as possible.

Pain can be another powerful influence on the way that risks are assessed by the patient. 'Do anything you like, doctor, as long as you stop the pain.' In this way pain can limit the choices of patients because of its intensity, and it can interfere with careful consideration of alternative risks. In these and other instances the doctor can never be perfectly certain that a patient has come to a fully adequate understanding.

COMMUNICATING AND UNDERSTANDING RISK

If the patient is properly to understand the risks associated with medical interventions, the lines and methods of communication must be open and free. Indeed, a serious hazard for the modern doctor is failure of communication.

Patients have two criteria for judging whether a consultation with their doctor is a good one. One criterion is good clinical decision-making. The other is good communication. Patients say that they like to be involved in the decisions which are made during the consultation, and yet Cartwright and Anderson (15) have shown that patients express more dissatisfaction with the information they receive from doctors than with any other aspect of medical care. Many patients do find it hard to talk to doctors, and this is only too often a mutual problem. Communication lies at the heart of medicine, and the success of the doctor–patient relationship depends very much on an open and frank discussion of under-standable risks. Because litigation does, sadly, result from failures in discussion and communication (sometimes years later), and because 'failure to warn' about risks is likely to be the allegation to support a claim of negligence, it is as well that the doctor make written notes that relevant warnings have in fact been given.

Perhaps in many ways patients have been led to expect too much from their doctors. Communicating risk should be in the mind of all medical staff, including doctors, during all their encounters with patients. Information given to patients in hospitals and doctors' waiting rooms should stress that the doctor will want the patient to know about the unwanted as well as the wanted effects of any test procedure or medical treatment. Often talking is not enough, and written information is fundamental to successful treatment. Patients are more likely to take important drugs if they have written information, and the risks of drug treatment are more likely to be understood and side-effects reported when the information has been presented in written form. A simple leaflet prepared for a variety of common conditions encountered by the particular doctor can be useful for handing to a patient.

When offered drug treatment, a patient may need to know the extent of the risk that the drug might adversely affect driving performance or decision-making, and whether there is a risk of interactions with alcohol or other drugs. When prescribing, the doctor needs to ask himself questions such as what does the patient believe about the risks of the drug, what has the patient been told about it, and what does the patient remember. In the future, computerized prescribing may be an advantage because bad handwriting would be avoided and a tear-off slip would provide information for the patient. There are also available a variety of publications that explain for non-medical people the effects and unwanted effects of medications, and to study how such publications present sometimes unpalatable information can be of great value to the doctor as well as to the patient.

Finally, the doctor should solicit feedback from the patient in order to assess the degree of understanding of risk that has been achieved, and be alert to facial and body expressions which may give a clue that the patient is confused or distressed in a way that has not been expressed verbally. Patients may be asked to restate in their own words what has been explained to them about the risks of treatment. Feedback within the doctor–patient relationship is an essential part of the mechanism for achieving understanding about risk. If there is still confusion, both the doctor and the patient must try again and again until mutual understanding—the basis of effective communication—has been achieved.

REFERENCES

1. Polani, P. 1983. The development of the concepts and practices of patient consent. Pp. 59–62, *in* Dunstan, G. R. and Seller, M. J. (Eds) *Consent in medicine, convergence and divergence in tradition*. King Edward's Hospital Fund, London.
2. Fitton, F. and Acheson, H. W. 1979. *The doctor–patient relationship*. HMSO, London.
3. Bergen, R. P. 1974. The confusing law of informed consent. *Journal of the American Medical Association* **219**: 229–325.
4. Action for negligence fails: principles restated. 1954. *British Medical Journal* **ii**: 105–106.
5. Sidaway v. Governors of Bethlem Royal Hospital and Maudsley Hospital. 1986. *Weekly Law Reports*, 8 March, 480.
6. United States Department of Health, Education and Welfare Code of Federal Regulations. 1978. Title 45, Public Welfare Part 46: 142.
7. Alfidi, R. J. 1971. Informed consent. *Journal of the American Medical Association* **216**: 1325–1329.
8. Hawkins, C. F. 1967. *Speaking and writing in medicine: the art of communication*. Charles C. Thomas, Springfield, Illinois.
9. Osler, W. 1961. *Aphorisms, from his bedside teachings and writings*, No. 256, 2nd edn. Charles C. Thomas, Springfield, Illinois.
10. Henderson, M. 1987. *Living with risk*. John Wiley & Sons, Chichester, and the British Medical Association.
11. Pochin, E. 1982. Risk and medical ethics. *Journal of Medical Ethics* **8**: 180–184.
12. Inman, W. H. W. 1986. Risks in medical intervention: balancing therapeutic risks and benefits. *In* Warden A. *et al.* (Eds) *The future of predictive safety evaluation*. MTP Press, Lancaster.
13. Slovic, P. 1987. Perception of risk. *Science* **236**: 280–285.
14. McNeil, B. 1982. On the elicitation of preferences for alternative therapies. *New England Journal of Medicine* **306**: 1259–1262.
15. Cartwright, A. and Anderson, D. 1964. *Human relations and hospital care*. Routledge, London.

39

Consent and the Doctor–Patient Relationship

JUSTICE MICHAEL KIRBY, AC, CMG

President of the Court of Appeal of New South Wales, Australia

PATIENT CONSENT IN A CONTEXT OF HUMAN RIGHTS

As a sign of the changing times we live in, it is as well to begin with the opinion of an elderly Scottish judge, ventured nearly a century ago, concerning a case brought by a patient against a doctor:

> This action is certainly one of a particularly unusual character. It is an action of damages by a patient against a medical man. In my somewhat long experience I cannot remember having seen a similar case before (1).

Times have certainly changed. Now it is common to read of the medical malpractice 'explosion' (2,3). Even discounting the more exaggerated and alarmist claims which are voiced about this phenomenon, it is certainly true that many more doctors and other health care workers are taken to court today than was the case even 40 years ago. What has happened in the past four decades to occasion this change?

Many explanations are given. They include the higher standards of general education enjoyed by members of the public; the consequential decline in the uniqueness of the position of professional advisers; and the tendency for unquestioning respect to be replaced by self-confident expectations of communication. So widespread is the public discussion of health, the latest drugs and technology and of alternative treatments that it is by no means uncommon to find amongst lay people a general appreciation of health care issues which was certainly absent in earlier generations. To treat such patients with condescension and paternalism not only creates a feeling of resentment; it also minimizes the opportunities for insightful discussion which may actually assist in diagnosis and in the treatment of the patient as a whole person: not just a person with a particular medical condition.

Everywhere around us we can see evidence of the changes which have come

Principles of Health Care Ethics. Edited by Raanan Gillon.
© 1994 John Wiley & Sons Ltd

about as a result of these social and technological developments. They have occurred at different rates in different countries, in harmony with general political and legal movements. Around the world we laugh at the television series 'Yes Minister', portraying the wily British civil servant with his attitude 'nanny knows best'. In many countries, including my own, the previous theory of ministerial responsibility held by such arrogant bureaucrats has given way to a more accessible and effective means to render public servants truly accountable to those they serve. We had to borrow the Ombudsman and notions of freedom of information from Scandinavia to achieve this end. In the field of health care, the last few decades have seen much parallel attention to the provision of improved procedures for making complaints and rendering doctors and others accountable for professional misconduct and neglect.

Yet in both the northern and southern hemispheres, intensive inquiries have revealed that an abiding complaint of patients in developed countries, otherwise quite satisfied with their relationship with their doctors, is that they are not allowed to participate sufficiently in deciding about their treatment nor given enough information to enable them to do so. This was the finding of the United States President's Commission in 1982 (4). On the other side of the world it was confirmed more recently by an Australian study which showed that 13% of patient complaints were about poor communication and 27% about poor attitude or behaviour on the part of health care providers (5) (see also *Australian Law Journal*, 64:383-385; 1990).

At the heart of the problem of consent and the doctor–patient relationship is the tension between the unquestioned need to respect the integrity and wishes of the individual patient (on the one hand) and the years of study and practical experience which go into the activities of medical diagnosis and treatment (on the other). Patients are infinite in their variety and in their inclination to know medical detail and in their capacity to understand it, if explained. Doctors and other health care workers are infinite in their variety: as in their capacity for communication, their inclination to spend the time necessary and their conviction about its utility.

Here, then, is the problem. Is it not better, the skilful diagnostician and busy surgeon may ask, to get on with the job doing the best possible for the patient according to the highest standards of the medical profession? If you want communicators and public relations experts who will make patients feel better— go to a therapist or tune into talk-back radio. You can *trust* the doctor to act by the best standards of his or her peers. Failure to do so will require an account to professional bodies and, possibly, in a civil action at law. Who knows what the patient would do if over-burdened with data about every conceivable risk of health care? Many patients would be frightened off beneficial treatment by exaggerating the risks and overlooking the far greater chances of benefit. So leave it to the professionals. Nanny knows best.

These arguments held sway in the common law of England until quite recently. They profoundly affected the approach of the courts of the many countries which derived their law from England. The principles stated were congenial to the judges who pronounced them. They reflected their own opinions about the circumstances in which other learned professions—including their own—should be rendered liable for want of care or want of communication to those seeking out their professional skills.

But the phenomenon of our age (apart from higher standards of education and technological advances) is the universal assertion of basic rights. In a sense it is a natural outgrowth of the social change which occasioned the American and then the French revolutions 200 years ago. It was no accident that those revolutions were accompanied by constitutional statements asserting what were then called the basic Rights of Man. The impact of United States power on the world of the twentieth century has helped to universalize this movement, with its roots as deep in English history as the *Magna Carta* of 1215 and the *Bill of Rights* of 1688.

The *Universal Declaration of Human Rights* was adopted by the General Assembly of the United Nations in 1948 in the aftermath of the Second World War. Its first Article declares that:

> All human beings are born free and equal in dignity and rights. They are endowed with reason and conscience and should act towards one another in a spirit of brotherhood.

One by one, the succeeding Articles of the Declaration confirmed this basic principle of universal respect for each precious individual human life. Article 3 promises:

> Everyone has the right to life, liberty and security of person.

Article 5 declares:

> No one shall be subjected to torture or to cruel, inhuman or degrading treatment or punishment.

In the special context of medical treatment the horrors of medical experimentation in Nazi Germany propelled the international medical community to a restatement at Nuremberg of the ethical principles governing health care (6,7). The Nazi Party had found sympathetic listeners in the medical profession. German doctors were not always the victims of the Nazi ideology but often active and responsible agents, committed enthusiastically to its principles of racial hygiene. Such recent and frightening evidence of the errors that can occur when a great profession loses its way necessitated the return to a basic restatement of the functions and limits of the doctor in relation to the patient. This takes the doctor, as it does any professional person, back to respect for the inviolable dignity of every human being, expressed in the *Universal Declaration of Human Rights* and the various other international, regional and specialist statements of basic rights which have been such a feature of the new world order developed around the United Nations since the Second World War.

It is therefore important to see the issue of informed consent as a tiny fragment of the mosaic of that order. One English Law Lord put it well:

> This illuminates the relationship between doctor and patient when they face one another. It is not fundamentally the expert instructing the ignorant, even though

those terms may accurately classify the respective parties. One free human being advises and helps another. The relevant law exists for the purpose of supporting that relationship (ref. 1, p. 11).

THE CHANGING APPROACH OF THE COMMON LAW

As a lawyer I necessarily approach the obligations of the doctor (with whom I include other health care workers) to secure the consent of the patient with the aid of the formulae by which that obligation has been expressed in legal decisions. But the reader should not rush away thinking that what will follow is an abstruse summary of cobwebbed books containing obscure legal rules. What follows is, in fact, a reflection on legal decisions in particular cases where doctor and patient have faced each other in a courtroom.

There are, of course, dangers in writing in general terms about consent of the patient as perceived by the law. The law is bound to particular jurisdictions. Even between England and Scotland it will differ. Expressed by judges in the diverse societies of England, Canada, the United States, Australia and elsewhere what is required will differ from one place to another and over time. Expectations of different societies and, within the same society at different times, will vary. Accordingly, the expression of what it is 'reasonable' to expect of the doctor in securing consent from the patient will vary. The basic starting point of the law in all of the places mentioned (and far beyond where the common law is daily applied) will be the same. But contrary to mythology and perhaps popular expectation, the law on this subject is not set in stone. Indeed, it is in the process of development. Unsurprisingly, it reflects the social and technological changes to which I have referred. Lately, it has also come to reflect the attitudes to basic individual rights which are reinforced in national, regional and universal statements of individual rights such as those I have mentioned. Even where these universal statements do not apply as a matter of strict law, they provide the intellectual environment in which lawyers (including judges) operate: performing their daily work. Inevitably, they influence (even subconsciously) the attitude that is adopted towards the rights of the individual patient and the duties of the individual doctor.

In some jurisdictions the local parliament has enacted a law obliging the doctor to secure consent of the patient in order to avoid the risk of criminal prosecution for performing on the body of a patient an unlawful trespass (8). But normally the obligation of consent, and the content and quality of the consent needed, depend upon the common law expressed by judges. Consent only becomes critical, in a legal sense, when the doctor is sued for damages or prosecuted for unprofessional conduct. In a moral sense, however, it is vital at all times to the relationship which is established between the doctor and the patient.

Very few cases, even of medical mishap, result in actions against a doctor. Fewer still come to court. Few indeed (viewed as a proportion of the medical procedures daily performed in their millions) are the cases leading to professional complaint. So it would be inappropriate to regard consent as only needed for cases falling within these relatively rare exceptions. The law states its standards. Although invoked rarely in a courtroom, such standards set the tone and nature of the relationship between the doctor and the patient. They pervade that relationship. That is why their content is so crucial.

The common law of civil wrongs is conveniently divided into various categories. When consent is important in the courts it is usually because the doctor has been sued for a civil wrong or for breach of contract. But what is ordinarily claimed against the doctor is that he or she is guilty of trespass to the person or of negligence. Each of these wrongs is provided by the law, in part, to ensure that remedies are available to a patient for wrongful conduct on the part of the doctor. If a doctor undertakes a medical procedure without the patient's consent, the doctor is guilty of an assault (a battery). In such a case the patient can bring an action. If want of consent is proved, the patient can recover damages.

Until recently it has been considered, in most common law jurisdictions, that actions of battery in respect of surgical or other medical treatment were confined to cases where no consent at all has been given or (emergencies aside) surgery has been performed or treatment given beyond that to which there was consent. More recently, however, as a reflection of the greater recognition of the fundamental right of the patient to control his or her own body and to give or withhold consent, courts have begun to go further. They have asserted that it is not enough that the patient has been told generally about the nature of the procedure:

> The patient had a breast reduction operation to diminish the size and weight of her breasts. She was concerned that the operation would cause scarring. The doctor assured her that scarring was unlikely and, if it occurred, it would be superficial and soon fade away. She consented to the operation. In fact, the breasts were grossly and permanently scarred. The nipples were relocated unevenly. She complained of pain and lasting embarrassment. She succeeded in a claim for damages for battery as well as negligence. The court held that her consent to the operation was not a true consent because the doctor had not told her about the procedure and risks involved (9).

More usually, however, the patient's complaint is about the doctor's negligence. Even a complaint of breach of contract will typically import considerations of negligence because what is asserted is a failure by the doctor to observe reasonable care in treatment of the patient. In such cases there is often no complaint about lack of information or want of consent. The only complaint is that the performance fell below the standards reasonably expected of a competent doctor. Failure to recover all of the swabs from an operation or the performance of an arthrodesis on the wrong knee are cases of this class.

An increasing number of cases are now coming before the courts where things have gone wrong and the patient includes, amongst the complaints, that the doctor did not provide full and adequate information about the nature of the operation and its risks. For a claim, so framed, to succeed two things must be shown:

1. that the doctor's failure to disclose the information was unreasonable in the circumstances; and
2. that this failure was the cause of the harm to the patient in the sense that he or she would not have consented to the treatment had a proper disclosure been made.

The second element is often difficult for a patient to prove in a court of law. The mere assertion by the patient that the operation or treatment would not have been had will not prove that it was so. Such assertions are often coloured by a great deal of wisdom after the event. Judges and juries realize that; hence, many such claims founder upon this principle.

But sometimes the patient's assertion will be accepted. The question then is what is the test to be applied relevant to procuring a proper consent from the patient?

THE BOLAM TEST AND ITS CRITICS

Upon this question it is fair to say that the law is in a state of active development. Different answers to the question would be given in different countries. In England the approach to be adopted was expressed in a passage of instruction to a jury in an important case of medical negligence. It became known as the *Bolam* test, after the plaintiff who brought the case:

> Mr Bolam, a manic depressive, was given electro-convulsive therapy. A danger was of seizures which would cause fractures of the patient's bones. Measures such as restraint and the provision of relaxant drugs reduced those dangers but Mr Bolam was given neither. Nor was he routinely warned of the danger of fracture or the availability of relaxants or restraints. He did not ask about these things. In the course of his therapy he suffered severe fractures of the pelvis and sued the hospital. Following Justice McNair's direction to the jury, Mr Bolam lost.

The critical passage in the judge's direction to the jury, stating the law, was:

> [The doctor] is not guilty of negligence if he has acted in accordance with the practice accepted as proper by a responsible body of medical men skilled in that particular art. . . . Putting it the other way around, a man is not negligent if he is acting in accordance with such a practice, merely because there is a body of opinion which would take a contrary view (10).

This test has been repeatedly criticized as just another illustration of the 'nanny knows best' attitude which has hitherto permeated English law and society. A recent critic in the United Kingdom itself has asserted that it provided the greatest obstacle to successfully suing doctors in negligence because it effectively allowed them to set their own standards of care. A doctor could not be found negligent so long as he or she had acted in accordance with the practice accepted as proper by 'a body of medical men' (11–13) (see also Giesen (1), pp. 317–405).

In the United States a different principle was long ago accepted. Doubtless this was so because the courts approached the matter with a less tender concern for the protection of the doctor, when sued, and with a greater appreciation of the fundamental right of the patient to make informed decisions about medical procedures affecting his or her body. This different attitude almost certainly derived from fundamental differences which exist (despite the unity of the common law) between the conception of the individual in society on the opposite sides of the Atlantic. A reflection of this difference is also seen, as Professor Giesen points out, in the modern European law on this topic.

Years before *Bolam*, Justice Cardozo in the United States laid down the basic principle which has permeated American law on this topic:

> Every human being of adult years and sound mind has a right to determine what should be done with his own body (14).

Upon the basis of this different starting point, American courts have repeatedly upheld the patient's right not to be given medical tests or treatment without informed consent. A patient has the right to be informed about the nature and implications of proposed procedures. The patient must be told of the material risks, complications and side-effects. Without such information the patient is considered as incapable of giving the consent necessary to authorize the medical procedure.

Defenders of this principle assert that it is less paternalistic, more respectful of individual bodily and spiritual integrity, more likely to promote the remedy of the constant complaints of lack of communication which bedevil the doctor–patient relationship and more likely to result in better medical procedures, based upon a fuller appreciation of the patient's viewpoint. Critics, on the other hand, suggest that it results in defensive medicine, posits a fundamental lack of trust between patient and doctor, confuses patients unnecessarily with detail they do not want or need, bombards them with information they cannot fully understand, alarms them needlessly about risks that are remote and takes up a great deal of time which could be better spent actually treating patients rather than talking to them.

In my own country there has been a gradual shift away from the *Bolam test*. In a leading case in my own Court, the new rule was laid down:

> It is not the law that if all or most of the medical practitioners in Sydney habitually fail to take an available precaution to avoid foreseeable risk of injury to the patients, then none can be found guilty of negligence (15).

This approach has also been followed in South Australia where the courts have refused to surrender the standards required to the practices of the medical profession. It is for the courts—representing the community—not doctors, to lay down the reasonableness of what should, or should not, be disclosed to a patient. The reason for this stand was explained:

> In many cases an approved professional practice as to disclosure will be decisive. But professions may adopt unreasonable practices. Practices may develop in professions, particularly as to disclosure, not because they serve the interests of the clients, but because they protect the interests or convenience of members of the profession. The court has an obligation to scrutinize professional practices to ensure

that they accord with the standard of reasonableness imposed by the law. A practice as to disclosure approved and adopted by a profession or section of it may in many cases be the determining consideration as to what is reasonable. ... The ultimate question, however, is not whether the defendant's conduct accords with the practices of his profession or some part of it, but whether it conforms to the standard of reasonable care demanded by the law. That is a question for the court and the duty of deciding it cannot be delegated to any profession or group in the community (16).

In England more recent decisions have included a stern defence of the *Bolam* test; but also telling criticism of it, notably by Lord Scarman (17). The cases have not, however, finally settled the controversies about the *Bolam* test because of the state of the evidence before the courts. Lord Scarman, with the benefit of a detailed review of the United States and Canadian legal authorities, preferred the adoption in England of a test expounded by the United States Court of Appeals (17). This test enunciated a number of propositions. The first of them was:

The premise is the concept that every human being of adult years and of sound mind has the right to determine what shall be done with his own body. The informed exercise of a choice, that entails an opportunity to evaluate knowledgeably the options available and the risks attendant upon each. The doctor must therefore disclose all material risks (886 ff).

In the way of the law, Lord Scarman's dissent on this point of informed consent has greatly influenced the development of the law in my own country. It has been preferred to adherence to the *Bolam* test and the majority view in the English House of Lords favouring its continuance (see, e.g., ref. 18). Not all Australian commentators applaud this trend away from *Bolam* (see, e.g., ref. 19); but I do.

The problem with the old test is that it is, in reality, a relic of an earlier time and of earlier ideas of the proper relationship between doctors and patients. The notion that doctors know best and that, by the standards of their profession, they can determine what patients ought to know, turns the nature of that profession on its head. It is not there for the good of doctors. It is there for the benefit of patients. The only authority and legitimacy of the doctor to intervene in the life and body of the patient is, respectful of the patient's individuality, with that patient's informed consent. That is why a proper development of the law, reflecting the age of basic human rights in which the law now operates, will start at the other end of the equation of consent: just as the Americans do. Ask not what your doctor can do for you. Ask rather what you agree should be done to you with your informed consent.

EXCEPTIONS AND CONCLUSIONS

In the nature of a brief discussion of consent in the doctor–patient relationship it is impossible to review the vast body of literature on this topic deriving from the courts, academics and universities. Law-reform bodies have emphasized that the best foundation for the proper development of an appropriate relationship between doctors and patients is to be found not in general expositions of legal or moral principles but in what actually happens in the doctor's surgery or the hospital casualty room or operation ward (this was the conclusion of VLRC 24; see ref. 19). We may find that what is actually happening in the dialogue between doctors and patients is rather different, when the empirical data are examined, from what we have assumed. So it was found in the case of police stations in their treatment of criminal suspects: although I would not wish to extend that analogy.

Whatever the law says, and moral precept requires, there will always be limits upon the amount of information which a doctor can press upon a patient. These limits will depend upon:

1. the personality and temperament of the patient and the patient's attitude to receiving such information;
2. the patient's actual and apparent level of understanding;
3. the nature of the treatment—obviously the more drastic the treatment the more information will be required;
4. the magnitude and likelihood of possible harm, the incidence of risk and the remoteness of the chance that things will go wrong.

Because risk is the inescapable companion of any professional endeavour, and especially in the context of medical treatment, a realistic law will have regard to the crises which doctors daily face. The notion of imposing an obligation on the surgeon who discovers an unexpected problem in the midst of an operation, to sew up the patient and wait for a consultation, is wholly unrealistic. So is the notion that a doctor must have express consent before attending to an accident victim or to someone suffering an emergency or in a state of unconsciousness. The variety of doctor–patient relationships, and of the problems which arise within them, are so great that care must be taken in expounding universal rules about patient consent. Nor is this an exhaustive discussion of the circumstances in which questions of informed consent may arise. Thus, I have not explored the possible need for a general no-fault system of compensation for the victims of medical mishaps, such as is now available in New Zealand and in Sweden to obviate actions for damages when mistakes occur. Nor have I examined the particular issues that have lately arisen in the case of consent to medical treatment by infants and minors (for a recent discussion see Uniacke (20) and Grant (21)); or the special problems which have arisen in the context of screening patients for the AIDS virus (22–27). The issue of consent in the doctor–patient relationship is one of great controversy, precisely because it is the very centrepiece of that relationship. It marks out the fundamental way in which the relationship will work.

So long as it is a relationship based upon perceptions of the profession's standards it will tend to continue in a condescending and paternalistic approach which is fundamentally inimicable to the rights of the patients and the proper limits of the intervention of the outsider, however skilled and however well intentioned. That is why the guiding star must come to be the express or imputed agreement of the patient to anything that affects a patient's life, body and psyche. With the great privileges of, and respect for, the health care professions go great responsibilities. The first may be to do no harm; but the second is to have to the greatest extent practicable the fully informed consent of the patient. The law, in varying degrees, demands it. Moral and ethical principles reinforce the law. Social and technological changes give new content to what law and ethics require.

REFERENCES

1. *Farquhar* v. *Murray* (1901) 3 F 859, 862 cited by Lord Kilbrandon, Foreword, *in* Giesen, D. (Ed.) *International medical malpractice law*. J. C. B. Mohr (Paul Siebeck), Tübingen.
2. De Wees, D. N., Trebilcock, M. J. and Coyte, P. C. 1991. Medical malpractice crisis: a comparative empirical perspective. *Law and Contemporary Problems* **54**: 217.
3. Danzon, P. M. 1990. The 'crisis' in medical malpractice: a comparison of trends in the United States, Canada, the United Kingdom and Australia. *Law, Medicine and Health Care* **18**: 48.
4. United States, President's Commission for the Study of Ethical Problems. 1982. *Making healthcare decisions*, Vol. 2 : *Empirical studies of informed consent*. USGPO, Washington, DC.
5. Victoria (Australia). Parliamentary Social Development Committee. 1984. *Final report upon complaints procedures against health services*. VGPO, Melbourne.
6. Victoria, Law Reform Commission. 1989. *Informed decisions about medical procedures*. Report no 24: Melbourne, (VLRC 24): 7.
7. Post, S. G. 1991. The echo of Nuremberg: Nazi data and ethics. *Journal of Medical Ethics* **17**: 42.
8. *Consent to Medical and Dental Procedures Act* 1985 (Sth Aust), section 7(2) (b) (i), discussed VLRC 24, 41.
9. *D* v. *S* (1981) 93 Law Soc (Sth Aust) JS 405 (Supreme Court of Sth Aust). Discussed VLRC 24, 33.
10. [1957] 1 WLR 582, 586 (Eng—Queen's Bench Div).
11. Murphy, J. 1991. Grey areas and green lights: judicial activism in the regulation of doctors. *Northern Ireland Law Quarterly* **42**: 268.
12. Kennedy, I. and Grubb, A. 1989 *Medical law: text and materials*, pp. 171–367. Butterworths, London.
13. Jones, M. A. 1984. Doctor knows best? *Law Quarterly Review* **100**: 359.
14. *Schloendorff* v. *Society of New York Hospital* (1914) 211 NY 125; 105 NE 92, 93 (NY Ct Appeals); see also *Canterbury* v. *Spence* 464 F 2d (1972) (US Ct Appeals—Dist Columbia).
15. *Albrighton* v. *Royal Prince Alfred Hospital* [1980] 2 NSWLR 542, 562 (NSWCA—Reynolds JA). See now *Rogers* v. *Whitaker* (1992) 67 ALJR (HC).
16. *F* v. *R* (1983) 33 SASR 189, 194 (Sth Aust Full Court—King CJ). See also VLRC 24, 16.
17. *Sidaway* v. *Board of Governors of the Bethlem Royal Hospital and the Maudsley Hospital and Others* [1985] 1 AC 871 (Eng—HL).
18. *H* v. *Royal Alexandra Hospital for Children* [1990] Aust Torts Reps 81-000 (SCNSW—Badgery-Parker J).
19. Cassidy, D. I. 1992. Malpractice—medical negligence in Australia. *Australian Law Journal* **66**: 67–86.
20. Uniacke, P. 1991. Children's consent to medical treatment—implications for the medical profession. *Law Society Journal (NSW)*, 56–57.
21. Grant, V. J. 1991. Consent in paediatrics: a complex teaching assignment. *Journal of Medical Ethics* **17**: 199-204.
22. Keown, J. 1989. The ashes of AIDS and the phoenix of informed consent. *Modern Law Review* **52**: 790-800.
23. Swartz, M. S. 1988. AIDS testing and informed consent. *Journal of Health Politics, Policy and Law* **13**: 607-621.

24. Closen, M. L. 1990. A call for mandatory HIV testing and restriction of certain healthcare professionals. *St Louis University Public Law Review* **9**: 421-438.
25. Tribe, D. and Korgaonkar, G. 1991. Testing for AIDS without consent. *Solicitor's Journal* **135**: 566-567.
26. Alexander, I. 1991. Informed consent: law or lore? *National AIDS Bulletin*, July 3–4.
27. Giesen, D. and Hayes, J. The patient's right to know—a comparative view. (1992) 21 *Anglo American Law Review* 101.

40

Consent, Research and the Doctor–Patient Relationship

CHRISTOBEL M. SAUNDERS, MB, BS, FRCS

Clinical Research Fellow, Royal Marsden Hospital, London, UK

MICHAEL BAUM, CHM, FRCS

Professor of Surgery, Royal Marsden Hospital, London, UK

JOAN HOUGHTON, BSc

Deputy Director, Cancer Research Campaign Clinical Trials Centre, London, UK

The practice of medicine has always been 'experimental': cures being tried on patients and the results observed. Traditionally therapeutic regimens were derived from anecdotal experience, and medical innovations were largely a matter of trial-and-error. Such was the discovery of Ambroise Pare in 1537 of a new dressing for gunshot wounds. Prior to this all authorities had taught that burning oil should be applied to the wound to counteract the poison. But in his first campaign he was so inundated with gunshot wounds that he was forced to use an alternative 'digestive' made of egg yolks, oil of roses and turpentine.

> That night I could not sleep at my ease . . . I raised myself very early to visit them, when beyond my hope I found those to whom I had applied the digestive medicament feeling little pain, their wounds neither swollen nor inflamed and having slept through the night. The others to whom I had applied the boiling oil were feverish with much pain and swelling (1).

With the coming of the eighteenth century scientific method began to creep into the 'art' of medicine and surgery, and controlled experimentation gradually became adopted by doctors as a method of testing their treatment regimens:

Principles of Health Care Ethics. Edited by Raanan Gillon.
© 1994 John Wiley & Sons Ltd

On the 20th of May, 1747, I took twelve patients in the scurvy aboard the Salisbury at sea. Their cases were as similar as I could have them .... . Two of these were ordered a quart of Cyder a day. Two others took twenty five drops of elixir vitriol .... Two others took two spoonfuls of vinegar .... . Two were put under a course of Seawater. Two others had each two oranges and one lemon given them each day .... The two remaining took the bigness of a nutmeg .... . The consequence was the most sudden and visible good were perceived from the use of the oranges and lemons (James Lind, 1753 (2)).

Thus the putative approach to medicine has been rapidly overtaken in the past 40 years by the empirical method, embodied in the randomized, controlled clinical trial. The randomized trial was initially developed for agricultural research by R. A. Fisher in the 1920s, but was used for the first time in medical practice in Britain in the 1940s to evaluate streptomycin in the treatment of TB. It is now recognized as the most powerful research tool in the biological scientists' armamentarium for evaluating new medical treatments, when the expected difference in outcome between the two treatments is small. This type of research, however, uniquely relies on the co-operation of large numbers of subjects, who should be aware of the role they are playing in the 'experiment', i.e. they must give their consent.

The first mention for the need for formal consent in medical research came from William Beaumont in 1833, and was enshrined in the personal code of ethics of the 'father of experimental medicine', Claude Bernard, in 1856.

But the public took little interest in the issue of consent, either in routine clinical practice or in research, until after World War II when the horrendous experiments performed by Nazi doctors on the inmates of concentration camps came to light. The public outrage and disgust engendered by these atrocities led to the formulation of the Nuremberg Code in 1947, laying out guidelines for experimentation on humans (3). This was followed in 1964 by the Helsinki Declaration, last revised in 1989, which remains the code of ethics for those engaged in medical research on humans (4). Later statements include those by the Medical Research Council, and the British Medical Association and the Belmont Report of the National Commission for the Protection of Human Subjects of Biomedical and Behavioural Research (5–7).

The principles underlying all these codes of ethics are the maintenance of patient autonomy and non-maleficence—the doctor above all has a duty to protect his patient against harm and to respect his right to self-determination.

DILEMMAS IN CLINICAL RESEARCH

The aim of science is not to open the door to infinite wisdom but to set a limit to infinite error (Brecht, *The Life of Galileo*, 1963).

Most innovations in medical treatment arise from tissue culture in the laboratory or experiments in rodents. It would be foolish, naive and dangerous to translate these experimental ideas directly into standard medical practice without carefully controlled development.

This development, although usually categorized into three phases, is a continuum from non-therapeutic to therapeutic research. The initial phase looks at drug delivery and toxicity in human volunteers. The second phase investigates the efficacy of treatment activity in a predetermined set of patients with a specific disease. There is little argument that fully informed consent is needed for the largely non-therapeutic phase I and phase II clinical trials as they are usually of no benefit to the individual. Phase III clinical trials usually compare two treatments: the standard 'best' treatment and a new one. Such trials are initiated only where there is uncertainty about the best way to treat a disease; in a situation where there is a trial in progress the doctor has the option to randomize appropriate patients to the trial or to recommend an alternative treatment if he feels this is more suitable. This is generally considered therapeutic research (it may be argued that because the treatment is not individually recommended by the patient's doctor, it is in fact non-therapeutic) and is known as the randomized controlled clinical trial.

The randomized clinical trial of a large number of patients is the most scientific way to establish causality and avoid bias when comparing the outcome of two treatments, the difference between which may be only marginal, but nevertheless of clinical importance. Drawing conclusions from a small number of patients allocated in a non-random way is analogous to violating Heisenberg's uncertainty principle in quantum mechanics—observation of any variable of a very small size inevitably alters this variable in an unpredictable way, and very large numbers of observations need to be made to negate this effect.

'Uncertainty' in the clinical trials setting governs eligibility for randomization— the doctor must be 'substantially uncertain' which treatment to recommend before entering his patient into any trial (8).

Issues that cause controversy and conflict in clinical research include the design of clinical trials—in particular randomization; the dual role of the doctor as investigator and carer, and its effects on the doctor–patient relationship; and the issue of consent in phase III trials.

CLINICAL TRIALS

Randomized controlled trials have been much criticized in recent years for being unwieldy instruments for measuring subtle differences between treatments, and for dehumanizing their participants (9). But the randomized controlled clinical trial remains the most reliable, scientific and, we believe, ethical way of comparing treatments; and furthermore protects the public from the hazards of uncontrolled adoption of therapeutic revolutions (10).

A league table of evidence can be advanced in favour of a particular therapy (11). The weakest and most insecure type of evidence comes from anecdotal reports of patients' responses to treatments. Higher up the league are case series with historical controls or controls retrieved from databases, and better still may be observational studies of outcome using case–control methodology. But at the solid base of this hypothetical pyramid rests meta-analysis of repeatable randomized controlled clinical trials based on worldwide experience (see Table 40.1).

Some would assert that a randomized trial is not research at all, but a way of

TABLE 40.1 From (11), with permission.

1. Anecdotal case reports
2. Case series without controls
3. Case series with literature controls
4. Analyses using computer databases
5. 'Case–control' observational studies
6. Series based on historical control groups
7. Single randomized controlled clinical trials
8. Confirmed randomized controlled clinical trials
9. Meta-analysis of trials based on worldwide experience

combining appropriate treatment with treatment assessment (12). This may be an extreme view, but it is well accepted that it is the risk reduction approach to controlled experimentation that serves to keep to a maximum the numbers of patients who receive optimum therapy at any point in the evolution of treatment. The popular myth that patients are at risk when participating in clinical trials has been exploded by Gilbert (as quoted by Silverman (13)) who looked at the outcome of 46 trials of innovations in surgery and anaesthesia and found, on balance, new treatments showed no net gain or loss when compared to standard management, although patients treated within a clinical trial generally fare better than those treated off-protocol (14,15).

Randomization is of prime importance in the clinical trials process as it eliminates bias in apportioning treatment, allows two treatments to be studied concurrently, avoids systematic error and guarantees the validity of the statistical tests of 'significance' that are used to compare treatments (16). 'Blinding' the patient and/or investigator helps to eliminate bias in the assessment of outcome.

To enter a patient into a clinical trial, the doctor must assume a dual role of carer and investigator, and the patient must be willing to undergo a treatment which may not be directly benefical (or forgo a treatment which may be, if in the control group), but will improve medical knowledge for future generations. Any personal preference on the part of the patient should be respected, and if this is the case he/she should not be entered into a clinical trial. To do so would be to violate the patient's autonomy and to dilute the outcome of the trial if subsequently the patient decided not to accept the allocated treatment.

These controversies have led to much discussion in the medical and lay press in recent years (15,17–20). Discussion and resolution of these very important issues is vital if doctors are to continue to undertake trials of new and existing treatments, but these arguments are best pursued by a multidisciplinary team.

So should all patients undergoing treatment for conditions in which there is no one clearly superior mode of treatment be entered into a clinical trial? Caplan argues this from the stance of fair play:

> Fair play seems to require that those who reap the benefit of greater treatment knowledge and skill that are derived from biomedical research should be called upon to bear the burden and costs of pursuing such activities. (As quoted by Mackillop and Johnston (15)).

Despite the visible advantages of research, many authorities would disagree with statements such as that of Caplan.

THE DOCTOR–PATIENT RELATIONSHIP

It is well recognized that in 'western' medical practice there has been a gradual shift in the doctor–patient relationship over the past 20 years, from the paternalistic model to the deontological one. The relationship is still based upon the principles of patient autonomy, non-maleficence, beneficence and justice, but the emphasis has swung from beneficence to patient autonomy. The latter includes the right of the patient to fully informed consent before undergoing any procedure. This is particularly poignant in the clinical research setting.

On entering a patient into a clinical trial the relationship between the doctor and his patient will almost inevitably change—the doctor will be faced with the dilemma of being the traditional 'patient friend', and being the investigator whose interest lies not solely with the patient. One view would insist that the researcher is 'simply a clinician with an ethical duty to his patients not to go on giving them treatments without doing everything possible to ascertain their true worth' (12). Others would insist that a doctor's main duty is to his patient's personal welfare, which must always be put before the interests of scientific enquiry; and that any trial design should be sacrificed to the individual's needs. This argument implies that no patients should be entered into clinical trials.

Thus emerges a conflict of obligations—both on the part of the doctor and of the patient.

It would appear that the doctor has the obligation to obtain fully informed consent from the patient before taking part in any clinical research in all but exceptional circumstances. It is these exceptions which cause many of the ethical dilemmas in clinical research, and we will try to explore some of these in this chapter.

CONSENT

I have no doubt whatever that there are circumstances in which the patient's consent to taking part in a clinical trial should be sought. I have equally no doubt that there are circumstances in which it need not—and even should not—be sought. (Sir Austin Bradford Hill, 1963 (21))

In the grave moral matters of life and death, of maiming or curing, of the violation of persons or their bodily integrity, a physician or experimenter is more likely to make an error in moral judgment if he adopts a policy of holding himself open to the possibility that there may be significant future permissions to ignore the principle of consent than he is if he holds this requirement of informed consent always relevant and applicable. (Paul Ramsey, 1970 (22)).

Informed consent is a voluntary, uncoerced decision, made by a competent or autonomous person, on the basis of adequate information and deliberation, to accept a specific treatment when fully cognizant of the nature of the treatment, its consequences and risks (23). This may be verbal or written. There should be no fundamental difference between the information given to a patient in a clinical trial and that given in daily practice (24,25).

If informed consent is to have meaning, then the patients need to be informed about the uncertainties within which doctors practise. This too should apply not only in the clinical trial setting but also to patients treated off-protocol, for, if not, the regrettably not uncommon situation will arise in which double standards are practised. The doctor is at liberty to prescribe whatever treatment he wishes outside a trial protocol, but within a trial the constraints imposed upon him by an ethical committee of complete disclosure of all aspects of the treatments may actually cause the doctor and/or patient to refuse to participate in the trial, thus denying the patient the possible benefits of the new treatment and damaging the prospects of the trial ever determining whether the new treatment is beneficial or indeed results in harm.

In giving permission for a treatment the patient does not surrender his rights and privileges. Lord Scarman states that 'If a patient is fit to receive information and wishes to receive it, the doctor must "brief" the patient so he can make a free and informed choice' (26). To fail to do this is endangering the fabric of the doctor–patient relationship, and the trust and veracity therein. Indeed, if the doctor fails fully to inform the patient of the intended treatment he may be liable to criminal charges of negligence or battery.

However, how much a doctor tells the patient about his disease, its prognosis and the treatment alternatives is open to interpretation. Part of a doctor's clinical freedom and professional responsibility is the ability to interpret information as he considers most appropriate in order to reach a clinical decision. Full disclosure of all possible risks may actually cause excessive anxiety for the patient, and full disclosure of all the alternatives of therapy, in an unbiased way, imposes a huge burden of responsibility on the patient which he may not feel able to cope with, particularly at the stressful time when the diagnosis of a serious and possibly fatal disease has just been revealed to him (27). It is assumption of this responsibility by the doctor that represents the beneficial aspects of the remnants of paternalism.

This conflict of disclosure takes on an even more ethically significant position in a clinical trial. Here the doctor has reached a personal and professional equipoise—he does not know which of the available treatments is most efficacious with least adverse effects, thus must decide whether to treat routinely or enter his patient into a trial of treatments.

In an ideal world, and some would argue even in this one, fully informed consent should be obtained in all clinical trials. This consent should include:

1. the purpose of the trial,
2. the benefits to the patient and to society,
3. possible risks of treatment,
4. alternative treatments available,
5. the right to refuse or withdraw from the trial at any time without prejudicing further treatment in doing so,
6. the implications of randomization.

This consent should be completely voluntary. In seeking willing consent the patient's autonomy will be established, and he will be protected from fraud and deception. The patient will also gain more insight into the disease which may improve compliance with treatment. A dialogue will be started which will improve mutual trust and understanding between the doctor and patient, and engender a positive attitude. The need to obtain consent forces the doctor/investigator to scrutinize his motives, and acts as a form of self-audit.

But what of the disadvantages of informed consent in clinical trials? Is a patient who has just been informed of a diagnosis of a life-threatening disease able to give informed consent—is he competent (27)? And if so does he feel obligated to the doctor to enter the trial?

Many doctors feel that explaining the concept of a clinical trial—the uncertainty of the best treatment, randomization and possible risk—imposes an unacceptable burden on the patient's already traumatized psyche—and is not compatible with the dictum 'do no harm'.

There is some support for this viewpoint from Taylor and colleagues, who looked at the reasons why there was such a poor accrual rate (16% of that expected) in a North American trial of breast conservation versus mastectomy in breast cancer patients (28). They found that only 27% of the doctors enrolled in the multi-centre trial entered all eligible patients, whilst 38% entered some, and 35% entered none at all. A questionnaire was sent to the latter groups of doctors to find out why their accrual rate was so poor: 73% reported that the trial was a threat to the doctor–patient relationship; 38% had difficulty with informed consent; 22% disliked open discussions about uncertainty and 8% said they would feel a personal responsibility if the treaments were found to be unequal.

A more serious result of the enforced requirement to obtain fully informed consent is illustrated by the ISIS-2 trial of streptokinase and aspirin in acute myocardial infarction (8). In this study acutely ill patients were randomized to receive either conventional treatment or the addition of streptokinase and/or aspirin (as a result of the trial now established as clearly beneficial treatment). In the UK consent procedures were largely a matter of judgement—the doctor was required to speak to the patient as seemed humanly appropriate. However in the US doctors were required to read a 'preposterously' long document and obtain written consent for every patient 'the aim [of which] was to protect the doctor, not to protect the patient, and that if the protection of the doctor from lawyers harmed the patient then that was the price one had to pay for doing studies in the US'. Perhaps partly because of this procedure, recruitment into the US trial was slow, and the trial ended some months later than may have been possible, thus preventing the saving of thousands of lives.

A few people have looked at how the patient feels about entering a clinical trial, (29) and found that, although the majority are willing to participate, the response of a significant minority of patients to the honest doctor, who tells them that he genuinely does not know which treatment is best, is to take their custom to one who does profess to know best! There is also some evidence that patients who have been informed of all possible risks of treatment display increased side-effects and decreased treatment efficacy; thus consent itself could be held responsible for modifying therapeutic response (30).

Perhaps the most difficult issue to discuss with the patient is the concept of randomization. A clinical trial relies on groups of 'similar' patients (balanced with regard to demographic and prognostic factors) being selected randomly for either treatment arm. Both patient and doctor often find it difficult not to assert preference for one particular treatment even with a lack of empirical evidence; yet the patient outside a clinical trial rarely has the luxury of alternative treatments—for example most surgeons will perform the operation they have most experience with for a specific complaint, and the patient remains unaware of the existence of other options. This is not regarded as unethical practice, yet allocating a patient to a specific treatment within a clinical trial setting without informing the patient of all the alternatives is usually considered unethical.

All doctors naturally wish to individualize all aspects of their patient's treatment. This is not possible in a clinical trial where the loss of validity of the trial design would be unacceptable, prolonging the trial and increasing the number of patients needed for significant results. So we must again question whether a patient should be entered into a trial, if informed consent may cause harm, yet waiving consent violates the patient's autonomy, and may compromise not only the investigator's relationship with the patient, but also that of the junior medical and nursing staff caring for the patient, and the patient's family, who must accept yet more responsibility.

We feel the answer is yes—the patient should be entered into a trial despite these problems—our duty as doctors is to offer all patients the best treatment, and if we do not know which is best, then we must strive to find out.

There are a number of practical solutions to some of the ethical problems discussed above. We will look at these in some detail shortly, but first it may be illuminating to study an example of the problems this kind of theoretical debate can pose in clinical practice.

THE UNINFORMED PATIENT

In 1980 a clinical trial was initiated by the Cancer Research Campaign Clinical Trials Centre. This was a multi-centre collaborative study looking at the use of adjuvant systemic therapy in early breast cancer. Patients would be randomized to receive conventional surgical treatment—which in 1980 did not include adjuvant therapy—or to surgery and tamoxifen. The clinicians entering the trial at King's College Hospital initially argued that informed consent should be waived to avoid causing unnecessary distress to the patient by making her aware of her exact prognosis and the uncertainty of the best treatment. The ethical committee refused to waive consent so the trial was started with each patient giving fully informed consent and receiving an explanatory leaflet. However, 2 months into the trial, at the behest of the nurse counsellor, the trial organizers again approached the ethical committee as they felt that the additional burden on patients—who had just learnt that they had cancer and needed a mastectomy—of having to consider whether to enter a trial, was causing undue stress and anxiety. Thus the need for consent was waived, but it was agreed that all patients would receive a full explanation of the rationale behind their treatment. Eighteen months later another trial was started at King's, to investigate a method of improving psychological adjustment of women to mastectomy by the intervention of a professional counsellor. Informed consent was not required for this trial. Because funding for only one part-time counsellor was available, it was arranged so that at fortnightly intervals patients who presented to the clinic had a 50:50 chance of meeting the nurse counsellor. Additionally any patients identified by the clinician as having psychological problems were referred for counselling. This randomization of a rare resource—in this case counselling time—is commonly used to maintain the principle of justice.

In 1982 Mrs E. T. was referred to King's College Hospital with carcinoma of the breast. She was entered into both the above trials, receiving what with hindsight was the optimum treatment of the time—mastectomy and tamoxifen. Mrs E. T., however, subsequently found out that her treatment, rather than being individualized to her, had been randomized as part of a clinical trial, and she had not given her consent to participate in this. She took this matter up in the form of a complaint to the regional health authority, and although all clinical staff involved were later absolved of any charges of professional or ethical misconduct, the case did cause considerable dialogue in both the professional and lay press (8,9)—in the latter there being a number of reports of 'uninformed human experimentation'.

This case raises a number of issues. Was Mrs E. T.'s treatment in any way compromised by the clinician's concern to improve the quality of cancer care for future generations of women? We can safely say, with hindsight, that she did receive optimum medical treatment (and it is only as a result of such trials that we know what the optimum treatment is!), but at the price of a loss of trust in her doctors. However, thousands of other women in the trial were spared the additional anxiety and responsibility of having to make a decision about entering the trial. Does this constitute humane treatment or unethical imposition of the doctor's set of moral values on his patients?

Mrs E. T.'s response to being entered into a clinical trial is in sharp contrast to that of Mrs Thornton (27), who argues strenuously that she would have been much better served if the burden of responsibility of choosing whether or not to enter a clinical trial had not been put upon her but had been taken by her doctors!

NEW WAYS AHEAD

The aims do not justify the method—the method must be justified in its own right (9).

There is an increasingly vocal lobby which feels that the goal of achieving certainty via randomized clinical trials is too high a price to pay in humanitarian and ethical terms (9). And yet the ethics of not researching into newer and better ways to treat illness are highly questionable indeed! Thus alternative ethical models are being explored. Perhaps the most important and fundamental of these is public education—an already informed patient is more likely to be both willing and able to understand and participate in a clinical trial. The potential trial participant should be given adequate time to understand all the information given, and make a considered decision without pressure or coercion.

This may involve one or two extra visits to hospital, and ideally discussion with an unbiased but informed 'patient friend' such as a nurse counsellor. Patient information sheets, or more complex algorithms explaining the rationale behind various treatments, are often useful, and may be developed into computerized 'decision-making trees'.

Small clinical trials in single hospitals, e.g. comparing two types of suture material, can almost always be guided by the local ethics committee. However, large multi-centre trials may well benefit from approval by a national ethics committee (17). This inevitably means extra bureaucracy and time for projects to be passed, but does avoid the potential bias of local committees. To safeguard patients' autonomy further a 'Patient's Bill of Rights' has been developed. In the United States this is a well established document which actually has legal standing in some states. A similar Bill of Rights has recently been issued by the UK Ministry of Health. This is a generalized document and makes only brief mention of a patient's right to refuse to participate in medical research (31).

Others have tried to develop completely new ethical models. Zelen in 1979 (32) proposed a new model for a randomized clinical trial comparing a 'best' standard treatment with an experimental one. The patient is randomized into one of the two groups before being informed. The patient in the group receiving best standard therapy (G1) does not need to give informed consent. The patient in the group receiving the new treatment (G2) is given detailed information regarding the treatment and asked if he is willing to enter the trial. If the patient refuses he is transferred to G1. This method was subsequently modified, where there is no clear-cut 'best' treatment, so that after 'uninformed' randomization, both groups of patients were informed about the trial and asked to participate. The Zelen proposals are very useful in practice, but do present some ethical problems: patients are still being randomized into a trial without their consent, and although G1 patients are getting the best standard therapy they are unaware of possible alternatives. This may be very relevant; for example a trial of surgery versus radiotherapy where the patient may have strong feelings about which treatment he would prefer. Even in the modified Zelen approach where both groups of patients are fully informed after randomization, the patient may feel somewhat coerced into agreeing to continue with the trial after he has already been entered, and the investigator may feel the need to give an over-enthusiastic endorsement to the treatment to which the patient has been allocated, rather than giving a more balanced view. Perhaps, however, this enthusiastic endorsement should be viewed as part of the therapeutic strategy, thus engendering a positive attitude that appears so important in the treatment of some patients (27).

Others recommend reverting to the Bayesian approach to experimentation (33), where the probability of a hypothesis being correct is calculated in the light of evidence available, using a test group and historic controls. This method, however, relies on the ability to fix prior probabilities—that is, how likely the investigator subjectively feels it is that a new treatment is better than the old. This is obviously wide open to investigator bias. Moreover, historical control groups have definitively been shown to be inferior to randomized controlled trials in comparing two or more treatments (34).

A completely novel approach to consent in randomized clinical trials has been suggested by one of the authors (J. H.). This model attempts to maintain intact the doctor–patient relationship, whilst increasing the accrual rate into clinical trials. When the patient's diagnosis has been confirmed by the doctor, the doctor also explains that he is part of a national research structure which is looking at the patient's particular disease, and to whom he would like to write with the patient's details. This separate research body will then send information about the patient's disease and its treatment to the patient, along with a simplified protocol of the trial. If the patient would like to participate he simply returns to his doctor and signs the appropriate consent form. This allows the patient to distance the image of his doctor—who is treating him as an individual—from the impartial investigator who is conducting the trial. It also allows the patient and his family time to consider the options. This could be linked to a counsellor service when the patient re-attends to see his doctor.

Overcoming the ethical hurdles of combining a humanistic interest in the individual with a utilitarian commitment to improving the standards of health care for future generations is a challenge all doctors involved in research need to face up to, in order to practise safer, more effective and more ethical medicine.

ETHICS OF THE USE OF PLACEBOS IN CLINICAL TRIALS

Some trials of treatments require that the study is either blind or double-blind, i.e. the patient, or patient and investigator, do not know into which arm of the study the patient has been randomized. If one treatment is being assessed against a 'no-treatment' control this frequently requires the use of a placebo. Use of placebos can be controversial—is it right to withhold potentially beneficial treatment from one group of patients? Some years ago it was suggested that the incidence of neural tube defects in babies was higher in those born to mothers deficient in folic acid. Thus a trial was instigated randomizing women at high risk of delivering a baby with a neural tube defect into those receiving folate supplements, or a placebo (35). This created much controversy, as it was argued that all at-risk women should receive the potentially beneficial vitamin supplement, even if the possible hazards of the vitamins had not been assessed, in case it may prevent the delivery of handicapped babies. This rather emotive argument stands up poorly to scientific logic (36,37).

The trial was delayed and would have been aborted, but for the persistence of the Medical Research Council in pressing ahead with the trial. Now it can be firmly recommended that folic acid supplementation should be given to all women who have had an affected pregnancy, around the time of their subsequent conceptions. Moreover, no harmful side-effects have been demonstrated; and it has been shown that other vitamin supplements are not useful in preventing neural tube defects.

ETHICAL CONSEQUENCES OF NOT DOING RANDOMIZED CONTROLLED CLINICAL TRIALS

When a new treatment is proposed there is inevitably much enthusiasm from its proponents, whose initial trials of the treatment often given unexpectedly and unrepeatably good results. This type of ancecdotal evidence for the efficacy of a treatment is especially rife in the world of 'alternative medicine'. It quickly becomes unethical not to use this new treatment which promises such excellent results. Yet this type of slavish acceptance of unproven therapies is precisely what we have tried to move away from in modern medicine, as the apparent efficacy of the new treatment may, with careful analysis, be shown to be due to selection or placebo effect, whilst in the meantime unfortunate side-effects may become apparent (38).

Thus it is vital that any new therapy—and indeed many of the current ones—be subjected to proper scientific evaluation in the form of the randomized controlled clinical trial.

SUMMARY

We have addressed a number of the problems implicit in the concept of informed consent in clinical research, and although we may not have provided answers, perhaps what is more important is an open dialogue about the issues in which all parties—patients, doctors, lawyers and 'ethicists'—can join.

What is imperative is that clinical research continues, both to develop new types of treatment and to invalidate inadequately tested and potentially hazardous procedures currently in vogue.

We believe that the randomized controlled clinical trial is the most efficacious way of minimizing this risk to individuals, as well as advancing medical knowledge, and that the resultant 'good science' breeds 'good ethics'.

REFERENCES

1. Packard, F. 1992. *Ambroise Pare*. Oxford University Press, Oxford.
2. Roddis, L. 1950. *James Lind*. Henry Schuman, New York.
3. *Trials of war criminals before the Nuremberg military tribunal under Control Council law*; 2 (10): 181–82. US Government Printing Office, Washington DC, 1949.
4. World Medical Association. *Declaration of Helsinki. Recommendations guiding medical doctors in biomedical research involving human subjects*, 1964. Hong Kong revision, 1989.
5. *Responsibilities in investigations on human subjects*. Report of the Medical Research Council for 1962–63. HMSO 2382, HMSO, London.
6. British Medical Association. 1981 *Handbook of medical ethics*. BMA, London.
7. *The Belmont report*. 1978. National Commission for the Protection of Human Subjects and Biomedical and Behavioural Research. DHEW Publications 578–001: 4–8. US Government Printing Office, Washington DC.
8. Colins, R., Doll, R. and Peto, R. 1990. Ethics of Clinical Trials: three main recommendations. Unpublished report, the Clinical Trial Service Unit, University of Oxford.
9. Faulder, C. 1985. *Whose body is it?* Virago Press, London.
10. Baum, M. 1986. Philosophy and ethics of randomised clinical trials. Francis Fraser Lecture at British Postgraduate Medical Federation Academic Assembly.
11. Green, S. B. and Byar, D. P. 1984. Using observational data from registries to compare treatments: the fallacy of omnimetrics. *Statistics in Medicine* 3: 361–370.
12. Brewin, T.B. 1982. Consent to randomised trials. *Lancet* 8304: 919–921.
13. Silverman, W.A. 1985. *Human experimentation: a guided step into the unknown*. Oxford Medical Publications, Oxford.

14. Stiller, C. A. 1989. Survival of patients with cancer. *British Medical Journal* **299**: 1058–1059.
15. MacKillop, W. J. and Johnston, P. A. 1986. Ethical problems in clinical research: the need for empirical studies of the clinical trials process. *Journal of Chronic Diseases* **39** (3): 177–188.
16. Peto, R., Pike, M. C., Armitage, P. *et al.* 1976. Design and analysis of randomised clinical trial requiring prolonged observation of each patient. *British Journal of Cancer* **34**: 585–607.
17. Baum, M. Zilkha, K. and Houghton, J. 1989. Ethics of clinical research: lessons for the future. *British Medical Journal* **299**: 251–253.
18. Schaffer, A. 1982. Ethics of randomised clinical trials. *New England Journal of Medicine* **307**: 718–723.
19. Brahams, D. 1988. Randomised trials and informed consent. *Lancet* **2**: 1033–1034.
20. Baum, M. and Houghton, J. 1988. Letter. *Lancet* **2**: 1194.
21. Bradford Hill, A. 1963. Medical ethics and controlled trials. *British Medical Journal* **1**: 1043–1049.
22. Ramsey, P. 1970. *The patient as person, explorations in medical ethics.* New Haven Press, Connecticut.
23. Gillon, R. 1985, Consent, pp. 113–118. *Philosophical medical ethics.* John Wiley, Chichester.
24. Blum, A. L., Chalmers, T. C., Deutsch, J. *et al.* 1987. The Lugano Statement on controlled clinical trials. *Journal of International Medical Research* **15**: 2–24.
25. Baum, M. 1989. Limitations of nonscience in surgical epistemology. *International Journal of Technical Assessment in Health Care,* **5**: 381–389.
26. Scarman, L. 1986. Consent, communication and responsibility. *Journal of the Royal Society of Medicine* **79**: 697–700.
27. Thornton, H. M. 1991. Breast cancer trials. *Lancet* **339**: 44–45.
28. Taylor, K. M. Margolese, R. G. and Soskoline, C. L. 1984. Physicians' reasons for not entering eligible patients in a randomised clinical trial of surgery for breast cancer. *New England Journal of Medicine* **310**: 1363–1367.
29. Cassileth, B. R., Lusk, E. J., Miller, D. J. and Hurwitz, S. 1982. Attitudes towards clinical trials among patients and the public. *Journal of the American Medical Association* **248** (8): 968–970.
30. Marsh, B. T. 1990. Informed consent—help or hindrance? *Journal of the Royal Society of Medicine* **83**: 603–605.
31. *The patients' charter.* 1991. Department of Health, London.
32. Zelen, M. 1979. A new design for randomised clinical trials: *New England Journal of Medicine* **300**: 1242–1245.
33. Urbach, P. 1987. Clinical trial and random error. *New Scientist* **1539**: 52–55.
34. Hooning, M. J., van Doogen, J. A., Hart, A. A. M. *et al.* 1992. Breast cancer: a study into the value of a historical control group as comparative material for new methods of treatment. *European Journal of Surgical Oncology* **18**: 23–26.
35. MRC Vitamin Study Research Group. 1991. Prevention of neural tube defects: Results of the MRC Vitamin Study. *Lancet* **8760**: 131–137.
37. Wald, N. J. and Polani, P. E. 1984. Neural tube defects and vitamins: the need for a randomised clinical trial. *British Journal of Obstetrics and Gynaecology* **91**: 516–523.
38. Kingman, S. 1986. Medical research on trial. *New Scientist* **1485**: 48–52.
39. CRC Working Party in Breast Conservation. 1983. Informed consent; ethical, legal and medical implications for doctors and patients who participate in randomised clinical trials. *British Medical Journal* **286**: 1117–1121.

41

Stringent and Predictable Medical Confidentiality

M. H. Kottow, MA (Soc), MD

Professor of Ophthalmology, University of Chile, Chile

A major reason for the persistent and to a large extent fruitless polemic on confidentiality lies in the disregard shown to Descartes' demand that ideas be clear and distinct. Many of us have used sloppy terminology and indulged in the inconsistencies of categorical confusions, which is the logical equivalent of adding pears and bananas. It seems worthwhile to go into some of these misconceptions before attempting to review the issue of confidentiality.

SECRECY VERSUS CONFIDENTIALITY

Religious and sectarian practices often include esoteric secrets that are shared only by the initiated. Harm can accrue in the wake of ritual practices, as occurred in the exorcism exerted on a young German girl, Anneliese Michel, who died after one especially turbulent session. This death has been attributed to the fact that ' . . . her need for medical help went unnoticed because of the secrecy in which the exorcism was conducted'. This is correct, but the conclusion reached, that ' . . . confidence can be used, here and elsewhere, as a shield for activities that could ill afford to see the day of light' is unwarranted (1). It was certainly unusual and pernicious to practise religious rituals whilst ignoring the medical needs of Anneliese, but this is a case of immoral secrecy where confidentiality is not at issue.

It may be of interest to recall within the religious context that Judaism presents its own and peculiar distinction between professional and everyday discretion where, curiously enough, secrecy and confidentiality appear conflated. Professional discretion (secrecy?), according to the Judaic doctrine, always subserves the common law, for the law is of divine origin and therefore unarguable (2). Everyday confidentiality is considerably stricter, disallowing any breach that has not been granted by the confider. According to this interpretation, confidentiality would be an absolute obligation in everyday life, and a *prima facie* one in

Principles of Health Care Ethics. Edited by Raanan Gillon.
© 1994 John Wiley & Sons Ltd

professional dealings. A distinction of this kind seems indefensible, for the common law, whether of divine or mundane origin, mandates both professional and everyday actions.

We tend to equate and confuse secrecy with confidentiality. Secrets are often encountered in everyday life but frequently the information kept secret happens to be of a trivial nature or is being overrated by the secret-holder. Of course, there also are secrets that must remain sealed to avoid nasty social consequences, but more often than not, secrets have a certain pettiness about them. Secrets are revealed willingly, often arbitrarily, or by accident, but always tied to the promise not to tell, and the person receiving the information is bound to discretion by the more general agreement that rules promise-making.

The kind of secret that is a bond in itself without being embedded in some other relationship beyond the general one of agreements, has been also called secret of promise (3). As is well known to secret-sharers, promises of secrecy are highly vulnerable, this feature contributing to the capriciousness involved in keeping, sharing or unveiling secrets.

The reason I dwell on secrecy is to separate it from confidentiality, also known as secret of trust (3), as it is the ingredient or by-product of some more ample interaction such as a confession, a legal context or a medical encounter. The main point is that confidences are always indulged in for some ulterior purpose; the information being passed on is instrumental to some goal, and the only reason for sharing this information is to better achieve that goal. In contrast to the arbitrariness involved in secrecy, confidentiality falls under what Aristotle would have called a virtue: it is the choice of an adequate means to reach some rationally acceptable end.

We handle secrets in accordance with commonsense, intuitive feeling, social tact or loving care, all of which cannot be applied without further ado to confidentiality. Such personal and social traits may contribute or even be necessary, but they are not sufficient ingredients for an adequate management of confidential situations, for confidentiality is a more complex situation that needs to be analysed in its own right.

ABSOLUTE CONFIDENTIALITY?

The main discrepancy concerning confidentiality has been whether to accept it as an absolute value or rather allow breaches for the sake of more important goals that would seem menaced by concealing information. The idea of absoluteness elicits a feeling of uneasiness, for contemporary thinking has preferred to develop views that are more contextual, perspectivistic or circumstantial. Absolute confidentiality is therefore an extemporaneous misnomer, since no social practice and no value will hold in every and all conceivable situations (4).

Current terminology should be reviewed, preferring to speak of stringent or strict confidentiality when our aim is to say that discretion has priority over many, perhaps most but not all other considerations, and that confidentiality is to be honoured in a predictable way. Most of what follows is an attempt to clarify these two points and help posit the issue in its medical context.

DUTY-BOUND VERSUS UTILITARIAN APPROACHES

Confidentiality enters the arena of medical ethics by way of the Hippocratic oath, but contemporary English translations are ambiguous about the meaning implied in the original. Whereas some translate the Greek text as an invocation to respect confidentiality within the limits of that 'which ought not to be spoken [of] abroad' (5), others give a more stringent interpretation of confidential information as that 'which on no account one must spread abroad' (6). Obviously there is no agreement as to the strictness attributed to medical discretion in Greek medicine, but it does appear as an important duty to be honoured.

Duty-bound ethics must postulate a fundamental and unassailable duty, which necessarily remains vague and inoperant, or they will fall prey to endless disputes over which specific duties are the more basic and universal. This has led to the notion of *prima facie* duties, that is, duties that hold as long as no overriding circumstances make them void. Confidentiality can hardly escape such treatment and can also claim no more than a strong *prima facie* status at best.

In view of these difficulties, moralists have turned to look at ethical issues in terms of consequences or utility. To be sure, utilitarian views are also subject to severe criticism, since it will not be easy to establish the kind of values to be preferred; nor has anyone been able plausibly to explain how the consequences of an act or moral rule are to be correctly predicted and weighted.

Medicine, being a practice and therefore concerned with actions designed to achieve certain goals, has been inclined to favour a consequentialist approach, medical ethics having developed the three widely accepted guiding principles of beneficence, autonomy and justice (7). Confidentiality needs also to be discussed within this context, and an educated guess may anticipate that stringent confidentiality is defensible in terms of patient beneficence and patient autonomy, but that justice may well require some sort of compromise.

CONFIDENTIALITY AND BENEFICENCE

The doctor–patient relationship is a typically and essentially fiduciary one, where the patient seeks the doctor trustingly, in the hope of finding relief and in the certainty of not being harmed. It is understood that the medical team adheres to the Hippocratic principle *'primum non nocere'*. Fiduciarity therefore obtains before confidentiality is called upon, and everything, discretion included, is expected to be managed in a beneficial or harm-averting way.

Inasmuch as the doctor respects the patient as a fully fledged person, he will accept that the patient's best interests are served by keeping confidential all information that is not meant to be divulged. Such a commitment also holds when the patient is mentally incompetent or otherwise a non-person, but appears represented by acceptable proxies. In all such instances the patient's interests demand stringent confidentiality to be honoured by the medical team, insofar as it abides by the principle of beneficence.

But the situation may arise where the patient or his representatives do not seem to be judicious, and the patient's interests appear to be better served by breaching confidential information. Take the doctor being informed that a patient has suicidal thoughts he does not wish divulged. The doctor nevertheless assumes that it would be a measure of safety to commit the patient, thus necessarily making public the depressive mood. Does the potential benefit of institutional treatment outweigh the benefit of honoured confidentiality?

In pondering such decisions the medical team must remember that it is comparing its own views and values with those of the patient and/or his representatives. If the doctor respects confidentiality he will be granting the certain benefit of his discretion, and perhaps fail to secure the purported benefit of institutionalizing the patient, at the same time avoiding the certain harm of injuring confidentiality. Now if an act is certain to harm but appears only potentially beneficial, it is not ethically legitimate because it transgresses the principle of non-maleficence. For this reason, paternalistic decisions that go against the expressed wishes of patients or their proxies are not justified.

Paternalistic breaches of confidence have been defended in such statements as '[N]o one would hesitate to reveal the secrets of a temporarily deranged person about to do himself irreversible harm' (1). This is true, but irrelevant to our concern for confidentiality, because a 'deranged person' is not capable of entering a fiduciary relationship and therefore cannot be disappointed by undesired disclosures. The benefits of confidentiality obtain only when the patient's interests are best respected by being candid with the doctor, at the same time making sure that this information will not go beyond the medical encounter.

In sum, the doctor is in no legitimate position to decide that patients' best interests may be better served by divulging confidential information. The principle of beneficence is therefore adequately adhered to by non-exceptional confidentiality.

CONFIDENTIALITY AND AUTONOMY

The best and simplest way to handle confidential material would be uncritically to respect the principle of patient autonomy in terms of respected privacy. The right to privacy has not remained uncontroverted, for both judicial and philosophical considerations have tried to atomize or reduce privacy to purportedly more fundamental rights. Nevertheless, the notion has emerged that personal information not available to others is private in its own right and subject to one's discretional administration (8). The sum of what each individual exclusively knows about himself is not open to others unless one willingly discloses it, or unless overriding reasons allow privacy to be invaded.

Because privacy is not amenable to the scrutiny of others it constitutes an unquestionable area of autonomy. What happens in each individual's private sphere is of no concern to others. The desire for privacy is not trivial, for it arises from the need to protect one's image or some other specific interest. No-one considers it private information to prefer veal over mutton, but to expound one's sexual phantasies might be disparaging to the image one wishes to convey, and such feelings are therefore kept private.

The private realm is totally autonomous because no-one is socially responsible for his private thoughts or feelings. When a patient decides to enter a clinical relationship, he may consider it advisable to unveil information or knowingly allow information to be revealed by the invasive and pervasive gaze of medicine. Such disclosures transfer private information to the clinical relationship in the understanding that no harm can accrue in such a protected fiduciary environment. In telling about his intimate life, the patient appears to be relinquishing portions of his autonomy, for he is now subject to the scrutiny and judgement of the doctor.

It is quite unlikely that someone would willingly give up degrees of autonomy unless for very strong motives. Patients who decide to disclose information they consider private will do so for two possible reasons. Part of their private life may have become an obstacle to their autonomy, as could conceivably occur to a hitherto undisclosed homosexual who becomes obsessed by the fear of contracting AIDS; or the patient believes that unveiling private information will enhance the efficiency of the clinical encounter as, for example, by confessing heavy drinking, to help manage an acute gastrointestinal haemorrhage.

In confiding in his doctor the patient is reshuffling his autonomy and transferring part of it, more often than not weakened, to the medical arena. This being a fiduciary environment, the patient may rely on it that his autonomy will not be further damaged by public disclosure. Should the doctor entertain the need to pass confidential information on, he would necessarily be injuring the patient's autonomy and disappointing the trust put in him to avoid harm.

The more disautonomous he feels, or the greater his need to relinquish autonomy, the more a patient will rely on the fiduciary and non-maleficent aspects of the medical context he is surrendering to. If confidentiality is breached and the patient's disautonomy thus becomes public, his trust in the protection and beneficence of medicine will be all the more shattered. Thus, not only beneficence but also the principle of autonomy remain unbruised only if predictable confidentiality is strictly honoured.

CONFIDENTIALITY: THIRD-PARTY AND PUBLIC INTERESTS

Confidentiality and Justice

Confidential material is often explosive, for it contains information that seems to anticipate harm to a third party or to society at large. The Tarasoff situation is a case in point, where the court explicitly decided that a murder could perhaps have been avoided if confidentiality had been opportunely and insistently breached (9), but it is doubtful whether some consistent form of assessing the risks and benefits of breaching confidentiality and devising preventive measures against potential harmdoers can be developed. As long as a plausible risk/ benefit analysis is lacking, breaches of confidentiality will continue to be a particular and arbitrary decision of each clinical encounter, therefore remaining an ethically indefensible practice.

The maxim has been coined that 'the protective privilege ends where the public peril begins' (10). A proposition of this kind has terms too vague to justify any strategy. What is to be understood as a 'protective privilege'? How is 'public peril' to be gauged or, for that matter, its 'begin(nings)' to be determined? By lacking specificity, such a maxim has only decorative use.

Doctors Under Contractual Responsibilities

A very common situation occurs when the patient is seen by a doctor who is under direct and explicit obligation to, say, a commercial company, a public institution, or some other patient who might possibly be affected by this medical encounter. The doctor may be under a contractual bond to screen a person who is applying for a job, requesting insurance, submitting to premarital testing or offering to donate biological material. Strictly speaking, this individual is seeking a relationship with the third party, and the doctor is the commissioned mediator in this candidacy and under obligation to his contractor, not to the occasional client. The individual being surveyed has no claim to a confidential relationship, because the doctor had previously subscribed a duty of loyalty and cannot break it in order to enter a circumstantial obligation of confidentiality. Of course, the individual under scrutiny must know this, and will have to decide how candid he wishes to be about his disclosures and how willing he is to run the risk of being found and exposed as in some way defective or untruthful.

Doctors as Moral Arbiters

Medical teams may have no formal commitment to third parties and yet feel themselves under moral obligation to bring forth any information that might be deleterious to someone not primarily involved in the medical encounter. This is not a specific medical quandary, for it reproduces the more familiar situation of the friend who feels compelled to tell the husband about his wife's adulterous activities. Such moral puritanism is distasteful at the least, and more so if the informant has gained his knowledge through the privilege of a confidence. The ungraciousness is compounded if occurring in a medical context, for here the patient has confided out of a need for help. HIV-positive bisexuals who do not spontaneously inform their families are behaving as indecently as adulterous wives, but it is not for the doctor to set himself up as moral arbiter and to cheat on confidentiality. Indecencies are not improved by compounding them, and doctors are not called upon to escalate in an immorality race that leads only to progressive pollution of the moral climate.

Doctors and Public Benefit

The most defensible reason for breaching confidentiality would be the stark utilitarian view that public harm could thus be averted but, again, consequentialism is weak on predicting the probabilities and magnitude of the effects it is expecting. Violating confidentiality has harmful effects that are certain: it disturbs the fiduciary doctor–patient relationship, it creates a climate of suspicion that invites patients to be secretive or to consult less, it therefore lowers standards of medical assitance. On the contrary, the purported benefits are merely hypothetical, the patient might have taken it upon himself to divulge the critical information, the threats issued by the patients may never materialize, the consequences of non-disclosure could end by being less severe than the doctor's fears, or the doctor may be simply overdramatizing.

But of course, it could be the other way round and failure to pass confidential information could well be disastrous. The Tarasoff case (9) again comes to mind, and every maniac who might consult a psychiatrist before running publicly amok in search of immortality would also substantiate the perils of stringent confidentiality.

We live in a risk-laden social order, and yet we resent intrusions into privacy for the sake of averting hypothetical harm. Preventive arrests are not legitimate, nor are citizens normally allowed to carry fire-arms in self-defence. We even engage in 'just wars' in awareness that a world-wide holocaust could ensue, nevertheless considering the defence of the cause more binding than the perils of global destruction. All these are examples of potentially harmful effects being risked for the sake of some socially cherished value such as liberty, public order or democracy. Similarly to safeguard individual autonomy and freedom of decision, it should not be permissible for doctors to try to reduce hypothetical hazards by harmfully infringing confidential relationships with patients, and thus polluting the medical encounter.

The same train of thought that precludes absolute confidentiality must also pervade here by disallowing potentially risky situations to gain the absolute privilege of disrupting interpersonal relationships or social institutions of trust.

Society is certainly justified in taking measures to protect its integrity and values, but it seems inconsistent that priests and lawyers should be granted the privileges of discretion which are denied to doctors. All these professions are dealing with weakened and vulnerable individuals who are confiding in the need to be helped out of their miseries. The social order must gracefully accept this situation, and seek information without disrupting such delicate relationships as those attached to clergymen, lawyers, psychotherapists and doctors.

COMPLYING WITH THE WRITTEN LAW

Is the doctor exonerated from guilt if he informs by his own decision but in strict obedience of the law? Not necessarily, for there have been monstrous laws; and doctors who have demurred under totalitarian regimes, even participating in torture because *de facto* martial law so demanded, may have been pitied but have certainly not been applauded. Laws are more often than not reasonable and consensually accepted, and if such a law requires disclosure the doctor has no reason to object. But such instances are publicly known, and no morally sound patient has the right to request the doctor to disobey the law he is in accord with. Now this is precisely the point, the only one to my mind, where the stringency of confidentiality must abide. If a sound law requires declaration or information, this should be amply known so that all patients are aware that certain matters cannot legitimately remain confidential. This is what I meant by the predictability of confidentiality: it cannot be absolute, but its limits can be known, so that at no point will the patient be betrayed.

It is to be hoped that medical practice will reach such levels of ethical sufficiency as to render legislation in matters of information transfer obsolete. At such a point it would possibly be a standard of good practice to offer stringent confidentiality and to rely on public knowledge as to when information must be divulged for strictly medical reasons. It should also be the patient's privilege to know that, when in doubt, the medical team will prefer to honour confidentiality rather than err on the side of arbitrary indiscretion.

CONCLUSIONS

Medical confidentiality merits as privileged a social status as does confessional or juridical discretion. Whereas it is not absolute, confidentiality should be as ample as possible, and its limits should be clearly and publicly established. It thus becomes a strong *prima facie* duty for the doctor, that where breaches are not a matter of private mores, they are bound by transparent professional policy.

Unless confidentiality is applied in a generous way it will mar the clinical encounter, reduce its efficacy, lead patients to confide less and, in the ultimate effect, subtract patients with socially critical derangements from adequate medical surveillance. Thus, confidentiality remains essential to the medical encounter, and whatever limitations it falls prey to will not only undermine good medicine, they will also end up by making inaccessible precisely those patients that society is trying to bring under control. Sexual perverts, sufferers from veneral diseases, child abusers, drug addicts, potential killers—all will cease to confide in indiscreet medical practitioners lest society search for some other way of reaching them.

REFERENCES

1. Bok, S. 1983. The limits of confidentiality. *Hastings Center Report* **13**: 24–31.
2. Freedman, B. 1990. An analysis of some social issues related to HIV disease from the perspective of Jewish law and values. *Journal of Clinical Ethics* **1**: 45–49.
3. Gonsalves, M. A. 1981 *Fagothey's right and reason*. C. V. Mosby, St Louis, Toronto, London.
4. Harris, J. 1991. *The value of life*. Routledge, London, New York.
5. Veatch, R. M. 1981. *A theory of medical ethics*. Basic Books, New York.
6. Edelstein, L. 1982. The Hippocratic oath. P. 21, *in* Beauchamp, T. L. and Walters, L. (Eds) *Contemporary issues in bioethics*, 2nd edn. Wadsworth, Belmont.
7. Beauchamp, T. L. and Childress, J. F. 1983. *Principles of biomedical ethics*, 2nd edn. Oxford University Press, Oxford, New York.
8. Parent, W. A. 1983: Privacy, morality and the law. *Philosophy and Public Affairs* 269–288.
9. Goldman, E. B. 1980. Confidentiality and the Tarasoff case. Pp. 237–244, *in* Basson, M. D. (Ed.) *Ethics, humanism and medicine*. Alan R. Liss, New York.
10. Adams, J. 1990. Confidentiality and Huntington's chorea. *Journal of Medical Ethics* **16**: 196–199.

42

Absolute Confidentiality?

SIR DOUGLAS BLACK

Since I have been allotted, and been glad to accept, the ostensibly negative role of denying that confidentiality in the doctor–patient relationship is absolute, I must pre-empt possible misunderstanding by emphasizing my adherence to two important positive positions, which may be summarily expressed thus:

1. The doctor–patient relationship is both so important and so potentially fragile as to require the support of a clear ethical framework, understood and accepted implicitly or even explicitly by both doctor and patient.
2. I accept both the general value of stated ethical principles, and in particular the validity of the principles indicated by the terms 'autonomy, beneficence, non-maleficence, and justice'.

What then can be my grounds for questioning the absolute character of what is undoubtedly a major ethical requirement in the relationships between doctors and patients? The detailed arguments and instances which I see as supporting these grounds should, of course, form the content of this chapter, but it may make the nature of my argument clearer if even at this early stage I indicate its general course in the form of three summary propositions:

1. The statement of an ethical position can be valid, valuable, and generally acceptable, without its having the qualities of universality in acceptance and application which would justify its designation as 'absolute'.
2. There are likely to be 'legitimate exceptions' in the practical application of ethical principles, even those which are soundly based and generally accepted.
3. There are practical situations, both in clinical medicine and in public health medicine, where two or even more agreed ethical principles would appear to be in conflict, in the sense that action dictated by one of them would be incompatible with courses of action dictated by the other or others.

Principles of Health Care Ethics. Edited by Raanan Gillon.

CAN ETHICAL PROPOSITIONS BE 'ABSOLUTE'?

Warned by the fate of the anti-hero who maddened himself by the quest of the absolute in Balzac's novel, it is not my ambition to define the absolute as a 'thing-in-itself'; but more modestly to raise the question whether the propositions of medical ethics are of such a nature that they can properly be described as 'absolute', in the sense in which that adjective is generally used—*'Die Bedeutung eines Wortes ist sein Gebrauch in der Sprache'*. The first definition of absolute given in *Chambers 20th–century dictionary* (1983) is 'free from limits, restrictions, or conditions', which I take to be the common usage. Later on there is another definition, qualified by *'(philos)'*, which reads 'existing in and by itself without necessary relation to anything else'—a usage which certainly could not be relevant to practical medical ethics. But could even the first, less 'free-standing', definition be sensibly applied to the type of proposition commonly made in medical ethics?

At the (commonly accepted) risk of putting words into the mouths of hypothetical others, I suppose a deontologist might argue that some such propositions might rank as 'categorical imperatives', in the sense that they would be willed by all intelligences; and might give 'Thou shalt not kill' as an example. But even in relation to that precept, and among those intelligences to which we can obtain limited access by observing their behaviour and actions, there is a disturbing lack of unanimity, with deviance all too overtly expressed by terrorists, by other murderers, and more legitimately perhaps by agents of the state—and of course the different ethical standards of different countries and societies indicate that there is no escape from individual aberration by resort to organized collectivity.

There have, of course, been attempts, still within a deontological framework, and without rushing to naked utilitarianism, to escape from the difficulty imposed by the extreme variability of observed human behaviour, often accompanied by bizarre attempts at justification, such as the Nazi defence of slaying the mentally handicapped, even before they embarked on wholesale murder on racial grounds. For example, a distinction has been made between *prima facie ethical principles* (which should prevail in the absence of conflicting obligations); and *absolute duty* (which presumably must govern conduct without exception, and which seems difficult to exemplify) (1). Another approach recognizes the general validity of moral principles, but would resolve such conflicts as may arise between them by having set them in a hierarchical or *lexical ordering*, such that the 'higher' principles be satisfied before observing those 'lower' in the imposed order (2).

In the later, more pragmatic, sections of this chapter I shall be illustrating what I believe to be justifiable transgressions of the general principle of confidentiality of information given in the context of health care by patients to doctors, and indeed to other 'health care professionals', to use the accepted if somewhat cumbrous phrase used to denote the many groups other than doctors who give a professional service related to health. If confidentiality in these situations were indeed 'absolute', all such transgressions would be illegitimate and immoral; and it would obviously be wrong even to discuss them without having attained a prior conviction that confidentiality is not in fact 'absolute'. That is certainly my own belief; it may be an intuitive one, though I have laboured in preceding paragraphs to give it some groundwork in theory.

Those who, like myself, have a mistrust of absolutes, or to put it more simply are chary of the words 'always' and 'never' in our ethical discourse, are quite likely to be considered as ethical reprobates by those who take the opposite view. Let me therefore lay it on the line that I believe in the formulation and study of ethical principles and of the practical precepts which may flow from them; and that they represent a norm of proper conduct, deviations from which require to be justified. To go further in the specific matter of confidentiality, it has both historical acceptance going back to the ancient world; and a very strong ethical base, involving at least two of the four *prima facie* principles which inform this whole volume—those of autonomy and non-maleficence. To elaborate on the ethical base, release of personal health information supplied by patients is a breach of their *autonomy*, unless of course they have given specific informed consent. The dissemination of health information, whether by careless leakage or deliberate malice, offends against the principle of *non-maleficence*. Further, confidentiality of health information is compatible in almost all circumstances with the principles of beneficence and of justice; although later I shall hope to produce instances in which the need for beneficence or for justice may override the obligation to maintain the confidentiality of personal health information.

Thus far the argument has been largely theoretical, hoping to establish that ethical principles in general are not 'absolute', in the accepted sense of the word; but they constitute valuable guides to attitudes, which will then conduce to ethically acceptable behaviour. Within this framework a duty to maintain the confidentiality of personal health information is clearly in accord with ethical standards, and to do so represents the norm of proper action. But, like other guides to ethical conduct, it does not stand detached from the situations which adorn or perplex our daily lives. Questions which remain to be considered are, What constitutes a breach of confidentiality? Are there legitimate exceptions to confidentiality in the ordinary run of clincial practice? What are the special problems of confidentiality of health records in public health medicine and in society?

WHAT CONSTITUTES A BREACH OF CONFIDENTIALITY?

Not every disclosure of personal health information represents a breach of confidentiality. With one important proviso, any disclosure of information can be legitimated by the patient's consent to the disclosure. The proviso is, of course, that of *adequately informed consent*. This means that, for any disclosure of importance, the patient must know what is to be disclosed, the purpose of the disclosure, the person or persons to whom the disclosure is to be made, and that his consent is 'specific', i.e. he is sanctioning, unless otherwise agreed, *one* disclosure of a *specified part* of his record. These are the strict requirements, perhaps more easily stated than fulfilled, and of such gravamen that they may be strictly appropriate to areas in which possible damage or hurt to the patient may be foreseen. But in any matter of possible moment the necessary rigour of consent should be judged by the patient, whose trust or ignorance is not something to be abused.

Legitimation by adequately informed consent is the most valid guarantee that a disclosure does not constitute a breach of confidentiality. But of course it is now the rule rather than the exception that health care is provided not by an isolated doctor, but by a team of health professionals, and also in many cases social workers. Transfers of information are a necessary part of the care of any major episode of illness; and it would be unrealistic to subject each such transfer to the formal sanctions of informed consent. In actual practice the assumption is made that the patient in his own interests would agree to transfer of information relevant to his care and hopefully cure; this assumption of what may be called *implied consent* is pragmatically useful, if not even necessary in the interests of reasonable efficiency. It is, however, ethically and perhaps even legally frail, in that it could be construed as a derogation from the patient's autonomy. There is one safeguard which should certainly be applied to pragmatic transfers of personal health information, that they should be made only to those who require the information to enable them to serve the patient's own interests—it is this which constitutes the criterion known as the *right to know*.

It is transfer of personal health information without the consent of the patient to those who do not need to know such information for purposes of legitimate health or social care, which constitutes a breach of confidentiality. A deliberate breach of this kind, with malicious intent, is a serious ethical offence, and may also be a criminal act. Consideration of the numbers of people who may, quite legitimately, become possessed of health information about a patient, must arouse some concern about leakage of information, not through malice, but through inattention to proper reticence, or to carelessness in the handling of records. The important safeguard here lies in professional adherence to codes of confidentiality, and to similar obligations laid on other employees as part of their terms and conditions of service.

CONFIDENTIALITY IN A CLINICAL SETTING

'All happy families are more or less like one another; every unhappy family is unhappy in its own particular way.' Without suggesting that clinicians are either unhappy or, like Tolstoy's Oblonsky family, in 'a complete state of confusion', it is important to recognize that the welcome recognition that 'all patients are different' might in justice be extended to their doctors, and not least in their ethical attitudes and behaviour. At the level of ethical principle, doctors in general would assent to the sentence in the Hippocratic oath which says, 'Whatever I see or hear, professionally or privately, which ought not to be divulged, I will keep secret and tell no one.' But it should be noted that this obligation comes well short of the absolute secrecy attributed to the clergy in the confessional; the phrase 'which ought not to be divulged' leaves room for the exercise of professionally informed ethical judgement. Freedom commonly opens the way to error, and the particular temptation here is to act according to our own ethical preconceptions, rather than to discover the patient's own judgement of what should or should not be told. Of course, common sense has to enter, in the recognition that in the majority of clinical settings no particular problems are likely to arise, particularly if for sound pragmatic reasons we assume that if a patient agrees, at our suggestion, to see a colleague for a further opinion, he will not simply agree, but will positively expect that we will pass on information about his state of health. Such an assumption comes naturally to me, as a doctor who practised in a hospital setting, and dealt with general medical problems in which the help of a colleague was often needed, and in relation to which 'stigmatization' was not a likely issue. Even so, from time to time things would come to light with a bearing on life insurance, on fitness for employment, on disease communicable in various ways, or even on accident associated with previous treatment. As a rest from the theory, let me recall two specific examples of the kind of thing which can arise even in the humdrum practice of a general physician.

> A train-driver, appropriately from Crewe, was referred to me with central chest pain of a few days' duration, made worse by exertion, but still present at rest, and associated with shortness of breath on quite slight effort. His clinically suspected 'heart attack' was confirmed on investigation. I explained the situation to him, and pointed out that if he continued his present occupation he might be endangering others as well as himself; and I asked his permission to notify the railway's own doctor, so that after he had recovered from his immediate illness alternative safer employment could be arranged for him, as is usually possible in a large organization. Fortunately, he accepted this advice. Had he not done so, I believe it would have been my duty to notify the occupational physician of the railway in any case, rather than risk both harm to the man himself, and a distinct risk to public safety.

> A patient came with a story of cough and chest pain of several months' duration, of sudden onset after previous good health. He fortunately mentioned that he had had a tooth out shortly before his trouble began; but the true state of affairs would have come out in any case, as the chest X-ray showed collapse of the right lower lobe, and a large molar tooth in the corresponding bronchus. This was removed by bronchoscopy, but again I saw no alternative to explaining the nature of the illness, and the dentist involved became the subject of a successful claim, which he did not contest.

Perhaps these two experiences are in some sort of balance, since in one I could be considered to have 'shopped' a patient, had the need arisen; and in the other I 'shopped' a dental colleague. In relation to the thesis of this chapter, 'absolute confidentiality' would have prevented me from notifying the railway doctor, but would have allowed me presumably, in the patient's interest, to do the second; while in each case another doctor might well have acted differently.

As I hinted, perhaps somewhat obliquely, at the beginning of this section, the attitudes and consequent behaviour of doctors in relation to confidentiality are likely to be affected by the type of practice in which they are engaged. My own perspective as a general physician may well be different from that of an occupational physician, who has a degree of responsibility to an employer as well as to a patient; and even more different from that of a venereologist, whose access to patients is critically dependent on perception by the prospective patient that confidentiality will be absolute. This emphasis on absolute confidentiality has largely dictated the conventional wisdom on the ethical dilemmas posed by

AIDS; but I personally share the view expressed in a statement made in relation to AIDS by the General Medical Council in 1988, that 'most doctors are now prepared to regard these conditions as similar in principle to other infections and life-threatening conditions, and are willing to apply established principles in approaching their diagnosis and management, rather than treating them as medical conditions quite distinct from all others'. Thankfully, the public health aspects of AIDS are to be considered in a later chapter; but at the clinical level I would be prepared, in the face of absolute refusal by the patient, to divulge to a spouse, with the promise of appropriate counselling, that her partner had AIDS; and I support the action of surgeons in testing patients for HIV, when there is a risk that they might pass on the virus to other patients—just as I would see it as the surgeon's duty to notify an infection which he had acquired. I think I am consistent at any rate with the thrust of this chapter in considering the principle of autonomy not as absolute, but capable in the right circumstances of having to yield place to the principle of non-maleficence.

CONFIDENTIALITY AND SOCIETY

Although considerations of confidentiality are of the utmost importance in clinical settings, such settings are so much a relationship between individuals, some of them idiosyncratic by nature or as a result of illness, that the general principles by which they are undoubtedly informed are not easily extracted from the complex scene for demonstration purposes. However, society, or rather the agents acting on its behalf, quite rightly ask for a more formal definition of principles and of practical safeguards. From my background of clinical practice (which I can only hope to have been ethical in the manner of Molière's M. Jourdain's prose, i.e. adequate in practice without prior conscious study of the rules), I was called to the chair of a committee set up at the initiative of the British Medical Association (BMA), and with the support of the Department of Health, to consider matters of confidentiality as they affected personal health information. The immediate context of this was the prospect of legislation designed to protect from improper access any information held generally in computerized systems; but our own remit was 'limited' to health information. Because of the variety of professions concerned in the provision of health care, and because of the interface between health and social care, the committee was both large and multi-disciplinary; it became known as the Interprofessional Working Group (IPWG). The large size and the number of different interests in the IPWG, and changes in representation over a number of years, did not make for rapid decisions; on the other hand, we were greatly benefited by the drive and enthusiasm of Dr John Dawson of the Science Board of the BMA, and by the legal expertise and clarity of mind of Paul Sieghart. The group held well over 50 meetings, spread over so many years that the Bill which stimulated its formation has long overtaken it, and has indeed been the Data Protection Act since 1984. I mention my long-standing involvement with the IPWG not either to commend my patience as a chairman or to expose my ineptitude; but to explain the stimulus and the background to my own thinking on these matters, and perhaps also to persuade you that the problems, even if they lack the infinite personal variety of clinical transactions, are not without a complexity of their own. The general shape of the problems, and the principles underlying them, had become clear at least five years ago, and we had produced guidelines and an explanatory handbook which satisfied almost everyone—but in ethical matters as in many others, the desire to please everyone without exception is an *ignis fatuus*, offering its followers a choice of morasses, in one or other of which the consultation processes of government have now submerged our efforts. However, we did owe largely to representatives from the Department of Health a wise and clarifying decision—that although the Data Protection Act itself was limited in scope to mechanically processed information, in the health field the same principles of confidentiality should equally apply to the much greater amount of personal health information held on ordinary paper—the so-called 'manual record'. So in what follows I shall be speaking of personal health information in general, irrespective of the manner in which it is recorded.

In these matters the general principle, and also the public expectation, is that when an individual provides or a doctor elicits information on that individual's state of health, such information will not be divulged. To do so would breach the *prima facie* principle of *autonomy*. I suggested at the beginning of this chapter that departures from conduct apparently dictated by *prima facie* ethical principles could be justified either by the recognition of *legitimate exceptions*, or by *conflict between principles*.

Legitimate Exceptions

The most obvious of these is when a patient voluntarily abrogates his own autonomy, by giving free informed consent to the release of health information contained in his record. When information is to be used for other than clinical purposes—e.g. for insurance, welfare or housing—the patient's consent should have been preceded by explanation of the possible consequences of release of his personal health information to the authority concerned. A less important gloss, at least most cases, on the release of information legitimated by consent is that a patient can abrogate his own autonomy but not, without the other's consent, someone else's. For example, if the record includes a family history attributing to relatives a condition which they might not wish generally known, their consent should formally be obtained to disclosure of that part of the record. Common sense might suggest, however, that sensitive matter of this kind is not frequent, and that when it does occur it may be less cumbrous to delete that part of the record than to go through a formal consent procedure with a distant relative.

It was suggested earlier that, in a clinical context, those looking after the patient in various ways could have legitimate access to his record either in whole or in necessary part; and more debatably perhaps, that such transfers might be legitimated by the consent implied in having had recourse to health care. But when we go outside the clinical field the possibility of release on a 'right to know' basis is limited in two particular ways, which can be expressed in the form of questions which should be answered before the information is released:

Who needs to know?

How much of the record is needed?

On the first of these questions, it is the *need* to know, and not just the *wish* to know, which confers the *right*. When the disclosure is made in the interests of the patient, his consent should still be sought. Even so, the transfer of information should still be made to a responsible individual, not broadcast to an institution. On the second question, it is often preferable to make a specific disclosure, appropriate to the particular need, than to adopt the inherently sloppy course of sending unedited material. To go back for an illustration to the clinical field, I have on occasion seen patients referred from other hospitals bringing with them their entire notes and X-rays, but no summary of the specific problem at issue. I felt sad for the patient sitting there while I ploughed through this material; but I fell short of my duty of *agape* to the referring registrar.

These are but examples of possible legitimate exceptions to the principle of confidentiality of health information. In any material case their legitimacy should rest on a considered decision, taken in the interests of the patient. But there are also cases of conflict between the interests of individuals, between individuals and society, and even conflict between principles themselves.

Conflict Between Principles

It is a matter of common observation that one man's autonomy may be at another's expense; banal examples in the health field are in the 'freedom' to transmit colds, or to smoke in public. Some such conflicts of interest reflect discordance not simply in the application of a principle, but between principles themselves. As examples, I will discuss first the conflict between 'autonomy' and 'benevolence', using as illustration the possible constraints on research; and then the conflict between 'autonomy' and 'non-maleficence', illustrating it by legal pressures to use health information in the detection or prevention of crime.

Research

In order to avoid an argument tangential to the main theme, let me join the good company of Thomas Jefferson, and say that 'I hold it to be a self-evident truth' that it is desirable to increase knowledge by carrying out research; and it is further beneficial if the results of such research can be applied to the prevention and cure of illness. Clinical research has its ethical problems, soluble in the main by truly informed consent; but they are not particularly those arising from disclosing information, rather perhaps arising from withholding it. But one very important branch of research is based on the use of records, with as a rule no direct interview between researcher and subject in which explanation can be given and consent sought. The academic and practical values of epidemiological studies are not in question; argument focuses on how the patient's right of confidentiality can be secured. One extreme position, strongly held by nursing organizations, is that any access to records must be preceded by explicit informed consent given by the patient; in other words, complete preservation of autonomy, at whatever cost to research or its possible fruits. There are not, of course, any advocates of the theoretical other extreme, which would be research without consent and without safeguards. The middle position, taken by the majority of the IPWG, is that any proposal for epidemiological study of records should be submitted to a research ethics committee; and that the results should be published in such a way that no individual patient could be identified—'anonymized publication', in the jargon. Much valuable epidemiological research is based in part on death certificates, for example the effect of smoking on heart disease and lung cancer; a rigid stipulation of 'consent' would prevent such research.

Law Enforcement

The principle of 'non-maleficence' would seem to favour the arrest of criminals and the detection of crime; but the criminal himself might see things rather differently, especially if health information volunteered by him for another purpose was made instrumental in his pursuit. Absolute 'autonomy' would preclude the use of such information—would indeed preclude either arrest or prevention. On the other hand—and not fancifully—rigid devotees of law and order have happily suggested that the immigration officer or the tax inspector might get some useful information from clinical records. But I think most people might see this as a matter of degree, giving the preference to autonomy for trivial offences, but becoming skewed to non-maleficence in case of terrorism or other serious crime. But in the practical world two specific problems arise, how to define 'serious crime'; and who is to make the disclosure.

On the first of these, the Police and Criminal Evidence Act (1985) gives some help, which wisely falls short of the categorical, but instances the 'security of the state', the processes of criminal investigation and trial, and the life and health of individuals as things worthy of protection, even at some cost to autonomy. Representative crimes include homicide, rape, treason and kidnapping.

Formal disclosures to the police of health information are not a daily occurrence, but authorities must have a mechanism for deciding on them. In family practice the onus is presumably on the individual doctor; and in hospital the doctor in charge of the patient is the first choice; but he or she may not always be available in an emergency, and it may then be necessary to fall back on an administrative arrangement—which should not, however, be the first choice, as administrators, however strong their personal integrity, are under no professional constraint, and have not got the traditions of confidentiality which medical training and practice should inculcate.

Where a doctor finds himself possessed of information which may be relevant to the detection or prevention of serious crime, he can as a rule make his decision as a free agent. But there are quite a number of statutory provisions which may variously require, permit, or prevent disclosure; and in some of these contexts the requirement is on the health authority, with or in some cases without the necessary awareness of the doctor. A doctor may also be ordered by a court of law to disclose health information on his patient, and he is then under a legal obligation to do so. It is unlikely, but not impossible, that a legal requirement would be in flagrant conflict with personal or professional ethics; but if it were, the damage to personal integrity would have to be balanced against the penalty likely to be imposed by the court.

RECAPITULATION

Doctors and other health workers should not divulge personal health information given them by patients. This is a norm of conduct, not a categorical ethical imperative. Disclosures can be legitimated by the informed consent of the patient, and by the 'need to know' of other health professionals directly involved in the care of that patient. For information to go outside the health care field and into society generally, stringent safeguards are needed; but even so, other ethical principles in particular contexts may take precedence over the principle of confidentiality based on autonomy. There are also statutory and legal constraints to be taken into account.

REFERENCES

1. Ross, W. D. 1930. *The right and the good*. Oxford University Press, Oxford.
2. Rawls, J. 1976. *A theory of justice*. Oxford University Press, Oxford.

43

Promise-keeping and the Doctor–Patient Relationship

JENNIFER JACKSON

Director, Centre for Business and Professional Ethics, Leeds University, UK

THE BEAUCHAMP AND CHILDRESS PRINCIPLES AND PROMISE-KEEPING

'A well-developed ethical theory provides a framework of principles within which an agent can determine morally appropriate actions', say Beauchamp and Childress (1). Outside any special context it is not clear what it means to describe actions as 'morally appropriate'—appropriate for what? To whom? Is any deed that is not morally impermissible 'appropriate'? Can one deed be more 'appropriate' than another, e.g. a supererogatory deed?

Be that as it may, in the context of health care the four fundamental principles singled out by Beauchamp and Childress do indeed seem to be 'appropriate' action guides in as much as each corresponds to a duty doctors have *vis-à-vis* their patients (and more generally, health carers *vis-à-vis* their clients): the duty to do them good (beneficence); to do them no harm (non-maleficence); to respect their rights of self-determination (autonomy); and to respect their rights generally (justice).

But might not these four principles be more perspicuously reduced to two? The principle to do no harm would seem either to fall under the principle of justice—if by 'harm' we understand 'wrong' or 'injustice', or to fall under the principle of beneficence—if we determine what counts as a 'harm' in relation to what is or is not a net benefit, e.g. a surgically necessary amputation is not a harm just because it is a net benefit. If doctors are bound to do good (by the principle of beneficence) they are already thereby bound to do no harms that are not of net benefit: we do not need the further principle of non-maleficence. And if the principle of justice covers our duties to respect other people's rights generally, why do we need to introduce a separate principle to correspond to just one of these rights, *viz.* the right of self-determination?

At any rate, whether the major principles or duties of health care are two or four, the duty which concerns us here, to keep promises, quite clearly falls under the principle of justice—if justice is a matter of giving people their due, the keeping of our promises is undeniably something we *owe* promisees.

PROMISE-KEEPING—WHY A DUTY?

It is important to note that the basis of the duty to keep promises is *only* that an undertaking has been given. Of course, we may have additional reasons for keeping particular promises, reasons which may independently bind us to do as we have promised—perhaps keeping the promise is 'for the best' and we are duty bound to do whatever is for the best; perhaps keeping the promise shows a proper respect for the promisee's rights of self-determination as we may be duty-bound to do.

It is particularly important to notice that the duty to keep promises to patients does not derive from the duty to respect their rights of self-determination, although often the latter duty will be an additional reason why doctors ought to do as they have promised their patients. Suppose, for example, that patients are within their rights in refusing food or blood transfusions even when without them they will die. Then, presumably, they are also within their rights in exacting promises from their doctors not to impose either at a later date (e.g. should they, the patients, become unconscious). In such cases the doctors who promised would be doubly bound *both* because they had promised and because the patients' refusals would constitute a legitimate exercise of their autonomy. If, on the other hand, patients' rights of self-determination do not include the right to refuse life-saving treatment but nevertheless patients persuade their doctors to promise to respect their wishes, then these doctors are still bound, but only by their having promised and not by their duty to respect their patients' autonomy.

Everyone rightly expects that promises sometimes may justifiably not be kept and sometimes must not be kept. Some promises cannot be kept, such as if keeping one necessitates not keeping another: a doctor has promised to be at the bedside of Ms A. when she is in labour and to be at the bedside of Ms B. when she is in labour; quite unexpectedly both are in labour simultaneously in different hospitals. The institution of promising has built into it an element of discretion and vagueness over the bindingness of most types of promise, and we have good reason to preserve this feature of promise-making: we both want to tie people to act as agreed, and not to tie them too tightly, since neither we nor they can foretell precisely what will happen and what may turn out to be desirable.

While everyone agrees that doctors are sometimes justified in not keeping their promises, deciding and agreeing on particular cases whether not keeping a promise is justified is another matter. Appeal to the Beauchamp and Childress principles is at this point no help—they may rather be (part of) the problem, since here they can be pushing us in contrary directions. In order to understand better the scope of doctors' obligations to keep promises and how they might legitimately be limited, it might help us to enquire more closely into the importance of promises in the context of health care; why keeping them matters.

THE NEED FOR TRUST

Doctors make promises to patients in order to get their co-operation, e.g. to follow a course of treatment, to alter their habits in diet or exercise, to become hospitalized, to undergo surgery, to divulge sensitive information to others. Unless patients are willing to co-operate, which often involves surrendering considerable powers of self-determination, doctors may be unable to help them. Patients co-operate on the basis of trust, and doctors' promises enable patients to extend their trust further than they otherwise would be prepared to do. But such further extensions of trust are possible only if there already exists between doctors and patients a modicum of trust on which to build. Trust, therefore, is a fundamental precondition of effective treatment.

The need for winning patients' trust varies according to the degree to which health carers depend on patient co-operation in achieving their aims. Once surgeons have pocketed their patients' consent forms and proceeded to operate on the patients, they may not have any need to engage the patients in further active co-operation. Accordingly, patients should not be surprised (nor miffed, bearing in mind the time constraints under which the consultants work) if they find that the same consultants who, before their operations, had all the time in the world to talk things over with them and answer their questions, after the operations, whisk by the foot of their beds with scarcely a nod.

While such patients continue in hospital recuperating, they are cared for by nurses. Do nurses need to win their patients' trust? Not always, perhaps. Where the balance of power is so unequal as between postoperative patients and their nurses, patients may have no rational option but to submit and do as they are told. Of course, whether nurses need to win their patients' trust in order to care for them properly, depends in part on what that care is meant to accomplish. Is it simply to get patients back on their feet and out as quickly as possible so as to make beds available for others? If one takes a broader view of what caring involves, winning trust becomes more important; e.g. in helping a patient to face the future, to leave hospital with the confidence to cope with increasing disablement or with the determination to follow a recommended regimen in diet or exercise.

While the need to win patients' trust varies according to circumstances, the need to maintain their trust, to prevent them from becoming disillusioned about the trustworthiness of their doctors or nurses, is more constant. You may not expect to see this patient again. But the next doctor or nurse who does may have to overcome the legacy of mistrust you have engendered. And then too there are the third parties, who are observing you, to consider: the patients' relatives, your fellow doctors, nurses, trainees and ancillaries, whose trust, or respect for trust as a virtue, may be undermined.

PROMISES OF PATIENTS TO DOCTORS

Promises between doctors and patients are not only one-way—doctors may want to exact promises from patients, e.g. before handing over to them dangerous or expensive drugs. Again, doctors can usefully exact promises only from patients whose words they already believe they can trust. For reasons of space we will confine our attention here to promises of doctors to patients; when they may justifiably not be kept. But we might note in passing that, at least on the face of it, betrayals of trust by doctors are a much more serious matter than betrayals by patients. Patients, after all, often have no choice but to put trust in their doctors, and they do so in circumstances of conspicuous vulnerability and dependency—which makes the unjust taking advantage of them the more objectionable. Doctors are not normally so significantly wronged by their patients' betrayals of trust. Such betrayals may frustrate the doctors' efforts to help their patients, but it is the patients themselves who should expect to suffer in consequence, not their doctors.

PROMISE-BREAKING—A WRONG NOT A HARM

The value of promising and of promise-keeping derives from the value of maintaining trust. Thus, I have addressed the question why promise-breaking matters in health care in relation precisely to the *utility* of trust in doctor–nurse–patient relations. It is important to recognize, though, that it is only if promise-keeping is seen as a requirement of justice, and requirements of justice are seen to be constraints on the pursuit of benefits (whether benefits for ourselves or for others), that promises can be rationally relied upon. We need to distinguish the question whether breaking a particular promise would do any harm (or net harm) from the question whether breaking the promise would be wrong. Geoffrey Warnock illustrates persuasively how trust would quickly evaporate if people ceased to recognize that doing a wrong (acting unjustly) is a reason not to break a promise independently of whether what would do wrong would also do harm (2).

Thus it does not follow that, simply because no harm will result (perhaps because no one will ever know) if you break a particular promise, that breaking it is innocent. A promise binds regardless of whether keeping it does good or harm. Again, the importance of our being made to view the duty to keep our promises (and other duties of justice) as directly binding is something to be explained, as Warnock does, in terms of social utility—or, as I would prefer to say—social necessity. But that is not to say that our ultimate *motive* in acting dutifully is after all at bottom consequentialist in character.

If you need to take regular exercise to keep fit, and take up swimming for that purpose, you might be advised to try to get to enjoy your swims. If you do succeed in putting yourself in the mood to enjoy your swims, you then have a new and independent motive for swimming. There is no need to suppose that your *real* motive just continues to be the original motive—to keep fit.

I do not mean by this analogy to suggest that conscientious persons necessarily enjoy acting dutifully—that may depend very much on circumstances (you may be duty-bound to impart bad news—it would be no sign of virtue if you enjoyed doing so). All I mean to indicate with this analogy is that you can have one reason for putting yourself (or others) in the way of having another kind of reason for acting in a certain way—which reason, it is important to note, can be genuinely free-standing and a sufficient rational motivation of your choice.

Thus even if you took up swimming only because you wanted to keep fit, you may now continue to swim merely for the pleasure of it, and maybe despite the fact that this activity has become hazardous, e.g. because of water pollution.

In order to justify the directly binding character we ascribe to duties of justice, we must give an account of the point, the need, the use, of viewing these duties as direct constraints on our choices—and not as mere rules of thumb for bringing about morally acceptable or desirable ends. We can provide such an account, I am suggesting, without in any way undermining the genuinely deontological character of the *motivation* of those who conscientiously confine their choices of action within the constraints these duties impose.

Prima Facie and Actual Duties

While we need to become directly attached to keeping our promises, to become motivated to do so independently of consequential considerations, it by no means follows that we need to consider ourselves to be *unconditionally* bound by them. To allow ourselves to become so attached is both unnecessary and absurd.

It is unnecessary: we want people to take their promises seriously but not *that* seriously—not usually, anyhow. We expect people to do as they have promised but still to exercise discretion, not blindly to carry out their promises 'come hell or high water'. Thus, in a sense, 'because you have promised' is not always 'end of story'; but it often is.

To consider ourselves unconditionally bound by our promises is, anyway, absurd. We can find ourselves in situations where the promises we have made conflict—there is no way of fulfilling one promise, as it turns out, that does not prevent our being able to fulfil the other. Assuming that we are not obliged to do the impossible, we must consider, therefore, that promises are only *prima facie* binding.

Of course, not only may the duty to keep one promise stand in the way of a duty to keep another promise, but the duty to keep a promise may stand in the way of other kinds of duties we have. The *prima facie* duty to keep a promise may be overruled in a particular case just because keeping the promise in the circumstances would cause harm of a kind or scale that we have a duty to prevent. In short, we may be bound *prima facie* in conflicting ways, and then our failure to fulfil the duty which in the circumstances is overridden is not unjust.

Because trust is fundamental to the doctor–patient relationship, and because trust is notoriously fragile and very difficult to repair, even occasional betrayals of trust are a serious matter. But there are circumstances, as we have noted, in which not keeping a promise is justified or even obligatory—circumstances, in other words, in which the failure to keep a promise does not involve a betrayal (i.e. the unjust taking advantage of) trust.

MISUNDERSTANDINGS ABOUT PROMISES

Not only, though, may we have difficulty in agreeing as to whether a particular promise ought to have been kept, but we may even have difficulty sometimes in agreeing as to whether a promise was actually made in the first place. Misunderstanding and uncertainty is especially liable to occur on this point between doctors and patients for two reasons:

1. The way in which undertakings, half-promises, intentions, wishes are intermingled and communicated in conversation and gesture is convention-bound and may vary subtly but significantly from one small circle in society to another (which is one reason why it is easier to trust friends than strangers). Thus doctors may unwittingly mislead their patients, e.g. on the crucial question of whether they are undertaking to see to it that things will turn out thus and so, or merely expressing the hope and expectation that things will turn out thus and so.
2. It is often difficult for patients to quiz their doctors directly on this point without appearing to be impudent and mistrustful. Patients may not know whether or not what they are asking of their doctors, e.g. to tell them the results of tests as soon as they are available, or to not tell the family the results, is just standard medical practice for which it should not be necessary to exact promises from conscientious doctors.

Where unquestionably a promise has been made, what kinds of justification might there be for not keeping it? I suggest there are two kinds of justification—one making it permissible, merely, not to keep a promise; the other making it obligatory not to keep it.

PERMISSIBLE PROMISE-BREAKING

A justification for not keeping some promises might be based on the obvious permissibility of not keeping promises from which promisees release us. Suppose we are unable to seek such release in advance, but have good reason to believe that our promisees would release us if they could be consulted in advance and will consent to our failing to keep our promises retrospectively, so to speak, when we later come to explain our reasons to them.

Such a defence is surely sound. Maybe, though, it is of pretty limited application since (a) we would be justified in seeking consent retrospectively only in circumstances which prevented our seeking it in advance, and since (b) we are justified in seeking it retrospectively only if we do have good reason to believe it will be forthcoming. Many factors may prevent our having good reason to believe this—we would need to estimate accurately the importance of the promise in question being kept to the promisee. That may be easy enough in some cases. You expect your neighbours to be less put out if you neglect to keep your promise to water their flowers while they are away on holiday than if you neglect to keep your promise to feed their pets or their children. But often it is easy to misjudge the importance of a promise to someone else—how much your keeping it means to them. At any rate this type of justification for promise-breaking at best establishes merely that a promise may be broken, not that it must be broken.

OBLIGATORY PROMISE-BREAKING

More commonly, the justification that we give for breaking a promise is the 'necessity' arising from some other duty which impinges, and which in the circumstances we believe overrides the duty to keep the promise.

In some cases a prior duty not only makes it wrong to keep a promise, it makes it wrong to have made the promise in the first place. Sometimes doctors may be pressured by patients or by patients' relatives into making promises they have no business to make. Suppose a doctor, wanting to respect a patients' right of self-determination, is asking a patient whether the patient would want to be resuscitated in the event of cardiac arrest—the doctor might rightly judge that if the patient says 'No', that wish should be respected. It would not follow, though, that if the patient says 'Yes', the doctor should promise to comply with *that* wish. In other words a patient may have the right to decline a treatment without necessarily having the right to insist on it. Perhaps doctors should not allow their patients to dictate in advance that they will be resuscitated if necessary—what if the patients' conditions meanwhile worsen so much as to render resuscitation futile? What if there are other urgent calls on the resuscitation team from which such promises might divert them? (see ref. 3, p. 210).

It may be every bit as difficult to judge whether a promise should be given to a patient as it can be to judge whether a promise should be broken and, of course, such judgements often have to be made without forewarning, on the spot and under pressure.

Suppose, for instance, relatives press you not to tell a patient bad news (see ref. 3, p. 211). Perhaps as a general rule you consider yourself duty-bound to inform patients of bad results as well as good—maybe doubly bound, both because patient autonomy requires that patients are informed and because beneficence favours openness. In that case you are not free to make the promise the relatives press upon you. On the other hand, the relatives may argue that they know this patient well, as you do not (which may be true: especially in a hospital setting, patients are often strangers to their doctors). The relatives may insist that such is the personality and previous experience of this particular patient that openness would cause real distress and confusion, and would not in this case be beneficent. If they are to be believed, you then have to weigh the duty of autonomy against that of beneficence (or of non-maleficence if that is a distinct duty).

Where one duty conflicts with another, whether the duties in question both fall under the same general duty, e.g. the duty to act justly, or fall under distinct general duties, e.g. to act justly and to act beneficently, which of the duties should be given priority cannot be determined at this level of generality. The general principles or duties enunciated by Beauchamp and Childress do not as such constitute a framework against which to resolve the dilemma that occurs when it appears that we have a duty to do X and a duty not to do X, e.g. to keep a promise and to break it. One might suppose that these principles are underpinned by, and derived from, something more general, the nature of which might be revealed by a moral theory, e.g. by utilitarianism. But there are well-rehearsed difficulties with that theory and alternatives to it, particularly if their role includes the frameworking of principles within some decision procedure that is supposed to enable us to resolve the dilemma of conflicting duties.

Rather than moving in the direction of some more general principle on which to ground such broad action-guiding principles as Beauchamp and Childress put forward, I suggest that we should seek the solution to dilemmas of conflicting duties by looking to more specific information about the particular case in hand. The kind of moral judgement we need to exercise in such situations is more like applying a practical skill than like applying a deductive science. Those who judge well have, and draw on, experience of many similar cases. They do not think crudely in terms of one type of duty pitted against another, but of the implications of giving one or the other priority in the very circumstances which present. As with the learning of practical skills, case study and simulation is instructive.

WRONGFUL PROMISING

Promise-breaking, I have argued, is wrong if it involves a betrayal of trust, i.e. the unjust taking advantage of someone's trust. We should note that even where a doctor takes care not to break promises the *making* of them may still involve a betrayal of trust. Suppose, for instance, in seeking a patient's consent to some course of treatment you promise that you will do X if Y occurs, although you know very well that Y will not occur. If Y will not occur you know that you can safely make this promise in as much as the question whether or not to keep it will not even arise. But if the patient's consent to a treatment is conditional on your making this promise, the patient is being misled, indeed tricked, into a consent that is relevantly misinformed. Here you would be taking advantage of the patient's trust by merely pretending to be respecting the patient's autonomy. You might of course defend such a strategy as necessitated by the duty of beneficence, arguing that in this particular case it overrode your duty to respect the patient's autonomy.

CONCLUDING REMARKS

Promise-breaking may not be a particularly common form of betrayal of patients' trust. Doctors may be understandably wary of making explicit promises. More often patients' trust will be taken advantage of under a veil of deception, evasion and secretiveness. As we have seen, there are other aspects to promising which can be equally morally problematic for doctors; other ways in which patients' trust may be taken advantage of than by failing to keep promises made, *viz.* in the actual making of a promise one has no business to make or in misleading a patient (whether deliberately or carelessly) into supposing that an undertaking is being given when no such is intended.

Whether taking advantage of a patient's trust in any of these ways is in a given case unjust depends on whether what is *prima facie* our duty is actually so, to answer which we should look not to some over-arching principle for guidance but to the judgement of the wise and good whose powers of discernment are based on wide experience of life. For, as Aristotle famously insists, ethics is not an exact deductive science and its methods are importantly dissimilar.

REFERENCES

1. Beauchamp, T. L. and Childress, J. F. 1983. *Principles of biomedical ethics*, 2nd edn, p. 19. Oxford University Press, New York.
2. Warnock, G. J. 1971. *The object of morality*, p. 33. Methuen and Co., London.
3. Thomas, J. E. and Waluchow, W. J. 1990. *Well and good*. Broadview Press, Peterborough, Ontario.

44

Truth-telling, Lying and the Doctor–Patient Relationship

Roger Higgs, MBE, MA, FRCP, FRCGP

Professor of General Practice and Primary Care, King's College School of Medicine and Dentistry, London, UK

> *Big Mama*: You told me an' Big Daddy there wasn't a thing wrong with him but—
> *Doctor Baugh*: Yes that's what we told Big Daddy. But we had this bit of tissue run through the laboratory, an' I'm sorry to say the test was positive on it. It's malignant.
> *Big Mama*: Cancer! Cancer! (Tennessee Williams, *Cat On A Hot Tin Roof*, Act III)

As Tennesse Williams sat creating the flamboyant character of Big Daddy, a slimmer, quieter man sat in a chest hospital in southern England. Just approaching his 50th birthday, H.A. had been struck down by a pneumonia taking him within an inch of his life before new antibiotics could bring him back. A shopkeeper, meticulous, careful and anxious, he smoked heavily, a habit shared with his younger wife. So the doctors were not surprised when, as he slowly recovered, sputum test results showed that he not only had a pneumonia but also an underlying lung cancer.

The story is confused at this point. Certainly an operation was advised: and certainly a lung was removed. Perhaps his wife was told, perhaps she was not. But the patient was told he 'had tuberculosis'. Recovering without having to take drugs, he felt 'more fortunate than others in the ward'. But the pressures were such that, when he finally got home and was back in work, he began to smoke again.

Fifteen years later a new doctor took over at his local surgery. The notes, once sorted through, were clear. H.A. had had lung cancer, but after an operation, had done well. Then, as he neared retirement, he began to have chest trouble again—recurrent bouts of bronchitis, which took him off work and meant repeated visits to the new doctor. They got to know each other well, but the new doctor's suggestion that H.A. should stop smoking for his health's sake fell on deaf ears. Grandparents now, both H.A. and his wife had more than enough to contend with, a struggle to work and to earn enough for a diabetic daughter

Principles of Health Care Ethics. Edited by Raanan Gillon.
© 1994 John Wiley & Sons Ltd

and a grandchild born with a hip defect. The new doctor was frustrated. At the third chest infection, he said, 'Excuse me, but I want to say something really important. You're the only person I know who's lived so long—completely cured in fact—after having had lung cancer. But you're still smoking. How is it you won't give it up? Do you realize you might run the risk of a cancer in the other lung?'

H.A. looked aghast. 'A cancer? When?' With a sinking heart the doctor realized that H.A. knew nothing of this. After an explanation and discussion, a shaken H.A. left the surgery, went home, and went to bed.

And stayed in bed.

Mrs A. was cross. The doctor visited, apologized and talked to them both. H.A. no longer smoked—though his wife still did. But he stayed in bed.

Three weeks and four doctor's visits later, he got up. Six weeks later he went back to work. But he was somehow different. The doctor felt somehow closer to him and his family. But it was no surprise when six months later he decided to retire.

The doctor was enormously relieved when H.A. got out of bed, and pleased that, by giving up smoking, his patient might also have bought himself some more years of life, and even some years less blighted by recurrent bronchitis and declining lung function. He was less sure about how things had turned out for the family in general. He was sure that H.A. had not been told the truth by his surgeon before the operation, and possibly had actually been told a lie. But what about his own actions? Was telling the truth the best for H.A.? Why had standards and behaviours changed so much in the intervening years? Was honesty and openness between a doctor and a patient really the best, or was this just another fashion?

CONTRASTS AND EVERYDAY LIFE

The contrasts in this story are stark. They lie between the naked public hustle and bustle of a busy surgical ward and the intimate world of the surgery and bedroom; between the striving, achieving man in his late 40s, a stranger to illness, and the chronic bronchitic facing retirement and his body's gradual failure; between the experimental optimism of the early 1960s, ('You've never had it so good') and the steadying realism of the last decades, as the money began to run out. And strongest of all, between the two attitudes to telling the truth, which made it right, as a considered policy, to operate on a man to save his life and tell a lie, and, 20 years later, to risk his health by revealing the truth.

We can be sure, in these contrasts, sit some of the most important questions facing doctors and patients. What sort of life do we want for ourselves? What are we expecting of health professionals? There is fashion, and current standards— but behind these there seems confusion, both in the public mind and in the minds of thinkers and policy creators. Are we to see telling the truth as the gold standard, the yardstick against which every communication is to be judged, actionable if not achieved? Or are there circumstances and situations where human beings cry out for comfort, which includes the comfort and kindness of deception?

What we can be sure of is that, unlike many other issues in medical ethics, deception is not a hard case on the margins of everyday experience. The temptations to lie are commonplace. The young woman whose last game of tennis was marred by blurred vision and a tingling in her serving hand thinks she might have multiple sclerosis. The man who cannot cope with work wants a week off with 'flu'. The single parent whose child is ill must have a statement that she, the parent, is ill, or risk losing the lifeline of a job and its earnings. The child itself asks the mother, before an injection, 'Will it hurt?'. The man with a positive HIV test asks that no mention be made of it to an insurance company. The woman who had two abortions wants no mention of this to be made to the specialist in case her new husband finds out. And the husband, when he gets a venereal infection, wants her treated without her knowledge. Every day, if a meticulous health professional examines his work, there are demands that the truth be bent, folded, redirected, or simply screwed up and binned. Mostly, he accepts that this is part of the job, sometimes to the point that the deception is no longer seen. It is actually part of a larger and more disreputable truth, that we all have to get by, somehow, some way, until the challenge becomes clear—an angry patient, a desperate relative, a complaint, a case in law. All of a sudden our personal and professional standards are on the line, and we have to decide: what, and how important, is telling the truth?

TRUTH AND MEDICAL SCIENCE

What the truth really is must be a challenge the doctor really relishes. The scientific clinician will at once ask of H.A.: 'Did he *really* have cancer? The story sounds unconvincing—living so long, with just a sputum diagnosis and no pathology confirmation in the notes. How can we be *really* sure?' At once a chasm opens up at our feet. Perhaps an operation, a crippled respiratory system, the agony of bad news, an early retirement, were all for nothing. Doctors as scientists are in a very powerful position. They may 'bury their mistakes', but they may also mistakenly create their own cases to treat. A second opinion is always there for the asking, but what if we've already reached the second opinion, or if the second opinion herself is deceived? A frightened patient is vulnerable, which means both 'easy to wound' but perhaps also 'looking for a wound'. A symptom or illness is there: this previously fit man has a pneumonia, so there must be an underlying reason. The scientist searches for a reason. She would be only human to search a little too hard, or accept something on just a shade too little evidence.

Before the whole edifice of 'scientific' medicine—of which there are critiques enough to be found—crumbles to rubble in front of our eyes, we meet the first essential idea. Although medicine itself is not really a science, it is built on science which is itself founded on the search for truth, and on truthful communication once that supposed truth has been found. Given human nature and the temptation to lie, it is extraordinary that more Piltdown Men are not discovered every day. Scientists may disagree and disprove the observations, but open lying in scientific work seems rare. The benefit that modern society derives from science depends on truthful communication.

The same can be said of many other fields of human endeavour, such as technology, journalism or commerce. Here the deceptions of advertising, politics or salesmanship stand out against a background of the truthfulness that we expect from our fellow-men. To imagine a land where communication was based on deception would be to imagine a country not of the blind but of the mad. If all Cretans really were liars, the results would be almost unthinkable.

But if honesty is a basic assumption, and is in particular demanded of a people in their professional roles, why should it be different in medicine? Doctors are considered, if anything, more dependable citizens than most. If a certificate is to be witnessed a doctor is almost as good as a lawyer. False certification is a heinous sin in the eyes of medical regulatory bodies. So how does it come about that, down the centuries, commentators within and without the profession have stated that doctors can lie for the benefit of their patients?

> For the past 2500 years, from the time of Hippocrates (5th century BC) until about 1960, it has been part of medical wisdom that the disclosure by doctors to sick patients of their medical details can lead to loss of hope and so to a worsening of their condition . . . it was regarded imprudent or even negligent to provide information to patients that might be badly received (1).

Certainly, medical codes which gave positive instructions to doctors ignored the issue right up to the American Medical Associations' Principles of Ethics of 1980 (2). This silence concealed the well-known fact that nearly all authorities, whatever their views on telling the truth in other contexts, could agree with Plato that in the hands of a doctor truth could be used as a medicine—to be given, or not, as the doctor directed, in the dose that was deemed most efficiacious.

Before we look at why this might be so, it is important to make the distinction between the two uses of truth in ordinary parlance—the objective, the sought reality of truth, in its discoverable certainty, and the truth as told or transmitted.

TRUTH AND TRUTH-TELLING

Fascinating though the debates might be, we can disregard much of what epistemologists have examined when discussing truth in the *abstract*. Although this is of importance, for us here it will be a distraction. For the testing question in medicine, initially at least, is clearly not that of Pilate, 'what is truth?', but the very different, but possibly equally problematic 'are you intending to deceive?' Sissela Bok laid this out in her study, *Lying*: the issue is about telling the truth, or its variations, the communication of information, and not about the state of the information itself. 'The moral question of whether you are lying or not is not *settled* by establishing the truth or falsity of what you say. In order to settle the question, we must know whether you *intended your statement to mislead*' (3).

DECEIT AND THE PATIENT'S BEST INTEREST

Yet though doctors have been searching for the truth about disease and how the human body and mind works, they still have seen themselves as being allowed to deceive their patients intentionally for the patients' own good (and have been encouraged to do so by most commentators on the profession's work). To deceive people otherwise is charlatanism, and perhaps every generation has its examples. But the doctor and the charlatan are quite separate. The surgeon who made the decision to deceive H.A. was no quack, and did so from the highest of motives: he really believed it was in H.A.'s best interest not to know he had cancer. There are many duties laid on a doctor (and on fellow-professionals) but the primary one must be the duty to care: to subjugate his or her own personal interests within a professional context to that of the patient. How far the altruism stretches, or how deeply planted it is in the individual when testing situations arise, does not disprove the reality both of the aim and of the telling. All human beings are capable of selfless acts of heroism, but the assumption, indeed the requirement, of doctors is that they be seen to put the patient first in a number of ways. Where there is the possibility of cure, a health professional is allowed (with consent or even on occasions without) to act in ways which would render other people open to a charge of assault. For the doctor *not* to do these things would bring the threat of law.

Readings change perhaps most obviously when there is no possibility, or little possibility, of cure. Here again, down the ages, the doctor's duty has been clear: to reduce suffering, to 'comfort always', to act as a valve that reduces the pressure on the patient to see just how hopeless her situation is or just how little life is left. Here this duty has been seen to provide a merciful ignorance, but the decision is undertaken in the knowledge that recovery is unlikely unless the patient herself desires it, hopes for it, struggles towards it. Modern psychology confirms the power of the mind in this context, either way: we see those who turn their faces to the wall and fade gradually, and we see those who deny, or who decide to conquer, achieving remarkable recovery. If hope is the only medicine, it is a cruel and ignorant doctor who dashes this from the patient's hand.

Yet the rhetoric of this sort of statement has become less easy to respond to. Hope implies a possible future goal. Within a Christian society or any other where there is seen to be a life after death, hope certainly makes sense— although so also does a more realistic analysis of a shortened lifespan. But in a pluralistic society, or one where the majority does not believe in a significant after-life, hope takes on a different meaning. It becomes an expression used to cover or deny nihilism, the observable 'fact' of personal decline, approaching dissolution, the 'absurd' human condition where we exist in a world deprived of purpose with our annihilation the only certainty. To look so openly into this abyss requires a special sort of courage, the defiance of Camus's Sisyphus (4), or Nagel's irony (5). For doctors and patients, hope has come to be what we hope will not happen, and the personal or subjective view of what will make sense of what's happening: what will supply meaning to apparent misfortune.

HONESTY AND CHOICE

H.A. must have looked into the abyss when his new doctor told him of his cancer. However many years later it was, the shock of death that might have been was seismic. Why did the doctor open this wound? Yet again the thinking was partly beneficent and consequentialist, the view of what might be best for H.A. with 'fewer than the average number of lungs', recurrently ill, facing a nasty future of breathlessness and immobility. Cigarettes were harmful to him: it was his doctor's duty to warn him, not just that they were harmful, but they were especially harmful to *him*. But unlike the operation on a lung in an immobilized and hospitalized patient, taking away the harm of cigarettes could not be achieved by a paternalistic decision. H.A. himself had to understand the depth of that harm, such that the harm of *not* smoking—the withdrawal feelings, the facing of tensions without nicotine, the distancing from his wife as she continued to smoke—could be set in the personal balance of it.

Some would see H.A. as being less in control of himself than he should be: his own field of choice diminished by his nicotine dependency, his autonomy of will compromised. Whether this is so or not, stopping smoking cigarettes could only be his choice, could only be done by respecting him as an autonomous being. The doctor took the view that he could only be set free by telling him the truth.

And thus we come to the big turning point, the watershed dividing a policy of paternalism from the currently prevailing view. In a patient still competent, even if his freedom of action is diminished by advancing bronchitis and his will shackled by chemical dependency, our modern view would wish to respect that autonomy still 'available' as being the way in which his health might be improved, as the vehicle of change. Health is no longer satisfactorily described as absence of disease. Few of us are without some form of handicap, yet we still mostly consider ourselves healthy: many of those with an obvious disease are not helped by feeling that health is now for them a mirage. The concept of being in control, to the degree that one wants to be in control, is merged with that of health: to gain more control over an illness feels like a step on the way to recovery, to become more ill puts one's autonomy further at risk. Seedhouse's concept of health as potential expresses this well (6).

But even if the link is made between health and nurturing freedom of choice, that choice cannot be exercised without access to the options and knowledge of them. To be in the dark, in the modern view, is to have one's growth stunted, one's potential reduced or its achievement blighted. In a legal sense this must be so: no modern surgeon could offer a competent patient a lung operation now without obtaining consent, and it would be hard to see how such a consent would be valid without the information on which to base the decision. But at an even more fundamental level, the choice as to whether to be a patient at all—to discharge oneself or stay in the ward, to visit the doctor or stay away, to take the pills or throw away the prescription—is one which depends on being told the truth about the position one is in.

Thus the duty to care, to provide the best for the patient, now includes the duty to involve the patient in deciding what is best. There may be many reasons why H.A. might have seen himself as being healthier as a smoker than as an abstainer. Anxiety or tension within the household might be a great creator of heart disease too. The decision has to be made on the basis of professional advice, but not just by the professional. It is seen as a shared decision-making process, a decision made with consent after open discussion.

Is this what patients want? Those involved in the debate about ethical issues are often chary of using social sciences to study problems, but here there is no doubt of the usefulness of surveys to challenge prevailing thought. In a series of studies those who have, might have or are told to imagine they have a serious diagnosis have been questioned as to whether they wish to be told the truth about their condition. In these, at the most a tiny minority wish to remain uninformed: the overwhelming majority is for openness between doctor and patient. The message for practice is clear. A professional must find a way of offering an escape clause for those who are unable or currently unwilling to hear: but once that is done, the modern western patient wants to hear the truth (7,8).

THE PRACTICE OF TELLING

This brings us to practice, and out of pure theory. There are ways of offering a truth which can be more harmful, or less. There are ways of communicating which can empower or destroy. Enough is known about the how, when and where of communication to show that, once a position has been taken, there are ways in which harm can be decreased. H.A.'s doctor could have left him in bed—but he followed him up. Just as in any other field of medicine, the continuing care is as important as the crisis intervention. Fidelity requires that, once a professional has set to work, the work is not stopped until it is completed. The harm of an operation would be incomparably increased if the chest was left open: in ethics where principles conflict, the one that 'loses out' still exists, must be acknowledged and the balance later corrected. This is no less so where truth is being told. People take time to adjust to new information, or may not hear it all at a time of anxiety. They may misunderstand or may forget. The harm of bad telling may be worse than the harm of caring silence. If it is our duty as professionals to explain, it is our duty to do it well.

Sometimes this may be very difficult indeed. Sometimes it may be in a situation of great risk such that special preparation is necessary. The critically ill accident victim, who wants to know the whereabouts of her family who died in the crash, is not helped by an overworked, clumsy neophyte who has just read a book on medical ethics: which is why good teams and good teamwork are also ethical imperatives in modern medicine.

Those who defend reticence and less openness in a clinical encounter have often stressed the harm that may ensue. H.A.'s doctor saw that too. Some hospitals had stories of patients committing suicide after being told bad news, but few if any of these accounts can be traced to documented sources. That any patient should take his or her life under medical care is a tragedy, and one which must make everyone examine carefully what was said and done, or what was not heard or left undone. But there is also the harm of lies, both the individual harm and the general 'poisoning of the wells' which happens when people begin to distrust one another. We documented in detail a case where a patient was lied to about her operation, as H.A. was, and lived in limbo for months waiting to get better before something in her made her realize she was dying, and she 'got permission' from her GP to go (9). It seemed like a case of 'obstructed death', and this has been extensively discussed in one of the journals. (10). Even if a patient chooses to know nothing, the choice is dynamic and may change. Relatives may not be able to cope with a more open policy, and may not encourage or signal a housebound patient's need. There can be little loneliness more intense than that of being cut off from anyone with whom to talk about an issue as great as this—what the future is, what the meaning of the symptoms is, what is the 'me which seems no longer me'.

It is hard in these terms to avoid the conclusion that there are few situations in which a patient is best served by lies or withholding the truth. Certainly, the presumption on veracity between doctor and patient seems strong, and a professional would need strongly to justify a policy of dishonesty in an individual case. But this cannot be seen as an absolutist stance. Human life is too complex for such a simple solution. One position has been to suggest that at either end of the 'spectrum' of seriousness, lying may be permissible—the white lie of social convention, or the desperately ill. Before considering individual cases, however, we should look at possible objections to the policy as a whole.

OPTIONS AND ACCESS

One criticism of the 'autonomy culture' of modern practice is that it wrongly assumes access to services. It is no good informing people of what is wrong, and what should be done, if the service or therapy is not available. A heart-rending cry from an overseas doctor puts this in perspective: a patient is suffering from a curable condition but the state will not pay for the treatment. Should the patient be told this? The history of medicine teaches that it is often because people hear about and demand certain treatments that the standards and the range of treatments increases. Whether one is interested in the idea of the market as a model of health care or not, the equitable delivery of that health care implies the spread of information about possibilities. There is, in the issue of truth-telling, ordinarily little incompatibility between respect for autonomy and fairness in the distribution of resources. In a democracy there is no way of having a proper debate about competing claims for funding without information: a society without open knowledge about health care availabilities could not even begin the first stages of an Oregon process (the assessment of priorities in the community, in Oregon State, USA).

On a personal level, however, obtaining resources for a patient may often tempt the professional to tell lies. There is the old lady who needs hospital care but who, in a time of a shortage of beds, has not got a particularly 'interesting' diagnosis, or the patient who needs a screening test but cannot afford the charge now made by the health authority. The purist would still claim that in a democracy nothing will change unless these, if they are indeed examples of inequity, are realized for what they are and faced openly in the political machinery available. But Nel Noddings, in her study of the ethics of caring, thinks that such claims become nonsensical when caring itself is the moral point of reference. Within a caring relationship the person is put before the principle (11).

Thus a moral framework which can be established seems inadequate unless seen within the relationship between the professional and the patient. Unless our more general view works at this level it risks being another fashionable creation which simply awaits demolition. What can we say about the doctor–patient relationship which sheds further light on the difficulties we face in practice?

THE DOCTOR–PATIENT RELATIONSHIP

One of the difficulties we face is that a standard of honesty we find ourselves moving towards, while laudable, seems at once to be out of step with the standards of life elsewhere. Health professionals, by creating around themselves an atmosphere of moral rectitude, may deter open communication from patients who fear, very really, not just the result of the diagnosis but also the effects of the doctor's moral judgement. Just as the practice of genito-urinary medicine presumes an open attitude about sexuality and sexual practice, so an understanding and 'holistic' approach to medicine must leave a professional's view of honesty in the desk drawer at least. But there the analogy fails to hold—as the patient in the GU clinic does not (we hope) expect to have sex with the doctor, but the patients who seek understanding about the broad issues of their lives may be asking a doctor to lie on their behalf.

If the doctor is to offer this service and preserve her own probity and honesty, there is a risk of self-deception. The study of paper cases often suggests that a reasonable problem-solving manoeuvre is often not seen for the deception it really is. Many doctors will deny that they use deception, yet choose strategies in care management that on any but the tightest criteria would be seen as less than honest (12).

In order to help professionals to see what they were doing, in a previous article, I wrote:

> that it does not matter morally whether a deception is achieved with an outright lie, or by equivocality, evasion, by being 'economical with the truth', or merely by refraining from correcting a misunderstanding. We may be silent, tactful or reserved, but if we intend to deceive, what we are doing is tantamount to lying.

For this confusion I was correctly taken to task by Jennifer Jackson, who points out that there are several forms of intentional deception which are not lying (13). She goes on to claim that we need not be so scrupulous about veracity within the clinical encounter:

> We practise deliberate deception on one another in a variety of ways which we believe pose no significant threat to trust; for example, by putting someone off the scent to keep a planned treat or surprise; a stratagem, it may be noted, which we play on our friends with whom we care most to preserve trust.

And Byrne, following up on a commentary on the 'obstructed death' case by Dunbar, makes a distinction between 'truth-telling' (understood as 'leaving no information and facts unsaid') and 'truthfulness'—being faithful in communication, in a relationship of trust. He too feels that friendship may be an important parallel, and suggests in addition, 'I do not deceive my eight-year-old if I respond to his desperate requests to know if Father Christmas is real by giving him the reassurance on this score he so obviously needs at this point in his childhood' (14).

But although such examples are useful (and disregarding for the moment an analysis of the framework of ethics in which these authors may be working) they will probably do us more service by distinguishing the doctor–patient relationship *from* those existing between friends and in families than they will by creating parallels. That trust is central to an established and continuing relationship of any sort is not in doubt, but a doctor should be no more encouraged to abandon honesty at the beginning of a relationship, before trust has been established, than we should be to play dishonest tricks on people we do not know in the street. The professional trust, once established, is different in form and kind from that pertaining to friends and relatives, by virtue of its qualities, its intimacy or lack of it, and the promises it makes. A friend whose party we are clandestinely arranging does not come to us distressed—and if he or she did, I suggest most of us would call off our plans for deceiving him. Even with 'routine' attendances at a doctor, it is hard to imagine patients enjoying a large measure of practical joking from the doctor. Professional relationships are of a different sort from friendships, and the establishing of a close friendship within the doctor–patient relationship may sometimes be cause for the ending of the professional one. Alastair Campbell and I have looked at the moral implications of 'getting the distance right' in professional relationships (15), and Campbell has analysed the way in which such professional relationships are, and are not, like the loving ones of our private lives (16). The Father Christmas analogy is particularly apposite. Whether or not we accept a measure of (weak) paternalism in medical consultations, the ultimate aim of consultations with all adults is to return them to full competence and control—as reasonable a measure of health as may be found, even though not complete by any means. We are not 'kidding them along' (note the verb) because that's all the relationship requires. Once again, equity suggests that the less someone understands, the more effort should be put into communicating. It is as alarming to come across an underlying assumption of the good to be found in deceiving children as it is to come across Donagan allowing the 'dup[ing of] children . . . and those whose minds have been impaired by age or illness for "benevolent purposes"' (17). This hardly seems like the recipe one would like to offer for those caring for vulnerable people. We are not best advised to use the images of trust to turn our more vulnerable patients into childlike dependency. The concept of respect suggests that we should look at them in every way possible as potential equals: and that of healing, that we should act in such a way as to encourage positive change.

Trust and truth-telling are intimately involved. Trust is unlikely to be established between two people who feel that they are not being open with each other. The facts of the relationship are that trust *first* has to be established by openness and honesty; when that has happened, the necessity for lies is greatly diminished, and the opportunities for growth from both parties (perhaps by taking some risks) are greatly increased. It is possible both to be close to someone emotionally, and to have developed a trusting relationship, but also to be open about one's own inability to take action in a certain way. Respect is thus a two-way process: just as the patient's choice is respected by the doctor, so is the doctor's autonomy respected by the patient. An implicit promise to care for someone does not, as some writing on the ethics of caring seems to imply, mean an abrogation of one's own standards, but that one's own standards are part of the dialogue and are for discussion within the context of the decision required. It makes no sense for a professional to pretend that his or her standards are higher than they really are, but it will make a great deal of sense to explain why some request cannot be acceded to, or why, in this situation, a deception is possible, whereas in another it might not be. In such a way we see that a study of deception within medicine may lead us to more honesty in daily lives outside. Within the practice of medicine, veracity may be seen to be integral to its processes and to the relationships which this work requires.

REFERENCES

1. Reiser, S. 1991. Reported by Greaves, D. in Lessons from Victorian medical ethics. *Bulletin of Medical Ethics* **65**:24.
2. American Medical Association. 1980. Text of American Medical Association New Principles of Medical Ethics. *American Medical News* **9**.
3. Bok, S. 1986. *Lying: moral choice in public and private life.* Quartet Books, Penguin, London.
4. Camus, A. 1955. *The myth of Sisyphus.* London.
5. Nagel, T. 1987. 'The absurd'. Pp. 45–59, *in* Hanfling, O. (Ed.) *Life and meaning.* Open University, Oxford.
6. Seedhouse, D. 1986. *Health: the foundation for achievement.* John Wiley, Chichester.
7. Higgs, R. 1985. On telling patients the truth. Pp. 187–202, *in* Lockwood, M. (Ed.) *Moral dilemmas in modern medicine.* Oxford University Press, Oxford.
8. Novack, D. 1986. Changes in physicians' attitudes towards telling the cancer patient. *In* Weir, R. (Ed.) *Ethical issues in death and dying.* Columbia University Press, New York.
9. Higgs, R. 1982. Truth at the last—A case of obstructed death? *Journal of Medical Ethics* **8**:48–50.
10. Obstructed death revisited. *Journal of Medical Ethics* **8**:154–156, 1982; and A case conference revisited: an obstructed death and medical ethics, Dunbar S. with commentaries by Byrne, P. and Higgs, R. *Journal of Medical Ethics* **16**:83–92, 1990.
11. Noddings, N. 1984. *Caring: a feminine approach to ethics and moral education.* University of California Press, Berkeley and Los Angeles, California.
12. Novack, D. 1989. Physicians' attitudes to using deception to resolve difficult ethical problems. *Journal of the American Medical Association* **261**: 2980–2985.
13. Jackson, J. 1991. Telling the truth. *Journal of Medical Ethics* **17**: 5–9.
14. Byrne, P. 1990. Comments on an obstructed death. *Journal of Medical Ethics* **16**: 88–89.
15. Campbell, A. V. and Higgs, R. 1982. *In that case.* Darton Longman & Todd, London.
16. Campbell, A. V. 1984. *Moderated love.* SPCK, London.
17. Donagan, A. 1977. *The theory of morality.* University of Chicago Press, Chicago.

45

Individual Rights in the Health Care Relationship

BRENDA ALMOND

Professor of Moral and Social Philosophy and Director of the Social Values Research Centre, University of Hull, UK

A curious sequence of events took place in a Dutch hospital. A young doctor was temporarily replacing an older consultant. A patient he was to care for had had a blood sample taken on the instructions of the consultant before he left. The consultant had asked for the blood to be tested for HIV infection, but as the patient had not been informed of this before the blood was taken, the young doctor decided that the patient should be asked to give his permission for the test at this later stage. The patient, however, was reluctant to agree, and in the end a compromise solution was reached. The blood would be tested for HIV but the patient, exercising his right not to know his HIV status, would not be informed of the result. All parties adhered to this agreement; the test was done; the result was negative; the patient was not informed.

The case is a curious one, since rights feature in an unusual way in the situation. They are, however, the crux of the matter, and it would be difficult to describe the ethical issues involved without recourse to the notion of rights. As a notion it is not without its critics, but in fact it is no more suspect or doubtful than any other moral concept. Rights provide a widely understood language for moral debate, and belong to a tradition of ethical reasoning that goes back to antiquity. (For an account of this tradition see ref. 1). Complex questions, then, may be raised concerning their analysis. They are, however, an essential part of our moral vocabulary and no more suspect than other moral terms. If it makes sense—important sense—to talk about duties and obligations, about good and bad, right and wrong, then it also makes sense to talk about rights.

One advantage of the vocabulary of rights is that it focuses attention on a problem from the point of view of a wronged person, rather than from the point of view of another person's duties. Very often, however, and particularly in the medical situation, talk about the rights of one party has clear implications for

Principles of Health Care Ethics. Edited by Raanan Gillon.
© 1994 John Wiley & Sons Ltd

the duties and obligations of the other. It should not be assumed, however, that rights belong exclusively on one side of the health care relationship. On the contrary, the issue of testing for HIV may also raise questions about the rights of health care workers themselves. Recently, for example, in Florida, USA, there has been an authenticated case of the transmission of HIV to patients by a dentist, and this has given rise to demands that patients should be able to obtain information about their dentist's or surgeon's HIV status, as a necessary aspect of giving their genuinely informed consent to treatment.

This illustrates the point that, in health care situations, rights are unlikely to be absolute. It will often be a matter of judgement as to which, or whose, right should take precedence in any particular situation. In relation to abortion, for example, it is a commonplace that the right of a woman to determine what should happen to her own body may conflict with the right to life of a developing fetus; but conflict within the health care relationship itself, for example between the right of surgeons or dentists to privacy and the capacity to earn their living, and the right of their patients not to be unknowingly put at risk, is potentially equally fraught.

Beauchamp and Childress define a moral right as a morally justified claim that should, *prima facie*, be respected by others (2). Rights have also been described as trumps (as in a card-game) (3) or side-constraints (4), which set limits to how others may treat you. They limit the pursuit of utilitarian objectives by setting moral boundaries to possible courses of action. Not all moral obligations can be expressed in terms of rights. Traditionally, for example, duties have been divided into *perfect* and *imperfect* duties; according to this classification, rights involve only what are called *perfect* duties—those which involve the notions of justice, autonomy and perhaps also non-maleficence—and impose specific obligations on identifiable people. Imperfect duties, on the other hand, are unspecific in their objects and so involve only general obligations such as charity or benevolence. Perfect duties with corresponding rights are of particular interest in the health care context, which is highly specific and closely linked to law. Beauchamp and Childress prefer the language of principles to the language of rights, but concede there is correlativity and correspondence between the categories of obligations, rights and virtues (ref. 2, p. 59).

With this background, let us return to the original example. It is an incident which must be set in the context of a broader controversy in the Netherlands about a recent (1990) legislative proposal (Wet Geneeskundige Behandelings-overeenkomst—Medical Treatment Agreement) which would require that a patient's informed consent be obtained before routinely collected clinical information (and samples of tissue and fluids) could be used for research by anyone other than the patient's own doctor. Some medical research workers there fear that this places too many limitations on medical research, making it too costly and time-consuming.

This raises the general question, can patients' rights be set aside for pragmatic reasons? On the one side there is appeal to the common interest; on the other to a right to confidentiality and a right also to be treated as a person and as a patient, not merely as a means to the attainment of other people's goals and objectives. The testing of blood samples may, in certain circumstances, appear to violate these rights. It is possible it may also be incompatible, for various practical reasons to be discussed later, with the duty of non-maleficence which a health care worker owes a patient.

Is what is involved here, then, just a matter of deciding which of these has more *weight*—the rights of the patient or some conflicting interest? In attempting to answer this question it is important to notice that a conflict between rights and interests may raise very different considerations, depending upon whether the interests involved are those of (a) the patient, (b) the health care worker, (c) other specific individuals or (d) society. In each case different reasons may be given for seeking information about HIV status.

THE PATIENT'S INTEREST VERSUS THE PATIENT'S RIGHTS

In the example given, there was clearly a problem of diagnosis. The patient was in hospital as a result of various troublesome symptoms, the cause of which had not been identified. One of a number of possibilities to consider was HIV infection. The patient could have refused to allow a blood sample to be taken, thus making it impossible for an HIV test to be carried out. But he recognized that his medical care would be more effective if his doctor had access to the most complete information about his condition possible. He wanted his *doctor* to have the information, but he did not want to be burdened with it himself. He had already voluntarily given his blood, but now he claimed a different right: that of remaining in ignorance about his test result. As long as the only interest considered is that of the patient, this seems a reasonable position. People in the early stages of a number of other diseases may prefer not to be given a premature diagnosis, but to live their lives without the shadow of knowledge of their condition and future prospects. Why should anyone else impose this burden on them?

Patients' rights and interests also play a part in the converse case, in which positions are reversed and a patient wishes to know the HIV status of, e.g. a doctor or dentist. The patient may, for example, be interpreted as claiming that his or her interest overrides the right to privacy of the health care professional. Nevertheless, the patient's case can be argued on the basis of rights as well as interests, for there is another right involved here, that of the patient to informed consent, interpreted here as meaning that consent to treatment is not fully informed if there are extraneous risks involved in treatment of which the patient is unaware.

As far as the case of the Dutch patient is concerned, it is clear that a patient's right may conflict with his or her own interest. This is particularly clear in another case, that of a woman at the onset of pregnancy, where reluctance to allow investigation of HIV status may lead at the very least to pointless treatment or unpleasant investigation of symptoms in the absence of this knowledge. In most cases, too, where HIV infection is present, it will inevitably mean the loss of the opportunity for early treatment with its potential benefits. But people cannot be forced to exercise a right to what others deem necessary for their comfort and, in any case, the compromise worked out between the Dutch patient and his doctor avoided these adverse consequences. If there is something unacceptable or problematic about the 'right to ignorance', then it is to be sought elsewhere, in broader considerations. However, in widening the discussion it will be useful to give separate consideration to the no less complex issue of the rights of health workers themselves.

THE RIGHTS AND INTERESTS OF HEALTH CARE WORKERS

In the case of the Dutch patient the doctor had a duty of care for the patient. Care could be effective only on the basis of full information. Hence the duty of the doctor could be seen as generating a right to the disputed information. It is possible that the patient involved in the incident recognized this right, which as a matter of fact follows from the widely accepted ethical principle put forward by Kant that 'ought' implies 'can'. In other words a person cannot be morally obliged to do what lies ouside his or her power. In assigning to doctors a duty to care, society also *ipso facto* assigns to them some rights, including a right to seek and obtain information essential to that purpose. It is, perhaps, necessary to remark that this is not to argue the case on the basis of *interest*, although it is true that for other reasons, such as the possibility of infection in the case of some procedures, there might also be an argument based on the health care provider's own interest.

In the converse case, in which what is at issue is the HIV status of the health care provider, patients' interest in knowing if they are at risk from their dentist or surgeon may be argued to be strong enough to generate a right. If it is a right, however, then it conflicts with rights health care workers may claim parallel to those claimed by their patients—rights to privacy and confidentiality, a right to refuse to provide a sample of blood, and a right to preserve their own ignorance, on grounds similar to those claimed by the patient in the Dutch case.

A compromise reached by the BMA (British Medical Association) is that if a health professional in a particularly risky area such as surgery knows he or she is HIV-positive, this should be revealed in confidence to colleagues and a change to another less risky area of work arranged. Others see the issue as resolvable on the basis of factual assumptions, e.g. that the risk of infection of patients by health care workers is negligibly small; or, second, independently of this assumption, on the basis of remedies which do not violate rights, i.e. universal blood and body fluid precautions. The latter solution is offered in a recent WHO (World Health Organization) publication based on a consultation on the transmission of HIV and HIB (hepatitis B infection) in the health care setting:

> experts conclude that the cornerstone of prevention must be universal blood and body fluid precautions. Universal precautions are based on the assumption that all blood is potentially infectious, regardless of whether it is from a patient or health care worker, and regardless of whether a laboratory test is positive, negative or not done at all. Components of universal precautions include handwashing, careful handling of sharp objects, proper sterilization/disinfection or disposal of instruments after use, and the appropriate use of gloves, masks, gowns etc., as required by the specific health care procedure (5).

Understood in practical terms, then, the proposal means that precautions are to be in the hands of the health care professional and left to his or her judgement. From this point of view it bypasses rather than addresses the new issues raised by the Florida case. It is more effective as a way of addressing the issue of patient to patient, or patient to health care worker transmission of infection. But as far as health care worker to patient transmission is concerned, it is, implicitly and tacitly, an assertion of the health care worker's right to the same freedom of manoeuvre demanded by the non-professional. The circumstances differ, however, in that the health care worker could not assert a right to ignorance once a test result actually became available. His or her 'right to ignorance', then, could be preserved only by not testing, a situation which makes this claimed right look at least problematic in the case of the health worker. For the patient, however, such as the one with whom this discussion began, this particular right has implications and consequences which cannot be confined to the individual concerned. On the contrary, the rights and interests of certain other specific individuals also play a part.

THE RIGHTS AND INTERESTS OF OTHER SPECIFIC INDIVIDUALS

It is a special feature of HIV infection that its implications are not confined to the health care relationship. In many other illnesses, whether infectious or not, a patient is treated in hospital and returns home recovering or recovered. HIV remains for life, and involves a risk for other people through sexual contact or blood-to-blood contamination most likely to be brought about by the sharing of needles in intravenous drug-taking. The question must therefore be asked, Does any individual who proposes to continue an active sex life, whether homosexual or heterosexual, have a right to ignorance? Does this postulated right not violate the rights of other specific individuals, i.e. those with whom the individual has such a relationship, or with whom he or she engages in other risky activities such as the sharing of needles in intravenous drug use?

A number of arguments are frequently advanced to support the view that, notwithstanding the rights and interests of these other individuals, establishing HIV status is unnecessary or even counterproductive:

1. Irrespective of the result of the test, whether positive or negative, the same advice is appropriate: that precautions should be taken and risky activities avoided. It may be added that routine testing could create a false sense of security and so reduce commitment to the taking of precautions.
2. There is a 'window' period between the original infection and its appearing as a positive result in an antibody test. The additional point may be made here that infection could arise immediately *following* the test, and there could be no way to know this, again generating a sense of *false* or *misplaced* security.
3. The psychological point is made that it is in fact unpredictable how any particular individual will react to knowledge. While some will see a positive result as a reason for care, others may abandon all restraint in a wave of resentment or despair.
4. It is pointed out that there are a number of adverse social consequences for

individuals as a result of testing positive. These include social problems such as stigma and rejection, and practical problems such as difficulties in obtaining insurance, maintaining employment and retaining accommodation.

5. Finally, it is often argued in favour of maintaining ignorance that only consensual activities are involved, in particular, sex, or drug-taking, so that individuals who participate in such activities with anybody at all may be taken to have consented to the risk of HIV infection. Where sex is concerned, this is taken to be so even in the case of a marriage partner, and is sometimes advanced as an argument against informing a spouse of known risk.

Before considering these arguments, however, it will be useful to take account of a final set of considerations that compete with a simple claim about individual rights in relation to these issues.

THE WIDER SOCIAL INTEREST

The community in general has a considerable interest in acquiring knowledge about the epidemiology of AIDS. Because of its long latency and resistance to treatment it represents a considerable community threat which needs to be monitored in the same way as any other medical threat.

There is also a clear public health interest in *combating* AIDS, and again openness and information are essential for this task. Where the disease is rife it is already clear that the social and economic consequences are extreme. AIDS affects people in the prime of life, and affects women in their child-bearing years. The loss of a middle generation is already a cause for concern in some parts of Africa where as many as a third of the population between the ages of 18 and 45 are affected. Not the least of the implications of this disease are its reproductive aspects, including the hazards it poses for pregnancy and childbirth.

With these points in mind it will be useful to return to the arguments in support of a right to ignorance. The first of these related to advice, and it is important to point out that advice to refrain from risky activities is somewhat facile: for example, insofar as this is a way of referring to unprotected sex, it is worth remarking that this particular risky activity is actually essential for the continuation of the human population. The salient point is that even unprotected sex is not risky with someone who is *not* infected. Knowledge rather than ignorance is therefore crucial in certain key situations, in particular in a marital or quasi-marital relationship.

As far as argument about the time lag is concerned, it is true that currently the most widely used tests have this disadvantage, although speedier tests are being developed. Meanwhile, however, there is still some considerable utility in knowledge which stops short of completeness by leaving a 'window' of uncertainty. This is still *less* uncertainty than that which obtains if there is no investigation at all.

The argument about the psychological uncertainties surrounding human reaction is important, but it is not clear why it should weigh on the negative side of the argument. Presumably, those who are interested in weighing the *ethical* aspects of these matters would respond responsibly to knowledge. Those who would not behave responsibly could not be relied on to do so even in a state of untroubled ignorance.

The argument relating to the social and economic consequences of AIDS is also extremely important, and rightly draws attention to the ethical point that discrimination does indeed violate rights. For this reason, each of the practical problems mentioned—insurance, housing, and so on—needs to be addressed in its own right. Such matters are best addressed directly, however, and not via a policy of concealment or social and community self-deception. Indeed, in seeking solutions to social problems, facts are of the essence.

As for the argument about consent, it must be said that consent to one thing cannot simply be extended to another. For example, although sky-diving is a risky sport, and to engage in it is to accept some risk, to consent to go for an afternoon's sky-diving is not to consent to be dropped from a plane with a parachute known by the supplier to be actually, probably, or even possibly, torn. Or, to change the example, someone might accept an offer of a lift or ride in someone else's car, unaware that the driver has been told that the car is unroadworthy. If an accident ensues and the person accepting the lift is injured, it would be absurd to argue that consent to accept a lift implied consent to be driven under predictably dangerous conditions.

It might seem that what all these arguments amount to is a balancing of the benefits and costs of different courses of action—a utilitarian calculation designed to produce the greatest good for the greatest number of people. If so, then it must be said that most of the factual assumptions that play a part in discussion of AIDS are inevitably doubtful, disputable and based on inadequate data, for the simple reason that AIDS is a new phenomenon, and one involving a time lag of years between infection and the onset of symptoms. It is significant that the language of those who base strong recommendations for practice on factual assumptions inadvertently betrays this uncertainty, rather than the assurance it is desired to project. The assurances are very often embedded in phrases like 'it is believed to be' and 'there is no evidence that'. A series of adverts about AIDS in the USA were striking in the use of the latter phrase. It has to be said, however, that humans cannot meet laboratory conditions, so the fact that there is no evidence that something happens is no proof that it cannot or does not happen. Extreme requirements are needed for proof, for example, that someone's infection was caused in a particular way, and a person's own claims about his or her personal history may have to be discounted. It is significant, for example, that the authenticated case already mentioned of dentist-to-patient transmission involved an older woman and a young woman whose religious background lent support to the view that neither sexual nor drug-related transmission could have been involved.

But although these factual issues are of great importance, and are clearly relevant to policy, it is worth pointing out that the 'public health' issue is not *only* a matter of interest; for society is made up of individuals, and the interest involved is in the end a matter of the avoidable illness and early death of individual members of society. While one has an *interest* in being alive, it is an interest superseded by a *right*—the right to life, which is in fact the most fundamental of political and moral rights. The common interest, then, may in this case be interpreted as a matter of individual rights. Most of the subsidiary rights involved in the health care issues that have provided the focus for this chapter, while important, are less pressing than the right to life, and in considering rights to patient autonomy, health worker's privacy, confidentiality and a right to ignorance or peace of mind, it is important to bear this salient point in mind. Rights are not tradeable against utility, but they may have to be traded against each other. This can only be a matter of judgement, carefully setting out and analysing the complex arguments on any particular issue. As an example of this complexity, the case of testing for HIV is both crucially important and difficult to resolve.

REFERENCES

1. Almond, B. 1991. Rights. Pp. 259–269, *in* Singer, P. (Ed.) *A companion to ethics.* Blackwell, Oxford.
2. Beauchamp, T. L. and Childress, J. F. 1983. *Principles of biomedical ethics*, 2nd edn, p. 56. Oxford University Press, New York.
3. Dworkin, R. M. *Taking rights seriously*. Duckworth, London.
4. Nozick, R. 1974. *Anarchy, state and utopia*. Blackwell, Oxford.
5. *Global AIDSnews*. 1991. Newsletter of World Health Organization Global Programme on AIDS, Geneva, Switzerland. Preliminary Issue, p. 8.

PART III

MORAL PROBLEMS IN PARTICULAR
HEALTH CARE CONTEXTS

46

Moral Problems in Particular Health Care Contexts— Introduction

Raanan Gillon

In this section a wide variety of ethical problems arising in specific types of health care contexts are addressed, often from diametrically opposed viewpoints. The majority of the contributions concern life-and-death decisions in different circumstances, and especially those arising at the beginnings and the end of the normal human life span. Perhaps one of the most important general themes to emphasize in relation to this subgroup of papers is that the source of radical disagreement between some of the authors is not over the nature of our moral obligations to each other but rather on their scope of application—who or what *counts* as 'each other'? It is not that those who believe abortion is morally permissible disagree about a general moral obligation to avoid killing each other, but rather that they disagree about whether the human fetus comes into the class of 'each other' for these moral purposes.

Mori's chapter sets the scene for this debate by looking at the disagreement within Roman Catholicism about whether the developing embryo/fetus is 'ensouled' at or after conception (which in secular terms can be translated roughly into the question is it a 'person' at conception or does it become a 'person' after conception). Although he argues that the embryo and fetus prior to development of a brain could not be a 'person' (on the grounds that a capacity for rationality is a necessary condition for personhood) he also argues that in fact the Roman Catholic prohibition does not depend on an answer to this question; for Roman Catholic theology allows exceptions to the general moral prohibition against killing even of innocent human lives. Instead, he argues, the issue within Roman Catholicism turns on whether or not there is an absolute obligation not to interfere with the 'intrinsic teleology of the reproductive

Principles of Health Care Ethics. Edited by Raanan Gillon.
© 1994 John Wiley & Sons Ltd

process'—and he suggests that addressing this issue may afford a fruitful basis for contemporary Catholic analysis of the abortion question.

Finnis, on the contrary, argues that the obligations of justice and non-maleficence ('rightly understood'—he and Fisher have offered such an understanding in Chapter 4) 'prohibit every abortion', precisely because from conception onwards a human embryo and then fetus *is* a human person. In a vigorous argument for this claim—an argument that he asserts is as relevant to non-Catholics as to Catholics—he states that the very youngest human embryo already has the capacities necessary for specifically human activities such as self-consciousness, rationality and choice—'rather as you or I have the capacity to speak Tibetan or Icelandic, though we lack the ability to do so'. This capacity resides in the embryo's genetic structure. Readers will decide for themselves, but it is worth pointing to an ambiguity in the phraseology of this particular and striking analogy; we do, *in a sense* have a 'capacity to speak Tibetan or Icelandic', even when we can't; but is this sense any different from the claim that we have *the potential* to speak those languages? The question is an important one for those who believe that the fetus's undisputed *potential* to become a fully fledged member of the moral community is—in a morally important way—different from (for example) the unconscious patient's *capacity* to be a self-conscious and rational agent; for they will undoubtedly wish to grant a right not to be killed to such a patient, on the grounds that all persons, whether temporarily unconscious or not, should have such a right; while being resistant to the claim that all human beings having (merely) the *potential* for such capacities should have such a right.

'THE ARGUMENT FROM POTENTIAL'

Philosophical aspects of the 'argument from potential' are addressed by Fagot-Largeault. First she points out that if the Roman Catholic argument that the earliest embryo is already a person is valid, then its right to life is precisely *not* derived from an argument from potential but rather from its actuality as a person (it being assumed that all persons have a right not to be unjustly killed). However such claims, that human embryos are *actually* persons, are unlikely to convince those who do not share their theological presuppositions, she points out. Distinguishing between different sorts of argument from potential, and finding them all 'never quite conclusive', she nonetheless acknowledges 'the persuasive force' of the fact that a human embryo/fetus normally has the potential to become a normal human person. Perhaps the best way of formulating the argument from potential, she suggests, is to see it as providing a *prima facie* obligation not to interfere with the development of a normal human embryo/fetus—a *prima facie* obligation that becomes stronger the longer the fetus has been developing normally. And she discusses the difficulties of that question of 'normality' in this context, adding a powerful counterargument to those who claim that abortion for fetal abnormality manifests a search for 'the perfect baby' (rather, she claims, it manifests a search for a *normal* baby). She suggests that most women with experience of pregnancy would subscribe to such an approach, though 'more for its "naturalness" than for its theoretical strength'. In a boldly stated alternative view, Lloyd avers that 'For me, and for many other feminists, "humanness" is a social construct' and 'to put it in the simplest possible terms, a fetus becomes a baby when the pregnant woman says it is a baby'. As she sees it, the abortion issue turns entirely on the woman's informed choice.

For Strong and Anderson (an intellectually challenging philosopher–physician combination) social role is only one of several morally relevant concerns in deciding on the moral status to be appropriately conferred upon the fetus. Discussing the problems of maternal–fetal moral conflict that can arise during pregnancies in which there is no intention to abort, they argue that the moral status that should be (socially) *conferred* on the third-trimester fetus should be of a 'moral standing having a strength that is close to, although not quite as strong as, that of persons in the strict sense'. Thus: 'Pregnant women are persons in the strict sense, while third-trimester fetuses have a conferred moral standing that is less strong'. Balancing concerns for beneficence, respect for autonomy and a *prima facie* obligation to avoid killing persons (and thus what might be called honorific persons, including third-trimester fetuses), 'it might be legally and ethically justifiable to override the woman's autonomy in rare, extraordinary situations provided two conditions are met'. The first of these conditions is that the treatment should pose no significant health risk to the woman, and the second is that there must be compelling reasons to override the pregnant woman's autonomy (which usually would involve a combination of reasons such as protecting fetal life, preventing serious harm to the 'infant-to-be', preventing the orphaning of other children, preventing harm or death of the pregnant woman, preserving the 'ethical integrity of the physician; and promoting the well-being of the community'.

PREMATURE AND HANDICAPPED NEWBORN BABIES

Whitelaw and Thoresen consider moral issues that concern not fetuses in their third trimester of development but babies born as they are about to enter the third trimester of development or shortly afterwards. They express disgust at the idea that newborn babies might be allowed to die because they are not persons, and state that from their perspective as neonatal clinicians the primary consideration is the golden rule of always treating others as we would like them to treat us. They indicate that for them decisions about withdrawing or withholding life-prolonging treatment must first be based on that rule (which is not unlike, they suggest, a consideration of whether more benefit than harm for the child would result if treatment was maintained). In addition, discussion and agreement between doctors and nursing staff involved is required; and then agreement between them as a united team and the child's parents is required. If a decision to withdraw treatment is made it should be implemented in a way that avoids suffering, and if necessary morphine should be given, for example if withdrawing ventilation in a conscious but severely and incurably diseased baby.

VERSIONS OF THE GOLDEN RULE

It is worth asking, in the context of the golden rule, alluded to in other chapters too, whether this version—'always treat others as we would wish them to treat us'—is either necessary or sufficient a basis for ethical behaviour. Suppose, as seems reasonable, that people have totally different views about the way they would wish to be treated and not treated in various contexts, and suppose they all simply assume that others would wish to be treated and not treated the same way. By applying this version of the golden rule would they not in effect be simply imposing their views on others? Surely that is not the morality intended to be encapsulated by the golden rule. The 'morally respectable' version of the golden rule is more like: 'do and avoid doing to others what (on reflection) they would wish you to do and avoid doing to them'; thus the relevant question is not what would I want if I were in his or her shoes, but what would *he or she* want in his or her shoes. This version of the golden rule implies respect for autonomy, it implies indirectly a concern to avoid harm and promote benefit (insofar as that is what most people would wish for themselves); but it does not address the question of non-autonomous beings (as in these cases); and it is equivocal on issues of justice. However, *if* by 'others' is meant 'all others', then the golden rule also implies some theory of justice so as to *adjudicate* between the preferences of particular people and the preferences of all. If this expanded interpretation of the golden rule is accepted, it is of course entirely compatible with the four principles that are the subtheme of this volume.

The discussion about handicapped fetuses and babies is extended in the chapters by Davis and Harris. Davis rejects analyses of these issues based on 'personhood' as 'simply a linguistic fiction designed only to enable those perceived as undesirable to be swiftly and efficiently dispatched'. For her 'human life has intrinsic, infinite value' rather than being instrumentally valuable, and 'a short life is as infinitely valuable as a long one, and a severely handicapped life is as valuable as one free from obvious disability'. 'True beneficence', she argues, requires 'maximizing the life chances of all babies who are not actually irremediably dying'. In opposition to this stance, Harris uncompromisingly argues that 'there is no justification for thinking of the human zygote or embryo or fetus or neonate as in any way morally equivalent to full human persons'; none has the capacities necessary to be a person and necessary to ground the moral status including the right to life of persons. Allowing a disabled newborn baby to die ('to kill it, in other words'!) is morally acceptable and, he argues, no more an attack against disabled *people* than is curing disability.

EUTHANASIA AND FORGOING LIFE—PROLONGING TREATMENT

At the other end of life the main specific issues addressed in this section are once again to do with whether or not to provide life-prolonging treatment, or in some cases whether or not to kill (as in the trenchant discussions for and against voluntary euthanasia by Nowell–Smith and Gormally, respectively). Goulden discusses the issue of do-not-resuscitate (DNR) orders, pointing out among other things that we know that in various types of medical circumstances the probability of benefit from cardiopulmonary resuscitation (CPR) is zero or very nearly zero. It is worth asking how the contemporary American medical culture, in which the assumption that CPR should be provided unless a DNR order is written, can possibly be justified (certainly it is hard to think of any other medical treatment that must be given unless otherwise specified). Goulden points out that net benefit for the patient is a necessary criterion for life-prolonging treatment of any sort, not just CPR. For example in the context of intensive care it is important to identify as early as possible those patients who will not survive even if they are given the most intensive care; for if no benefit can arise it is important (a matter of distributive justice) not to waste valuable resources on what can be reliably predicted, by methods such as the APACHE scoring system, to be futile interventions. But he adds that even life-prolonging treatments that would be beneficial and desired may sometimes be too expensive to be provided, either to all who might benefit or to any; one way or another 'rationing there must be'.

Dame Cicely Saunders writes from the polar perspective of hospice care, not about rationing of life-prolonging treatments but of provision of care for those who are dying, given ethical and legal assumptions that intentional killing is impermissible. Amongst many valuable reminders she points out that adequate pain relief very rarely has the widely assumed effect of shortening life, though in any case adequate symptom control is the primary consideration; and she warns against 'the nihilistic statement still sadly heard' that 'there is nothing more I can do'—a statement that, given the enormous development of palliative medicine 'is hardly ever true'.

In the context of clinical decisions concerning life and death Gillett expands his ideas about 'the pause'—that internal invitation to pause for reflection that arises typically just when such choices are required. In a characteristically subtle discussion he pursues the interrelationships of awareness of and commitment to moral principles on the one hand and intuition, moral emotion, moral experience, moral empathy and sensitivity and other aspects of 'moral psychology' on the other, and their necessary amalgamations in actual moral judgements. He concludes: 'the pause without the principles is blind and the principles without the pause are empty'.

CHILDREN AND PARENTAL PROXY CONSENT

Another theme in this section involves the moral issues that arise when patients or clients have impaired autonomy. The principle of respect for autonomy, in any case qualified by the need for equal respect for the autonomy of all potentially affected by such respect, is also modified when the subjects of moral concern either have no autonomy (for example babies) or have inadequate autonomy (for example young children, severely mentally ill or impaired people, including the mentally impaired elderly). Implicit in much of the discussion about babies is the assumption that parents are the proper guardians for their children. With babies and very young children the basis for such guardianship can only properly be what the parents perceive as the child's best interests (and in medical contexts such perception is likely to be heavily influenced by the advice of the medical and nursing team, as Whitelaw and Thoresen make clear). Such an assumption is now grounded in British law, and applies to health care professionals too, in their duty of care to their child patients. However, as children mature and they develop their capacity for autonomous action major moral tensions can arise if a child's understanding and opinions about his or her best treatment differ from the parents' views—a particularly difficult dilemma if the doctor agrees with the child rather than the parents. These issues are discussed by Graham, who reminds us that, both legally and ethically, the role of the parent is to make decisions on behalf of and in the interests of the child, so long as the child has not developed sufficient maturity to decide for himself or herself. Beyond that point 'parental rights yield[ed] to the child's right to make his own decisions'. (Graham also proposes the use of the Rawlsian device of the 'veil of ignorance' for purposes of allocating health care resources. Were it to be used, instead of current systems of power politics, adults would, he believes, be far more generous in their allocations to child health!).

IMPAIRED AUTONOMY AND PSYCHIATRIC ETHICS

Fulford and Hope also address the issue of impaired autonomy, but in the context of psychiatric ethics. Arguing for the inherently value-based nature of disease concepts, made more obvious in the context of psychiatric disease because the incorporated values are often highly contentious, they see psychiatric illness as impairment of intentional action as well as impairment of function. Addressing the central psychiatric moral issue of compulsory treatment they acknowledge that issues of autonomy and beneficence are generally of importance. Yet somewhat surprisingly they argue that the peculiar relevance of severe psychotic symptoms as a justification for compulsory treatment in cases of psychiatric illness is not easily encompassed by consideration of these two moral concerns. Perhaps this is because they assume that clinical decisions about compulsory treatment will turn 'crucially on the trade-offs between beneficence and autonomy'. On that basis if, in a particular case, compulsory treatment would produce sufficient benefit then autonomy ought to be overridden to achieve that benefit, and clinical decisions would be expected to reflect this. But ordinary experience and their empirical survey show that this is not the case.

However, there is no need to assume that such moral conflicts have to be, or are normally, settled by 'trade-offs' in particular cases. On the contrary there is a widespread moral assumption that people's autonomy ought to be respected even when they reject medical interventions that would be clearly highly beneficial, perhaps even life-saving. Those interested in justifying such non-intervention on the basis of utilitarian trade-offs (and the need for this is in no way entailed by the Beauchamp and Childress framework) are likely to do so by looking at the over-all long-term utility of such norms, even where in the short term respecting them does not maximize utility. But the question still remains, who counts as an adequately autonomous agent, who falls *within the scope* of respect for autonomy? Those who do not may well be treated paternalistically, whether they are children of sufficiently immature autonomy or the psychiatrically ill of sufficiently impaired autonomy.

Thus a different way of looking at the cases summarized by Fulford and Hope is to ask first, is the autonomy of this patient severely impaired by psychiatric illness? If no, the question of compulsory treatment does not arise, because of respect for the patient's autonomy. If yes, (i.e. if the patient no longer falls within the scope of the principle of respect for autonomy where such respect would conflict with his or her interests) can substantial benefit be provided to the patient by compulsory intervention, or does the patient afford a significant threat to others from which they can be protected by compulsory medical intervention? On this analytic basis severe psychotic features, as in the two cases described, do indeed provide a very firm basis for intervention, because they afford very good evidence that a person's autonomy is severely impaired by psychiatric illness and because there is good reason to believe that the patient can be substantially benefited by intervention. (In addition others may be protected if the psychotic behaviour is harming others.) Thus, *pace* Fulford and Hope, there is no need to invoke some additional morally relevant concern encompassed in severe psychosis, over and above the very relevant fact that it impairs a person's autonomy sufficiently for respect for his remaining autonomy to become subservient to moral concerns of beneficence (and justice too—one might for instance wish to argue that such patients should have a *right* to such compulsory treatment).

WHY PSYCHOTHERAPISTS MUST NOT HAVE SEX WITH THEIR CLIENTS

In an interesting variant Holmes and Lindley, discussing ethical issues arising in psychotherapy, argue the explicit case against therapists having sexual relationships with their patients/clients. One part of their argument is the standard one that health care workers have an obligation not to harm their patients, and that such sexual relationships are generally harmful. A second part of their argument is that such sexual relationships are deceitful—for there is an implied (and in the case of doctors, explicit) undertaking not to have sexual relationships with clients/patients. The third and specifically psychoanalytic component of their argument is that the process of the analysis itself can involve considerable—albeit temporary—undermining of the patient's autonomy—and also of the therapist's—within 'a bipersonal transferential field' such that the emotional autonomy of both the patient and therapist are severely impaired. Thus sex in such a context is in effect *not* sex between autonomous consenting adults but more like child abuse by an emotionally impaired adult.

THE ELDERLY AND THE DEMENTED

Autonomy can be severely impaired as people become old, and both Muir Gray and Norberg consider the ethical issues that then arise. In a contribution that emphasizes the importance of listening to and trying to understand patients' life stories (a theme that unsurprisingly appears in many contributions to this volume), Norberg argues that the objective in care of the elderly with dementia should be to try to benefit the patient precisely by trying, to the extent that is possible in the circumstances, to respect his or her autonomy. 'The caregiver needs an ethical attitude of caring and concern as well as creative imagination so that she or he can see the patient's situation, firstly as the patient would have seen it, had he or she been healthy, i.e. from the perspective of the patient's life story and the project she or he her- or himself has set. Secondly the caregiver must be able to perceive the situation as the patient perceives it in the present and help her or him to find ways to come as close to her or his life plan as possible despite the disease.'

In the preceding chapter Muir Gray warns against generalizing about 'the elderly' or even 'the demented' or 'people with Alzheimer's'. While there is a statistical correlation between increasing age in the elderly and the adverse events that lead to impairment of autonomy, both mental and physical, Muir Gray inveighs against the 'ageist belief' that 'all older people are incompetent' and the resulting paternalism towards the elderly as a class. And he argues that many of the disablements that the elderly are afflicted with are the result of the behaviour of younger people, whether individuals including 'care professionals' in contact with them, or by social actions, attitudes and policies. Moreover, he argues, recognition that this is the case leads to guilt, and guilt leads to resentment, and resentment to inadequate care on the one hand and paternalistic incarceration on the other. (He adds an interesting speculation on why the elderly have been and perhaps still are so often cast into the role of witch.)

Among the measures to improve care of the elderly, including the prevention of unwarranted paternalism, discussed by Muir Gray are an awareness by caring professionals that they can become just as 'institutionalized' as their patients, and the introduction of volunteers to act as advocates for the elderly, especially for those whose competence is diminished by Alzheimer's disease and who have no relatives. And just as Graham is keen to redistribute resources towards care of children, Muir Gray is keen to remove the prevalent poverty of old age. One approach, he suggests, would be to halve the salary of every public servant and reallocate the savings 'to another group who benefit[ed] from the public purse, namely old age pensioners dependent upon state support'.

AN UNRELATED TRIO: INFERTILITY, MEDICAL EDUCATION AND MEDICAL PUBLISHING

Three of the contributions to this section on moral issues arising in particular health care contexts do not pursue the scope of application themes discussed above. The Snowdens, both sociologists, discuss ethical problems arising in the context of infertility. In a wide-ranging survey (which could also be profitably read in the context of gynaecologist Braude (Chapter 84) in the section on scientific advances) they defend 'planned and purposeful' disclosure of their origins to children born as a result of donor insemination. Among their various arguments the main one seems to be that it 'is extremely difficult to keep secrets secure for a lifetime and children who learn accidentally of their origins are much more likely to be damaged by such a revelation than are children who are told purposively'.

In their chapter on medical ethics education Hope and Fulford argue for medical ethics to be taught throughout the clinical training of medical students, and to be taught as a 'practice skill' alongside and integrated with the teaching of medical law and communication skills. Their underlying theme is that for good ethical judgements to be made in clinical practice—the objective of medical ethics teaching in medical schools—not only must the medical student or doctor be able to think clearly about the ethical issues involved; he or she must also have a working knowledge of the relevant legal background within which the decision must be made; and be able to understand the relevant experiences of the affected people, primarily the patient but also relatives and members of the health care team.

Finally, in this section, Nylenna and Riis address ethical issues that arise in the context of medical publishing. Among their many concerns, as they address the perspectives of authors, editors, referees, publishers and owners, readers, research subjects and society as a whole, are fraud and excessive publishing. The latter, which has led to the scientific publications mountain, needs serious attention at all levels, the authors argue. This includes the scientific academic establishment as a whole, which by giving weight to *numbers* of publications when appointing and promoting scientists, encourages many of the undesirable practices currently afflicting medical publishing. Among the possible remedial actions they consider are limits on the number of publications that are eligible for consideration in appointments and promotions procedures and (less seriously?) even a limit on the total number of papers that any scientist should be allowed to publish during his or her lifetime! In general the authors urge that the activity—one might say the industry—of medical publishing needs to catch up with the contemporary 'ethical awakening' that has affected the rest of medicine.

47

Abortion and Health Care Ethics I: A Critical Analysis of the Main Arguments

MAURIZIO MORI

Via XI Febbraio 25, 26100, Cremona, Italy

Before the 1960s abortion was illegal in most western countries and its immorality was undisputed. In the span of a few years the situation changed drastically: people asked for a more liberal legislation and the moral prohibition was challenged. The request for a liberal legislation was successful and abortion is nowadays legal in most western countries. However, on the moral issue there is a lively controversy, and it is not even clear what is the root of disagreement. Without taking any stand on the morality of abortion as such, I will attempt to clarify the arguments advanced for the main positions.

THE 'CURRENT VIEW' (CV)

Current ethical debate on abortion began in the late 1960s when some important books and papers were published on the subject (for example, refs 1–4). They framed the subsequent debate, establishing what I call 'the current view' (CV). According to the CV, in order to decide the morality of abortion it is necessary to answer the 'fetus question', i.e. to take a stand on when human life begins or on whether the fetus is or is not a human being, where 'fetus' here indicates the process from fertilization to birth, and 'human life' and 'human being' are equivalent to 'person'. Those who give a *positive* answer are 'anti-abortionists', because they say that the fetus is a person and abortion a kind of homicide which ought to be prohibited. Anti-abortionists disagree on whether or not abortion is morally right in 'tragic situations' (when a woman's life is at stake or in case of pregnancy after rape), distinguishing between two different positions: (1) forbids abortion absolutely; and (2) allows abortion only in tragic situations. Tragic situations being nowadays relatively rare, (1) and (2) are *practically* equivalent. Those who give a *negative* answer to the fetus question

Principles of Health Care Ethics. Edited by Raanan Gillon.
© 1994 John Wiley & Sons Ltd

are 'abortionists', because—even if they would rather abortion did not occur—they usually permit it in many circumstances. Abortionists disagree on the limits within which abortion can be permitted, distinguishing between two positions: (3) allows abortion only for 'social reasons', or to protect women's 'health' in the broad sense, including psychological factors; and (4) allows abortion always, i.e. on women's demand. As it is difficult to control these matters socially, often (3) and (4) are *practically* equivalent. However, these positions are conceptually different, as shown by Figure 47.1, representing the logical frame of the abortion debate according to the CV.

The CV is strongly supported by anti-abortionists, who emphasize that abortion is a kind of homicide and its prohibition a matter of basic equality among human beings. Abortionists tend either to avoid the fetus question, stressing other aspects such as back-street abortion, or to reject it openly, remarking that in the modern world law and morality are separated, so that it is possible to give a positive answer to the fetus question and also to permit abortion legally, or that the fetus question is relevant only within a theological debate on infant baptism and ensoulment. Anti-abortionists admit that sometimes unwanted pregnancies raise difficult problems, but think that the fetus's right to life takes precedence over women's autonomy or social indications. They recognize also that law and morality are different, but they observe that the law cannot be so grossly immoral as to discriminate between human beings. Finally, they say that the fetus question is not limited to the theological problem of ensoulment (or animation) because the problem of ensoulment itself is *equivalent* to the problem of when a person comes into being, a problem which is crucial for any just society.

Anti-abortionists seem right in saying that the law cannot be morally repugnant, and also their claim concerning the centrality of the fetus question must be carefully considered. Given the former equivalence it is important to remember that in the theological debate there is a person only after ensoulment, and that 'ensoulment' indicates the act by which God directly infuses the 'rational soul' into the human body, adequately formed. According to the 'mediate animation theory' (typical of the Aristotelian–Thomistic view) this can occur only some time after fertilization, when the body is already animated by a vegetative and a sensitive soul. The idea that the rational soul is infused directly by God may be interpreted as indicating that persons are *qualitatively* different from the rest of organic nature: even if rooted in nature, persons are

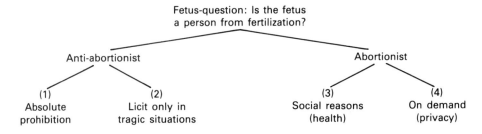

FIGURE 47.1 Frame of the abortion debate according to the CV.

'non-natural objects', objects which 'transcend' organic matter or are 'emergent' from it. For this reason the study of 'persons' is not merely 'scientific' but it pertains to philosophy. This non-naturalistic conception of the person is deeply entrenched in western culture. Even if it is possible to criticize it, I do not consider this possibility, both because anti-abortionists strongly defend it, and because such a criticism implies a deep revision of the whole western world-view.*

The CV has two parts: the *conceptual* one claims that the answer to the fetus question is a necessary condition for stating the morality of abortion; and the *historical* one claims that the fetus question has always been at the centre of the issue.† The historical claim is interesting because it seems to provide a strong support for anti-abortionism, and for this reason I will examine it first.

THE HISTORICAL PART OF THE CV

Standard historical analyses of the moral debate on abortion are devoted to showing that, up to the 1970s, abortion's prohibition had been 'an almost absolute value in history'. Abortion and infanticide were permitted in the pagan Graco-Roman world because the fetus was considered as being part of a woman, and the father was free to dispose of his offspring. Opposing this view, early Christianity proclaimed the absolute prohibition of abortion, which was undisputed up to the 1450s. Arguing on the basis of the limited knowledge of Aristotelian biology, from the 1450s to 1750s some casuists permitted abortion in some cases, thinking that 'the subhuman character of the unensouled fetus authorized man to prefer other values to its existence' (ref. 5, p. 29). Such a tendency was promptly condemned by papal authority, but a much stronger opposition came from a new doctrine of 'immediate ensoulment', i.e. the theory according to which the rational soul is infused immediately at fertilization. Such a theory began in the seventeenth century, and slowly matured to have 'an ultimate significance for the view of abortion' (ref. 5, p. 34). Early diffusion of the new theory was facilitated by a movement of liturgical devotion to the Immaculate Conception, but decisive support came from the advancement of biology. Leaving aside minor disagreements, this historical scheme is widely accepted so that the general idea conveyed is that after the casuistic pause, the reaffirmation of the absolute prohibition depends on the new biological knowledge which supports immediate animation. In this sense, holders of mediate animation are portrayed as either endowed with a poor biology or engaged in futile and tricky 'cosmetic semantics'.‡ For this reason the historical part of the CV favours anti-abortionism.

---

* This 'non-naturalistic' conception of the person is compatible both with the view that the qualitative difference depends on the presence of a soul conceived as a spiritual substance different from matter, and the view that the difference depends on the fact that psychological phenomena are 'emergent' from, and irreducible to, organic matter (even though not a different substance).
† As Noonan (5) says, 'the most fundamental question involved in the long history of thought on abortion is: How do you determine the humanity of a being?' (p. 51).
‡ See Iglesias (6); other authors who seem to accept, at least in general, this historical view, include G. Grisez (2). However, Dunstan (7) claims that the Catholic tradition took a radical turn only in 1869, while Noonan and others think this change began earlier.

Being unable to examine the historical scheme in full here, I will at least consider the three major steps which are supposed to show the steady ascension of immediate animation since the 1750s: the statement of the dogma of the Immaculate Conception in 1854; Pius IX's Constitution *Apostolicae Sedis* in 1869; and the great advancement in biological knowledge of recent centuries.

The Dogma of the Immaculate Conception

This affirms that Mary was conceived free from sin 'in the first instant of her conception'. Since the feast of the Immaculate Conception is on 8 December and Mary's nativity on 8 September (exactly nine months later), it is claimed that the statement of the dogma presupposes the immediate animation theory. Noonan says that 'the new dogma dealt the old formula [of mediate animation] a glancing if not a fatal blow' (ref. 5, p. 38). However, those who think that the dogma supports immediate animation are probably misled by the language of the dogmatic definition: in English, as in most modern languages, the word 'conception' is equivalent to 'fertilization', but in the Latin theological language *conceptio* (conception) is a technical term with a different meaning. We have to distinguish between (1) *conceptio activa* (active conception), indicating the generative act of the parents (the sexual act), and (2) *conceptio passiva* (passive conception), indicating the effect of the sexual act. At this point again: (2a) *conceptio passiva inchoata* (incompleted), occurring before the infusion of the rational soul, and (2b) *conceptio passiva consummata* (completed), occurring in the same instant in which the fetus is ensouled.* Since 'each word of the definition'—as it appears from the preparatory works—'was accurately thought and pondered' (9), the correct conclusion is that it is the *person* of Mary that is privileged by the Immaculate Conception 'in the first instant of her passive completed conception, or in the same instant in which the fetus is animated by rational soul. About the true instant in which the soul is infused in the body ... in the definition nothing is said or hinted, and this intentionally' (ref. 8, p. 20).

To explain why the Church celebrates the feast on 8 December it is necessary to look at the history of liturgy, where we discover that the feast probably began in the East in the eighth century, so that it existed 'before one was clearly aware of any theological implications at all'.† Since in Latin theological language *conceptio* is still a technical term, the statement of the Congregration for the

---

* These distinctions are clearly presented in Roschini (8). It is interesting to note that the distinction between *conceptio activa* and *passiva* goes back to P. Lambertini (who was to become pope Benedictus XIV), for whom *conceptio passiva* indicated only rational ensoulment, or the *conceptio hominis*, and disregarded the *conceptio carnis*, as it is sometimes called. Furthermore, this distinction is mentioned by the General Procurator of the Dominican order, F. Gaude, *Sullo immacolato concepimento della madre di Dio e sulla dogmatica sua definizione in rapporto specialmente alla scuola tomistica ed all'istituto dei PP. Predicatori*, Cumbo, Malta, 1855, in particular pp. 110 ff.

† See Bowman (10), p. 113. Other interesting remarks can be found in Messenger (11), where Canon De Dorlot remembers that the object of the *cultus* was defined in 1661 (when mediate animation was dominant) by Alexander VII, whose words show that 'it is not the *historical* fact that is commemorated, but [that] the feast is *in honour* of the Conception of the Virgin' (p. 324).

Faith that 'human life must be absolutely respected and protected from the moment of conception' (12) must be carefully interpreted.

Pius IX's Constitution 'Apostolicae Sedis'

This states that 'those who procure abortion, when the effect occurs' are excommunicated *latae sententiae*, dropping the traditional distinction between ensouled and unensouled fetus. Noonan (5) observes that 'an implicit acceptance of immediate ensoulment was found in the action' (p. 13), Dunstan remarks that former moral tradition 'was repudiated by Pope Pius IX in 1869' (13), and Sutton says that the dropping of the traditional distinction 'was a reflection of the progress of embryology' (14). So this change in canonic law is considered a decisive turning point which led Catholic theology to immediate animation. Considering the great importance attributed to it, it is a bit surprising to discover that in Pius's Constitution abortion is one of about 40 cases deserving excommunication *latae sententiae*. The Constitution's aim was not to regulate abortion, but to bring order in the canonical rulings concerning this kind of excommunication, rulings which were different from diocese to diocese: it individuates clearly the specific cases deserving such a penalty, and lists them according to the authority to which the excommunicated had to apply for absolution: the Pope, the Bishop, etc. Abortion was just one of the three cases reserved for the Bishop.* Once set in its proper historical context it is clear that this change in canonic law is irrelevant to the philosophical issue concerning animation. This is confirmed *historically* by major contemporary commentaries of the Constitution: they devote only scattered remarks to abortion, and only in passing mention the dropping of the traditional distinction, a fact which shows how little theoretical significance was attributed to it.† Except in a peculiarly long commentary, in which an anonymous author remarks that even if the traditional distinction was abandoned for excommunication, it was not abandoned for other canonical penalties: 'since the Constitution did not introduce any change concerning irregularity and other sanctions established in the former legislation, this distinction [concerning the ensouled/unensouled fetus] is still valid for these penalties; somebody will incur them only when such a crime is accomplished on an ensouled fetus'.‡ Moreover, contrary to what Dunstan seems to think, Pius IX himself supported mediate animation theory, as is clear from a letter that he sent to the President of the Medico-philosophical Academy of St Thomas Aquinas, in which he explicitly approved the Thomistic position

---

* The other two cases are that concerning priests who married without being authorized, and that concerning those who intentionally falsify Apostolic letters or cooperate in such a practice. Moreover, it must be observed that in general most of the Constitution's attention was devoted to free-thinkers and to masonry.

† Other problems widely examined were the two following ones: first that concerning how to decide when the effect actually occurred, since the law required it; and secondly the problem concerning who were to be considered 'cooperators', and mainly whether or not the woman who aborted was to be subjected to excommunication. This problem was widely discussed, and raised the so-called *quaestio elegans*.

‡ See Anon (16). It is also interesting to observe that this Commentary (pp. 307–332) criticizes the other anonymous author quoted by Noonan in support of his thesis (see below).

held by G. M. Cornoldi SJ concerning the soul's and body's union, a position vigorously defended also by other thomists such as M. Liberatore SJ (15). Also *conceptually* there is no argument showing that such a change in canonic law presupposes a change at a philosophical level: in favour of this alleged change Noonan (5) quotes an anonymous author saying that otherwise the law would be 'more onerous, which is contrary to the intent of the Constitution' (p. 39). But by doing so Noonan does not prove that the anonymous author is right, he simply assumes it. However, there might have been other good reasons justifying the new penalty, such as a willingness to repress abortion when the possibility of performing it was becoming wider, and the anonymous author might have been wrong. Noonan does not even consider this possibility because— *presupposing* that the ensoulment question has always been (either explicitly or implicitly) at the centre of the long history of the abortion debate—he states a sort of *logical* connection between the quantity of penalty and the kind of crime (homicide or not). However, this connection is not logical, as Noonan presupposes, but *social*, because when a legislator establishes a penalty he has to consider many factors, such as common estimation of the act, the expected influence of the punishment, the possibility of scandal, etc. Therefore, from a change of penalty one cannot directly infer anything about the kind of crime.

As counter-proof of the fact that the change of the canonic rule did not affect the philosophical position of the Catholic Church on ensoulment, the Holy See in 1884 condemned Rosmini's immediate animation theory, and in 1917 issued the 24 Thomistic propositions, some of which clearly support mediate animation.* These acts would have been logically inconsistent if the Holy See had implicitly accepted the immediate animation theory.

The Progress of Biological Knowledge

This is supposed to be the most important factor for the reaffirmation of the absolute prohibition after the casuistic pause. Noonan (5) remarks that as early as the eighteenth century 'medical opinion had rejected' the Aristotelian biology and its theory of mediate ensoulment; in the nineteenth century also 'educated European opinion' in general refused it; and in the present century almost everyone did, even if 'vigorous champions of the old theory could still be found. The most influential was Arthur Vermeersch' (p. 39). The basic idea of this

---

* Antonio Rosmini (1797–1855) was an Italian theologian and philosopher who tried to synthesize some tenets of Kantian philosophy with Catholicism, and in his general philosophical–theological system also defended immediate animation. In 1884, in the Decree *Post Obitum*, the Holy See condemned 40 of his propositions, and four of them concern immediate animation theory. For an interesting analysis of Rosmini's position of immediate animation, cf. A. Luciani (17). Luciani was to become Pope John Paul I, and this work can be read in his *Opera Omnia*, vol. I. Unfortunately this edition does not include the text of the first edition (1950) of the book, which is quite different from the second edition. In general I can remark that in 1958 Albino Luciani still rejected the immediate animation theory and vigorously defended the mediate animation theory.

For the 24 Thomistic propositions, cf. E. Messenger (11), and in particular E. Hugon (18). Noonan seems to understate these issues because he assumes that the reaffirmation of the absolute prohibition of abortion after the casuistic pause was not just a mere repetition of past arguments, but 'a development' of a new doctrine.

argument is that mediate animation depends on poor scientific knowledge, and that the few authors (such as Vermeersch) who defend it are simply ignorant in matters relating to biology: as Iglesias says: 'in the light of our present biological information, we cannot avoid concluding that Aquinas today would have considered the human embryo from conception a *homo*, . . . a human person' (Iglesias (6), p. 109).

This view of a progressive ascension to the truth is appealing, but misleading for our issue: it is true that in the eighteenth century 'medical opinion' rejected the Aristotelian biology, but this happened because—trusting those who claimed to have seen 'exceedingly minute forms of men, with arms, heads and legs complete, inside the spermatozoa under the microscope' (19)—biologists accepted 'preformism' with its idea of a *homunculus* hidden in the gametes. Now we know that preformism is wrong, and that biological development is not just growth in size of what is already there, but is 'epigenesis', i.e. emergence of new characteristics. Again, it may be true that in the nineteenth century 'educated European opinion' in general rejected mediate animation, but this happened because positivism banished all 'philosophical' problems, saying that scientists must only describe reality. Since the fetus question is a *philosophical* one, positive scientists' 'authority' as such is not decisive. On the other hand most of those who examined the problem *philosophically* defended mediate animation, as confirmed by the many debates on evolution theory.* As for the first half of the present century, we have still many positivists saying that biologists should only look *at* embryos, but also a lively philosophical discussion, stimulated by the many biological discoveries which, by the 1930s, led to a fairly good understanding of the reproductive process.† If we look at *these* discussions, surprisingly enough, we realize that the majority of those who wrote specifically on the problem of ensoulment agreed that 'modern science has resuscitated the old theory of successive animation of the human embryo'.‡ Authors such as Vermeersch were not so few in number, and included many authors well-read in biology and providing sound arguments. The fact that many *moralists*, in their general manuals, accepted immediate animation can be easily explained—noting that it is much easier to show the gravity of abortion if it is described as a kind of homicide.

---

* It is interesting to remember that the issue of animation at the time was mainly discussed not in relation to abortion (which was in any case prohibited) but in relation to the problem of evolution theory and the origin of man, or the transmission of original sin, and other problems. For a good survey of the discussion, cf. Liberatore (20) and Farges (21).

† For a fairly good clear presentation of the state of the art in the 1930s, see J. Rostand (22). Leaving aside some minor questions such as the number of chromosomes (thought to be 48 instead of 46), this book shows that in the 1930s the basic mechanism of reproduction was already understood.

‡ See Zalba (23), p. 92. Among other authors holding a similar position I can mention here only the following: Lanza (24), p. 303 (which is certainly the most thorough analysis of the problem that I know of); in English the most relevant book is Messenger (11). Other authors include Hugon (25), Sertillanges (26), Gedda (27), Josia (28), Hering (29) and Hudeczek (30). I could list many others, but for further information a good, neutral survey of the discussion can be found in Gentili (31).

Conclusion

The historical part of the CV, with its idea of a steady ascension to immediate animation, is grounded in poor historical analysis. Anti-abortionism can still have strong arguments in its favour, and I will now examine the three major arguments which constitute the conceptual part of the CV.

THE CONCEPTUAL PART OF THE CV

As already mentioned, progress in scientific knowledge is supposed to be the most important argument for immediate animation. Usually anti-abortionists do not specify which piece of knowledge is crucial for their thesis, but sometimes they say that it is the DNA discovery of 1953, which provides decisive evidence that 'whatever powers we have now . . . [they] are a *manifestation* or a *development* of the powers we had from the beginning' (Iglesias (6), p. 79): the fetus is a person because from fertilization it is endowed with the genetic information of the person. This idea is intuitively appealing because at fertilization two 'things' (sperm and ovum) fuse together and give origin to a new 'thing' (the fetus), which often grows up to become a person. However, such an idea is misleading because persons are not mere 'things', but are peculiar 'non-natural objects', and this fact compels us to change our commonsense view: first, if it were true that the whole person was already in the genetic code, then—since the DNA formed at fertilization is a string of *material* molecules—we would have to conclude that persons are mere 'natural objects', which is inconsistent with our premise concerning persons. Secondly, if it were true that the whole person was already in the genetic code, then we would have to espouse a version of pre-formism in which the *homunculus* is hidden not in gametes but in the genetic combination formed at fertilization.*

Pre-formism seems acceptable because it is simpler than epigenesis, but such a simplicity is deceptive: 'although the instructions of the developmental processes are "pre-formed" in the genes, in the same sense as the instructions for a computer are in the perforations of the computer tape, the development of the embryo is epigenesis, formation of a new body which was not present earlier as an individual' (33). In brief, scientific knowledge of DNA does not support immediate animation. Moreover, if we hold an adequate epigenetic view of biological development, it is easy to defend the mediate animation theory, saying that in embryological development there is a change of different *levels* of existence: first a vegetative life, then a sensitive one, and finally the rational life (as in the Aristotelian tradition). Since a formed and functioning brain is a necessary condition for rationality, if there is no brain there is not even the *capacity* for rationality, and therefore up to then the fetus certainly is

---

* The idea that many contemporary anti-abortionists presuppose a sort of new version of pre-formism is clear in cases such as that of Angelo Serra SJ, when he writes that 'already from the first moment . . . are contemporarily present and are developing the central structures which will appear at a certain point as the primitive streak. At any point of development there already exists the unity which later will be defined as the fetal–placental unity', in Serra *et al.* (32). T. Iglesias, in the passage that I have quoted, also seems to presuppose a sort of process/product fallacy.

not a person. It is difficult to state exactly *when* rational life begins, but this is a different problem which cannot be examined here.

At this point one may wonder why so many people accept the idea that biological knowledge supports immediate animation, and in order to explain this fact we have to look back in history. Part of the answer depends on the cultural background underlying the fetus question in the early 1970s, when it was formulated in terms of 'When does human life begin?'. This question appeared meaningful also because at the time Haeckel's 'recapitulation theory', according to which each human individual in its embryological development passes through the stages of the evolutionary process (first a plant, a fish, a mammal, etc.) so that 'ontogenesis recapitulates phylogenesis', was still influential. This theory was taken as a 'scientific truth', and even if vigorously criticized since the 1930s, its influence was so profound that as late as 1952, in the great *Enciclopedia Medica Italiana*, it was stated that in the second period of its development (after the third week) 'the embryo ... does not present the characteristics which are proper to the *human species*', and only later can it be considered 'as belonging to the *human species*'.* Data on DNA then appeared decisive for the fetus question, because this clearly showed the falsity of Haeckel's theory: 'from the time of fecundation there is no genetic change. *But without genetic change there can be no change of species*'.† However, Haeckel's theory was also sometimes interpreted as 'scientific' evidence for the mediate animation theory, and therefore the falsity of the former was taken as a sign of the falsity of the latter. Yet this inference is invalid: even if in the embryological process there is no change analogous to the change of species, there can be another significant kind of change such as a change of *levels* of existence. In the 1970s this possibility was not immediately perceived, and so the idea that biological knowledge supports immediate animation gained consensus, this process being facilitated by various factors such as an uncritical acceptance of the 'authority' of some scientists, an attitude inclined to refuse the 'old subtleties' of traditional philosophy, an urge for a vivid platform against abortion, etc. However, scientific knowledge does not support the immediate animation theory.

Just a few words on the second argument advanced by anti-abortionists, who say that from fertilization the fetus deserves protection because it is a *potential* person. If 'potentiality' is used in its proper meaning the argument's invalidity becomes manifest: in the Aristotelian view *potentiality* is the mirror-image of the *teleology* intrinsic to reality: each thing tends to its specific goal and, before reaching it, it has the *potentiality* of doing so. Therefore, to say that an X is a potential Y is equivalent to saying that X is not Y, even if it has an intrinsic capacity to become Y in future. If we say that the fetus is a potential person,

---

* See Andreassi (34). For criticism of Haeckel's theory, cf. De Beer (35). Rostand's remarks (22) on this topic are also interesting.

† See Miller (36), p. 76. This problem is also mentioned in the influential paper by A. Bompiani (37). Moreover, the Italian biologist Giuseppina Pastori, a pupil of Father Agostino Gemelli, the founder of the Catholic University in Italy, in the early 1970s observed that not many years before 'in a climate of Darwinistic enthusiasm it was common to say that the human embryo passed through the stages of little fish, of little bird, of mammal, in order to comply with the thesis that ontogenesis recapitulates phylogenesis' (38).

we *implicitly* admit that the fetus is not a person, even if it has an intrinsic capacity to become a person. This was Vermeersch's point: how can you properly speak of 'homicide' if the fetus is not a person? We can still claim that we ought to protect potential persons, but this alleged new duty on the one hand is different from the duty to protect actual persons, and on the other hand it would also protect gametes already located in a woman's body, because like the fetus they also are potential persons (at an earlier stage). Certainly we do not know which gametes will become a person, but this is an epistemological problem, and does not affect gametes' potentiality to become persons.*

The last argument concerns mainly Catholic theology. Even if many Catholics defend the CV, the Catholic magisterium forbids abortion *absolutely* and without taking any stand on the fetus question.† So it is unclear which argument justifies such a prohibition, and some think it is the following: in Catholic moral tradition there is a distinction between 'doubts of norm' (*dubium juris*), about whether or not there is a norm prescribing a certain action, and 'doubt of fact' (*dubium facti*), about whether or not one's situation is that regulated by the norm. To explain this distinction the following example is usually presented: if Titius, a hunter, sees something moving beyond a bush and does not know whether it is a rabbit or a man, he faces a *dubium facti*, because he knows that there is a norm prescribing not to kill people, but he doubts whether or not it applies to his specific situation. In the case of *dubium facti* the Catholic tradition obliges us to take the safer option, and Titius ought not to shoot. If he does, he is in any case *guilty* of homicide, because by shooting he shows that he was, in his heart, ready to kill a man (even if actually he killed a rabbit). Analogously in the case of abortion: it is dubious whether or not the fetus is a person, and facing a *dubium facti* we ought to treat the fetus *as* a person.‡ The first objection to this argument is that when the fetus has not even the *capacity* for rationality, there is no doubt that it is not a person. Moreover, the argument shifts from the objective level about the *act's rightness* to the subjective level about the *agent's guilt*: if beyond the bush there is a rabbit, Titius' *act* is *not* a homicide, but Titius is *guilty* of homicide (at least in the sight of God) but if he shoots at a plastic target desiring to kill a man, because in his heart he is ready to kill a man. This shift shows that the rabbit example is inadequate, because it presents a situation in which it is *easy* for Titius to abstain from acting: what if, instead of a rabbit, beyond the bush there might be an armed enemy? In this case Titius ought not to grant the benefit of the doubt to the moving object and refrain from shooting. In the case of *dubium facti* it is not always one's duty to take the safer option, because otherwise we ought never to drive over 20 km/h,

---

* Some think that fertilization constitutes a radical difference because they assume that, before fertilization, sperm and ovum are merely *parts of the bodies of the man and woman respectively*. This description is misleading, because gametes are not mere body-part cells; they have a special intrinsic teleology and are directed to generate new individuals, even if, as a matter of fact, statistically, most of them die.

† Declaratio De Abortu (1974), note 19, where explicitly The Sacred Congregation of the Faith states: 'This declaration expressly leaves aside the question of the moment when the spiritual soul is infused .... It is a philosophical problem from which our moral affirmation remains independent'.

‡ Congregation for the Doctrine of the Faith, Instruction *Donum Vitae*, I, 1.

being always likely to kill somebody.* This shows that the rabbit example conceals a further premise, i.e. the idea that sexual activity (like hunting rabbits) is something unnecessary and superfluous, something that persons can easily do without. But then, abortion's prohibition does not depend on the *dubium facti* situation, but on the idea that life's transmission has special rules to be respected.

There is no sound argument showing that from fertilization the fetus is a person. If the CV were adequate, anti-abortionism would have to be rejected. But our historical analysis and the official position of the Catholic Church show that the answer to the fetus question is not at all a necessary condition for the morality of abortion, and therefore we can reject the CV itself. The whole debate on abortion must be re-framed.

A MORE SOLID BASIS FOR THE DEBATE ON ABORTION

Holders of the CV claim that if the fetus is not a person, then there is no duty towards it. However, this idea is wrong because we have duties not only towards persons, but also towards other things. In this sense our central problem now is to know *whether* or not there is a duty to the fetus and *why* there is or is not such a duty. On this issue the real distinction is not between utilitarians and deontologists, as many may think, but between two different more general views that I would like at least to outline.

The Absolute Duty View

According to this view there is a duty to the fetus, and it prohibits abortion *absolutely*, i.e. without any exception at all, even in tragic situations. This implies that this duty is different from, and does not depend on, the duty not to kill, because this last duty admits exceptions, at least in self-defence.† Therefore, abortion's prohibition depends on a more general duty prescribing not to interfere with the intrinsic teleology of the reproductive process. This duty forbids not only abortion, but also contraception, voluntary sterilization, artificial insemination, homosexuality, etc. The basic idea implicit in this view is that reproductive powers are primarily devoted to transmitting life, and any interference with the process is absolutely illicit. Given that the process of life's transmission is continuous, the only acceptable dividing point is the free act by which persons decide to activate their reproductive powers: persons are free to decide whether or not to activate sexual powers, but, if they do, they ought not to interfere with reproductive intrinsic finalism and let nature (with its potentiality) have its course. Probably the only reason which can justify such an *absolute* duty is the idea that biological teleology reveals a natural or a divine

---

* For a development of this criticism cf. Mori (39, 40). For a different kind of criticism of the argument see the enlightening paper by C. A. Tauer (41).
† It is not even 'don't kill the innocent', because sometimes even this duty admits exceptions: because of his insanity a mad-man trying to kill me is innocent, but nevertheless I am allowed to kill him in self-defence. On this point see Messenger (11), pp. 301–312; also Bender (42).

design. However, the problem of justifying an absolute duty is quite different from the problem raised by the fact that, according to this view, the absolute duty is violated by any interference with biological finalism. In this sense both abortion and contraception are acts 'which offend God's design about the transmission of life'.* Even if conceptually these acts are of the same kind, the quantity of penalty attached to singular crimes may of course be different, for the reasons previously mentioned.

The Non-absolute View

This view includes both various kinds of utilitarians and *prima facie* deontologists; even if differing on other significant points these ethical perspectives converge in saying that one's main duty is to minimize suffering, because when two *prima facie* duties conflict the 'reasonable' solution is the minor evil. This means that both *prima facie* deontologism and utilitarianism agree that morality (like language and other man-created institutions) is a social enterprise aimed at satisfying the wants and needs of sentient beings. On the contrary, in the absolute view, morality is not at all a social creation, because the absolute duty is independent of human will and does not vary according to circumstances in order to meet wants and needs, but these ought to be regulated according to the requirement of the absolute duty. For further information on this distinction see Mori (44). To admit just one exception to the absolute duty is not just to soften the view in order to avoid extreme tragic situations, but to abandon it completely, and change the whole conception of morality itself: it is to produce a sort of *Gestalt shift* in morality and change the point of view. If we do so, we must be ready to re-describe the whole situation on the basis of the new viewpoint, and in our case this implies a re-description of the reproductive process as such: if we abandon the absolute duty, sexual organs are not any more primarily devoted to the transmission of life, but they become organs like others, organs whose function is to serve the individual's well-being. This is the profound intuition underlying Thomson's celebrated violinist's example: a woman does not violate a violinist's right to life if she unplugs the connection established during the night without her consent, between hers and a violinist's liver, even if the act causes the violinist's death. Analogously a woman does not violate a fetus's right to life if she disconnects the link between her body and an unwanted fetus. The counter-intuitive aspect of this example depends on the fact that we continue to assume that sexual organs have a peculiar

---

* See Montini (43). Cardinal Montini was to become Pope Paul VI a few years later. In this sense our former remark about the meaning of *conceptio* may be relevant. Moreover, at the end of his long and detailed analysis, A. Lanza writes the following: 'The evaluation of the crime of abortion must be different, both morally and legally, before and after the infusion of rational soul: after animation it is a real violation of the person's right to life; before animation, however, one cannot speak of such a violation, because there is no rational soul. However, it is a violence which is *always illicit*, inflicted to the order established by nature, a violence that from a moral point of view can be reduced to the same level of anticonceptional practices and can be considered as a crime against the family' (Lanza (24), p. 297). Finally, in the index of the papal teaching on 'matrimony', abortion and contraception were classified as crimes of the same kind; this at least before the sexual revolution of the 1970s.

function which makes them radically different from the liver. But if we abandon the absolute view, and look at things from the new viewpoint, we will realize that Thomson's analogy is sound, and that contrary to commonsense intuition, if the fetus were a person, abortion would be permitted in most situations, because the duty to continue pregnancy is not a duty of justice, but a duty of beneficence.* Therefore, different positions on abortion have to be represented as shown in Figure 47.2.

Position (1) is the only really anti-abortionist one, because it is the only one forbidding abortion on principle. All the other positions are 'abortionist' in the sense that they do not forbid abortion on principle, even if they may prohibit it for other reasons. In this sense the non-absolute view is complex, and within it we must distinguish between two positions: that in which reproduction is a *social* problem, and that in which it is an *individual* one. In the first case we have a variety of possibilities: (1*) is extensionally equivalent to (1) because both forbid abortion *always*, even if for completely different reasons. In (1) abortion's prohibition depends on the absolute *principle*, while in (1*) it depends on *empirical* considerations, for example the fact that in the given historical circumstances abortion always leads to disastrous social consequences. Position (2) is the one which allows abortion only in tragic situations, and Figure 47.2 makes it clear that (2) is not just a softer version of (1), but a different kind of position: in (1*), as in (2), prohibitions and exceptions are justified by empirical considerations, such as the fact that in such historical circumstances a given exception minimizes suffering. Position (3) is the one which allows abortion also for 'social indications', including psychological and economic factors, and it is now clear that (3) is just an extension of (2): once an exception is admitted it is possible to widen its field according to circumstances' requirements. Position (4*) is extensionally equivalent to (4), because both permit abortion *always*, even if for different reasons: (4*) presupposes that reproduction is a social problem, and

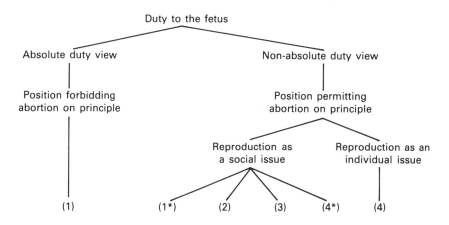

FIGURE 47.2 Adequate frame for a debate on the morality of the abortion.

---

* See Thomson (45). For further analysis on this implicit assumption of the Thomson argument see Mori (46), also see Mori (47).

permission is justified by *empirical* considerations: for example in circumstances in which a private 'contragestative' such as RU 486 would be easily available, any social limit to abortion may be found too onerous. Finally, position (4) justifies permission *on principle*, because here reproduction is a 'private affair' and abortion a woman's 'right'.

In position (1) there is no room for a woman's (or a couple's) autonomy, because its exercise is limited to the free act by which the person decides to activate his/her reproductive capacities. Once the reproductive process has started, the absolute duty forbids any interference with it, and therefore also abortion. This position is nowadays counter-intuitive, and even many Catholics charge it with so-called 'biologism', i.e. a naive assumption of biological teleology as a moral rule. I do not think that this criticism can be justified, because the absolute duty view is internally coherent: assuming that the reproductive process has a special intrinsic teleology (which is an 'empirical' statement), one can claim that there is an absolute duty not to interfere with it in any circumstances. It may be difficult to justify such an absolute duty, but on the one hand this is a different problem (as we have already pointed out), and on the other hand one can say that such a duty depends on the respect due to natural or divine design (known by reason), or on empirical considerations showing that only when people are educated to such a respect can we have socially responsible people. Even if, particularly in tragic situations, the absolute duty seems to disregard people's well-being, holders of the absolute view can claim that it allows society to achieve more real and solid well-being in the long run, because it avoids any 'individualism' typical of the non-absolute view. Here I cannot examine the claim that only the absolute view can guarantee the level of education which is required for people living in a just society, but the idea that the non-absolute view is in itself individualistic is certainly misleading. It depends on the presupposition that morality is not a social enterprise, a claim which should be proved and not presupposed. Only (4) is 'individualistic' in some meaningful sense, because in (4) women's right to autonomy has on principle precedence over any other consideration, so that abortion is a purely 'private affair': no social considerations can limit women's autonomy. Without examining the problem whether or not individualism is acceptable (and why), those who consider reproduction a social issue avoid any individualistic position, and have many different practical solutions on abortion, according to social wants and needs in different historical circumstances. A change of circumstances such as population number, or the spread of deadly sexually transmitted diseases, etc. may change the balance between autonomy, beneficence and justice. The problem of finding a proper solution is a crucial empirical question requiring interdisciplinary cooperation.

GENERAL CONCLUSIONS

I have shown that the CV is untenable both conceptually and historically: far from going along with the traditional views of the matter, we should realize that 'the current debate departs notably from that of the past', because in the past 'the time of animation was never looked on as a moral dividing line between permissible and immoral abortion' (47). Since it is false to say that Catholic reaffirmation of the absolute prohibition after the (alleged) casuistic pause depends on the immediate animation theory (as holders of the CV claim), it may turn out that the CV itself is just a short parenthesis in the long history of the morality of abortion, a parenthesis which can be explained historically as a consequence of the 'culture shock' deriving from the challenge of what seemed to be a self-evident axiom of morality. Since there are no sound arguments showing that from fertilization the fetus is a person, the time is ripe to go back to a more traditional debate, and justify our position on abortion either on the basis of the absolute duty or the non-absolute view, according to different circumstances.

REFERENCES

1. Callahan, D. 1970; *Abortion: law, choice and morality.* Macmillan, New York.
2. Grisez, G. 1970. *Abortion: the myths, the realities and the arguments.* Corpus Books, New York.
3. Noonan, J. T. Jr (Ed.). 1970. *The morality of abortion.* Harvard University Press, Cambridge, Mass.
4. Feinberg, J. (Ed.). 1984. *The problem of abortion,* 2nd edn. Wadsworth, Belmont, CA.
5. Noonan, J. T. 1970. An almost absolute value in history. *In* Noonan, J. T. (Ed.) *The morality of abortion.* Harvard University Press, Cambridge, Mass.
6. Iglesias, T. 1990. *IVF and justice,* p. 95. Linacre Centre for Health Care Ethics, London.
7. Dunstan, G. R. 1988. The human embryo in the western moral tradition. Pp. 38–57, *in* Dunstan, G. R. and Seller, M. J. (Eds) *The status of the human embryo.* King Edward's Hospital Fund, London.
8. Roschini, G. 1948. *Summa mariologiae,* vol. II, p. 21. Berdaletti, Rome.
9. Roschini, G. 1969. *Maria Santissima nella storia della salvezza,* vol. III, p. 10., M. Pisani Editori, Isola del Liri.
10. Bowman, C. A. 1958. The Immaculate Conception in Liturgy. Pp. 113–159, *in* O'Connor, E. (Ed.) *The dogma of the Immaculate Conception.* Notre Dame University Press, Notre Dame, Indiana.
11. Messenger, E. C. 1952. *Theology and evolution.* Burnes & Oates, London.
12. Congregation for the doctrine of the faith, *Instruction donum vitae,* 1987, p. 12.
13. Dunstan, G. R. 1990. Introduction: text and context. P. 4, *in* Dunstan, G. R. (Ed.) *The human embryo: Aristotle and the Arabic European traditions.* University of Exeter Press.
14. Sutton, A. 1990. *Prenatal diagnosis: confronting the ethical issues,* p. 91. Linacre Centre for Studies of Ethics of Health Care, London.
15. Cornoldi, G. M. 1878. *La conciliazione della fede cattolica con la vera scienza ossia Accademia filosofico-medica di S. Tommaso d'Aquino,* 2nd edition, Mareggiani, Bologna (in an appendix of this book at pp. 109–111 is published Pius IX's letter dated July 23rd, 1874).
16. Anon. 1879. Commentaire sur la constitution *apostolicae sedis* de Pie IX. *Nouvelle Revue Théologie,* **11**: 331.
17. Luciani, A. 1958. *Il problema dell'infusione dell'anima in A. Rosmini,* 2nd edn. Editrice Gregoriana.
18. Hugon, E. 1921. Les vingt-quatre thèses thomistes. *Revue Thomiste,* pp. 276–301 and 356–384.
19. Needham, J. 1959. *A history of embryology,* p. 205. Cambridge University Press, Cambridge.
20. Liberatore, M. (SJ) 1862. *Del composto umano.* Civiltà Cattolica, Rome, p. 573.
21. Farges, A. 1908. *La vie et l'évolution des especes,* 7th edn. Beche et Tralin, Paris, p. 335.
22. Rostand, J. 1936. *Dal germe al neonato,* translated into Italian by O.F. and revised by Carlo Foá. Hoepli Editore, Milan.

23. Zalba, M. (SJ) 1966. The Catholic Church's viewpoint on abortion. *World Medical Journal*, pp. 88–93.
24. Lanza, A. 1940. *La questione del momento in cui l'anima razionale è infusa nel corpo.* Edizioni Universitarie, Rome.
25. Hugon, E. 1934. *Philosophia naturalis*, vol. II, pp. 508–516. Desclèe, Paris.
26. Sertillanges, A. D. 1947. La creazione dell'anima umana. *Quaderni di Roma*, vol. 1, pp. 301–308. Sansoni editore, Rome.
27. Gedda, L. 1949. La questione dell'infusione dell'anima nei gemelli. Now reprinted in Gedda, L. 1963. *Problemi di frontiera della medicina*, pp. 93–99. Borla, Turin.
28. Josia, C. G. 1951. Infusione dell'anima umana nel feto. *Perfice Munus*, pp. 15–30.
29. Hering, H. M. 1951. De tempore animationis foetus humani. *Angelicum* **28**: 18–29.
30. Hudeczek, M. M. 1952. De tempore animationis foetus humani secundum embryologiam hodiernam. *Angelicum* **29**: 161–181.
31. Gentili, E. 1964. Il momento dell'animazione razionale. Studio sistematico. *La scuola cattolica*, pp. 221–240.
32. Serra, A., Sgreccia, E. and Di Pietro, M. L. 1991. *Manipolazioni genetiche e nuova embriologia*, p. 82. Vita e Pensiero, Milan.
33. Dobzhanski, T. 1969. *The biology of ultimate concern*, p. 29. Rapp & Whiting, London.
34. Andreassi, G. 1952. Entry 'Embriologia umana', *in Enciclopedia Medica Italiana*, col. 1659. Sansoni, Firenze.
35. De Beer, G. 1951. *Embryos and ancestors*, 2nd edn. Oxford University Press, Oxford (1st edn published 1939).
36. Miller, C. E. 1970. Abortion: good science = good morals. *The Homiletic and Pastoral Review* pp. 759–763.
37. Bompiani, A. 1972. Individualità biologica e dignità umana del concepito. *Rivista del clero italiano*, p. 197.
38. Pastori, G. 1972. Intervento, *in* Polli, E. and Bettinelli, C. (Eds.) *L'aborto: diritto o crimine?* p. 150. Ferro Edizioni, Milan.
39. Mori, M. 1988. *La fecondazione artificale: questioni morali nell'esperienza giuridica*, pp. 265–279. Giuffrè, Milan.
40. Mori, M. 1987. Aborto: divieto del V o del VI comandamento? *Prospettive Settanta*, p. 102–144.
41. Tauer, C. A. 1984. The tradition of probabilism and the moral status of the early embryo. *Theological Studies* **45**: 3–33.
42. Bender, L. 1953. Ius in vita. *Angelicum* **30**: 50–62.
43. Montini, Cardinal G. B. 1961. Famiglia cristiana. *Lettera pastorale alla diocesi di Milano.* Reissued by Editrice Sales, Rome, 1965.
44. Mori, M. 1991. 'Etica', *in Grande dizonario enciclopedico*, pp. 276–285. UTET, Turin.
45. Thomson, J. J. 1971. A defence of abortion. *Philosophy and Public Affairs* **1**: 44–66.
46. Mori, M. 1990. Il feto ha il diritto alla vita. Pp. 735–840, *in* Lombardi Vallauri, L. (Ed.) *Il meditevole di tutele.* Giuffrè, Milan.
47. Mori, M. 1990. La bioetica. Pp. 186–224, *in* Viano, C. A. (Ed.) *Teorie etiche contemporanee.* Bollati-Boringhieri, Turin.
48. Connery, J. (SJ) 1977. *Abortion: the development of the Roman Catholic perspective,* pp. 304, 305. Loyola University Press, Loyola.

48

Abortion and Health Care Ethics II

JOHN FINNIS, FBA

Professor of Law and Legal Philosophy, Oxford University; Fellow and Tutor, University College, Oxford

If the unborn are human persons, the principles of justice and non-maleficence (rightly understood) prohibit every abortion; that is, every procedure or technical process carried out with the intention of killing an unborn child or terminating its development. In the first part of this chapter I argue that the only reasonable judgement is that the unborn are indeed human persons. In the second I explore the ways in which the principles of justice and non-maleficence bear on various actions and procedures which harm or may well harm the unborn. The right understanding of those principles, in the context of 'the four principles', is sketched in an earlier chapter, 'Theology and the Four Principles: A Roman Catholic View I' but the considerations which I set out in the present chapter in no way depend on Catholic faith; they are philosophical and natural-scientific considerations valid and, in my view, properly decisive for everyone, quite independently of any religious premises.

MOST PEOPLE BEGIN AT FERTILIZATION

Leaving aside real or supposed divine, angelic and extraterrestrial beings, the one thing common to all who, in common thought and speech, are regarded as *persons* is that they are *living human individuals*. This being so, anyone who claims that some set of living, whole, bodily human individuals are not persons, and ought not to be regarded and treated as persons, must demonstrate that the ordinary notion of a person is misguided and should be replaced by a different notion. Otherwise the claim will be mere arbitrary discrimination. But no such demonstration has ever been provided, and none is in prospect.

Among the most serious attempts to provide a demonstration is Michael Tooley's argument that personhood is gradually acquired by development; it concludes that not only the unborn but also newborn babies are not persons

---

(1). But Tooley's argument begs the question by simply *assuming* two basic but unargued premises: (a) that abortion is morally acceptable, and (b) that an active potentiality or capacity which is not being actually exercised cannot be the defining property of personhood even when it is a capacity really possessed by an individual (2–4).

Some contemporary neo-Aristotelians, notably Joseph Donceel, have argued that personhood is dependent on sense organs and a brain, and that the early embryo, though a living human individual, is only a pre-personal entity which changes into a person (is 'ensouled'), not gradually but by a sudden, substantial change that occurs when the brain first begins to develop; *thereafter*, the personal soul shapes the development of the whole entity (5). (By 'substantial change' is meant the change which occurs when an individual entity of one kind changes into an individual entity of a different kind, as typically occurs, for example, in a chemical reaction.) But Donceel's view, like its mediaeval predecessors, is inconsistent with the biological data and with itself (3,6,7). The beginning of the brain's development does not yet provide a bodily basis for intellectual activities, but provides only the precursor of such a basis; so if this precursor is sufficient for 'ensoulment', there is no reason why earlier precursors should fail to suffice. In fact each embryonic human individual has from the outset a specific developmental tendency (involving a high degree of organization) which includes the epigenetic primordia of all its organs. The hypothesis of a substantial change by ensoulment at some time after the forming of the zygote is an unncessary multiplication of entities, to be eliminated by Occam's razor, i.e. the scientific principle of economy in explanations.

The biological basis for the mediaeval view that specifically human ensoulment takes place some weeks after conception has completely disappeared. Mediaeval Aristotelians such as Thomas Aquinas depended upon the biology then current, which taught that life originates from semen and menstrual blood, that neither of these is alive, and that the very limited active instrumental power in the semen organizes the blood into a body which can begin to grow and nourish itself first in a plant-like way and then in an animal-like way. If the mediaeval Aristotelians had known about the organic life which organizes the roughly one billion items of molecular information in the one-cell conceptus with a self-directing dynamic integration that will remain continuously and identifiably identical until death, they would have concurred with the view of their successors (and almost everyone else) since the eighteenth century (8). On this later view the fertilized human ovum is specifically human (not merely vegetable), and even the youngest human embryo already has a body which in its already specified (but quite undeveloped) capacities, its epigenetic primordia, is apt for understanding, knowing and choosing. Rather as you or I have the capacity to speak Tibetan or Icelandic, though we lack the ability to do so, so even the youngest human embryo *already* has the biological capacity appropriate to supporting specifically human operations such as self-consciousness, rationality and choice (given only time and metabolic transformations of air, water and other sustenance). The active potential which he or she already has includes the very capacities which are distinctive of persons (9). So he or she is a human being and human person with potential, not a merely potential human person or potential human being.

The most serious contemporary effort to show that there is no lasting human *individual* (and therefore no person) until about two weeks after conception, is by Norman Ford (10). Unlike Tooley and Donceel, Ford holds that personhood begins when an individual with a truly human nature emerges. But the conclusions of his argument are so radically opposed to any biological understanding of human development that they turn out to offer no serious alternative to the standard view: an individual with a truly human nature begins at fertilization. For detailed analysis, refutations and bibliography, see (refs 3, 11–13). Still, Ford's argument is worth tracing, because it attempts to take seriously certain claims often unreflectively uttered, such as that until implantation, or the formation of the primitive streak, or the loss of toti- or pluri-potentiality among the embryo's cells, or the end of the period during which twinning may naturally occur, the conceptus is 'not individuated'.

Ford proposes that at fertilization an ontologically individual and biologically human entity, the zygote, begins, but that (whatever biologists may think) this is never the same individual as the one which (with the same genetic constitution and gender) will begin about 16 days later and will thereafter survive as one and the same individual until death perhaps many decades later. For, according to Ford, the ontologically individual and human zygote is replaced at the first mitotic division by two ontologically individual beings, which in turn are replaced by four, the four by eight, the eight by 12 and 16, these by 32 and 64, and so forth, until by day 14 there are many thousands of ontologically entirely distinct individual human beings (even though all biologists think there is still, unless there has been twinning, only one individual human being). Then these thousands of individuals all suddenly cease to exist when God forms them into 'one living body'.

What drives Ford towards this remarkable conclusion is, on the one hand, his imagination, which finds nothing that looks human in shape until the spatial axes of future somatic development emerge around day 15, and on the other hand the classic puzzle about twinning and mosaics (hypothetical combination of two embryos into one). However, his own theory makes twinning unintelligible, since it occurs at a time, around day six or seven, when, on his view, there is not one individual to become two, but hundreds to become . . . how many? (Ford does not even try to apply his theory to the facts about twinning, facts which he has earlier treated as decisive against the standard view.)

What, then, should be said about twinning, and about the assumed possibility of human mosaics? Simply that, biologically, one always finds just individuals. If these split, or combine to form a mosaic, one then simply finds one or more different individuals. Twinning is an unusual way of being generated; the relationship between the earlier and the later generated individuals is an unusual form of parentage. Being absorbed into a mosaic would presumably be an unusual way of dying. Common thought and language has not had to categorize these events, but there is little or no intrinsic difficulty in doing so.

Nor should one here substitute one's imagination for one's reason. Domination of thought and argument by imagination and conventional associations occurs at various places in the debate. Many people, for example, allow themselves to be dominated by the assumption that no single organ can be larger than all the other organs of an animal, and/or that no major organ can be transient and disposable; they therefore refuse to take seriously the biological data and philosophical considerations which establish that the placenta is an organ of the embryo. Or again, many people (not least some theologians) argue that personhood or ensoulment cannot begin at conception, because they feel it intolerable to suppose that a high proportion of human persons never get beyond the earliest stage of existence as persons. Now that supposition may indeed challenge the imagination. But it is not intolerable to reason, for (a) in every era hitherto, *infant* mortality has been very high, often as high as the rate of pregnancy losses in modern western society; (b) many pregnancy losses are due to chromosomal defects so severe that the losses are not of human beings, but only of beings which (like hydatidiform moles) had a human genome but lacked the epigenetic primordia of a human body normal enough to be the organic basis of at least some intellectual act; and (c) as Ford himself reflects (ref. 11, p. 181), it is presumptuous to suppose that we know how God provides for those who never have any intellectual life, and what are the limits of his provision.

Any entity which, remaining the same individual, will develop into a paradigmatic instance of a substantial kind already is an instance of that kind. The one-cell human organism originating with the substantial change which occurs upon the penetration of a human ovum by a human sperm typically develops, as one and the same individual, into a paradigmatic instance of the rational bodily person, the human person; in every such case, therefore, it is already an actual instance of the human person. In the atypical case where a *genetically* human zygote lacks the epigenetic primordia needed to develop any brain, there is no human being and so no human person, no unborn child (14). And there is another atypical range of cases: some people, including some or all identical twins, were never activated ova, because their life began during the two or three weeks after fertilization, by others dividing or perhaps also others combining.

In all this, what is decisive is not the possession of a unique human genome, but rather the organic integration of a single, whole bodily individual organism. That organic integration, whether the developing organism has one cell or many and whether those cells are toti-potential, pluri-potential or fully specialized, is found from the inception of fertilization. On all biologically and philosophically pertinent criteria that event marks substantial change (in the sense explained above), and no subsequent development or event can be identified plausibly as a genuine substantial change. If there remain biologically and/or philosophically unresolved questions about identity (individuation) in the exceptional cases of embryos which are about to twin, this no more affects the identity of the remaining 97% of embryos than the puzzles about the identity of some adult Siamese twins affect the identity of the rest of us.

Of course, our imagination balks at equating the intelligent adult with a one-cell zygote smaller than a full stop and weighing only 2 mg. But imagination also balks at differentiating between a full-term child just before and just after birth. And *reason* can find no event or principle or criterion by which to judge that the typical adult or newborn child or full-term or mid-term unborn child is anything other than one and the same individual human being—human person—as the one-cell, 46-chromosome zygote whose emergence was the beginning of the personal history of that same child and adult.

In short, science and philosophy concur in the conclusion: every living human individual must be regarded as a person.

JUSTICE, BENEFICENCE AND NON-MALEFICENCE FOR MOTHER AND CHILD

Every attempt to harm an innocent human person violates the principles of non-maleficence and justice, and is always wrong. Every procedure adopted with the intention of killing an unborn child, or of terminating its development, is an attempt to harm, even if it is adopted only as a means to some beneficent end (purpose) and even if it is carried out with very great reluctance and regret. Such procedures are often called 'direct abortions'. But here 'direct' does not refer to physical or temporal immediacy, but to the reasons for the procedure: whatever is chosen as an end or (however reluctantly) as a means is 'directly' willed (15–17). What is only an unintended side-effect is 'indirectly' willed. Using this terminology, one can rightly say that 'direct abortion' is always wrong, while 'indirect abortion' is not always wrong. But it would be clearer to reserve the word 'abortion' (or 'induced abortion' or 'therapeutic abortion') for procedures adopted with the intent to kill or terminate the development of the fetus, and to call by their own proper names any therapeutic procedures which have amongst their foreseen but unintended results the termination of pregnancy and death of the fetus.

The ethics governing therapeutic procedures which impact fatally on the unborn can be summarized as follows:

1. The direct killing of the innocent—that is, killing either as an end or as a chosen means to some other end—is always gravely wrong. This moral norm excludes even the choice to kill one innocent person as a means of saving another or others, or even as a means of preventing the murder of another or others.
2. Every living human individual is equal to every other human person in respect of the right to life. Since universal propositions are true equally of every instance which falls under them, *equality in right to life* is entailed by the truth of two universal propositions: (a) every living human individual must be regarded and treated as a person, and (b) every innocent human person has the right never to be directly killed.
3. The unborn can never be considered as aggressors, still less as unjust aggressors. For the concept of aggression involves action. But it is only the very existence and the vegetative functioning of the unborn (and not its animal activities, its movements, its sensitive reactions to pain, etc., real as these are) that can give rise to problems for the life or health of the mother.

So the concept of aggression extends only by metaphor to the unborn. Moreover, the unborn child, being in its natural place through no initiative and no breach of duty of its own, cannot be reasonably regarded as intruder, predator or aggressor; its relation to its mother is just that: mother and child (18).

4. Provided that bringing about death or injury is not chosen as a means of preserving life, an action which is necessary to preserve the life of one person can be permissible even if it is certain also to bring about the death or injury of another or others.
5. Not every indirect killing is permissible; sometimes, though indirect, it is unjust, e.g. because there is a non-deadly alternative to the deadly procedure which could be used for preserving life.

A just law and a decent medical ethic forbidding the killing of the unborn cannot admit an exception 'to save the life of the mother'. Many of the laws in Christian nations used to include exactly that exception (and no others), but there are two decisive reasons why a fully just law and medical ethic cannot include a provision formulated in that sort of way. First, that sort of formulation implies that, in this case at least, killing may rightly be chosen as a means to an end. Second, by referring only to the mother, any such formulation implies that her life should *always* be preferred, which is unfair.

However, a just law and a decent medical ethic cannot delimit permissible killing by limiting its prohibition to 'direct killing' (or 'direct abortion'). For this would leave unprohibited the cases where indirect killing is unjust (e.g. because it could have been delayed until the time when the unborn child would survive the operation; or because it was done to relieve the mother of a condition which did not threaten her life).

Where the life of mother or of the unborn child is at stake, the requirements both of a decent medical ethic (including the four principles) and of just law can be expressed in the following proposition:

> If the life of either the mother or the child can be saved only by some medical procedure which will adversely affect the other, then it is permissible to undertake such a procedure with the intention of saving life, provided that the procedure is the most effective available to increase the overall probability that one or the other (or both) will survive, i.e. to increase the *average probability* of their survival.

This proposition does not say or imply that killing as a means can be permissible. It does not give an unfair priority to either the mother or the child. It excludes any indirect killing which would be unfair.

Nevertheless, it may seem at first glance that the proposition would admit direct abortion in certain cases. For people often assume, and many Catholic theologians argue, that any procedure is direct abortion if in the process of cause and effect it *at once* or *first* brings about the damage to the unborn child.

But even amongst Catholic theologians who reject every kind of compromise with secular consequentialism and proportionalism, there are some who propose an alternative understanding of direct killing, using the framework of Thomas Aquinas's analysis of acts with two effects and of Pope Pius XII's interpretation of 'direct killing' as an action which aims at the destruction of an innocent human life either as an end or as a means (19,20). The directness which is in choosing a means is to be understood, according to these theologians, not by reference to immediacy or priority in the process of cause and effect, as such, but by reference to the intelligible content of a choice to do something inherently suited to bring about intended benefit.

The proposition I have set out above requires that any procedure which adversely affects the life of either the mother or the unborn child be intended *and inherently suited* to preserving life (both lives) so far as is possible. It thus falls within an acceptable understanding of Catholic teaching on direct abortion. At the same time it demands that any such procedure satisfy the requirements of justice (fairness) which are conditions for the moral permissibility of indirect abortion. The most obvious and likely application of the proposition is in cases where four conditions are satisfied: some pathology threatens the lives of both the pregnant woman and her child; it is not safe to wait, or waiting will very probably result in the death of both; there is no way to save the child; and an operation that can save the mother's life will result in the child's death. Of these cases the example most likely to be met in modern health care is that of ectopic pregnancy (assuming that the embryo cannot be successfully transplanted from the tube to the uterus).

Abortion to 'save the life of the mother' because she is threatening to commit suicide (or because her relatives are threatening to kill her) obviously falls outside the proposition and is a case of direct, impermissible killing. It is neither the only means of saving her life (guarding or restraining her or her relatives is another means), nor is it a means suited of its nature to saving life; of itself, indeed, the abortion in such a case does nothing but kill.

RAPE

A woman who is the victim of rape is entitled to defend herself against the continuing effects of such an attack and to seek immediate medical assistance with a view to preventing conception (21). (Such efforts to prevent conception are not necessarily acts of contraception, for they seek to prevent conception not *as* the coming to be of a new human life but rather *as* the invasion of her ovum as a final incident in the invasion of her body by her assailant's bodily substances.) But the possible presence of an unborn child changes the moral situation notably. Even if a procedure for terminating pregnancy were undertaken without any intention, even partly, to terminate the development and life of the unborn child, but *solely* to relieve the mother of the continued bodily effects of the rape, that procedure would be unjust to the unborn child, who is wholly innocent of the father's wrongdoing. For people are generally willing to accept, and expect their close friends and relatives to accept, grave burdens short of loss of life or moral integrity in order to avert certain death. So imposing certain or even probable death on the unborn child in these circumstances is an unfair discrimination against the child.

However, if a procedure such as the administration of the 'post-coital pill' is undertaken for the purpose only of *preventing* conception after rape but involves some *risk* of causing abortion *as a side-effect* (because it is not known at what stage of her cycle the woman is), there can be no universal judgement that the adoption of such a procedure is unjust to the unborn. For there are many legitimate activities which foreseeably cause some risk of serious or even fatal harm, a risk which in many cases is rightly accepted by upright and informed people as a possible side-effect of their choices to engage in those activities (22, 23).

PRENATAL SCREENING AND GENETIC COUNSELLING

Examinations and tests done with the intention of, if need be, treating the unborn or preparing for a safe pregnancy and delivery are desirable and right when undertaken on the same criteria as other medical procedures. Examinations and tests done to allay anxiety or curiosity are justifiable only if they involve no significant risk to the child. But anyone who does or accepts a test or examination with the thought of perhaps suggesting or arranging or carrying out an abortion if the results show something undesirable, is already willing, conditionally, abortion, and so is already making himself or herself into a violator of the principles of non-maleficence and justice.

Health care personnel who respect those principles have a responsibility not only to refrain from recommending or conducting tests or examinations with a view to seeing whether or not abortion is 'medically indicated', but also the responsibility of telling a woman within their care which of the various tests she may be offered by others are done only or mainly for that immoral (but widely accepted) purpose and which are done to safeguard the health of the unborn child (24).

PARTICIPATION

Anyone who commands, directs, advises, encourages, prescribes, approves, or actively defends doing something immoral is a cooperator in it if it is done and, even if it is not in the event done, has already willed it to be done and thus already participates in its immorality. So a doctor who does not perform abortions but refers pregnant women to consultant obstetricians with a view to abortion wills the immorality of abortion.

On the other hand, some people whose activity contributes to the carrying out of an immoral act need not will the accomplishment of the immoral act; their cooperation in the evil is not a participation in the immorality as such. Their cooperation is often called 'material', to distinguish it from the so-called 'formal' (intended) cooperation of those who (for whatever reason and with whatever enthusiasm or reluctance) will the successful doing of the immoral act. Formal cooperation in immoral acts is always wrong; material cooperation is not always wrong, but will be wrong if it is unfair or a needless failure to witness to the truth about the immorality or a needless giving of a bad example. So a nurse in a general hospital who is unwilling to participate in abortions but is required by the terms of her employment to prepare patients for surgical operations (cleaning, shaving, etc.) may prepare patients for abortion without ever willing the killing or harming of the unborn child; she does only whatever she does towards any morally good operation; so her cooperation can be morally permissible *if* in all the circumstances it is not unfair and a needless occasion of scandal (morally corrupting example to others). The surgeon, on the other hand, must will the harm to the unborn, since that is the point of the immoral abortion and he or she must will the operation's success; so he or she is a participant, indeed a primary participant, in immorality, even if he or she too is doing so only in order to retain employment or gain medical qualifications (25). Hospital managers who want every patient to give written and full consent to operations must want women who come to the hospital for abortions to consent precisely to abortion; so these managers willy-nilly encourage the women's immoral willing of abortion; indeed, the managers' immoral commitment of will may well be greater than that of women whose consent is given in a state of emotional upheaval and distress.

All health care personnel have a moral right (and duty) of non-participation in wrongdoing. This right is not in essence one of 'conscientious objection', since it is founded not on the sheer fact of having made a good-faith judgement of conscience—which might be mistaken—but on the basic human duty and corresponding right not to participate in what really is a moral evil. But where the state recognizes a legal right of 'conscientious objection' to participation in abortion, health care personnel have the moral right and duty to avail themselves of that legal right wherever they would otherwise incur any kind of legal obligation or institutional responsibility to cooperate 'formally' (i.e. intentionally) in abortion. They should take the appropriate steps in good time (but even if they have culpably failed to take those steps, should still refuse all formal cooperation in any of the immoral activities now so widespread in the practice of health care).

EMBRYO EXPERIMENTATION

What has been said above about abortion applies, of course to embryos living *in vitro*—understanding by 'embryo' any human individual from the beginning of fertilization. Any form of experimentation on or observation of an embryo which is likely to damage that embryo (or any other embryo which it might engender by twinning), or to endanger it by delaying the time of its transfer and implantation, is maleficent or unjust or both, unless the procedures are intended to benefit that individual itself. Any form of freezing or other storage done without genuine and definite prospect of a subsequent transfer, unimpaired, to the proper mother is unjust unless done as a measure to save the embryo in an unexpected emergency. Any procedure whereby embryos are brought into being with a view to selecting among them the fittest or most desirable for transfer and implantation involves a radically unjust and maleficent intention, however good its further motivations (26–28).

BENEVOLENCE AND AUTONOMY

The open acceptance of abortion into reputable medical practice during the past quarter of a century—an ethical and civilizational collapse of historic magnitude and far-reaching effects—creates a profound challenge for all who remain willing to adhere to the proper meaning of non-maleficence and justice. They need a proper sense of their own autonomy, as upright moral subjects who preserve and respect the truth amid a social fabric of untruths and rationalizations. They also need to retain and live out a full respect for the principle of beneficence. By refusing their participation in abortion they show beneficence to the unborn (even though these will almost certainly be killed by others); and to the mothers of the unborn (however little they appreciate it at the time); and to all whose lives are endangered by the spread of an ethos of 'ethical killing' in the name of compassion or autonomy. They retain a full responsibility for the compassionate care of pregnant women and for women whose pregnancy was terminated by abortion, no less than of women threatened by or suffering in or after miscarriage or stillbirth. They should be aware of the very real special needs and vulnerabilities of those who have had an induced abortion, even though those needs and sequelae are widely denied by those who promote abortion and produce rationalizations for doing and undergoing it.

REFERENCES

1. Tooley, M. 1983. *Abortion and infanticide.* Clarendon Press, Oxford.
2. Hurst, G. 1977. *Beginning lives*, pp. 107–111. Basil Blackwell/Open University, Oxford.
3. Grisez, G. 1989. When do people begin? *Proceedings of the American Catholic Philosophical Association* **63**: 27–47.
4. Atkinson G. M. 1977. Persons in the whole sense. *American Journal of Jurisprudence* **22**: 86–117.
5. Donceel, J. F. 1970. Immediate animation and delayed hominization. *Theological Studies* **31**: 76–105.
6. Ashley, B. 1976. A critique of the theory of delayed hominization. Pp. 113–133, *in* McCarthy, D. G. and Moraczewski, A. S. (Eds) *An ethical evaluation of fetal experimentation: an interdisciplinary study.* Pope John XXIII Medical–Moral Research and Education Center, St Louis, MO.
7. Gallagher, J. 1985. Is the human embryo a person? *Human Life Institute Reports*, No. 4, pp. 22–26. Human Life Research Institute, Toronto.
8. Heaney, S. J. 1992. Aquinas and the presence of the human rational soul in the early embryo. *Thomist* **56**: 19–48.
9. Wade, F. C. 1975. Potentiality in the abortion discussion. *Review of Metaphysics* **29**: 239–255.
10. Ford, N. M. 1988. *When did I begin?* Cambridge University Press, Cambridge.
11. Fisher, A., O. P. 1991. Individuogenesis and a recent Book by Fr. Norman Ford. *Rivista di Studi sulla Persona e la Famiglia Anthropotes*, no. 2: 199–244.
12. Fisher, A. 1991. 'When did I begin?' revisited. *Linacre Quarterly*, August, pp. 59–68.
13. Tonti-Filippini, N. 1989. A critical note. *Linacre Quarterly* **56**: 36–50.
14. Suarez, A. 1990. Hydatidiform moles and teratomas confirm the human identity of the preimplantation embryo. *Journal of Medicine and Philosophy* **15**: 627–635.
15. Pius XII, Pope. 1944. Address of 12 November 1944. *Discorsi & Radiomessaggi* **6**: 191–192.
16. Congregation for the Doctrine of the Faith. 1974. *De abortu procurato*, para. 7. Declaration on Abortion of 18 November. Catholic Truth Society, London.

17. Finnis, J. 1991. *Moral absolutes*, pp. 40, 67–77. Catholic University of America Press, Washington, DC.
18. Finnis, J. 1973. The rights and wrongs of abortion: A reply to Judith Thomson. *Philosophy and Public Affairs*, **2**: 117 at 138–143; reprinted in Dworkin, R. 1977. *The philosophy of law*. Clarendon Press, Oxford.
19. Zalba, M. 1977. 'Nihil prohibet unius actus esse duos effectus' (Summa theologica 2-2, q.64, a.7) Numquid applicari potest principium in abortu therapeutico? Atti del Congresso Internazionale (Roma-Napoli, 17/24 Aprile 1974), *Tommaso d'Aquino nel suo Settimo Centenario*, Vol. 5, *L'Agire Morale*, pp. 557–568, esp. 567–568. Edizioni Domenicane Italiane, Naples.
20. Grisez, G. and Boyle, J. M. 1979. *Life and death with liberty and justice*, pp. 404–407. Notre Dame University Press, South Bend, IN, and London.
21. Catholic Archbishops of Great Britain. 1980. *Abortion and the right to live*, para. 21. Catholic Truth Society, London.
22. Catholic Bishops' Joint Committee on Bio-ethical Issues. 1986. The morning-after pill: some practical and moral questions about post-coital 'contraception'. *Briefing* **16**: 33–39.
23. Catholic Bishops' Joint Committee on Bio-ethical Issues. 1986. The morning-after pill—a reply. *Briefing* **16**: 254–255.
24. Sutton, A. 1990. *Prenatal diagnosis: confronting the ethical issues*, pp. 1–188. Linacre Centre, London.
25. Grisez, G. 1984. *Christian moral principles*, pp. 300–303. Franciscan Herald Press, Chicago, IL.
26. Fisher, A., O. P. 1989. *IVF: the critical issues*. Collins Dove, Melbourne.
27. Catholic Bishops' Joint Committee on Bioethical Issues. 1983. *In vitro fertilisation: morality and public policy*, part II. Joint Committee on Bioethical Issues, Abingdon.
28. Congregation for the Doctrine of the Faith. 1987. *Donum Vitae. Instruction on respect for human life in its origin and the dignity of procreation.* Catholic Truth Society, London.

49

Abortion and Health Care Ethics III

Leonora Lloyd

National Abortion Campaign, London, UK

The 1967 Abortion Act requires the permission of two doctors before an abortion can be performed in Britain (excluding Northern Ireland, where the Act has never applied). The Act also lays down the conditions which the doctor must satisfy himself or herself the patient fulfils before that permission can be given.

The Act was the culmination of a process whereby doctors confirmed their control over the circumstances under which abortions took place. Initially, their concern was to prevent illegal abortions, both for the sake of women's health, and to ensure that as professionals they managed the procedure according to their own rules, spoken and unspoken.

John Keown, in *'Abortion, doctors and the law'* (1), shows the extent to which doctors' organizations influenced the law.

> The profession was . . . firmly opposed to any reform which compromised clinical freedom either by taking the final decision out of the hands of the medical attendant or by specifying the indications for abortion too exactly.

Doctors had been warning of the dangers of abortion even before the 1803 Act. Quacks ('irregulars') used all sorts of noxious substances and dangerous instruments, even when there was no certainty the woman was pregnant. Before quickening, in any case, there was no certain method of proving pregnancy.

However, as Keown and others acknowledge, of at least as much importance was the necessity for the newly emerging medical profession to differentiate themselves from the 'irregulars'. The same process took place in America, where abortion was the key issue used by doctors to professionalize themselves (2).

Doctors and their attitudes played an important part in the formation of law relating to abortion from 1803 onwards. The Ellenborough Act of that year was the first explicitly to make abortion illegal. The law on abortion was unclear, and it was felt to be inadequate to contain a widespread problem. Increasing

scientific knowledge meant that conception and pregnancy were better understood, and doctors could use this new knowledge to justify restrictions on
abortion. Whilst women who committed infanticide were subject to execution,
abortions generally went unpunished.

A number of amendments were made to the law over the next few years,
usually as a result of the influence of the increasingly powerful medical
profession. For example, the Ellenborough Act dealt only with abortions using
drugs. In 1828, Lord Lansdowne's Act made the use of instruments to procure
abortion illegal. The original Act had been criticized by medical practitioners
for this omission, not least because drugs were rarely effective, whilst the use
of instruments was.

The earlier Acts distinguished between abortion before and after 'quickening'
(the point at which the woman felt the fetus move) and this was amended in
the Offences Against the Person Act, 1837, again as a result of pressure from
doctors, who did not accept 'as scientifically sound the popular belief that
quickening marked the inception of fetal life' (1).

The 1861 Offences Against the Person Act made yet further changes in the
law. Self-abortion by the pregnant woman was made an offence. Supplying of
means to commit an abortion was made a misdemeanour (which did not stop
the continued advertising of 'ladies' aids' in the popular press). In addition, it
confirmed an earlier court ruling that the woman did not have to be actually
pregnant for an offence to have been committed. It was enough that a third
party had simply attempted to procure an abortion.

This does not mean that doctors felt that abortions should never take place, nor
that in practice they treated fetal life as inviolate. I would argue that the key issue
was one of control, rather than ethics. Abortion was treated (and in theory still is)
as a matter of health: so long as doctors could assure themselves that they were
doing abortions in the interests of women's health, then they were justified. What
was important was that they retained control over the process.

The 1967 Abortion Act did not substantially change this situation. Doctors
retain that control. As I shall discuss later, in practice it allows doctors who
want to do so to permit abortion 'on demand', but some doctors can and do
refuse to allow women to have abortions.

Since the 1967 Act was passed, there have been around 17 attempts to change
the law, only two of which would have resulted in further liberalization. Proposals
have included requiring that at least one of the doctors giving permission must
be a consultant, or have been qualified for a certain number of years.

Many of these attempts to restrict abortion have been accompanied by massive
campaigns on both sides, in which a declared objective by anti-abortion groups
has been to influence public opinion and reduce the demand for abortion.
Neither of these objectives has been achieved. The actual practice of women
shows considerable support for legal abortion: by 1991 it was estimated that 42
per cent of British women had had or could expect to have an abortion at some
time (3). There is little sign that the abortion rate, at its highest ever in 1990 at
15.83, is likely to drop very much in the near future.

On 21 of June 1990 (4), during the passage of the Human Fertilisation and
Embryology Act, the House of Commons for the first time debated proposals

TABLE 49.1 Abortions on women resident in England
and Wales by number and rate

Year	Number	Rate per 1000 women is 15–44*
1970	75 962	7.97
1975	106 224	11.00
1980	128 927	12.62
1985	141 101	13.11
1990	173 900	15.83

*This rate is based on abortions at all ages in relation to
the population of resident women aged 15–44.
Source: 1990 Abortion Statistics, OPCS, HMSO.

which would have required either the permission of only one doctor up to 12 weeks gestation, or that a single doctor agreed that the pregnancy had not exceeded 12 weeks (in effect, abortion on request). The latter proposed clause attracted 159 votes in support, but was lost by 105 votes. The former, less sweeping proposal, lost by only 28 votes.

These proposals were in line with current public thinking, as shown by public opinion polls (all material on polls of public and medical opinion from ref. 5 and from a poll conducted in 1991). Earlier public opinion polls asked 'Do you think that the choice as to whether or not to continue a pregnancy should or should not be left to the woman in consultation with her doctor?' but in recent years (1988 and 1990 polls) this was amended to: 'Do you think that women should have the right to choose an abortion in the first months of pregnancy?' The results over the years can be tabulated as shown in Table 49.2.

Doctors have also been polled for their opinions on abortion. By 1977 there had been at least eight polls, some of GPs, some of gynaecologists. In seven polls the question asked was 'Should the Act be changed to become more liberal, left as it is, or changed to become more restrictive?' Further surveys of medical opinion since then have shown solid support for the Abortion Act and slowly growing support (but still a minority) for women having choice. Between 1977 and 1988 the proportion of gynaecologists agreeing with abortion 'on demand' grew from 18 per cent to 23 per cent, whilst a poll conducted by the anti-abortion organization, the Society for the Protection of the Unborn Child (SPUC) in 1988 showed that only 3 per cent of obstetricians and gynaecologists believed that abortion 'should never be allowed in any circumstances'.

The debates in Britain are echoed internationally in the nature of laws on abortion. Whilst in practice some countries prohibit abortion in life-threatening situations, the biggest single block of laws are those permitting abortion only when the woman's life is in danger (Table 49.3). The idea that women themselves can make the abortion choice is however a reality in many parts of the world. This is surely in line with respect for the principle of autonomy. There is no reason to believe that women in Britain are less well educated, less moral or less able to make important decisions about their own lives than women

TABLE 49.2 Summary of public opinion polls (see text)

	1979	1980	1982	1983	1985	1987	1988	1990
Should	76	76	80	74	79	79	80	81
Should not	14	11	15	17	11	11	15	10
Don't know	10	13	5	10	10	11	5	9
Percentage who favoured the right to choose								
Sex								
Male	71	75	81	72	76	73	78	78
Female	81	78	79	75	81	84	81	84
Social Class								
Upper Middle (AB)	73	82	82	73	83	83	*	82
Lower Middle (C1)	77	72†	84	76	77	78†	*	86
Skilled WC (C2)	80		80	76	79		*	82
Semi/unskilled (DE)	73	73	77	70	77	74	*	81
Age group‡								
16–24	70	77	81	73	73	78	83	90
25–34	79	72	80	70	83		89	82
35–44	79	77	81	70		78	80	
45–64	80	79	81	77	83	78	80	79
65+	72	71	77	75	69	80	70	77
Religion								
Church of England	75		85				86	
Catholic	72		69				67	
Free Church	73		70				74	
None	85		81				85	
Politics								
Conservative	77	80	82			84		
Labour	77	74	82			76		
Democrats	81	83	79			79		

*Not classified in this year.
† C1 and C2 amalgamated.
‡In 1987 the age groups were: 15–34, 35–44, 45–54 and 55+; in 1990 the age groups were: 18–24, 24–44, 45–64 and 65+.

elsewhere in the world. But in Britain it is clear that the attitudes of doctors can make a big difference to the chances of a woman getting an abortion on the National Health Service. In the Northern Regional Health Authority, for example, over 83 per cent of women were able to obtain an abortion in the NHS within their own region in 1990, whilst in the West Midlands RHA under 14 per cent of women managed to do so (Figure 49.1). These sorts of discrepancies are overwhelmingly due to the attitude of the consultants responsible for providing an abortion service.

Overall, fewer than half of all women in the UK can get an NHS abortion, and this is clearly as a result of medical decisions. Whilst the demand for abortion has grown and public opinion has increasingly supported abortion rights, public provision has actually reduced (Table 49.4). The attitude of anti-abortion doctors clearly does not stop women getting abortions. Where it does, it discriminates against younger, poorer and less educated women, who do not

TABLE 49.3 Abortion laws worldwide, by number of countries and share of world population (6)

Legal conditions	Countries* Number	Share of world population Percentage
Life endangerment†	53	25
Other maternal health reasons	42	12
Social and socio-medical reasons	14	23
No mandated conditions‡	23	40

*Countries with populations of at least 1 million.
†Technically in some countries in this category abortion is prohibited without exception.
‡Includes some of the world's most populous countries (China, the countries of the former Soviet Union, and the United States (although this is no longer the case in some states)).

Source: Stanley K. Henshaw, Induced abortion: a world review, 1990, *Family Planning Perspectives*, March/April 1990.

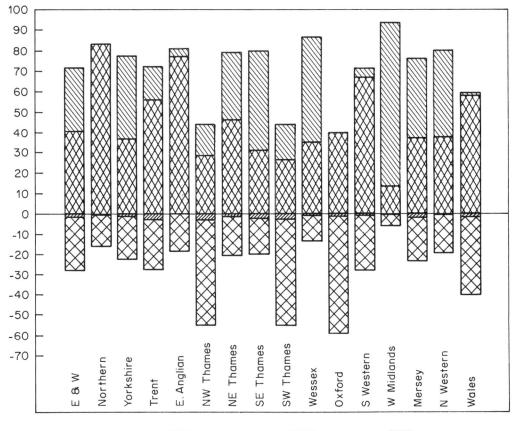

FIGURE 49.1 Abortions, 1990 (*Source: Abortion Statistics,* OPCS, 1990)

TABLE 49.4 Percentage of women having NHS and non-NHS abortions (residents)

Year	NHS	Non-NHS	Agency*
1970	62.4	37.6	
1975	48.0	52.0	
1980	47.0	53.0	
1985	46.2	49.6	4.2
1989	41.5	53.1	5.4
1990	42.3	52.2	5.5

*Agency abortions are those paid for by the health authority, performed in private or charitable clinics, and free to the patient.

Source: based on *Abortion Statistics, 1990*, OPCS (HMSO).

know their way around the system or are too poor to use the private/charitable sector. In most cases it merely results in delay. If the doctor's aim is to save fetal life, therefore, it generally fails to do so.

Different doctors make different decisions, based on subjective views about their patient's age, marital status and class. This is clearly not in accord with the principle of justice. For example, Macintyre (7) showed that single women who were nurses, students or professionals at the time of requesting an abortion were successful in nearly 62 per cent of cases, whilst skilled, unskilled and clerical workers succeeded in only 18–28 per cent of cases.

Macintyre (8) also found that doctors were asking single women far more questions about their past sexual history and use of contraception, and possibly classifying their patients into different moral categories: 'normal-as-if-married', 'promiscuous, or bad, girl' and 'nice girl who made a mistake'. Abortion under these circumstances is an 'award' given or withheld by a kind (or not so kind) doctor, with no regard to the reality of the woman's life, the prospects for her future or the future of her child.

Far from being beneficial to patients, anti-abortion doctors or those who select to whom they will give consent, in most cases add to the woman's distress and can cause positive harm by delaying the time at which she has the abortion. For example, haemorrhage is seven times more likely in abortion after 12 weeks than before (9). In addition, a large body of research shows that the greatest distress for most women seeking abortion occurs between the time pregnancy is discovered and the time when the abortion is done, after which levels of distress are quickly reduced (for a more detailed treatment of this, see ref. 10). Clearly, operating on the principle of beneficence, a doctor would act to reduce distress and stress, by reassuring the woman that her request would be granted, helping the woman to find a trained counsellor if she needed to talk through her feelings, and ensuring that the abortion was performed as soon as possible.

THE DOCTOR'S ROLE IN ABORTION

In law, only qualified doctors can give permission for an abortion and perform abortions. Doctors may also be involved in some form of counselling process.

Medical students get very little training for any of these roles. I have questioned a number of doctors of different ages, most of whom qualified after 1967, and in every case they recall having only brief tuition in methods of abortion and 'about half an hour on the ethics'. For some of them, particularly women, this proved to be quite distressing. One, who trained at Liverpool, told me: 'The gynae consultant who lectured us was most offensive in his attitudes towards women, almost prurient. He was violently anti-abortion and his remarks about women seeking termination made me feel quite sick.' Certainly, none of the doctors I spoke to had any training whatsoever in counselling. This includes those who go into general practice—the woman quoted above was a general practitioner, who also worked as a locum with the Pregnancy Advisory Service, from whom she did get training. However, the PAS, in common with other private and charitable services, has specially trained counsellors, who do most of this work.

This lack of training is evident to women who go to their general practitioners to ask for an abortion, and who then go on to seek an NHS abortion. Doctors show their own prejudices and ask questions rather than initiate open-ended discussions.

As a result of this unsatisfactory process, doctors then have to make a decision, based on the grounds allowed under the Act. As one doctor put it, they become 'arbiters between the mother and the fetus' (11). The vast majority of women having abortions are perfectly healthy and their pregnancies, if allowed to continue to term, would result in the birth of a perfectly healthy baby. Under the terms of the 1967 Abortion Act, which requires there to be a 'medical condition' of some sort, it could be said that those abortions are in fact illegal.

The Act's supporters argue that what is known as the 'statistical clause' makes these abortions legal. The Act allows an abortion where it is safer to terminate than to continue with the pregnancy, and statistically that is always the case. (The relevant part of the Act before amendment read: 'that the continuance of the pregnancy would involve risk to the life of the pregnant women, or of injury to the physical or mental health of the pregnant woman or any existing children of her family, greater than if the pregnancy were terminated'. As amended, the meaning remains the same.) However, the regulations require a medical condition to be specified and in 1990, out of a total of 173 900 abortions, 159 587 (nearly 92 per cent) cited 'mental disorders', including over 112 000 'neurotic disorders'. In other words, perfectly healthy women are being stigmatized as mentally unstable. The Act requires doctors to tell lies and demeans women.

The current regulations came into effect in 1981. Until then, the Act's provision that doctors could take into account the woman's 'current or foreseeable circumstances' was reflected in the fact that over 19 per cent of notifications did not include a 'medical condition', whilst by 1990 this had fallen to under 7 per cent. At the time of the change a number of doctors were threatened with prosecution for not including the required 'medical condition' in their notification forms.

Whilst there are many doctors more than happy to relinquish the control they have over the abortion decision, particularly those who are members of Doctors for a Woman's Choice on Abortion, others disagree. They may argue that their role is to 'save life', not to destroy it, and that the fetus has an inalienable right to life. Others will argue that abortion is dangerous to women—if not physically, then mentally—and that the doctor must therefore aim to restrict terminations to those few in which the doctor believes the benefits will outweigh the disadvantages.

I would argue that both these arguments are irrelevant today. Doctors opposed to abortion on principle are very much in the minority; their beliefs are not held by most people, and it is unethical for a small group of people to impose their views on others over whom they happen to have some power.

In recent years women have argued for the right to determine questions relating to their fertility on their own behalf, and this has gone hand in hand with changing attitudes to medical decisions generally. Patients are now seen as equal partners in the decision-making process, as autonomous beings. Only with regard to abortion is this not so in law for adults. Even patients with limited mental capabilities are rightly regarded as having some capacity for taking decisions about their own lives—but not in connection with their reproductive capacities.

In addition, pregnant women are generally not ill. Whether they wish to continue with their pregnancy or not, they wish to be treated as healthy women with a specific problem. They do not need 'treatment' in the generally understood sense, and as intelligent human beings are able to make ethical and moral decisions on their own behalf.

The only justifications for doctors retaining their role in the decision-making process would be if they had special knowledge unknown and unknowable to the patient concerned, or if they had special qualities which fitted them for making decisions, which were not possessed by their patients. I would argue that even if this was true at some point in time, it is certainly not true now.

The two areas which doctors might feel they have special knowledge about are the effects of abortion on women's health and the development of the fetus.

DOCTORS AND WOMEN'S HEALTH

I said above that one reason given by doctors who are either essentially anti-abortion, or more concerned about retaining control than about the fetus, for refusing all or some abortions is the effect of abortion on women's health. This concern is clearly misplaced as far as the physical effects are concerned.

Legal abortion in the UK is a very safe operation. In 1988, four women in every thousand who had an abortion had some kind of complication, a total of 761 (this figure includes women from outside England and Wales). One woman died. A total of six women have died between 1984 and 1988 as a result of abortion. During this time there have been 1 044 099 abortions in the UK; so less than one woman in every 100 000 has died.

In 1988 there was a total of 41 deaths as a result of 'complications of pregnancy' (12), including one from legal abortion, four as a result of ectopic pregnancy, and two from spontaneous abortion. A further 17 were from complications mainly related to pregnancy, five because of problems during labour, and a further 12 from the after-effects of pregnancy. As there are about 5 times as many births as abortions in the UK, we would have expected only six deaths from pregnancy altogether if the likelihood of death was the same for all causes—induced (deliberate) abortion and all the other causes—as the rate of death from induced abortion on its own. So we could conclude that pregnancy and childbirth are eight times as dangerous as legal abortion in the UK.

However, this is only true if there was a death every year from abortion. In fact, in the 5 years 1987–1991 there were only two—which means that abortion is around 20 times as safe as pregnancy.

There is also a very low rate of morbidity from abortion, but anti-abortion doctors who delay women can actually increase women's ill-health, as the later the abortion the more likely there are to be complications.

The question of women's mental health is more complicated (see ref. 10). In 1989 USA Surgeon General Koop (who is a self-declared anti-abortionist) published the results of a survey of over 200 pieces of research, which confirmed the physical safety of legal abortion, and which also showed that there was no evidence that women's psychiatric health suffered as a result of abortion. In Britain a long-term prospective study (9), started in 1976, confirms this finding.

When compared with the alternative, that is continuing the pregnancy, the health risks of abortion are minimal. For example, according to a report in the 12 January 1992 *Observer Magazine* there are 1000 new cases of postnatal depression a week in Britain. Depression amongst women can occur as a result of childbirth, premenstrual syndrome, menopause or oral contraceptives. Abortion was not even mentioned as a possible cause of depression in this article. It could therefore be argued, on the basis of available evidence, that to persuade a woman, against her will, to have a baby she does not want could result in positive harm to her health, and therefore goes against the principle of non-maleficence.

THE DEVELOPMENT OF THE FETUS AND ITS CLAIMS TO HUMANITY

A common argument amongst anti-abortionists is that many women 'do not know' that what they are doing is 'killing their baby', and that if they did know they would not have an abortion. In the early 1980s, anti-abortion organizations ran what was known as the 'glass tummy' campaign, which featured a woman with a 'see-through' uterus containing a well-developed fetus. If only, the ads said, women could see their developing baby, they would know it was a real baby, not just a piece of tissue, and they would not have abortions.

This is still an important theme in their propaganda. For example, the first bulletin of the newsletter of 'British Victims of Abortion' (13) quotes a woman saying: 'If I knew then what I know now, you would never have died, my child'. (BVA is affiliated to the Society for the Protection of the Unborn Child.)

In support of their argument that the fetus is a baby, anti-abortionists point to the way in which the fetus develops. One of their most quoted texts is Valman and Pearson's article, 'The first year of life' (14), published in the *British Medical Journal* of 26 January 1980, photocopies of which are available at public meetings of anti-abortion groups.

This short article makes bald statements about the development of the fetus. There is no indication in the article as to what status the authors accord the fetus, although they do sometimes refer to him [sic] as a 'baby'.

Anti-abortionists also frequently state that life begins at conception, and that at that point 'the genetic make-up of the new human being is complete—the colour of hair and eyes, build, gifts and talents are all established at this point' (15). It is clear that they have a very specific attitude to human development when 'gifts and talents' are equated with eye colour.

These simplistic descriptions of fetal development contrast with those of Johnston and Grobstein (16,17). The former makes it clear that other than purely genes affect the development of the fetus:

> Biologists suspect that somehow certain molecules (probably proteins) become differentially attached to particular genes, depending on whether these genes are in sperm or egg. These molecules in turn will affect the various genes to which they are attached—but they do so only after fertilisation.

Whilst anti-abortion literature states that a unique human individual exists at conception, which has only to grow, some theorists are more sophisticated. Thus John Mahoney, in *Bioethics and belief* (18), in the chapter on abortion, discusses at length at exactly what point the soul enters the human embryo. He argues that it cannot be at conception because of the problems raised by, for example, division of the conceptus into twins.

I assume from this discussion that, for Mahoney, personhood requires a soul, and it is this which differentiates us from other animals. However, anti-abortionists increasingly claim to base their arguments not on religious theory, but on science. If there are any doubts, they say, then they must be resolved in favour of the 'unborn child'.

There has been a recent explosion of information about the development of the fetus, as technology enables pictures to be taken at every stage of pregnancy, and the majority of women—including many who have abortions—have scans during their pregnancies. Well-educated women are just as likely to have an abortion as the less well-educated. Yet the abortion rate continues to rise. Women are clearly not having terminations out of ignorance. By suggesting that they are, anti-abortionists are showing the contempt for women that underlies their paternalistic stance.

THE IDEOLOGICAL CONTEXT

Abortion has always existed, in every society that has been studied. In Greek and Roman society abortion was openly practised. Laws and religious ideology simply drove the practice underground.

The Bible does not refer to induced or elective abortion at all. There is a reference in the Old Testament as to how the law would regard an accidental abortion caused by a man striking a pregnant woman. If the woman is unharmed, then the attacker is simply fined, the amount to be determined by the husband, who is the one deemed to have suffered the loss. Only if the woman herself dies as a result has a capital crime been committed.

Clearly, as Jewish commentators accept (19), the fetus is not a person in the sense that the woman is a person. What is also interesting in the light of the present discussion is the fact that the loss is the husband's and not the wife's: 'any of her products, whether through work or pregnancy, are the property of the husband. The text in Exodus 21 indicates that in biblical law a fetus has the status of an object, not of a person.' This understanding applies even to non-accidental abortion in Jewish law. Abortion is allowed to save the life of the mother and this applies even during birth 'because her life takes precedence over its life'.

The same text was used by Christians (20) to prohibit abortion, because of the way in which it was translated. The Jewish text reads: 'But if other misfortune ensues, the penalty shall be life for life.' The Christian translation of the word for misfortune is 'form' and is applied to the fetus rather than to the mother. (It would be interesting, but pointless, to speculate whether this was an error or a deliberate mistranslation.) For many centuries there was debate within the Church as to when the fetus came to be 'formed', at which time the soul entered the body; at times there was belief in immediate ensoulment, at others that it took place after 40 days in the case of a male and 80 days in the case of females.

Abortion was seen as particularly sinful when performed to cover up an illicit relationship, with both partners liable to punishment. It was not the status of the fetus which was of concern to the early Church; for them, abortion was a sexual sin like masturbation, adultery and homosexuality.

It was not until 1869 that the Roman Catholic Church finally determined that 'ensoulment' began with conception, and that from that point on a person exists. Even now, that is not an infallible teaching.

The Church was (and is) opposed to both contraception and abortion, because it sees sex as something that happens only between husband and wife for the purposes of procreation. Women are seen primarily as child-bearers. 'I want to remind young women that motherhood is the vocation of women .... It is women's eternal vocation', said Pope John Paul II in his weekly general audience on 10 January 1979.

Little has changed since Augustine wrote: 'I don't see what sort of help woman was created to provide man with, if one excludes the purpose of procreation. If woman is not given to man for help in bearing children, for what help could she be?' Augustine believed that the use of contraception turned wives into harlots. Today, the Church still believes that, in the words of *Humanae Vitae*:

> It is also to be feared that the man, growing used to the employment of anti-conceptive practices, may finally lose respect for the woman and, no longer caring for her physical and psychological equilibrium, may come to the point of considering her as a mere instrument of selfish enjoyment, and no longer as his respected and beloved companion.

Underlying such sentiments is the idea that sex is something done by men to women, albeit with love as the motive. Sex as an equally shared and desired experience has no place in this theory, much less sex for pleasure and recreation. For women, child-care and housework must take the place of sex.

Clearly, the roots of anti-abortion ideology are to be found, not in concern for fetal life—that merely provides the theoretical excuse—but in anxiety over the status of women and a very particular view of (especially female) sexuality.

Protestant fundamentalist groups also see sex and (particularly) women's sexuality as dangerous forces which, if unleashed and given full reign, will damage society. Despite their carefully formulated public pronouncements the underlying philosophy of the anti-choice groups differs little from that of the religious hierarchies.

These views have to some extent informed medical opinion, particularly in the nineteenth century when religious ideas were more important in the formation of medical ethics than in today's more secular society.

IS ABORTION ETHICAL?

Whilst it is true to say that abortions have always occurred, in historical terms they have often done so in conditions of secrecy, illegality and disapproval. But it is also true to say that until recently women's voices on this, and most other things, were silent. The laws and morals of the time were determined, not by women, but by men.

A pregnant woman has consciousness, a history, maybe an existing family, and has made plans for the future. All that counts as naught because of a philosophy that characterizes the fetus as 'innocent' or 'helpless'. The Church attempts, by involving itself in the political process, to impose these views on all of us, regardless of our personal beliefs. In recent years, in particular, the Catholic Church has intervened in Ireland, America and Poland to influence policy on abortion.

With the increasing secularization of society, however, anti-abortionists have not been able to rely solely on their religious arguments, but have had to resort to the arguments outlined in the previous section.

Clearly, non-religious people and even atheists can be anti-abortion. But few are active in the various groups, and even fewer are also anti-choice. There is some distinction between these two expressions: those who are anti-choice are always anti-abortion, but not all those who are anti-abortion for themselves are also anti-choice for others.

Feminists and others have also discussed the issue of 'when does human life begin?' (see, for example, ref. 2), and have come to rather different conclusions. They recognize that the fetus is alive, that it is of the human species and that if left alone may well develop into a normal human baby. But the descriptions given of development are purely physical, and can be applied to any mammalian fetus. The definition of 'humanness' is not clarified by these descriptions.

For me, and for many other feminists, 'humanness' is a social construct. It is our humanity which has enabled us to form societies. Within this society we make relationships and are dependent emotionally and physically on each other. The fetus is totally dependent on the pregnant woman for its nourishment and oxygen, whilst the woman develops an emotional relationship with her expected child. As long as the fetus remains within the body of the woman it cannot form a relationship with anyone else.

This has certain problems (as do all theories of humanity), in that what it implies is that an individual is human if other humans say it is. This opens the door to allowing dominant groups of humans to classify others as non-human, or sub-human, or in other ways not quite as human as themselves, as we have seen in the past. But this is a political, and not a philosophical, question, and requires a political answer, not one based on religious dogma.

In terms of the status of the fetus, however, what it means is that, to put it in the simplest possible terms, a fetus becomes a baby when the pregnant woman says it is a baby.

This is reflected in the language women use about wanted and unwanted pregnancies, and about their pregnancies at different stages.

> Women all over the world recognise three stages. First they say 'My period is late' and I think nearly all will accept anything that will bring it on. Secondly they say 'I am pregnant' and I think most will accept an early abortion if appropriate. Thirdly a woman says 'I'm going to have a baby', and then I think she is very ambivalent and probably is not going to end the pregnancy unless she perceives an extreme threat (21).

This mirrors women's changing attitudes to their expected baby and their feelings about it. Despite the fact that the majority of wanted pregnancies today will end in the live birth of a healthy baby, women still have a fear of the effects of pregnancy on their health, and the possibility of disability or death for their new baby.

When the pregnancy is, or may be, unwanted, then the feelings are even more complex. All women's life experiences and the circumstances leading to the pregnancy are different, which is why only the individual woman, and no-one else, can finally determine the outcome of the pregnancy.

The definition of 'humanness' given above overcomes a problem which is often discussed when considering the ethics and morality of abortion: if there is no physical point during the development of the fetus after which abortion is not allowed, what is the difference between abortion and infanticide? If one accepts the 'social being' definition of humanness, then clearly before birth the fetus can only have a social connection with the mother, but after birth this social connection can be with anyone. It therefore also deals with another anti-abortion argument: they say that if abortion is allowable on the grounds of the dependence of the fetus on the pregnant woman, then this devalues other (born) dependent human beings. But these other human beings are not only already part of the social fabric in a way that an unborn fetus is not, they are also not dependent on just one other person tied to them whether she wants to be or not.

Clearly, for many women having an abortion, their problem is two-fold: they do not want a baby, but also they do not want to be pregnant. For others, the pregnancy is not so much of a problem as the baby itself, and for them adoption might be a better option than abortion. Adoption is not, however, a clear-cut option, and for many women would pose as many, if not more, problems as abortion. For these women, the thought of carrying a child for nine months, only to give it away, would not be possible.

This dichotomy is reflected in the way women describe their experience of unplanned pregnancy. Time and again, one hears them say: 'I was initially quite pleased to be pregnant, because it proved my body worked', or some such thing. Then they start to consider the three options open to them: to have and keep the baby, to have the baby adopted, or to abort.

The idea that women can determine for themselves whether or not their fetus is to become a baby will obviously strike anti-abortionists with horror, but even those holding more permissive views may react negatively, worried about what this means in terms of time limits for abortion. Yet in practice this view is likely to result in earlier, rather than later, abortion. Comparisons of practice in countries such as Holland, the United States and Britain, show that where women have choice they are more likely to have abortions earlier than in countries such as Britain where doctors make the decisions.

The other aspect to be considered is the effect of making abortion illegal or very restrictive. Women's desire to control their fertility is very strong, one might say instinctive, so widespread and pervasive is the use of contraception, abortion and even infanticide. All the research shows that women denied this control will seek illegal abortion at whatever risk to their life and health. It has been estimated by the World Health Organization that some 200 000 women die every year as a result of illegal abortions. One-fifth to a half of maternal deaths could be prevented if all women had access to safe, legal abortion (6).

In addition, it does not seem as if making abortion illegal reduces its incidence; often quite the opposite, especially as in many countries where this happens, contraception is also either illegal, too expensive or too difficult to obtain. Often this is because of religious or political opposition to fertility control as such.

So forbidding abortion will not save fetal life, and in addition will take a tremendous toll of women's lives and health. In countries with poor infrastructures, where traditional extended forms of family are breaking down, the death of the mother may also lead to the early death of existing children. There is little that is 'pro-life' about anti-abortion practice.

WHAT SHOULD THE DOCTOR'S ROLE BE?

Under the current law, doctors can delay a woman, or even prevent her having an abortion. I would argue that this is immoral, given that abortion gets more dangerous with increased gestation, and the trauma increases. Not only does the woman become more aware of her pregnancy, but she has to cope with the problems caused by the doctor's refusal to help her. Whilst a small minority of women may be grateful for being in effect forced to continue with an unwanted pregnancy, in practice the women most affected will be the poor, the very young, or those ignorant of the system. The example of the Republic of Ireland shows that determined women will find a way, even when it is illegal for them to have access to reliable information.

But the problem remains that some doctors object to having anything to do with abortion. These doctors are not fools, and know full well that the majority of their patients seeking terminations will get them. Yet these same doctors are often part of organizations which seek to prevent women making the abortion decision for themselves. The fact is that women's access to abortion services is not dependent on their own beliefs and attitudes, but on those of their doctors.

It is no part of the argument from those who are pro-choice that doctors (or other medical personnel) should be forced to take any part at all in a procedure that they find abhorrent. Far from it. It is not in the interests of women if this happens.

I would argue that, as long as doctors retain their current powers, they have the duty to explain where they personally stand on abortion. But the evidence shows that some doctors do not do this, and are even prepared to tell outright lies about the law, the woman's rights, the availability of abortion or the dangers to the woman. For example, the doctor may tell the woman that she is 'too late' at nine or 12 weeks. Alternatively, the doctor may employ delaying tactics, requiring another pregnancy test, or sending the woman to a consultant known to be anti-abortion.

The result is that women seeking abortion are in effect forced to take part in a macabre game of snakes and ladders, in which the lucky ones throw sixes every time and always land at the bottom of the ladder, until they reach the desired end, whilst the less fortunate find themselves at the starting square. What the anti-abortion doctor does is at worst to force women to become mothers regardless of their own desires, at best to delay them and increase their difficulties.

If abortion became available 'on demand', doctors would still probably be the first port of call for many women wanting confirmation of pregnancy. They would need to confirm that there was no evidence of ectopic pregnancy. Under an amended law, women would then go to clinics (within and without the NHS) for their abortion, where they could obtain counselling if they wanted it. Or women could bypass their GP altogether and go straight to the clinic.

The majority of abortions could be performed by trained paramedics under local anaesthetics, or by non-surgical means—the first of these, RU486, is already in use in the UK. Those requiring abortions at a later stage might need general anaesthetics or other medical help. All the paramedics, nurses and doctors working in the clinics would be there by choice, so no problems would arise in terms of conscience.

I foresee the day when early abortions could be obtained by the woman obtaining a pill from a chemist or clinic after an ectopic pregnancy had been ruled out, and choosing to have the abortion at home. There is nothing very startling in this idea, as it is exactly what happens in millions of cases when and where abortion is illegal. The difference is that it would be much safer and more certain.

Doctors would, of course, be involved (as they are now) where the abortion failed or was incomplete, or where there were some complications, and further treatment was required.

In addition, there might be cases where the abortion was considered because of a doctor's recommendation. In general, just as I am opposed to doctors attempting to influence a woman against having an abortion which she wants, I am opposed to doctors trying to influence a woman to have an abortion even by suggesting it—the idea must originate with the woman. But where the continuation of the pregnancy would endanger the woman's health, then the doctor has a duty to suggest that the woman consider abortion. Even in this situation, even when her life is at risk, the final decision must be hers. The doctor has no right to impose his views on her if her religious or other beliefs forbid abortion altogether.

When a later abortion is being performed, the doctor's duty is to use the method which is best for the woman. It is important to remember that the desired outcome, even in a later abortion, is a dead fetus, not a live baby struggling to survive. Methods which ensure that the fetus is killed *in utero* are therefore to be preferred.

Three other special cases deserve consideration. First, that of the young girl or of a woman with limited mental capacity. There is a real problem in these cases, in that the idea of having a baby may be very appealing, although the reality is (particularly with young girls) the pregnancy could seriously endanger their health, their child has a higher than average chance of being stillborn or dying soon after, and the capacity of the girl or woman to look after their own child may be negligible. Even in these cases, however, the doctor and other people involved have a clear duty to ascertain the views of the woman and to try and take them into account, to explain in the simplest possible way what the risks and options are, and to attempt to come to a decision that is in the best interests of all concerned. Particularly in the case of women with limited mental capacity, it should not be assumed that they cannot care for their own child, albeit with some support, or that conversely they do not understand what an abortion involves. In both cases there would need to be some consideration of the views of those involved in the patient's day-to-day care. I would also argue that a doctor who was against abortion in any situation should not allow himself to be involved, but should pass his patient on to another doctor.

The second 'special' case is that of the pregnancy which is initially wanted, until disability is diagnosed. In 1990, disability was mentioned in less than 1 per cent of cases, and this proportion has been going down in recent years, despite increasing use of screening techniques.

There have been some attempts to restrict abortion on grounds of disability. Anti-abortion groups have claimed to have ready bills for this purpose, which if passed would have the effect of allowing abortion of 'healthy' fetuses (i.e. ones in which no abnormality had been detected or tested for) but not those which might be born dead, or die a few seconds after birth. Attempts to reduce

TABLE 49.5 Abortions on grounds of handicap*

Year	Number†	Percentage
1980	1900	1.47
1985	1921	1.36
1988	1732	1.03
1989	1651	0.97
1990	1589	0.91

*These are abortions on ground 4 of the 1967 Abortion Act: allowing abortion if two registered medical practitioners believe that 'there is a substantial risk that if the child is born it would suffer from such physical or mental abnormalities as to be seriously handicapped'.
†This includes all mentions of ground 4, which is sometimes taken in conjunction with other grounds.

Source: Abortion Statistics, OPCS.

the time limit have had similar motivation, although in practice the proposers of such measures have to amend their own bills to allow exceptions for disability in order to give them a chance of passing. Various public opinion polls have shown that disability, along with rape, is the most popular justification for abortion.

Recently, the burgeoning disability rights lobby has been debating this issue again, but the split between those who think the woman's right is paramount, whatever her reason for the abortion, and those who want to see some controls, is echoed in this group as it is in society in general. For example, an article in the feminist journal *Spare Rib* (22) by disability activist Jenny Morris, calls for a time limit of 24 weeks, on the ground that abortion after viability is discrimination against the disabled. In practice, however, if this was to happen, whilst some 20 women having abortions on grounds of their health would be prevented from so doing, only three abortions on grounds of disability would not take place. If abortion on the grounds of the woman's health remained legal after 24 weeks, these three women might well get abortions on the grounds of the effects of carrying a baby which might well die at birth or shortly after on their own health. Clearly, this is not an easy issue, but for me the main question still remains: someone has to decide, someone has to make the choice, and when there is a conflict the woman's wishes are paramount.

A third dilemma is posed around the question of 'sex selection' abortions. Whilst not a particular problem in the UK, abortions of female fetuses do occur after amniocentesis in countries such as India and China. But even in the West, questionnaires show that the majority of couples would want a boy if they had only one child, or for the first child to be a boy. As research shows that first children have advantages over second and later-born children, there could be serious consequences for women in particular and humanity in general if sex selection—whether through abortion or otherwise—was generally practised.

The answer is not to attempt to restrict abortion, but to raise the status of women. Sex-selection abortions take place where women are seen as inferior to men. Women's desire to have boy children is a reflection of the reality: that boy babies get fed better and are therefore more likely to survive; that they get better education, and are more likely to work; when they get married, they will bring their wife to the parental home, together with a dowry; and they will help to provide for their parents' old age, whilst girls leave home to live with their husbands, and their dowries can cripple the family financially.

In addition, a woman who does not produce a son can be cast out from her home and lose her existing children. In societies where marriage is the only way in which a woman can be assured of a reasonable standard of living and status, this could be disastrous for her. It is therefore very difficult to condemn a particular woman who decides to have an abortion because she is carrying a female. It is impossible to separate the woman from the society she lives in, and its expectations. This is not to approve sex-selection abortions, particularly as the women who resort to them cannot be said to be acting as a result of their own freely arrived-at decision. To oppose them by preventing abortions in general could, in fact, ensure the continuation of women's inferior role, whilst simply transferring the problem to infanticide of baby girls, as has happened in China. The answer is much more complicated and requires structural, political changes, not attacks on abortion.

SUMMARY

Women are no less likely than doctors or others to be people capable of making moral, ethical decisions about their own lives. No-one is more affected than the woman concerned—not doctors, priests, politicans, or even her partner (whose views she will often take into account when making her decision in any event). To deny her the right to make this decision is to deny her full personhood and humanity—which cannot be gainsaid—in the name of the humanity of the fetus, which is less certain.

Doctors in the UK have no more claim to moral certitude than doctors elsewhere, who appear to have accepted their role as technicians rather than power brokers in abortion decision-making. I look forward to the day—which must surely come very soon—when women have the right to make this choice for themselves.

REFERENCES

1. Keown, J. 1988. *Abortion, doctors and the law: Some aspects of the legal regulation of abortion in England from 1803 to 1982*. Cambridge University Press, Cambridge.
2. Petchesky, R. P. 1986. *Abortion and women's choice*. Verso, London.
3. Botting, B. 1991. Trends in abortion. *Population Trends*, Summer, OPCS.
4. *Hansard*, vol. 174, no. 126.
5. Francome, C. and Lloyd, L. 1989. *Abortion and public opinion*. Abortion Law Reform Association/National Abortion Campaign. NOP Poll by Colin Francome, September 1991.
6. Jacobson, J. L. 1990. *The global politics of abortion*. Worldwatch Institute, Washington, USA.
7. Macintyre, S. 1977. *Single and pregnant*. Croom Helm, London.
8. Macintyre, S. 1976. Who wants babies? The social construction of instincts. *In* Barker, D. and Allen, S. (Eds) *Sexual division and society*. Tavistock, London.
9. Frank, P. 1985. Sequelae of induced abortion. Ciba Foundation Symposium: *Abortion: medical progress and social implications*. Pitman, London.
10. Lloyd, L. 1992. *Abortion and after abortion: myths and reality*. National Abortion Campaign.
11. Aitken-Swan, J. 1977. *Fertility control and the medical profession*. Croom Helm, London.
12. *Mortality statistics for 1988*. HMSO, London.
13. British Victims of Abortion newsletter, Autumn 1990.
14. Valman, H. B. and Pearson, J. F. 1980. The first year of life: what the fetus feels. *British Medical Journal*, 26 January.
15. SPUC membership leaflet, 1983.
16. Johnson, M. 1989. Did I begin? *New Scientist*.
17. Hall, E. and Grobstein, C. When does life begin? *Psychology Today (USA)*.
18. Mahoney, J. 1984. *Bioethics and belief*. Sheed & Ward, London.
19. Jakobovits, I. 1959, republished 1975. *Jewish Medical Ethics*. Bloch, New York.
20. Coates, M. 1992. *Christianity and abortion*. National Abortion Campaign.
21. Potts, M. 1985. Medical progress and the social implications of abortion: summing up. *In* Frank, P. (Ed.) *Abortion: medical progress and social implications* (see ref. 9).
22. Morris, J. 1991. Abortion: whose right to choose? *Spare Rib*, September.

50

Abortion and Arguments from Potential

ANNE FAGOT-LARGEAULT, PhD, MD

Université de Paris-X, Département de Philosophie, Nanterre, France

One argues from potential, either when one justifies therapeutic abortion of severely defective fetuses through saying that they do not have the potential to develop into full human persons, or when one derives an (at least *prima facie*) right to life of fetuses from the recognition that they are 'potential human beings'. Arguments from potential are never sufficient to imply a moral decision, but they are interesting arguments, because they testify to our attempts at grounding our moral judgements into the nature of what there is.

Arguments from potential are ontological arguments, that is, arguments from the nature of beings. They are relevant to moral issues on abortion to the extent that questions such as: 'What *is* that fetal life I want (do not want) interrupted?' and 'Who *am* I to decide to interrupt (not to interrupt) my pregnancy?' are relevant to an investigation of questions such as: 'Is it right (wrong) to have an abortion?'. We are assuming here that queries about what should be done are not independent of any queries about what there is.

The notion of potentiality (or potency) is an old philosophical notion. Aristotle (1) said that it can be grasped by analogy (*Metaphysics*, IX, 6, 1047a37). 'Man generates man, and plant generates plant' (*Parts of animals*, I, 2, 646a35). An acorn is a potential oak tree: it is not an oak tree, but it has the (inner) capability, under favourable circumstances, to develop into an oak tree (not into a poplar or a pine tree). A fertilized chicken egg is a potential chicken: it will not always develop into a chicken, but if it gets a chance to develop, it is likely to develop into a chicken, not into a cuckoo or a toad. Similarly: if the human zygote and early embryo I once was, in actuality was 'nothing but a collection of cells' (2), those were human cells with the potential to develop into the human person I am now.

Aristotle used the concept of potentiality as a rather descriptive notion, to mean that, when a living entity develops, although it is the same subsisting entity (organism) developing throughout, in the process of development some

---

Principles of Health Care Ethics. Edited by Raanan Gillon.
© 1994 John Wiley & Sons Ltd

features get actualized at some point, that were not there before. Take for example the heart of the embryo: first, it is not there (it is only potential), then it is there (it is actual). Thus the organism may in the course of time acquire essential properties that it did not actually possess earlier.

How is this relevant to a discussion of moral issues about the human embryo? Kuhse and Singer (3) said in a rather crude way, somewhat reminiscent of Aristotle, that in its early development the human embryo has the moral status of a lettuce or other vegetable, then with organic differentiation it takes the moral status of an animal, and later on, finally it acquires the status of a rational being. According to them, the moral obligations we have towards the human fetus can only be obligations towards what is actually there. There is no moral duty not to inflict suffering when the capacity to feel pain is not there. There is no moral duty to respect autonomy when the capacity to make autonomous decisions is not there. In brief, there is a gradation of obligations relative to the progressive actualization of new essential properties.

That, however, is not enough to solve the ethical problem of abortion. It implies that some methods of abortion should be prohibited, for example, as Kuhse and Singer have pointed out, it implies that, after the fetus has become capable of feeling pain, no abortion should occur without anaesthesia. But it does not say if and when abortion is right or wrong. To answer that sort of query, it seems that we have to question the presupposition that there cannot be any moral obligations towards what has not yet been actualized: don't we have moral obligations toward the potentials?

There are two types of arguments from potential. Let us call them the maximal argument, and the minimal argument.

When in England the Committee chaired by Dame Mary Warnock (4) described the human embryo as a 'potential human being', the Roman Catholic Church retorted that the embryo was 'a human being with a potential'. When in 1984 in France, the National Ethics Committee (5) declared that the human embryo must be recognized as 'a potential human person', again Roman Catholic bishops made it known that they disagreed with such a characterization: the embryo was not a 'potential person', it was an actual person, and as any actual person does, it had potentials.

It is sometimes claimed that abortion is morally wrong because the aborted fetus might have the potential to be a genius: you might be murdering a future Mozart or Einstein. That is a maximal, and indeed, very poor argument from potential. For the potential genius might as well be a potential tyrant, or 'a mediocrity' (6). There is certainly no moral obligation to let every potential of a human being develop. Gardeners know that good gardening takes cutting, trimming, pruning. Even a very liberal education of human children has among its objectives repressing potentials for violence, aggression and hatred, and selecting in favour of altruistic tendencies. And if an echographic test in the course of pregnancy reveals that the fetus has a diaphragmatic hernia, obstetricians nowadays will tend to recommend a surgical cure of the hernia, rather than letting the malformation develop (7). In other words, interrupting the actualization of potentials is not always wrong. The possibility (how probable? should we make estimates and set thresholds?) that some egg's potentials might be outstanding could theoretically yield a motive to give it a chance to develop, at least in the eyes of the supporters of 'positive eugenics'. But as we currently know virtually nothing about the positive potentials of any fetuses, trying to dissuade a pregnant woman from seeking abortion when she has good reasons to do so, through evoking the possibility that her fetus might be endowed with wonderful talents, is a treachery.

Note that the Roman Catholic Church did not commit the above fallacy. It argued that abortion is wrong because it is the killing of an actual human person. That the actual person has potentials is then irrelevant for the anti-abortion argument. The important point is that the human being is substantially the same throughout its lifetime: he/she cannot acquire new essential properties, new emergent properties have to be pre-formed in some way. It takes a special (in this case, theological) assumption to enable one to hold that a human egg is an actual person from the time of conception. Short of believing that God has a project on this humble germ, and that He calls it from its very beginning in its mother's womb to be a 'partner of Himself' (ref. 8, Intro. § 5) (that is, without a relational ontology of personhood complementing your substantial ontology), you may find it hard to recognize that this minute bunch of cells is a human being, or a person, especially if you know that a very early embryo may yield two or more individuals.

Here we need a crucial distinction between being 'something human', and being a 'human being' or a 'person'. Human embryos and fetuses are indeed human, just as human gametes (germ cells) are human, and just as human body cells or organs are human: they belong to human (genetic) lineage. This is not to say that all living cells or organic systems within a human lineage should be endowed with the dignity of human beings or persons. Take any one of your body cells, say a liver cell: you do not treat it as a person, even though current cloning techniques make it theoretically possible for that cell to initiate the development of a full human being with a genotype identical to yours (in other words, another person, a 'double' of your self). We expect 'another person' to be a moral and social partner, someone we can (at least minimally) communicate with, someone with an (at least minimal) sense of being an 'I', and (maximally) a subject capable of taking responsibility for himself and making rational decisions. Let this crude and intuitive characterization guide us here, without going back to the history of the philosophical and legal notion of person (9,10) and without reviewing recent research on the criteria of 'humanhood' or 'personhood' (see refs. 11 and 12, and ref. 13, sections 2 and 3). Observe that the radical view that any human embryo is an actual person with an absolute right to life, is a minority view in the western moral tradition (14).

Should you at this point persist, as a matter of faith, in saying with conservative Roman Catholics that the human embryo or fetus is not merely something human, but an actual human being, you might still claim that it does not follow from such a doctrine that abortion is morally indefensible. You could argue, as Judith Jarvis Thomson forcefully did (15), that the actual human person the fetus or embryo is, has no right to use his mother's body without her full consent, particularly when his/her life is a threat to the mother's own life. But then, you would not use an argument from potential, you would argue in terms of conflicting rights, that is, in terms of justice. On the other hand, should you reckon that the human egg, at least in its early stages of development, cannot in any reasonable sense be considered a full human person, you could still take a conservative view on abortion, by arguing that this human life is precious and should be preserved, because it is the life of a 'potential human person'. Claiming that abortion is morally wrong because it cuts short the development of a 'potential human being' and prohibits its actualization, is quite another argument from the (maximal) argument above. Call this one the minimal argument from potential. It does not allude to whatever potentials you may think of. It concentrates on a very basic or generic potential, one that we (current human persons) all possessed as embryos, whatever our potential talents were. The argument says that although the embryo or fetus is not (yet) a human person, its life has an absolute value, to the extent that it has the potential to develop into a full human person.

The (minimal) argument from potential may be used, either against voluntary (elective) abortion of presumably normal fetuses, or in favour of therapeutic (eugenic) abortion of severely defective fetuses. Therefore it seems crucial for the use of this argument to elucidate what a 'normal' human potential is. In the following we shall successively envisage the pro-life use, and then the pro-choice use, of the argument.

The recognition that human embryos and fetuses are potential human beings is not morally neutral. There is a mystery of life there, apt to inspire a feeling of the sacred. In fact, more generally, the recognition of the power of any seed or animal egg to develop into a complete individual of its own species has had moral and religious implications in many cultures. The question is, how far do such implications go, and are there special implications relative to the human race?

When the National Ethics Committee in France discussed the acceptability of using fetal tissue for therapeutic purposes (see ref. 5, 1984a, 1990b) it made it very clear that the fact that fetuses are recognized as 'potential human persons' implies that fetal tissue should not be considered as mere 'laboratory material', that the tissue should be removed after the fetus has been pronounced dead, and that the project of a therapeutic use should have no bearing either on the woman's decision to interrupt her pregnanacy, or on the abortion technique, etc. It did not prohibit using fetuses from voluntary terminations of pregnancies. In other words, it derived moral implications from the potentiality thesis, but the implications did not go so far as a ban on elective abortion.

There may be legal implications as well as moral implications. In most countries with abortion laws, the legal limits within which an abortion is permissible vary with the motive. When the mother's life is threatened by her fetus, the life of the fetus may in general be terminated at any time during pregnancy, in agreement with the intuition that the life of an actual person is more precious than the life of an (only) potential person. The legal limit allowed for terminating a pregnancy at the request of the pregnant woman is usually much stricter than the legal limit for terminating a pregnancy for a therapeutic motive, that is, when a malformation of the fetus has been diagnosed, in agreement with the intuition that late abortions of presumably normal fetuses are morally worse than early abortions, and that the termination of a defective fetus is more acceptable than the termination of a healthy fetus of the same age. That which is potential, said Aristotle, is indeterminate. Common intuitions embedded in legislations suggest that fetal cells, at first toti-potential, then multi-potential, then progressively actualizing into an individual human being become more precious as their destination becomes more individualized and determined, and that the life of fetuses calls for more protection as fetuses get closer to emerging as human persons.

At first sight, therefore, the potentiality thesis may (weakly) imply a principle of the sanctity of human life, or of all life, it may (weakly) imply a moral rule to the effect that fetal life should be in general protected, and better protected when the fetus approaches its actualization as a full being of its own species, but it does not seem to imply that the potentiality, in the case of a potential human being, should never be frustrated. 'It is logically possible to recognise the pre-embryonic cells as having the potential of the human species without attributing to them full protection proper to the actual embodiment of the human species; and, given the right indications, it is morally possible also' (16).

What would it take to conclude from the human potential of the embryo to its inviolability? Either the implication is postulated, or the argument needs additional premises. Postulating that any potential human being, although not ontologically equal, should be granted an equal moral status with the actual human being, is possible, but arbitrary. Such a principle, besides being of doubtful philosophical soundness, could lead to impractical consequences: should a healthy woman, whose pregnancy is a result of a rape, go to court if she wants an abortion, should she seek an advocate to speak for her fetus, and how should the case be judged in terms of equal rights? We had better look for additional premises, to strengthen the implication at least in some cases.

Michael Tooley challenged the 'potentiality principle'; that is, the principle that, if there is an essential property possessed by adult human beings, which of itself endows them with 'a serious right to life', then 'any organism potentially possessing that property has a serious right to life even now, simply by virtue of that potentiality' (17). Tooley's thesis is that 'only an organism that conceives of itself as a continuing subject of experience has a right to life' (*ibid.*), yet the property of self-consciousness cannot be potential, which ruins the potentiality principle. Tooley's demonstration is based on a sharp opposition between psychological properties such as the desire not to suffer pain (presumably possessed by many animals), and the unique property of self-consciousness (Locke's criterion of personhood). He illustrates his thesis through an example which shows its plausibility: while we feel it is worse to torture a kitten than to kill it, we feel it is worse to kill a human being that to torture him/her. Assume, however, as Fleming has argued (18), that there is continuity rather than discontinuity, from the desire not to suffer pain, or from any desire, to the desire to go on living. Then you might argue that in normal human fetuses, from the moment there are desires and appetites, a desire to continue existing is potentially implied, and so the potentiality principle would be valid at least from then.

An alternative additional premise is suggested by Thevoz (19). He acknowledges that potential personhood does not directly imply the moral status of actual persons. Indirectly, however, as the fetus is recognized by its parents as a future person, it is granted the status and dignity of that person by anticipation through the relationship established with its genitors (this is another case of a relational principle completing an otherwise incomplete argument, where parents are the substitutes of God).

Another additional premise might be that, each time a potential human being is denied the opportunity to actualize and thrive, the beauty of a unique and irreplaceable experience is missed for the whole of the universe, and there is a moral obligation to minimize the spilling and waste of human resources. That premise is, however, very weak in the face of concrete overpopulation problems.

It has also been argued that the natural waste of human embryos (two out of three of all fertilized eggs in the human species abort or miscarry spontaneously during the first weeks of pregnancy) entails a presumption in favour of preserving the remaining eggs. That is a rather paradoxical stand, for in the eyes of most observers the huge natural waste of eggs makes by comparison the extra waste due to elective human abortion look negligible. Yet A. Suarez (20,21) has claimed that most eggs eliminated by nature are not 'actual embryos', for they have 'serious chromosomal or structural anomalies' which render them incapable of developing and coming to term. Nature does the sorting out for us. Actual embryos, that is, embryos which prove capable of surviving, *a priori* have complete human potentials. They may in confidence, and according to Suarez they should, be granted in advance the moral status of persons.

As none of those possible additional premises is entirely convincing, the argument from potential is never quite conclusive. However, it carries some persuasive force in the light of any of those premises. Note that all premises put an emphasis on some favourable circumstance of human development: the embryo is not monstrous, it is developing smoothly, there are loving parents waiting for the child, it is going to be an ordinary self-conscious and rational human being. Thus, perhaps it is best to formulate the pro-life argument from potential conditionally. If an embryo is presumably normal (which may be guessed from the fact that it has not spontaneously miscarried, and the pregnancy is medically unproblematic), then there is a *prima facie* moral obligation to respect its development. Such an obligation is negative: it is a *prima facie* obligation not to interfere. Let us put the argument in positive form: it takes good and strong moral reasons, and careful moral deliberation, to overturn the *prima facie* obligation, and to justify terminating a presumably normal fetus. Not any slight motive of convenience can do. And as the likelihood that the fetus has a normal human potential increases with duration of pregnancy, there may come a time during pregnancy after which no motive is strong enough, save new evidence that the fetus does not, in fact, have a 'normal' human potential.

Most women with an experience of pregnancy would probably subscribe to the argument put in that form, more for its 'naturalness' than for its thoretical strength. It is in agreement with common intuitions, also embedded in legislation. For example, the French law of 17 January 1975 on termination of pregnancy states that respect is due to human beings 'from the very beginning of life', that the legal limit for elective abortion is the end of the 10th week of fetal development (12th week of pregnancy), that the intervention must be performed by a medical doctor, after the woman has been fully informed of the risks and of her rights should she decide to keep the child, and after she has consulted with a social worker. The woman's written consent is accepted only after a delay of one week. Women under 18 years of age need the consent of their legal guardian. In other words the legislator has wanted to ensure that early elective termination, although permissible, will not be got too easily, that some amount of deliberation will have taken place, and that the motives will have been weighed.

The same French law of 1975 states the conditions under which voluntary termination of pregnancy may be performed at any time during pregnancy for a 'therapeutic motive'. The therapeutic necessity (threat to the health of the mother, or high probability that the child will suffer from a serious and incurable disease) must be certified by two trained medical doctors, one of whom must be registered on a list of 'experts' by a Court of Justice. As soon as there is 'scientific' evidence of a serious handicap, it seems that the minimal argument from potential turns pro-choice.

Between 1985 and 1988 Grenier (22) conducted a survey of the acceptability and consequences of prenatal diagnosis (PND). Her hypothesis was that, as PND becomes commonplace, the position of children or adults born and living with one of the defects which are the targets of PND must necessarily deteriorate because they bear traits against which society has chosen to discriminate (for a classification of malformations detectable through PND, see Henrion *et al.* (23), pp. 290–291). Observations did not confirm the hypothesis, but that is besides our point here. Grenier interviewed 246 persons in France and in Québec, either parents with a Down's syndrome child, or women who in the course of a pregnancy had had amniocentesis aimed at the detection of Down's syndrome, or families who had had both experiences. As the researcher was concerned with PND becoming available perhaps too easily, and termination of pregnancy being implicitly viewed as the standard outcome where the fetus was found defective, she systematically asked the question, or rather proposed the statement: 'In requiring PND, you were asking for the perfect child'. The virtually unanimous reaction she got was: 'We did not want him perfect, we wanted him normal'. Comments are suggestive of a sharp distinction drawn between 'perfect' and 'normal', that is, of a rejection of the maximal argument from potential, and the adherence to the minimal argument from potential.

Comments went like this: 'Amniocentesis is meant to detect defects, not to plan for perfection; planning for perfection is another story altogether'; 'We all dream of the perfect child, we know it won't be perfect'; 'The stereotype of the perfect child is a utopia, it's a cliché, it's promotional'; 'The important issue was: we wanted it healthy, we did not want it handicapped'; 'We wanted it to get a fair chance'; 'We wanted it able to progress, develop, become autonomous; Above all, become autonomous'; 'You are responsible for what you beget' (Grenier (22) II, 3, 5: 219–223).

To sum up: those couples with a concrete experience of having a defective child, or trying to prevent having a defective child (or another defective child) deemed it 'absurd' to screen for perfection, and at the same time they went along with the argument that the detection of a severe abnormality in a fetus may be sufficient reason to justify terminating the fetus, when the recognition of the abnormality amounts to a prediction that this fetus will not be able to develop into a full human person. Admittedly, the Down's syndrome case is a borderline case, to the extent that Down's syndrome individuals, unless they are afflicted with other malformations, are capable of biological autonomy, if not of complete social autonomy. There are clearer cases of potentials less than fully human, such as the case of anencephalic fetuses. There are also more doubtful cases, such as the case of Huntington's disease. The criterion of a 'normal human potential' is not a straightforward criterion when used in moral arguments. 'Normal is not a static or peaceful concept, but a dynamic and controversial concept', said G. Canguilhem (24, 1966, p. 1). When defining a deontology of PND, French obstetricians (25) tried to draw a line between 'medically justified indications' (serious and incurable diseases which meaningfully shorten life expectancy, or ruin the quality of human life) and those which are 'not medically justified' (a benign or curable anomaly, such as hexadactylia, for example). The philosopher Canguilhem (23) and later the biologist F. Gros (26, p. 8) have warned that biological norms tend to be reinterpreted in the light of social norms, and that one should resist sliding from arguments in terms of biological normality to arguments in terms of social acceptability. But that is also a reason not to pretend that we should let 'nature' decide for us what defects are compatible with a humanly acceptable human life, and what defects prohibit the thriving of a human person. As difficult as it is to make thoughtful decisions about the fate of defective fetuses, it seems that refusing to take a stand may sometimes be morally worse than accepting one's responsibilities. In such deliberations, although it is of fragile use because it presupposes a judgement on what a meaningful human life is (Goffi (27), p. 112), the minimal argument from potential is of some help.

The argument from potential, in the case of PND and termination of pregnancy ('negative eugenics'), may also be applied to parents. A father of a family who chose to keep and raise a Down's syndrome child expressed both satisfaction at having developed fully his child's limited potential, and melancholy at having invested so much love and energy to get such a modest result: 'Of course I would have been happy, had he been able to enter the polytechnic school, but anyway—we've reached his maximum' (Grenier (22), p. 222). Some parents argue that it takes 'more than an ordinary human potential' to take care of a severely defective child. Human decency is a moral requirement; heroism is not. The decision to terminate a defective fetus, 'rather than having the child and beating him up', as one of the parents said (Grenier (22), p. 218), may in some cases be the right decision. At any rate, no parents should be blamed for acknowledging that they do not have the makings of angels.

To conclude: an ontological argument such as the (minimal) argument from potential is not in general sufficient to support a moral claim. From the fact that a human fetus is seriously defective (that it does not have the potential to develop into a full human person) it does not (logically) follow that it should not be allowed to live, and from the fact that a human fetus is presumably normal (that it has the potential to develop into a normal human being), it does not (logically) follow that it has a right to life. To draw the moral conclusion, it takes at least one additional moral premise, stating what we think is good and should be promoted. In fact, in our moral deliberations we usually bring in several (possibly conflicting) moral premises, such as the premise that the woman's autonomy of decision is an important moral value, and should be respected, or such as the premise that the life of a human fetus is precious, and should be protected. There is always some amount of arbitrariness in the moral premises we adopt, and in the value orderings implied in the ways we rank them. We would not be the moral agents we are, or try to be, if we did not take responsibility for that arbitrariness, rather than evading it. However, we do not like to think that our moral premises are entirely arbitrary. We like to ground them, to some extent, in the silent order of nature. That is what arguments from potential are meant to achieve.

REFERENCES

1. *The basic works of Aristotle*, edited by Richard McKeon, 1941. Random House, New York.
2. Warnock, M. 1987. Do human cells have rights? *Bioethics* 1: 1–14.
3. Kuhse, H. and Singer, P., 1985. *Should the baby live? The problem of handicapped infants*. Oxford University Press, Oxford.
4. Warnock, M. 1984. *Report of the Committee of Inquiry into Human Fertilisation and Embryology*. HMSO, London; translated: *Fécondation et embryologie humaines*. La Documentation Francaise, Paris.
5. Comité Consultatif National d'Ethique pour les sciences de la vie et de la santé (CCNE). 'Avis et rapport sur les prélèvements de tissus d'embryons ou de foetus humains morts à des fins thérapeutiques, diagnostiques et scientifiques' (1984a). 'Avis et rapport sur les problèmes éthiques nés des techniques de reproduction artificielle' (1984b). 'Avis et rapport sur les problèmes posés par le diagnostic prénatal et périnatal' (1985). 'Avis et rapports (scientifique, éthique) relatifs aux recherches sur les embryons humains in vitro et à leur utilisation à des fins médicales et scientifiques' (1986). 'Avis et rapport sur l'utilisation de la mifepristone (RU 486)' (1987). 'Avis sur les recherches sur l'embryon soumises à moratoire depuis 1986, et qui visent à permettre la réalisation d'un diagnostic génétique avant implantation, accompagné d'un Rapport, et d'un Document sur les conditions des recherches sur l'embryon humain in vitro' (1990a). 'Avis concernant les greffes intracérébrales de tissus mésencéphaliques d'embryons humains chez cinq malades parkinsoniens dans un but d'expérimentation thérapeutique' (1990b). 'Avis sur les réductions embryonnaires et foetales' (1991), In: *Rapport 1984, Rapport 1985, Rapport 1986, Rapport 1987, Rapport 1990, Rapport 1991*. La Documentation Française, Paris.
6. Hartshorne C., 'Concerning abortion: an attempt at a rational view', *Christian Century*, 21 Jan 1981.
7. Fellous, M. 1991. Echographie, foetus, personne. Pp. 189–220, in Novaes, S. (Ed.), *Biomédecine et devenir de la personne Seuil*, Paris.
8. *Donum vitae. Instruction sur le respect de la vie humaine naissante et la dignité de la procréation*. Cerf, Paris.
9. Ladrière, P. 1991. *La notion de personne, héritière d'une longue tradition*. Pp. 27–85, in Novaes, S. (Ed.) *Biomédecine et devenir de la personne*. Seuil, Paris.
10. Fagot-Largeault, A. and Delaisi de Parseval, G. 1987. Les droits de l'embryon (foetus) humain et la notion de personne humaine potentielle, *Revue de métaphysique et de morale*, **87(3)**: 361–385; reprinted with modifications in 1989: Qu'est-ce qu'un embryon? Panorama des positions philosophiques actuelles, *Esprit* **151** (6): 86–120.

11. Fletcher, J. 1972. Indicators of humanhood: a tentative profile of man, *Hastings Center Report*, **2**(5).
12. Smith, P. A. 1983. The beginning of personhood: a Thomistic perspective, *Laval théologique et philosophique* **39** (2): 195–214.
13. Bondeson, W. B., Engelhardt, Jr, H. T., Spicker, S. F. and Winship, D. H. 1983. *Abortion and the status of the fetus*, Reidel, Dordrecht.
14. Dunstan, G. R. 1988. The human embryo in the western moral tradition. In Dunstan, G. R. and Seller, M. J. (Eds) Pp 39–57, *The status of the human embryo. Perspectives from moral tradition*. Oxford University Press, Oxford.
15. Jarvis Thomson, J. 1971. A defence of abortion, *Philosophy and Public Affairs* **1** (1): 47–66.
16. Dunstan, G. R. 1990. *The moral status of the human embryo*. Bromham, D. R., Dalton, M. E. and Jackson J. C. (Eds) Pp. 3–9 *in Philosophical ethics in reproductive medicine*. Manchester University Press, Manchester.
17. Tooley, M. 1972. Abortion and infanticide, *Philosophy and Public Affairs* **2** (1): 37–65.
18. Fleming, L. 1987. The moral status of the foetus: a reappraisal. *Bioethics* **1**: 15–34.
19. Thévoz, J.-M. 1985. Un statut moral pour l'embryon? Recherche protestante, *Le Supplément* **153**: 113–124.
20. Suarez, A. 1988. Ist der Menschliche Embryo eine Person? Ein rationaler Beweis, *Schweizerische Ärztezeitung* **24**: 1030–1033.
21. Suarez, A. 1990. L'embryon est une personne, si l'adulte qui dort est une personne. Une démonstration en partant des môles hydatiformes, des tératomes et des chimères, *Médecine et Hygiène*, 28 November: pp. 3458–3462.
22. Grenier, Y. 1990. *Le diagnostic prénatal—ses implications psycho-sociologiques et éthico-philosophiques. Une étude comparée France-Québec*, Thèse de doctorat: Université de Paris-XII.
23. Henrion, R., Dumez, Y., Aubry, J.-P. and Aubry, M.-C. 1987. *Diagnostic prénatal et médecine foetale*. Masson, Paris.
24. Canguilhem, G. 1943. *Essai sur quelques problèmes concernant le normal et le pathologique*. Faculté des lettres, Strasbourg. Reprint followed by: 'Nouvelles réflexions sur le normal et le pathologique', under the title *Le normal et la pathologique*. PUF,Paris (1966).
25. Maroteaux P., *et al*, 1984. A propos de l'Avis du CCNE sur le diagnostic prénatal et périnatal, *Archives Françaises de Pédiatrie* **41**: 445–448; reprinted (1986) *in Lettre d'information du CCNE* **3**:5.
26. Gros, F. 1988. Les progrès de la biologie contemporaine. *Diogène*, April–June, no. 142.
27. Goffi, J.-Y. 1991. Le diagnostic prénatal et la valeur de la vie, *Studia Philosophica* **50**: 87–114.

51

An Ethical Framework for Issues During Pregnancy

CARSON STRONG, PHD

Associate Professor, Department of Human Values and Ethics, University of Tennessee, Memphis, Tennessee, USA

GARLAND D. ANDERSON, MD

Professor and Chairman, Department of Obstetrics and Gynecology, University of Texas Medical Branch, Texas, USA

In 1989 a Florida jury found Jennifer Johnson guilty of two felony counts arising from her use of crack cocaine during pregnancy. She was prosecuted after two successive children born 14 months apart tested positive for cocaine at birth. The charges on which she was convicted were child abuse and delivery of drugs to a minor, based on the transplacental passage of a cocaine derivative. She was sentenced to 15 years probation, 200 hours of community service, and mandatory drug treatment. In the event she becomes pregnant again, she must notify her probation officer and comply with a court-approved prenatal care program (1–3).

This case involving use of law to control maternal behaviour is not isolated. A 1987 report identified 18 cases of court-ordered treatment of pregnant women (4), and there have been at least 50 attempts to prosecute women in the United States for using drugs or alcohol during pregnancy (5). Maternal–fetal conflict has emerged as an ethical issue partly because advances in obstetric technology have resulted in the fetus increasingly being regarded as a patient. Monitoring the health status of the fetus and intervening if necessary have become routine in obstetric practice. Possible interventions include labour-arresting drugs, Cesarean section for fetal indications, and in some cases surgical fetal therapy (6). These developments have presented a number of new questions. Is it ethically justifiable to compel a woman to undergo treatment needed for the fetus? Is it right to control aspects of lifestyle such as drug abuse in order to protect fetuses?

Principles of Health Care Ethics. Edited by Raanan Gillon.
© 1994 John Wiley & Sons Ltd

In addition, advances in ultrasonography and prenatal testing have improved the ability to detect fetal anomalies *in utero* (7). When malformations are detected before viability, abortion is legally available in the United States based on the 1973 Supreme Court decision in *Roe* v. *Wade* (8). However, anomalies sometimes are not detected until later in pregnancy, and even when found before viability the woman sometimes chooses to continue the pregnancy. In these cases yet other ethical questions arise. What are the obligations of mother and doctor to intervene aggressively for the sake of a fetus with anomalies? Is abortion of a fetus with severe malformations ever justifiable during the third trimester?

Resolution of the above questions requires an ethical framework suited to issues during pregnancy. One component of such a framework consists of ethical principles such as those discussed in the present volume. However, such principles alone do not suffice for a framework dealing with pregnancy. A second needed component is a justifiable view concerning the moral standing of the fetus. Ethical issues during pregnancy involve uncertainty about the fetus's moral standing, leading to disagreements over how to weigh conflicting ethical principles that apply to mother and fetus. This chapter will attempt to provide a justifiable ethical framework that contains both components. The framework then will be applied to cases raising prominent issues, in an attempt to reach reasonable conclusions concerning the doctor's professional responsibilities in specific situations.

MORAL STANDING OF THE FETUS

Arguments concerning the moral standing of the fetus can be religious or secular, but this chapter focuses on the latter. Two main approaches have been taken in secular arguments. According to the first approach the fetus becomes a person when it acquires some special characteristic during gestation. Various characteristics or 'indicators' of personhood have been proposed, including viability (8,9), having the potential to become a rational self-conscious individual (10), membership in an intelligent species (which begins at conception) (10), having the basic anatomical structure of human beings (11), and sentience (12). However, serious objections have been raised against the view that viability is grounds for personhood (10,13). Similarly, persuasive arguments have been given against having the potential to become rational and self-conscious (12,14), membership in an intelligent species (12,15), having the anatomical structure of human beings (10,15), and sentience (16). Thus, none of the arguments that personhood begins during gestation have been successful (17). Moreover, there is a widely held view implying that *any* attempt to locate the beginning of personhood during gestation is mistaken. On this view, self-consciousness is a necessary and sufficient condition for personhood. This is a characteristic lacking in fetuses and newborns and acquired by human beings at a later stage in development.

The second approach recognizes that no characteristics acquired during pregnancy give rise to personhood, but asks whether the fetus has a moral standing based on considerations in addition to its own characteristics. Several authors have suggested that conferring moral standing on fetuses might be justified by the *consequences* of doing so. For example, Benn suggests that one reason for treating infants with tenderness and consideration is the good consequences this might have for the persons they grow up to become. Failure to provide tender care to some might also lead to callous unconcern for others. As Benn puts it: 'But if a case like this can be made for infants, it may apply equally well to fetuses; or at least, to fetuses at a stage of maturity at which we can reasonably associate the way we treat them with the way we treat babies' (18). Feinberg agrees with this approach, and suggests that it is the fetus's *similarity* to real persons that makes the consequentialist argument plausible (19). Engelhardt agrees that self-consciousness is necessary to be a 'person in the strict sense', but suggests that we might confer upon infants and others who are not persons in the strict sense the status 'person for social considerations'. He identifies additional good consequences of doing so: promoting important virtues such as sympathy and care for human life; protecting against the uncertainties as to when exactly humans become persons in the strict sense; and protecting persons from various vicissitudes of competence and incompetence (15). According to Engelhardt, it is because infants occupy a *social role* that these consequences are likely to follow from conferring moral standing upon them. Another good consequence suggested by Warren is that the desires of many would be promoted, since most people care deeply about infants and wish them to be treated well (16).

The above considerations enable us to formulate a justifiable view concerning the moral status of fetuses. In focusing narrowly on social role, Engelhardt overlooks that it is the overall similarity with persons in the strict sense that undergirds the consequentialist argument. The closer an individual is to the paradigm of a human being who is a person in the strict sense, the more likely it is that consequences of the sort identified will occur, and thus the stronger the argument for conferred moral standing. Social role is but one aspect of that similarity. Each of the 'indicators' mentioned above constitutes a morally relevant way in which an individual can be similar to paradigmatic persons—to human beings who are persons in the strict sense (17). For infants who possess all the indicators mentioned, including social role, there is a relatively strong argument for conferred moral standing. By contrast, for embryos and fetuses in early gestation the argument is considerably weaker because such individuals lack the basic anatomical structure of human beings, sentience, viability, and a significant social role. They are much less similar to the paradigm.

According to this framework, for any given stage of gestation we should consider the degree of similarity to the paradigm of human beings who are persons in the strict sense. Let us consider the implications for fetuses during the third trimester. They are members of an intelligent species, normally have the potential to become persons in the strict sense, and have the basic anatomical structure of human beings. They have reached viability, a point that today normally occurs during the late second trimester, and data concerning neurological development (20) and responses to stimuli suggest that they are sentient. In addition, several considerations indicate that they occupy a social role to some degree (17). First, the pregnant woman can purposefully act in ways that benefit her fetus; she can eat nutritious meals and seek medical care for conditions that can adversely affect the fetus, such as hypertension and diabetes. Second, increasingly obstetricians can monitor the health status of the third-trimester fetus and offer interventions when needed. Third, parents often have a deep psychological attachment to the fetus by this time. One can reasonably conclude that the similarity with the paradigm is sufficiently close to justify some type of conferred moral standing, based on the consequentialist argument.

The question arises concerning how strong the conferred moral standing should be. Let us begin with infants. Our moral intuitions tell us that infants normally should be regarded as having a moral standing comparable in strength to that of persons in the strict sense, including a right to life. This view appears to be widely, although not universally, held. It has been a prominent view expressed, for example, in debates concerning the 'Baby Doe' issue (21,22). The fact that it is widely held is reflected in the law, which considers newborns to be legal persons. The consequentialist argument supports these intuitions and provides a justification for them. Admittedly, this conferred standing of infants is less secure, resting as it does on consequentialist arguments, rather than the moral standing of persons in the strict sense. If there were a situation in which a conferred right to life conflicted with the right to life of a person in the strict sense, then it would be plausible to give priority to the individual who is a person in the strict sense. However, outside of such exceptional cases, the conferred rights of infants should be regarded as full-bodied. Conferring a serious moral standing upon infants might very well promote the good consequences identified, but it is doubtful that conferring a weak, easily overridden moral status would do so. Thus the justification for the conferred moral standing of infants is itself undermined if the conferred standing is regarded as weak.

The consequentialist argument for third-trimester fetuses is nearly as strong as that for infants. The difference in strength lies in the fact that infants typically are more involved in a social role. This difference, however, is not great enough to claim that birth constitutes a sharp dividing line between those who should and those who should not have moral standing. Thus, the moral standing of fetuses in the third trimester should be regarded as a serious one. Its strength should be regarded as very close to, although perhaps not quite as strong as, that of infants.

This view has at least two main strengths. First, it is consistent with and helps justify several widely held moral intuitions: that late abortion is morally much more problematic than early abortion; that near-term fetuses have a moral standing that is very close to that of infants; and that newborns should be regarded as having serious moral standing. Second, it is helpful in addressing ethical issues during pregnancy, as we shall see below.

A possible objection is that serious moral standing cannot be conferred upon fetuses near term without at the same time denying the personhood of women. Warren, for example, has expressed concern that giving near-term fetuses legal rights that are equal to those of women would deprive pregnant women of the rights to personal autonomy, physical integrity, and sometimes life itself (16). In response, the proposed view confers upon near-term fetuses a moral standing having a strength that is close to, although not quite as strong as, that of persons in the strict sense. Thus, it does not necessarily follow from the proposed view that fetuses near term should have legal rights *equal* to those of women. Moreover, even if fetuses and women had equal legal rights it would not necessarily follow that forced treatment or other control of pregnant women would be ethically or legally justifiable. Consider the fact that although parents and children have equal legal rights, the law does not condone forcing parents to donate organs for transplantation needed by their children. From the assumption that a pregnant woman morally ought to do, or refrain from, certain actions, it does not necessarily follow that the law may justifiably be invoked to coerce her. Moreover, even if there are exceptions in which forced behavior is ethically justifiable, the wholesale overriding of women's interests envisioned by Warren would not occur, provided the exceptions are few.

ETHICAL PRINCIPLES

Three ethical principles are especially pertinent to ethical issues during pregnancy. The principle of *autonomy* implies that the pregnant woman has a right to make decisions concerning her medical care, and that the doctor has an obligation to inform her concerning the medical options. Proposals to control the woman's behaviour for the fetus's sake are problematic, in part, because her autonomy would be violated. The autonomy of the doctor also is a consideration. It implies that the doctor has a right to practice medicine in accordance with acceptable standards of the profession, including a right to refuse to perform unethical or illegal acts.

The principle of *beneficence* applies to all parties involved in ethical conflicts during pregnancy. It implies that the doctor has an obligation to the pregnant woman to preserve and promote her health and avoid causing her harm. When conferred moral standing is justifiable, the doctor has an obligation of beneficence towards the fetus. Sometimes the duty of beneficence towards the fetus conflicts with duties of autonomy or beneficence towards the mother. How these duties should be balanced depends in part on the *strength* of the duty of beneficence to the fetus, which in turn depends on the strength of the consequentialist argument given the characteristics of the fetus in question. The principle of beneficence also applies to others who might in some cases be involved, such as the father of the fetus and other family members, but the well-being of such parties usually is less central to the conflict than that of mother and fetus. In addition, the well-being of the doctor should not be overlooked. It is especially relevant when a proposed action involves serious legal risks to the doctor, for there are limits to the legal risks to which doctors are reasonably expected to expose themselves for the sake of patients.

The principle of *avoiding killing* is relevant because procedures that can cause fetal death are sometimes considered, such as early termination of pregnancy or cephalocentesis to deliver a hydrocephalic fetus (17). Although there is debate concerning when, if ever, killing is ethically justifiable (23,24), clearly there is a very strong presumption against killing persons in the strict sense. When conferred moral standing is ethically justifiable, there is a strong presumption against killing the fetus.

For some authors the principle of avoiding killing falls under the more general principle of non-maleficence (25), which in turn is regarded by some as coming under the principle of beneficence (26). However, it is not clear that killing always harms the one killed, since there might be genuine cases of mercy killing. Also, harm to the one killed does not exhaust the moral significance of killing, as there might also be adverse social consequences. We identify avoiding killing as a separate principle for these reasons, and because it proves useful in discussing the issues to be considered.

The implications of the framework can be illustrated by applying it to representative cases. One test of the validity of the framework is its helpfulness in dealing with such cases.

MATERNAL BEHAVIOR HARMFUL TO THE FETUS

The case of Jennifer Johnson discussed above illustrates the coercion of pregnant women for the sake of fetuses. Such action is motivated by the view that fetuses and newborns have moral worth and deserve protection. The view that third-trimester fetuses have serious moral interests is supported by our ethical framework, which argues for conferred moral standing. However, our framework also gives due consideration to maternal autonomy. A number of authors have defended the view that the woman's rights should *never* be overridden (27–34). One concern is that forced treatment might open the door to further intrusions of the liberty of pregnant women (32). Scenarios have been depicted involving widespread regulation of the lives of pregnant women (30). Forced treatment would disrupt the woman's relationship with her doctor, possibly interfering with her receiving needed care (35). A policy of routinely controlling pregnant women might drive many away from health care, with resulting harm for mother and fetus (34). Moreover, if the patient steadfastly refuses, forcing treatment upon a struggling resistant patient would be difficult and brutish (32,36). The difference in moral standing of mother and fetus is also important. Pregnant women are persons in the strict sense, while third-trimester fetuses have a conferred moral standing that is less strong. We suggest that these arguments support a presumption in favor of the woman's autonomy and well-being that is very strong but not absolute. It might be legally and ethically justifiable to override the woman's autonomy in rare, extraordinary situations provided two conditions are met (36). The first is a restriction established by legal rulings in the United States. Based on Supreme Court decisions, it has been argued that it is unconstitutional for courts to require a woman to undergo increased medical risks for the sake of her fetus (4,27,28,34,36,37). Thus, the first condition is that the treatment poses insignificant or no health risks to the woman or would promote her interest in life or health. The second condition is that there must be compelling reasons to override the mother's autonomy. Maternal–fetal conflicts often are discussed as though the only interests involved are those of mother and fetus, but other considerations can sometimes be relevant. Compelling reasons might vary depending on the case, and usually would consist of a combination of factors. Such factors might include, but are not limited to: protecting fetal life, preventing serious harm to the infant-to-be, preventing the abandonment of other children due to maternal death, preventing harm to the mother's health, protecting the mother's life, preserving the ethical integrity of the doctor, and promoting the well-being of the community. Some of these factors alone might never justify court-ordered treatment, but several in combination might do so in exceptional cases. An example of such a case was suggested by one of the authors (36).

Other issues arise over lifestyles that harm fetuses, such as drug abuse during pregnancy. Studies indicate that from 8 to 17 per cent of pregnant American women are substance abusers (38–41), and these figures might be conservative due to under-reporting. Cocaine use can cause spontaneous abortion, *in utero* strokes, and *abruptio placentae* (42–45). It also is associated with preterm labor and delivery (46–51), intrauterine growth retardation (46,47,50–52), congenital anomalies (53) including cardiac (54), urinary (55), and neural tube defects (42), and increased infant mortality (42). Cocaine-exposed infants often have withdrawal symptoms including irritability, restlessness, inability to sleep, incessant shrill crying, and in severe cases convulsions (56–58). Long-term effects are believed to include learning disabilities (42,57).

An example of a clinical dilemma posed by drug abuse is the following.

Case 1. The patient was an 18-year-old woman at 25 weeks' gestational age with a chronic placental abruption that had resulted in two bleeding episodes. She also had premature rupture of the membranes and a history of cocaine abuse. She was admitted to the hospital and given three units of packed red blood cells. Steroids were given in an attempt to promote fetal lung maturation. Continued hospitalization was considered necessary in order to closely monitor several problems. First, the abruption could result in another bleeding episode. Heavy bleeding could cause serious complications for mother and fetus, including fetal exsanguination, and would require emergency Cesarean delivery. Second, ruptured membranes increase the risk of fetal infection. These reasons for staying in the hospital were explained to the patient, but after several days she left against medical advice. It was suspected that she left in order to obtain cocaine. The doctors were faced with several options: they could seek court-ordered hospitalization; they could offer early delivery on the theory that the risks of premature birth would be less than the risks due to maternal behavior; or they could try to persuade the woman to return for continued hospitalization.

Some have advocated that pregnant addicts be held in state custody in detoxification centers (59). One problem with this approach is that health care providers would be involved in reporting patients to authorities. If routinely followed, this approach would likely drive drug-using women away from prenatal care (5,42). The approach also would highly invade the liberty of women, but because injury might already have occurred the degree of benefit to the fetus would be unclear (42). Another problem in the United States is the shortage of facilities to provide such treatment. Many drug rehabilitation programs refuse to accept pregnant women due to fear of liability for injured babies (60,61). Moreover, coerced treatment of drug addiction sometimes does not receive the cooperation of the patient (5). These considerations indicate that detention is not an acceptable approach. In Case 1 hospital incarceration should be ruled out.

Whether to offer early delivery in Case 1 is a difficult question. Delivery at approximately 25 weeks' gestational age would involve significant risks of neonatal complications including brain hemorrhage, lung disease, and death. On the other hand, the fetal risks associated with non-intervention are difficult to quantify because the mother's behavior is unpredictable. Perhaps her absence from the hospital would be of short duration. If early delivery results in infant death or injury, the doctor will have contributed causally to the harm. Because there is a significant chance that the principle 'do no harm' would be violated by early delivery, this approach does not appear to be the best. Efforts should be made to persuade the woman to return to the hospital.

MANAGEMENT OF FETAL ANOMALIES

The autonomy of the pregnant woman gives rise to the doctor's obligation to help her make informed decisions when fetal anomalies are detected. This obligation requires the doctor to explain the possible management options to the woman. There seem to be four main approaches in such cases. One option is abortion, but in most localities in the United States it is not legally available after viability. The doctor should inform the woman of the limited access to abortion (62) and discuss its legal availability in her locality. A second approach involves continuing the pregnancy in a manner that attempts to optimize the well-being of the fetus. This *aggressive* approach utilizes procedures involving increased maternal risks when needed for the fetus, including tocolysis (use of labor-arresting drugs) and Cesarean delivery. The third option resolves conflicts between maternal and fetal well-being in favor of the woman. This *non-aggressive* strategy avoids interventions that pose increased risks for the mother. Fourth, there is an intermediate approach to weighing the interests of mother and fetus. This approach would permit the woman to be exposed to increased risks in some, but not all, situations. In this *balancing* approach, individual decisions would be based on factors such as the degree of risk to the woman posed by a particular procedure, as well as the degree and likelihood of potential benefits for the fetus. Discussing these four approaches would be an appropriate way to carry out the professional obligation to inform the woman of her options.

It might be objected that abortion need not be mentioned when it is not locally available, or seems beyond the means of a particular patient. In reply, knowing about the limited availability of abortion might help the woman think through her decision. Also, the patient might have resources of which the doctor is unaware, such as a source of borrowed funds to obtain abortion in another locality. Given these considerations, respect for the woman's autonomy suggests that it is better to inform than not inform. Another objection is that doctors who oppose abortion need not mention it as an option. In response, conscientious objection would justify the doctor in withdrawing from a case and referring the patient to another doctor who does not object to discussing abortion. However, conscientious objection would not be grounds for continuing the doctor–patient relationship in a manner involving failure to carry out professional duties to inform (63).

The question arises concerning what recommendations, if any, the doctor should make concerning the options. We suggest that the appropriate recommendations will depend on a number of factors, including the strength of the argument for conferred moral standing in a given case. Another factor is the degree to which the principle of beneficence can be promoted for a given fetus, which in turn depends on fetal prognosis with and without proposed interventions. Additional factors include the reliability of the fetal diagnosis, the maternal risks posed by interventions, the likelihood that such risks would materialize, and whether the procedures used would constitute killing. How the doctor's recommendations and management might vary with these factors can best be illustrated by applying the ethical framework to selected case examples.

> *Case 2.* An ultrasound examination performed to estimate gestational age revealed fetal anencephaly. This diagnosis was confirmed by amniotic fluid measurements of alpha-fetoprotein and acetylcholinesterase at approximately 32 weeks' gestational age. The parents were informed that the prognosis for the fetus was extremely poor. Anencephalic fetuses lack a functioning cerebral cortex. The majority are stillborn, and most that are born alive die within 24 hours of birth. Death almost always occurs within two weeks. The parents were very upset over the news about their fetus. Throughout the following week the mother was distressed over the thought of continuing the pregnancy, and returned to the doctor requesting an abortion. This raised the question of whether a third-trimester abortion in this case would be ethical and legal.

The doctor's response in this case should be based on an analysis of fetal and maternal interests. Fetal anencephaly can be diagnosed *in utero* with a high degree of certainty (64). Its lack of a cerebral cortex entails that the fetus is unable to experience pain or other sensations. Because it lacks sentience, the fetus cannot be said to have interests (65), and it lacks the capacity to be benefited or harmed in any way by management decisions. Thus, the mother's interests clearly should be the primary consideration. Because there is no chance of benefiting the fetus, the aggressive and balancing approaches would not be appropriate. The choice between abortion and non-aggressive management should be left to the woman. The ethical justification of abortion is based on several considerations. The fetus will have a short non-sentient existence regardless of what is done, so a prompt death associated with abortion would not deprive it of any benefit. Moreover, the abortion itself could not cause pain or suffering to the fetus, due to the absence of awareness. Abortion would be ethically justifiable if it promoted the autonomy or well-being of the woman.

It might be objected that third-trimester abortion is wrong despite the above considerations, because it violates the principle of avoiding killing. In response, the fetus's lack of sentience, viability, and potential for personhood in the strict sense reduces the degree of similarity with the paradigm and weakens the argument for conferred moral standing. This does not mean that abortion should be taken lightly in this case, but it provides reasons for claiming that the principle of avoiding killing has diminished force in such circumstances.

The legality of abortion in this case might be an issue, but in the United States a legal defense is possible based on recent Supreme Court rulings. The court has stated that before viability the woman has a constitutionally protected right to abortion (8). In addition, states may not define viability by drawing a line at any particular gestational age or birth weight (66). Instead, the assessment of viability is left to the judgement of the doctor in each individual case (66). Moreover, the court has held that viability involves the capacity for continued extrauterine survival beyond a brief period (66). Thus, given the prognosis doctors can reasonably judge that anencephalics are not viable, in the sense in which that term is used by the court. Because they lack viability, abortion is legal.

Case 3. A fetus at 28 weeks' gestational age was found by ultrasound examination to have an occipital encephalocele (herniation of brain and meninges through a defect in the skull resulting in a sac-like structure) and microcephaly (abnormally small head). The size of the herniation was relatively large, being more than half the diameter of the fetal head. The diagnosis was believed to be reliable, in part because the skull defect was itself visualized in the examination. During counseling, the mother was informed that fetuses with such large herniations usually die, and in the occasional case of long-term survival there almost always is minimal cognitive development.

Like anencephalics, this fetus lacks the potential for cognitive development necessary for personhood in the strict sense. The doctor should recommend against the aggressive and balancing approaches. Non-aggressive management is ethically justifiable because the magnitude and likelihood of potential fetal benefit from aggressive interventions is small and significant maternal risks would be avoided. Unlike anencephalics, this fetus should be regarded as viable and presumably it is sentient. Thus, the legal and ethical justification of abortion would be less strong than in cases involving anencephalic fetuses. The principle of avoiding killing is weightier, and a false-positive diagnosis is possible. Thus, abortion in this case would not be ethically justifiable unless necessary to prevent serious harm to the mother.

Case 4. A 24-year-old woman, gravida 3, para 2, was found by ultrasound at 29 weeks' gestational age to have a fetus with hydrocephalus (abnormal accumulation of cerebrospinal fluid within the ventricles of the brain) and lumbar meningomyelocele. Follow-up ultrasound examinations at 31 and 33 weeks revealed no other anomalies, but showed that the fetal head was larger than normal and progressively increasing. Chromosome analysis yielded no abnormal findings. During counseling the parents were informed that the fluid build-up can raise intracranial pressure and enlarge the head, making normal passage of the fetus through the pelvis impossible. If persistently high, the pressure destroys white matter and causes mental retardation. A decision would be needed concerning method of delivery. One approach would involve delivery as soon as the fetal lungs were mature, using Cesarean section if necessary to avoid fetal head trauma. This method aggressively attempts to promote the interests of the fetus by permitting prompt postnatal evaluation and treatment of the hydrocephalus. The doctor explained that with aggressive treatment the fetus would have approximately a 70% chance of surviving, but about half of survivors were mentally handicapped in varying degrees. A disadvantage of this approach is exposure of the mother to risks associated with surgical delivery. An alternative approach avoids Cesarean section by waiting until labor begins spontaneously. If at that time the fetal head is too large to pass through the pelvis, a needle could be inserted into the cranium and cerebrospinal fluid extracted to reduce head size. However, this cephalocentesis almost always results in stillbirth or neonatal death within several days, due to the rapid head decompression or needle-induced hemorrhage.

In this case one must choose between the aggressive and non-aggressive approaches, where the latter might involve cephalocentesis. The doctor should strongly recommend the aggressive approach, based on several considerations. First, the potential harm to the fetus associated with cephalocentesis is great. Although the child will be handicapped, there is a significant potential for cognitive development. Despite the handicaps, continued life would be in the child's interests. Second, performing cephalocentesis likely would violate the principle of avoiding killing (17,67). The principle is weighty in this case because a reasonable argument can be made for conferred moral standing. A choice by the woman for Cesarean delivery should be fully supported by the doctor. If the patient prefers vaginal delivery, the doctor should continue counseling in an effort to persuade her to choose the other approach.

CONCLUSION

We propose an ethical framework for problems during pregnancy that gives prominence to the principles of autonomy, beneficence, and avoiding killing. The framework includes an ethically justifiable view concerning the moral standing of fetuses and infants. This view confers upon third-trimester fetuses a moral standing having a strength close to, although not quite as strong as, that of persons in the strict sense. The framework also recognizes important moral arguments supporting maternal autonomy. These arguments suggest that in weighing maternal and fetal interests there should be a strong presumption in favor of maternal autonomy. However, this presumption can be overriden in rare, exceptional circumstances. When fetal anomalies diminish the similarity with the paradigm, this fact can play a significant role in weighing maternal and fetal interests and making management decisions. When applied to specific fetal anomalies the framework appears helpful in clarifying the doctor's professional obligations concerning making recommendations and carrying out management decisions. To the degree that the framework is helpful, added support is given to it.

REFERENCES

1. Chavkin, W. and Kandall, S. R. 1990. Between a 'rock' and a hard place: perinatal drug abuse. *Pediatrics* **85**: 223–225.
2. Garcia, S. A. 1990. Birth penalty: societal responses to perinatal chemical dependence. *Journal of Clinical Ethics* **1**: 135–140.
3. Moss, K. 1990. Substance abuse during pregnancy. *Harvard Women's Law Journal* **13**: 278–299.
4. Kolder, V. E. B., Gallagher, J. and Parsons, M. T. 1987. Court-ordered obstetrical interventions. *New England Journal of Medicine* **316**: 1192–1196.
5. Chavkin, W. 1991. Mandatory treatment for drug use during pregnancy. *Journal of the American Medical Association* **266**: 1556–1561.
6. Harrison, M. R., Golbus, M. S. and Filly, R. A. (Eds). 1991. *The unborn patient: prenatal diagnosis and treatment*, 2nd edn. W. B. Saunders, Philadelphia.
7. Filkins, K. and Russo, J. F. (Eds). 1990. *Human prenatal diagnosis*, 2nd edn. Marcel Dekker, New York.
8. *Roe v. Wade*, 410 US 113 (1973).

9. Zaitchik, A. 1981. Viability and the morality of abortion. *Philosophy and Public Affairs* **10**: 18–26.
10. Devine, P. E. 1978. *The ethics of homicide.* Cornell, Ithaca.
11. Becker, L. C. 1975. Human being: The boundaries of the concept. *Philosophy and Public Affairs* **4**: 334–359.
12. Sumner, L. W. 1981. *Abortion and moral theory.* Princeton University Press, Princeton.
13. Fost, N., Chudwin, D. and Wikler, D. 1980. The limited moral significance of 'fetal viability'. *Hastings Center Report* **10**: 10–13.
14. Kuhse, H. and Singer, P. 1982. The moral status of the embryo: two viewpoints. Pp. 57–63, *in* Walters, W. and Singer, P. (Eds) *Test-tube babies.* Oxford University Press, Melbourne.
15. Engelhardt, H. T. Jr. 1986. *The foundations of bioethics.* Oxford University Press, New York.
16. Warren, M. A. 1989. The moral significance of birth. *Hypatia* **4**: 46–65.
17. Strong, C. 1991. Delivering hydrocephalic fetuses. *Bioethics* **5**: 1–22.
18. Benn, S. I. 1984. Abortion, infanticide, and respect for persons. Pp. 135–144, *in* Feinberg, J. (Ed.) *The problem of abortion.* Wadsworth, Belmont.
19. Feinberg, J. 1984. Potentiality, development, and rights. Pp. 145–150, *in* Feinberg, J. (Ed.) *The problem of abortion.* Wadsworth, Belmont.
20. Anand, K. J. S. and Hickey, R. R. 1987. Pain and its effects in the human neonate and fetus. *New England Journal of Medicine* **317**: 1321–1329.
21. Caplan, A. and Cohen, C. B. (Eds.) 1987. Imperiled newborns. *Hastings Center Report* **17**: 5–32.
22. President's Commission for the Study of Ethical Problems in Medicine and Biomedical and Behavioral Research. 1983. *Deciding to forego life-sustaining treatment.* US Government Printing Office, Washington.
23. Gaylin, W., Kass, L. R., Pellegrino, E. D. and Siegler, M. 1988. Doctors must not kill. *Journal of the American Medical Association* **259**: 2139–2140.
24. Vaux, K. L. 1988. Debbie's dying: mercy killing and the good death. *Journal of the American Medical Association* **259**: 2140–2141.
25. Beauchamp, T. L. and Childress, J. F. 1979. *Principles of biomedical ethics.* Oxford University Press, New York.
26. Frankena, W. K. 1973. *Ethics*, 2nd edn. Prentice-Hall, Englewood Cliffs.
27. Nelson, L. J. and Milliken, N. 1988. Compelled medical treatment of pregnant women: life, liberty, and law in conflict. *Journal of the American Medical Association* **259**: 1060–1066.
28. Nelson, L. J., Buggy, B. P. and Weil, C. J. Forced medical treatment of pregnant women: 'Compelling each to live as seems good to the rest.' *Hastings Law Journal* **37**: 703–763.
29. Purdy, L. M. 1990. Are pregnant women fetal containers? *Bioethics* **4**: 273–291.
30. Field, M. A. 1989. Controlling the woman to protect the fetus. *Law, Medicine and Health Care* **17**: 114–129.
31. Johnsen, D. 1987. A new threat to pregnant women's autonomy. *Hastings Center Report* **17**: 33–40.
32. Annas, G. J. 1982. Forced cesareans: the most unkindest cut of all. *Hastings Center Report* **12**: 16–17, 45.
33. Elias, S. and Annas, G. J. 1987. *Reproductive genetics and the law.* Year Book, Chicago.
34. Gallagher, J. 1987. Prenatal invasions and interventions: what's wrong with fetal rights. *Harvard Women's Law Journal* **10**: 9–58.
35. American College of Obstetricians and Gynecologists Committee on Ethics. 1987. *Patient choice: maternal–fetal conflict.* ACOG committee opinion no. 55. American College of Obstetricians and Gynecologists, Washington.
36. Strong, C. 1991. Court-ordered treatment in obstetrics: the ethical views and legal framework. *Obstetrics and Gynecology* **78**: 861–868.
37. Rhoden, N. K. 1986. The judge in the delivery room: the emergence of court-ordered cesareans. *California Law Review* **74**: 1951–2030.

38. Chasnoff, I. J. 1989. Drug use and women: establishing a standard of care. *Annals of the New York Academy of Sciences* **562**: 208–210.
39. Neerhof, M. G., MacGregor, S. N., Retzky, S. S. and Sullivan, T. P. 1989. Cocaine abuse during pregnancy: peripartum prevalence and perinatal outcome. *American Journal of Obstetrics and Gynecology* **161**: 633–638.
40. Chasnoff, I. J., Landress, H. J. and Barrett, M. E. 1990. The prevalence of illicit-drug or alcohol use during pregnancy and discrepancies in mandatory reporting in Pinellas County, Florida. *New England Journal of Medicine* **322**: 1202–1206.
41. Frank, D. A., Zuckerman, B. S., Amaro, H. *et al.* 1988. Cocaine use during pregnancy: prevalence and correlates. *Pediatrics* **82**: 888–895.
42. American Medical Association Board of Trustees. 1990. Legal interventions during pregnancy: court-ordered medical treatments and legal penalties for potentially harmful behavior by pregnant women. *Journal of the American Medical Association* **264**: 2663–2670.
43. Handler, A., Kistin, N., Davis, F. and Ferre, C. 1991. Cocaine use during pregnancy: perinatal outcomes. *American Journal of Epidemiology* **133**: 818–825.
44. Chasnoff, I. J., Burns, W. J., Schnoll, S. H. and Burns, K. A. 1985. Cocaine use in pregnancy. *New England Journal of Medicine* **313**: 666–669.
45. Dombrowski, M. P., Wolfe, H. M., Welch, R. A. and Evans, M. I. 1991. Cocaine abuse is associated with abruptio placentae and decreased birth weight, but not shorter labor. *Obstetrics and Gynecology* **77**: 139–141.
46. MacGregor, S. N., Keith, L. G. and Chasnoff, I. J. 1987. Cocaine use during pregnancy: adverse perinatal outcome. *American Journal of Obstetrics and Gynecology* **157**: 686–690.
47. Oro, A. S. and Dixon, S. D. 1987. Perinatal cocaine and methamphetamine exposure: maternal and neonatal correlates. *Journal of Pediatrics* **111**: 571–578.
48. Chouteau, M., Namerow, P. B. and Leppert, P. 1988. The effect of cocaine abuse on birth weight and gestational age. *Obstetrics and Gynecology* **72**: 351–354.
49. Little, B. B., Snell, L. M., Klein, V. R. and Gilstrap, L. C. III. 1989. Cocaine abuse during pregnancy: maternal and fetal implications. *Obstetrics and Gynecology* **73**: 157–160.
50. Chasnoff, I. J., Griffith, D. R., MacGregor, S., Dirkes, K. and Burns, K. A. 1989. Temporal patterns of cocaine use in pregnancy: Perinatal outcome. *Journal of the American Medical Association* **261**: 1741–1744.
51. Evans, A. T. and Gillogley, K. 1991. Drug use in pregnancy: obstetric perspectives. *Clinics in Perinatology* **18**: 23–32.
52. Hadeed, A. J. and Siegel, S. R. 1989. Maternal cocaine use during pregnancy: effect on the newborn infant. *Pediatrics* **84**: 205–210.
53. Bingol, N., Fuchs, M., Diaz, V., Stone, R. K. and Gromisch, D. A. 1987. Teratogenicity of cocaine in humans. *Journal of Pediatrics* **110**: 93–96.
54. Lipshultz, S. E., Frassica, J. J. and Orav, E. J. 1991. Cardiovascular abnormalities in infants prenatally exposed to cocaine. *Journal of Pediatrics* **118**: 44–51.
55. Chavez, G. F., Mulinare, J. and Cordero, J. F. 1989. Maternal cocaine use during early pregnancy as a risk factor for congenital urogenital anomalies. *Journal of the American Medical Association* **262**: 795–798.
56. Doberczak, T. M., Shanzer, S., Senie, R. T. and Kandall, S. R. 1988. Neonatal neurologic and electroencephalographic effects of intrauterine cocaine exposure. *Journal of Pediatrics* **113**: 354–358.
57. Dixon, S. D. 1989. Effects of transplacental exposure to cocaine and methamphetamine on the neonate. *Western Journal of Medicine* **150**: 436–442.
58. Lindenberg, C. S., Alexander, E. M., Gendrop, S. C., Nencioli, M. and Williams, D. G. 1991. A review of the literature on cocaine abuse in pregnancy. *Nursing Research* **40**: 69–75.
59. Parness, J. A. 1983. The duty to prevent handicaps: laws promoting the prevention of handicaps to newborns. *Western New England Law Review* **5**: 431–464.
60. Chavkin, W. 1990. Drug addiction and pregnancy: policy crossroads. *American Journal of Public Health* **80**: 483–487.

61. Connolly, W. B. Jr and Marshall, A. B. 1991. Drug addiction, pregnancy, and childbirth: legal issues for the medical and social services communities. *Clinics in Perinatology* **18**: 147–186.
62. Chervenak, F. A. and McCullough, L. B. 1990. An ethically justified, clinically comprehensive management strategy for third-trimester pregnancies complicated by fetal anomalies. *Obstetrics and Gynecology* **75**: 311–316.
63. Chervenak, F. A. and McCullough, L. B. 1990. Does obstetric ethics have any role in the obstetrician's response to the abortion controversy? *American Journal of Obstetrics and Gynecology* **163**: 1425–1429.
64. The Medical Task Force on Anencephaly. 1990. The infant with anencephaly. *New England Journal of Medicine* **322**: 669–674.
65. Feinberg, J. 1974. The rights of animals and unborn generations. Pp. 43–68, *in* Blackstone, W. T. (Ed.) *Philosophy and environmental crisis*. University of Georgia, Athens, Georgia.
66. *Colautti* v. *Franklin*, 439 US 379 (1979).
67. Strong, C. 1991. Maternal rights, fetal harms. *Hastings Center Report* **21**: 21–22.

52

Ethical Problems in Infertility Treatment

ROBERT SNOWDEN, BA, PhD, DSA

Professor of Family Studies, Sociology Department, University of Exeter, Devon, UK

ELIZABETH SNOWDEN, SRN, BEd(HONS)

Research Assistant, Institute of Population Studies, University of Exeter, Devon, UK

INTRODUCTION

It is generally accepted that in the UK approximately one couple in ten will have problems in conceiving a child when they wish to start a family. However, it is difficult to find empirical data to support this often-quoted figure. A somewhat higher figure (up to 16%) is given by Hull (1), who assessed the demand for infertility investigation and treatment within the catchment area of his city-based hospital in the UK and concluded that as many as one couple in six may need medical help at some stage in their reproductive life in order to achieve a pregnancy. If it is accepted that the accurate figure lies somewhere between these estimates it would appear that the potential demand for infertility treatment on a national basis is considerable. When such findings are linked to the deep-felt needs of most couples afflicted with the problem of subfertility or infertility a rich 'market' becomes discernible. Reproduction and the relationships associated with it contain powerful feelings of a subjective, emotional and personal nature at one level, while at another level the topic is characterized by important qualities affecting all members of a given social or cultural group. In the absence of reproduction, and the sexual behaviour of individual women and men which normally precedes it, there would be no society. Put this way there is probably no other topic which links so obviously the private behaviour of individuals and the maintenance of the social system of which those individuals are a constituent part. Perhaps this serves to explain the close interest society has always had in matters associated with who reproduces by whom and under what circumstances. At no time in recorded history has reproduction (and sexual behaviour) been left entirely to happenstance; the presence of social control of reproduction of some sort is a feature of all known societies.

Justification for the social control of private sexual behaviour and the reproduction which results from it is not hard to determine. The channelling of the human sex drive in directions that do not unduly disrupt the well-being of the social group is a sensitive task which in the past has relied more on gradually evolving mores than on sudden insights based on newly discovered technical advances. The introduction of contraception to the mass market (generally related to the discoveries associated with the vulcanization of rubber in the mid nineteenth centry) is a case in point. Even today, 150 years after this event, western societies are still finding it difficult to come to terms with the changes in personal and social behaviour which result from the ability to separate the experience of sexual intercourse from the experience of reproduction. For some, the availability of contraception has a direct link with what they believe to be socially disruptive factors arising from uncontrolled sexual behaviour; sexual promiscuity, extramarital affairs, cohabitation, single parent families, a rise in the rates of sexually transmitted diseases and a deterioration in the relationships between the sexes and the generations. For others the availability of contraception is seen to provide freedoms unknown to previous generations; freedoms which provide openings for equal opportunity for both women and men—but especially for women—to exert greater control over their own lives. While change inevitably produces a measure of stress, the management of that stress raises ethical questions at a number of levels ranging from a consideration of personal rights to matters associated with present and future social coherence.

Contraceptive behaviour—or the preferred term 'fertility-regulating behaviour' which encompasses a wider range of behaviour than that confined to pre-conception activities—is behaviour undertaken to prevent or interfere with the natural consequences of sexual behaviour. This is in contrast to behaviour which attempts to redress the inadequacies of a pre-existing condition. Treatment for infertility differs from contraceptive practice in important ways despite both being directly associated with 'family planning'. Whereas one seeks to prevent reproduction from taking place the other encourages reproduction which otherwise would not have taken place. The ethical dilemmas associated with the availability and use of contraceptive technology and infertility services are not the same, but they play an important role in the relationships between individuals at a variety of levels. The link between the individual and society is one based on such relationships, and any procedure likely to affect this link is worthy of close examination.

The ethical dilemmas surrounding the treatment of infertility reflect this individual/societal link, and four areas of major concern can be identified. These relate to the need for assurance at societal level that infertility services and the scientific procedures associated with them are conducted responsibly and in accordance with agreed rules of conduct, the need to consider the welfare of the infertile person or couple receiving treatment, the person willing to donate part of his/her own genetic inheritance and the person who is created as a result of the treatment provided. While it is admitted that the categorization of issues into their consequences at social, recipient, donor and child levels unduly simplifies the relationships which undoubtedly exist between each and all of them, it does permit the presentation of a framework within which this complex topic can be addressed.

SOCIAL FACTORS

It is not so much the *experience* of infertility which raises issues of social concern; no doubt a level of infertility has been present throughout human history and across all cultural groups. It is in the manner of its *treatment* in terms of social reaction and practical help, that ethical issues are likely to arise. The way in which barren women have been treated (and still are treated in some societies) raises important questions concerning human rights and personal autonomy. But in more recent times 'cures' for infertility have tended to replace reactions to an experienced condition. These cures are seldom direct and, in some respects, may be better described as the use of technology and technical skill to deal with the problems of childlessness rather than the alleviation of the infertile condition. It is in the debates surrounding whether or not such practices should take place that ethical considerations have most force.

During the present century, and with increasing speed as it comes to its close, technological advances in association with the development of new medical skills have resulted in two major changes in the process of human reproduction. The first relates to the ability to separate reproduction from the act of sexual intercourse, and the second to the fertilization of human gametes external to the female body. Taken together, these developments have the potential to alter human relationships in ways that are hardly foreseeable at the present time. In terms of human reproduction western societies have embarked on a journey of almost science-fiction proportions where parent/child, partner, kinship and even societal relationships as we know them can no longer be assumed. Presented this way, the new techniques in the treatment of infertility have epoch-making relevance at the very centre of human experience.

Debates have taken place in many countries concerning the central problem of whether or not infertility treatment requiring the use of donated gametes or procedures involving external human fertilization should be allowed. Nowhere has this been more fully debated than in the United Kingdom, which was the first to introduce comprehensive regulation of these practices in the form of nationally agreed laws. Among other topics (including experimentation on embryos and the timing of permitted abortion) the Human Fertilization and Embryology Act (HF&E Act) 1990 specifically regulates infertility treatments which involve the use of donor gametes or external fertilization, and provides for a code of practice in the management of relevant services.

It is not the intention to repeat here ethical issues raised in debate about whether or not such treatment and research should be allowed; these issues have been discussed over a number of years. Now that regulation is in place, debate tends to be more narrowly focused on the share of resources to be taken up by infertility services and on the implications for those directly involved.

The Allocation of Resources

In the allocation of increasingly scarce resources within a comprehensive health care system what degree of priority should be given to the treatment of the involuntarily childless couple to achieve a pregnancy? Some would argue that the 'need' to have a child does not warrant treatment in the conventional sense, especially when the person being treated is often the fit member of a partnership. What is being described is not a true need in a medical sense nor a disease amenable to traditional medical treatment; this type of need could more accurately be described as a 'want' on the part of those unfortunately afflicted, and therefore must remain on the periphery of professional medical intervention. Such a view is reinforced when other applicants for medical support who are suffering from disease traditionally treated within the health service are believed to be disadvantaged owing to a lack of resources necessary to support appropriate treatment. Others present their opposition to the use of scarce resources in this way in terms of the national and global problems associated with overpopulation. Put bluntly, the argument goes that in an overpopulated world it is selfish and foolish to use scarce and expensive resources actively to encourage an increase in the number of babies being born.

These views tend to ignore the evident distress and personal suffering of infertile couples. Even within the individualistic age in which we live there remains a strong assumption that the birth of children is a natural consequence of marriage or of a loving relationship; couples who do not conform to this norm are still liable to be marginalized in our society and to feel themselves to be 'as strangers from life as it is normally lived' (2). The pain of an involuntarily childless lifestyle can be great, and the resultant feeling of loss and lack of purpose among those who face what has graphically been described as 'genetic death' (3) is often difficult to bear. Clearly, the right to the use of scarce resources can be in conflict with the right to reproduce.

What brings this dilemma into closer focus is the discovery and availability of techniques which have opened up new possibilities for the treatment of infertility. Where once infertile couples might have resigned themselves to an acceptance of their condition, the possibility of a 'cure' is now likely to drive couples to 'leave no stone unturned' in the quest for a child of their own. However, it would appear that in terms of health service provision the treatment of infertility is not usually afforded a high priority. The 1991 UK report of the Interim Licensing Authority for Human In-vitro Fertilization and Embryology reported that 'funding of IVF clinics continues to be a problem' (4). Only three clinics were found to be wholly funded by the UK National Health Service (NHS) and therefore providing treatment free of charge to the patient; some clinics were partially funded by the NHS with the additional costs of running the unit being met by those being treated, but the great majority of the clinics required the full cost of treatment to be met by the patient. Those few centres able to offer free treatment had long waiting lists and were obliged to limit treatment to those living within the hospital's catchment area. This, in effect, limits access to the newer treatments to couples who are affluent enough to meet the financial costs involved.

The Involvement of Science

Recent advances in the treatment of infertility have been due to significant developments in biological knowledge (e.g. the process of fertilization), to the adaptation of scientific techniques developed for other purposes (e.g. cryopreservation and the manufacture of precision instruments) and to the acquisition of new skills (e.g. microinjection of single sperm, etc.). This scientific complexity is present at a number of levels and inevitably contributes to the cost of the treatment being offered. It has also contributed to a situation where the advancement of careers (and professional status) has become associated with the scientific advances being made. In some respects the subject has become one in which the scientific imperative is in danger of promoting the means taking precedence over the ends in terms of helping an infertile individual or couple to conceive.

The newer infertility treatments are relying on advanced scientific techniques which are being developed at a pace which allows little time for an adequate assessment of their social and ethical implications. The HF&E Act provides evidence of this difficulty. When the legislation was enacted in 1990, the then Secretary of State for Health was able to declare with confidence that 'in my view it (the Act) is the most comprehensive measure of its kind in the world'. Yet within months of this statement doubt was being expressed about the relevance of the Act to the control of infertility treatment involving the sex selection of embryos and the possible use of immature eggs obtained from aborted fetal tissue. Scientific advances which have made possible what was previously unthinkable (and therefore unknowable), are so far ahead of their social consideration that suggestions for their control inevitably appear reactionary, and an interference with scientific progress in an area that cries out for a resolution of the distressing condition of infertility. What can be done is moving at such a pace that questions of what should be done sometimes appear to have little relevance.

The social concern evidenced in the call for regulation at the level prescribed in the HF&E Act demonstrates clearly that reproduction is perceived as being more than simply a biological process occasionally requiring technical and medical assistance; such a process has profound social and psychological implications at both personal and societal levels. Upon the biological base of reproduction is built an edifice of psychological and social factors which influence a constellation of past, present and future human relationships. For most women and men the birth of their own child is one of the most important social events in their lives. The description of the child as 'our own' is usually based on an abstract notion of the family line, involving a genetic linkage of some sort. Here the subjective feelings associated with what Back calls lineage consciousness (5) meet a more objectively determined genetic link. For most people such a combination presents the mixture which informs the basic structure of social life.

THE COUPLE SEEKING TREATMENT

Apart from the uncertainty surrounding the use of both financial and scientific scarce resources, and assuming that the ethical considerations present in any professional/client relationship are appropriately observed, additional ethical issues do not normally intrude where infertility treatment leads to the birth of a child who is genetically linked to those seeking treatment. All that has occurred is the intervention of specialist procedures to enable the couple to have their 'own' child in all senses of that description. It is when a disruption occurs between the genetic (objective) and the social (subjective) creation of the child that additional ethical issues become apparent. The parent–child relationship is normally based on a combination of genetic and social factors, and any attempt to separate them does not result in a clear division with genetic factors on one side and social factors on the other; each is profoundly intermingled with the other and a simple dichotomy is not possible. However, when the process of fertilization and reproduction is viewed merely as a *biological* event devoid of psychosocial implications, the use of sperm and ova from whatever genetic source is seen as comparatively unimportant. To the clinician facing the problem of attempting to achieve a pregnancy for his/her patient, the use of donor gametes is an obvious alternative to the use of defective or poorer-quality gametes being produced by the couple seeking treatment. Many of the new infertility treatment techniques make use of donor gametes, and whereas to the clinician this use might be the next obvious step in the treatment programme, to the couple the step to the acceptance of donor gametes has profound social and psychological implications. A child will be born to them who does not possess genetic links with one or other parent, or perhaps neither nurturing parent. It might be argued that the relative importance of genetic versus nurturing links favours those responsible for nurturing the child, but few would argue that the genetic link is of no importance whatsoever. Whilst the saying 'blood is thicker than water' is difficult to define precisely, most appreciate its meaning, and few would argue against the validity of the message it conveys. It is therefore of great importance that couples are given sufficient time to consider together (and with others who might be affected) the implications of accepting donor gametes, so that they are able to give considered and informed consent to such treatment. If such treatment is successful the implications for themselves, other family members and for the resulting child will be both far-ranging and enduring. The provisions of the HF&E Act (6) specifically draw attention to the need to make available 'proper' counselling for couples seeking treatment involving use of donated gametes, and for those donating the gametes to be used for this purpose. Such counselling is proposed with the aim of ensuring that those providing and using donated gametes have considered the personal and social implications of their participation in relevant treatment.

Selection of Couples

The provisions of the HF&E Act also require that 'a woman shall not be provided with treatment services unless account has been taken of the welfare of any child who may be born as a result of the treatment (including the need of that child for a father), and of any other child who might be affected by the birth' (7). This implies that some degree of selection of couples should take place, and that the needs of the potential child should be balanced against the needs and wishes of the couple seeking treatment. The Code of Practice (8) issued by the Human Fertilization and Embryology Authority (HFEA—set up by the HF&E Act), states that neither consideration is paramount over the other, and that the subject should be approached with great care and sensitivity. Couples requesting infertility treatment tend to be hostile to selection procedures and to any suggestion that their suitability for parenting should be assessed. They assert that couples conceiving children in the normal way, whatever their degree of suitability or unsuitability as parents, do not have restrictions placed upon their freedom to conceive. However, it has been argued that we all are free to exercise our autonomy only so far as this is consistent with everyone else's freedom to exercise their autonomy. The rights of other individuals must be considered (9). In the case of infertility treatment the autonomy of perhaps the most important person—the resulting child—creates a peculiar difficulty, mainly because at the time of treatment the child does not exist! Clearly, a potential child is not in a position of being able to speak up for his/her own rights. As Matthews has remarked 'yet to be designed is a consent form which the unborn child can sign' (10). The treatment team has the unenviable task of being required to balance the needs of the child yet to be conceived with those of the individual or couple seeking treatment. This balance can be difficult to achieve when the clinician is, in practice, dealing with the strongly felt desires of the childless couple. The couple's needs are those with which the clinician is immediately faced, whereas those of the child can only be based on an abstract notion of what might happen in the future.

The requirement of the HF&E Act that the welfare of the resulting child 'must be taken into account' is sufficiently imprecise to permit a flexible judgement based on the specific circumstances surrounding the couple at the time they seek treatment, but the stipulation clearly implies that parental selection of some sort is to be undertaken. On what basis should this selection take place and who should decide? In the case of child fostering or adoption, detailed regulated procedures involving specially trained independent assessors have been identified, developed and agreed over decades of experience. When infertility treatment using donor gametes is undertaken, even where neither parent is directly genetically linked to the child, the only stipulated restriction is that based on the vague wording of an Act referring to the need to take the resulting child's welfare into account. The HFEA Code of Practice does provide some guidance in the interpretation of this requirement, but adherence to this code is not mandatory and is confined to advising those providing a licensed service to 'bear in mind' certain factors. These include the parents' commitment to the child, their age and medical histories, their ability to deal with possible multiple births, any possible risk to the child to be born, the attitudes of other family members and the possible effect of the birth on other children of the family. The couple must also be offered counselling in order to explore the implications of these factors, but there is no obligation on the potential parents to take up this offer.

The clinician responsible for the provision of treatment must also be afforded his/her own right to autonomous decision-making. As Gillon points out (9), the doctor is not obliged always to do what the patient wants (pp. 75–76). Self-respect for one's own autonomy is proper, and there are some actions one may refuse to take if they are believed to go against one's own moral principles. However, a decision to refuse treatment could well be seen in a negative light by the couple seeking treatment. It may be particularly difficult for the potential parents to accept that a child's needs and welfare might not always be consistent with their own desires. Clearly, the reasons for any refusal to treat the infertile couple will need sensitive presentation.

Information Provision

Before the participants in regulated infertility treatments can properly exercise their autonomy in decision-making it is necessary for them to receive adequate information. For many couples the experience of infertility is seen as a crisis period in their lives. The decision to have a baby (a decision in which their own fertility was almost certainly taken for granted) has been frustrated. This leaves many couples with a feeling of being out of control of their own lives. Medical consultation may increase this feeling; the couple are now dependent upon a clinician to investigate and discover any cause which might underlie their infertility. Investigative procedures may appear repetitive, lengthy and disorganized, and cause considerable stress. The couple need to gain a sense of control over what is happening to them; adequate information plays an important role in enabling them to regain this sense of being in control and of being able to make appropriate choices about treatment options. At a time of stress, information presented orally may be only partially absorbed, and it is important that information is also available in written form so that the couple can read it away from the stress of a medical consultation.

In addition to factual information the couple will need time to consider the meaning and implications which their infertility and specific treatment options might have for their marital and other family relationships. This goes farther than a discussion of the likely consequences and outcomes of the treatments available in terms of success and failure, and is likely to require the input of a skilled counsellor. Counselling is of particular importance if the use of donor gametes is contemplated (11). While donor procedures might enable childlessness to be overcome, the underlying infertility remains unresolved, and the implications of this for the infertile individual, the couple and the child need careful consideration.

Treatment Implications

In Vitro Fertilization

Human *in vitro* fertilization and embryo replacement had its first successful outcome in 1978 with the birth of Louise Brown. Following this momentous event much research effort was put into improving the success rate of this extremely complex and difficult procedure. However, the marked improvement in success rates which was hoped for has not come about. Whilst some centres of excellence have improved their success rates the general level of success remains disappointing. Neither has there been an agreed definition of what constitutes 'success'; this has varied between centres, with some centres quoting pregnancy rates per embryo transfer rather than live-birth rates. The rate of spontaneous abortion following embryo transfer is relatively high and a considerable number of pregnancies do not end in a live birth. Clearly the couple's interpretation of success is not merely based on the achievement of a pregnancy, but on the relative likelihood of their taking home a live baby. A further complication in interpreting the likelihood of success for each couple is caused by the relatively high incidence of multiple births. The birth of twins or triplets to some couples means that when the success rate is expressed in terms of the number of live babies born, the number of successful couples will be fewer than that stated. It is important that a consistent and clearly understood definition of successful treatment outcome, allowing comparability between treatment centres, is presented to potential clients.

Reading and Kerin (12) have argued that whilst the likelihood of failure remains greater than that of success, outcomes should more properly be presented to the patient in terms of failure rates as well as success rates. Couples hear the word 'success' and may convince themselves that they will be one of the successful couples; their attention is directed away from the failure that is statistically much more likely. Reading and Kerin have also pointed out that a type of gambling behaviour, resulting from a partial-reinforcement schedule, can be observed among couples undergoing treatment. Even though the majority fail, couples are aware that a few are rewarded with the birth of a baby. This observation can cause couples to undertake repeated treatment cycles in the hope that they will be one of the lucky couples who 'hit the jackpot' next time. IVF is a complex procedure on which couples expend much nervous energy and financial commitment, and failure can cause much stress.

Superovulation and Surplus Embryos

Because of the high failure rate associated with IVF the procedure of superovulation was introduced in order to maximize the chances of successful treatment. This means that following the administration of superovulatory drugs to increase the number of eggs which develop, a dozen or more are collected and inseminated. External fertilization of the eggs is the relatively successful part of the procedure. The greater chance of failure lies in the second part of the procedure when the fertilized eggs are placed in the uterus in the hope that they will implant and establish a pregnancy. The chances of a pregnancy being established are increased if a number of embryos are replaced; but this also increases the chance of multiple pregnancy with all its attendant disadvantages. Regulations therefore permit only three embryos to be transferred to the uterus.

Because there are frequently more than three embryos which have resulted from the external fertilization process, an excess of embryos is likely to remain. These embryos, surplus to the couple's present need, can be frozen for future transfer, donated to another couple for treatment, donated for research or be allowed to perish. All these four options pose difficult ethical problems and a complex choice for the couple.

To the couple these embryos are precious; this is often the nearest they have ever been to having a baby of their own. The couple have together produced one or more fertilized eggs; from a lay point of view they have 'conceived'. If any embryos are freeze-stored, the couple may see them as possible future children held in a state of suspended animation. Clearly this is a possible source of much stress. The failure of these embryos to implant when placed in the uterus some time in the future may be perceived as a miscarriage with the attendant grief that this kind of bereavement can cause. Recent incidents in the USA illustrate other problems which can occur when embryos are freeze-stored; if couples divorce they may come to conflicting decisions about what should happen to the embryos; if a couple die as the result of an accident the stored embryos become 'orphans'.

Surplus embryos can be donated to another couple for whom external fertilization of their own gametes is not possible or has failed. This procedure has been called 'pre-natal adoption'. Whilst in earlier years most adoption research paid attention to the adopted child it has more recently been recognized that the relinquishing mother often suffers a prolonged period of grieving over the loss of her child. It may well be that couples donating embryos may also grieve over these 'lost' potential children, particularly if their own IVF treatment is unsuccessful and they remain childless. They may suffer the added torment of imagining some other couple giving birth to 'their' child.

The ethical implications of experimentation on human embryos have been well rehearsed and it is not appropriate to examine these here. It is sufficient to accept that almost everyone would agree that these implications are complex. A couple having to decide whether or not to donate their surplus embryos for research have to make what can only be described as a difficult decision. Likewise a decision to allow any spare embryos to be discarded raises still more complex ethical issues. These embryos, given the right environmental conditions, contain the potential for development into a human individual. The role of superovulation in the production of 'spare' embryos therefore raises many complex ethical issues.

The practice of superovulation is problematical in other ways. The use of superovulatory drugs in an attempt to increase the success rate of IVF makes the treatment process more complex, exposes the woman to the possibility of adverse, drug-induced side-effects and makes the treatment much more expensive. The role of pharmaceutical companies which produce these drugs in the setting up of infertility treatment centres may also be questionable. Some treatment centres are now moving away from the use of superovulatory drugs, preferring treatment based on 'natural cycle' IVF in the hope that this less expensive treatment may become more widely available to couples who would otherwise be unable to afford treatment.

GAMETE DONORS

Because donors are required to remain anonymous it is very easy for others involved in the treatment process unintentionally to depersonalize them completely and so not to recognize the need which donors have for information and counselling about the implications of their actions. Several aspects of donation may prove problematical for the donor. For example, the possibility inherent in donor insemination for the spread of HIV infection means that all donors should undergo tests for HIV. Even if the donor has no cause to fear a positive result this test may have implications for such things as personal insurance cover. The possibility that the donor after initial semen analysis might himself prove to be sub-fertile may also cause stress. In addition the donor is being asked to play an important part in the creation of a child about whom he will be given no information and for whom he will take no responsibility. Such a child will, of course, have nurturing parents who are likely to care for the child lovingly; and yet in later life, perhaps as his own children are growing up, a donor might find himself disturbed by the thought that he has other unknown offspring. This concern might be thought to be irrational. But human beings are not simply detached rational beings; they also have strong emotions and a history of many generations of socialization which stresses the responsible nurture of one's offspring. Donors have in the past been discouraged from thinking too closely about the consequences of their donation in the belief that this attitude of detachment is in their best interests (13). Not only is it unrealistic to assume that a donor in later life will always remain detached and untroubled by his earlier action, but the ethics of encouraging a donor to give formal consent to the donation of gametes without adequate consideration of the consequences must also be questioned.

Gamete donation also has implications for the donor's relatives in that the donation might lead to them also having unknown kin. For example, a donor's own child might have unknown half-brothers or sisters conceived as a result of their father's donation; to an adolescent child knowledge of this possibility can be profoundly disturbing.

It is widely recognized that the recruitment of a sufficient number of men willing to act as sperm donors often proves difficult. It is important that individuals who are approached to become donors should not feel themselves under an obligation to the person making the approach. For example, medical students, in the process of being socialized into their chosen profession, may well find it difficult to question or to refuse a request coming from an established member of their chosen profession.

The recruitment of egg donors is likely to be even more difficult as the collection of eggs is an invasive procedure and also involves the administration of superovulatory drugs. The donor is therefore at some risk of harmful side-effects. For this reason relatives or close friends of the infertile woman have in the past been asked to donate eggs. Finch (14) has suggested that such a request goes beyond the bounds of what families see as reasonable mutual support between relatives; nevertheless a sister might feel herself pressured to respond positively to such a request. Likewise women about to undergo (or having undergone) gynaecological or infertility treatments themselves might feel under an obligation to respond positively to a request for donor eggs. It is important that the freedom of potential donors to refuse, or to withdraw or vary the terms of, their consent is respected.

The difficulty in obtaining donor eggs has led some scientists to consider obtaining them from the ovaries of cadavers or from aborted fetal ovaries. While the practical advantages associated with the collection of eggs from such sources (including their almost limitless supply) may appear obvious, the ethical issues surrounding the ownership of this genetic material, and who can give consent for its use, are far from resolved. Such a source of supply, when viewed from the resulting child's perspective, also raises questions about the potential psychological effect of having a deceased woman or an aborted fetus as a genetic mother, and in the case of abortal tissue, a grandmother who acquiesced to the abortion.

CHILDREN CONCEIVED AS A RESULT OF TREATMENT

The HFEA is required to keep registers of donors and of any children who might be born following regulated treatment. The provisions of the 1990 HF&E Act ensure that the gamete donor remains anonymous, however certain non-identifying information may be given to a 'child' on reaching the age of 18 years (or earlier if marrying with the consent of parents) provided an opportunity for the 'child' to receive proper counselling has been given. A 'child' can enquire of the Registrar whether the person she/he intends to marry might be related to him/her. This provision is intended to prevent the possibility of half-siblings marrying each other unknowingly. However, the Act specifically prohibits the giving of information which may identify any gamete or embryo donor. It could be argued that this restriction of the information which may be given to children conceived as a result of regulated treatments is not in the best interests of the children. The HFEA's Code of Practice acknowledges a child's potential need to know about his/her origins (15), and yet the legislation restricts the amount of information which legally may be given. This apparently contradictory position may well be challenged in future years by these children as they attain the age of majority. It is not difficult to imagine the frustration which could be generated by the knowledge that information about oneself is held in official records, and that one is denied access to these records.

Confidentiality and Secrecy

Certain infertility treatments, particularly donor insemination, have traditionally not been discussed openly. The majority of couples, and some practitioners providing this service, have felt it advisable that recourse to such treatments should be afforded a degree of secrecy. Doctors have tended to regard this as a matter of the confidentiality associated with medical practice. However, if the restriction of information which surrounds treatments using donor gametes is examined more closely it can be seen to have at least three component parts; firstly, the confidentiality of the consultation between the doctor and the infertile couple; secondly, the anonymity of the donor; and finally, the pretence by the couple that the child is the result of a natural conception. The confidentiality of consultations with members of the medical profession is essential and entirely proper, but arguments can be presented both for and against maintaining the anonymity of gamete donors. Some believe donor anonymity to be an essential mechanism designed to protect the integrity of the recipient family by preventing the development of conflicting emotional ties between family members and the gamete donor; anonymity is seen as a mechanism which will create a protective barrier between the donor and the recipient couple (16). Others argue that such anonymity restricts the rights of the child to have knowledge of the identity of his/her genetic forebears; an identity which appears in an official register to which he or she is denied access (17). Lusk (18) suggests that rather than thinking in terms of the resulting 'child' it is more helpful to think in terms of the resulting adult. Consideration of the adult situation (which the child will eventually attain) is more likely to encourage consideration of this topic in terms of human rights. The third component of secrecy, which supports the pretence that the child has been conceived naturally, denies information to those who might be thought to have a legitimate interest in such knowledge. Secrecy deceives family members about their ties with close relatives and can undermine the trust on which family relationships are presumed to be founded. This deception may be carried out with the intentions of sparing the couple, the child, and other relatives the distress which disclosure may cause. However, when viewed from the perspective of the persons being deceived, such behaviour is likely to be seen quite differently; they usually feel wronged and let down. The belief that it is better not to acknowledge treatment, but to pretend to everyone that the pregnancy has occurred naturally, can also carry implications that recourse to donor insemination is in some way shameful and should therefore be denied.

It is encouraging that some couples are now willing to be more open with significant others about their recourse to donor insemination. Recent legislative changes which enable the child to be registered legally as the child of the couple have contributed to this willingness. But other factors influencing the couple not to acknowledge their recourse to such treatment remain. The stigma which surrounds male infertility, and the still-controversial nature of the donor insemination process itself, operate to make the couple hesitant about the reactions of others. It is hoped that a more favourable climate of understanding about donor insemination can be fostered among society in general. Couples are also understandably uncertain about the reaction of their child were he/she to be told of the manner of his/her conception. Preliminary studies indicate that children do not react adversely to such knowledge when they are told in a planned and purposeful way (19). But more research into ways of telling children, and of their reactions, is urgently needed. It would be fatuous to assume that all children will react positively and that problems will never arise as a result of greater openness about the children's origins. What does seem clear, however, is that children who are not told are in danger of finding out accidentally. Even couples who assert that they have told no-one often will qualify this statement by agreeing that they have, in fact, confided in at least one other person. It is extremely difficult to keep secrets secure for a lifetime and children who learn accidentally of their origins are much more likely to be damaged by such a revelation than are children who are told purposively.

When considering treatment options the specialism of infertility treatment shares with the specialism of obstetrics the problem that there is not one patient but two to be considered in any decision which is made. The best interests of the mother, or the couple, must be balanced against the best interests of the child. In certain instances these interests conflict and cannot both be met in full. Assisted conception techniques which make use of donor gametes open up new possibilities for solving the problem of couples who are faced with childlessness. However, in solving the couple's problem by the use of donor gametes, some burdens are inevitably placed on the shoulders of the child. The child will be born into a situation where one or other (or perhaps both) nurturing parent is not that child's genetic parent. This is an abnormal situation which holds the potential to cause distress to the child.

However carefully and skilfully the situation is dealt with the child is at some risk of experiencing psychological disturbance. While it is to be hoped that the majority of children will find little difficulty in coping with such a situation it is inevitable that not all will do so. Further research into the outcome of the new infertility treatments in terms of the child so produced is urgently needed. This research should not be directed solely at the physical and developmental outcomes for these children; implications for their social and psychological well-being within a family setting must also be investigated.

REFERENCES

1. Hull, M. G. R. 1986. Infertility: nature and extent of the problem. *In* Bock, G. and O'Connor, M. (Eds) *Human embryo research: yes or NO?* Ciba Foundation. Tavistock Publications, London.
2. Payne, J. 1978. Talking about children: an examination of accounts about reproduction and family life. *Journal of Biosocial Science* 10(4): 367–374.
3. Snowden, R. and Snowden, E. 1984. *The gift of a child.* George Allen & Unwin, London.
4. *Sixth report of the Interim Licensing Authority for Human In-vitro Fertilization and Embryology.* 1991. P. 12. London.
5. Lindahl, M. W. and Back, K. W. 1987. Lineage identity and generational continuity; family history and family reunions. *Comparative gerontology, B,* 1: 30–34.
6. Human Fertilization and Embryology Act. 1991. Section 13(6) and Schedule 3.
7. Human Fertilization and Embryology Act. 1990. Section 13(5) and Schedule 3.
8. Human Fertilization and Embryology Authority. 1991. Code of Practice, para. 3.3 (p. 3i).
9. Gillon, R. 1985. *Philosophical medical ethics,* pp. 56–57. John Wiley & Sons, Chichester.
10. Matthews, C. D. 1980. Artificial insemination—donor and husband. Pp. 260–281, *in* Pepperell, R. J. (Ed.) *The infertile couple.* Churchill Livingstone, London.
11. Report of the King's Fund Centre. 1991. *Counselling for regulated infertility treatments,* p. 5. London.

12. Reading, A. E. and Kerin, J. 1989. Psychologic aspects of providing infertility services. *Journal of Reproductive Medicine* **34**(11): 861–871.
13. Daniels, K. R. 1986. Psychological issues associated with being a semen donor. *Clinical Reproduction and Fertility* **4**: 341–351.
14. Finch, L. 1988. Implications for the donor (unpublished paper). Conference on Egg Donation, Interim Licensing Authority, King's Fund Centre, London.
15. Human Fertilization and Embryology Authority. 1991. Code of Practice, Paragraph 4.41, (p.4.ii).
16. Haimes, E. V. 1990. *Family connections: the management of biological origins in the new reproductive technologies.* PhD thesis, University of Newcastle-upon-Tyne, pp. 126–127.
17. McWhinnie, A. M. 1988. The child, the family and society. Pp. 11–15, *in* Bruce, N. (Ed.) *Truth and the child.* Family Care, 21 Castle Street, Edinburgh.
18. Lusk, T. 1988. The importance to children of having knowledge about their parents. Pp. 16–18, *in* Bruce, N. (Ed.) *Truth and the child.* Family care, 21 Castle Street, Edinburgh.
19. Snowden, R., Mitchell, G. D. and Snowden, E. M. 1983. *Artificial reproduction: a social investigation.* George Allen & Unwin, London.

Editor's note For a chapter complementary to this one, see also Chapter 84 in this volume.

53

Ethical Dilemmas around the Time of Birth

ANDREW WHITELAW, MD, FRCP

Associate Professor of Neonatology, National Hospital, Oslo, Norway

MARIANNE THORESEN, MD, PHD

Neonatal Research Fellow, National Hospital, Oslo, Norway

Doctors and nurses working in neonatal intensive care units frequently have to decide whether it is right to start, continue or stop life support to a newborn infant in critical condition. In one London hospital such a dilemma was faced, on average, every month (1). The decision as to whether to start resuscitation usually has to be made very rapidly, but the decision to discontinue life support may require days or weeks of assessment and discussion. In Britain and in Norway the responsibility for these decisions is usually taken by the senior medical staff with the agreement of the parents and nursing staff.

Ethics as presented by philosophers have made relatively little impact on neonatologists, nurses or parents. The communication gap was illustrated for us by a lecture audience of neonatal nurses who were outraged and mystified by a philosopher telling them that it was ethically acceptable to let some infants die because babies were not 'persons'. The purpose of this chapter is to consider the three commonest types of ethical dilemma in neonatal medicine:

1. The very immature infant born before 26 weeks gestation.
2. The infant who has acquired severe neurological damage.
3. The infant born with severe congenital malformations.

We shall describe, from our own experience, the kind of principles and arguments actually used when the infants have been considered. In addition we shall discuss the application of the four ethical principles: respect for autonomy, beneficence, non-maleficence, and justice.

Principles of Health Care Ethics. Edited by Raanan Gillon.
© 1994 John Wiley & Sons Ltd

THE PRINCIPLES OF OUR OWN PRACTICE

1. The first requirement has been accurate diagnosis and detailed assessment of prognosis based on up-to-date information.
2. We have found it hard to improve on the golden rule of always treating others as we would like them to treat us (2). Is there a realistic chance of giving the infant an active and happy life to experience love, touch, communication, beauty, humour and the pleasures of good food and drink?
3. As responsible clinicians, our treatment of patients has had to be compatible with the law and public opinion.

THE VERY IMMATURE INFANT UNDER 26 WEEKS GESTATION

Chances of Survival

Developments in mechanical ventilation, intravenous nutrition, drug therapy, physiological monitoring and blood product transfusion have made it possible to achieve survival rates (not just for the first week but actually to go home) of up to 64% at 25 weeks gestation, up to 39% at 24 weeks and up to 14% at 23 weeks gestation (3). This has been achieved in selected patients at university hospitals with concentration of dedicated staff and equipment. When whole populations have been surveyed, survival has been lower, for example 14.6% at 25 weeks in Holland and no survivors at 24 and 23 weeks (3). A recent very large survey in the US reported 5% survival to 28 days at 23 weeks gestation but 36% survival at 24 weeks (4).

Chances of Impaired Survival

A major worry has been the high frequency of major impairments in survivors below 26 weeks. In Liverpool, for example, 45% of survivors at 25 weeks were impaired, e.g. cerebral palsy, visual loss, hearing loss, epilepsy or developmental delay, with 25% having multiple impairments (3). Large neonatal centres in North America, Australia and Europe have consistently reported major disability rates well above 10% in the survivors below 26 weeks. Periventricular leukomalacia (ischaemic injury to the white matter), intraventricular haemorrhage with parenchymal involvement, post-haemorrhagic hydrocephalus and retinopathy of prematurity are major pathologies leading to impairment in this age group.

Cost of Survival

The economic cost of survival for these infants is large. As virtually every organ system in the body is immature, many weeks of life support are often required. One study in Cleveland, Ohio, in the 1980s, reviewed infants weighing less than 750 g (roughly equivalent to less than 26 weeks) and found the average cost to be US$ 158 800 (range $72 110 to $524 110) (5). When one considers that more than 10% of the survivors will have serious disability requiring long-term therapy and support, and that a significant number of the mothers are young, unsupported, and socially disadvantaged, one can appreciate that society, as well as the family, is paying a very high price for the survival of each of these infants.

Orientation of the Mother

We try to talk to the mother before she gives birth at 23, 24 or 25 weeks to inform her of the prognosis and treatment possibilities, and hear her attitudes and wishes. The position of a well-educated, married, 39-year-old woman who has undergone 10 years of infertility and has finally become pregnant with twins after *in vitro* fertilization (IVF) is very different from that of a 17-year-old who becomes pregnant while under the influence of drugs at a party, and who wants an abortion but discovers she is pregnant too late for termination. For the 39-year-old it will probably be her last chance to have a baby. She may be willing to accept any burden to have a surviving child to love and care for. A child with cerebral palsy or visual loss may thus benefit from having a family with both personal and material resources. The 17-year-old may feel herself not ready to take on the role of mother, and may have few personal or material resources, particularly if she is not supported by the father, who may be equally young.

Assessment of the Infant at Delivery

It has been our policy to have at least one paediatrician present at the birth, with sufficient experience to assess the infant and carry out resuscitation. The obstetric estimation of maturity can be significantly wrong, especially if the mother has not had an early antenatal examination. On the other hand, after IVF the maturity is known with absolute certainty. If the infant appears to be very immature (less than 24 weeks) with transparent red, almost jelly-like, skin and in very poor condition from asphyxia, infection or birth trauma with no sustained breathing and only a slow heart rate, all cases have died within a few days even with maximum treatment. Thus we do not resuscitate.

If, however, the infant appears to have some vitality in terms of spontaneous movements or efforts to breathe, then full support is given and the response carefully monitored. Nearly always is it necessary to intubate the trachea and mechanically ventilate. Having started treatment it must be whole-hearted, but there is always the option of withdrawing intensive care if circumstances change greatly. Much will depend on whether the baby develops the complications: respiratory distress syndrome, pneumothorax, intraventricular haemorrhage, septicaemia, necrotizing enterocolitis or bronchopulmonary dysplasia, as they have a major influence on survival and long-term morbidity. Knowledge is constantly advancing. The use of surfactant therapy and better treatment for chronic lung disease may improve the outlook even further at this low gestation. We have not discontinued support on grounds of severe lung disease, as we do not feel that we can predict early which infants will ultimately develop fatal chronic lung disease.

THE INFANT WHO HAS ACQUIRED SEVERE NEUROLOGICAL DAMAGE

Preterm Infants

Among preterm infants intraventricular haemorrhage and periventricular leuko-malacia are the two most important processes leading to neurological disability. It is important to stress that an accurate prognosis can be reached only after careful and repeated assessment using clinical examination, high-frequency cranial ultrasound and, in some cases, neurophysiological studies, particularly EEG.

Intraventricular Haemorrhage

Intraventricular haemorrhage, even if large, may not involve the brain parenchyma and thus may have a very good prognosis, if hydrocephalus does not follow. However, a parenchymal echodensity on ultrasound may indicate infarction as 'extension' from a haemorrhage (grade 4 intraventricular haemorrhage). Many infants with intraventricular haemorrhage, complicated by unilateral parenchymal extension, have gone on to good overall function with normal intelligence despite having hemiplegia (6).

Periventricular Leukomalacia (PVL)

Extensive bilaterial cystic PVL has a very bad prognosis with virtually 100% cerebral palsy rate but, in addition, many of the infants have mental retardation, blindness and epilepsy (6). Children who have survived with severe PVL are amongst the most pitiful and joyless we have seen, and several sets of parents have said that, had they known what would happen, they would have asked the doctors to stop intensive care early on. Our policy has been to advise against intensive care life support for babies with extensive bilateral cystic periventricular leukomalacia.

Full-term Infants with Birth Asphyxia

Despite advances in obstetrics a small number of infants continue to develop brain damage after fetal hypoxia. In spite of immediate intubation, mechanical ventilation, correction of hypovolaemia, acidosis and hypoglycaemia, a minority go on to develop encephalopathy with convulsions and altered tone and consciousness. Intensive care can result in the survival of some infants who will later go on to develop spastic quadriplegia, microcephaly, mental retardation, blindness and epilepsy.

Assessment of Prognosis

It is possible to assess prognosis at various stages. For example, full-term infants who fail to establish spontaneous respiration, despite resuscitation, within 30 minutes have a 100% chance of developing severe cerebral palsy and mental retardation if they survive (7). Thus it is common practice to stop active resuscitation if an infant has not started to breathe after 30 minutes. Clinical and neurophysiological assessments of the encephalopathy give help with the prognosis. Several days of deep coma with absent brainstem reflexes and persistent seizures on EEG with a flat background are predictive of severe handicap or death (8). In such cases we have advised against further intensive care life support.

INFANTS WITH SEVERE CONGENITAL MALFORMATIONS

Down's Syndrome

In Britain during the 1970s it was common for infants with Down's syndrome and duodenal atresia not to receive life-saving surgery, but to be sedated to relieve suffering until they died from dehydration or aspiration. This was, of course, carried out only in cases where the family and all the nursing staff agreed. This was done in the belief that life with Down's syndrome was so meaningless and limited that it was not being 'kind' to the infant to go through the discomfort of surgery in order to survive. The burden of care on the family, in some cases, influenced the decision. Attitudes have changed. Individuals with Down's syndrome are now much more part of the community, and it is clear to most people that a child with Down's can experience love and most of what goes to make up 'happiness' even if full independence and a long lifespan are not achieved. If a Down's syndrome baby in the 1990s has duodenal atresia alone with no cardiac abnormality, there is rarely any argument about whether the duodenal atresia should be operated. The attitude now is that the child should not be denied a chance of happiness for want of a simple operation.

Legal Precedents in England

This change in attitude was influenced by legal cases. In 1981, in London, the parents of an infant with Down's syndrome and duodenal atresia decided against surgery. Through the action of the local authority social services, the Court of Appeal eventually ordered that she have the operation, and this was carried out against her parents' wishes. She was then cared for by a foster family. Another infant with Down's syndrome, but no clinical evidence of a life-threatening abnormality, was rejected by the parents. Dihydrocodeine was prescribed in repeated doses, and the infant died after three days. The paediatrician was tried for attempted murder and, although he was acquitted, many paediatricians believe this was largely because severe life-threatening pathology was discovered at autopsy. Thus the law in England has taken the view that the handicap of Down's syndrome is not sufficient reason for allowing a baby to die with no attempt at life-saving treatment.

Legal Precedent in the USA

In the USA, law and government have been more closely involved with these decisions. In 1983, following the death without surgery of 'Baby Doe', who had Down's syndrome and tracheo-oesophageal fistula, in Bloomington, Indiana, a national outcry prompted a federal directive that infants were not to be discriminated against because of handicap. Any hospital found to be denying customary medical care to a handicapped infant could have federal funding withdrawn.

A later federal ruling allowed doctors to exercise 'reasonable medical judgement' in deciding which treatments would ameliorate the baby's condition. The regulation (9) acknowledged that withholding treatment was not neglect if:

1. the infant was chronically and irreversibly comatose;
2. the provision of such treatment would merely prolong dying;
3. the provision of such treatment would be virtually futile in terms of the survival of the infant.

Spina Bifida and Hydrocephalus

Selective surgical treatment has also been advocated by Professor John Lorber for newborns with spina bifida and hydrocephalus, the unoperated infants generally receiving sedation and having a short survival (10). Lorber's criteria have come in for criticism as a more positive attitude to rehabilitation of children with spina bifida has developed. Although some infants with spina bifida, hydrocephalus and other malformations are not actively treated nowadays, many paediatricians and paediatric surgeons ignore Lorber's criteria, and treat actively virtually every case, as the prospects for an independent and happy life are better than previously thought.

Trisomy 18

While Down's syndrome babies generally receive active treatment, this is not the case in more severe chromosome disorders. Professor David Smith, one of the fathers of the study of malformations, advised that infants with Edwards' syndrome (trisomy 18) should not receive surgery or intensive care life-support (11). This advice was based on the observation that all such infants have serious heart defects, are severely mentally retarded and 90% die before 12 months of age. This policy is still generally applied. Because Edwards' syndrome may be recognized with considerable confidence in the delivery room, discussion and decision-making can begin before the chromosome results arrive days later. The perception is that the life of babies with trisomy 18 is so limited and joyless that prolonging life is not prolonging happiness. Surgery, on the other hand, undoubtedly causes some pain. Some time ago we diagnosed a baby as having both trisomy 18 and tracheo-oesophageal fistula (TOF) on the day of birth. Using Smith's argument, it was felt by the nursing and medical staff that it was inappropriate to carry out the necessary surgery for TOF, which is considerably more complicated than that required for duodenal atresia. The infant required the mouth and pharynx to be suctioned continuously to prevent saliva from obstructing her breathing, but she did not require mechanical ventilation. She also had a serious heart defect. Her parents were Roman Catholics and we wondered what their reaction would be to our medical view that curative treatment was not possible, and neither surgery nor intensive care was indicated. They did not take the view that all life was sacred and to be preserved at all costs. Their concern was to prevent unnecessary suffering. They understood and agreed to our policy of not using intravenous feeding. Furthermore, it was agreed that if suctioning her pharynx and comforting her in the normal way, by stroking and holding her, did not relieve distress, she could be given morphine. She did receive one dose of morphine and died within two days.

There are a number of congenital malformations and syndromes which have a hopeless prognosis but some are beginning to move from the hopeless to the treatable category with advances in therapy (for example hypoplastic left heart). A decision to withdraw life support must be made on a certain diagnosis with the most up-to-date information on treatment and prognosis.

Werdnig Hoffmann Disease

A floppy infant, respirator-dependent from soon after birth, was investigated for congenital neuromuscular disorders and found by clinical examination, nerve conduction, electromyography and muscle biopsy to have the severe infantile form of spinal muscular atrophy (Werdnig Hoffmann disease). Experience is totally consistent that improvement does not occur in this situation. After a number of unsuccessful attempts at weaning him from the ventilator over a period of two months, it was the feeling of the parents, doctors and nursing staff that the discomfort of mechanical ventilation should stop. He was unable to move a muscle against gravity but had wide alert eyes and an expressive face. It was felt that to be disconnected from the ventilator and gradually suffocate while conscious would be very unpleasant for him. A generous intravenous dose of morphine was given before he was extubated, and he died apparently without suffering.

Thanatophoric Dwarfism

We recently investigated a newborn with short limbs, a small chest and ventilator dependence. After carefully reviewing the clinical features and radiographs with genetic and radiological colleagues, the diagnosis of thanatophoric dwarfism was agreed on. This has a hopeless prognosis for survival without ventilator support, and he was extubated after a dose of morphine.

APPLICATION OF THE FOUR ETHICAL PRINCIPLES

Beneficence

The ethical principle of beneficence, or doing good, is very close to our interpretation of the golden rule: always treat others as you would like them to treat you. If it is realistic to make a real improvement and allow a little more happiness to that individual, it should be done. Applying the principle of beneficence, then clearly, from the baby's point of view, a chance (although small) of healthy survival to enjoy a normal life is better than no chance at all. Thus every effort should be made to save a potentially normal child such as a 25-week premature, even with a high risk of hemiplegic cerebral palsy from a unilateral parenchymal haemorrhagic infarct, but good prospects for intelligence. The life of children with extensive bilateral cystic PVL is so limited that one can question how much joy remains. Prolonged crying, irritability and feeding difficulties are the rule. This early phase is then often replaced by loss of vision and fits at about six months of age. Tight tendons, limb and spinal deformities then follow unless active physiotherapy and splinting are used.

Non-maleficence

If one applies the principle of non-maleficence, or not causing harm, one can appreciate that prolonged intensive care and intravenous nutrition involves suffering from innumerable re-intubations of the trachea, venous and arterial punctures, not to mention pleural drains, lumbar punctures and surgery in some cases, as well as relative isolation from normal close family contact. This is the argument used against the prolonged intensive care or surgery for babies with trisomy 18, extensive cystic PVL, thanatophoric dwarfism, or a 23-week infant. What of the mother? Should a 16-year-old uneducated girl be burdened with the responsibility of a multiply impaired child when she should herself be going to school and growing up? Are her prospects for education and independence being damaged by the survival of an unplanned and handicapped child?

Respect for Autonomy

Respect for autonomy is difficult to apply to a 23-week infant, or indeed any neonate. We would replace the term with 'respect for a fellow human being'. Clearly the infant has no way of expressing his/her decisions. In this respect he or she is different from an older child or adult who has experience of life, knows something of the meaning of survival and of pain, and can weigh up two sides of a decision. The middle-aged man with acute myeloblastic leukaemia who decides not to go through with chemotherapy and possible bone marrow transplantation is able to consider the alternatives. The newborn infant cannot. Is it possible to imagine what goes on in the mind of such an infant? The will to survive seems to be a basic characteristic of all mammals and, in addition, even infants of 23 weeks are capable of showing pain and stress. What of respect for the autonomy of the parents? Does it mean that the parents should have the sole right to decide on starting or stopping intensive care? It is the parents who will have to live with the consequences in a way that the medical and nursing staff will not.

Justice

Parents' Right to Decide

One of the universal human rights is the right to life, i.e. not to be unjustly killed. The parents' right to decide about their child is not absolute. Refusing necessary medical treatment for a child can be justification for the law to intervene and take away the rights of the parents. Parents may not, in most countries, refuse life-saving blood transfusion to their child on religious grounds. The same principle applies to any other life-saving treatment including mechanical ventilation and surgery. The statistics on non-accidental injury and sexual abuse indicate that parents' wishes for their children are not necessarily always in the child's best interest. The parents' wishes have to make sense looked at from the child's point of view.

Discussion Between Parents and Doctors on Withdrawal of Life Support

It is vital that the parents have the opportunity to voice their feelings about the treatment of their child. A decision to withdraw treatment has to be unanimous among the doctors and nurses concerned with the infant. This medical assessment can then be presented to the parents. The discussion with the parents should not take the form of 'Do you want treatment stopped so that your baby will die?' Rather, the whole medical history, the infant's current status and the prognosis should be explained. The pain and fear associated with continued intensive care can be pointed out if the infant is conscious. It can be suggested that intensive care is not restoring health but merely prolonging an uncomfortable life or postponing death. Since the intensive treatment is ineffective, the medical decision is to stop the intensive treatment and change to relief of suffering. The doctor should then listen to the parents' response. In most cases they indicate understanding and acceptance of the medical assessment with the doctors taking responsibility. If the baby is on a ventilator, the endotracheal tube and most of the monitoring and intravenous equipment can be removed and the parents can then hold the baby in their arms.

Morphine to Relieve Terminal Distress

Once the decision to extubate and relieve suffering has been taken, one can consider whether morphine should be given to relieve distress in a conscious infant dying of respiratory failure. Morphine does have a respiratory depressant effect in large doses, and thus may shorten the process of dying. We have not used muscle-relaxant drugs in this situation and it would be quite illogical to use one on its own as they leave the patient fully conscious but paralysed. It is obvious that the whole process of assessment and unanimous decision-making must be completed before one gives morphine and then extubates. Everyone must be quite clear that the morphine is being given to relieve suffering in a patient who is dying from natural causes.

Parents' Insistence on Continued Life Support

If the parents do not want treatment stopped, it should be continued while further investigation and discussion take place. Even if the medical staff think the prognosis so poor that they do not advise continued active treatment, if the parents wish to take responsibility for the care of a mentally retarded quadriplegic child at home, they must be allowed to do so. It is their child. Such children do not always tear the family apart, but may indeed act as a focus of love and caring. We have been humbled by seeing the occasional families who have shown us that life can be meaningful even with devastating cerebral damage.

Justice in Allocation of Resources

The concept of justice also includes proper allocation of benefits and burdens. Should one child be entitled to very expensive medical treatment when health care resources are limited and the same amount of money could be used to benefit many more individuals, e.g. by hip replacement or preventing and treating blindness in the Third World? The question of allocation of resources does not present itself in this way to the individual clinician and individual patient. If the equipment and staff are available when the child is born, the decision will be made on consideration of that individual child, regardless of the suffering of others. If, on the other hand, all available nurses and ventilators are used to full capacity, some infants will not receive intensive care however much the doctors and parents may wish it. This form of rationing has occurred for many years in the London area, with the large central regional neonatal intensive care units turning away scores of critically ill infants referred from other hospitals every year. The decision to accept or refuse cannot usually be made on the basis of medical prognosis because two infants rarely present at exactly the same time. If one has just filled one's last intensive care incubator with a 24-week infant with a poor prognosis, and is then offered a 28-week infant with a good prognosis from another hospital, one does not stop treating the first infant so that he will die quickly and so provide facilities for the second infant. Having admitted the first (24-week) infant to their unit, the doctors and nurses would feel a professional duty to provide care based on medical indications.

QUESTIONS WE HAVE TO ASK OURSELVES

Our approach to these decisions about whether to use or not use intensive care life support or surgery in newborns has generally been one of interpreting the golden rule of always treating others as we would like them to treat us, i.e. putting ourselves in the position of the individual baby. What would we want if we were lying there in the incubator, intubated and connected to a ventilator?

If there were even a small chance of achieving a happy healthy life would we not take it? If there were a good chance of surviving with a handicap that is limited (cerebral palsy of the hemiplegia or diplegia type) would we not take that chance of survival? Similarly if we have to survive with Down's syndrome would we not prefer that to death? On the other hand, if prolonged and painful treatment were necessary to achieve vegetative survival without the possibility of participating in the world, would we not refuse treatment?

The paediatrician has a crucial duty to make sure the diagnosis and prognostic information is as thorough as possible. Without that, no decision can be rationally based. Furthermore, the paediatrician's experience of children who have survived with different kinds of disability or malformation facilitates a balanced and informed discussion with the parents about how treatment decisions should be taken.

REFERENCES

1. Whitelaw, A. 1986. Death as an option in neonatal intensive care. *Lancet* **2**: 328–331.
2. St Matthew. The Sermon on the Mount. P. 13, *in New English Bible: New Testament.* Oxford University Press, Oxford (1961).
3. Cooke, R. W. I. 1988. Outcome and costs of care for the very immature infant. Pp. 1133–1151, *in* Whitelaw, A. and Cook, R. W. I. (Eds) The very immature infant less than 28 weeks gestation. *British Medical Bulletin* **44**.
4. Phelps, D. L., Brown, D. R., Tung, B., Cassady, G., McClead, R. E., Purohit, D. M. and Palmer, E. A. 1991. Twenty-eight day survival rates of 6676 neonates with birth weight of 1250 grams or less. *Pediatrics* **87**: 7–17.
5. Hack, M. and Fanaroff, A. A. 1986. Changes in the delivery room care of the extremely small infant (< 750 grams): effects on morbidity and outcome. *New England Journal of Medicine* **314**: 660–664.
6. De Vries, L. S., Dubovitz, L. M. S. Dubowitz, V. *et al.* 1986. Predictive value of cranial ultrasound in the newborn baby: a reappraisal. *Lancet* **2**: 137–140.
7. Steiner, H. and Nelligan, G. 1975. Perinatal cardiac arrest. Quality of survivors. *Archives of Disease in Childhood* **50**: 696–702.
8. Sarnat, H. B. and Sarnat, M. S. 1976. Neonatal encephalopathy following fetal distress. *Archives of Neurology* **33**: 696–705.
9. Moreno, J. D. 1987. Ethical and legal issues in the care of the impaired newborn. *Clinics in Perinatology* **14**: 345–360.
10. Lorber, J. 1972. Spina bifida cystica. Results of treatment of 270 consecutive cases with criteria for selection for the future. *Archives of Disease in Childhood* **47**: 854–873.
11. Smith, D. 1982. *Recognisable patterns of human malformation*, 3rd edn pp. 14–15. Saunders, Philadelphia.

54

All Babies Should Be Kept Alive As Far As Possible

ALISON DAVIS

INTRODUCTION

The treatment of newborn handicapped babies has been at the centre of health care ethics debates in recent years. The main arguments have been about surgical treatment for those with life-threatening conditions and/or serious disabilities, and two schools of thought have emerged; those who believe 'quality of life' decisions must dictate which babies are so treated, and those who stress the 'value of life', believing that all babies should receive treatment appropriate to their medical condition, regardless of residual disability.

The aim of this chapter is to demonstrate that disability cannot ethically be a factor in determining treatment for the newborn, and to suggest that babies with an obvious disability should be treated using the same ethical code as would be applied to any other child.

Ethical medical care constitutes a continuum from cure at one end to palliative care at the other, depending on the condition of the patient. Thus the question is not 'whether to treat' (with the implication that 'non-treatment' will mean death), but rather 'how to treat' each baby. The four *prima facie* principles of respect for autonomy, beneficence, non-maleficence and justice may be difficult to apply directly to the newborn, since others will always have to make decisions on their behalf. However, it is possible to develop a code of practice whereby the principles can be exercised on behalf of babies and others incapable of expressing consent. I suggest that this can best be done by assessing 'beneficence' on the basis of one positive and one negative obligation—namely the positive duty to protect life, and the negative duty not directly to destroy or injure life.

I will concentrate on the questions most frequently before the public eye—the treatment of babies with Down's syndrome and spina bifida—to demonstrate these principles in practice. My contention is that every baby, however handicapped and however rejected by the parents, is of infinite value and worth,

Principles of Health Care Ethics. Edited by Raanan Gillon.
© 1994 John Wiley & Sons Ltd

and that residual handicap is not in itself a reason to deny life-saving or life-enhancing surgery. Life is 'a good' which ought to be protected, and 'quality of life' decisions made by able-bodied people on behalf of handicapped newborns have no place in rigorous ethical thought.

This does not mean that I am advocating futile treatment, given in a vain attempt to prolong the act of dying. Rather, I am suggesting that dying handicapped babies be treated in the same way as would be ethical for dying adults—that once it has been established that continued aggressive surgical or medical treatment is futile, palliative care must be substituted. 'Allowing the dying to die' must never mean, however, that doctors, in the name of 'beneficence', institute treatment regimens the purpose of which is to hasten death. Neither must it mean that they may cause the deaths of babies who are *not* actually dying. Decisions about who is irremediably dying are the proper realm of medical ethics. Decisions about who is 'worth saving' are not. Death-conducing decisions masquerading as 'beneficence' are unequivocally unethical, and are counter-productive to the human rights and dignity of all vulnerable people.

WHAT VALUE DOES HUMAN LIFE HAVE?

It is impossible to consider questions about appropriate treatment for newborn babies, handicapped or not, before first defining what actually constitutes human life, and then committing oneself to one of two mutually exclusive positions:

1. that human life has intrinsic, infinite value;
2. that human life should be valued primarily for its instrumentality (i.e. that its value lies only in what it enables its possessor to do, or in the status accorded to it by some significant other).

I define 'human being' as meaning any living, genetically human individual from the moment of conception to the moment of brainstem death. That any such being is both 'living' and 'human' is indisputable. What has been disputed however, is the value such life has.

The view currently in the ascendancy is that human life without 'relevant capacities' is valueless. According to the Australian philosopher Michael Tooley, this means that 'an organism possesses a serious right to life only if it possesses the concept of a self as a continuing subject of experiences and mental states, and believes that it is itself such a continuing entity' (1). Jonathan Glover derives from this argument the conclusion that 'questions about killing should be decided by considering the autonomy of the person whose life is at stake, the extent to which his life is worth living, and the effect of any decisions on other people' (2). This kind of philosophy leads inexorably to the conclusion of Peter Singer and Helga Kuhse that 'some infants with severe disabilities should be killed' (3).

Those who share the utilitarian view, and value human life only in instrumental or relative terms, regard *any* newborn child as less valuable than an adult, because newborns are incapable of acting autonomously, and are presumed to have no concept of the self; yet it is interesting to note that they use this argument only to justify killing those with disabilities. The basis on which this judgement is made is always that handicapped lives are inherently less valuable, less worth living and generally 'burdensome' to those human beings (generally the parents) deemed to be more deserving of consideration. I regard this as a false premise, which leads to prejudicial judgements about the lives of those with severe disabilities.

Peter Singer maintains that 'the greater an infant's potential for a happy and worthwhile life, the stronger the reason against killing it' (3). He claims that decisions about happiness and 'worthwhileness' can be judged on the basis of disability, an assumption which presupposes that the lives of severely disabled people are totally predictable and determined solely by their physical or mental condition, whereas those of the able-bodied (whose potential for 'happiness' is never assessed) are not. Upon closer examination it transpires that some doctors are claiming an ability to be able to assess not only the potential for happiness for handicapped babies, but also the likelihood of their achieving an independent life, employment, marriage and 'self-assurance' (4). Peter Singer goes so far as to say that mistakes in these calculations do not matter—that it is worth destroying one life he considers to be 'potentially worthwhile' in order to eliminate any number of others judged 'worthless' (3).

My own view is that such calculations are possible only if one accepts the underlying assumption that the value of a child's life can be computed on a calculus applicable to all the other values being weighed against it—i.e. only if the value of life itself is comparable to such values as bodily comfort, ease or freedom from responsibility. I do not believe that it can ethically be weighed in this way, since I regard every human life as being of infinite value. Since infinity is implicit in itself, it cannot be multiplied or divided, and thus a short life is as infinitely valuable as a long one, and a severely handicapped life is as valuable as one free from obvious disability. Any grading of human beings according to 'value' is both repugnant and highly dangerous, since once one human life is judged worthless or expendable, all are inevitably reduced from an absolute to a relative value.

Current efforts to designate the newborn handicapped as inherently less valuable than the able-bodied are morally equivalent to the Nazi ethic, as stated in the 1920 book by Karl Binding and Alfred Hoche entitled *The destruction of life devoid of value* that 'we doctors know that in the interest of the whole human organism, single less valuable members have to be abandoned and pushed out' (5). The views of more powerful individuals, be they doctors, parents or philosophers, about what constitutes a 'worthwhile life' are irrelevant to the infinite value human lives actually possess. This infinite value is inherent in being human, and is not conferred by either a particular person or by the state. As Teresa Iglesias says, 'what human beings can do is a manifestation of what they are. It is what they are that determines what they can do, not the other way about' (6).

I believe that all human beings share the right not to be deliberately killed, and that neither size nor state of health affects the infinite value of human life.

SHOULD SEVERELY HANDICAPPED BABIES BE REGARDED AS HAVING 'MERE BIOLOGICAL EXISTENCE' OR AS BEING 'PERSONS WITH RIGHTS'?

As we have seen, opinions vary as to whether severely handicapped infants have infinite value, no value at all, or a value relative to the opinions of certain others. An additional argument hinges around the question of 'personhood' as opposed to 'humanity', with certain philosophers suggesting that the newborn handicapped, though undeniably alive, are not 'persons' and thus need not be granted the rights reserved for human beings thus designated.

Singer, Kuhse and Tooley believe that rights are dependent upon an individual having a concept of the self, and of being the subject of experiences and desires. It is this same belief which leads Glover to say 'a defective baby is better replaced by a later normal one, as a more worthwhile life is the result' (2). This view, in effect, gives handicapped babies less than 'no value at all'—a negative value, in which a non-existent potential life has greater value than the actual life of the handicapped child.

Although utilitarian philosophers assume that 'persons with rights' must possess certain qualities, it is a matter of subjective judgement whether or not babies have such qualities, and whether the presence of a disability should affect their treatment. The very concept of, for example, 'self-determination' (one of a number of arbitrary terms, like autonomy or rationality, which are used to assess 'personhood') involves not just an actual act of such determination, but also the nature which provides the potential for the act—human nature. As Jenny Teichman says, 'one can have a rational nature even if one happens to be quite irrational . . . this does not appear to me to be any more intrinsically problematic than the idea that all cattle are mammals, even the bulls' (7).

Babies certainly do have *some* concept of self and *some* desires for the future. They cry when hungry, expecting the result to be satisfaction of that hunger; and if this is 'mere instinct' then so too are our own appetites and desires for food, from cordon bleu cookery competitions to the appalling consequences of unsatisfied hunger in Africa.

The implications of distinguishing between 'life with rights' and 'biological existence without rights' become clear when one considers statements like that made by Francis Crick, joint Nobel prizewinner for the discovery of the double helix of DNA, who said 'no newborn infant should be declared human until it has passed certain tests regarding its genetic endowment, and if it fails those tests it forfeits the right to live' (8). This view accords perfectly with that of Peter Singer, who believes that killing a 'defective' infant is not only not equivalent to killing a person, but not actually wrong at all.

My own view is that 'human being' and 'person' are interchangeable terms, and that no qualifications other than belonging to the human race are necessary for an individual to enjoy the basic right not to be killed. In the past many marginalized people have been declared 'non-persons' in order to justify denying them the full benefits of personhood; for instance slaves, Jews, women, any 'enemy' in any war. It seems quite ironic that systems discriminatory to some oppressed groups, for instance the apartheid system in South Africa, are being dismantled at the very time when fatal discrimination against those with disabilities is being justified and even praised.

'Human rights' only have any real meaning when they are universally applied to all human beings, while 'personhood' is simply a linguistic fiction designed only to enable those perceived as undesirable to be swiftly and efficiently dispatched. Denying rights to those who are weak and vulnerable is not merely the beginning of a 'slippery slope'; it is a judgement which ultimately condemns the whole human race to oblivion.

HOW SHOULD NEWBORN HANDICAPPED BABIES BE TREATED?

It is likely that neonatal killing of the handicapped has always gone on to some extent, often under the guise of 'stillbirth', but it is only in relatively recent years that the philosophy underlying the practice—that the handicapped are better eliminated—has been overtly stated. The most stark and uncompromising statement of this view was during the period of the German Third Reich, when 70 000 mentally and/or physically handicapped people were killed at six clinics, with the pretence that it was simply granting them a 'merciful release'. The attempt to project this practice as benevolent was clearly belied by Dr Arthur Guelt, Director of Public Health, who stated (in 1935) that 'the ill-conceived "love of neighbour" has to disappear, especially in relation to inferior or asocial creatures. It is the supreme duty of the state to grant life and livelihood only to the healthy' (9). The current mask of beneficence which doctors use to justify killing the newborn handicapped (i.e. Dr Garrow of High Wycombe Hospital called the killing of a spina bifida baby 'the loving thing to do' (10)) is equally belied by the evidence, which reveals many examples of deliberate killing by doctors using eugenic or economic arguments, or both, to justify their actions.

The 1967 Abortion Act, under which the unborn lost their right to protection from harm, really provided a turning point in attitudes to the very young, because it enshrined in law the concept that the weakest human beings have relative, not absolute, value. Since that time eugenic attitudes have become increasingly prominent, and there is no doubt that the 1990 ruling to allow abortion up to the moment of birth on grounds of fetal disability (contained in the Human Fertilization and Embryology Act) will contribute to an increasing disregard for the value of handicapped lives.

Neonatal killing of the handicapped is often described as allowing babies to die', though if any group other than the handicapped were being so treated it would undoubtedly be termed 'murder'. Rationalizations of the practice include claims that it removes a burden on society and the family, and that it is 'kinder' for the child, the assumption always being that life with a disability is 'intolerable'. Two main groups of infants have been affected by these decisions:

1. Those with Down's syndrome who have an additional condition which would be lethal if left untreated.
2. Those with spina bifida, where an operation would reduce disability, but would not normally be necessary to save life.

For the first group of babies there are two main treatment options: (a) to operate, as would be done routinely in the case of a non-handicapped baby with the same potentially lethal condition, or (b) to refuse surgery, which would eventually result in the death of the child. For the second group the two options would be (a) to operate to reduce the disability and minimize the chance of infection if the baby's general condition was such that this could be achieved, or (b) not to operate which, contrary to popular opinion, would *not* necessarily result in the death of the child. In the case of both groups in recent years an additional 'option' has been gaining ground; sedation of those 'selected' to receive no operation, and giving them only water instead of milk, to ensure an early death.

Professor John Lorber of Sheffield has been among the most outspoken of many doctors who have claimed the right not just to make medical decisions about handicapped lives, but to make an additional moral judgement that those not actively treated should die. He says 'the main object of selection is not to avoid treating those who would survive with severe handicaps ... there are babies we do not operate on because we want the babies dead; that is absolutely clear' (11). An anonymous letter in *The Lancet* explained how such deaths would be brought about, saying that the babies would be given 'careful and loving nursing, water sufficient to satisfy thirst, and increasing doses of sedative' (12). It is often said that the parents have a 'right to choose' whether or not their child will be subjected to this, but again it is only ever viewed as an ethical choice when the child is handicapped. In such cases the child is seen as a threat to the parents' well-being, rather than as a person in his own right, and the death may be referred to as 'letting nature take its course', even though the whole point of medicine as a discipline is to prevent nature taking its course.

It is interesting to note that all such decisions ultimately hinge on a negative value judgement about the lives of disabled people. In this respect a distinction is very often made (for instance in the 1988 BMA Euthanasia Report) that while people with a handicap acquired later in life can be rehabilitated and enabled to live fulfilling lives, the congenitally handicapped are substantively different and may be viewed as dispensable because of 'the harm that many such infants do to the families into which they are born and the often blighted and miserable lives which they lead' (13). It is difficult to escape the conclusion that the reason for this discrepancy in attitude lies in the fact that it would be inconsistent for doctors to have a positive attitude to handicapped newborns, while simultaneously supporting the option of abortion for similarly handicapped unborn children.

Such distinctions only serve to highlight the fact that inconsistency and moral action are incompatible. The view that human lives are of infinite value, which I suggest *is* both consistent and moral, dictates that all babies, whether or not their condition permits a life-saving or life-enhancing operation, should be fed, nurtured and loved, even if their lives will be very short. Babies with Down's syndrome are entitled to the same treatment as would be given to a non-handicapped child, while in the case of spina bifida, operations should be done at the optimum time for each child to minimize the disability and maximize life chances. Those for whom an operation is not immediately appropriate should be cared for at home, if possible, and given an operation later if their condition permits it. None should be deliberately killed.

Assessing 'potential misery' is impossible, as quickly becomes apparent if one imagines trying to make the same assessment for a non-handicapped child. In any case, much of the 'misery' associated with congenital handicap is caused not by the disabling conditions themselves but by the attitudes prevalent in a society which would demonstrably rather kill the disabled than care for them. If people with disabilities are ever to achieve equal status with the able-bodied, they must begin to be seen as whole people with the same infinite value as everyone else, not merely as collections of malfunctioning body parts.

If handicapped babies are 'persons'—as I believe they are—then the degree of handicap, or the presence or absence of loving parents, makes no difference to their right to be treated in the same manner as other 'persons'. Anecdotal evidence of 'miserable lives' lived by disabled people cannot justly be extrapolated to the whole disabled community, since no finite number of observations can logically entail a universal conclusion; neither can arbitrary distinctions between congenital and acquired disability be logically sustained. In fact, what evidence there is points to the opposite conclusion—that most people with disabilities value their lives, and would *not* rather be dead.

We have a clear moral duty to respect the value of life, rather than attempting to establish a sliding scale of human worth. In other words we need first to establish what is the morally correct way to treat human persons, and then act upon those principles with respect to *all* human beings.

As Dr Richard Cook says, 'Sedation and starvation, though apparently based on compassion, not only denies the unique and unpredictable value of human life, but fails to recognise that real love cannot run counter to moral principles' (14).

TREATMENT DECISIONS MADE ABOUT HANDICAPPED NEWBORNS

The British Medical Association's *Handbook on medical ethics* (1982) states that 'a decision by society that an individual either against his will or without his consent should have his life terminated is totally abhorrent to the medical profession'. However, the practice of selecting some handicapped newborns for death is commonly occurring despite this apparent prohibition. A consideration of decisions made on behalf of babies with Down's syndrome and spina bifida (the two most common immediately apparent congenital disabilities), as well as for those with multiple handicaps, will suffice to make the facts clear.

In the case of Down's syndrome, decisions have been inconsistent, indicative of the fact that the treatment such babies receive depends more on the views of doctors and parents about the value of their lives than on their actual medical condition.

In 1981 Baby Alexandra was born with Down's syndrome and an intestinal obstruction which would have been surgically treated as a matter of routine for a non-handicapped baby. Her parents initially rejected her, and refused the necessary surgery. However, the director of her local social services department took the case to court, where the operation was approved. Alexandra recovered and, interestingly, was subsequently accepted by her parents.

Later in 1981, however, Dr Leonard Arthur was brought to court accused of murdering his patient John Pearson—a Down's syndrome baby who was apparently in good health. John Pearson was also rejected by his parents, but he needed no operation to survive, and would have lived given ordinary care. Dr Arthur nevertheless put him on a course of 'treatment' which resulted in his death three days after birth. He was given water only, not milk, and the pain-killing drug DF118, which is not recommended at all for use in infants, was administered in doses sufficient to kill an adult.

Dr Arthur was eventually acquitted even of the reduced charge of 'attempted murder', which provoked comments from other 'eminent' doctors in support of his actions. Typical of these were Sir Douglas Black, President of the Royal College of Physicians, who stated that in the case of 'a child suffering from Down's syndrome and with a parental wish that it would not survive, it is ethical to terminate life', while Professor Alexander Campbell of Aberdeen said 'we believe that choices for death, whether by active or passive means, should be permitted' (15). The general conclusion seemed to be that it was unthinkable that any 'eminent doctor' could be guilty of acting unethically, regardless of the undoubted facts of the case.

Death-making decisions continue to be made about babies with Down's syndrome. Some 30% of such babies have an additional atrioventricular defect of the heart, and in 1988 Maria Hinds, a Down's syndrome baby with this defect, was declared 'inoperable' by her local hospital in Yorkshire. Her mother then took her to Toronto Children's Hospital in Canada, where 80% of the operations for this defect are done on children with Down's syndrome with a success rate of 90%. Maria had the operation and is now alive and well, but the fate of the other 300 or so Down's babies born with this defect every year in Britain is uncertain. Presumably, most of their parents are also being told that their child's condition is 'inoperable', since out of nine paediatric cardiac units in Britain only one, in Liverpool, routinely carries out atrioventricular canal defect repair on babies with Down's syndrome, although all will operate on a similarly affected non-handicapped child (16).

The other group of children most commonly subjected to selection for life or death are those with the myelomeningocele form of spina bifida. Towards the end of the 1960s a debate arose among paediatricians in Sheffield, which polarized around two men—Professor Lorber, who was in favour of 'selective treatment' on the basis of the degree of residual handicap predicted, with those not selected for active treatment being 'encouraged to die', and Professor Zachary, who favoured active treatment for all whose medical condition permitted it.

Professor Lorber's criteria for 'non-treatment' (17), based on the assumption that the lives of severely handicapped people had a negative value, were:

1. degree of paralysis,
2. presence of hydrocephalus,
3. degree of spinal curvature,
4. additional congenital abnormalities.

The clear objective for those not operated upon was, as has already been clearly seen, an early death. This philosophy, and the prejudicial view of disabled people which underpinned it, was shared and promoted by others, notably by Dr G. C. Lloyd Roberts, who said in 1972, 'At 13 [the spina bifida child] has usually reverted to a wheelchair in which he sits, obese, odiferous, acneiform and impotent, contemplating a sorry future with justifiable melancholy ... neglect, which includes the withholding of antibiotics, will usually resolve the dilemma' (18).

A letter in the *British Medical Journal* in 1990 made it clear that such 'selection' is still going on. The author, Mary Seller, suggested the future possibility (when a 'reliable anatomical prognostic indicator' was found) that the same selection criteria might be used on the unborn as well as the newborn with spina bifida (19).

Professor Zachary set out his entirely different criteria for treatment in an article in the *British Medical Journal* in 1977 (20). He divided babies with myelomeningocele into three categories, the first two of which would not receive an immediate spinal operation:

1. Those judged likely to die very soon, for whom surgery would have no bearing on whether they lived or died.
2. Those with a lesion so wide that the chances of primary healing after surgery would be small, and for whom the risk of wound breakdown was greater than the risk of no operation. For this category, simple protection of the spinal lesion was advocated.
3. Those considered to have a good chance of wound healing. Babies with some movement of the legs would receive an immediate operation to preserve muscle function, while those with no perceptible leg movement would be operated on within 24–48 hours to minimize the possibility of infection.

The main differences in approach between Professors Lorber and Zachary in fact lay in the decisions made about those *not* selected for an operation. Professor Zachary advocated giving them treatment for hydrocephalus, renal tract and orthopaedic problems with the aim of maximizing their life chances, and left open the possibility of a later spinal operation if the baby's condition improved. Professor Lorber, on the other hand, stressed the need 'not to yield to the temptation to treat hydrocephalus as [it] is an important cause of death', and death was his objective for the non-treatment group (17).

Professor Zachary explained that the babies Professor Lorber was selecting for 'non-treatment' were in fact sedated with chloral hydrate, so that they were too sleepy to cry for food, and thus starved to death. It was by using this very regimen that Dr Donald Garrow admitted killing a spina bifida baby named Louise, by 'a combination of infection which we weren't treating, dehydration and starvation' (10). Claims that spina bifida babies not operated on will die spontaneously are belied by such admissions—the truth is that they are being pushed into death by doctors who want this outcome.

More recent cases of death-making decisions have concerned multiply handicapped children. In 1989 Mr Justice Ward ruled that a hydrocephalic baby ('Baby C') should be 'treated to die' and need not be fed. This ruling was, fortunately, overturned by the Appeal Court, and Baby C was cared for until she died naturally (21).

In October 1990 the High Court ruled that 'Baby J', who was brain-damaged, paralysed and possibly deaf/blind (although uncertainty was expressed about the exact extent of his disabilities) should 'not deliberately be given life-saving treatment' because he had the prospect of only an 'intolerable existence'. In support of this judgement Dr Richard Nicholson, Editor of the *Bulletin of Medical Ethics*, commented that the condition of Baby J would be similar to that of children with severe spina bifida who were 'not now kept alive, because doctors realized their quality of life would be appalling' (22). He went on to say that 'allowing' the newborn handicapped to die was increasingly common practice— a statement backed up by Dr Malcolm Chiswick of Manchester and Professor Peter Dunn of Bristol, who both admitted to 'allowing' on average one handicapped baby to die every month (23).

It is thus apparent that decisions about handicapped babies actually involve a choice for life or death, based on the unsubstantiated hypothesis that the value of life is inversely proportional to the degree of handicap. I regard such judgements about the lives of disabled people as discriminatory, untenable and unethical, and believe that all babies should be treated to maximize their life chances unless they are actually in the process of dying.

In fact, once one begins to take a more positive attitude to disability it becomes apparent that appropriate intervention can significantly reduce the degree of impairment. For instance, an article in the *New England Journal of Medicine* (1991) found that delivering spina bifida babies by Caesarean section, rather than vaginally, avoided pressure on the exposed nerve roots, which was causing additional neural damage. At two years of age, children who had been delivered by Caesarean were found to be 2.2 times less likely to have severe paralysis than those delivered vaginally, a discovery which will be of real benefit to disabled babies (24).

Those babies for whom early death is inevitable, and for whom aggressive treatment is thus inappropriate, can still be cared for (either at home or in a children's hospice), in a way which will enable them truly to 'die with dignity'. Genuine relief of terminal pain for any patient who is dying is aimed not at *causing* death, but at accepting the reality and inevitability of imminent natural death. Such relief of suffering may foreshorten the dying process, but it does not involve deliberate killing, neither does it exhibit a maleficent motivation, which I suggest *is* present in policy decisions that certain categories of people are 'better off dead'. In fact, judiciously used, pain relief can *extend* life, by removing the physical and mental stress associated with severe pain.

'Wantedness'—that is, acceptance or rejection by the parents, or by society in general, does not dictate human value, and should have no bearing on the treatment of any human being. The fact that the Nazis did not 'want' the Jews or the handicapped did not make the holocaust morally neutral, neither does the rejection of some handicapped babies by their parents justify their being 'encouraged to die'. True beneficence lies in valuing all human beings as individuals who deserve the best possible treatment because of what they are—

infinitely precious people—not because of what they may or may not one day achieve.

ECONOMICS AND JUSTICE

It has often been suggested that eliminating the handicapped by neonatal killing or eugenic abortion is 'cost-effective'. The implication in such calculations is always that money spent on disabled people would be better diverted to those who are perceived as having lives of greater value and worth.

The Sunday Times calculated in 1981 that the cost of caring for the Down's syndrome baby Alexandra throughout her lifetime would be in the region of £100000, and went on to say that 'there is also increasing concern at the pressure on care facilities because of the growing number of severely handicapped children being kept alive' (25).

More recently, economic arguments have been frequently used in connection with prenatal screening tests, designed to detect handicapped babies and destroy them at an earlier age. Professor Nicholas Wald of St Bartholomew's Hospital Department of Environmental and Preventive Medicine said in 1989, for example, 'screening for spina bifida is highly cost effective. On average just over 1/3 of spina bifida babies will live beyond the age of 5, and 4/5 of these will be severely handicapped ... the cost of looking after such children is far higher than the cost of detecting cases. It is not a finely balanced equation, but a very clear one' (26). This appears to me to be so close to the Nazi philosophy as to be indistinguishable from Hitler's view that 'Society as a great authorised agent of life must be made responsible for every unsuccessful life; it has to pay for it, so it must prohibit it' (27). Maybe my opponents will refute this link, but in that case they must be prepared to point to exactly where the difference lies.

Such calculations, whenever they are made, inevitably rest upon an evaluation not of 'who can be saved' but of 'who is worth saving'. In view of this I think a new, more positive attitude is needed towards disability, which recognizes firstly the real value of human beings, and secondly the need to establish a just social system of priorities based on the realization of that value. How far we are from achieving this is apparent by considering the fact that in 1977 the following calculation was made—if every child with Down's syndrome in the USA were institutionalized (which would actually be the most expensive and least appropriate care for them) their keep would cost about 1/10 of what Americans spend every year on dog food (28). The reality is in fact that most handicapped children will live either with their natural families or with adoptive families, so that such 'worst-scenario' economics tend to be wildly inaccurate. An even more fundamental objection than their inaccuracy, however, is apparent to those who value human life: is a child not worth more than dog food?

If, as I believe to be the case, the only just social system is one which recognizes the infinite value of all human beings, care and appropriate treatment must be given according to need, not according to size, power, strength or any other arbitrary measure. If resources are limited they should be allocated on the basis of the weakest and most in need having the highest priority (a concept easily recognizable in the example of a sinking ship, where the unwritten rule is 'women and children first').

The assumption that human lives have relative rather than infinite worth is implicit in every decision deliberately to cause the death of a handicapped child. It is the same assumption which has been used to justify the abuse of human beings throughout history, from the Roman galleys, to Auschwitz, to Soweto, to present-day hospitals where unborn and newborn disabled babies are killed. The solution to all such injustices is apparent—to acknowledge the real value of human life, and then to treat all human beings accordingly.

CONCLUSION

'Allowing severely handicapped babies to die'—an apparently beneficent phrase—has become a euphemism used by doctors to mask the fact that they are deliberately causing the deaths of babies they believe would have lives 'not worth living'. This is totally contrary to true beneficence, which would involve maximizing the life chances of all babies who are not actually irremediably dying.

Since most people think that doctors are 'the experts' who know best, and who can be trusted, the fact has been overlooked that doctors are not uniquely qualified to judge human worth. Disabled people might rather not be disabled, it is true, but that is not equivalent to saying that, in the absence of cures, they would be 'better off dead'. Disability can cause misery, but so can being a black South African, being mentally ill, or having AIDS. The answer is to legislate for a legal and ethical system based on the equal innate value of all human beings and to provide an adequate support network for those in need. To seek to eliminate vulnerable people who are viewed, for whatever reason, as 'undesirable' is to collude in the fallacy that power and human worth are synonymous. It is bad medicine, bad politics and the ultimate denial of basic human rights.

In defence of the 'non-treatment' of Baby J, Dr Richard Nicholson of the *Bulletin of Medical Ethics* compared the baby's condition with that of children with severe spina bifida, saying 'very severely handicapped children tend to commit suicide in their teens, because at that stage weight changes make it impossible for them to get around, and they realise they will spend the rest of their lives in wheelchairs. On top of that they are nearly all incontinent, and face a lifetime of operations' (29). It is time, at last, to state my personal involvement in this debate. I was born with spina bifida and am disabled to just the extent described by Dr Nicholson. I do not, however, share his view that having such a disability predisposes one to suicide.

I do not believe there is an ethical option deliberately to cause the death of a handicapped child, however severe the disability, and I cite my own life as evidence that neonatal predictions of 'misery' are unfair, unjust, inaccurate and highly dangerous. I believe that babies should be given appropriate treatment aimed wherever possible at preserving life, in the same way as non-handicapped babies, and I regard the current 'fatal selection' decisions as demonstrating the ultimate discrimination against my people. My philosophy accords with that of Albert Schweitzer, who said 'Reverence for life reveals to me the fundamental principle of morality, namely that good consists in maintaining, furthering and enhancing life, and that destroying harming or hindering life is evil' (30).

REFERENCES

1. Tooley, M. 1973. A defence of abortion and infanticide. P. 51, *in* Feinberg, J. (Ed.) *Problems of abortion*, Belmont.
2. Glover, G. 1977. *Causing death and saving lives*. Pelican, Harmondsworth.
3. Singer, P. and Kuhse, H. 1985. *Should the baby live?* Oxford University Press, Oxford.
4. Professor John Lorber. 1978. Radio interview with Ian Kennedy, 18 October.
5. Binding, K. and Hoche, A. 1920. *The destruction of life devoid of value*. Felix Meiner, Leipzig.
6. Iglesias, T. 1990. *IVF and justice*. Linacre Centre, London.
7. Teichman, J. 1985. The definition of a person. New Hall Cambridge. *Philosophy* **60**: 175–185.
8. Crick, F. 1980. Quoted in *Whatever happened to the human race?* by Schaeffer, F. and Everett-Koop, C., Fleming, H. Revell, Old Tappan NJ.
9. Guelt, A. 1935. The structure of health. Quoted in Supplement to *Humanity Journal* 7/1980. Epsom, Auckland, NZ.
10. Garrow, D. 1979. Interview on ITV programme 'Jaywalking', 15 January.
11. Lorber, J. 1978. Comment in discussion at the 1975 Skytop Conference, recorded in C. A. Swinyard (Ed.) *Decision making and the defective newborn*, Springfield, Illinois, pp. 111–120; 231–258; 304–311; 344–356; 562–586; 598–617.
12. Anonymous letter. 1979. *Lancet* **2**: 1123–1124.
13. *BMA Euthanasia Report*, 1988. BMA, London.
14. Cook, R. 1981. *God and the handicapped child*. Christian Medical Fellowship, London.
15. Judge's summing up in the trial of Dr Leonard Arthur, 5 November 1981, London.
16. Down's baby who beat all the odds. *Daily Mail*, 9 October 1988.
17. Lorber, J. 1978. Selection—the best policy available. *Nursing Mirror*, 14 September.
18. Lloyd-Roberts, G. C. 1972. Developments in orthopaedic surgery. *Nursing Mirror*, 8 August.
19. Letter from Mary Seller, Guy's Hospital Division of Medical and Molecular Genetics. 1990. *British Medical Journal*, 4 August.
20. Zachary, R. 1977. Life with spina bifida. *British Medical Journal* ii: 1460–1462.
21. Child can be allowed to die, judges say: treatment to ease pain rather than prolong life. *The Times*, 21 April 1989.
22. Chiswick, M. 1990. Doctors facing monthly life or death dilemma. *Sunday Telegraph*, 21 October.
23. Dunn, P. 1990. Head of 'Life' offers to look after Baby J; senior doctors praise Appeal Court's 'compassionate' ruling. *Sunday Correspondent*, 21 October.
24. Luthy, D. A., Wardinsky, T., Shurtleff, D. B. *et al.* 1991. Cesarean section before the onset of labor and subsequent motor function in infants with meningomyelocele diagnosed antenatally. *New England Journal of Medicine*, **324**: 662–666.
25. Council faces £100 000 bill for mongol child. *The Sunday Times*, 9 August 1981.
26. NHS test denied to mothers. *Observer*, 2 April 1989.
27. Hitler, A. 1923. *Mein Kampf*. Reprinted and published by Radius Books (Hutchinson) 1969.
28. Diamond, E. 1977. The deformed child's right to life. *In* Horan, D. J. and Delahoyde, M. (Eds) *Infanticide and the handicapped newborn*. Brigham Young University Press, Provo, Utah, 1982.
29. Nicholson, R. 1990. Quoted in Handicapped baby may be left to die say judges. *Daily Telegraph*, 20 October.
30. Schweitzer, A. 1929. *Civilisation and ethics*, 2nd edn, p. 210 A. & C. Black, London.

55

Not All Babies Should Be Kept Alive As Long As Possible

JOHN HARRIS

Professor of Applied Philosophy and Research Director of the Centre for Social Ethics and Policy, University of Manchester, UK

This volume is dedicated to the idea that all problems of bioethics can be fruitfully elucidated by reference to a set of moral principles that have sometimes been characterized as the 'Georgetown mantra'. This title refers to the vigorous use of at least three of these familiar principles in the writings of Tom Beauchamp and James Childress, who work at Georgetown University.

There is no doubt that respect for autonomy, the idea that we should help others and that we should not harm them, and finally that we must be just in our dealings with them, are important parts of any morality. However, seeing all ethical problems in terms even of so prominent a set of principles has its dangers. For one thing there is a tendency to use them as a checklist, and the tendency to put ticks in boxes is inimical to thought, let alone to reasoning. We may be tempted to think that if we have considered a problem from the perspective of these four principles we have done all that may reasonably be required of us as moral beings, whether or not we have resolved the problem or come to a decision as to what to do. However, since these principles can conflict, we may have a further duty to try to prioritize them, to see which are more important. If we fail to do this we may find that the four principles yield no obvious solution or course of action, and there may then be a tendency to think that, having rehearsed the principles, we are now free to decide on our intuition or feelings.

Or we may need to attempt to see whether all or some of the principles are in fact expressions or dimensions of some prior and more fundamental principle, and to try to discover what this principle is. Moreover, the Georgetown mantra may incline us to feel that resolving conflicts of principle is beyond our terms of reference; that it is enough if we simply note what each principle has to say about a particular dilemma.

Finally, as in the present case, the crucial issue may lie in what we might call

Principles of Health Care Ethics. Edited by Raanan Gillon.
© 1994 John Wiley & Sons Ltd

the scope of these and other principles. We may need to decide whether these, or indeed other principles, apply at all in the present case, or apply to the sorts of creatures we are considering. Disputes about whether or not this is so cannot be reconciled by reference to the principles but must be solved by other means. What these might be, the differences between this and Chapter 54 may well reveal.

WHAT IS A BABY?

A first issue to sort out is the question of what precisely we are talking about. I know that Alison Davis, for example, the author of Chapter 54, agrees with me that there is no moral difference between the newly fertilized egg, the zygote, and the newly born baby, the neonate. For both of us there will be no significant difference between the ethics of failing to sustain the life of the zygote and failing to sustain the newborn. Where I'm sure we part company is that for me there is no morally significant difference between the unfertilized egg and the zygote. We will also differ crucially in what follows from our agreement about the continuum between the zygote and the neonate. For whereas she believes that the zygote and the neonate and everything between are as morally important as adults like herself and me, I think that from egg to newborn the emerging human individual is significantly less important than self-conscious adults; that it is, in short, of a different moral status.

HOW CAN SUCH A DISAGREEMENT BE RESOLVED?

In what follows I shall try to trace the natural history of an argument, a hypothetical argument between what I imagine is accepted by someone who believes as Alison Davis does and what is maintained by someone who sees things rather as I do. By an argument, of course, I do not mean a heated exchange of prejudices. Rather I mean to explore how the attempt to defend our respective positions might advance through various stages. Of course I will not be content merely to present the stages. Like all those who engage in rational argument I believe that I am closer to the truth than those with whom I disagree. What I hope is that you, the reader, will not simply take sides from what you now believe, but will decide where the weight of good argument lies.

If we are to decide whether or not all babies should be kept alive as long as possible we need to know many things. We need to know what sorts of creatures babies are, what obligations are owed to them, what rights they possess; in short, what their moral status is. We also need to know what will happen if we do keep them alive. Will they suffer? Who else will suffer? Are there any competing rights or obligations, and which are stronger?

WHAT SORTS OF MORAL CREATURES ARE BABIES?

I believe it to be a scientifically demonstrable fact that each individual life, human by virtue of its genetic code, begins at fertilization and continues thereafter in an unbroken line through the stages of the embryo, fetus, infant, toddler, teenager etc. until death, natural or unnatural, intervenes. I do not believe there is any logically significant point other than fertilization at which life can be said suddenly to commence. That being so, the whole concept of rights, what they mean and how they should be exercised, becomes a matter of crucial importance.

If human rights are to have any meaning, they must apply equally to all human beings (1).

These are the words of Alison Davis, and of course she is aware that 'there are several possible standpoints from which to decide whether one gains human rights when one begins to live, or when one begins to be a "person" or indeed whether these two events are one and the same thing' (2). Davis identifies three such standpoints as the principal runners—the utilitarian, the Kantian and the pro-life. Davis rejects the utilitarian position because: if 'one takes a utilitarian approach, the weakest will inevitably lose out, since they are powerless and "useless", in economic terms at least'. Davis believes that utility commits us to the view that those less 'perfect' are vulnerable to the claims of those more 'perfect'.

It would also justify using me as a donor bank for someone more physically perfect (I am confined to a wheelchair due to spina bifida) and depending on our relative worth, it would justify using any of us as a donor if someone of the status of Einstein, or Beethoven, or even Bob Geldof, needed one of our organs to survive.

Next Davis dismisses the 'Kantian' view.

Kant himself believed that we must treat entities morally only when they are rational (or potentially so) because our being able to do so is itself a rational judgement . . . . But why is rationality so important? None of us are rational when we are asleep, neither can we be certain our rationality is only temporarily in suspension then. What if we die before waking? What about the mentally ill and mentally handicapped people, and animals (ref. 2, p. 151).

Finally Davis summarizes the pro-life view which she accepts:

I believe the pro-life view, that rights accrue to all living human beings, and that that and 'personhood' are interchangeable terms is not only a humane but also a logically consistent philosophy. In my view there can be no sound differentiation between the two, and that being so, I believe individual rights begin—at conception—and should be protected from then on (ref. 2, p. 151).

The pro-life view taken by Davis is certainly logically consistent. Whether it is humane is another matter to which we will come. But what else might be wrong with it? How does it compare ethically with its rivals? What do we need to know in order to answer this question?

One first step to take might be to ask to what does such a position commit us? What follows from holding it? Then we might need to know whether the rival positions characterized by Davis are as unattractive as she makes them appear, and whether these are the only or most plausible rival positions? For she is surely right when she says that 'we can only ethically base our treatment of specific cases on a sound general theory'. Then we must ask whether Davis's characterization of the scientific facts is accurate. Finally we must decide which of the possible positions on the question is most consistent, most defensible and most attractive from an ethical point of view. I shall now try to say something in answer to all these questions.

WHAT FOLLOWS FROM BEING PRO-LIFE?

A number of moral imperatives follow from being pro-life in Davis's sense. The first is that abortion is never justifiable, not even to save the life of the mother, nor however disabled the fetus is and the child which it will become will be. On such a view the mother's life is of no more importance than the doomed fetus, and so both must be equally respected. Indeed it looks as though this will be true even if the child will live inevitably only a few pain-racked weeks after delivery. For on the pro-life view the embryo is from conception of equal moral importance, and neither the degree of disability nor the life expectancy of the fetus or child is relevant. And again, this must be true and abortion ruled out even if the fetus will have no chance of being carried to term and the mother will die if it is not aborted. For the embryo has the same rights from conception as anyone else. The most a pro-life view could do in such a case is toss a coin as to whether to save the life of the mother or preserve that of the fetus.

Or again, suppose in an *in vitro* fertilization (IVF) clinic six eggs have been fertilized and four are severely anomalous and likely to be disabled, or are diagnosed as having crippling and terminal genetic diseases. The pro-life view must be that it would be wrong automatically to implant the two healthy embryos, for all have equal rights. Indeed all should be implanted even if this will almost certainly mean that none will survive.

If a woman in an IVF clinic has only two eggs fertilized, and one is severely disabled, she must on the pro-life view have both implanted, and it would be unethical for a doctor to do other than this whatever the woman wanted.

If these are less than attractive options we have a motive for a closer examination of the merits of the pro-life view and the merits of possible alternatives to it. The acquisition of such a motive by examining precisely to what a moral position commits us is often a useful first step in moral reasoning.

However, those who find the above possibilities by no means disquieting may still need to be satisfied as to whether the general theory which generates them is sound.

Let us turn next to the facts.

WHEN DOES HUMAN LIFE BEGIN?

We can start by recalling Davis's firm statement, typical of many such views. 'I believe it to be a scientifically demonstrable fact that each individual life, human by virtue of its genetic code begins at fertilization . . .'. This is as a matter of fact false, but interestingly not in a way that advances the argument much on either side. Conception may result in a hydatidiform mole, made of human tissue but which can turn into nothing but a large and life-threatening bundle of cells. Conception, even when it is not on the right lines, does not immediately result in a human individual. The fertilized egg becomes a cell mass which eventually divides into two major components, the embryo and the trophoblast. The embryo or inner cell mass becomes the fetus, and the trophoblast develops to form the fetal part of the placenta and the umbilical cord.

But already I have gone too fast. After fertilization the single cell divides into two and then subdivides into four, eight, 16 cells and so on. At this stage all, say 16, cells are totipotential, that is to say they have the power to become anything that a human cell can become. If the 16-cell embryo were divided into two eight-cell clumps, each clump could then become a separate embryo and in principle develop normally to term if placed in the right environment. These two separate eight-cell embryos could be recombined into one again. Is the 16-cell embryo *an individual* or *two individuals*? As division continues to the blastocyst stage (around 64 cells) the outer cell mass, the trophoblast, loses its totipotentiality and becomes cells which can only form elements of the placenta. The inner cell mass, the embryo, remains at this stage totipotential or at least pluripotential and, as we have noted, if the embryo is split at this stage it can still become two or possibly more different embryos which could in principle be re-combined again.

Now there is an important sense in which the early zygote is not an individual human being but a number of different, distinct though not entirely separate cells which may grow separately (if the number of cells in each clump reaches a 'critical mass'—at least four)* into a number of 'individuals', individual zygotes that is. Each of these so-called 'individuals' will eventually consist of an embryo and a trophoblast, distinct though not separated elements, with different potential.

SOME METAPHYSICAL QUESTIONS

Interesting questions arise for those who believe that individual life begins at conception. If, as late as the blastocyst, we have the potential to create two new individual lives rather than one, are we not needlessly sacrificing a human life if we don't help the blastocyst to achieve its potential to be twins? Could we, having successfully divided a blastocyst, be justified in combining it again and snuffing out one human embryo? If we would not be justified in re-combining it, why isn't there some moral imperative to divide it if we can?

Most metaphysical of all. What wrong is done if we take an eight-cell embryo, separate the cells and combine each with a different embryo? No cell has been destroyed or even damaged and yet an embryo has disappeared.

Part of what I have described can only be observed in laboratory conditions, of course, and the division of the embryo into two requires manipulation in the laboratory. However, even in normal human conception *in vivo*, the zygote may

---

* I understand that it is currently accepted that totipotential cells require other cytoplasm of some indeterminate critical mass in order to have the chance to develop as embryos. It seems that four cells probably provide sufficient mass for these purposes. The blastocyst stage is currently as far as experiments in animal embryology have gone in dividing the blastocyst into two separate embryos.

become two individuals (or possibly three) and this splitting into twins or triplets can happen* as late as two weeks after conception. However, I neither wish to split hairs nor zygotes, and I am happy to grant that the zygote is human; the fact that it is not necessarily an individual is morally irrelevant since twins or other multiples are as important or unimportant as individuals.

But this said, the unfertilized egg and the sperm are also human and alive, although like the zygote they are not yet beyond a peradventure an individual. There is a real sense in which, both from the point of view of their potential and for what they are, they are analogous to the zygote. The sperm and the egg are distinct individuals together forming the potential to become a zygote and together possessing all the potential of the zygote. The zygote at the two-cell stage is two distinct individuals, each having the potential for separate development, and if remaining conjoined having the potential to become either the embryo or the trophoblast.

As I have indicated, I see no reason to deny the description 'human being' to the zygote as long as we bear in mind that this leaves all questions about its moral status open. It is human as far as it is a member of any species and it is a being, that is, it is alive, in being and capable of further development and 'being' under the right conditions. We must also remember that the use of the term 'it' does not imply that 'it' is an individual. In all the above senses the unfertilized egg and the sperm are also human beings.

We are here, of course, in the realm of metaphysics. What is an 'individual' what is a 'being'? The language we use is attenuated at best when applied to what we know about early human development. The term 'human being' is unproblematic in its paradigms—Alison Davis and myself. It is highly problematic when applied to a single cell. We have to argue from analogy or potential. Is it more like a *this* or more like a *that*, is it potentially a *this* or potentially only a *that*?

And if parthenogenesis proves possible,† then the human egg by itself is a human being for what that's worth. And of course this is the crucial question: what's it worth to be human? Instead of asking is the egg or the embryo or the infant analogous to a paradigm human being or potentially a paradigm human being, we need to ask what makes a paradigm human being morally important. For if we can answer this question we will know whether or not the egg or the embryo or the infant has what it takes, or enough of what it takes to be morally important. The crucial issue here is whether human rights, or as I would prefer to say, full moral status, is to be accorded to the human egg or the human zygote or the infant.

The belief that if 'human rights are to have any meaning, they must apply equally to all human beings' requires a theory to show why this is so. It does not simply follow from the fact that the egg or the zygote is human and is a

---

* Or at least can be observed as late as 14 days after conception.
† Parthenogenesis is the process whereby the egg can be stimulated to grow without fertilization. This process can be artificially initiated in human eggs; but as yet it does not seem likely that such parthenogenetic embryos, although they have developed to the stage of a detectable heartbeat, can be successfully implanted and carried to term in a human host.

being. But of course there is an important sense in which neither the egg nor the embryo are human beings in the fully fledged sense in which we normally understand the term. They are rather human *becomings*. However, again I do not positively object to the term 'human being' as applied to the human egg or the human conceptus. The crucial question is whether all human beings are of the same moral status.

It is at this point that we must look at one or two theories about why individuals acquire or possess moral importance.

THE PROBLEM

The problem we must remember is two-fold. It is first to know what we should think about our obligations to, and the rights of, the human being or the human organism at various stages of its development. If we can be confident about this we will be able to address the subject of this pair of chapters, namely whether or not all babies should be kept alive as long as possible. The second part of the problem is to know what if any theory or general justification can be given for our answer.

The Problem and the Four Principles

To put the problem in terms of the four principles we can simply ask the question: when, why and to whom do the four principles apply? Whom or what do they or should they protect?

Speciesism

Alison Davis has outlined a consistent view of the matter, namely that rights accrue to all living human beings and that human beings begin at conception. But why do rights accrue to human beings? In virtue of what precisely about us is this so, if it is? Why, for example, are animals excluded if they are? In her criticism of the view she characterized as 'Kantian', Davis gave animals a passing thought. Criticizing the idea that rationality was what was morally important about humans she stated 'none of us are rational in our sleep', and asked rhetorically: 'what about the mentally ill and mentally handicapped people, and animals?' If it is relevant to ask why animals are excluded if rationality is highlighted, we must ask the same question when species membership is highlighted. What justifies our prioritizing a particular species and according its members the protection of a system of rights?

Aside on Moral Argument

Now there are circumstances in ethics when it is legitimate to make grand assumptions like the present one that human beings are important. It is often both a good and an efficient strategy in moral argument to go back to a point of agreement and then argue forward. So, if all are agreed that rights attach simply to human beings, then all that has to be accomplished in argument is to show that the disputed case falls under the general rule and the argument is won. Hence if all human individuals are protected from the moment they begin then if we want to know whether or not the fetus or the zygote or the child has rights, all we need to establish is whether or not they are human.

The problem is, of course, that those whose intuitions tell them the zygote is ultimately valuable will want to argue that it is human. Those who do not feel that the zygote or the embryo or the fetus are morally important, or as morally important as adults or children, will want to argue that these are not fully human or are pre-human or pre-persons. It is at this point that the argument is apt to become sterile in the extreme, with increasingly implausible considerations adduced to 'prove' that the zygote is or is not a human being properly so called. It is at this point that we need to accept that the requisite agreement about what is important cannot be achieved, and press the point further, asking a more ultimate question. In this case: what is so important about being human? For if we ask this question we may find a way through. For if we know *why* humans are morally important we may know if and whether the zygote, for example, is important in this way, whether or not it may plausibly be called a human being or a full human being or a new human individual or whatever.

SPECIESISM REVISITED

There are three possible positions that might be held by those who believe that rights accrue to all living human beings. They all give moral importance to the idea of humanity—it is *being human* that counts. But in each case precisely what is meant by 'humanity' is rather different. In one case it is simply membership of the human species that counts; this prioritizing membership of a particular species *per se* is speciesism properly so called. The second idea is that it is an individual's humanity in some richer sense that counts morally. That is, it is a set of capacities or features that human beings possess that makes them morally important, and they are important because they possess these features, these human characteristics. The third position combines the two, arguing that while it is human characteristics and not species membership that is morally important, it is justifiable or necessary to extend the protections that go with these features to the class of beings which standardly possess them, namely members of the human species, whether or not in the particular case they actually possess these features.

We must look a little longer at all three types of speciesism.

Species Membership

I hope it is obvious that asserting moral importance for members of a particular group simply because they are members of that group without any attempt to specify why such membership confers rights or is morally significant in any way, is prejudice pure and simple.* It is like asserting membership of a race,

---

* Mary Warnock seems to take this sort of view both in the Warnock Report and in her various glosses upon it. See for example Mary Warnock, *A question of life*, Basil Blackwell, Oxford, 1985.

or gender, or religion, or nation state, or geographical region makes people of that race, gender, etc., morally important on that account alone. It is to claim a distinction without a difference.

Human Values

In this sense it is the nature of humans that is claimed to be morally significant. They are morally important because of their humanity understood as an evaluative term encompassing the typical morally important features of human beings; their intelligence perhaps, their capacity to feel sympathy and compassion, their autonomy and so on. This 'humanity' refers to the things that relevantly distinguish the Sunday diner and the Sunday dinner, that make humans more morally important than turkeys or roast potatoes. I ought to keep you alive as long as possible if that's what you want, but I do not have the same obligation to the turkey, because of things you possess, things about you, not shared by the turkey. You differ from the turkey in morally relevant ways, not simply because you are a member of one species and the turkey a member of another, not simply because you are a featherless biped and the turkey a feathered one.

Typical Humans

The third view is developed to solve the problem about what to do with human beings who do not possess those features identified as associated with human values, with the value of being human.* Creatures like human embryos or human newborns. The problem with human embryos and human newborns is that they do not yet possess any of the sorts of features plausibly referred to above under the heading 'human values'. True they are alive, human, sentient, aware of their environment in some senses, but so are cats and canaries. They are not, however, self-aware, autonomous, or at this stage capable of valuing their own existence. The argument here is that although they do not possess morally relevant capacities, that is capacities that relevantly distinguish them from cats or canaries, they are members of a species whose typical members do possess these features, and *this* is what makes them morally important.

Now this claim might be interpreted in two different ways. If it is the claim that they are members of a species whose typical members are morally distinguishable from cats and canaries, and that they will themselves in fact develop the capacities that relevantly distinguish them, then this becomes the potentiality argument and we will look at it separately in a moment. It becomes the argument that they are not valuable for what they now are but for what they will become.

If it is taken as saying that whether or not they ever develop morally relevant capacities they are now valuable because they are members of a species whose typical members possess these capacities, then I must say that I for one fail to see the force of the suggestion. It would be like arguing that Fred who is tone

---

* This view is taken among others by Rosalind Hursthouse see her *Beginning lives*, Basil Blackwell, Oxford, 1987; especially Chapter 6.

deaf and musically illiterate, but who comes from a family of musical prodigies, whose parents are famous virtuosi and whose siblings are all concert musicians, should be valued *as a musician* for the musical ability possessed by typical members of his family but not by him.

We are still struggling to discover what it is or might be about humans that makes them morally important. We have, I hope, reached the point where we can see that the resonant claim that 'if human rights are to have any meaning they must apply equally to all human beings', is far from unproblematic. We have seen that each of the three senses we might give to valuing humans as such fails morally relevantly to distinguish humans from animals. We are left with the problem of how to justify our intuition that if the house is on fire (whether or not we are vegetarian or animal rights activists) we should save the baby before the cat and the canary. The last chance is the argument from potentiality.

HUMAN POTENTIAL

The argument from potentiality involves the idea that we are not valuable for what we are but for what we will become. The structure of this argument involves a fallacy, and even if this were not true it embraces too much. It is a commonplace that acorns are not oak trees, and that destroying an acorn is not the moral equivalent of cutting down an oak tree. We are all potentially dead meat but this (I trust) affords no-one a reason to treat another person as if they were already dead meat.

We have seen that the argument embraces too much, for if it means that we must protect and accord rights to whatever has the potential to become a human person then the unfertilized egg and the sperm, ununited, have that potential. Consider Figure 55.1: *A* clearly has the potential to become *B* if anything does, and *B* has the potential to become *C*, so *A* has the potential to become *C*. The ethic that requires us to protect and try to instantiate all human potential has much to recommend it. However, it is an exhausting ethic, particularly for women, and one fraught with environmental dangers. Only those prepared fully

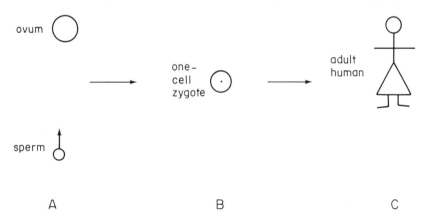

FIGURE 55.1

to embrace it, and not embarrassed by the fallacy of the potentiality argument, can be happy with its conclusion.

NOT ALL BABIES SHOULD BE KEPT ALIVE AS LONG AS POSSIBLE

I hope that we have reached a point at which it will be clear that newborn babies, neonates, share whatever moral status fetuses, embryos and zygotes have.* If abortion is justified then so is infanticide.

There are a number of reasons for this. I will review these briefly then deal with the question of the meaning of infanticide for disability and of whether or not it constitutes discrimination against those with disability or denial of their full status and dignity as persons.

DO BABIES DIFFER FROM FETUSES?

The answer to this question is clearly 'no' or rather 'not necessarily'. We must ask what is so significant about birth? How can it affect the moral status of the individual born? If a fetus was not significantly different from cats or canaries before birth what has changed? The answer, of course, is nothing about the nature of the individual itself. True it has obtained an existence independent of its mother, but so what? There will come a time when human creatures can exist both without birth and even without 'untimely ripping'. We will, I suppose, eventually develop ectogenesis, the artificial womb which will allow embryos created *in vitro* to emerge into the world from glass rather than from flesh and blood. Such embryos will always have an existence independent of their mother, as do *in vitro* embryos now.

True a fetus may become *viable* at a particular if variable point, but again so what? Viability as it is currently used means in effect not 'capable of sustaining its own life' (which of us not living in a state of nature can do that?); rather it must mean 'can be kept alive outside the womb'. But again we must ask what moral difference does geography or technology make? Why is an individual more important if being kept alive in an artificial incubator two metres to the south of its mother than in a human one two metres to the north of the artificial incubator? Moreover, viability is notoriously geography- and technology- dependent. If it is true that a baby has a good chance of being viable at 23 or 24 weeks if it lives near enough to a first-class premature baby unit, but will only be viable at 30 weeks in another location, then viability might lead us to conclude that there was a significant moral difference between one baby and the other at 24 weeks.

The *Human Fertilization and Embryology Act 1990*, for example, permits abortion for fetal abnormality at any time prior to birth. This means that an obstetrician who aborts, say, at 28 weeks for fetal abnormality commits no offence if he kills

---

* The arguments necessary fully to address this issue are much more complex than we have space for here. I have tried to deal with them elsewhere, and readers who remain understandably dissatisfied with the argument so far will find arguments and references to pursue in my *The value of life* (3), Chapters 1–4.

the fetus *in utero*, but does commit an offence if seconds or minutes later he kills the infant after delivery.

THE ARGUMENT SO FAR

I have argued that there is no justification for thinking of the human zygote or embryo or fetus or neonate as in any way morally equivalent to full human persons. I have suggested that what makes someone a person properly so called is whatever it is that relevantly distinguishes persons from animals. I have not here offered a positive account of what precisely this is, and I will not do so now. This is fully set out in my book *The value of life* (3). I have indicated, however, that it is likely to involve some combination of self-consciousness, and fairly rudimentary intelligence. We have also seen that human rights, if they attach to humans, do so not in virtue of their humanity but in virtue of what makes human nature (among other possible natures) morally different (when it is morally different) from the nature of birds, beasts and plants when they are morally different.

DISABILITY AND THE DISABLED

It is often said by those with disability that abortion for disability, or failure to keep disabled infants alive as long as possible, constitutes discrimination against the disabled as a group. It is tantamount to disvaluing them as persons. Davis herself identifies this view with utilitarianism and takes the idea further, commenting, 'it would also justify using me as a donor bank for someone more physically perfect'. This is not necessarily so. On the view I have elaborated above, all persons share the same moral status whether disabled or not. To decide not to keep a disabled baby alive (to kill it, in other words) no more constitutes an attack on the disabled than does curing disability. To set badly broken legs is not an attack upon those confined to wheelchairs. To prefer to remove disability where we can is not to prefer the non-disabled as persons.

If a pregnant mother can take steps to cure a disability affecting her fetus she should certainly do so, for to fail so to do is deliberately to handicap her child. She is not saying that she prefers those without disability as persons when she says she would prefer not to have a disabled child.

The view defended here would neither permit the sacrifice of Ms Davis, nor indeed of anyone else, to preserve the life even of Bob Geldof, let alone Einstein. It does, however, suggest the lives of non-persons of whatever species are worth less than those of persons, and may legitimately be sacrificed to protect the interests of persons.* In particular it would permit abortion and infanticide, and the use of, for example, anencephalic babies and individuals in persistent vegetative state as organ donors. These suggestions will doubtless worry many people, and I do not have the space here to attempt to show why I believe such worries to be misplaced. However, I do not believe that even *prima facie*, such

---

* Other things being equal, of course; among which other things are the requirement that we do not inflict pain on other sentient creatures except in the gravest of emergencies.

conclusions are morally more disturbing than the prospect of sacrificing a healthy young mother so that her fetus can survive *in utero* for an extra few months.

ACKNOWLEDGEMENT

I am indebted in this chapter to my colleague Dr Susan Kimber, of the Department of Cell and Structural Biology in the University of Manchester, for her invaluable advice on the early embryo.

REFERENCES

1. Davis, A. 1986. Informed dissent: the view of a disabled woman. *Journal of Medical Ethics* **12**: 75–76. (See also Chapter 55, this volume.)
2. Davis, A. 1988. The status of anencephalic babies: should their bodies be used as donor banks? *Journal of Medical Ethics* **14**: 150–153.
3. Harris, J. 1990. *The value of life*. Routledge, London.

56

Children: Problems in Paediatrics

Philip Graham

The Hospital for Sick Children, Great Ormond Street, London, UK

Health care for the growing child raises ethical issues that require separate consideration for two particular reasons: (a) development of competence, and (b) proxy consent and the role of parents.

THE DEVELOPMENT OF COMPETENCE

The competence of children to take part in decision-making where investigation and treatment is concerned increases with age. It is widely accepted that when procedures involving children are to be carried out, these should be explained to children in terms that they understand, no matter how young they may be. It could be argued that it is pointless to enter into verbal explanations with babies and very young children. But when babies are about to undergo new experiences—for example tasting a new food, meeting a strange relative for the first time—parents intuitively talk to them even when they are only a few weeks old. So it seems reasonable to encourage the same reassuring behaviour where health care procedures are involved. A sudden unexplained assault on a baby for a venepuncture is more likely to produce prolonged distress than a similar procedure preceded by a soothing explanation. So *explanation* is a universal right for children.

The *assent* of children to health care procedures can obviously only be meaningfully in question when the child can understand its nature. Assessing a child's competence to understand may not be an easy matter and, in past years, there has been a consistent tendency to underestimate the capacities of children in this respect. Eiser (1) (1985) has reviewed evidence concerning children's knowledge and understanding of medical treatment. She suggests that children between 6 and 7 years may view treatment as punishment. Between 7 and 10 years, although children become aware that the purpose of treatment is to make them better, they often do not understand the reasons why doctors and nurses may need to cause pain. By 10 years, children have a more mature understanding of the nature of treatment.

Principles of Health Care Ethics. Edited by Raanan Gillon.

With such evidence available, it would seem reasonable for health care professionals to seek assent from children of 10 years and above. However, age is only a rough guide to level of understanding. Children of a particular age vary in their levels of cognitive development. As a rough guide to the degree of variation, if one takes 100 children aged 10 years and administers a verbal test involving comprehension, it is likely that about 15 will show an understanding level of an average 8½-year-old or less, and two or three will show a level of understanding of 7 years or less. About 15 will show a level of understanding at or better than an average 11½-year-old, and between two and three at or better than an average 13-year level. So those seeking consent from a child need to be able to make an individual judgement of a child's understanding. This need not be such a complicated matter as it sounds. If, before embarking on an explanation, a health professional asks a child what he already understands about his condition and its treatment, she is likely to be able to gauge the level of the child's understanding as well as know the words the child already uses to describe his problem. If, however, an individual assessment of this kind is not practicable (and it is difficult to see why this should ever be the case), then an explanation may need to be given that is appropriate for an average child of that particular age. It is important to remember that some aspects of investigation and treatment are far easier to understand than others.

A further issue arises when a child's assent is sought, but not obtained. It could be argued that seeking assent from a child is not meaningful unless the child's dissent is taken seriously. Taken to its extreme this argument would indicate that where a child's assent was not forthcoming, but the child was regarded as competent to understand the issues in question, the investigation or treatment should not be performed without going through the same legal process as would be the case if the patient were an adult, and refused the procedure. However, most would argue that, where young children are concerned, it is important to seek assent even if the procedure is still to be undertaken if the child dissents. This issue will be discussed further under the heading of autonomy.

PROXY CONSENT AND THE ROLE OF PARENTS

When an investigation or therapeutic intervention is to be performed on a child, parents are required to provide proxy consent, permission on behalf of their child. The principles involved in seeking consent from parents are the same as those that would be involved if the patient were an adult (Part II, Chapter 39), but certain issues need particular stress where children are concerned (2). Proxy consent can be satisfactorily obtained only when parents are in receipt of full information. In serious cases this may well need an open discussion of the risk of death, even if this is low. The balance between possible benefits and possible harm needs to be discussed, as well as the way in which this balance might change as the child's condition improves or deteriorates. The giving of consent needs to be seen not as a once-for-all procedure, but as part of a process in which parents are consulted about the on-going course of their child's illness.

The degree to which this is achieved can be judged only in the context of how health care staff encourage or restrict family-centred care.

The degree to which health care professionals inform parents fully of the risks of any procedures to be undertaken on their children is a matter of concern. Brahams (3) reported a case occurring in Scotland in which the Sheriff to a Fatal Accidents and Sudden Deaths Inquiry gave it as his opinion that parents had a greater right to have such information about their children than adult patients to information about procedures carried out on themselves. He argued that parents and no-one else had a legal duty to act in the best interests of their children, and they could not do this unless they were in full possession of the facts. It has been demonstrated (4) that, regrettably, parents often do not have full information provided to them. In a sample of 150 parents of children seen in the accident and emergency department of a children's hospital in England, 57% of blood samples were taken and 89% of treatment regimens instituted without parental permission. The reasons for over half the blood tests and 31% of the drug treatments were not explained. It is, of course, likely that the situation would be less unsatisfactory in relation to consent for more serious procedures such as surgical operations.

In most cases it can reasonably be assumed that parents are the people who know their child best, have their child's best interests at heart, and are the people most likely to act for the benefit of their particular child. Consequently, in the normal course of events it is the duty of child health professionals such as doctors and nurses to support parents wholeheartedly in the decisions they may wish to make for their children. However, a substantial minority of parents act to the detriment of their children. These include not only those who physically, sexually and emotionally abuse their children. A significant number of children are over-protected by their parents and fail to achieve anything like as autonomous a life as they might (5).

AUTONOMY

J. is a 13-year-old girl of average intelligence with congenital heart disease. She was operated on in infancy, and remained well for 10 years, but for the last three years her condition has very slowly deteriorated. She is still in good physical condition and would be able to withstand a further operation well, but there is a 10% chance of mortality at or around the time of the operation. Without the operation she will continue to deteriorate at a slow rate. If she survives the operation she is likely to have at least 15 years' good-quality life. In about two years' time her condition will remain operable, but it is likely that the risk of operation would rise to between 15% and 20% mortality. Following this it is likely that the risks of operation would rise unacceptably. Her parents, who are both anxious people, wish to delay the operation. J., who is regarded as fully competent to understand the issues involved, wishes to have the operation now, and J.'s view is shared by the surgeons who, however, wish to leave the decision with the parents. The operation is not performed.

In this situation there is a difference between parents and child in the judgement of the value of two years' reasonably healthy life. It is the child's life, not the lives of the parents that is in question, but the parents may be seen as exercising their rights as trustees of the girl's welfare to the best of their ability. The surgeons do not have the right to operate without parental consent. If the surgeons refer the case to the social services department as an issue involving child protection, it is highly likely that the social workers would not wish to intervene. Clearly if the risk of operation were much lower now, but much higher in two years' time, the situation concerning child protection would be very different, and social workers would be likely to take a different view. There are therefore situations in which it may be difficult to respect a competent child's autonomy in relation to decisions concerning her own body. Similar situations arise in relation to elective cosmetic surgery when, for example, the parents of a child with a facial disfigurement wish an operation to be performed, but the child, quite competent to make her own decision, does not. One positive step that can be taken in such circumstances is to offer counselling to parents and child separately and together. A desirable outcome of counselling would be that parents and child reach an agreed decision with no-one involved feeling that pressure has been exercised to achieve a consensus.

A highly controversial ethical issue relating to the autonomy of children and health care arises in relation to contraception. Do adolescents regarded as under-age (16 years in the UK) for sexual activity have the right to contraceptive advice from doctors without their parents being informed? On the one hand, parents are responsible for their daughters' health and behaviour, and a doctor giving contraceptive advice in these circumstances can be seen as undermining their legitimate right to use every means possible from preventing their daughters from engaging in what they would regard as premature sexual activity inimical to emotional and possibly physical health. It is certainly possible, though perhaps not likely in most cases, that some girls would not engage in sexual activity if they were not given the means of contraception by their doctors. Further, the mere giving of contraceptive advice by a doctor might be regarded as authoritative permission to engage in intercourse.

On the other hand, a physically mature under-age girl who goes to a doctor for contraceptive advice can also be seen as a person unusually responsible for her age. Realistically she is likely to engage in sexual activity whether or not she receives such advice. If she does not use contraception the risk of unwanted pregnancy with the consequent risks of ill-health and emotional damage due to therapeutic termination or carrying the pregnancy to term are not inconsiderable.

The legal situation in the UK has been clarified and the principle of adolescent autonomy supported by a judgment of the House of Lords in the Gillick case (6). The case arose when the mother of an under-age teenage girl started proceedings against the Department of Health to prevent its employees providing contraceptive advice to her daughter without her knowledge. A Department of Health circular had indicated that, in some circumstances, such advice might be given. The application was dismissed in the High Court, but an appeal was unanimously allowed at the Court of Appeal. In a divided (3 to 2) judgement the House of Lords upheld the Department of Health position. In his judgement Lord Fraser gave his view that doctors could provide contraceptive advice without communicating with parents providing the girl understood the advice and refused to allow her parents to be informed, that it was likely that intercourse would happen anyway in these circumstances, that the girl's health was likely to suffer if she did not receive advice, and that it was in the girl's interest that she should receive such advice.

The principles underlying this case, and others like it, were enunciated with admirable clarity at the same time by Lord Scarman. He said that parental rights were derived from parental duty and existed only so long as they were needed for the protection of the person and property of the child. Parental right yielded to the child's right to make his own decisions when he reached a sufficient understanding and intelligence to be capable of making up his own mind. The application of the principle of autonomy in the care of children could surely not be more clearly stated.

K. is a 14-year-old girl with anorexia nervosa. She is 5 ft 5 in tall (165 cm) and weighs 4 stone 10 lb (K 30). She has been losing about 2 lb (K 1) a week for the past six weeks as a result of dieting and over-exercise. Family meals are characterized by constant shouting by the parents to get K. to eat. The psychiatrist seeing the family believes that K.'s psychological problems are centred around her need to achieve autonomy from her parents who, she feels, have pressurized her in school work and music lessons. If she continues to lose weight at the present rate she will be in physical danger in about a further month. A period of two months' outpatient treatment has been unsuccessful. Previous experience with other teenagers has led the psychiatrist to believe that most youngsters, once admitted to her unit, start to eat soon after admission. However, some do not and these require tube feeding if they are to survive. The psychiatrist offers admission to hospital. The parents agree, but K. refuses. She says if she is not admitted she will begin to eat, but she has said this throughout the previous two months and has nevertheless continued to lose weight rapidly.

This type of problem has been helpfully discussed by Freeman (7) in the light of a US Supreme Court decision in the case of *Parham* vs. *JR*. The Supreme Court ruled that parents had a right to commit their under-aged child to a mental institution even if the child refused. The court argued that the child had a right to a pre-admission hearing, but that the doctor involved in the case could be regarded as the neutral party filling this role. Freeman criticizes this decision, concluding that the psychiatrist cannot be regarded as a neutral party. He argues that a court hearing should occur in such cases, but the judicial implications of this policy might make it impracticable. One complicating issue in cases of this type that are not at all uncommon, is that the child's disorder cannot be viewed in the same terms as a purely physical condition such as cancer or heart disease. The child's symptoms are, at least to some degree, related to parental behaviour, so those who may be partly causing the condition are also those taking responsibility for decisions about its management.

In England and Wales, under the Mental Health Act 1983, the position of children under the age of 16 who are regarded as competent (in terms of emotional maturity, intellectual capacity and psychological state) to make decisions about the treatment of their own condition, are in the same position as adults. Even if their parents disagree, they cannot be admitted to hospital informally against their will. Compulsory admission can be arranged only if the criteria for adult patients are met. Official guidance (8) suggests that, in circumstances such as those described in the above example, one needs to take into account a range of factors in addition to the child's competence. These include consideration of the necessity for treatment, and the viability of treatment at home. When parental behaviour in relation to a child's mental state is thought to be significantly harmful, for example by refusal to let a child obviously in need of inpatient treatment receive it, the provisions of the 1989 Children Act become relevant and, to achieve satisfactory care, it may be necessary to discuss with social workers the possible need to apply for an emergency protection order, a care order, or a child protection order.

The issues surrounding autonomy in the above example are very complex. K. is striving for autonomy, but is doing so in a maladaptive manner, certainly dangerous to her health and perhaps for her survival. The psychiatrist wishes to help her to achieve autonomous functioning, but in a more adaptive manner. Her parents, who have restricted her autonomy in the past and, without counselling, will continue to do so in the future, are nevertheless in accord with the psychiatrist as to the treatment plan. K. is not allowed to exercise her autonomy in the way she wishes. Her parents and the professionals involved, doubtless with the best intentions, take her right to choose away from her and, ethically, when viewed either from a deontological or a utilitarian perspective, this seems the right decision. K. is admitted to the psychiatric unit as an informal patient; action justified on the perhaps contentious grounds that her psychological state has rendered her incompetent to make a decision on her own behalf.

NON-MALEFICENCE

The principle of non-maleficence (not doing harm) is most likely to be questioned in children in the conduct of research (both therapeutic and non-therapeutic) and in the prolongation of life at a level that might be regarded as valueless or worse than death.

Research

Ethical issues in relation to research in children have been comprehensively discussed by Nicholson (9) and Campbell (10). *Non-therapeutic research* is undertaken when studies are carried out in a systematic fashion with the aim of advancing knowledge, but without any intended benefit to the subject. Examples would include the taking of a blood sample by finger-prick in order to establish normal values of a chemical substance, or the interviewing of a sample of adolescents drawn from the general population about their mood swings in order to compare them with a group of children of similar age admitted to hospital with suicidal behaviour. The conduct of non-therapeutic research is essential to advance certain types of knowledge. This does not, of course, mean that scientists have a right to carry out any non-therapeutic research they wish. In general it is agreed that such research should be carried out only when there is a less than minimal risk to the subject, that is a risk no greater than might be met by the child in everyday life. Non-therapeutic research in children can, it is argued, be justified only when the risk is at or below this level regardless of the possible benefits to other children (9).

The legality of consent in the UK to non-therapeutic research in infants and young children has been discussed by Dworkin (11). His view was that although, strictly speaking, it was unlawful for parents to give consent for this type of research on their children, the UK courts had not ruled on this matter and, if they did, they might take a less strict view. The courts might well allow a parent to weigh up various possibly conflicting interests and give permission in certain circumstances. The advantages to the child subject in experiencing a sense of achievement in having undergone minor inconvenience for the benefit of others might be one such consideration. The triviality of the research procedure (e.g. taking an extra 2 ml of blood from a group of ill children who were going to have a venepuncture for other reasons anyway) might be another.

The writer was involved in an example of non-therapeutic research which might be regarded as on the borderline of acceptability (12). The example brings up issues of consent as well as the principle of non-maleficence. It was regarded as desirable to know more about the sexual knowledge and behaviour of normal children in order to provide a clearer perspective in the investigation of children who had possibly been sexually abused. A sample of normal 4–16-year-old children was identified from general practice age/sex registers, and parents were contacted by letter requesting an appointment at home with them. At that point they were told only that their help and the help of their children was needed to assist in the diagnosis of children seen in hospital departments. At the personal visit that followed, they were told that the research team wished to investigate ordinary children by interviewing them and their families about family behaviour in relation to nudity, bathing, sexual behaviour and knowledge. The information was necessary to assist in the diagnosis of sexually abused children. Children would be interviewed separately about some of these matters. However, they would not be given any new information they did not already have, and they would be encouraged not to answer questions they did not wish to. About 85% of the families originally approached consented to this procedure.

At the beginning of the interview with the child, the research interviewer 'empowered' the child to refuse to answer questions by coaching the child to say 'No, I don't want to answer that', in answer to a question, and proceeded only once it was clear that the child understood her right to do this and could exercise it. The interviewer exercised her judgement whether or not to proceed with questioning if the child seemed upset.

One week after the research interview, parents were interviewed by telephone (or sent a postal questionnaire if they did not have a telephone) about possible adverse effects of the interview. The great majority of children appeared not to have been upset in any way, but about 3% did show subsequent behaviour that might be regarded as briefly upset, though none in a serious way. The most serious was a 13-year-old girl who suffered a headache she attributed to the interview for a few hours after it, but was subsequently back to her normal self.

The conduct of this study points to the need to be able to make as clear a judgement as possible of harmful adverse effects before the research is undertaken.

If this is not possible, usually because similar work has not previously been carried out, then the research team has a duty to monitor for adverse effects and to stop the procedure if it becomes clear that these are more than minimal. In some circumstances, possible harmful effects have been monitored with children. Thus Smith (13) looked at the responses of 96 seven-year-olds from whom a blood sample had been taken for non-therapeutic research. About 8% were mildly upset, but none moderately or seriously so. These findings cannot, however, be generalized to other procedures, to older or younger children administered the same procedures, or to an apparently similar procedure carried out with greater or lesser technical skill and psychological preparation.

The issue of consent to non-therapeutic research procedures is also raised by this example. The concepts of assent and consent have been considered earlier in this chapter. It would seem reasonable to suggest that the need for explaining procedures to younger children and obtaining their assent, and obtaining the consent of older children, is at least as important in therapeutic and non-therapeutic research as it is in clinical investigation and treatment.

Therapeutic research, the systematic application of investigation or treatment procedures in sick children to advance knowledge, is also essential to improve paediatric care. The risks that may be taken can, however, be greater than with non-therapeutic research, because the aim is to benefit the individual child involved, as well as others who may suffer from the same condition. Acceptable risks cannot be quantified because these will depend on the seriousness of the condition from which the child suffers and the potential benefit of the procedure to the child, as well as the risk of the procedure. Thus a significant operative mortality of 5–10% may be acceptable with children who otherwise have an expected mortality of 100% over the next year.

The main ethical concern in relation to therapeutic research relates not to its frequency, but to the rarity with which it is conducted when new treatments are introduced. Perhaps paradoxically, a surgeon who wishes to undertake a new type of operation may do so without impediment, providing she does so in an unsystematic manner without scientific monitoring and, of course, providing she is acting with the best interests of the child in mind, and in the knowledge that at least a proportion of her colleagues would regard the procedure as good practice. If, however, she wishes to evaluate the effectiveness of treatment, using a randomized allocation design, she must obtain the permission of an ethics committee.

Both therapeutic and non-therapeutic research require the agreement of research ethics committees before they can be carried out. There are a small number of special considerations relating to ethics committees where research with children is concerned. It is recommended (9) that the membership of ethics committees dealing with research on children should include a parent and at least one child health professional. Committees should ensure they pay particular attention to the degree to which children's assent and consent are obtained as well, of course, as to issues of parental consent. There is, of course, a whole range of other issues relating to the ethics of research that affect children but also adults, and these are dealt with elsewhere (Part II, Chapter 40).

The Prolongation of Valueless Life in Children

This issue is discussed in several contributions to Part III of this book. Clearly there are certain special considerations in relation to children. The full involvement of parents in decisions concerning, for example, the termination of life support in children who are brain-dead is, of course, essential. The situation is more complicated where the child is, at least to some degree, competent to participate in decisions that are to be taken. The involvement of the child in decision-making has many advantages, but most would agree that the issues are complex (14). The degree to which children can participate will be closely linked to the knowledge they have about the life-threatening nature of their condition. From a clinical point of view, the most important component of care is the availability of an adult within the health care team who has the trust of both parents and child. Such a person can be alert to the fact, for example, that a young teenager who has shown no signs of wanting to know the truth about the future, is now beginning to want to talk about it. Similarly, she can help the child who does not want to talk about his illness for fear of upsetting his parents by communicating his concerns to the parents.

Children cannot make advance directives to indicate they do not wish to be kept alive in circumstances where life-saving techniques will achieve only a valueless, painful existence. Their parents have to make such decisions for them as trustees of their welfare. In general, if parents and paediatric nursing and medical staff are in good communication, this does not lead to difficulties. However, the presence on the paediatric nursing or medical staff of individuals who take a different view from the majority, or parents who retain a belief in the possibility of a miracle long after this seems within the realms of possibility to the medical staff, present complex situations sometimes not at all easily resolvable. The principle of non-maleficence may be inevitably contravened if parents insist on life being preserved when the hospital staff are convinced that, to keep a child alive, they are inflicting suffering when the child has no meaningful future, or, in contrast, when parents insist on a child's life being maintained when hospital staff, responsible for day-to-day care, believe the child's existence is worse than valueless. Both situations have been widely reported in the United States.

BENEFICENCE

The duty to engage in health care activities that are beneficial to children, and the rights of children to beneficial health care, are in no way different in nature from those in adulthood. If anything, the rights of children to health care may be seen as more imperative than those of adults because of the longer period of life-span that benefits will be enjoyed. However, the application of the principle of beneficence to children does raise special problems. All these relate in some way to the fact that parental beliefs, attitudes and behaviour are either causing ill-health or preventing the child from receiving the health care he needs.

Child Abuse

Children suffer from three main types of abuse at the hands of their parents. Physical abuse may occur at any level of severity from unusually severe bruising to injuries sufficient to cause death. (An unusual but by no means rare form of physical abuse is known as Munchausen's syndrome by proxy; in this situation a parent, virtually always the mother, treats her well child as if ill and instigates or administers physical treatments that are harmful.) Sexual abuse takes many forms, from indecent exposure, through inappropriate fondling to partial or complete intercourse—such behaviour often involving fathers or step-fathers and their daughters. Emotional abuse involves constant belittling, denigration and hostile behaviour of parents towards a child—often only one child in a family is picked on and scapegoated in this way. Unfortunately, all these types of abuse are very common with, for example, about one in 10 adult women reporting having been sexually abused within the family in childhood.

Parental Refusal of Treatment of Children for Positive Reasons

Some parents hold firm religious or other beliefs that prevent their children receiving appropriate health care in particular circumstances. Thus children from families where the parents are Jehovah's Witnesses may not receive blood products even if they suffer from exsanguination or disorders of blood clotting. Increasingly, parents with faith in homoeopathy or other forms of alternative medicine are reluctant to allow their children to receive conventional medical treatments. Of course, in some circumstances the benefits of conventional remedies are highly questionable, and such parental behaviour may well be in the interests of the child or at least not inimical to it. However, there are many situations involving, for example, the use of antibiotics in some infectious diseases, and blood transfusions where serious operative procedures are undertaken, in which the benefits of conventional medicine are not seriously questionable.

Parental Neglect Leading to Poor Health Care for Children

Children may suffer from parental neglect from the stages of early fetal development through childhood to adolescence. In pregnancy the mother may neglect herself, smoke heavily, drink alcohol, eat an inadequate diet and fail to obtain available pre-natal care. In infancy the baby may again be fed inadequately and not taken to health facilities when sick. Low immunization rates and poor compliance with necessary treatment (e.g. diet in coeliac disease and phenylketonuria, medication in diabetes and asthma) are commonly due to parental behaviour. In some circumstances the benefits of compliance are uncertain, but in many others they are again not really in question.

In all these situations, application of the principle of beneficence is complicated by virtue of the fact that there is conflict between two desirable approaches—the approach involving cooperation with parents who are agents and trustees acting on behalf of the child and in the child's best interests, and the approach involving delivery of health care to children that gives them the best chance of a rich quality of life. Reconciliation of these two approaches is not always possible. It seems reasonable, however, to suggest principles that can be applied in these circumstances. Confrontation and disagreement with parents will inevitably be necessary in some situations as part of the process of caring for the child. In emergencies, for example, when a child's life is at risk, if he is not transfused, he may need to be given blood even if this is against his Jehovah's Witness parents' wishes, though as new substitute blood products become available, even this may not be necessary. Parents who deny they have caused an injury may need to be confronted when there is clear evidence that this is not the case, e.g. when there are cigarette burns on the child's skin, or adult bite marks. However, such confrontation should be limited in duration, and a partnership with parents resumed as soon as possible. In some circumstances it becomes clear that parents are never going to be able to provide adequate care for their child. In these hopefully unusual situations the principle of beneficence will involve health professionals working with staff from social services or social welfare departments to find new parents (foster-parents or, to achieve permanency, adoptive parents) to act as more effective trustees for the child's welfare. However, even in these circumstances the child's best interests may often be served by retention of some contact with their parents and, in England and Wales, the 1989 Children Act insists on the parents retaining a degree of responsibility, even if their children are not living at home temporarily or permanently.

A further dilemma exists when a parent, perhaps because of the presence of mental illness, cannot look after her child. It may be in the child's best interests for a complete or partial separation to occur, but it might be in the mother's best interests for her to retain contact with her child. In these circumstances it is generally agreed, both in law and by general consensus, that the child's interests must be regarded as paramount.

THE PRINCIPLE OF JUSTICE

Children do not have a vote, and consequently do not participate in the democratic process. Consequently they have no direct say in the distribution of scarce resources that might be directed towards them. In these circumstances it seems particularly appropriate to use a Rawlsian 'veil of ignorance' model (15) to consider how resources might fairly be distributed to this non-enfranchised group of the population. This model proposes a hypothetical discussion between people before they embark on their life journey. At the time they have their discussion they do not know how their life chances are to be distributed. In a capitalist society some will become rich, others will be poor. In any society some will enjoy good health, others suffer poor health. How will they decide on fair ways to distribute and redistribute the limited resources to which the population in question has access? On the basis of their hypothetical decisions a fair means of resource distribution might be devised, and the principles used in coming to conclusions might be used in real-life situations.

The situation *is* hypothetical, but it is interesting to speculate how children would be viewed if a group of mature adults pretended to exist in a pre-life situation and discuss the distribution of resources. It seems to me reasonable to suppose the following. First, resources would be allocated preferentially to children rather than adults on the assumption that they would live longer to enjoy the benefits (see above). However, this presupposes an equivalent quality of life in the years that are lived by children and by adults. Secondly, resources might be allocated preferentially to those children with a reasonable prospect of autonomous, independent living (in terms of relationships, marriage, parenthood, employment) rather than to those with limited or absent prospects for autonomous life. Third, resources would be allocated according to their cost-effectiveness. Thus, at one end of the scale, cheap, effective remedies would be preferred to expensive, ineffective remedies.

Let it be said at once that there are both moral and practical problems with this approach. From a moral point of view it might be regarded as offensive to view the life of a child who is not going to achieve autonomous living as less valuable than a child who is. Parents of children with learning difficulties would certainly take strong exception to this view, and some people would regard as unacceptable any attempt to compare the values of individual lives (16). Further, the Rawlsian model implies a moral consensus among a group of people who do not actually exist. Is it reasonable to base a system of distributing resources upon a fiction?

From a practical point of view the approach also has major problems, but many of these might be overcome. For example, there is at the moment no satisfactory quality of life measure for children, so that it is not possible to compare the effectiveness of one treatment against another within one condition, or to compare the cost benefit of similar resources used for different conditions. Further, many investigations and types of treatment remain either uncosted or only unsatisfactorily costed. Finally, the effectiveness of a treatment is often unpredictable in the individual child. Rapid scientific development of new treatments makes it quite possible that some form of palliative care, thought only to be of minor value at the time it was applied, might become of major significance if a new effective treatment for the condition in question comes on the scene.

These moral and practical dilemmas that the Rawlsian model raises are formidable, but it may nevertheless be desirable to consider an allocation of resources along these lines. This might be preferable to the present situation in which resources are clearly allocated unfairly, often to the more powerful clinicians with the most influential contacts, and clinical decisions are made equally arbitrarily by clinicians using criteria they would often find difficult to articulate. Those working with children sometimes think that the young would benefit considerably if there were greater attempts to allocate resources using clearly defined ethical judgements.

CONCLUSION

The ethical issues concerning the health care of developing children often at the threshold of competent understanding of their condition, are complex. Health care professionals looking after children are often heavily stressed by the nature of their work, by inadequate resources, and by poor management of those resources that are available. Consequently it is not surprising that their practice in relation to issues covering, for example, proxy consent for therapeutic and research procedures, is sometimes questionable. Very significant improvements could occur if health care professionals, especially nurses and doctors, were more aware of these issues, felt secure in their professional behaviour and the principles guiding them (but able to be flexible in individual cases), were knowledgeable about the law and, perhaps most important of all, had time to spend with parents and children listening to their views.

REFERENCES

1. Eiser, C. 1985. Changes in understanding of illness as the child grows. *Archives of Disease in Childhood* **60**: 489–492.
2. Alderson, P. 1990. *Choosing for children: parents' consent to surgery*. Oxford University Press, Oxford.
3. Brahams, D. 1986. Exploration and disclosure of risks in the treatment of children. *Lancet* **1**: 925–926.
4. Fell, J. M. E. and Rylance, G. W. 1991. Parental permission, information and consent. *Archives of Disease in Childhood* **66**: 980–981.
5. Graham, P. J. 1991. *Child psychiatry: a developmental approach*. Oxford University Press, Oxford.
6. Dyer, C. 1985. Contraceptives and the under sixteens. House of Lords Ruling. *British Medical Journal* **291**: 1208–1209.
7. Freeman, M. D. A. 1983. *The rights and wrongs of children*. Frances Pinter, London.
8. Department of Health and Welsh Office. 1990. *Code of practice. Mental Health Act 1983*. HMSO, London.
9. Nicholson, R. (Ed.) 1986. *Medical research with children: ethics, law and practice*. Oxford University Press, Oxford.
10. Campbell, A. G. M. 1988. Ethical issues in child health and disease. Pp. 215–253, *in* Forfar, J. (Ed.) *Child health in a changing society*. Oxford University Press, Oxford.
11. Dworkin, G. 1978. Legality of consent to non-therapeutic medical research on infants and young children. *Archives of Disease in Childhood* **53**: 443–446.
12. Smith, M., Grocke, M. and Graham, P. 1993. *Normal family sexuality and sexual knowledge in children*. Monograph Series, Royal College of Psychiatrists (In press).
13. Smith, M. 1985. Taking blood from children causes no more than minimal harm. *Journal of Medical Ethics* **11**: 127–131.
14. Lansdown, R. and Goldman, A. 1988. The psychological care of children with malignant disease. *Journal of Child Psychology and Psychiatry* **29**: 555–567.
15. Rawls, J. 1972. *A theory of justice*. Oxford University Press, Oxford.

57

Ethics and Psychotherapy

Jeremy Holmes, MRCP, FRCPsych

Consultant Psychiatrist/Psychotherapist, North Devon District Hospital, UK

Richard Lindley, PhD

Solicitor, formerly Lecturer in Philosophy, University of Bradford, UK

In this chapter we shall be concerned with those therapies which, not content simply with the removal of unpleasant symptoms, aim for bigger game. Many, if not most psychotherapy patients (and their therapists) are, overtly or unconsciously, hoping that therapy will lead to a happier, more fulfilled, less trammelled life: to feel more free and to achieve deeper and more secure relationships. Thus psychotherapy requires a scrutiny of the most intimate and personal aspects of people's lives, and can potentially turn a person's world upside-down.

Given that psychotherapy may lead people completely to re-evaluate their ways of life and relationships it is perhaps surprising what scant attention has, with a few notable exceptions (1–3), been devoted to psychotherapeutic ethics. This is in part no doubt due to Freud's wish to establish psychoanalysis as a science and his extreme scepticism when it came to spiritual or moral matters, confining himself, as he preferred to say, to the foundations of the building of psychoanalysis, rather than loitering in its airy upper chambers where he saw the existentialist Binswangler and the later Jung.

With the recent upsurge of interest in ethical issues in medicine and the other professions, however, this is changing (4–5); For example most psychotherapy organizations now consider it necessary to have a code of ethics by which their members should abide. In this chapter we make no attempt to cover the whole field of psychotherapeutic ethics, but concentrate specifically on two aspects in which analytical psychotherapy has a particular contribution to make to the general understanding of medical ethics. The first concerns the autonomy, a vital, but often misunderstood goal of psychotherapy. We shall consider the account given by analytical therapy of the developmental origins of autonomy,

Principles of Health Care Ethics. Edited by Raanan Gillon.
© 1994 John Wiley & Sons Ltd

and how psychotherapy may enhance the autonomy of its beneficiaries. The second considers the ethical problem of sexual relations between therapists and their patients. We approach this by looking at how the phenomenon of *transference*—the distortion of present feelings, perceptions and experiences by relationships and experiences from the past, especially infancy and early childhood—may be an obstacle to autonomy and how it may interfere with and influence the behaviour, 'ethical' or otherwise, of therapists and doctors.

Ethical problems in psychotherapy can conventionally be considered under three headings. The first concerns the general conduct of the therapy—its arrangements, boundaries, contractual agreements and so on. Secondly there is the question of the underlying values which inform and guide the therapy—its aims and general philosophy of life. Thirdly there is the issue of the specific way in which therapists handle and behave towards clients within a session, this being largely the practical application of items one and two, but nevertheless a topic which merits consideration in its own right.

MEDICAL AND PSYCHOTHERAPEUTIC ETHICS

Ethical issues in the first area include such matters as informed consent, financial or sexual exploitation of patients by unscrupulous therapists, and the problems of maintaining confidentiality in psychotherapy. Most ethical codes in psychotherapy focus on these questions, and are based on comparable principles that have been evolved to tackle them within medical ethics.

An important principle underlying such codes is that of *autonomy*, and therapists, like medical practitioners, are enjoined to do nothing which might compromise a patient's autonomy: they should, for example, avoid attempts to coerce, control or cajole them into courses of action, even when motivated by a benevolent desire to prevent patients from acting against their best interests.

And yet this anti-paternalistic principle is not without exception. Many of the interesting dilemmas in medical ethics arise from the question of how to give proper weight to the autonomy of patients. Nowhere is this more acute than in psychiatry where, through mental illness, a patient's capacity to act autonomously may be severely impaired. Occasionally it *is* in a patient's best interests apparently to have her autonomy removed, as in the case of suicidally depressed patients.

In evaluating such apparent violations of autonomy it is necessary to make careful distinctions. There is, first of all, the question of whether the (overall) autonomy of the patient is being sacrificed out of concern for some other value, for example a belief in the intrinsic value of longevity. Second there is the question of whether short-term autonomy is being sacrificed for greater long-term autonomy. Third is the question of whether the patient's current state of mind is so impaired that preventing him from doing what he currently wants to do is not a serious assault on his autonomy.

Dilemmas surrounding autonomy are similarily important in psychotherapy, since patients' distress and, through transference, their devotion to a therapist, may lead them to make bad choices about therapy, or to being exploited sexually or financially by their therapist (5).

THE AIMS OF PSYCHOTHERAPY

In the underlying philosophy which underpins psychotherapy we find that autonomy again looms large. In *The values of psychotherapy* (5) we argued that a major aim of therapy is the promotion of autonomy, and that, since autonomy has, at least from the time of John Stuart Mill, been thought of as socially desirable, psychotherapy, as an autonomy-enhancer, should also be seen as beneficial. This was how we put it then:

> What *is* autonomy? Autonomy literally means 'self-rule', and has its origins in the ancient Greek city states, where granting a dependent state *autonomia* meant allowing it a degree of devolved self-government. The term has been transposed to apply to individual people as well as collectivities. Autonomy in the context of psychotherapy implies taking control of one's own life. The deep-seated desire for autonomy is captured in this statement by Isaiah Berlin:

> 'I wish my life and decisions to depend on myself, and not on external forces of any kind. I wish to be the instrument of my own, not of other men's acts of will. I wish to be a subject, not an object; to be moved by reasons, by conscious purposes, which are my own, not by causes which affect me, as it were, from outside. I wish to be a somebody, not a nobody, a doer—deciding, not being decided for, self-directed and not acted on by external nature, or by other men as if I were a thing, or an animal, or a slave incapable of playing a human role, that is, of conceiving goals and policies of my own and realising them. ... I wish, above all, to be conscious of myself as a thinking, active being, bearing responsibility for my choices and able to explain them by reference to my own ideas and purposes.'

> In this statement Berlin, writing as a political philosopher, posits a distinction between an 'internal' self or agent striving for autonomy and 'external' forces which may control or thwart this wish. The importance of his account for psychotherapy is that many people, especially those seeking emotional help, are frustrated not by their circumstances but by themselves. The 'external nature' by which they feel controlled comprises their own impulses and feelings; the 'causes' which affect them are internal, though they may be experienced as alien and unwanted. Psychotherapy enhances autonomy because it brings these internal 'external' forces within the orbit of the acting, thinking, feeling, responsible self. This idea is contained in Freud's famous imperative definition of the aim of psychoanalysis as 'where id is, there ego shall be' (Freud (6)), or in Bettleheim's (7) re-translation 'where *it* is, there *I* shall be'. This state can be called 'emotional autonomy'.

> Emotional autonomy does not mean isolation or avoidance of dependency. The opposite of autonomy is heteronomy, not dependency. The lonely schizoid individual who preserves his 'independence' at all costs may well be emotionally *heteronomous*, unable to bear closeness with another person because of inner dread and confusion. A similar state of emotional heteronomy affects the psychopath who is unaware of the feelings of others. The emotionally autonomous individual does not suppress her feelings, including the need for dependence, but takes cognisance of them, ruling rather than being ruled by them. In Freud's important rider to his principle he likens the ego to a horseman and the id to the mount, and points out that at times, in order to control one's horse, it has to be given its head.

> Psychotherapy helps its patients by promoting their emotional autonomy. It produces a 'man that is not passion's slave'; not someone who is emotion-less, but rather someone who is no longer enslaved by emotion-generated heteronomy. This is part a developmental process, providing an opportunity for emotional growth towards maturity to occur; in part an educational process, coming to understand what emotional forces are at work within one; and in part a moralizing process, effectively giving one the strength to do what one really judges to be best.

This psychotherapeutic concept of 'emotional autonomy' recasts autonomy *in relational terms*. A person's autonomy depends on the way in which he or she relates to the world, and in particular to his/her significant others. An optimal state of emotional autonomy would imply, for example, a balance between closeness yet separateness that has been shown to be associated with marital harmony (8), while both overdependence, and emotional isolation and compulsive individualism, are correlated with marital distress and breakdown.

Psychotherapy can be costly both financially and in terms of the challenges it can pose to a patient's existing way of relating to the world. We would argue that these costs are worth paying because the prospect of improved autonomy is a prize of inestimable value. However, to justify itself, psychotherapy needs to offer an explanation of how *it* is particularly equipped to promote emotional autonomy. To meet this challenge it is necessary to ask how autonomy arises, and how it may be fostered and developed.

OBJECT RELATIONS THEORY AND THE ORIGINS OF AUTONOMY

Object relations theorists—a diverse group of mainly British psychoanalysts who include Klein, Fairbairn, Winnicott, Balint and Bowlby—provide an account of infant development that describes the conditions under which emotional autonomy develops, and conversely those under which it founders, resulting, it is hypothesized, in neurosis and breakdown in later life. Through psychotherapy these pathological developmental pathways may be overcome, leading through the development of personal growth and insight, to greater emotional autonomy.

For Bowlby (9) the precondition of emotional autonomy is, paradoxically perhaps, secure attachment. The child whose parents provide a secure base feels free to explore the world (including his or her own feelings) and to develop a sense of an autonomous self. On the basis of this secure emotional environment the child develops 'internal working models' of secure attachment figures which enable him to withstand anxiety and to develop his or her own identity without excessive reliance on the support or opinions of others.

Bowlby's ideas were developed by looking at the after-effects of major disruptions of parenting such as those that result from bereavement or prolonged separation in childhood. Winnicott (10) considers how autonomy may be compromised even within an apparently secure relationship, showing how the growing infant may become *compliant*, bending to the needs of the mother, rather than satisfying his own wishes and desires. This leads, he believes, to the development of a *'false self'*, lacking in real autonomy and spontaneity, concealing a needy or depressed self that craves expression and may manifest itself in pathological ways. Winnicott's experiences as a paediatrician before becoming a psychoanalyst enabled him to study in great detail the minutiae of mother–infant interaction and to show how their mutual *play* can either foster or inhibit the growing infant's sense of autonomy.

The implications of Winnicott and Bowlby's work are that emotional autonomy can be compromised by anxious attachment, schizoid detachment, or by compliance and the development of a 'false self'. The task of psychotherapy is to help overcome these defensive manoeuvres. Both were pupils of Melanie

Klein (11) who emphasized *splitting* as a fundamental defensive mechanism in infancy. Later Kleinian writers, especially Bion (12), have shown how splitting is a precursor to *projective identification*, a defence in which the infant's split-off anxieties, or potentially overwhelming feelings of rage and frustration are projected into the mother, who *contains* them in her state of 'maternal reverie' in such a way that they are transmuted into a manageable form, and how they can, with the help of the 'thinking breast', be reintegrated into the infant's growing psyche as development proceeds.

INTEGRATION AND CONTAINMENT

Underlying the idea of emotional autonomy therefore is the concept of *integration*. The individual who is divided against himself, who has to keep true self and 'false self' separate at all costs, or who has disowned parts of himself and projected ego ideal or unwanted aggression in to the environment cannot act in a truly autonomous way (13, 14).

Projective identification can be healthy or pathological. The capacity to identify, to empathize, to understand the world depends on our ability to put ourselves out of ourselves and into someone else's shoes. In pathological states this process becomes compulsive and unconscious. The outside world contains and reflects back split-off mood states. The paranoid person experiences the world as persecutory: the angry and rejecting husband feels that his wife is hostile and uncaring. The task of the therapist is, by neutrality, containment and reflection, to break the vicious circle in which the world continually confirms what is projected into it.

Implicit in psychotherapy then is an ethic which values a harmonious relationship between container and contained in which that which is contained is securely held, but not trapped; in which what is held is whole and not internally divided; and in which there is easy interplay between container and contained. The healthy individual is able to remain separate yet fully connected to the world.

Psychotherapy is not moralistic in the sense of trying to lay down a particular ideal of good conduct. Unlike the doctrines of religion it does not purport to resolve moral dilemmas. It aims to enable its participants to make their own choices, unfettered by the chains of neurosis.

THE ETHIC OF THE SESSION

Students of psychotherapy learn their craft in a number of ways—from observing their own therapist's behaviour, from sitting in with experienced therapists in assessment sessions, from audiotapes and videotapes, from their supervisors, and from the process of trial-and-error as they work with their own patients. Discussion of how therapists approach patients, their attitude and manner, as well as the question of when and how and in what way they 'intervene', come usually under the heading of 'technique'. In *The values of psychotherapy* (5) we argued that many of the apparent ethical dilemmas of analytic psychotherapy—how much the therapist should reveal of herself in response to direct questions, whether to make special allowances for patients who are disadvantaged or traumatized, whether it was ever justified to deceive patients in their best interests—are in reality not ethical dilemmas at all, but can be resolved technically through the understanding of transference and countertransference.

There is, however, a deeper layer to therapy upon which these transferential issues rest, which is a precondition of successful therapy, and which raises genuine questions of ethics which lack a purely technical solution.

According to the Rogerian school the essential attributes of a successful therapist are empathy, honesty, and non-possessive warmth (15). It is generally agreed that some degree of personal maturity and balance is needed in candidates for psychotherapy training (16). *Balance,* an essential feature of maturity, can be expressed in a series of dichotomies. The therapist should be reliable but not robot-like; stable but humanly frail; non-judgemental but not collusive; present to the patient, but not intrusive; compassionate but reserved; self-renunciative but not passive; non-exploitative but not self-sacrificing; not goody-goody but always good enough.

Ferenczi (17) challenged the view that change in therapy derives merely from intellectual understanding and technique with the statement 'it is the analyst's love which cures the patient'. Subsequent analysts have been somewhat wary of this approach, especially in the light of Ferenczi's possible sexual involvement with his patients. The issue turns on what are meant by 'love' and 'understanding'. Love can be subdivided into sexual love, conjugal love, protective love (of parents for their children for example), and compassionate love. Most loving relationships contain a mixture of all these elements in varying degrees. Therapeutic love is compassionate in the sense that the therapist empathically puts herself in the patient's shoes in order to appreciate and recognize her suffering.

These distinctions are not always easy to recognize, and the boundaries between the different kinds of love are not clearly marked. Nowhere are the ethical dilemmas of psychotherapy more acute than over the question of circumscribing the love which therapists should show for their patients. Ethical difficulties arise if the boundaries are crossed and, rather than compassion, the therapist offers sexual or 'conjugal' (i.e. interminable) love.

SEXUAL INVOLVEMENT BETWEEN THERAPIST AND PATIENT

Sexual involvement between the therapist and patient has been a troublesome problem since the early days of psychoanalysis. With the increasing awareness of sexual abuse in society generally several studies (18, 19) have focused on therapeutic abuse, which occurs mainly but not exclusively between male therapists and female patients, and have established the relative frequency of this phenomenon. According to Gartrell at least 5% of therapists in the United States have abused patients at some time.

Unlike victims of child sexual abuse, however, psychotherapy patients who enter sexual relationships with their therapists are not children. Such relationships are universally condemned by psychotherapeutic codes of ethics. But providing there is no element of coercion, what is *wrong* with such relationships? They may well be emotionally damaging but the same, after all, could be said of many sexual relationships between adults which society is quite happy to condone.

There are at least three ways of answering this challenge. The first points to the inherent inequality between patient and therapist. The patient is often in a state of distress and severe emotional need, and is therefore not in a position to make rational choices about whom she wishes to go to bed with. The job of the therapist is to help her to understand the roots of her distress and, by providing a secure and trusting atmosphere of non-sexual intimacy, help her to achieve a more balanced and autonomous state of mind. In this respect therapists should adopt the role of 'good-enough' parents who create for their children conditions for healthy emotional growth, and who do not abuse the power and intimacy which their role as parents gives them to gratify their own sexual needs. The therapist should, like a responsible parent, recognize his patient's emotional and sexual needs without responding to them emotionally or sexually.

The sexually abusing therapist is exploiting the patient for his own needs rather than hers, and although this may make him no worse than many other males in our society we expect particularly high standards of ethical behaviour in those with whom we entrust the emotionally wounded, no less than we do for the physically wounded.

A second consideration is the question of *deception*. The sexually abusing therapist, when first entering into a psychotherapeutic contract is unlikely to advertise the fact that he may to try to 'help' his patient sexually. This is hardly surprising since, as we shall see, he himself is probably unaware of his intentions. A distinction should be drawn between therapists who explicitly offer 'surrogacy' as part of the therapy for, say, sexual problems, and the sexually abusing therapist in the course of normal therapy. The sexually abusing therapist is harming his patient (and the evidence suggests that sexual involvement between therapist and patient almost always is harmful to the patient) not just by sexual exploitation, but also because, by offering one thing, i.e. therapy, and providing another, i.e. sex, he is deceiving her.

Deception is, in any event, wrong because to deceive someone is to treat him or her, in Kant's expression, 'merely as a means to an end'. It is particularly wrong in psychotherapy because, as we have argued, the overall aim of therapy is to increase emotional autonomy. Deception is antithetical to autonomy, and indeed a major part of the task of therapy is to expose the feelings and impulses of which the patient is unaware, but which nevertheless influence her, and these can in a sense be seen as forms of (unconscious) self-deception. It was only because he was unaware of who his real parents were that Oedipus came to kill his father and to marry his mother. The tragedy of therapeutic sexual abuse is that, at the moment of abuse, both parties may genuinely believe that what they are doing will be beneficial.

This brings us on to what, from the point of view of analytic psychotherapy, is the central issue in therapeutic abuse. This is the influence of unconscious transferential forces which affect both patient and therapist, and which create a 'bipersonal transferential field' (20) which provides the context for the abuse. This viewpoint postulates not just a damaged patient who turns to the therapist in search of the tenderness she lacked with her father and the nurturance and protection she sought in vain with her mother, but also a therapist who has projected all his own pain and longing for intimacy into his patient, and who unconsciously through his 'help' hopes to overcome his repressed feelings of helplessness and loneliness. In the timeless moment of sexual abuse the 'rules' of therapy are abolished no less than they are when the sexually abusing father or step-father obliterates the mother who has failed to protect her child. The patient who has been sexually abused as a child will be particularly vulnerable to therapeutic abuse because of the unleashing of these transferential forces.

An example is now presented which had all the potential for the development of therapeutic abuse. It exemplifies a minor form of 'frame violation' (20) falling far short of abuse, but nevertheless with considerable, albeit temporary, damaging effects on the progress of the therapy and the well-being of the patient.

A woman in her 40s, divorced, without a partner, who had been sexually abused by her father in childhood developed a strong erotic transference in which she daydreamed of being married to her therapist, of making love with him, but *dreamed* that he put his arm protectively around her in a non-sexual way so that she felt, as she never normally felt, safe and secure and at peace. A holiday break was approaching which the therapist sensed would be very difficult for the patient. As they were parting at the end of the session he found himself shaking her by the hand, an action usually reserved for his first encounter with a patient and not repeated until therapy comes to an end. The moment he did so he realized that it was a mistake, driven by his own counter-transferential guilt about the break. She grasped at the hand with both of hers as though she were drowning, and gazed intently at him, for a brief moment. On his return from holiday she revealed that she had developed a paralysis of her hand! She was convinced that this was 'psychological', brought on by *her* guilt at having achieved what she so dearly wanted, i.e. physical contact with her therapist. He, on the other hand, felt sure that she had developed multiple sclerosis and imagined that she would become progressively more and more dependent upon him and that she could never be discharged from therapy. On reflection he was able to understand this as a counter-transferential projection of her feeling that she was an unbearable burden to her carers. This derived from her childhood experience of premature separation from her mother who sent her to a boarding school at the age of five, and which constituted her way of explaining her mother's inability to protect her from the sexual abuse by her father. Eventually she consulted a neurologist; the paralysis turned out to have a physical but not life-threatening cause due to cervical spondylosis, and after a few weeks she made a full recovery.

Therapeutic abuse remains an ever-present possibility in psychotherapy given the intimacy of the therapeutic relationship, the fact that a large proportion of patients seeking therapy have difficulties with intimate relationships, and that a not-insignificant proportion of those who are drawn to the therapy profession may also be beset with their own emotional difficulties. There is a need therefore for a set of safeguards which are likely to ensure the ethical practice of psychotherapy. These include personal therapy for therapists, regular supervision for therapists at all levels, and the organization of a properly regulated and recognized psychotherapy profession (5). Such measures will not be watertight. Patients and therapists will occasionally fall in love, and not always with disastrous results. No doubt sexual and other forms of therapeutic exploitation will also continue in spite of all these measures, but at least they will ensure that an atmosphere of good practice prevails, that there are agreed standards against which deviant behaviour can be measured, that disciplinary procedures exist for the censure and if necessary expulsion of erring therapists, and that the public can have some legitimate confidence in a profession whose basis must always be that of a trusting and secure relationship.

CONCLUSION

Autonomy is a central preoccupation of medical ethics. In this chapter we have tried to show how a sense of autonomy may be enhanced or hindered in the course of emotional development, and how the intimacy of the therapeutic relationship may evoke transferential forces which may lead therapists to compromise their patients' autonomy, and what safeguards are needed to minimize this possibility.

The past few years have seen a huge expansion in the volume, range and public awareness of the psychotherapies. This expansion has itself raised ethical questions, for instance that of informed consent and the need for patients to be aware of the possible alternative forms of treatment before embarking on a particular course. It has also thrown into public scrutiny a set of ethical issues that had hitherto lain undisturbed within the somewhat arcane and marginal realm of psychotherapy. Some critics have responded to this expansion by continuation of the, by now, discredited attempts to dismiss the therapy profession as a whole (21), but despite this it seems likely that psychotherapy will continue to establish itself a significant cultural force and a practice of distinct efficacy. The associated ethical and moral issues that it raises have only been touched on in this survey. There is little doubt that in future they will be actively debated both within and without the emerging profession of psychotherapy.

REFERENCES

1. Michels, R. 1976. Professional ethics and social values. *International Review of Psychoanalysis* 3: 377–384.
2. Rieff, P. 1979. *Freud: the mind of the moralist*. University of Chicago Press, London.
3. Shafer, R. 1976. *A new language for psychoanalysis*. Yale University Press, London.
4. Lakin, M. 1988. *Ethical issues in the psychotherapies*. Oxford University Press, New York.
5. Holmes, J. and Lindley, R. 1989. *The values of psychotherapy*. Oxford University Press, Oxford.
6. Freud, S. 1923. *The Ego and the Id*. Hogarth, London.
7. Bettleheim, B. 1983. *Freud and man's soul*. Chatto, London.
8. Beavers, W. and Hampson, R. 1990. *Successful families*. Norton, New York.
9. Bowlby, J. 1988. *A secure base*. Routledge, London.
10. Winnicott, D. 1965. *The maturational processes and the facilitating environment*. Hogarth, London.
11. Klein, M. 1950. *Contributions to psychoanalysis*. Hogarth, London.
12. Bion, W. 1970. *Attention and interpretation*. Tavistock, London.
13. Hinchelwood, R. 1989. Therapy or coercion: psycho-analytic considerations on ethics. Freud Memorial Lecture, University College London, January.

14. Storr, A. 1965. *The integration of the personality.* Penguin, London.
15. Truax, C. and Carkhuff, R. 1967. *Towards effective counselling and psychotherapy.* Aldine, Chicago.
16. Storr, A. 1979. *The art of psychotherapy.* Oxford University Press, Oxford.
17. Ferenczi, S. and Rank, O. 1925. *The development of psychoanalysis.* Nervous and Mental Disease Publishing Co., New York.
18. Gartrell, N. *et al.* 1986. Psychiatrist–patient contact. *American Journal of Psychiatry* **143**: 1126–1131.
19. Rutter, P. 1990. *Sex in the forbidden zone.* Unwin, London.
20. Langs, R. 1976. *The bipersonal field.* Jason Aronson, New York.
21. Masson, G. 1985. *The assault on truth.* Penguin, London.

58

Psychiatric Ethics: a Bioethical Ugly Duckling?

K. W. M. FULFORD

Research Fellow, Green College, Oxford, UK; and Honorary Consultant Psychiatrist

TONY HOPE

Leader of Oxford Practice Skills Project, The Medical School, University of Oxford, UK; and Honorary Consultant Psychiatrist

INTRODUCTION

Psychiatry has a paradoxical place in biomedical ethics. As a practical discipline it is perhaps more problematic ethically than any other branch of medicine—so much so that some have argued that mental illness is really a moral rather than medical concept (1). Yet until recently, with the appearance of some important benchmark publications (2–5), psychiatry has been relatively neglected by mainstream medical ethics.

In this chapter we explore some of the reasons for the neglect of psychiatric ethics. The nature of psychiatric ethics is first outlined briefly, and then illustrated with a more detailed exploration of the problems raised by involuntary psychiatric treatment. This shows that traditional bioethics, and the four-principles approach in particular, has assumed a scientific, value-neutral model of disease to which ethical principles can be applied. This approach works well enough in the 'high-tech' areas of medicine with which bioethics has been mostly concerned. But in psychiatry it stops short of the specifically medical ethical difficulties raised by the subject. In psychiatry the concept of disease is itself ethically problematic.

It is this feature of psychiatry which, we argue, has distanced it from traditional bioethics. But it is this feature, also, which points directly to the need for a more complete model of disease, one in which the evaluative element in its meaning is taken as seriously as the factual. This in turn provides a framework

Principles of Health Care Ethics. Edited by Raanan Gillon.
© 1994 John Wiley & Sons Ltd

for medical ethics in which the principles approach can be supplemented by a sensitive engagement with the concrete details of the individual case. This turns out not to be an argument for situational ethics as such, however. Situational ethics alone provides no more secure a foundation for psychiatric ethics than undiluted principles. In pointing the way to a new medical ethics, therefore— an ethics in which principles and practice, concept and case, are fully reconciled— psychiatric ethics is transformed from a bioethical ugly duckling into a clinical–ethical swan.

THEORY AND PRACTICE IN PSYCHIATRIC ETHICS

The gap between theory and practice in psychiatric ethics is well illustrated by the structure of Beauchamp and Childress's *Principles of biomedical ethics* (6) (we will sometimes refer to this just as the *Principles*). In the main text, psychiatry is largely eclipsed by AIDS, abortion and other stalwarts of the standard bioethical portfolio. A number of important psychiatric topics are there, certainly: for example, the possibility of rational suicide; the place of involuntary treatment for depression and addiction; and the limits of confidentiality in psychotherapy. But compared with other topics psychiatry is writ small. This is illustrated by the American Medical Association being given 37 page references in the index, whilst the American Psychiatric Association gets only one! Moreover, other important topics in psychiatric ethics are not mentioned at all: contentious treatments, such as ECT, neurosurgery, and the chemical modification of sexuality; conflicts of loyalty in family therapy; research with patients incompetent to give consent; and so on. When we turn, however, from theory to practice, from the main text to the appendix of clinical cases, the emphasis is reversed. Here, psychiatry, far from being eclipsed, is actually dominant, no less than 20% of cases being concerned directly with psychiatric patients.

At first glance there is no shortage of possible reasons for the neglect of psychiatry by much of bioethics. In the first place the issues with which psychiatric ethics is concerned, although pervasive, are mostly low profile. Psychiatry has its *causes célèbres*: abuses of compulsory treatment (7,8), for example; and, conversely, failures to prevent patients from harming themselves or others (9). By and large, though, compared with, say, reproductive medicine, there are few headlines in chronic schizophrenia, mental handicap and dementia. Then again, the subject-matter of psychiatric ethics is for various reasons relatively inaccessible: it is diverse, there being no unifying theme (like the status of the embryo in reproductive medicine); and it is arcane, many important symptoms of mental illness (e.g. thought insertion) being unfamiliar outside psychiatry.

Closer inspection, however, shows that these features of psychiatry, far from resolving the paradox of its neglect, actually sharpen it. If ethical problems in psychiatry are low profile, this is because they are firmly embedded in day-to-day practice. They are so familiar that they are simply not noticed for what they are. Even compulsory treatment, a relatively prominent area of ethical concern, is not confined to a few specialists (as is *in vitro* fertilization, for example): it is part of the everyday clinical work of psychiatrists, psychiatric nurses and social workers. Furthermore, the practice of psychiatry raises the full range of traditional bioethical concerns, often in highly pertinent and novel ways: autonomy and beneficence, as we will see in the next section, are crucially involved in compulsory treatment; dementia raises issues of personal identity; hypomania raises problems about well-being; and so on. Indeed the very diagnostic concepts employed in psychiatry provide a bridge between medicine and morality, these concepts running from the organic disorders, through depression and phobias, to hysteria (problematically differentiated from malingering), and on to behavioural disorders (sometimes, as in DSM-III (10) actually defined by reference to social-evaluative norms). The diversity of psychiatric illness, therefore, should have increased its interest to ethicists, and not only to ethicists but also to other philosophers. As Glover (11), Wilkes (12) and others (13,14) have indicated, much of the subject-matter of descriptive psychopathology is the subject-matter also of philosophy—emotion, affect, perception, identity, volition, thought and action, intention, belief and desire!

We need to look deeper, therefore, for the reasons for the relative neglect of psychiatry by bioethics. In the next section we pursue these reasons by considering the issues raised by compulsory psychiatric treatment. These will be illustrated by a case-vignette questionnaire study. In the section after that we apply the *Principles* approach to the results of this study. The two sections taken together will show that the four principles, although providing a useful framework for describing and analysing the ethical problems raised by compulsory treatment, stop short just where the key practical problems for psychiatric ethics begin. This will be shown to be because the *Principles* approach assumes an exclusively value-free model of the medical concepts. This will in turn lead to our conclusions about the place of the four principles in medical ethics generally.

INVOLUNTARY PSYCHIATRIC TREATMENT

Involuntary (or compulsory) psychiatric treatment is a central topic of concern for psychiatric ethics (14). The justification of such treatment rests broadly on the idea that someone who is seriously mentally ill may be treated against their express wishes if this is in their best interests (or sometimes for the protection of others). This idea has been widely held, in many different cultures, and from earliest historical times. Yet it is highly contentious. Objection to the notion that fully conscious adult patients of normal intelligence should be treated against their wishes in their own interests, lies behind much of the opposition to the very notion of mental illness. Compulsory treatment, it is felt, whatever its humanitarian objectives, is an abuse of human freedom and dignity. Certainly it is vulnerable to abuse. Sporadic abuses occur periodically and institutionalized abuse was widespread until recently in the former Soviet Union (7). The critics of psychiatry may have made too much of such cases. But its supporters, perhaps, have underestimated the risks of misuse, of inadvertent wrong uses of involuntary treatment.

The difficulties here are nicely illustrated by the results of a recent case-vignette questionnaire study carried out in Oxford. The study is described in more detail elsewhere (15). Essentially, 22 psychiatrists were asked to consider a series of case-vignettes and to indicate whether or not they thought the patients concerned should be treated if necessary on an involuntary basis. The results are shown in Figure 58.1. There was more or less complete agreement on 12 of the 14 cases: against involuntary treatment in 10 cases and in favour of it in cases 4 (hypomania) and 9 (schizophrenia). There was disagreement, however, about cases 1 (anorexia) and 3 (depression).

There are, of course, limitations to studies of this kind. The case-vignettes are brief and invite filling out. Furthermore the sample size is small and restricted to psychiatrists from one university department. But all this surely makes it the more remarkable that the results should reflect so directly both the strength and weakness of the intuitive ethical basis of compulsory treatment. The strength of the intuition is reflected in the fact that even under these artificial and restricted conditions there was more or less complete agreement (both for and against compulsory treatment) on all but two cases. The weakness is evident in the fact that among just 22 psychiatrists, all from the same clinical department, there was significant disagreement over the remaining two cases. Thus, even ignoring radical objections to compulsion as such, and occasional gross abuses of psychiatry, it would seem that there is an important grey area in which ethical intuition alone is an insufficient basis for decisions about involuntary psychiatric treatment. The question that arises, then, is the extent to which the four principles contribute to understanding in this area.

INVOLUNTARY TREATMENT AND THE FOUR PRINCIPLES

Among other possible approaches, the four principles provide a helpful framework for exploring the difficulties involved in involuntary treatment. What is at issue is a balance of the patient's autonomy against the obligations of the doctor to act beneficently, or at any rate non-maleficently. This is no less than a statement of the *prima facie* dilemma posed by cases 1 and 3 in our study.

Within the framework provided by the principles, moreover, other philosophical insights help to sharpen our understanding. Thus, Beauchamp and Childress draw on Joel Feinberg's concept of 'weak paternalism' to help specify the intuitive basis of compulsory treatment. Strong paternalism involves overriding a patient's express wishes in their best interests even though they are capable of autonomous decision-making. But it is weak paternalism that is involved in the psychiatric case. Compulsory psychiatric treatment is justified only where the patient is *not* capable of autonomous decision-making. This in turn leads to an account of autonomy. Again, Beauchamp and Childress, drawing on various philosophical sources, supply this. Autonomy requires understanding, intention, and freedom from external controlling influences. Competence, in turn, is a threshold condition for autonomy. People are competent to make an autonomous decision if they are capable not only of understanding what is involved but also of deliberating on the decision in a coherent way.

All in all, then, there is a useful package of ideas here, useful as a framework both for setting out and for clarifying the issues raised by involuntary psychiatric treatment. Sometimes, indeed, this package is sufficient to resolve questions of involuntary treatment, or at any rate to justify decisions made about such

CASES	Likelihood of Involuntary Treatment (%)
1. Miss A. N. Age 21 student. Four-year history of intermittent anorexia. Currently seriously underweight, exercising and using laxatives; amenorrhoeic. Refusing admission on the grounds that she is 'too fat'.	25
2. Mr O. C. Aged 27. Bank clerk. Three-year history of progressive slowness at work. Referred with depression and anxiety following suspension from work. Shows severe and progressive obsessional checking which he agrees 'is something wrong with him'. However he drops out of treatment.	10
3. Mr S. D. Aged 48. Bank manager. Presents in casualty with biological symptoms of depression and nihilistic delusions. History of attempted suicide. Asking for something to 'help him sleep'. He refuses to stay in hospital when he is told that he may be suffering from depression.	50
4. Miss H. M. Aged 25. Novice nun. Brought by superiors for urgent outpatient appointment as they are unable to contain her bizarre and sexually disinhibited behaviour. Shows pressure of speech, grandiose delusions and auditory hallucinations. Refusing to stay.	100
5. Mr B. Aged 16. School boy. Seen by GP at parents' request with failing vision in one eye. Despite progressively impaired vision refuses to accept that he is unable to see with that eye. Diagnosis of optic atrophy but refuses investigation through fear of hospitals.	< 5
6. Mr A. Aged 50. Doctor. Developed thickening of lips, hoarse voice, and enlargement of skull over several years. Refused to accept that these changes were anything other than age-related and rejected his colleagues' diagnosis of acromegaly. Refusing investigations.	0
7. Miss H. P. Aged 30. Secretary. Admitted to neurology ward and transferred to psychiatry under protest. Unable to use right hand (patient right-handed). Paralysis 'non-anatomical'. History of self-injury. Rejecting psychological diagnosis and planning to discharge herself.	< 5
8. Mrs C. R. Aged 47. Housewife. Refusing investigation of breast lump discovered on routine screening. Understands that she does not have to accept treatment if the lesion is found to be malignant. Normal mental state.	0
9. Mr S. Aged 18. Student. Emergency psychiatric admission from his college. Behaving oddly. Showed thought insertion (Mike Yarwood 'using his brain'). Complaining that people were talking about him. Refusing medication and planning to leave hospital.	100
10. Mrs H. F. Aged 51. Shop worker. Complained to general practitioner of hot flushes and irregular periods. Had developed backache and X-rays showed osteoporotic change. Refusing HRT despite full explanation of the implications.	0
11. Mrs A. G. P. Aged 25. Housewife. Progressively housebound over two years with agoraphobic symptoms. Refusing behavioural treatment despite threat to job and marriage.	0
12. Mrs M. Aged 46. Nurse. Withdrawing from marital therapy because she resents the implication that their 'problems' are in their relationship. Says her husband is 'sick'. Her husband has been violent in the past and is now threatening to kill her.	< 5
13. Mr P. P. Aged 23. Unemployed man. Seen in casualty by the duty psychiatrist. Brought in by a girl friend because he is angry and threatening to kill a rival. Has been drinking. History of criminal assault. No other symptoms. Refusing to stay.	< 5
14. Mr S. C. Aged 60. Retired. Recent diagnosis of bronchial carcinoma. Normal mental state. Wants repeat prescription of sleeping tablets. GP knows him to be a supporter of euthanasia and suspects he intends to kill himself.	< 5

FIGURE 58.1 A case-vignette study of involuntary psychiatric treatment. The case-vignettes shown in the left-hand column were presented in a questionnaire study to 22 psychiatrists. The percentage figures in the right-hand column reflect the degree of agreement about the use of involuntary treatment. The results fall into three broad groups: 100% agreement on the use of involuntary treatment for cases 4 and 9; significant disagreement about its use for cases 1 and 3; more or less 100% agreement that it should not be used for the remaining cases.

treatment, in actual practice—as in case 9 described by Beauchamp and Childress. This case describes an elderly lady with periods of confusion caused by arteriosclerosis. She was confined against her express wishes in a mental hospital on the grounds, first, that it was in her best interests (she was at risk of serious injury during periods of confusion), and, second, that her impaired cognitive functioning, although intermittent, rendered her incompetent to make a genuinely autonomous decision about confinement in hospital. We may disagree with the decision made in this case, but even disagreement would have to be framed within the package of ideas outlined in Beauchamp and Childress's *Principles*.

That the package is not *generally* sufficient, however, can be illustrated by examination of Figure 58.2. What this shows, broadly, is that, although the principles of beneficence and autonomy are indeed involved in questions of involuntary treatment, they fail to explain the distribution of results of our questionnaire study. Thus the cases from our questionnaire study are shown in this figure in the left-hand column, listed in descending order of likelihood of involuntary treatment—that is, those most likely to be treated involuntarily are at the top (hypomania; schizophrenia), those least likely at the bottom. Next to each of these cases is shown the *prima facie* weights of beneficence and of the elements of autonomy and competence as outlined by Beauchamp and Childress. A number of assumptions have had to be made in attributing these weights, of course: beneficence, consistently with standard medical–ethical thinking, relates to serious risk of more or less immediately life-threatening consequences for the patient or others; lack of understanding is assumed not to mean simply that the patient disagrees with the doctor. But the attribution of weights to the four principles is in practice always subjective. As Beauchamp and Childress emphasize, even judgements of competence, although not generally recognized as such, are heavily value-laden. Hence, if clinical decisions about involuntary treatment turned crucially on the trade-off between beneficence and autonomy, as a four-principles analysis suggests, we should expect the plus signs in Figure 58.2 to cluster at the top of the table. That is to say, we should expect those patients who are *most* likely to be treated against their wishes to be those who are *most* at risk of life-threatening consequences, and, at the same time, *least* capable of autonomous decision-making (16). This, as Figure 58.2 also shows, is true of case 9 described by Beauchamp and Childress. But it is not generally true of the patients in our questionnaire study. There is at best a poor correlation between the elements of beneficence and autonomy and the likelihood of compulsory treatment.

It seems, then, that clinical decisions about involuntary psychiatric treatment are driven by some factor (or factors) other than, or in addition to, the principles of autonomy and beneficence, at least as they are analysed by Beauchamp and Childress. One candidate factor is the presence of psychotic symptoms. There are arguments of a general kind to suggest that these are important (14). What these arguments amount to is that it is not just irrationality which is material to involuntary treatment, nor even irrationality as illness, but the particular kind of irrationality by which psychotic disorders are characterized. This conclusion is consistent with the results of our questionnaire study. As the right-hand column of Figure 58.2 shows, where other criteria fail to correlate with the

Cases	Likelihood of involuntary treatment (%)	Beneficence (life-threatening)	Autonomy			Competence		Psychotic symptoms
			Not intentional	Lacks understanding	Controlling influences (external)	Lacks deliberative capacity	Incoherence	
4. Hypomania	100			+		+	+	++
9. Schizophrenia	100						+	++
3. Depression	50	+						+
1. Anorexia	25	+	?					?
2. Obsessional disorder	10		?			.		
7. Hysteria	<5		+	+				
5. Optic atrophy	<5			+				
12. Marital problems	<5							
13. Personality disorder (drunk)	<5	+	+	+		+	+	
14. Bronchial carcinoma	<5	+		+				
6. Acromegaly	0			+				
8. Breast lump	0	+						
10. Osteoporosis	0							
11. Agoraphobia	0							
Case 9 dementia (Beauchamp/Childress)		+	+	+		+	+	+

FIGURE 58.2 Correlation between the results of the case-vignette study and (a) the principles of Beneficence and Autonomy, and (b) the presence of psychotic symptoms. The cases described in Figure 58.1 are shown here in descending order of probability of involuntary treatment. Case 9 from Beauchamp and Childress has been added. The order of cases is compared with the elements of beneficence and autonomy (which includes competence) as analysed by Beauchamp and Childress. The poor correlation with these elements is contrasted with the good correlation with the presence of psychotic symptoms.

intuitive selection of patients for involuntary treatment, the presence of psychotic symptoms matches this selection exactly.

The conclusion, therefore, which is suggested by this analysis of the results of our questionnaire study, is that the justification of involuntary treatment rests on a notion of irrationality—instantiated centrally by psychotic symptoms—which is not captured by the standard analyses of autonomy and competence, as in Beauchamp and Childress's *Principles*. This may have wider significance for medical ethics. There is a tendency in philosophical accounts of irrationality to assume that the significance of psychotic symptoms is carried simply by their being a non-specific instance of a general notion of incompetence. On this view, psychotic symptoms, indeed illness as such, can in effect be written out. But what we have tried to show in this section is that a notion of incompetence which is specifically related to the concept of psychotic mental illness is required to justify the specifically medical intervention of involuntary treatment.

THE FOUR PRINCIPLES AND THE 'MEDICAL' MODEL

We have taken the poor correlation between the 'four-principles' approach and the results of our case-vignette study to suggest that this approach stops short of a factor which is crucial to ethical reasoning, at least in relation to involuntary psychiatric treatment. However, our further suggestion that this factor is or involves the concepts of illness and disease, specifically the concept of psychotic mental illness, might seem to indicate a quite different conclusion—namely, that the failure of this correlation indicates a point of intersection between morals and medicine, between the ethical theory incorporated in the *Principles* approach and a body of empirical knowledge of disease by which medicine, as an essentially scientific discipline, is constituted. On this view, then, the key issues in the case of involuntary treatment—the issues which, however we interpret them, are reflected in the results of our questionnaire study—are not ethical at all but empirical.

This interpretation implies a particular model of the medical concepts, one which has become known as the 'medical' model. Boorse (17), Kendell (18) and others have developed explicit versions of this model. Medical expertise is taken to rest on a body of scientific information about disease, which is either in its own right value-free, or capable of reduction to value-free criteria of biological functioning. It is sometimes argued that this view of medicine is no longer widely held (19). But the soubriquet '*medical* model' says it all. Sociologists (20, 21), philosophers (22), and some doctors (23,24), have long recognized the essentially value-laden nature of the medical concepts. But most doctors still believe that disease theory, at least, is, in Boorse's phrase (17), 'continuous with theory in biological and other basic sciences'.

At all events, there are clear indications that a scientific model of the medical concepts is implicit in Beauchamp and Childress's *Principles*. There are hints of this in repeated references to the pre-eminence of the doctor's specialist knowledge: autonomy can mean acceptance of authority (p. 69); the authority of the doctor is modelled on that of a parent (pp. 212–213); a patient's (autonomous) wishes may be overridden where these amount to 'poor choices about courses of action recommended by their physicians' (pp. 211–212). The most explicit indication, however, comes in the discussion of rationality as a component of competence. Beauchamp and Childress argue that judgements of rationality, like other elements of competence, often involve references to (highly contestable) value judgements about what a rational person would do (p. 84). But they then go on to contrast the evaluative nature of judgements of rationality with medical judgements. Balancing autonomy with beneficence is said to be a 'moral *not a medical* problem' (p. 84, our emphasis). Moreover, 'if precise, nonevaluative criteria were available for making such determinations of competence, the [problem of deciding whether someone's choices are rational] would vanish'; as it is 'moral judgements and policy choices . . . cannot be avoided' (p. 84, our bracket).

All this suggests, then, that Beauchamp and Childress assume a standard 'medical' model of the medical concepts in which they are, at root, value-free. The model is only implicit, however. Indeed it is significant that there is no discussion of the meanings of illness and disease in the *Principles*. The four principles represent a general ethical theory applied to what is in effect taken to be a value-neutral area of technical expertise. No wonder, therefore, that their analysis of the ethics of involuntary treatment does not extend to the particular medical concept of psychotic mental illness. Our interpretation, on the other hand, suggests that this concept, and with it the concepts of illness and disease generally, are essentially value-laden. It is to the significance of this alternative model that we turn next.

THE FOUR PRINCIPLES AND AN ALTERNATIVE MODEL

It should come as no surprise that the *Principles* assume an essentially scientific model of the medical concepts. After all, bioethics was developed directly in response to the ethical problems generated by technical and scientific progress in medicine. Moreover, in many areas of physical medicine the model is appropriate up to a point, ethically speaking (though as we will see in the last section, it is never entirely appropriate). This is because even if, as a value-based model of the medical concepts suggests, value judgements are implied when a condition is construed as a physical disease, the criteria for the value judgements in question are by and large uncontentious (14). They are not disputed and hence are not problematic diagnostically (25). It is for this reason that the concept of physical disease has largely factual connotations. It appears to be a descriptive concept, not because it is value-free, but because the evaluative element in its meaning is generally unproblematic, and, hence, goes largely unnoticed. The 'medical' model of disease as a purely scientific concept can thus be understood as a simplified model, one in which the evaluative element is just ignored.

By the same token, though, this simplified model is not appropriate in psychiatry. Thus, recapitulating the argument just given, the concept of mental illness has overtly evaluative connotations because, where the criteria for the value judgement expressed by disease are uncontentious when applied to physical conditions, they are often highly *contentious* when applied to mental conditions. This is true not only of notoriously problematic conditions such as psychopathy and sexual disorders, but also of more mundane conditions such as anxiety and depression. As one of us has argued elsewhere, there is far wider variation in the criteria by which we judge a condition of anxiety or sadness to be good or bad, than, say, a condition of (physical) pain (14). Hence, the simplified science-based view of the medical concepts, which works well enough in physical medicine, can be positively misleading when transferred to psychiatry. This is no mere theoretical possibility. In several important areas—in respect of abuse (8), in relation to the classification of psychiatric disorders (25), and in a variety of other contexts (26)—a failure to recognize the evaluative element in the meanings of the medical concepts has led to significant adverse practical consequences. Merely recognizing this element is of course in itself not to handle it better. But it is a step in this direction. As Gillon (19) has pointed out, at the very least it leads to a positive role for team-work, allowing a balancing of evaluative considerations in such contentious areas as involuntary psychiatric treatment.

In relation to psychiatric ethics, then, the traditional model of the medical concepts as essentially value-free is not only inappropriate but incomplete. This is not a criticism of the four-principles approach as such. Beauchamp and Childress make no claim to completeness. In relation to involuntary treatment, in particular, they emphasize that the notion of weak paternalism raises deep difficulties about the assessment of autonomy and the proper role of health professionals (pp. 224–225). The burden of the present argument is rather that, where these difficulties extend to the meanings of the concepts of illness and disease, they are themselves ethical, rather than merely empirical, difficulties. We have shown this here for involuntary treatment and much the same is true of a wide range of other ethical problems in psychiatry (27). What is needed in psychiatric ethics, then, according to this argument, is not an alternative to the four principles, but an account of the evaluative nature of the medical concepts which will serve as an addition or supplement to them.

A good deal is required of such an account. In particular it must extend to the particular kind of value that is expressed by the medical concepts, namely medical rather than, say, moral or aesthetic value: illness is *prima facie* different from, for example, both wickedness and ugliness. The point is well made by involuntary treatment. The basis of specifically *medical* intervention is not that someone who is suicidal is in a bad condition, or that they are simply irrational, but that they are in a condition which is appropriately construed *as* an illness. The corresponding key issue in forensic cases is the familiar 'mad versus bad' distinction.

The analysis of the particular kind of value expressed by the medical concepts takes us from ethics as such into the philosophy of action. The importance of this was anticipated by Flew (28). The key idea is that, where the traditional science-based view focuses on the analysis of disease in terms of failure of function, a value-based view focuses on the closely related (but distinct) analysis of the patient's experience of illness in terms of incapacity, or failure of intentional action. A number of authors have explored this approach (14,29,30). Its outcome, again, is not anti-scientific. What it provides is a more whole or complete picture of the medical concepts, one in which the evaluative element in their meaning has as central a place as the descriptive; in which the patient's experience of illness is given equal prominence with medical knowledge of disease; and in which the analysis of this experience in terms of action–failure complements and extends traditional accounts of disease in terms of failure of functioning.

This expansion of our view of the medical concepts is illustrated in Figure 58.3. The traditional science-based model is not, as some of its critics have argued, wrong. But it is hemianopic. And as one of us has shown in detail elsewhere, a full-field view is required to explain the remarkable range of phenomena subsumed by the concept of mental illness. Psychotic disorder, in particular, so resistant to definition in right-field terms (31), yields directly to a left-field analysis, both of the general clinical concept of 'loss of insight' (14) and of the specific symptoms of delusion, hallucination and thought insertion (15). This full-field analysis, moreover, turns out to be directly relevant not only to psychiatric ethics but to medical ethics as a whole.

PSYCHIATRIC ETHICS AND MEDICAL ETHICS

We have argued here that our analysis of the basis of involuntary psychiatric treatment shows the value of the *Principles* as a framework for medical ethical reasoning. An account of the evaluative nature of the medical concepts is required as well, but one which is complementary to, rather than displacing, the principles approach. From the perspective of the critics of the four principles, however, it may seem that our analysis has shown up its weaknesses. Certainly, in the language of our two-fields diagram, where the principles approach is predominantly a right-field ethical theory, the elements required of a left-field theory—closeness to the patient's actual experience of illness, sensitivity to the value-systems not only of the patient but of the other key participants including nursing staff and relatives, and the corresponding importance of the multidisciplinary team—all these are elements which are emphasized by the various forms of situational ethics. These elements, indeed, are essential in particular to casuistry, recently advocated by some as an alternative to the principles approach (32,33). As a method of ethical reasoning this approach, at least as applied to actual clinical cases, relies on a detailed understanding of the 'lived experience' of those involved. It is no coincidence, then, from this perspective, that the recent rise of interest in psychiatric ethics should have paralleled a renewed recognition of the value of situational ethics.

Psychiatric ethics, however, if showing the limitations of the principles approach, also shows up the weaknesses of situational ethics. Situational ethics, unsupported by a framework for discursive reasoning, is open to manipulation and abuse. This is the fate which, since Blaise Pascal's attack on it in the seventeenth century, mediaeval casuistry has been widely thought to have suffered (32); and the motivation behind the development of meta-ethical theory was precisely the attempt to secure a rigorous foundation for ethical reasoning (34). There have been trenchant reminders recently of the limitations of the analytical

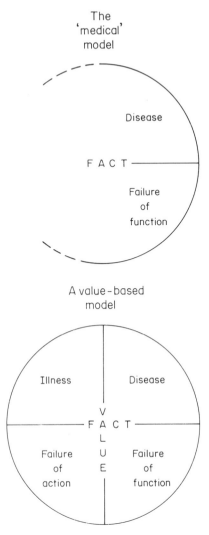

FIGURE 58.3 The conventional 'medical' model of medicine as a science is shown here as a half-field or hemianopic view. In contrast, a value-based analysis of the conceptual structure of medicine generates a full-field view. In the latter the experience of illness, analysed in terms of failure of action or incapacity, is as important as the (conventionally emphasized) knowledge of disease analysed in terms of failure of functioning. A full-field view provides a framework for developing a specifically *medical* ethics in which the principles approach and situational ethics are fully reconciled. (From Fulford (27) by permission of Oxford University Press.)

method in ethics (35). But in psychiatric ethics, at least, there is a danger that the baby will be thrown out with the bathwater.

This is well shown by casuistry. As a method for clarifying ethical issues, even for reaching agreement, casuistry is a powerful addition to the medical ethical armamentarium. In general medicine it is, sometimes, sufficient for the resolution of, say, decisions about abortion or terminal care. The point correctly made by modern casuists is that while we often disagree about the basis of our ethical decisions we nonetheless commonly agree on what should be done in particular concrete cases (32). But this can only be because, whatever our differences of interpretation, we have a shared system of values. And mental illness, as we have seen, differs from physical illness (overall) *precisely* in that our values are *less* widely shared—the criteria by which we judge mental conditions to be good or bad being open and problematic where the corresponding criteria for physical conditions are (relatively) closed and unproblematic. In psychiatry, therefore, casuistry alone would be at best insufficient, at worst manipulative. Certainly, casuistry would in itself have been no defence against the abuse of psychiatry in the former USSR. The argument of this chapter suggests that a principles approach, too, would not have been sufficient, an account of the evaluative element in medical diagnosis also being required. But a skilled casuist of Marxist–Leninism would surely have been no less successful than his mediaeval counterparts in justifying the suppression of dissent.

Psychiatric ethics thus requires both; principles as well as patients, discursive reasoning as well as attention to the details of the particular case; left-field as well as right-field thinking. Yet this is surely no less than what is required for medical ethics generally. Throughout medicine, if doctors have a shared ethic, it is one which, as the growing dissatisfaction with medicine directly indicates, is not always shared by other health care professionals (36,37), nor even, perhaps particularly (27), by patients. The need for a balanced ethic, for a full-field ethic rather than either a right-field or left-field hemianopia, is thus more transparent in psychiatry but it is there in medicine as a whole.

CONCLUSIONS

In this chapter we have explored the place of the four principles in psychiatric ethics by considering the particular difficulties raised by involuntary psychiatric treatment. An analysis of the results of a case-vignette study in terms of the four principles suggested that they failed to address the specifically *medical* ethical issues raised by treatment of this kind. This in turn has been shown to be because the four principles, as set out by Beauchamp and Childress, assume a traditional 'medical' model in which the concepts of illness and disease are essentially value-free. The four principles thus provide a helpful framework for ethical analysis in psychiatry but one which, being a general ethical framework, is incomplete. On the other hand situational-ethics alternatives to the four principles are also not sufficient as a basis for psychiatric ethics. What is required is, rather, a balance of the two. We have argued that the basis for such a balanced ethic is a 'full-field' view of the medical concepts themselves, one in which value is incorporated on an equal basis with fact.

In all this, however, we have suggested that psychiatry merely points the way for other areas of medical ethics. This is why psychiatric ethics may be emerging from its traditional role as the ugly duckling of bioethical enquiry. But if this is right, the stakes are considerably raised. For the development of a balanced ethic for everyday clinical practice, involving as it does analytical as well as empirical considerations, will be dependent as much on philosophical as scientific medical research. There is a long-term programme here (38), therefore. More immediately, though, the requirement for full-field rather than right-field thinking in medicine presents a challenge for medical education. It is to this that we turn in Chapter 59 of this book.

REFERENCES

1. Szasz, T. S. 1960. The myth of mental illness. *American Psychologist* **15**: 113–118.
2. Bloch, S. and Chodoff, P. 1991. *Psychiatric ethics*, 2nd edn. Oxford University Press, Oxford.
3. Kopelman, L. M. 1989. Moral problems in psychiatry. Pp. 253–290, *in* Veatch, R. (Ed.) *Medical ethics*. Jones and Bartlett, MA.
4. Hope, R. A. 1990. Ethical philosophy as applied to psychiatry. *Current Opinion in Psychiatry* **3**: 673–676.
5. Anzia, D.J. and La Puma, J. 1991. An annotated bibliography of psychiatric medical ethics. *Academic Psychiatry* **15**: 1–7.
6. Beauchamp, T. L. and Childress, J. F. 1989. *Principles of biomedical ethics*. Oxford University Press, Oxford.
7. Bloch, S. and Chodoff, P. 1977. *Russia's political hospitals*. Camelot Press, Southampton.
8. Fulford, K. W. M., Smirnoff, A. Y. U. and Snow, E. 1992. Concepts of disease and the abuse of psychiatry in the USSR. *British Journal of Psychiatry* (forthcoming).
9. Grinstead, P. 1992. Patients slips through legal loophole. *Hospital Doctor*, 12 March, p. 43.
10. American Psychiatric Association. 1980. *Diagnostic and statistical manual of mental disorders*, 3rd edn. American Psychiatric Association, Washington, DC.
11. Glover, J. 1988. *I: the philosophy and psychology of personal identity*. Penguin, London.
12. Wilkes, K.V. 1988. *Real people: personal identity without thought experiments*. Clarendon Press, Oxford.
13. Braude, S. E. 1991. *First person plural: multiple personality and the philosophy of mind*. Routledge, London.
14. Fulford, K. W. M. 1989. *Moral theory and medical practice*. Cambridge University Press, Cambridge.
15. Fulford, K. W. M. 1992. Thought insertion and insight: disease and illness paradigms of psychotic disorder, *in* Spitzer, M. (Ed.) *Phenomenology, language and schizophrenia*. Springer-Verlag (forthcoming).
16. Eastman, N. L. G. and Hope, R. A. 1988. Ethics of enforced medical treatment: the balance model. *Journal of Applied Philosophy* **5**: 49–59.
17. Boorse, C. 1975. On the distinction between disease and illness. *Philosophy and Public Affairs* **5**: 61–84.
18. Kendell, R. E. 1975. The concept of disease and its implications for psychiatry. *British Journal of Psychiatry* **127**: 305–315.
19. Gillon, R. 1986. *Philosophical medical ethics*. John Wiley, Chichester.
20. Parsons, T. 1951. *The social system*. Free Press, Glencoe, IL.
21. Sedgwick, P. 1973. Illness—mental and otherwise. *Hastings Center Studies* **1** (3): pp. 19–40. Institute of Society, Ethics and the Life Sciences, Hastings-on-Hudson, New York.
22. Farrell, B. A. 1979. Mental illness: a conceptual analysis. *Psychological Medicine* **9**: 21–35.
23. Agich, G. J. 1983. Disease and value: a rejection of the value-neutrality thesis. *Theoretical Medicine* **4**: 27–41.
24. Reich, W. 1991. Psychiatric diagnosis as an ethical problem. Pp. 101–135, *in* Bloch, S. and Chodoff, P. (Eds) *Psychiatric ethics*, 2nd edn. Oxford University Press, Oxford.
25. Fulford, K. W. M. 1992. Closet logics: hidden conceptual elements in the DSM and ICD classifications of mental disorders. *In* Sadler, J. Z., Schwartz, M. and Wiggins,

O. (Eds) *Philosophical perspectives on psychiatric diagnostic classification.* Johns Hopkins University Press, Baltimore, MD (forthcoming).
26. Fulford, K. W. M. 1990. Philosophy and psychiatry: points of contact. *Current Opinion in Psychiatry* **3**: 668–672.
27. Fulford, K. W. M. 1991. The concept of disease. Pp. 77–99, *in* Bloch, S. and Chodoff, P. (Eds) *Psychiatric ethics,* 2nd edn. Oxford University Press, Oxford.
28. Flew, A. 1973. *Crime or disease?* Barnes & Noble, New York.
29. Nordenfelt, L. 1987. *On the nature of health: an action–theoretic approach.* D. Reidel, Dordrecht, Holland.
30. Toulmin, S. 1980. Agent and patient in psychiatry. *International Journal of Law and Psychiatry* **3**: 267–278.
31. David, A. S. 1990. Insight and psychosis. *British Journal of Psychiatry* **156**: 798–808.
32. Jonsen, A. R. and Toulmin, S. 1988. *The abuse of casuistry: a history of moral reasoning.* University of California Press, Berkeley, CA.
33. Kass, L. R. 1990. Practicing ethics: where's the action? *Hastings Center Report,* 20, (Jan./Feb.), pp. 5–12.
34. Moore, G. E. 1980. *Principia ethica.* Press Syndicate of the University of Cambridge, Cambridge.
35. Williams, B. 1985. *Ethics and the limits of philosophy.* Fontana, London.
36. Alderson, P. 1990. *Choosing for children: parents' consent to surgery.* Oxford University Press, Oxford.
37. Marsden, C. 1990. Ethics of the 'doctor–nurse game'. *Heart and Lung* **19**: 422–424.
38. Fulford, K. W. M. 1989. Philosophy and medicine: the Oxford connection. *British Journal of Psychiatry* **157**: 111–115.

59

Medical Education: Patients, Principles and Practice Skills

TONY HOPE

Leader of the Oxford Practice Skills Project, The Medical School, University of Oxford, UK; and Honorary Consultant Psychiatrist

K. W. M. FULFORD

Research Fellow, Green College, Oxford, UK; and Honorary Consultant Psychiatrist

INTRODUCTION

The Pond Report on the teaching of medical ethics in Britain was published in 1987 (1). Its recommendations start confidently with this statement: 'Medical ethics is central to the practice of medicine and its implications should be made explicit throughout medical education.' The report was widely influential and gave further impetus to the already burgeoning teaching of ethics in medical schools throughout the UK. Yet much of this activity has remained marginalized. There have been many initiatives: but these have been mostly those of a few enthusiasts, local to each medical school, rather than among clinical teachers as a whole. Similarly, there has been much support at a political and administrative level: but the actual place of medical ethics in the curriculum has remained secondary. It continues to be an addendum, an extra course squeezed in at the margins. There is as yet no sense of a coherent discipline fully integrated into all aspects of medical education as envisaged by the Pond Report.

In our chapter on psychiatric ethics we outlined a model of medicine in which evaluative considerations have as central a place as descriptive or scientific considerations. This model was shown to generate a conceptual framework within which principles and situational ethics could be combined to provide an effective basis for tackling some of the specifically *medical* ethical issues which

---

Principles of Health Care Ethics. Edited by Raanan Gillon.

arise in the practice of psychiatry. However, we indicated that the model had wider significance for medicine generally, and in this chapter we consider its implications for medical education. Specifically, we describe a model of medical ethics education derived as the practical counterpart of the theoretical model developed in our earlier chapter. In this model, medical ethics is not taught in isolation. It is combined with medical law and communication skills in a series of clinically centred seminars. These 'practice skills' seminars, moreover, are not run as a separate module. They are spread across the three years of the clinical curriculum, fully integrated into existing teaching arrangements. We will first give an account of the course itself and then consider the place of the four principles in courses of this kind.

ETHICS AND PRACTICE SKILLS

In the terms of the model of medicine described in our earlier chapter, the marginalization of medical ethics is an aspect of right-field thinking. So long as medicine is thought to be essentially a science, medical education must focus on imparting scientific knowledge. Good practice depends on knowing what to do in a given clinical situation, and this in turn depends on a sound grasp of nosology, clinical pharmacology, anatomy, physiology and other scientific subjects which, rightly, figure prominently in medical education. But full-field thinking reminds us that good practice requires more than this. Good *practice* in medicine requires not only a knowledge of what to do but also the skills necessary for the successful application of that knowledge. To put the point slightly differently, in a given clinical situation we need to know not only what to do but how to do it. And knowing how, according to the model described here, includes, centrally: (1) a sensitivity to the ethical aspects of a situation and an ability where necessary to think sensibly about them, (2) an understanding of the legal framework within which the situation is set, and (3) an awareness of the patient's actual experience, and the experience of others involved (members of the health care team as well as the patient's relatives), as the basis of the communication skills necessary to pull all this together in an effective treatment package.

The relative importance of each of these practice skills varies from case to case. That they are nonetheless inseparable in the practice of medicine can be seen by considering an example widely discussed in the standard medical ethics literature, that of the under-age girl who asks her family doctor for contraceptive advice while refusing to allow him or her to involve her parents. Empirical considerations are clearly relevant; for example, the facts about the benefits and harms of different forms of contraception for young women, and for this patient in particular. The key difficulties, though, are, on the face of it, ethical. In the standard medical ethics literature these have been discussed in general terms. The four principles in particular provide a helpful framework for setting out the issues—balancing the autonomy of the patient, and the doctor's duty of confidentiality, against his or her obligations to her parents; weighing the potential harms from entering a sexual relationship prematurely against the perhaps greater benefits of good contraceptive advice; and so on. These issues, moreover, have to be considered within the context of the legal framework governing not only the doctor's general responsibilities but also the patient's age and other aspects of consent. No decision in this case can be taken in the UK without regard to the legal judgement in the Gillick case, for example (2). In practice, though, none of these considerations can be separated from the way in which the doctor actually handles the situation. Of course, the best communication skills in the world will not suffice in the absence of an appropriate grasp of the relevant considerations, empirical, ethical and legal. But these considerations, too, will not suffice in the absence of a sensitive appreciation of how the girl, her parents, and not least the practice nurse, all feel about the situation, together with a willingness and the ability to give time to coming to an appropriate conclusion. Thus, if ethics is to affect practice, it is inseparable from communication skills (3,4).

Recasting medical ethics in this way, as no more than a component of practice skills, may seem to result in a new marginalization of the subject. Instead of being marginalized at the periphery, it might be thought, it is now marginalized in the centre—an internal exile in place of its former external exile. Moral philosophers, in particular, are inclined to take a somewhat lofty view of the suggestion that medical ethical problems can sometimes be resolved by so practical a communication skill as 'giving time'. Yet it is clear, from the pattern of medical complaints if in no other ways (5,6), that it is precisely where communication skills are lacking, rather than in the breach of some high-flown moral principle, let alone through actionable tort, that dissatisfaction with medical practice most commonly arises. Absorbing medical ethics into practice skills, therefore, is not to marginalize it at all. It is to place it firmly where it belongs, at the heart of everyday clinical practice.

THE OXFORD PRACTICE SKILLS PROJECT

The Oxford Practice Skills Project represents a conscious attempt to reflect the above considerations in a course for clinical medical students; that is, students who have completed their pre-clinical training (mainly in basic medical sciences), who are now learning clinical medicine and hence are in day-to-day contact with patients, but who have not yet qualified as doctors. The practice skills approach is clearly relevant to other groups: postgraduate doctors, nurses and other health care workers, and indeed anyone involved in professional work with people. In the case of medical students, however, our impression is that over the period of their clinical training, the sensitivity of student doctors to ethical issues, and indeed more widely to the feelings and concerns of patients, actually decreases. This is no doubt in part an effect of 'exam pressure'. But if so, this too is a reflection of the hegemony of right-field thinking in medicine. The challenge, then, to medical education, is to match our effectiveness in imparting knowledge with an equally effective promotion of practice skills. We will examine the implications of this for three areas of course design and development: the practical arrangements for teaching, seminar content and syllabus, and appraisal.

Teaching Arrangements

The practical arrangements for teaching medical ethics, and other elements of practice skills, has received scant attention in the literature. Yet they are fundamental. Much medical ethics teaching has been carried out by philosophers, theologians, lawyers, or 'expert' doctors, brought in to provide a separate course. But such arrangements reflect and, more seriously, reinforce right-field thinking. They convey, in the body language of medical education, at best that ethics is a specialist medical discipline, the province solely of special consultants in much the same relationship to medicine as cardiologists or rheumatologists; at worst that, like medical law, it is not really part of medicine at all.

One objective of the Oxford Practice Skills Project is to develop a course which is woven as far as possible seamlessly into the existing arrangements for clinical teaching. We have tried to achieve this in two principal ways. First, instead of a separate 'block', the course is organized as a series of seminars strung together across the three years of the students' clinical training. This is shown in Figure 59.1. Second, apart from introductory and concluding sessions, the aim is for most of the seminars to be run, not by the project team in isolation, but in partnership with other clinical teachers. Thus seminars on 'do not resuscitate' orders are organized with each of the medical teams in the student's first clinical attachment; seminars on consent with the surgical teams; and so on. Clearly, these arrangements are not in themselves sufficient to ensure that medical ethics, as an element of practice skills, becomes part of everyday clinical work. There is still a problem of generalization, of transferring attitudes and behaviour adopted in practice skills sessions to clinical practice in general. Similarly, there is a need for clinical teachers other than members of the project team to be involved in day-to-day practice skills training as well as in specific sessions. Once the course is well established we hope to develop a 'cascade' method for training clinical teachers in practice skills—that is, training one group, the members of which each train a further group, and so on. But we believe that the existing arrangements have already given a strong *de facto* signal of the central place of practice skills in everyday clinical care.

Seminar Content and Syllabus

Just as the practical arrangements for practice skills training are crucial to their integration into medical education, so, too, is the content of the seminars themselves, both individually and as they build up into a syllabus for the course as a whole. The core seminars in the Oxford Practice Skills Course are all clinically centred. This is industry-standard in medical ethics teaching (7–9). Like others, we involve not just doctors but also all members of the clinical team, as well as patients. Our practice skills seminars, however, differ from many other approaches to teaching medical ethics in that the focus of each seminar is not always directly on ethics. The focus is on the practical problem of providing good clinical care for patients and their relatives. This in turn leads to a recognition of the importance of medical ethical considerations as part of effective practice skills. Medical ethics, even including (in varying degrees)

	Title	Group	Time	Setting
INTRODUCTION	YEAR 1			
(i)	Explaining structure of practice skills	LG	30 min	Introductory course
(ii)	Introduction to practice skills	LG	45 min	Introductory course
(iii)	Introduction to English and Welsh Law	LG	45 min	Introductory course
CORE SEMINARS				
1	'Do not resuscitate', allowing patients to die	SG	2 hours	General medicine
2	Testing for HIV	SG	2 hours	General medicine
3	'Have we got a consent form?'	SG	2 hours	General surgery
4	Post mortems	LG	2 hours	Pathology
5	'Is my smear normal?' 'Yes, but . . .'	LG	1 hour	Pathology
	YEAR 2			
6	The incompetent patient	SG	2 hours	Psychiatry
7	We're desperate for a baby	SG	2 hours	O & G
8	Coping with anger and violence	SG	2 hours	Accident service
	YEAR 3			
9	Death and transplantation	SG	2 hours	Surgery
10	Patients as subjects of research: 'Are you willing to enter our trial?'	SG	2 hours	Medicine
11	'We haven't got a bed': the allocation of resources	SG	2 hour	Medicine
CONCLUDING SEMINAR				
12	Preparing for your first house job	LG	1 hour	Revision course

FIGURE 59.1 The Oxford Practice Skills course is based on a series of seminars (the 'core seminars') which are spread through the three years of the clinical syllabus. Most are small group sessions (SG = 15–20 students); some are large groups, involving the year as a whole (LG = 100 students).

philosophical medical ethics, is thus discovered by the students themselves, along with other disciplines relevant to the development of their practice skills, at the heart of their everyday clinical work.

An important strength of the clinically centred approach is that it is never merely gestural. Whatever the philosophical ramifications of a particular case, however important these may be in their own right, there are always in principle definite practical decisions to be made. A weakness of this approach, on the other hand, is that it can become somewhat diffuse. In order to give clear direction, the policy decisions made about the aims of the course should always be translated into well-defined elements of a specific syllabus. The four principles, as we discuss in more detail later, can be helpful in this regard. They provide a coherent framework of clinically relevant considerations capable of generating a syllabus with a clear overall structure and definite content. But whatever approach is adopted, the basis of 'street-cred' in medical ethics education, to pragmatically minded students as well as their clinical teachers, is a clear indication of the scope and extent of what there is to learn. The more stretching and demanding the better! A simple device for identifying and controlling the syllabus content, while retaining a clinically centred approach, is the use of a grid. Part of our grid is shown in Figure 59.2.

Appraisal

For most technical skills in medicine the criteria of success are not contentious: the suture *holds*, the bone heals *straight*, the heart murmur turns out to *be* mitral, and so on. Similarly, along with well-defined criteria go relatively straightforward assessment methods. In the case of practice skills, on the other hand, both the criteria and methods of appraisal are highly problematic. The proper aim of medical ethics teaching, in particular, is itself a medical-ethical issue. In the narrowest of tautologies good practice skills means good practice; though even this cannot be taken for granted. The aim could be, for example, to ensure that there are some doctors who can engage in dialogue with lawyers, politicians and philosophers, able to give the medical perspective coherently. Then, as regards methods, some believe that medical ethics is of its nature too subjective, too personal, to be assessed in any formal way. Certainly there is no consensus in the literature about the methods by which either students or, indeed, courses in medical ethics should be assessed. Indeed, there have been only a few pioneering attempts at formal assessment of courses (10–12).

For all the difficulties, however, we believe appraisal is essential to the eventual integration of practice skills into medical education. Without appraisal there can be no development of a syllabus, of teaching methods, of an established 'corpus' of expertise comparable with the scientific content of medical education. A first step in this direction is suggested by the educationalist John Wilson (personal communication). He argues that statements of general aims in any educational enterprise should be cashed out in terms of specific elements each of which is justified (i.e. *prima facie* relevant to good practice), discrete, and specified operationally (i.e. in a form in which it can be assessed). Thus good practice in medicine involves (*inter alia*) showing care, attending to the patient's wishes, courtesy, awareness of ethical concepts, and so forth. Similarly, if these and other elements make up the final goal of good practice, there will be a number of intermediate aims: awareness of ethical issues, an ability to think coherently about them, the development of appropriate attitudes, the acquisition

SYLLABUS	SEMINARS 3 — HAVE WE GOT A CONSENT FORM?	4 — POST-MORTEM PERMISSION
ETHICS		
Active euthanasia		
Organ donation		+
Informed consent	++	+
Quality of life		+
LAW		
• Consent	++	
Informed consent	++	+
Children	+	
• Organ and tissue donation	++	++
Coroner system		++
Human Tissues Act		
COMMUNICATION SKILLS		
• Giving risk-benefit information	++	++
• Giving emotionally sensitive information		++

FIGURE 59.2 Part of a grid which relates the seminars in the Oxford Practice Skills course to the elements of each of the three main syllabus areas of ethics, law and communication skills.

of knowledge, and, ultimately, change of behaviour. We discuss these in more detail in the next section, specifically in relation to the four principles.

If the aims of appraisal—defined in the way Wilson suggests—are an asset for integration, so too are the methods. This is true both of student assessment and of appraisal of the course itself. Thus, students should be assessed for their competence in practice skills, not separately, but in whatever context they are assessed on their clinical competence generally. So far as ethics is concerned, this arrangement further reinforces its place as part of everyday clinical work. Course appraisal is equally important. Here the standard methods of questionnaire, structured interview, and so on, can be helpful. More important, though, are methods based on active involvement: direct feedback from patients, participant observer studies, and 'action research' techniques employed by students themselves. These latter methods are intrinsically relevant to skills development, they stimulate vital feedback on the content and design of the course, they contribute to the process of integration of practice skills into clinical training, and, perhaps most significant of all, they provide an object lesson in the essential practice skill of continuing self-assessment.

THE FOUR PRINCIPLES AND PRACTICE SKILLS

It is remarkable, though perhaps a reflection of the 'pre-paradigmatic state' of the discipline, that through all the recent debate about the four principles their role in medical education has been almost entirely ignored.

Nonetheless the general arguments adduced in this debate are relevant. Those arguing in favour of the principles point out that they provide a coherent framework for bioethics, largely independent of cultural background and moral and religious affiliations, and yet incorporating an uncontentious view of the commitment of health care professionals to the welfare of their clients (13). Those who are against the principles, point, severally, to the limitations of a 'principles' analysis of medical-ethical issues; to their tendency to reinforce the unequal power relationship between professional and client (14); and to a tendency to divorce ethical thinking from the (ethically) substantive detail embedded in real cases (15).

To the supporters of the four principles, the arguments of their opponents often seem misdirected. That the four principles should have been misperceived is, however, itself a reflection of their close connection with right-field (doctor-led) thinking. Situational ethics, on the other hand, advocated by some opponents of the four principles, is, correspondingly, left-field thinking—concerned as it is with the patient's actual experience and with (often indeterminate) ethical and legal considerations arising from the muddle and disorder of real clinical situations. We argued on theoretical grounds in our earlier chapter that what is needed is not a shift from right-field to left-field thinking, from principles to situational ethics, but a coherent synthesis of the two. It seems reasonable, then, to expect that this will be true of medical ethics education. The practice skills approach reflects and is designed to encourage full-field thinking. Whether or not it succeeds in this is one of the questions we hope to test. There are nonetheless *a priori* grounds for believing that it will. In the remainder of this section we examine these briefly under each of the three aspects of course design and development considered above.

TEACHING ARRANGEMENTS

An important feature of the practical arrangements for practice skills training is that seminars should be run jointly by the project team and the clinical teachers in individual specialties. One advantages of the four principles in this regard is that they amount to a 'theory' of medical ethics which is structurally compatible with the background and expectations of scientifically trained doctors. The principles have a clear structure, are directly relevant to clinical decision-making, and they provide a framework within which detailed analyses of medical-ethical problems can be carried out. In these respects the four principles mirror corresponding scientific 'theories' of disease. For shared teaching, they thus provide a resource with which everyone can feel more or less comfortable.

On the other hand it is against precisely this feature of the four principles, their 'professional format', that some of its most pertinent criticisms have been directed. As Alderson has pointed out, the principles approach can place patients at a double disadvantage, deprofessionalized first by the technical expertise of doctors, and now by a new ethical expertise (14). The balancing factor here is the detailed attention to the actual experience of the patient (and significant others) implicit in the requirements for situational ethics. But this, too, tackled with the central practice skills objective of clinical decision-making firmly in mind, need involve no cognitive dissonance. For doctors are familiar with the need to attend carefully to a patient's symptoms in making a diagnosis (though often we fail to do this!). The practice skills approach requires the same detailed attention to how the patient (and others) feel in implementing treatments.

Seminar Content and Syllabus

Similar considerations apply to both the content of individual seminars and the overall course syllabus. As with the practical arrangements for practice skills training, the four principles can provide a valuable link with the more familiar scientific aspects of medical education. They need to be set in a wider context, however, to avoid the dehumanizing effects of a purely theoretical ethics. Even in our introductory seminars we introduce the four principles by showing how they are implicit in, and can help to make clear the nature of, the dilemmas posed by a particular case. And even here it is important to make clear that they are not to be used algorithmically for 'mathematical' problem-solving. They help us to understand the difficulties, and this can contribute to resolving practical problems. But there is more even to the ethical part of the problem than just this—there is the relevant detail; there may be issues not usefully subsumed to the four principles; and there are aspects which are not ethical at all, as traditionally conceived—medicolegal aspects, and, crucially from the practical point of view, good communication skills.

The four principles are thus implicit in medical ethics as part of practice skills training, rather than a 'taught element' in their own right. This is reflected in the syllabus grid: there is no horizontal element of, say, autonomy; but autonomy is a key issue in a number of the elements specifically identified (confidentiality, for example).

Appraisal

As we should expect in the present stage of the development of medical ethics education, it is when we come to appraisal that we get the clearest indications of the strengths and weaknesses of the principles approach. Following Wilson's precept we will summarize these briefly in relation to the four intermediate aims of practice skills training listed earlier, and to the final aim of behaviour change.

Awareness

It is a truism that medical ethics education cannot get started as a practical discipline unless there is awareness of the problem in the first place. The generality of the four principles, although sometimes the basis of objections to them, makes them a powerful heuristic teaching aid in this respect. They are not essential, of course. Indeed we find that groups of students can generate many ethical issues relevant to a given clinical situation without referring to the four principles. Nonetheless explicit use of the principles can help to suggest aspects of a problem which have been missed. Moreover, once an issue (confidentiality, say) has been identified as involving a conflict between principles (perhaps autonomy and beneficence), then the discursive analyses available in texts such as Beauchamp and Childress (16) can help to deepen understanding. The danger is that this can degenerate into legalistic or algorithmic thinking, divorced from the experience of the patient and others concerned. But properly followed through in the way that Beauchamp and Childress suggest, it points firmly to the need to embed clinical decisions in a given case in a sensitive awareness of the patient's perspective. This is, of course, one of the many respects in which the involvement of patients and patient groups in practice skills training is essential. There is no more powerful way of raising awareness than the direct accounts of their experiences of health care provided by those on the receiving end.

Thinking Skills

The process of deepening our understanding of an ethical issue is part of the thinking skills emphasized by most teachers of medical ethics as an essential aim of professional training in this area. The discursive approach adopted by Beauchamp and Childress can be helpful in this respect, provided arguments are developed out of real cases. As Campbell and Higgs noted (17), in a book which epitomizes the very best of case-based ethical discussions, the skills of philosophical analysis are an important defence against the abuses of language by which so much unethical practice is disguised.

Casuistry offers a different approach. In one sense of the term—the application of principles to particular cases—there is no conflict with the principles approach. However, Jonsen and Toulmin (15) have pointed out that there is often agreement on what is right in a particular case even though there is disagreement on why it is right. Hence they suggest that reasoning about ethics should proceed by direct comparison of cases, with variation of the relevant details, rather than from general principles. This can be a powerful approach with students. Moreover, it is consistent with the way in which doctors come to decisions in the scientific side of medicine. Much of diagnosis, for example, is based on pre-conscious comparisons with a store of cases actually experienced, rather than by algorithmic deduction.

Here, however, as elsewhere, the two approaches—deductive and casuistic—are complementary rather than mutually exclusive. Even in diagnosis the weakness of 'experts' is that they tend to miss aspects of a clinical presentation which, though fully apparent, are inconsistent with prior expectations. In practice skills, similarly, comparison of cases within a group of like-minded people can compound, rather than expose, prejudice and preconception. Both ways of thinking are thus likely to turn out to be important practice skills.

Attitudes

There is a view of practical ethics which regards the development of correct attitudes as the prime objective of ethical training. This has been emphasized by recent work reviving interest in the virtues (18). As May has argued, many of the traditional virtues translate readily into attitudes which are crucial to good practice (19). These virtues, moreover, are capable of definition with a degree of specificity often lacking from other areas of ethical enquiry, and this could be important for appraisal. Attitude-change, however, is contentious as an aim of medical ethics education because the choice of attitudes to be encouraged necessarily reflects a substantive moral position. Broad attitudes—such as taking the moral dimension in medicine seriously, advocated by Kahlke and Reiter-Theil (20)—raise no special difficulties. But we have already noted that more specific objectives are necessary if medical ethics education is to be capable of adequate appraisal.

The four principles imply specific attitudes, of course, such as respect for autonomy. But the effects, specific and non-specific, on student attitudes of teaching the four principles are unknown. It is possible, as some of the critics of this approach have argued (14), that it could encourage an overly intellectual approach to ethical problems. On the other hand, emphasis on, say, autonomy, could lead to enhanced respect for the feelings and wishes of the patient. There are many variables here. But it seems to us that some attempt to measure attitudes and attitude change is integral to the appraisal of practice skills training, and it could be that the specificity of the virtues will prove helpful in this respect.

Knowledge

Although we have emphasized the skills aspects of practice skills training, there is clearly a substantial amount of plain information with which students should become familiar. Less clear, though, are the boundaries between what is essential and what is optional. This is true, notably, of traditional moral philosophy. There are arguments for and against a greater or lesser familiarity with traditional discussions of key issues, such as the distinction between schools of moral theory (consequentialist versus rights-based, for example), elements of moral reasoning (the doctrine of double-effect), meta-ethical theory (the meaning and implications of moral terms—wants, needs, duties, etc.), and so on. The four principles offer a helpful compromise. They stand between 'raw' cases and abstract theory, they encompass and give context to the relevant legal principles, and they are presented in a form which leads naturally to philosophical theory for those students who wish to develop their understanding in this direction. Of course, knowledge of the four principles should not be presented as an end in itself. The guiding principle throughout should not be the internal concerns of moral philosophy, but the ways in which it can be harnessed to the needs of the practice skills necessary to good clinical care.

Behaviour

The ultimate aim of all skills training is change of behaviour. Awareness, thinking skills, attitudes and knowledge are all directed towards this end. It is, though, a reflection of the undeveloped state of medical ethics training that there are so few indications of its effects, good or bad, on actual practice. The four principles, in particular, could help or hinder. As principles which are *'prima facie* relevant', each principle counting to some degree in a given clinical situation (16), they could provide a dynamic basis for action, open and responsive to the contingencies of the particular case. As such they could help to avoid the arrogant assurance which is so widely resented in the behaviour of doctors. On the other hand, a preoccupation with the conflicting ethical aspects of a case, rather than acting on clear (if illusory) certainties, could paralyse action. We simply don't know.

CONCLUSIONS

In this chapter we have extended the theoretical model of medicine outlined in our chapter on psychiatric ethics to the practical problem of professional training in medical ethics. The 'full-field' model of the conceptual structure of medicine outlined in that chapter suggests that medical ethics should be taught, not as a separate subject, but embedded in the practice skills necessary for the successful application of scientific medical knowledge in everyday work with patients. This brings medical ethics in from the cold. The structure of teaching arrangements for practice skills training, the content of individual seminars and of the overall syllabus, and the aims and methods of appraisal all help to shift ethics from its present position at the margins of medical education into a central position. The particular role of the four principles in relation to practice skills remains to be established. Nonetheless we have shown that there are *a priori* grounds for believing that in each aspect of course design and development they are likely to be helpful, though not in themselves sufficient. We have indicated some of the ways in which our experience thus far suggests that this will indeed turn out to be so where ethics is taught as part of practice skills.

REFERENCES

1. Pond, D. 1987. *Report of a working party on the teaching of medical ethics*, p. 35. IME Publications, London.
2. Kennedy, I. and Grubb, A. 1989. *Medical law: text and materials*. Butterworths, London.
3. Grant, V. 1988. Good communication vital for ethical practice. *IME Bulletin* **44**: 13–17.
4. Culver, C. M., Clouser, K. D., Gert, B., Brody, H., Fletcher, J., Jonsen, A., Kopelman, L., Lynn, J., Siegler, M. and Wikler, D. 1985. Basic curricular goals in medical ethics. *New England Journal of Medicine* **312**: 253–256.
5. Cleary, P. D. and McNeil, B. J. 1988. Patient satisfaction as an indicator of quality of care. *Inquiry* **25**: 25–36.
6. Aharony, L. and Strasser, S. 1992. Patient satisfaction—what we know about what is still unexpected (submitted).
7. Miles, S. H., Lane, L. W., Bickel, J., Walker, R. M. and Cassel, C. K. 1989. Medical ethics education: coming of age. *Academic Medicine* **64**: 705–714.
8. Pellegrino, E. D. 1989. Teaching medical ethics: some persistent questions and some responses. *Academic Medicine* **64**: 701–703.
9. Gillon, R. 1990. Teaching medical ethics: impressions from the USA. Pp. 89–115, *in* Byrne, P. (Ed.) *Medicine, medical ethics and the value of life*. Wiley, Chichester.
10. Howe, K.R. 1985. Evaluating medical ethics teaching. University Microfilms International, no. 8520529 (300 N. Zech Rd., Ann Arbor, 11 Michigan 48106).
11. Hébert, P., Meslin, E. M., Dunn, E. V., Byrne N. and Reid, S. R. 1990. Evaluating ethical sensitivity in medical students: using vignettes as an instrument. *Journal of Medical Ethics* **16**: 141–145.
12. Self, D. J., Wolinsky, F. D. and Baldwin, D. C. Jr. 1989. The effect of teaching medical ethics on medical students' moral reasoning. *Academic Medicine* **64**: 755–759.
13. Gillon, R. 1986. *Philosophical medical ethics*. Wiley (for the *British Medical Journal*), Chichester.
14. Alderson, P. 1990. *Choosing for children: parents' consent to surgery*, pp. 203–204, 207. Oxford University Press, New York.
15. Jonsen, A. R. and Toulmin, S. 1988. *The abuse of casuistry: a history of moral reasoning*. University of California Press, Berkeley, CA.
16. Beauchamp, T. L. and Childress, J. F. 1989. *Principles of biomedical ethics*. Oxford University Press, New York.
17. Campbell, A. V. and Higgs, R. 1982. *In that case*. Darton, Longman & Todd, London.
18. MacIntyre, A. 1985. *After virtue: a study in moral theory*. Duckworth, London.
19. May, W. F. 1992. The virtues in a professional setting. Ch. 6, *in* Fulford, K. W. M., Gillett, G. R. and Soskice, J. M. (Eds) *Medicine and moral reasoning*. Cambridge University Press, Cambridge.
20. Kahlke, W. and Reiter-Theil, S. 1992. Ausbildung in medizinischer Ethik—Stand und Perspektiven in Deutschland. *Wiener Medizinische Wochenschrift* (submitted).

60

The Health Care of the Elderly

J. A. MUIR GRAY, MD, FRCPS(GLAS), MRCGP, FFCM

*Specialist in Public Health Medicine, Oxford Regional Health Authority,
Oxford, UK*

The objective of this chapter is to discuss the relationship between the general
principles of health care ethics and care of elderly people.

In looking at the chapter headings for this book it is obvious that the list
consists of topics from a number of different types of categories. Different
approaches can be used to categorize the topics included in the list of chapters,
but one obvious distinction between two different types of topic is that some
topics concern the particular context in which ethical problems arise, for example
in the care of a terminally ill patient or in decision about abortion. Another
group of topics relate to particular groups of patients, notably those with mental
illness, mental handicap, children and the unborn, and this chapter relates to
this particular category, although the two different categories of topic obviously
inter-relate.

INCOMPETENCE AS A FOCUS OF ETHICAL CONCERN

Some of the groups that are a particular focus for concern have been listed in
the previous section, but what is it that the topics in this category have in
common? Why is it that a book on health care ethics, or indeed articles on
health care ethics, focus on these groups rather than on other groups in the
health service, for example people with broken legs or people having elective
operations or people with streptococcal infection of the throat?

The groups which are the focus of ethical concern are presumed to be
vulnerable principally because a belief prevails that they are not fully competent
and able to look after their own affairs, which means that they are at greater
than average risk of manipulation by professionals, albeit well-intentioned
manipulation, and that they need outside agencies to consider their welfare and
take appropriate action for them either as individuals or as groups. Elderly
people are classified with the mentally ill, mentally handicapped and children
because it is presumed that they are incompetent. This presumption is particularly

Principles of Health Care Ethics. Edited by Raanan Gillon.

marked when elderly people are referred to health or social services as being 'at risk'.

ELDERLY PEOPLE 'AT RISK'

Social work offices and general practice frequently receive referrals from people other than the elderly person who is deemed to be 'at risk'. The risks run by elderly people vary. The elderly person may simply be perceived as neglecting him or herself, or there may be a risk of a specific health problem, for example hypothermia, malnutrition, falls or fire.

In the 'at risk' referral there are three main players—the professional to whom the referral is made, the elderly person and the anxious other—and it is usually, but not always, the anxious other who makes the referral. The anxious other may be a neighbour, friend, relative or another professional, but the principal reason for referral is that the other person is anxious about the elderly person. Almost always the elderly person referred as being 'at risk' is in fact at higher than average probability of sustaining some adverse health event, but this is not the principal reason for a referral. The main reason why elderly people are referred as being 'at risk' is that the elderly person either refuses to accept that he or she is at risk, or is refusing to take what the anxious other, or others, define as appropriate action.

Similar referrals are not made concerning people who are smoking 40 cigarettes a day or drinking heavily, provided those people are not elderly. It is age, and the assumption that the person is incompetent, an assumption made whether or not the person is suffering from Alzheimer's disease, that leads to the referral. The most striking example of this approach to elderly people deemed to be at risk is provided by the legislative powers of compulsory removal of older people which were included in the National Assistance Act in the United Kingdom.

Section 47

Section 47 of the 1948 National Assistance Act gave the Medical Officer of Health the power to apply to a magistrate for the compulsory removal of persons who '(a) are suffering from grave chronic disease or being aged and infirm, or physically incapacitated or living in insanitary conditions and (b) are unable to devote to themselves and are not receiving from other persons proper care and attention'. The Medical Officer of Health was also given power to remove persons to prevent 'Injury to the health of or serious nuisance to other persons'.

These powers had been introduced by a number of local authorities in England in the preceding 20 years, but were introduced nationally by the National Assistance Act. The powers are still available and are used about 200 times a year, mostly to remove very elderly people. At no point in the evolution of these powers was the ethical issue discussed. It has been assumed throughout that the people in these circumstances are incompetent, the evidence for their incompetence being the circumstances in which they live. Incompetence, however, should be defined with respect to an individual's intellectual ability and not with respect to circumstances alone.

DEFINING INCOMPETENCE

Incompetence is a legal term used to define a person's inability to make particular decisions. In legal use it is not a global term, and people are not defined as being generally incompetent, because even an individual with a severe degree of Alzheimer's disease retains some abilities. Incompetence refers to specific contexts, for example incompetence to make a will, or incompetence to manage financial affairs.

Much of the ethical concern about elderly people is based on two premises concerning their competence.

The first is that all very elderly people are *ipso facto* incompetent. Some people, although not holding this extreme view, believe that all older people with Alzheimer's disease are *ipso facto* incompetent, but this is not necessarily the case.

The second belief is that if an older person develops any evidence of incompetence, for example evidence of an inability to manage his or her finances adequately, it is assumed that such people are unable to look after themselves in any way and therefore require institutional care.

The concept of incompetence should not be used in a global sense with elderly people, and the reasons why older people are presumed to be incompetent will be discussed in more detail in the next section of this chapter.

BELIEFS ABOUT INCOMPETENCE IN OLD AGE

Older people are statistically more likely to suffer many of the adverse events which are the source of concern of people who believe that older people are incompetent, and that paternalistic decision-making is justified when dealing with older people. The principal reason they do so is that people assume they are incompetent. The objective of this section is to examine the factors supporting this belief.

The Decline in Intelligence

Certain aspects of intelligence decline with age. However, those aspects of intelligence which decline with age, principally short-term memory and the ability to think quickly, are not those aspects of intelligence which allow one to make competent decisions.

Alzheimer's Disease

People who suffer from Alzheimer's disease may be incompetent in certain contexts, but the diagnosis of Alzheimer's disease does not necessarily mean that such people are *ipso facto* necessarily incompetent to look after themselves, and even if incompetence is revealed in some aspects of their life Alzheimer's disease does not result in global incompetence until an advanced stage.

ATTITUDES TOWARDS ELDERLY PEOPLE

Attitudes shape beliefs, and certain attitudes towards elderly people are important in influencing beliefs and in determining the attitude that condones paternalistic intervention in older people, thus necessitating special legal powers to protect their liberty.

Firstly, some people are moved by the plight of older people and their reaction to older people in difficulty is to wish to care for and protect them. If this attitude is also accompanied by the belief that all older people are incompetent, what has been called an ageist belief, then paternalistic intervention against the wishes of the old person will be considered to be justifiable. There are, however, two other attitudes which are also relevant—guilt, and confusion about the relative responsibilities of the neighbour and the state—and these will be discussed in subsequent sections.

Guilt as a Source of Concern

Some of the difficulties faced by older people result from ageing and the increasing incidence of disabling disease that occurs with age. However, it is obvious that many of the problems are caused by poverty. The principal cause of poverty in old age is the decision taken by those in power in society that this should be their position. Those in power, however, should be regarded not only as politicians but also the electorate as a whole. Subsections of the electorate, for example various professional and working groups, have been able to improve their standard of living by industrial action or the threat of industrial action, but older people have no such levers of power, and although older people are relatively better off than they were, they are still impoverished when compared with the working population.

Younger people understand this, consciously or unconsciously. They may seek to alleviate their guilt by providing tokens of their esteem for older people, for example the 'Christmas bonus' for pensioners or food parcels or gifts for older people at Christmas, but these gifts, which many people see as symbols, can also be viewed as token offerings given by one group who feels guilty towards another group that engenders guilt. Guilt can lead to constructive action, but it can also lead to certain types of displacement activity; for example one response to the guilt generated by being aware of an old person who is cold and at risk of hypothermia is to offer practical assistance to increase that old person's income and warm the dwelling; an alternative is to request that person's removal to residential care.

The part that guilt plays in creating problems for older people is illustrated by the history of witchcraft in the United Kingdom.

Old People as Witches

The typical witch was not a young person with hysteria or schizophrenia, but a poor old person who made the neighbours feel guilty.

The sequence of events leading to an accusation of witchcraft in seventeenth-century England was typically that an old person made certain people in a village feel guilty, either by requesting help from them or simply by generating feelings of guilt, and it has been argued that witchcraft accusations were a feature of Post-Reformation England because in Post-Reformation England there was no means of resolving the guilt through confession.

When some adverse event occurred in the life of the person feeling guilty he had to seek some explanation for this, because at that time explanations for adverse events other than chance were more commonly sought. Two possible alternatives offered themselves to the afflicted individual. One was that God had sent the affliction as a punishment; the second was that a curse had been put upon that person, and when thinking of the source of the curse it was possible to identify the person who caused the feelings of guilt, particularly if that person had been turned away from the door when seeking help, and had uttered some curse or given a hostile look when so turned away.

As Keith Thomas stated, in his seminal study on witchcraft,

> The tensions which produced witchcraft allegations were thus those generated by society which no longer had a clear view as to how its dependent member should be treated; they reflected the ethical conflict between the twin and opposing doctrines that those who did not work should not eat, and that it was blessed for the rich to support the poor (1).

Some of the hostility that formerly focused on older people now focuses on those who provide health care, particularly if they are seen to be allowing older people to continue to live at risk.

Part of the reason why this tension existed, and exists today, was the confusion about the relative responsibilities of the neighbour or family member, on the one hand, and the state on the other.

The Confusing Role of the State

The need for intervention of the state, or of a service provided or supported by the state, is sometimes unequivocal, as for example when an old person fractures a hip, but the classic health care problems associated with an ageing population are not only these acute and clear-cut problems but also multiple disease resulting in physical handicap or psychological disability or both.

Another reason why witchcraft accusations developed in the seventeenth century is considered to relate to the introduction of the Poor Law in England at that time. Before 1601 taxes had been levied specifically for the support of dependent members of society, and as the traditions of mutual charity died away individuals were less willing to offer help, but were often still troubled by feelings of guilt.

In providing health care for older people the uncertain role of the family or of the neighbour is a source of tension. Relatives and neighbours may feel guilty that the old person is in a predicament or is suffering, but also be confused about their own contribution. This confusion is not helped by the use of the word 'care', which can mean anything from intensive care with a ratio of seven nurses to one patient to the type of neighbourly assistance that one old person can provide for another.

Although many relatives are grateful for the help they receive from health and social services there are others who are hostile, or potentially hostile, to professional carers. This is often combined with an expressed wish that the institution should 'do more' for older people and conflicts are common between professionals who believe that an old person can be rehabilitated, causing discomfort to the old person in the process, and relatives who believe that it is kinder to push the old person in a wheelchair. This type of conflict is more common in social services than in health service settings, for two reasons.

The first is that people going into hospital are known to go into a hospital for treatment as well as care, and treatment is known to involve discomfort or degree of risk. It is accepted that harm may have to be done, for example a surgical operation, or a risk may have to be borne to produce a benefit. People who are admitted to social services are not, in the eyes of the public, admitted for rehabilitation or treatment, although they are to be 'cared for', and 'care' may mean doing everything for the old person. The second reason is that the old person admitted to a social services setting may engender more guilt than the old person admitted to hospital, because the family perceive that other people will think them uncaring for allowing this admission to take place, whereas an admission to a hospital service has always the apparent justification that the admission was necessary for treatment.

In those health care systems in which hospital treatment is free, whereas social service care has to be paid for, even greater tension is created between relatives and professional carers.

COPING WITH INAPPROPRIATE LEVELS OF GUILT

The text so far has painted a bleak picture of society, but the focus has been on the counterproductive aspects of the general attitude called caring. This should not obscure the fact that the majority of people who care for elderly people do so for altruistic reasons, and not as a means of coping with guilt. Often relatives have quite inappropriate levels of guilt, and it is common for professionals to have to help younger members of the family disengage from their emotional over-commitment and from providing more support than the old person actually needs.

SHOULD COMPULSORY REMOVAL CONTINUE?

In this chapter the compulsory removal of old people, using the powers of Section 47 of the National Assistance Act, has been taken as a paradigm of paternalistic attitudes towards older people and the ethical issues involved in the management of an old person deemed to be 'at risk'. Most professionals are unhappy with the existence of Section 47, and believe that some change should take place, but what type of changes should take place to base the legislation on sounder ethical principles than the shaky foundation on which Section 47 is currently based?

Repealing Section 47

Some people have called for the repeal of Section 47. They have done so because they believe that Section 47 infringes the liberty of older people. Many of the specialists in public health medicine who use Section 47 powers would argue that Section 47 can equally be seen as a means of preserving the liberty of older people. They would cite two pieces of evidence to support this claim.

Firstly, the majority of people referred are not removed, and removals are only made usually after those primarily involved in the case have decided that compulsory removal is the only answer. The specialist in public health medicine may, however, argue that the old person who has been referred, and is only receiving domiciliary care on three days a week, needs in fact seven-day care rather than compulsory removal.

Secondly, public health physicians would argue that Section 47 can be seen as a defender of liberty because it lays down clear rules for the admission of older people to a home. In some parts of the country Section 47 is never used, principally because the professional culture in those parts of the country believes that Section 47 has no part to play in the care of elderly people. In those populations therefore there is never any compulsory removal. It should not be assumed, however, that all removals which are not based on legal compulsion are voluntary. Many older people go into residential care unwillingly due to a combination of inadequate domiciliary services and concerted gentle pressure. It could be argued that Section 47 should be used more often than it is used at present, in those situations in which elderly people are unwilling to be admitted to residential care, because if these powers are not available then other steps may be taken, for example increasing the old person's medication until she is unable to argue her case coherently, or simply putting the person under so much psychological pressure that she succumbs and agrees to admission.

If Section 47 were to be retained there is little dispute that it should be amended, for it is now over 60 years since it was drafted.

Changing the Context

Individual professionals, teams of professionals and services operate in context, and the two most important aspects of the social context which influence the way 'at risk' referrals are handled were identified in the first part of this chapter as being, firstly, confusion between the social responsibilities of the state and the neighbour and family and, secondly, guilt.

Clarifying the role of the State

Ideally, the role of the state should be clearly defined and the role of the neighbour and family would therefore be unambiguous, but this will never be possible, particularly where old people simply need large amounts of general care of the sort that they would receive if they had children living nearby who were able and willing to help. Where the old person receives technical help of the sort that cannot be provided by family members the function of the state and its servants is clear, but when the main needs are for shopping or housework, or help with personal care, then there is an inevitable confusion between the function of the state and the function of the neighbour and relative.

This confusion may be further complicated if neighbours and relatives are hostile towards public services, hostility often understandable, for well-paid public servants are regarded with justifiable envy by people whose economic position is precarious or deprived. 'You are paid to care' is not uncommonly said to professionals faced by angry neighbours or relatives, and this charge is true, but the big question remains unclear what is actually meant by the word 'care'.

Minimizing Guilt

Poverty is common among older people and that poverty results from collective decisions taken by society and expressed through its legislators. Much of paternalism stems from guilt, but to remove the cause of this guilt would be to remove poverty in old age. It is not impossible. If the salary of every public servant were halved the gap between the income of public servants and elderly people could be significantly reduced if that money were reallocated to another group who benefited from the public purse, namely old age pensioners dependent upon state support.

It is essential that professionals recognize that they too are part of the problem of poverty, and it is not simply neighbours responding in a certain way because of guilt; professional practice is also influenced by the fact that professionals responsible for 'caring for older people' are at least as dependent on older people as older people are on them.

Thus, the 'at risk referral' and the complex ethical issues involved in the management of these individual cases will continue to pose challenges for professionals, and even more for the older people who are referred as being 'at risk'.

Amending the Procedure

If Section 47 were to be retained many of the procedures would need to be modified to ensure that the rights of the older person were protected.

More Effective Training

Professional training for those who work with elderly people has improved in the past 20 years, and although there is no scientific evidence, those who have been working with older people for 20 years or more can be in no doubt that professionals who work with them now are more aware of ageism and its implications, and are less likely to make paternalistic assumptions and do not respond so readily to social pressures based on the assumption that disabled older people, or older people with Alzheimer's disease, are all incompetent.

There is, however, a limit to the effects of professional training, in part because individual professionals, after training, go to work in institutions and become institutionalized. The term 'institutionalization' is almost always used to refer to patients, but professionals also become institutionalized, as does anyone who lives within a framework of beliefs and attitudes.

The effects of institutionalization can be prevented by professional development and continuing education but are very powerful. Steps other than professional training and continuing education must be taken to prevent paternalism, and one of the most important means of doing this is by increasing the power of the elderly person by encouraging advocacy.

Introducing Advocates

The elderly person referred because he or she is deemed to be 'at risk' often has to cope with a large number of different professionals. Typically, a general practitioner, a community nurse, social worker, home help organizer and one or more home helps may be involved. The old person may be visited by these people serially, or have to meet with them in groups, together with visits from neighbours and family in which more forceful attempts are made to persuade the old person to see what is commonly called 'the reality of the situation', even if the old person is expressing his or her view clearly, or has written it down in a form of 'living will'.

Often the professionals stand up for the liberty of the individual against family and neighbours, and sometimes one professional in particular—for example the psychogeriatrician or social worker—stands up for the liberty of the old person in the face of pressure of other professionals. In the majority of cases referred the public health physicians, who act as Proper Officers for the District Council in the discharge of Section 47 powers, act on behalf of the older person by refusing to use Section 47 powers because the majority of cases referred are not moved. However, it should not be assumed that professionals can always act in the best interests of older people, and attempts are being made to train volunteers to act as advocates for older people, particularly for those older people whose competence is limited because of Alzheimer's disease and who have no relatives. Old people with these characteristics in residential care are particularly vulnerable, and have been the focus for most attempts to introduce advocacy schemes, which will undoubtedly develop during the 1990s.

CHANGING COHORTS

The main force for change will, however, come from old people themselves. The new cohorts of people who are becoming old today are more assertive, healthier, better educated and better organized than those who are already very old. As new cohorts enter old age they will challenge and change social attitudes towards old age, and thus change the context in which care is given, but old frail people will continue to evoke powerful and confused feelings of guilt and sympathy, so the type of ethical problems described in this chapter will continue to exist as a problem both for professionals and those old people they are trying to help.

REFERENCE

1. Thomas, K. 1971. *Religion and the decline of magic*. Weidenfeld & Nicholson, London.

61

Ethics in the Care of the Elderly with Dementia

ASTRID NORBERG, RN, PhD

Professor, Umeå University, Umeå, Sweden

In the care of the demented elderly, caregivers meet special ethical problems. How they deal with these problems is connected with their philosophy of life. Thus caregivers in Israel reason in another way than caregivers in Sweden (1). A comparison based on interviews from 1980 to 1984 suggested that caregivers in Israel gave priority to the ethical principle of sanctity of life which is central to Judaism, while caregivers in Sweden were more prone to give priority to the ethical principles of beneficence and non-maleficence when reasoning about feeding decisions for the severely demented. Interviews with nurses in Sweden in 1988 showed that their overall attitude to ethics was to give priority to the ethical principle of autonomy, but when faced with a problematic feeding situation they tended to change their priority to the ethical principle of beneficence (2). The nurses also stressed that the way they act would depend on the concrete situation at hand. Since the expression of ethical attitudes seems to be coloured by the specific perspectives on care held by different professionals (3) it should be emphasized that this chapter is written from a nursing perspective.

In the care of the demented the main interest is that caregivers not only reason but also act in an ethically good and right way towards their patients. Thus there is a need for a theory on ethics in practice.

In this chapter the ethics in the care of elderly with dementia will be discussed from a narrative relation ethics perspective. Relation ethics answers questions like: How should I meet this patient? How can I be a good nurse? Narrative ethics states that ethics is embedded in stories that are told and lived by people.

NARRATIVE RELATION ETHICS

Narrative relation ethics deals with the question of how we can fulfil our roles and relate to others as positively as possible (cf. ref. 4). The notion of the

Principles of Health Care Ethics. Edited by Raanan Gillon.

ultimately good for man (a nice life story) is the starting point for Aristotle's ethics (5). I think it should be the starting point also for ethics applied to the care of the demented.

When we find ourselves in a situation it is already 'ethically delineated', i.e. it was created by people's choices, preferences and evaluations which have crystallized themselves into 'causes to be defended, ideas to be realized, tasks to be performed', 'values which play the role of rules of action' (6). Another way to express this is that we create and tell our stories within stories that others have already told. When we narrate we order actions into the past, the present and the future. Our understanding of life can be expressed in stories answering the questions: what, who, how, with whom, against whom, for whom. People are simultaneously involved in many stories, that of their families, their countries, their professions, mankind and so on. There is also a personal story. The person tells and is told (7).

Narrative ethics does not exclude the use of ethical principles. However, the principles have another function than in, for example, deontological ethics. They become principles of a fundamental ethical attitude that is expressed through our narrative competence (create, participate in, tell and understand stories of human conduct) (6).

Narrative ethics is believed to present a fundamental unit of cognitive, emotional, and conative dimensions of human life as well as to take into account situational factors (circumstances). The story a person tells about her- or himself shows her or his actions, feelings and thoughts in a concrete context, i.e. together with co-actors in a situation that has already been created. The story illustrates how the story-teller perceives the situation.

In order to come to a conclusion about how to act in an ethically difficult care situation we have to interpret the situation and act in accordance with our interpretation. In situations where we have co-actors we also have to find arguments for our interpretation as well as listen to others' interpretations in a genuine dialogue. At best we come to a shared interpretation. If not we may at least understand each other's versions of the story and agree about how to handle the disagreements.

THE CARE OF THE DEMENTED

Dementia Disease

Dementia denotes a number of progressive diseases leading to a deterioration of intellect, personality and communication (cf. ref. 8). The course of dementia contains various stages (9) which have been described as representing a general regression towards more primitive experience and behaviour (10). In the last stage of dementia the diseased have lost most of their verbal (11) and non-verbal (12) communicative competence.

Being demented means having problems relating to oneself, others and the world. The demented react to all kinds of contact with primitive types of anxiety such as anxiety for annihilation and separation. They lose their experience of wholeness and meaning (cf. ref. 13).

Ethical Problems

Parallel to the course of the dementia disease different ethical problems appear in the care. During the first stages of the disease family members often care for the patients. Before the very last stage of the disease patients are often institutionalized and mainly cared for by professional caregivers.

In the earlier stages of dementia the patients change gradually. The family members meet sides they have not seen before. This of course leads to relational problems which at worst cause abuse and neglect (14), problems that are very difficult for caregivers to recognize and handle (15). When the patients have reached the last stage of the disease their family members have often accepted that they have changed. Sometimes they experience the diseased as dead although still alive (16). This poses ethical problems regarding how to relate to the patient.

The quality of the demented person's life appears to be very poor (17,18). An important challenge for caregivers then becomes the improvement of the quality of life. Related to the question of the patient's quality of life is the question of the meaning of life. There are family members and professional caregivers who think that the life of the demented person has no meaning (19,20).

Another problem is the refusal-like behaviour that the patients may exhibit, for example refusal-like feeding behaviour. Caregivers feel uncertain whether to interpret the behaviour as an expression of the patient's wish or as involuntary behaviour relating to symptoms such as agnosia and apraxia (21).

The demented person's behaviour has often been described as 'behavioural disturbances' (22). Examples of this kind of behaviour are vocally disruptive behaviour (23) and wandering (24). There are many ethical problems connected with the question of how to handle this kind of behaviour.

NARRATIVE RELATION ETHICS IN THE CARE OF THE DEMENTED ELDERLY

During the course of dementia the patient's psychological defence mechanisms become weaker (cf. ref. 25). This means that the patient becomes more and more vulnerable. The demented elderly easily feel threatened not only from the outside but also from their own psyche. The caregivers have great power to hurt them or to protect them. A careless conversation can, for example, easily arouse anxiety reactions in the patients. When they cannot recognize their environment and make decisions about what is good or bad for them there is a risk that they will take actions violating their own integrity. Then caregivers have to act to protect the patient against her- or himself. The patient's family members may act as vicarious decision-makers. In institutions professional caregivers have the same function concerning everyday matters. This, of course, makes it vital for the caregivers to understand the patient's experience in order to judge what actions would be in line with the patient's wishes at present, with her or his previous values (cf. ref. 26) or what will be best for her or him (cf. ref. 27).

The most important question is how the caregivers see the demented patient; is the patient seen as a subject worthy of close contact or is the patient seen as an object to be manipulated (cf. ref. 20). People give meaning to their experiences by narrating them (29). When we try to understand other people's peculiar actions we often place them in a narrative context to make them appear meaningful. 'He did this and that because he intended to . . .'. The fact that we talk about the demented person's actions as 'disturbing behaviour' means that we cannot see the meaning, i.e. we have not been able to see the story wherein the behaviour is a meaningful component. We communicate this understanding to the patient and there is a risk that the patient accepts our views.

Human behaviour can be seen as expressions of experiences (30). Thus so-called behavioural disturbances can be seen as expressions of the demented person's experience. It is an important task for the caregiver to find the personal meaning of the behaviour on behalf of the person. This is a prerequisite for the caregiver's improving the demented person's quality of life.

Being able to experience episodes of our lives as whole and meaningful stories is an important aspect of our narrative competence. The demented person gradually loses this competence. The caregiver then has an important task helping her or him experience wholeness and meaning.

Aristotle's ethics (5) is connected with the idea of the good life which should be realized in the life course. It stresses that it is not single actions *per se* but single actions in relation to the life as a whole that are important. Based on this view it is suggested here that there is an ethical demand that the caregiver has an overall perception of what was the life plan and the good life of the patient, i.e. knows the patient's life story so that s/he is able to make an individual care plan for the patient. The task for the caregivers is to help the patient create nice little everyday stories contributing positively to the overall life story. However, it has been revealed that there are caregivers in dementia care in Sweden who have very poor knowledge about their patients' lives prior to hospitalization (18).

Severely demented patients have been said to regress to primitive ways of functioning and to exhibit childlike reactions (31). This might mean that they also regress to a functional stage prior to narration (cf. ref. 32), i.e. to a stage where they are not able to express their experiences through telling stories. Instead they live in an undifferentiated world of emotions. They react to the emotional atmosphere although they cannot explain and justify their reactions. This suggestion seems congruent with the observation that caregivers and the severely demented share meaning without verbal communication taking place (33,34). It should be noted that the healthy person does not abandon his or her primitive skills but covers them. Therefore healthy caregivers with good contact with their primitive experiences can communicate with the severely demented patient on this undifferentiated emotional level.

Interpreting the Patient's Story

Our identity is rooted in our very personal story. If we lose this story we lose our identity. This is what happens to the demented. They feel uprooted and homeless when they cannot remember their past, recognize their present and foresee their future (cf. ref. 13).

Empathy is an important ingredient of narrative relation ethics. Reading facial expressions and the tone of voice of the other for instance stimulates it (cf. ref. 35). The person identifies with the other and sees the situation from the other's perspective. This is a problem in the care of the demented. In order to see the patient's world it is necessary to communicate. When the demented person's ability to communicate verbally decreases caregivers have to rely more and more on their interpretation of non-verbal cues. When the patient's communicative non-verbal as well as verbal cues become extremely unclear and weak some caregivers seem to stop seeing the patients as human beings while others impute meaning into their cues (28,34).

Asplund (36) suggested that there is a connection between the caregiver's experience of 'an overall meaning in life, the experience of meaning in the care of the severely demented and the experience of meaning in the patient's communicative cues'. Although some patients produce neither speech nor whole patterns of facial expressions (31) there are caregivers who feel they understand their patients. They seem either to impute meaning into the patient's cues or to grasp a meaning prior to any imputation. When caregivers impute meaning into the severely demented person's unclear and weak cues they exert great power over their patients. The caregivers may, for example, interpret the patient's refusal-like feeding behaviour as a demand to be given help to die or as a demand to be force-fed because of the inability to understand the situation and act accordingly (cf. ref. 21). This presupposes that their overall ethical attitude demands that they act in accordance with the ethical principle of autonomy. Their ethical attitude could also tell them to use their understanding of the situation to decide what is best for the patient and act according to the ethical principle of beneficence (cf. ref. 27) (2).

Because it is so difficult to understand the demented person's communication it is important to work very hard to improve their caregivers' hermeneutic competence. Here some suggestions of what the severely demented experience will be made. They are based on interpretation of observations of action and of fragmentary utterances by the patients seen as parts of whole situations (13), and interviews with experienced caregivers (34).

Interviews with experienced caregivers about demented patients' experience (34) were based on the assumption that emotions can be transferred between people without any conscious attempt being made by either party. The patient projects emotions on the caregiver who processes them and sends them back in a form that can be contained by the patient. Therefore caregivers in lasting and close contact with vocally disruptive demented patients were thought to be able to tell what their patients experience by describing the emotions evoked in themselves when caring for these patients. The caregivers described what they thought the patients experience when screaming, e.g. anxiety for abandonment—'being abandoned and deserted, not belonging to anyone/ anything and being helpless, longing for someone/something like one's mother'; anxiety for dissolution—'feelings of emptiness and meaninglessness of the situation, dissolution of the ego and an expression of chaos and despair'; anxiety due to threats to and loss of autonomy—'experience of restriction and confinement related to such as being fettered in a chair, imprisoned in his own body by his apraxia and not being allowed to or not being able to make his own decisions'.

It is, of course, an ethical issue to be able to perceive the patient's situation in a way that would be accepted by the patient, had she or he been able to express acceptance.

The interviews with caregivers of vocally disruptive demented patients thus revealed that the caregivers saw their patients as anxious, very lonely and needing human contact. This view, however, did not result in care actions aimed at relieving the perceived anxiety and spending time with the patient. On the contrary, observations on the wards where these patients were cared for, showed that they were even more isolated than the demented who did not exhibit vocally disruptive behaviour (37). This can be explained by the caregivers' emotional reactions in the situation. They described how they felt a need to help the patients but how they also felt powerless and insufficient (34). In order to handle this kind of situation it seems reasonable to believe that defence reactions are aroused in them. By reducing the amount of contact with the patients the emotional reactions of powerlessness and insufficiency were also reduced.

Translating Understanding into Action

The investigation described above highlights the well-known fact that the relationship between ethical thinking and action is complex (38). Feelings seem to be an important link, but the circumstances of the situation at hand also interfere, for example, the opportunity to receive support from co-workers or superiors. It seems necessary to apply ethics that helps caregivers not only perceive the situation, feel and reason in a good and right way, but also to find the means and the courage to perform the good and right actions. This is a complex process that calls for a complex ethical theory.

On the basis of Aristotle's ethics (5) it is believed that people need practical wisdom in order to be able to do good and right things. This wisdom develops through experience reflected upon and integrated in the personality. If this is the case, it seems urgent that caregivers in dementia care have support and time to reflect upon their personal experience together with the demented. When asked about their reasoning in an ethically problematic care situation in dementia care (2) there were caregivers who said that a certain episode in their personal life or in their care work had led to a change in their perception of the care of the severely demented. Such experiences were, for example, their own mother's death. These research findings are in line with theories stating that persons can use paradigm cases and maxims based on their personal experience almost in the same way as theorists use theories (cf. ref. 39). If this is true it is important that caregivers receive help to reflect upon and organize their experience so that they can develop practical wisdom to help them translate their good intentions into action. An important aspect of this is the need of shared experience and support (cf. ref. 40). Caregivers act in a complex social system and need to act together. It seems reasonable to assume that it is easier to obtain consensus on the ethical attitudes that should guide the minute-by-minute work if caregivers are given an opportunity to share each other's experience of the care work and reflect on similar as well as on different experiences.

Promoting an Experience of At-homeness

An outstanding problem in the life of the moderately demented elderly is the fact that they do not feel at home in life (13). They regress. They search for the homes of their childhood or for the homes where their little children were taken care of. It was apparent that six investigated demented women expressed experiences of being at home only when they were in close contact with a 'significant other' in a calm atmosphere. Feeling at home included experiences of being related to themselves—they knew who they were; being related to others—they knew who the others were; being related to events and objects—they knew what they did and recognized the objects present in their environment; and being present in time and place—they knew when things occurred and where they were. Their perception of reality, however, did not always coincide with that of their caregivers. Patient and caregiver could dwell in a different time and in different places.

The patients investigated sometimes seemed to feel at home, but suddenly made a transition in time and tended to go back to their past homes. It seemed that such behaviour was elicited by things that threatened the patient, for instance too heavy demands, and being left alone. It became evident that the demented person's experience of feeling at home is easily destroyed. This means that there are ethical demands on the caregiver to handle the patient's at-homeness with care and work to protect and promote it. When the patients expressed their being at home they seemed 'being present', 'being related' and 'being part of', i.e. feeling whole and connected with their past and future.

It seems reasonable to suggest that the feeling of being at home is analogous with the experience of integrity (wholeness and meaning) as described by the Erikson (41) theory of 'eight stages of man'. According to this theory a prerequisite for a positive solution of the crisis 'integrity versus despair' (phase-specific in old age) is that the person can also resolve the preceding crises at the present stage of development; 'trust versus mistrust', 'autonomy versus shame and doubt', 'initiative versus guilt', 'industry versus inferiority', 'identity versus identity confusion', 'intimacy versus isolation', and 'generativity versus stagnation'. Positive solutions are threatened by the dementia disease. It is not easy to trust people when you do not recognize them; to act autonomously when you have problems performing voluntary actions; to take initiative when you have forgotten your future; to be industrious when you have lost an acquired skill such as eating; to experience identity when you do not remember your personal story or recognize your own body; to experience intimacy when you have lost most of your communicative skills; to experience generativity when you depend on others for help with everyday matters, or to experience integrity when you cannot connect what happens to your life philosophy as you have lost your ability of abstract thinking.

With this interpretation of the patient's experiences it becomes urgent for caregivers to work very hard to promote those important experiences that the patient needs and has such problems to receive. The caregiver needs an ethical attitude of caring and concern as well as creative imagination, so that she or he can see the patient's situation, firstly, as the patient would have seen it, had he or she been healthy, i.e. from the perspective of the patient's life story and the project she or he herself or himself has set. Secondly, the caregiver must be able to perceive the situation as the patient perceives it in the present, and help her or him find ways to come as close to her or his life plan as possible despite the disease. To accomplish this the caregiver must be sensitive to the patient and creative enough to find ways to create and tell a nice story about the patient. As time goes by the dementia will progress and the patient will become less and less able to grasp the full time span. In the late stages of the disease the goal for the caregiver must be to create nice little stories about everyday matters such as a good dinner or a nice rest. Integrity-promoting care has been tried in a nursing home in Sweden. It leads to an improvement in the demented patients' psychological (42), neurochemical (43) and social (44) functioning.

Conflicting Realities

Ethical problems may occur when the patient's and the caregiver's realities conflict. The patient is treated like an object when the caregiver does not care enough to take the patient's experiences seriously. This may mean that the caregiver does not make any attempts to share the patients' reality by trying to understand them or trying to explain her or his reality to them. The caregiver leaves the patients in their distorted world without trying to understand what they experience. The confused world may be experienced as a safe place—the patients feel at home (cf. ref. 13) but it might also be experienced as a frightening place (cf. ref. 45). There is an ethical demand that the caregiver tries to understand what the patient experiences, whether the patient will violate or promote her or his own integrity and act accordingly. It also seems vital that the caregiver is honest with the patient in order to enhance the patient's trust in the caregiver. It can be as uncaring to correct the patients and orient them to the caregiver's reality as to leave them alone in their own reality. Brännström (45) argued that a weak paternalism is needed in the care of confused and demented persons, i.e. caregivers care for their patients enough sometimes to act for their best by letting them hear an 'adequate no' (cf. ref. 46). The caregivers will need practical wisdom to enable them to find out what is best in the situation at hand.

The Caregiver in Dementia Care

Referring to Lögstrup's (46) ethics, Asplund (36) suggested that the way caregivers experience the severely demented is connected with their own outlook on life. If they see life as intrinsically meaningful, as a gift and an ethical demand and the relationship between people as more essential than single individuals they can more easily experience the care of the severely demented as meaningful. If, on the other hand, they experience life as meaningful only to the extent that people impute meaning into it, they may have serious problems experiencing any meaning in their care for the severely demented. These patients cannot fill their lives with meaning by their own production.

Care activities such as feeding patients, can be seen as some kind of medical treatment. Care activities can also be seen as ends in themselves. Feeding has, for example, been described as an expression of love and concern. This means that feeding can never be withdrawn but does not necessarily lead to any results (cf. ref. 47). Asplund (36) suggested that the outlook on life as a gift and an ethical demand is connected with a view of care activities as meaningful ends in themselves, while they are seen as mere means towards ends in the outlook on life as a neutral raw material.

When the patient no longer responds to the caregiver's communicative attempts the caregiver (and the patient) may feel lonely and rejected (cf. ref. 34). The loneliness may threaten the caregiver's commitment and the patient may be treated like an object (18). Interviews in dementia care have shown that caregivers may experience powerlessness (48), and meaninglessness (20). Burnout was found to be more common among caregivers in dementia care than among other caregivers (49).

The patients and the caregivers are interdependent. This means that what the caregivers do to the patients they also do to themselves (cf. ref. 50). If caregivers see patients as objects they become objectified themselves. When caregivers do not see any meaning in the patient's life they do not see any meaning in their care for the patient either. If the patient is left homeless the caregiver will become homeless too, i.e. feel alienated in her or his work in dementia care. Caregivers feel estranged from their patients and thus also from themselves.

CONCLUSION

This chapter has illustrated how narrative relation ethics could be used in the daily care of the demented. It has also been said that caregivers need an ethical attitude of care and concern as well as practical wisdom to help them imagine new ways to help the demented feel at home in life. This will also lead to positive experiences for the caregivers themselves. The Golden Rule (51) seems an appropriate maxim: 'Do to others as you would have them do to you'.

REFERENCES

1. Norberg, A. and Hirschfeld, M. 1987. Feeding of severely demented patients in institutions. Interviews with caregivers in Israel. *Journal of Advanced Nursing* **12**: 551–557.
2. Jansson, L. and Norberg, A. 1992. Ethical reasoning among registered nurses experienced in dementia care. Interviews concerning the feeding of severely demented patients. *Scandinavian Journal of Caring Sciences* **6**: in press.
3. Udén, G., Norberg, A., Lindseth, A. and Marhaug, V. 1992. Ethical reasoning in nurses' and physicians' stories about care episodes. *Journal of Advanced Nursing* **17**: in press.
4. MacIntyre, A. 1985. *After virtue. A study in moral theory*, 2nd edn. Duckworth, London.
5. Oksenberg Rorty, A. (Ed.) 1980. *Essay on Aristotle's ethics*. University of California Press, Los Angeles.
6. Kemp, P. 1988. Toward a narrative on ethics: a bridge between ethics and the narrative reflection. *Philosophy and Social Criticism* **14**: 179–201.
7. Tappan, M. B. 1989. Stories lived and stories told: the narrative structure of late adolescent moral development. *Human Development* **32**: 300–315.
8. American Psychiatric Association. 1987. *Diagnostic and statistical manual of mental disorders (DSM III-R)*, 2nd edn. APA, Washington, DC.

9. Reisberg, B., Ferris, S. H. and Franssen, E. 1985. An ordinal functional assessment tool for Alzheimer's type dementia. *Hospital and Community Psychiatry* **36**: 593–595.
10. Nolen, R. N. 1988. Functional skill regression in late-stage dementias. *American Journal of Occupational Therapy* **42**: 666–669.
11. Bayles, K. L. and Kaszniak, A. W. 1987. *Communication and cognition in normal aging and dementia.* Little-Brown, London.
12. Asplund, K., Norberg, A., Adolfsson, R. and Waxman, H. 1991. Facial expressions in severely demented patients. A stimulus-response study of four patients with dementia of the Alzheimer type. *International Journal of Geriatric Psychiatry* **6**: 599–606.
13. Zingmark, K., Norberg, A. and Sandman, P. O. 1992. Experience of at-homeness in patients with Alzheimer's disease. *American Journal of Alzheimer's Care and Related Disorders and Research* (accepted for publication).
14. Pillemer, K. A. and Wolf, R. S. (Eds). 1986. *Elder abuse. Conflict in the family.* Auburn House, Dover.
15. Saveman, B. I., Norberg, A. and Hallberg, I. L. 1992. The problems of dealing with abuse and neglect of the elderly. Interviews with district nurses. *Qualitative Health Research* **2**: 208–223.
16. Levine, N. D., Gendron, C. E., Dastoor, D. P., Poitras, L. R., Sirota, S. E., Barxza, S. R. and Davis, J. C. 1984. Existential issues in the management of the demented elderly patient. *American Journal of Psychotherapy* **38**: 215–223.
17. Hemsi, L. 1982. Living with dementia. *Postgraduate Medical Journal* **58**: 610–617.
18. Ekman, S.-L., Norberg, A., Viitanen, M. and Winblad, B. 1991. Care of demented patients with severe communication problems. *Scandinavian Journal of Caring Sciences* **5**: 163–170.
19. Farran, C. J., Keane-Hagerty, E., Salloway, S., Kupferer, S. and Wilken, C. S. 1991. Finding meaning: an alternative paradigm for Alzheimer's disease family caregivers. *Gerontologist* **31**: 483–489.
20. Norberg, A. and Asplund, K. 1990. Caregivers' experience of caring for severely demented patients. *Western Journal of Nursing Research* **12**: 75–84.
21. Norberg, A., Bäckström, Å., Athlin, E. and Norberg, B. 1988. Food refusal among nursing home patients as conceptualized by nurses' aides and practical nurses. An interview study. *Journal of Advanced Nursing* **13**: 478–483.
22. Sandman, P. O., Adolfsson, R., Norberg, A., Nyström, L. and Winblad, B. 1988. The long-term care of the elderly. A descriptive study of 3600 patients in different institutions in the county of Västerbotten, Sweden. *Comprehensive Gerontology A*, **2**: 120–133.
23. Hallberg, I. R., Norberg, A. and Eriksson, S. 1990. Functional impairment and behavioural disturbances in vocally disruptive patients in psychogeriatric wards compared with controls. *International Journal of Geriatric Psychiatry* **5**: 53–61.
24. Hope, R. A. and Fairburn, C. G. 1990. The nature of wandering in dementia: A community-based study. *International Journal of Geriatric Psychiatry* **5**: 239–245.
25. Hallberg, I. R. 1990. Vocally disruptive behaviour in severely demented patients in relation to institutional care provided. *Umeå University Medical Dissertations*, New Series no. 261.
26. Veatch, R. M. 1984. An ethical framework for terminal care decisions: a new classification of patients. *Journal of the American Geriatrics Society* **32**: 665–669.
27. Ekman, S.-L. and Norberg, A. 1988. The autonomy of demented patients. Interviews with caregivers. *Journal of Medical Ethics* **14**: 184–187.
28. Athlin, E., Norberg, A. and Asplund, K. 1990. The caregivers' perceptions and interpretations of severely demented patients during feeding in a task assignment care system. *Scandinavian Journal of Caring Sciences* **4**: 147–156.
29. Tappan, M. B. and Brown, M. L. 1989. Stories told and lessons learned: Toward a narrative approach to moral development and moral education. *Harvard Educational Review* **59**: 182–205.
30. Laing, R. D. 1967. *The politics of experience*, pp. 15–38. Penguin, Harmondsworth, Middlesex.

31. Asplund, K., Norberg, A. and Adolfsson, R. 1991. The sucking behaviour of two patients in the final stage of dementia of the Alzheimer type. *Scandinavian Journal of Caring Sciences* 5: 141–147.
32. Stern, D. N. 1991. *Diary of a baby*. Fontana, London.
33. Sandman, P.-O., Norberg, A., Adolfsson, R., Axelsson, K. and Hedly,V. 1986. Morning care of patients with dementia of Alzheimer's type. A theoretical model based on direct observations. *Journal of Advanced Nursing* 11: 369–378.
34. Hallberg, I. R. and Norberg, A. 1990. Staff's interpretation of the experience behind a vocally disruptive behaviour in severely demented patients and their feelings about it. *International Journal of Aging and Human Development* 31: 297–307.
35. Vitz, P. C. 1990. The use of narratives in ethical development. New psychological reasons or an old education method. *American Psychologist* 45: 709–720.
36. Asplund, K. 1991. The experience of meaning in the care of patients in the terminal stage of dementia of the Alzheimer type. Interpretation on non-verbal communication and ethical demands. *Umeå University Medical Dissertations*, New Series no. 310.
37. Hallberg, I. R., Luker, K., Norberg, A., Johnsson, K. and Eriksson, S. 1990. Staff interaction with vocally disruptive demented patients compared with demented controls. *Aging* 2: 163–171.
38. Locke, D. 1983. Doing what comes morally. The relation between behaviour and stages of moral reasoning. *Human Development* 26: 11–25.
39. Jonsen, A. R. and Toulmin, S. 1988. *The abuse of casuistry. A history of moral reasoning*, pp. 250–265. University of California Press, Berkeley.
40. Björkhem, K., Olsson, A., Hallberg, I. R. and Norberg, A. 1992. Caregivers' experience of providing care for demented persons in their homes. *Scandinavian Journal of Primary Health Care* 10: 53–56.
41. Erikson, E. H. 1982. *The life cycle completed*. W. W. Norton, New York.
42. Bråne, G., Karlsson, I., Kihlgren, M. and Norberg, A. 1989. Integrity-promoting care of demented nursing home patients: psychological and biochemical changes. *International Journal of Geriatric Psychiatry* 4: 165–172.
43. Widerlöv, E., Bråne, G., Ekman, R., Kihlgren, M., Norberg, A. and Karlsson, I. 1989. Elevated CSF somatostatin concentrations in demented patients improved psychomotor functions induced by integrity promoting care. *Acta Psychiatrica Scandinavica* 79: 41–47.
44. Kihlgren, M., Kuremyr, D., Norberg, A., Bråne, G., Engström, B., Karlsson, I. and Melin, E. 1992. Nurse–patient interaction after training in integrity promoting care at a long-term ward. Analysis of video-recorded morning care sessions. *International Journal of Nursing Studies* (accepted for publication).
45. Brännström, B. 1991. Care of the acutely confused elderly hip-fracture patient. Empirical studies and an ethical model of care. *Umeå University Medical Dissertations*, New Series no. 324.
46. Løgstrup, K. E. 1971. *The ethical demand*. (Danish original 1956). Fortress Press, Philadelphia.
47. Lynn, J. and Childress, J. F. 1983. Must patients always be given food and water? *Hastings Center Report* 13: 17–21.
48. Åkerlund, B. M. and Norberg, A. 1990. Powerlessness in terminal care of demented patients: An exploratory study. *Omega* 21: 15–19.
49. Åström, S., Nilsson, M., Norberg, A. and Winblad, B. 1990. Empathy, experiences of burnout and attitudes towards demented patients among personnel in geriatric care. *Journal of Advanced Nursing* 15: 1236–1244.
50. Hegel, G. W. F. 1967. *The phenomenology of the mind* (German original 1807), p. 228. Harper & Row, New York.
51. Luke 6:31. *Holy Bible*, New International Version, Classic Edition. Hodder & Stoughton, London, 1989.

62

Non-treatment Orders, including Do Not Resuscitate (DNR)

PAUL GOULDEN FRCANAES

Consultant Anaesthetist, Dewsbury District Hospital, UK

The subject of withdrawing or not providing treatment to certain patients falls easily into two areas: firstly treatments which, if not provided for whatever reason, lead to a bad outcome or even death for the patient at some time in the future, and secondly procedures which, if not undertaken, lead to immediate death, in particular the process of active resuscitation following a cardiac arrest.

To deal with the second situation first, for many years attempts had been made to resuscitate the suddenly collapsed or recently drowned by various techniques of artificial respiration and by squeezing the heart through a suitable surgical incision (1,2).

In so far as these techniques were applied, with varying degrees of success to apparently previously fit people collapsing, for instance under anaesthesia, they do not seem to have raised any moral question (perhaps beyond the metaphysical ones about all medical practice).

There was little to do for patients dying in the ward and their passing, although tragic, was regarded as a natural end-point. This began to change in 1960 when Kouvenhoven in Baltimore (3) described impressive recoveries after cardiac arrest with the new technique of closed-chest cardiac massage, coupled if necessary with the newly described defibrillator. This seemed to be an effective technique which could be undertaken by any doctor or even paramedical or lay person with a modicum of training, but no special surgical skills or equipment.

Over the next 10 years virtually all large acute hospitals in Europe and North America set up rapid-response 'crash teams' to bring resuscitation skills to the bedside of anyone suddenly dying in hospital. Although no-one was able to produce results as good as those described by Kouvenhoven in a published series there is no doubt that many lives have been saved. Resuscitation teams are a fact of life, and in an effort to reduce the mortality from coronary artery disease acute resuscitation by closed-chest compression and ventilation has

Principles of Health Care Ethics. Edited by Raanan Gillon.
© 1994 John Wiley & Sons Ltd

extended into the ambulance service and even (very effectively in some schemes) to trained lay people in the community.

As the active management of cardiac arrest became commonplace, situations arose, especially in large North American institutions, where it was virtually impossible for a patient to die in hospital from any cause without the application of active resuscitation. Increasingly this attitude converted what might have been a peaceful passing away of a patient with a poor quality of life, or short-term prognosis, into an ineffective aggressive charade, perhaps allowing the patient to survive a few more hours in one of the newly developing intensive care units.

Recognizing the inappropriateness (not to mention the expense) of this course of action individual hospitals, particularly in the United States, began to develop policies on the withholding of active resuscitation in certain patients.

To do this in a blanket way at the very best smacks of paternalism, and at a time when much more consideration was being given to the autonomy of individuals it was obviously much more logical to find out what they wanted. Unfortunately the circumstances of a cardiac arrest preclude any discussion with the patient, so reliance has to be placed on knowledge of his or her pre-existing views, hopefully expressed as some form of living will.

An increasing number of states in the USA have recognized a person's autonomous right to determine what should be done with his/her body even at the moment of death, and have passed legislation accepting the legally binding status of a suitable formulated declaration of the patient's wishes ('living will').

In the United Kingdom the living will has no legal force, and medical practice in this area continues to be dominated by paternalistic attitudes in which the patient's relatives often connive, although the paternalism is often justified by an appeal to the concept of non-maleficence by suggesting that it will be harmful to patients to know that they might die, so we won't tell them.

However, even in the United States living wills cover only a small proportion of patients in whom the question of a 'Do Not Resuscitate' order might be appropriate so practitioners are thrown back to 'rule of thumb'.

Do not resuscitate orders continue to raise difficulties (4,5). Problems include doctor ambivalence about who should be consulted before a DNR order is put in place (patient, spouse, children, siblings, nurses?) particularly if the patient is not competent; identification of the true competence of a patient who may have had sedative drugs, and the frustration of nurses and resident doctors asked to continue possibly complicated or invasive therapy in a patient for whom there is to be no active resuscitation.

Youngner *et al.* (6) found that 14% of patients in one intensive care unit had DNR orders in place.

Thomlinson and Brody (4) divide the indication for writing DNR instructions into three groups, each of which poses slightly different ethical problems. First, where the treatment is of no medical benefit (futile treatment). Here it is suggested that doctors are under no ethical obligation to provide therapy shown to be generally ineffective (even if the patient wants it). Blackhall (7) reviewed a number of studies on the outcome of cardiopulmonary resuscitation (CPR). Taking as the desired outcome survival to leave hospital, only one in seven of the cases of Bedell *et al.* in Boston (8) survived, and no patients with metastatic carcinoma, acute stroke, generalized sepsis or pneumonia left hospital after a cardiac arrest despite maximum therapy.

Other large studies confirmed these findings. Blackhall suggests that to offer CPR to patients in these categories offers a cruelly false hope, implying potential benefit where there is none. This clearly appeals to the concept of non-maleficence. What he is saying is that as CPR is of no benefit to these patients, it should not be considered as part of the treatment. A national consensus could be reached on the basis of carefully analysed published studies for conditions in which CPR has been shown to be ineffective, and the beneficent doctor should have no ethical difficulty in issuing a DNR order in these cases.

A second group of patients (described by Thomlinson and Brody (4)) are those in whom the quality of life after cardiopulmonary resuscitation is likely to be unacceptably low. The benefits of survival would not outweigh the burdens. An example is a patient disabled after a previous arrest. It can be predicted that even after a successful resuscitation the disability would be increased, possibly converting a marginally acceptable quality of life into an intolerable one. The value judgements required here are enormous, and can probably only really be made in consultation with the patient.

Potentially the largest and most difficult group of patients for whom a DNR order might be appropriate are those with a very poor quality of life before their cardiac arrest, for instance because of immobility, breathlessness or constant pain.

If the patient is content with his/her quality of life, and wishes life to continue no matter what, respect for life and the autonomy of the patient should rule out the possibility of a DNR order. If, however, the patient indicates that he/she would be better off dead, it is necessary to consider whether respect for his/her autonomy should outweigh considerations of prolonging life. If it does there is no problem with a DNR order. The problems arise firstly in finding out what patients really want at a time when, if they have not made 'a living will', their competence may be in doubt, and secondly in addressing the question whether, if the patient is better off dead than alive, is the moment of cardiac arrest the critical moment or should this conclusion influence earlier management?

Leaving aside the thorny question of assisted suicide or euthanasia, if a man is not to be resuscitated when he has a cardiac arrest, is there any point in prolonging his intolerable life by perhaps even more intolerable treatments, such as ventilation or dialysis, or should a decision to 'let nature take its course' be taken much earlier in the course of the patient's decline?

This of course leads us from DNR orders to the more general question of non-treatment, which will be discussed later.

Youngner *et al.* (6) found that all the interventions commenced before writing DNR orders were continued in at least 70% of patients. They were not quickly transferred out of the intensive care unit, and continued to consume levels of resources at least as great as patients in whom cardiopulmonary resuscitation was to be attempted. The implication of this, of course, is that additional therapies may have been introduced even after the DNR decision.

Ventilation was the most frequently continued intervention, presumably because in most cases the patients had respiratory failure, and withdrawal of the ventilator would produce death often within minutes in a way not seen by, say, withholding antibiotics.

The issue of discussing DNR orders with patients with a poor quality of life is so bound up in difficulties that it is very tempting either not to make a decision, and possibly rob a dying patient of dignity or, recognizing the undesirability of this, to fall back on the paternalistic 'doctor knows best'.

In the early days of 'living wills' Jackson and Youngner (9) identified examples of a number of situations in which it may be difficult clearly and validly to determine the wishes of a patient.

1. The patient may be ambivalent, with views that change from day to day.
2. There may be clinical depression (indeed proponents of the life-at-all-costs school would argue that a wish not to live for the longest possible time could be diagnostic of depression).
3. The patient may see his 'death with dignity' as a way out of another problem possibly amenable to help, such as a carer who cannot cope unaided, or he may have unjustified fears of certain lines of treatment which are amenable to sensitive explanation.
4. The patient may feel unable to express his own views because they conflict with contrary views held by members of his family and, of course, there is the question of competence; often a problem in some of the most tragic cases.

If it is impossible to ascertain the views of the patient, is paternalism acceptable?

Possibly it is, provided it is informed, logical and coherent. A paternalistic decision taken in the interests of a patient by a health carer is probably at least as valid from both the moral and legal viewpoint as seeking the views of the relatives. Although they may be able to shed some light on the patient's previously expressed views, they do not have any valid locus in their own right and may have their own agenda, from relief at being free of a burden, to guilt at not doing enough in the past. However, if a paternalistic viewpoint has to be adopted there are many caveats. Age, for instance, is not an accurate predictor of either survival or function after a cardiac arrest (10). Also a quality of life intolerable to a young man, for instance being bedbound, may be quite acceptable to an old person who has become used to it or expects less. Indeed if we are considering suffering, the young person may suffer much more if he survives a cardiac arrest than an old person, simply because he would expect to live longer. We would, for example, routinely ventilate a young sportsman with a high quadriplegia but have grave reservations about undertaking this line of treatment in the old, but the logic may be perverse.

In general then, DNR orders would seem to have a valid place in modern medical practice.

Where resuscitation attempts would be futile they could be imposed paternalistically, but where there are quality-of-life considerations it is of the greatest value to know the views of the patient, and to this extent pre-existing instructions in the form of a 'living will' are potentially of great benefit.

However, if the question is whether a patient in severe distress would be better off dead than alive, discussion should move away from the management of cardiac arrest into the broader arena of non-treatment decisions.

Is it ever acceptable not to offer a treatment, and if so in what circumstances? Presumably in practice there must be some limits placed at present, otherwise it would be possible to commit ever-increasing resources of both personnel and money to staving off death for hours or days, and even societies which believe that life is a gift from God and every moment is to be treasured, do not seem to do this.

If, however, treatment is to be limited, what is the moral basis of doing this? The overwhelming question would seem to be the resource issue, tragically highlighted in the developing world but not to be ignored in the rich west. That said, there could be circumstances in which, even if resources were available, treatment would be inappropriate. An example of this is the use of futile treatments, and this has been explored by Schneiderman and colleagues (11). They point out that the benefit of a treatment is to be judged not just by its physiological effect but by its ability to help progress the patient in the direction of an acceptable quality of life. Therefore the fact that, for instance, dialysis will correct the plasma electrolytes is irrelevant if having normal electrolytes will not help a patient wean from a ventilator. They do not regard merely getting a patient into a state where he is surviving with a total preoccupation with and dependence on medical treatment and monitoring to the extent that he cannot achieve any other life goals as a reasonable aim, so treatments which can only achieve this are in their view futile, and not therefore morally obligatory.

What, then, of treatment which would undoubtedly prolong life in a patient who had a very poor quality of life? An example might be the use of dialysis for renal failure in a quadriplegic.

There is no doubt that dialysis would prolong the life of the patient, and if this is what he wanted, and resources permitted, it is obviously entirely appropriate that it should be used. However, if the patient has already decided (or it has been decided on his behalf) that because his life was intolerable, being dead was better than being alive, is it necessary to wait for a cardiac arrest before implementing a DNR order, or does the decision not to resuscitate remove the need to provide dialysis?

Of course this leads us into a vicious spiral; if we are not obliged by our duty of beneficence to provide an expensive and invasive treatment such as dialysis for these patients, what about cheap and non-invasive therapy such as antibiotics? If we are not going to add therapies which will prolong life, what about procedures currently in place? Should we discontinue antibiotics if we are not going to dialyse? It is not far from here to the murky waters between killing and letting die (12). Rachels has argued persuasively that there is no difference (13), but it has to be accepted that doctors function within a framework of legal and social rules which go beyond the rules of their particular profession (14). In particular the action of killing someone is perceived generally as a crime in all circumstances where illogically an inaction which allows that person to die may not be strongly censured.

To use an example, if I see a patient with respiratory failure I may or may not put him on a ventilator. The appropriateness of my action will generally be judged in the light of all the circumstances, the patient's wishes, my skills in that particular technique, the facilities available and so on. If, however, I put a pillow over his face to suffocate him I would be regarded as having done wrong no matter what the circumstances.

There is an almost universal reluctance in the medical profession to countenance active killing except, at present, in The Netherlands, where there seems to be a tacit acceptance of euthanasia in certain situations. It is perhaps as well for the integrity of the medical profession that this is so. Even in The Netherlands doctors seem to have a reluctance to use methods of euthanasia which are immediately effective, such as barbiturates and muscle relaxants, preferring to use methods where death comes in hours rather than off the end of the needle.

Although consent to the non-introduction or withdrawal of treatment is of the greatest assistance to a doctor who has the courage to broach the subject with the patient, in many cases the patient will be incompetent. In that case, as with DNR orders, it is not necessary to take lack of consent as refusal, and it may be appropriate for the doctor to act paternalistically, taking all the relevant facts into consideration. At present almost one-fifth of deaths result from a non-treatment decision (15).

A particular difficulty is posed by the question of what to do about nutrition. Whereas the use of a ventilator or dialysis, or even the administration of antibiotics, is clearly a medical intervention, what of food and drink? Are these such basic requirements that they should be provided come what may, even if this involves tube-feeding, gastrostomy or even parenteral nutrition? The instinctive feeling is that nutrition is something so basic that it should be provided. The obvious risk is of seeming to prolong a life which can be of no value or an intolerable burden to the patient.

If we can deal in a logical manner with patients who find life an intolerable burden, where does that leave us with patients who may have every wish to go on living, but who need treatment beyond our resources?

If health care is regarded as a basic human right on a global scale, we are immediately in some difficulty, as it seems futile to talk of the use of treatments of limited efficacy and great expense while patients in Africa are dying of appendicitis. It is more comfortable, at least from a western perspective, to regard health care, although something we value highly, as something to be determined to a large extent by local economic activity. Therefore in a given country or region we have a parcel of resources (primarily cash but also people) which can be devoted to health care. The size of the parcel is a political decision; the doctor's problem is who gets what? (16,17) To try to cut the cake we have to try to decide what we want to achieve. Various goals might include avoidance of pain, avoidance of function-reducing disability and prolongation of life in a form acceptable to the liver. If we have effective interventions to achieve all these aims and we can afford them, fine. The problem is we haven't, and can't.

To be specific, there are a large number of conditions for which there is no effective treatment although they are seriously life-shortening, for instance AIDS, and treatments which, although apparently effective in achieving the aims, cannot be deployed on a wide enough scale in any society which has to look to its other priorities such as education and housing.

How then do we use what we have? What we are getting into here is a system of rationing. Hopefully this should not be a burden on individual practitioners working out their obligation to their patient within the limits imposed on them by external forces such as their employers or insurers, but rationing there must be. Rationing seems to appeal to the principle of justice. As expressed by Aristotle, this means that equals shall be treated equally and unequals unequally in proportion to the relevant differences. In health terms who are equals, what is equal treatment and what are relevant differences? Clear water, a safe environment and immunization against infectious diseases might be considered a basic ration for all, but beyond this health interventions are very needs-specific.

Perhaps a starting point is that all members of a given society are equal and no treatment should be available to one which is not available to all (18). While treatment is cheap and easy this is a persuasive argument, because it is only necessary to look at the 'up' side. In the UK everyone should be able to get a broken leg set or diabetes controlled. However, when treatments are expensive, difficult to apply or in some other way limited (say by a shortage of donor organs), a rigorous application of this rule would mean some people who might benefit from treatment not having it because not everyone could.

Therefore we must consider whether it is possible to construe some relevant differences between members of the group and construct sub-groups who could be treated differently on a just basis. This could be done, for instance, by identifying a group with greatest life-expectancy (the youngest) or with dependants on a benefit-maximizing basis (a utilitarian answer to a deontological problem). The most ill could be done first, on the basis of greatest need, although with some interventions such as heart transplants all potential recipients are gravely ill.

Some form of assessment of social worth could be used, but this form of assessment is notoriously subjective. Clearly age alone is not a relevant difference if the procedure offers only a limited survival for all patients, but for a curative procedure it may well be.

The range of possible medical interventions is vast, and few individuals are going to require more than a handful. How then is it possible to allocate a just proportion of resources to various aspects of treatment if it is not possible to do everything? Health economists, particularly Williams in the York group, adopt a utilitarian, benefit-maximizing approach. Their measure is the Quality Adjusted Life Year (19). They recognize that if prolonging life at all costs were the most appropriate health intervention we would devote all our efforts to increasingly arcane methods of staving off death, ventilating and dialysing the moribund whilst sacrificing treatments that had no effect on length or survival (indeed because of operative risk may have a negative net effect) but are devoted entirely to improving quality of life.

This does not seem to be what society desires, or indeed what happens in practice. In order to provide a comparison between different treatments, Williams has described the QALY, which is obtained by multiplying the years of survival (appropriately discounted) by a matrix-derived factor for quality of life. The treatments which should be undertaken are those which obtain most QALYs per unit of expenditure. Using the QALY system an intervention which produces perfect health for one year followed by death (score 1×1) would rate less well than one producing two years survival with moderate discomfort (score 2×0.9).

The matrix used in the QALY system recognizes that life may be a burden worse than death, so some states, such as survival, bedbound and in constant pain, rate negative scores. Any treatment which prolongs this state is automatically a worse buy than anything else, even heroic treatments with poor chance of survival. Of course the system is inherently paternalistic. Individual bedbound patients are not asked about their quality of life; the system makes generalizations.

The QALY system is ingenious, but is it ethically sound? While it stands up on a utilitarian basis, for the deontologist autonomy and beneficence seem to be ignored. All resources are allocated irrespective of individual patients. What of justice? If you are dying is the cost of your QALY a relevant difference, meaning that you might get a kidney transplant but not a heart transplant?

A difficulty in even contemplating a system of resource allocation based on QALYs is that, because medical treatment has grown in a serendipitous way, some therapies such as maintenance haemodialysis or aggressive surgery for certain cancers are a very poor buy but would be almost impossible to discontinue.

At an individual patient level it is very difficult for the clinician to use a value-for-money method of deciding treatment, particularly if the treatment is available in the hospital. For instance, if you have no dialysis facility (and no possibility of transferring the patient) his renal failure becomes of rather academic interest. If, however, you have the facility but are advised not to use it in a particular patient because for that particular patient the QALY score is too low (say because the patient is bedbound for another reason), the decision is much harder. In the critically ill the doctor may be much more focused on getting the patient to survive until tomorrow than taking the long view.

It is in the treatment of the critically ill, and in particular in intensive care units that the question of committing extensive resources to a single patient is most sharply drawn into focus. Intensive care is still a growth area of modern medicine. Patients often have multiple organs system failure, and whilst it is true that many patients survive who would have had no chance 30 years ago, in-unit mortality may be as high as 40% (depending on admission policy) and cost can be enormous. Typically a bed in an intensive care unit costs 10 times as much as a bed in a regular ward.

If anything, the resources expended on non-survivors are greater than those who survive. It is very tempting for the intensive care doctor to fall back on the position that his only ethical responsibility is to the patient he is treating here and now, and to deploy every drug and physiological intervention that is available in the hope that it may improve the outcome. He appeals to respect for life, beneficence and a doctor's duty to his patient to justify his position. However, even if resources are not severely limited at a given time they are finite, so if the doctor deploys them on some patients he may be denying them to others.

If the purpose of the exercise is to help patients survive (hopefully with a good-quality survival) who would not do so without the intensive care unit, rather than spending a lot of money in an interesting way, presumably it would be better to get more patients to survive.

If it is possible to identify patients who will certainly not survive whatever is done, treatment is obviously futile and therefore not morally obligatory. Resources could be redeployed from non-survivors to potential survivors. In addition it is not very dignified to be 'intensive cared' to a certain death, and while wanting every chance of survival it is quite possible that if most people were asked they would not want this. It is therefore perfectly acceptable to invoke non-maleficence, beneficence, respect for autonomy, justice and the whole hand of deontological principles in favour of not treating certain non-survivors. The problem is identifying them, preferably at as early a stage as possible. Here the work of Knaus *et al.* in Washington has given us a clue (20). Knaus and colleagues realized that it was impossible to compare the results achieved in intensive care units using the best therapy without knowing the severity of illness of the patient. A simple diagnosis such as multiple trauma was obviously of no help. He and his colleagues have devised scoring systems based on the degree of derangement of a number of physiological parameters, together with points for age and chronic health status, to produce a numerical APACHE Score (acute physiological and chronic health evaluation). This has been refined to a second and third version over the past few years. The higher the APACHE score the more ill the patient.

By amalgamating the results from a number of intensive care units in the USA Knaus *et al.* were able to establish a large database of patients and their scores. By looking at the outcomes of those patients who were having the best available therapy it was possible to predict the mortality rate for certain scores. If patients are certain to die whatever is done, should they be treated at all, beyond what is needed to make them comfortable? Initially it was suggested that the APACHE methodology was not applicable to individual patients, but as confidence in the database has grown it seems that it may be.

Chang, using a combination of absolute values of the score and the change over a period of time, was able to predict the deaths of 109 out of 831 intensive care patients with no false predictions. (Of the 722 whose predicted outcome was uncertain 181 others also died (21).)

Once the prediction of certain death has been made using this sort of method, it seems perfectly sensible to stop all treatment; the only exception being some new, experimental therapy which is additional to or different from established best therapy. The subject of not treating patients is a difficult one for any health professional. For resource allocation and the provision of certain categories of treatment it is easy enough to hide behind the politicians and economists, and hope that their methodology is sound, ethically justifiable and does not bear too hard on our particular special interest. Faced with the individual patient the decision is much more difficult. It is not possible to do everything for everybody and in some cases it may be wrong to do so.

We must temper our respect for life with considerations of respect for the patient's autonomy, beneficence and non-maleficence and justice, and hope that we can strive to reach an ethically tenable position in each case.

REFERENCES

1. Flagg, P. J. 1919. *The art of anaesthesia*, 2nd edn. J. B. Lippincott, Philadelphia.
2. Lee, J. A. 1947. *A synopsis of anaesthesia*. John Wright & Sons, Bristol.
3. Kouwenhoven, W. B., Jude, J. R. and Knickerbocker, G. G. 1960. Closed-chest cardiac massage. *Journal of the American Medical Association* **173**: 1064–1067.
4. Thomlinson, T. and Brody, H. 1988. Ethics and communication in do-not-resuscitate orders. *New England Journal of Medicine* **318**: 43–46.
5. Veatch, R. M. 1985. Editorial. Deciding against resuscitation, encouraging signs and potential dangers. *Journal of the American Medical Association* **253**: 77–78.
6. Youngner, S. J., Lewandowski, W., McClish, D. K., Juknialis, B. W., Coulton, C. and Bartlett, E. T. 1985. 'Do not resuscitate' orders. *Journal of the American Medical Association* **253**: 54–57.
7. Blackhall, L. J. 1987. Must we always use CPR? *New England Journal of Medicine* **317**: 1281–1285.
8. Bedell, S. E., Delbanco, T. L., Cook, E. F. and Epstein, F. H. 1983. Survival after cardiopulmonary resuscitation in the hospital. *New England Journal of Medicine* **309**: 569–576.
9. Jackson, D. L. and Youngner, S. 1979. Patient autonomy and 'death with dignity'. *New England Journal of Medicine* **301**: 404–408.
10. Charlson, M. E., Sax, F. L., Mackenzie, C. R., Fields, S. D., Braham, R. L. and Douglas, R. G., Jr. 1986. Resuscitation: how do we decide? *Journal of the American Medical Association* **255**: 1316–1322.
11. Schneiderman, L. J., Jecker, N. S. and Jonson, A. R. 1990. Medical futility: its meaning and ethical implications. *Annals of Internal Medicine* **112**: 949–953.
12. Editorial. 1984. *Journal of Medical Ethics* **2**: 59–60.
13. Rachels, J. 1975. Active and passive euthanasia. *New England Journal of Medicine* **292**: 78–80.
14. Kennedy, I. McC. 1976. The Karen Quinlan case: problems and proposals. *Journal of Medical Ethics* **2**: 3–7.
15. Van der Maas, P. J., Van Delden, J. M. M., Pijnenborg, L. and Looman, C. W. M. 1991. Euthanasia and other medical decisions concerning the end of life. *Lancet* **338**: 669–674.
16. Mooney, G. 1984. Medical ethics: an excuse for inefficiency. *Journal of Medical Ethics* **10**: 183–185.
17. Black, D. 1991. Paying for health. *Journal of Medical Ethics* **17**: 117–123.
18. Harris, J. 1985. *The value of life*. Routledge & Kegan Paul, London.
19. Williams, A. 1985. The value of QALYs. *Health and Social Services Journal*, 18 July, Centre 8 (a pullout insert in Supplement 3). (See also Chapter 71, this volume.)
20. Knaus, W. A., Draper, E. A., Wagner, D. P. and Zimmerman, J. E. 1985. APACHE II: A severity of disease classification. *Critical Care Medicine* **13**: 818–827.
21. Chang, R. W. S. 1989. Individual outcome prediction models for intensive care units. *Lancet* **2**: 143–146.

63

The Pause and the Principles

Grant Gillett

Bioethics Research Centre, Otago, New Zealand

In clinical practice it soon becomes evident that the ability to identify principles which bring order to the analysis of a problem in medical ethics is invaluable. Such principles capture and systematize insights about what matters to human beings, and they help us to think about the ethical conflicts in clinical care. The clarity brought to a problem by the principles is, however, no more than a way-station on the road to an adequate grasp of the practical medical ethics. In fact the most difficult problems in clinical ethics are often taxing precisely because they involve a *conflict* of principles. Thus, for instance, one struggles with the problem of defective neonates.

> Baby A was born with *spina bifida*. The spinal defect was at the thoracolumbar junction and was open. It was clear that baby A would never walk or achieve bladder control. In the first few days of life she also developed marked hydrocephalus with a thin cortical mantle and was, on this count likely to be quite badly mentally defective (although the doctors could not make a firm prognosis). Mr and Mrs A were quite clear on their wishes; they did not want to raise or have to watch the lifelong struggle of a child with severe mental and physical handicaps. Dr B agreed with them and was willing to give the baby comfort feeds only, without antisepsis or antibiotics for the spinal defect so as to allow a meningitis to develop. Dr C was indignant. He claimed that one could not harm a human being in this way, and that the proposed course of action was tantamount to child murder.

This case is challenging because it shows the strengths and weaknesses of two very different elements of moral judgements in medicine. Both doctors may well have acted according to the same principles. Let us say that Dr B thought *beneficence* required him to spare baby A a life of suffering, and *autonomy* required him to accede to the wishes of baby A's proper surrogate decision-makers—Mr and Mrs A. What is more, he claims that *justice* demands that we consider the opportunity costs of supporting baby A's unsatisfactory life because the health care system has many other worthy needs to meet. Dr C thought that beneficence required him to save baby A's life and that autonomy required that he protect baby A from those who would override the proper respect due to

Principles of Health Care Ethics. Edited by Raanan Gillon.
© 1994 John Wiley & Sons Ltd

her as an individual human being. He thought that justice would not allow us to disregard the life of one individual on the basis of the needs of others.

This conflict is clearly problematic and not easily resolved. The principles themselves have been part of its genesis. Higher-order principles such as *'autonomy always outweighs beneficence and justice'* neither command widespread agreement nor do they help us decide between the competing arguments. Therefore we need to discover some other means of engaging morally with the realities which are being conceptualized so that we can grasp them sufficiently clearly to make sound moral judgements. This need can be addressed by considering the related and somewhat neglected topics of *moral sense* and *moral judgement*. Nowhere are these more in evidence than when ethical decisions have to be made about hard cases arising in clinical medicine. Such cases give rise to what I have called *'the pause'*. I shall discuss this phenomenon and then spell out why I think it is a legitimate part of moral understanding (in two sections which are more of theoretical and philosophical interest than clinical use). I shall then return to a more practical discussion of clinical intuitions and their role in clinical ethics.

THE PAUSE

In many clinical situations life-and-death choices have to be made. These decisions are never easy but their moral weight is particularly evident where a clinician must, on the basis of careful judgement, take a decision which ends a human life. This often gives one pause; in fact, one could say (with apologies to T. S. Eliot), 'between the thought and the action comes *the pause'*. This pause does not influence a moral decision in either direction, but rather commends to the agent some deeper reflection on her decision and its moral content. It alerts one to the fact that the statable reasons and the ethical decision that results can fail to capture the moral reality that is involved. On reflection, it may emerge that one's moral reasoning and judgements have captured all that requires consideration; but in some situations there are features that are difficult to locate in a clearly premised argument or syllogism, yet which ought to influence our moral decision. I have argued that this is the case with many requests for euthanasia.

A doctor faced with a euthanasia request may well feel uncertain even though the patient's wishes and her own detached clinical judgement tell her that the future holds very little for him. I would argue that this pause is based on a sense that something important is at stake which may not have appeared in one's moral reasoning. In the case of euthanasia, for instance, it may point us towards unspoken psychological features of dying that can go unrecognized. The patient may have unmet needs (e.g. for pain relief or company) in his terminal care, or he may want reassurance that he is still valued although he feels himself to have become worthless, or he may be fearful of the future, short as it may be (1). The pause may also indicate an intuitive awareness of the dangers, for the doctor herself, of acting as both life-giver and death-bringer within the same *persona*. The sensitivity that gives rise to these worries and uncertainties, even if they are groundless in particular cases, is surely part of the moral structure of a person who can be trusted as a healer.

A sense of moral challenge or uncertainty is, in fact, all too common in real ethical dilemmas. It is not, however, universal. It tends to accompany life-and-death decisions in particular and to reflect an intuitive awareness of the importance of what is at stake. The weight that one's own clinical judgement must bear in such cases—for instance, in ceasing resuscitative efforts for a 22-year-old admitted with a devastating subarachnoid haemorrhage—is hard to bear. The moment of the decision makes one conscious of the frailty of the human mind which has made it. If, however, the decision is not so weighty, or if the reasoning is absolutely watertight, one's clinical intuitions rest easy with the ethical analysis and there is no pause. For instance, if a doctor were about to introduce a group of students to a patient when he realized that he had not gained the patient's consent for student teaching, he might still go ahead without hesitation (perhaps on the basis of a sketchy and very approximate utilitarian calculus). Here we may be uncertain about the values and variables that need to be considered but, because very little hangs on the decision, the pause is inappropriate. Imagine a different situation in which a child is being denied life-saving treatment because of some odd religious belief held by her parents. Again we are in no doubt about our response; the parents' right to decide is based on the presumption that they will act to safeguard the best interests of the child (according to reasonable or common-sense conceptions of best interests). Because their decision indicates that they have a different agenda and set of commitments from those we are prepared to accept as commensurate with the best interests of the child, we withdraw our moral deference to them and rest the power to make that decision in hands we regard as more reasonably informed. Here, I suggest, most clinicians would be in no doubt about their moral grounds and would act according to ethical principles without feeling the pause.

The pause seems to rest on a sense that there is something in a situation which may not have been taken into account, and that the decision is weighty. It indicates a significant conflict between intuition and argument. Our arguments may tell us one thing and apparently 'cover the field' in their consideration of morally relevant factors, but our intuitions tend in another direction so that we feel there is something we are missing, something which is being undervalued in the ethical analysis. But does this mean we are stuck with emotivism in medical ethics even though general ethics jettisoned it long ago? To explain why this is not so takes us a little further into the foundations of moral thinking.

MORAL CONCEPTS, MORAL SENSE AND MORAL JUDGEMENT

Moral concepts are the currency of moral reasoning. A typical moral syllogism is full of them.

1. Cruelty is wrong.
2. It is cruel to inflict gratuitous suffering on sentient beings.
3. That is a sentient being.

4. That suffering serves no defensible purpose and is therefore gratuitous.
5. Action A' which causes that suffering is cruel.
6. Action A' is wrong.

Notice that to apply concepts like 'cruel', 'suffering', 'sentient' we must recognize that certain states of affairs exhibit certain features evident to suitably equipped observers. Williams calls concepts like these 'thick' moral concepts because they have both factual and evaluative content inextricably mixed with them; 'the way these notions are applied is determined by what the world is like . . . and yet, at the same time, their application usually involves a certain valuation of the situation, of persons or actions'(2). (I shall return to the dual—recognitional and action-guiding—aspects of these judgements in due course.) To recognize these states and successfully conceptualize their features so that they can enter into our moral thought is a matter of judgement. In general, one judges that a thing is thus and so (i.e. instances a given concept), by learning the technique of picking out the conditions which ground the application of the concept being used. This takes practice. For instance, trainees in neurosurgery must learn to detect instances of the concept 'berry aneurysm' both in X-rays and in operating theatre if they are to master the techniques of detecting and treating aneurysmal haemorrhages in the brain. They learn to make the necessary judgements by being shown berry aneurysms (in X-rays and in operations) by their supervisors. After a certain amount of training, which imposes agreement in judgements (3), they become equipped not only to provide a definition of a berry aneurysm but also to pick 'the critters' out in practice.

How do we develop the ability to recognize those states of human beings which underpin moral concepts like cruelty, kindness, consideration, distress, and so on. Using these moral concepts clearly rests on our natural propensities to empathize with one another, to feel what another person feels, and their use is refined by experience. We learn that this is anger, this is pain, this is loneliness, and so on through our interactions with others, and through the discourse we share with them we articulate our sensitivities or intuitions concerning 'how it is' with human beings in certain situations. These meaningful judgements about 'how it is' with others are part of the attributions of cruelty, love, and so on that we come to learn. Thus empathy and the judgements it enables lead to a human being becoming engaged in the interpersonal and relational nexus which creates and signifies moral attributions. In this sense moral concepts and their understanding rest on intuitions.

A moral agent is formed by participation in this nexus of activity. And the moral formation of the agent runs very deep into the agent's mental life. Different kinds of interaction between the agent and others impinge upon *what matters* to one of the people involved, and are linked to moral attributions or clothed with moral significance; for instance, if I hit you that is not just an action I have done but also involves a *harm* or *hurt* that you have suffered and which has moral significance. Such exchanges and their components are *signified*— picked out and conceptualized by using signs—in our moral discourse. The content of these attributions—of harm, care, kindness, help, and so on is accessible on the basis of the empathy which underpins all interpersonal relationships (and indeed our learning of concepts in general) (4). That content depends on the many natural ways in which we find ourselves empathically moved by certain situations, and it is articulated by using the terms which form moral discourse. This articulation makes connections between the deeds and feelings signified and the ways one *ought* to act. The ability to apply moral concepts and then make these connections is the basis of moral reasoning.

We could define *moral sense* as the ability to apply and use moral concepts. Moral sense, on this view, enables one to recognize that certain morally important features are present in a situation but also involves a tendency to be moved by (feel the conative (will-involving) force of) these perceptions. Both aspects of moral sense—the ability to see that certain conditions (empathically grasped) ground morally relevant ascriptions to other creatures and the tendency to feel imperatives to act thus and so (i.e. to be moved to action) are essential to moral thought. Two examples can be used to show that if one lacked either capacity, one would not know what one was talking about in moral discourse.

> Ernst has been reprimanded on several occasions for hurting others. He is found having tied up his small cousin and, despite the pleading and evident distress of the little girl, is burning her feet with a live coal. When he is taken to task he admits freely that it is wrong to be cruel to others and that cruelty involves making others suffer gratuitous pain or distress, but denies that he was aware of this being the case with his little victim.

It is almost impossible to know what to say about Ernst. One is inclined to think that there is some deep disturbance in his psyche. I would argue that we believe this because the recognition that others are hurt or suffering in various ways seems so basic to human thought and behaviour. In fact, if we regard mental ascriptions as having shared and communicable meaning then, as Strawson has noted, the ascription to self is necessarily linked to ascriptions to others (5,6). Thus, as long as we recognize that statements such as 'He is in pain' and 'I am in pain' essentially involve a common shared concept—here 'pain'—then it becomes an *a priori* truth that we can and do appreciate the grounds on which such statements are made about self and others (7). Thus there is a deep incoherence between Ernst's claims and the rationally structured attributions we feel we ought to make to any human subject.

A complementary example concerns the practical or conative role of morally relevant ascriptions.

> Freda is sitting in the same room as her father who is gasping and tearing at a string net which is strangling him. When asked about her apparent indifference, Freda answers that she is well aware that her father is suffering, she knows that he might die, she knows that in general one ought to help others in need if one can, but is unable to connect these thoughts in such a way as to be moved to act by her father's plight.

This, again, is a deeply puzzling situation. One tends to regard the 'being moved' or conative aspect of the thoughts Freda avows as inseparable from a proper understanding of them. We feel compelled to invoke a hidden agenda

('She hates her father and wishes him dead') or a mental defect ('She is demented or mentally impaired') rather than accept her words as a sincere statement by an intact human agent. This is, again, best explained by the fact that the conative role or force in practical reasoning of morally relevant ascriptions (such as 'suffering', 'need', or 'help') is part of one's understanding of them.

It appears, then, that we can jettison neither the idea that understanding moral concepts involves the ability to judge that others are in need, nor the idea that such understanding in a particular case moves one (defeasibly—in that one may choose not to) to act. The best explanation for these features of moral concepts derives from the fact that we learn moral judgements through interactions with other human beings on the basis of natural empathy.

This last point uncovers another foundation of our moral attitudes to human beings. Our empathy for each other suggests that there are certain ways of living that are not worthwhile. Most people express this by remarks like 'He would never want to be left like a vegetable' or 'Don't ever let me get like that!'. Such remarks indicate a widespread sense that there is a level of function below which a human life is not worth living. This is such a widely shared intuition that, absent any implication that one might actively terminate life (and therefore violate 'sanctity of life' dogmas), most people admit that, at a certain point in the decline of function caused by disease, it is better to 'let nature take its course'.

These aspects of our moral psychology must, however, be related to moral justification or principled judgement. How do intuitions become incorporated into moral reasoning?

MORE THEORY: MORAL JUSTIFICATION AND REASONING

Justification is the process of demonstrating consistency with commitments underpinning an area of thought. Thus one justifies a truth claim for a logical statement through logical analysis and the principle of non-contradiction. A different set of basic commitments underpins scientific justification. Scientific analysis relates sets of observations to a theoretical base which might change over time or with paradigm shifts in scientific discourse but, in general, commands convergence in its methods of reasoning. We therefore need to ask how moral reasoning can accommodate the 'moral sentiments' that seem to underpin it.

Recall that concept-using beings make moral judgements such as 'that is cruel', the content of which has an implicit conative force in that it moves us to commend certain types of conduct and condemn others. And this content can (indeed *must* if the link between self- and other-ascription holds good), to some extent, be grasped by those 'who participate to any degree in human relationships or experiences with others requiring some interaction or response' (8). Moral content informs our conception of right conduct and concerns the moral phenomenology of a given experience—what it is like to be in various subjective positions within that experience and how those perspectives are clothed by moral discourse so that they mesh with our moral reasoning. The appreciation of these aspects of a situation constitutes the facts on which an ethical decision is made.

One of the most basic features of moral sense is the ability to recognize that another creature is a *morally significant being*, and therefore that certain things *matter* to it and are morally relevant. It is obviously futile to reason about many of the things that happen to a being to whom nothing matters. Thus a failure of moral sense at this basic level gets moral reasoning off on the wrong foot. But our moral sense also picks up the threads of a problem when we are trying to appreciate what matters to another person.

In moral reasoning we have to choose a resolution of the problem that respects the moral realities. These realities concern the feelings and vulnerabilities of the human beings affected by the decisions taken. To reason about them we have first to register what they are, then conceptualize them in ways that do them justice and finally we have to resolve the problem in the way that pays best regard to any conflicts inherent within it.

> Consider Greg, a 21-year-old patient who is half-way through a difficult course of adjuvant therapy for a recurrent cancer. He is feeling tired, unwell and nauseated. He is sick of being in hospital and of losing his hair. He knows that the treatment is going well but one day announces that he has had enough. We ask whether we are morally justified in persuading him to continue (according to the principle of beneficence) or whether we should abide by his decision in the name of autonomy? Here we must weigh and balance principles so as to produce a reasonable response to his need.

A resolution of this situation requires moral reasoning of a more real kind than any carefully constructed syllogistic problem. It requires, among other things, an assessment of Greg's autonomy in the light of his current experience. We cannot just accept a bald statement of his opinion without asking whether it really does reflect what he would want if he were able to make the best judgement of his own situation. This will colour one's presentation of the options that are open to him because that will have a marked effect on his perception of them. His personal response to his crisis is likely to emerge from his present physical and psychological state and his reaction to how we and others relate to him. To decide on a course of action and advice which enables the patient to respond in a way that really meets his needs in a situation like this calls for both sensitivity and wisdom. And the process of 'mapping' a concrete situation on to the basic principles—of autonomy, beneficence, non-maleficence and justice—is part of reasoned clinical ethics. Therefore it is impossible to separate moral sense and moral judgement from the process of justifying moral decisions.

Moral sense and moral judgement enable one to discern, for instance, when 'the cake is worth the candle', whether the patient can exercise significant autonomy, how much moral weight to put on different probabilities or outcomes, when we have a person to deal with and when we do not, and these are all essential to well-grounded moral reasoning. The best analogy to the wisdom or skills that arise with moral sense is the knowledge of when and where and how to use techniques such as finding the square root or the highest common factor in mathematical problem-solving. Absent such techniques, the reasoning involved cannot find its way about in real situations.

A POTTED VERSION OF THE MORAL THEORY

1. Moral reasoning involves moral concepts.
2. Moral concepts rest on judgements that things are thus and so, and that one ought to do something about those things.
3. The sensitivity and skills of judgement or intuitions which ground moral concepts underpin the ability to make reasoned responses to real ethical problems.
4. Moral reasoning is predicated on developed moral intuitions.

This suggests that, when we turn to those real situations involved in medical ethics, clinical judgement and experience and therefore clinical intuitions may be important.

CLINICAL INTUITIONS AND MEDICAL ETHICS

Clinical intuitions are developed over the course of a clinical life. They give one a sense of the right direction to head in investigating a clinical problem, and the weights to put on different aspects of a situation when medical decisions must be made. The ability to do this well is called 'clinical acumen' and it is a special case of the practical wisdom that Aristotle holds to be a general characteristic of ethical behaviour; 'not knowing that dispositions are attained through actually doing things is the sign of a complete ignoramus' (9). The reflective clinician incorporates in his clinical wisdom a sense of the applicability and aptness of certain ethical considerations in any given situation. Thus clinical experience not only leads to practical medical wisdom but can also give rise to ethical wisdom if the clinician is open and sensitive to the personal and moral issues at stake in her practice. In fact, if (after Aristotle) practical wisdom is the ability to assess a situation and act well in the light of that assessment we would expect the skills of assessment and management that inform clinical acumen to be very useful in ethical analysis. The opinion of a wise or practised clinical agent, for instance, may be of great help in those life-and-death situations where the pause is evident. Faced by the enthusiastic interventionalism of juniors in an elderly patient with a devastating illness she might remark: 'I don't think Mrs H would want to go through all that'. She could probably follow this with a discussion of the burdens of treatment and the poor probabilities of good outcome that would make her decision look to be the only reasonable one in the circumstances. We should always remember that an interventional decision is a decision to harm and ought only to be undertaken when the patient stands to gain some *substantial benefit*. The difficulty is that we need to be careful about whose notion of benefit is in play.

To overcome this problem and, indeed, clarify our thinking about such decisions, we can define substantial benefit as '*An outcome which now or in the future the patient would regard as worthwhile'* (10). This definition is very interesting. It is patient-centred but will often require imaginative identification with or empathy for the patient in order to guide us properly in our dealings with the patient. The ethical reasoning in a case tries to capture our awareness of this basic reality but often does so quite inadequately. The experienced and sensitive clinician tends to get it right because she has been 'through the hoops' with many patients, and therefore the insight that shines through her comments reflects accumulated practical wisdom. Her discussion should show that she is a competent judge of the situation because it should show her to appreciate the moral issues at stake, act with recognizable and endorsable moral sensitivities, and be sincere (11). These features, which characterize the response of a moral agent with integrity, emphasize that clinical intuitions are complementary to and consonant with informed ethical discussion because each of them is 'filled out' or given substance by cumulative experience of clinical cases.

In the example with which we began, two doctors were arguing over the fate of baby A. They completely disagreed even though both appealed to the same principles to justify his stand. A person of sound clinical intuitions and wisdom would bring certain perceptions to bear on the ethical problem. She would have a sense of the type of outcome to be expected in baby A and the type of costs, in terms of pain and suffering, that those outcomes would require. All these considerations tend to be based on a multitude of inconclusive indicators and are not easily fitted into calculi with specifiable components (this is, in fact, the kind of judgement that human beings are good at but computers are not (12)). She would have a sense of what a person would go through in having the necessary interventions and the likelihood that they would lead to further interventions and/or complications which would not only prejudice the outcome in the case but also have their own 'knock-on' costs to the patient and his relatives. She would see hope where that was justified, and get a sense that things were going irredeemably wrong when that was the case. She would be able to make a judgement of the type 'You can't win Monopoly on Whitechapel and Old Kent Road' when that was indicated. In fact, one repeatedly has to make this type of judgement in neonatal intensive care situations and many others where the pause is prominent. This and the many other considered and balanced judgements that go into applying the principles aright in clinical life are consistent with, but not given by, the principles. They can be made only on the basis of clinical experience and intuitions, and they amount to a kind of practical wisdom which, in Greek thought, was the essence of ethical conduct. In fact, at least one moral philosopher has recognized the need for philosophical analysis to pay regard to applied experience and remarks: 'Such willingness to learn, to become less of an intellectual judge and more of an apprentice participant, is to be found among contemporary moral philosophers less in the theorists than in those who *have* become associates of the non-philosophers, in other professions' (13).

CONCLUSION

The pause, I have argued, is the phenomenological marker of moral sense and should alert us to a moral challenge inherent in an ethical dilemma. That challenge may, of course, have been met quite adequately by the ethical discussion in a given case. But the pause is felt most acutely when the ethical challenges are not fully captured by the discussion that has occurred. When this happens we may need to dig a little deeper, to range beyond the narrow terms of moral debate that we have defined for ourselves and to seek new insights. A valuable source of these insights are those who have lived reflectively through clinical problems and have, thereby, accumulated a store of medical and ethical wisdom which is relevant to the principled resolution of difficult problems. Therefore, when a sensitive appreciation of what is at stake is the key to informed ethical debate we draw equally on an understanding of certain principles and a developed moral sense.

This implies that the tendency to feel the pause, which I have claimed is an indicator of an informed moral sense, is indispensable in moral reasoning. Moral sense tells us what it is that moral concepts are actually about, and therefore why ethical principles matter. Indeed, it would be fair to say that the principles are given content by moral sense. But moral sense also enters the picture when the principles are weighed and balanced so as to arrive at a moral judgement in a particular situation. Such a judgement rests on our sense of what is at stake, and how it is with the human beings enmeshed in a situation. In clinical situations this understanding, which is the result of thinking and acting in accordance with moral sense, gives rise to clinical intuitions. These intuitions are central in the ethical analysis of clinical problems because they reveal the moral realities with which we are dealing.

I will therefore, yet again, adapt a saying of Kant's and remark that *the pause without the principles is blind and the principles without the pause are empty.*

REFERENCES

1. Gillett, G. 1988. Euthanasia, the pause and letting die. *Journal of Medical Ethics* **14**: 61–68.
2. Williams, B. 1984. *Ethics and the limits of philosophy*, pp. 129ff. Fontana, London, pp. 129ff.
3. Wittgenstein, L. 1953. *Philosophical investigations*. Blackwell, Oxford, no. 242.
4. Gillett, G. 1987. Concepts, structures and meanings. *Inquiry* **30**: 101–112.
5. Strawson, P. 1959. *Individuals*, p. 99. Methuen, London.
6. Gillett, G. 1992. *Representation, meaning and thought*. Oxford University Press, Oxford.
7. Gillett, G. 1991. The neurophilosophy of pain. *Philosophy* **66**: 191–206.
8. Mason, J. K. and Meyers, D. W. 1986. Parenteral choice and selective treatment of deformed newborns: a view from mid-Atlantic. *Journal of Medical Ethics* **12**: 67–71.
9. Aristotle, *Nicomachean ethics* (ed. R. Bambrough, 1963) New American Library, New York Bk III.5, p. 324.
10. Campbell, A., Gillett, G. and Jones, G. 1992. *Practical medical ethics*. Oxford University Press, Auckland (In press).
11. Gillett, G. 1989. Informed consent and moral integrity. *Journal of Medical Ethics* **15**: 117–123.
12. Gillett, G. 1982. Representations and cognitive science. *Inquiry* **32**: 261–276.
13. Baier, A. 1985. *Postures of the mind*, p. 238. Methuen, London.

64

In Favour of Voluntary Euthanasia*

PATRICK NOWELL-SMITH

Honorary Vice-President, Voluntary Euthanasia Society, and Past President, World Federation of Right-to-Die Societies

The word 'euthanasia' literally means a good death, and is nowadays used to mean a serene and peaceful death, the kind of death we would wish for ourselves and others. In many cases such a death occurs naturally; but very often it does not, so that the word has come to be used solely for the act of bringing about such a death when it does not occur naturally. When death is brought about by an action, such as the injection of a lethal dose, it is called 'active'; when it is brought about by inaction, such as non-resuscitation after cardiac arrest, it is called 'passive'. This distinction has played a large part in discussions of the subject, though as we shall see its importance has been greatly exaggerated.

Euthanasia is called 'voluntary' when it is administered to people who have requested it or given their informed consent. As this chapter is about voluntary euthanasia it will not discuss important questions about the proper treatment of newborn babies, very young children, and older children and adults who are for one reason or another unable to express their wishes. Still less will there be any discussion of the objections raised by those in whose minds euthanasia is associated with Nazi atrocities. They are irrelevant because their victims did not choose to be killed.

'When a person has a distressing and painful terminal disease, do you think doctors should or should not be allowed by law to end the patient's life if there is no hope of recovery and the patient requests it?' When this question was put by the Roper Organization of New York in 1988 58% of the replies were 'Yes' and 27% were 'No' (1). In Canada, Great Britain, France, and Holland the proportion of 'Yes' answers to similar questions has been consistently over 70%

---

* This chapter includes material from an article written by the author called 'the right to die', first read at the ICUS conference in 1986. Reproduced by permission of the International Conference on the Unity of the Sciences.

Principles of Health Care Ethics. Edited by Raanan Gillon.

in recent years. Before 1935 when the first Voluntary Euthanasia Society was formed in London such a question had been rarely, if ever, asked. Before confronting the moral and legal issues it is important to understand why the topic of euthanasia should have become so frequently discussed, and why support for euthanasia has so dramatically grown.

In the distant past most people who escaped the diseases of childhood and violent death died either peacefully or from such diseases as plague, cholera, typhus, smallpox, tuberculosis or pneumonia. By 1935 all these except the last had been virtually eliminated in western societies. Pneumonia was known as the 'dying man's friend' because it brought release to people who thought their lives no longer worth living. The first of the antibiotics by which pneumonia is now controlled came on the scene in the thirties, and the most common causes of premature death today are heart diseases, stroke, cancer, and the various degenerative diseases. Death from these causes can hardly be described as serene and peaceful.

Apart from its role in the prevention and cure of diseases, medical science and technology have enormously increased our power to keep people in a purely biological sense 'alive' almost indefinitely whether they like it or not. Sometimes these people are conscious and suffering; sometimes they are irreversibly unconscious as a result of which they have no thought, no feeling, no possibility of human communication. The best known case is that of Karen Quinlan who became unconscious in 1975 and died well after a court permitted her life-support systems to be removed 10 years later. In England the best known case is of Tony Bland, who went into persistent vegetative state in 1989 and whose artificial feeding and hydration were withdrawn in 1993 after the House of Lords ruled such withdrawal to be 'not unlawful'.

The social changes that our society has undergone since the Second World War, though less often mentioned than the technological, are at least as important for the purpose of explaining the increased interest in euthanasia. A good death is most likely to be experienced by people who die in their own familiar homes where they can enjoy the support of family, friends, and neighbours. There are two reasons why such a death is much less frequent than it used to be. Patterns of family loyalty have changed and children often live far from their parents and cannot often visit them when they are dying. Moreover, because the main causes of death are what they are, three-quarters of us will die not in our own homes, but in a hospital or old people's home where conditions are often cheerless and sometimes horrendous.

The second reason why growing anxiety about what is in store for them has led to an increased demand for euthanasia is connected with the distinction between active and passive. In the days when most people died at home active euthanasia was regarded by many doctors as good medical practice. The doctor would sign the death certificate as due to natural causes, and unless there were serious grounds for suspicion the certificate would not be questioned. We do not know how widespread the practice was because, then as now, active euthanasia was treated by the law as murder and doctors would naturally keep quiet about it. In 1936, when the Voluntary Euthanasia Society presented its first bill to legalize the practice into the House of Lords, the royal doctor, Lord

Dawson, spoke against the bill on the grounds that 'good doctors do it anyway'. But now, in an institutional setting, active euthanasia cannot be administered without the knowledge of colleagues and paramedics. So doctors have to be more cautious.

THE MORAL CASE FOR VOLUNTARY EUTHANASIA

Discussion of the moral issues is complicated by the fact that the law in Britain treats active euthanasia as murder and, except in Scotland, makes assisting suicide a crime carrying a penalty of up to 14 years in prison. So, for the moment, let us imagine that no such laws existed. Is it morally permissible for a doctor to administer euthanasia in the circumstances envisaged by the Roper Poll? For centuries the fundamental principle of medical ethics has been the principle of beneficence: doctors should always act in the best interests of their patients. So what should the doctor do in the following typical case?

> A woman is dying of terminal cancer of the throat. She is no longer able to take food and fluids by mouth and is suffering considerable distress. She would be able to live for a few more weeks if medical feeding by way of a nasogastric tube were continued. However, the woman does not want the extra two or three weeks of life because life has become a burden which she no longer wishes to bear. She asks the doctor to help her die. The doctor agrees to discontinue medical feeding, removes the nasogastric tube, and the woman dies a few days later (ref. 2, p. 611).

There are three things the doctor in this story could do. First, he could continue the nasogastric feeding, if necessary by force; secondly, he could, as he actually did in the story, discontinue the feeding and keep the woman comfortable until she died of the cancer, or he could agree to the woman's request and end her life then and there. The first course is immediately ruled out by the principle of beneficence, though some doctors in the past used to take it. The second course is passive euthanasia. Since 1967 the hospice movement has championed the idea that people who are dying without any hope of recovery should be recognized as such. While it is morally wrong to shorten their lives, no attempt should be made to prolong them; they should simply be kept physically and mentally as comfortable as possible. 'The usual practice in the UK is to employ the minimum of measures necessary to make the patient comfortable and not to worry if some of these measures ... shorten the dying process through respiratory repression or malnutrition' (3). Our question, however, is not about what current practice is but about what it ought to be, and since the two or three weeks of life left to the woman if the doctor chooses the second option will be spent either in pain or under heavy sedation, the principle of beneficence requires the doctor to choose active euthanasia. Their medical training has given doctors a competence in diagnosis and in predicting the likely outcome of different kinds of treatment which the average patient lacks. But does this competence extend to knowing what is in the patient's best interests? The concept of 'best interests' is not an easy one, but the United States President's Commission for the study of ethical problems in medicine and biomedical and behavioural research did attempt to spell it out. 'All patients', it said, 'have an interest in well-being and in addition to this, normal adult or competent patients also have an interest in self-determination . . . in the capacity to form, revise and pursue his or her plans for life' (ref. 2, p. 612).

Given the emphasis which the Commission puts on self-determination as an ingredient in a person's best interests, an emphasis with which few people in this country would disagree, it is clear that the principle of autonomy also points to active euthanasia as the appropriate course for the doctor to take. What is surprising is that the Commission came to the quite different conclusion that patients should be *allowed to die* when, from their point of view, life has become an intolerable burden.

So far we have only heard one side of the case; so we must now consider what reasons there might be for denying a person's moral right to active euthanasia.

1. *Playing God.* It is said that only God has a right to determine the time and manner of a person's death; but this is really a most extraordinary argument. For if we took it seriously we should have to say that no doctor has a right to try to prevent the death of a person whose life he could save!

2. *The sanctity of life.* The idea that no human life should be taken because all human life is sacred is also religious in origin, since it comes from the idea that life is a gift from God. In this form people who have no religious belief can only agree to differ, but many of them do hold that there is something special about human life for which 'sacred' is not a bad name. But without its religious background sacredness is a rather vague concept. Precisely what is involved in treating other people's lives as sacred? In a discussion of voluntary euthanasia we have to consider only competent persons, and the idea that their lives are sacred must at least include the idea that their interests and requests should be treated with respect. If so, the argument from the sanctity of life, used by itself, is ineffective; for to refuse their requests when there are no other good reasons for refusing is surely not to treat them with respect.

3. *The slippery slope.* People who advance the sanctity of life argument may well do so because they believe that if once we treat all human life as less than sacred we take the first step down a moral slippery slope that may lead to clearly unacceptable consequences. This is a type of argument that has frequently been used against changes in the moral climate of our society and changes in the law. In most cases the fear has proved groundless, and it seems to be groundless in this case also. In this case the fear is that 'assisting death on patients' requests might lead to a slide down a moral slippery slope towards unrequested ending of the lives of unconscious, demented, or mentally handicapped patients. Such a moral slide seems improbable. Except in cases of irreversible unconsciousness, . . . disapproval of involuntary termination of patients' lives is strongly entrenched in the concepts of most doctors and laymen' (4).

4. *Erosion of trust.* It has been argued that patients would not trust a doctor who is known to practise active euthanasia. This objection misses the point that what is at issue is *voluntary* euthanasia. There is no question of doctors being

allowed to administer euthanasia to patients without their knowledge and consent, and it is much more likely that the open practice of voluntary euthanasia would actually increase patients' trust in their doctors. 'At present many patients fear that their doctors, using modern technology, may prolong their lives against their wishes. This may erode their trust as much as any fear that their doctors might end patients' lives without being asked to do so' (4).

5. *Pressure on the elderly.* The most serious objection to voluntary euthanasia is that it might not in all cases really be voluntary. Subtle pressures to sign their own death warrants might be put on old people by greedy heirs, and even if there is not much to inherit, the care of an old person day after day, perhaps for many years, is a burden which many people might find intolerable. This objection does not claim that euthanasia itself is morally unacceptable, but it shows that moral wrong-doing is likely to occur, even if only rarely, if it were made legal. Any revised law must be hedged about by sufficient safeguards to prevent this abuse.

THE CASE FOR LEGISLATION

In the United Kingdom and in all broadly similar countries active euthanasia is treated by the law as murder because the intention of the agent is to kill. In most countries it makes no difference at the trial stage if the motive for killing was compassion, though the motive becomes important when it comes to sentencing. Until very recently this was the case in the United Kingdom also, but under our present law, if a person is guilty of murder the judge has no option but to impose a sentence of life imprisonment. As we shall see this can lead to great injustice, and there are grounds for hoping that this law will be repealed so that UK practice can return to that of other civilized countries.

When Section 1 of the Suicide Act (1961) abolished the crime of suicide, assisting suicide automatically ceased to be criminal, leaving a gap which needed to be filled. It would be all too easy to commit a murder, for example by drugging the victim's drink, and then to escape punishment by claiming that this was done at the victim's request. For since the victim himself raised the glass to his lips the death was a suicide and no crime had been committed. To prevent this, Section 2 of the Act made assisting suicide a crime.

If a doctor prescribes an analgesic drug at a sufficient strength to control the patient's pain, even though he knows very well that the patient will shortly die, he does not commit murder because his intention is not to kill the patient but to relieve the pain. The same is true if he orders non-resuscitation after cardiac arrest because his intention is to prevent further suffering. So these and other forms of passive euthanasia are not murder and, indeed, are not crimes at all provided that the doctor has conformed to standards of good medical practice set, not by the law, but by the medical fraternity. To many people the distinction between intending to kill someone and doing something that you know will kill him seems to be a distinction without a difference.

So much for the law as it stands on paper. Opponents of legal reform argue that its apparent harshness towards mercy killers, medical and lay, is an illusion. 'Our legal system', said the Law Reform Commission of Canada, 'has internal mechanisms which offset the apparent harshness of the law. It is possible that in some circumstances the accused would be allowed to plead guilty to a lesser charge ... Finally in truly exceptional circumstances, the authorities have it within their discretion not to prosecute' (5). All this is as true in Britain as it is in Canada. Only five doctors have been prosecuted for mercy killing in England since the beginning of this century (6,7), and in 1992 Dr Nigel Cox received a suspended sentence of one year on conviction for attempted murder (7); and although there are about a dozen cases of mercy killing by lay people every year reported in the media these cases are usually treated with great leniency. An unknown but probably large number of mercy killings by doctors and lay people go unreported either because no suspicion arises or because the authorities decide not to prosecute.

In non-medical cases the mercy killer is almost always a spouse or very near relation. A typical case is that of Phillipa Monaghan who gave up her job in London and took her children to Wales so that she could look after her mother who was dying of motor neurone disease. After many urgent pleas from her mother for release Mrs Monaghan gave her sleeping pills, smothered her with a pillow and told the police what she had done. When she pleaded guilty to attempted murder, the trial judge said: 'I am not going to send you to prison. I think you've suffered enough. You're obviously a caring and loving person. You did what you did because you couldn't bear to see your mother suffering. She wanted to die and brought great emotional pressure on you to help her terminate her life.' Mrs Monaghan was placed on probation for two years which, in the circumstances, was tantamount to an absolute discharge (8).

The idea that we need not worry about the harshness of the law on paper because the law in action is more lenient is tempting, but fallacious. The circumstances in which people ask for help in dying are even today not 'truly exceptional', and as the population ages and the power of medical technology increases they are likely to become even more common. It is cold comfort indeed for doctors to be told that if they do what their patients ask they *may* not be prosecuted, and that even if they are, they *may* not suffer any penalty. And it is cold comfort for people who want medical help in dying to tell them that they must find a doctor who is prepared to break the law and to risk prosecution.

The case of Mr Anthony Cocker (9) was from a moral point of view exactly like that of Mrs Monaghan except for the fact that it was his wife whom he smothered. Since the principle of justice requires that like cases be treated alike he should have been treated as Mrs Monaghan was. Unlike her, however, he had pleaded guilty to murder and a technicality in the law required the judge to sentence him to life imprisonment. In such cases the Home Secretary can exercise the royal prerogative of mercy to quash or reduce the sentence. But the process is a slow one, and Mr Cocker spent almost four years in prison for his compassionate crime.

ASSISTING SUICIDE

Suicide is no longer a crime, and it is right that people who want to commit suicide because they are temporarily depressed should not be allowed assistance. But many people want to end their lives because they see no end to an existence which has become intolerable to them, and they want to use a method as little distressing as possible to their survivors. The most common methods used to be the gas oven and a combination of alcohol and barbiturates. But since natural gas replaced coal gas, and barbiturates have been replaced by less lethal soporifics, these methods are no longer available. Between 1975 and 1986 the rate of suicide by self-poisoning in the United Kingdom fell by about 30% (10). A technique much recommended and much used today is to take a sufficient dose of sleeping pills and then to have a plastic bag tied over the head in case the pills alone prove ineffective.

In December 1984 an 84-year-old lady who had many reasons for ending her life decided to commit suicide by taking an overdose of barbiturates. This she had a legal right to do, but fearing that the attempt might not be successful, and that she would wake up in worse shape than before, she asked a friend, Mrs Charlotte Hough, to sit with her and to put a plastic bag over her head when she had fallen asleep. Mrs Hough did what she was asked and told the police what she had done. She was initially charged with murder, but because it was uncertain whether the death was due to the drug or to the plastic bag, she was charged with attempted murder. On pleading guilty she was sentenced to nine months imprisonment. The judge said that although he had great sympathy for Mrs Hough a prison sentence was necessary to uphold the law. On this *The Sunday Times* commented:

> Mrs Hough's crime was compassion and it served to underline once more the need for better legislation governing voluntary euthanasia and the dangers of being without it. People should be allowed to die on their own terms and, as Barbara Wootton once wrote, 'not on those of nature's cruelty or doctors' ingenuity' (11).

Is it just that Mrs Hough should have been sent to prison when many others who did what she did were not? Suicide, if it is not to be committed in gruesome ways that most of us would wish to avoid, is a lonely business, and most people would like to be comforted in their last moments by the presence of a relative or friend. By forbidding this our present law offends against the principle of benevolence.

ACTIVE AND PASSIVE

There is certainly a difference between killing and letting die, between the injection of a lethal dose and the withholding of a life-support system. But is there always a significant moral difference which the law rightly marks by treating the one as murder and the other as in some cases good medical practice? Until recently most people have assumed that there is. 'Thou shalt not kill', wrote the Victorian poet Arthur Hugh Clough, 'but needst not strive officiously to keep alive.' In spite of the fact that the Roper Poll showed that 60% of the people polled who were affiliated to a religious body were in favour of active euthanasia, most religious leaders still condemn it while supporting passive euthanasia.

But the idea that there is always a great *moral* difference between killing and letting die, and that it is always in favour of letting die, is wholly fallacious. Is a parent who locks a child in a cupboard until he starves morally better than one who strangles a child? And whatever the law may say, the plain man does not regard mercy killing as murder and realizes that, as in the case of the woman dying from cancer of the throat, killing is often better than letting die.

Medical opinion appears to be divided. In its 1984 *Handbook of medical ethics* the BMA said that 'the profession condemns legalized active euthanasia' (12). The report of its 1988 working party is less downright but still argues against it, mainly on the grounds that it 'goes against the intuitions . . . of most medical and nursing personnel', 'is at variance with all their training and inclinations' and 'runs counter to settled and informed medical opinion' (13). The present writer has examined these arguments and found them insufficient (14).

The BMA's view of current medical opinion in Britain is not backed by any evidence, and runs counter to such evidence as there is. A poll of general practitioners taken by NOP Market Research Ltd in 1987 asked the following question: 'At the moment euthanasia is illegal. Suppose the law was changed to permit voluntary euthanasia and there was a patient on your list, whose case you knew well, who suffered from an incurable physical illness that was intolerable to them. If that patient made a signed request that you end his/her life would you consider doing so or not?' Thirty-five per cent of GPs polled said that they would definitely consider it, and a further 10% said that they might possibly do so. This is a substantial minority, and it shows that the BMA's view that euthanasia is condemned by the profession as a whole is exaggerated (15).

A working party set up by the Institute of Medical Ethics in 1989 went further. 'The majority view of the IME working party may be formulated as follows. A doctor, acting in good conscience, is ethically justified in assisting death if the need to relieve intense and unceasing pain or distress caused by an incurable illness greatly outweighs the benefit to the patient of further prolonging his life' (16). The dramatic stories reported in the media always involve painful and incurable diseases, and it is often said that since pain can be controlled active euthanasia is not necessary. The IME's working party did well to mention distress as well as pain. Paralysis, incontinence, and dyspnoea are not, in the strict sense, painful, but they can cause intense distress. So, above all, does loss of dignity, independence, and autonomy.

The authors of the IME working party report may, perhaps, be criticized for not going far enough. Why should the availability of euthanasia be limited to people suffering from a terminal and incurable disease? Why not extend it to people who, although not suffering from such a disease, already find their condition intensely distressing, and who know that because they will not be getting any younger there is no remedy for this condition except death? Perhaps they did not consider such cases because, as doctors, they are reluctant to accept the layman's idea that such people are simply 'dying of old age'. Perhaps they wanted to limit their proposals to what seems at present politically possible.

But the extension deserves to be considered since it plays a large part in the motivation of people who join voluntary euthanasia societies.

The present writer is convinced that this is true from his experience on the committees of voluntary euthanasia societies in two countries. Here is a letter typical of many written to *Dying With Dignity* in Canada.

> I am seventy-nine years of age in relatively vigorous health and constantly amused with life while it lasts. But I saw my father and my mother, years apart, in the same chronic care hospital suffering helplessly for months when they might have been quietly released; and this makes me dread a similar fate unless the law is changed so that one can choose, if still able, to slip away in dignity from the inhumane methods many hospitals employ today to keep one from dying a natural death.

In all cases in which a doctor has to make a decision as to how to treat a patient whose life is near an end in painful or distressing circumstances the crucial question is not the question usually put: 'Shall I prescribe palliative care only, as a way of keeping the patient as comfortable as possible while nature takes its course, or shall I end the patient's life as quickly as possible?', but 'Is there any realistic hope that the patient will recover and be able to lead a life which seems to him or her worth living?'. Once that question has been answered in the negative active euthanasia must be the morally right answer, and it is to be hoped that it will one day be a legally permissible answer.

CONCLUSIONS

We saw earlier that the most important objection to the practice of active voluntary euthanasia is that requests for euthanasia might not always really be voluntary, because pressure might be put on people to sign their own death warrants. We also saw that if active voluntary euthanasia is to be legalized the revised law must contain safeguards against this abuse. No legal safeguards against abuse can be 100% effective, but the system of legal control in Holland makes it extremely unlikely that any such abuse can occur. According to Section 293 of the Dutch Penal Code 'Any person who terminates the life of another person at the latter's express and urgent request is liable to a term of imprisonment not exceeding twelve years.' But gradually since 1973 the Dutch courts, in collaboration with doctors and the prosecuting authorities, have developed a system in which doctors will not be prosecuted if they conform to the following rules:

1. The request for euthanasia must come only from the patient, and must be entirely voluntary.
2. The patient's request must be well considered, durable and persistent.
3. The patient must be experiencing considerable (not necessarily physical) suffering with no prospect of improvement.
4. Euthanasia must be a last resort. Other alternatives to alleviate the patient's situation must have been considered and found wanting.
5. Euthanasia must be performed by a doctor.
6. The doctor must consult with an independent doctor colleague who has experience in this field (17).

In a system which requires such investigation and consultation cases of abuse must be very rare indeed. But it is the fact that, while active euthanasia is practised furtively in the UK and in other countries, it is practised *openly* in Holland that gives it such advantages, for both doctors and patients, as far to outweigh the remote possibility that it might be abused. For doctors—and they are the majority—who are compassionate and wish to act in the best interests of their patients it has the advantage that they know they will not be prosecuted if they follow the rules, and since most cases are not published in the media, they need not fear being stigmatized even by the minority of people who disapprove of all euthanasia.

For patients the main advantage is that they know that euthanasia will be available when they feel that the time has really come for it. Many old people are afraid of insomnia and ask their doctors for sleeping pills. Then, when they have them in the cupboard, they don't use them because they know that if they do not fall asleep at once they need not lie distressingly awake. In the same way people suffering from a degenerative disease, and people who are simply growing old, are fearful that one day they will want a peaceful end and not be able to get it. This anxiety may last for many years and deny them the enjoyment of those years which would be theirs if they could be confident that such a death will be available when they want it.

The availability of medical euthanasia will also greatly reduce the incidence of amateur mercy killings. This, as we saw, is usually the killing of a spouse or near relative, and it is always an act of love. So imagine, if you can, just what it is like to have to choose between having to refuse the last, urgent request of someone you love and killing that person with your own hands. If medical euthanasia were available, this agonizing choice would no longer be necessary.

REFERENCES

1. Poll taken for The National Hemlock Society, Eugene, Oregon, 1988.
2. Kuhse, E. 1985. Euthanasia—again. *Medical Journal of Australia* **142**: 611.
3. BMA working party report. 1988. *Euthanasia*, p. 47. BMA, London.
4. Institute of Medical Ethics working party report. 1990. *Lancet*, 8 September, p. 611.
5. *Euthanasia, Suicide, and Cessation of Treatment*. H.M. Stationery Office, Ottawa, 1984.
6. VES *Newsletter* No. 39, May 1990, p. 1.
7. Brahams, D. 1992. Euthanasia: doctor convicted of attempted murder. *Lancet*, 26 September, pp. 782–783.
8. *The Times*, London, 15 July 1989.
9. VES *Newsletter* No. 37, September, 1989, p. 2, and No. 45, May 1992, p. 4.
10. *Mortality Statistics for England and Wales*. H.M. Stationery Office, London.
11. *The Sunday Times*, London, 16 December 1984.
12. *The handbook of medical ethics*. 1984. BMA, London.
13. BMA working party report: *Euthanasia*. London, 1988, pp. 15, 18–19.
14. Nowell-Smith, P. 1989. Euthanasia and the doctors. *Journal of Medical Ethics*, **15**: 124–128.
15. VES *Newsletter*, No. 31, September 1987.
16. IME working party report. 1990. *Lancet*, 8 September, p. 613.
17. Dr Else Borst-Eilers, VES *Newsletter*, No. 38, January 1990, p. 7.

65

Against Voluntary Euthanasia

LUKE GORMALLY, LicPHIL

Director, Linacre Centre for Health Care Ethics, London, UK

INTRODUCTION

This chapter is mainly devoted to presenting a case for holding that *no* choice intentionally to bring about a person's death for euthanasiast reasons can be right. It will also be briefly argued, later, that voluntary euthanasia should not be legalized.

While the considerations which underpin the case here presented against euthanasiast killing are of quite general relevance it is important to recognize their special significance for the doctor–patient relationship. That relationship is at the heart of the practice of medicine. Needing health care, patients are dependent on the doctor's knowledge, skill and commitment to their medical good (1). But patients require more than that from doctors. Because of their vulnerability, patients are often not well placed to prevent their ill-treatment or exploitation. So we need doctors to have a clear sense of what is owing to human beings in the way of respect, care and distributable goods. This formula about *what is owing to others* by way of *action and restraint*, is shorthand for the requirements of justice as that concept is understood in the classical tradition of moral philosophy (2). Willingness to deal with others in accordance with those requirements is the virtue of justice. This virtue is for all of us fundamental to living well in our relationships with others, but the dependency and vulnerability of patients makes justice a peculiarly indispensable disposition in doctors. How this bears on the practice of euthanasia by doctors will emerge in the course of this chapter.

WHAT COUNTS AS VOLUNTARY EUTHANASIA?

'Voluntary euthanasia' is here taken to mean: *(a) the intentional causing of a patient's death or, more plainly, the intentional killing of a patient, (b) in the course of medical care, when (c) the killing is carried out at the patient's request and (d) the doctor believes that, because of the patient's mental condition and quality of life, death would be a benefit to the patient and killing him would therefore be justified.*

Principles of Health Care Ethics. Edited by Raanan Gillon.
© 1994 John Wiley & Sons Ltd

There are four elements to be considered:

1. What is at issue in considering euthanasia is *intentional* killing. This occurs when a doctor aims to bring about a patient's death either by something he does (e.g. injecting a lethal dose of a toxic substance) or by something he deliberately *omits* to do *precisely with a view to securing the patient's death*. He may, for example, withhold necessary life-prolonging treatment, which he had an obligation to provide, precisely for the sake of the patient's death. So one can intentionally kill a patient by deliberate omissions just as much as by positive deeds. To kill someone is simply to bring it about that a person dies.

   It is generally acknowledged that deliberate killing requires to be justified, so the justification of euthanasia has to meet whatever basic conditions require to be met for the justification of intentional killing.
2. The killing of the patient is *in the course of medical care*. People other than doctors can kill patients for euthanasiast reasons, but proponents of voluntary euthanasia are particularly interested in having doctors kill patients *as an accepted part of clinical practice*.
3. The killing is carried out at the patient's request. Proponents of voluntary euthanasia place great emphasis on the free rational choice of the patient; and some of them insist that they have no wish to promote non-voluntary euthanasia (i.e. the killing of patients, such as the demented, who are incapable of giving consent) or involuntary euthanasia (i.e. the killing of patients contrary to their wills). It will emerge, however, that the 'voluntary' character of voluntary euthanasia is not decisive for its justification, and that what does appear to be decisive in that respect could equally well justify non-voluntary euthanasia.
4. The doctor believes that, because of the patient's mental condition and quality of life, death would be a benefit to the patient and killing him would therefore be justified. The existence of the request suggests that the patient believes he has good reason to be killed by a doctor. But it is the doctor who is to do the killing and who is answerable for it. The doctor, therefore, needs to be satisfied that he has good reason to kill the patient. If his satisfying himself on this score consists of little more than ascertaining that the patient himself firmly believes his life is no longer worthwhile then precisely *that* judgement on the patient's life becomes the practical basis for the doctor's action. Doctors who carry out euthanasiast killings are not robotic agents of patients, and cannot forswear responsibility for the practical judgements which provide the reasons for killing. In particular, they are responsible for the judgement that death is a *benefit* to the patient, since the case for killing is that it is allegedly beneficial to the patient rather than to others.

WHICH KILLINGS MAY BE JUSTIFIED?

It is fundamental to human well-being in society that human beings should enjoy protection from lethal attack. So the right to life—understood as a right not to be unjustly killed—is the most basic human right. But any such formulation of a right to life leaves unclear what could justify killing and so what killing would not be contrary to the requirements of justice.

In seeking to determine what killings might be justified, and therefore not inconsistent with justice, it is important to be clear about the basis on which human beings enjoy fundamental human rights, such as the right not to be unjustly killed. The tradition of common morality holds that *all* human beings enjoy such a right because, *simply in virtue of their humanity*, they possess an equality of dignity. The notion of dignity that is being employed here implies that an objective, ineliminable value belongs to human lives in virtue of the fact that they are the lives of human beings. Since there is no such thing as being more or less a human being, we are *equal* in the dignity or worth we possess in virtue of being human.

That equality of dignity means that each human being has a claim to be recognized as a subject of justice and other moral duties.

The worth or value which we refer to by speaking of basic human dignity must be incommensurable with other important values if it is to feature in deliberation as the *ineliminable* basis of the claim that each human being is to be treated as a subject of justice. If that value were commensurable with the goods which can be enjoyed and the evils which can be suffered *in* a life, aggregation of them all could seem to reduce certain lives to negative value. If that type of calculation were *in principle* possible then there would be scope for rationalizing many kinds of killing, since those to be killed would seem no longer to have a claim to be regarded as subjects of justice.

If we try to dispense with the assumption that human dignity belongs to every human being in virtue of his or her humanity we are left without a rationally defensible understanding of justice.

It is well known that precisely this assumption is widely rejected by advocates of abortion, infanticide, euthanasia and other types of medicalized killing. A number of them argue that human dignity (and basic human rights) depend on possession of *presently exercisable capacities* of a kind characteristic of developed human beings: capacities for understanding, choice and rational communication. Others argue that human dignity depends on actually enjoying an acceptable quality of life.

Any such position requires us to make *choices* about *what* degree of *which* abilities give a person rights, or what kind of quality of life does so. If one behaves towards other human beings on that basis one cannot avoid being *arbitrary* about where to draw the line between those one recognizes as possessing rights and those one reckons not to possess basic human rights. But where the determination of who are the subjects of justice is arbitrary, one simply lacks a recognizable framework of justice. If we are to have a defensible understanding of the domain of justice (i.e. one which ensures that whom we treat justly is not a matter of choice) then we have to assume that just treatment is owing to all human beings in virtue of the dignity and worth which belongs to their humanity.

This assumption is not only indispensable but also reasonable in itself. It is true that what makes it clear that human beings possess a distinctive dignity and value (which makes them superior to other animals) is the exercise of abilities for understanding, choice and rational communication. But that dignity and value do not belong exclusively to those individuals in whom distinctive human abilities have already developed. We need to recognize that these abilities are acquired in virtue of a capacity inherent in our nature to develop just such abilities. If we set great value by the developed abilities then all the more should we value the nature in virtue of which we come to possess those abilities. Human worth and dignity may be appropriately manifested in our distinctive behaviour as human beings. But there could not be such behaviour without the powers inherent in the nature which all of us possess. Hence there is a dignity and a worth we all possess just in virtue of being human.

Since the dignity which attaches to our humanity is the basis of what we most fundamentally owe to each other in the way of respect, recognition of that dignity is the precondition of human beings treating each other properly. Any purported justification of killing must then at the very least be *consistent* with recognizing the dignity of every human being.

Whatever else may be said about traditional justifications of killing in capital punishment and killing of unjust aggressors in warfare, those justifications are arguably at least consistent with recognition of the dignity of the persons whose killing is justified. The killing of capital punishment should be justifiable on the grounds that the criminal to be killed *deserves* that punishment. To say that someone deserves death is to entertain a high conception of the dignity of the criminal, for he can be said to deserve such punishment only if he knowingly chose to do what he did, and so made himself answerable for it.

Similarly the commonly recognized justification for killing in warfare is to put an end to a grave injustice perpetrated by people who could have acted otherwise. (To refuse to fight *is* possible even in face of duress, as we see in the case of Franz Jägerstätter) (3). As with capital punishment, the reason for the killing is not inconsistent with recognition of the human dignity of those who are killed.

Both justifications—of capital punishment and of the killing of unjust aggressors in warfare—yield a common formula stating the basic norm in regard to killing: one ought never intentionally to kill the 'innocent': those not guilty of crime, which it is one's task to punish, or of unjustified violence, which it is one's office to resist.

WHY JUSTIFICATIONS OF EUTHANASIAST KILLING FAIL TO MEET THE BASIC REQUIREMENT

The rationale of the absolute prohibition on the intentional killing of the innocent is to exclude any killing inconsistent with recognition of the human dignity of the person to be killed. (Why precisely 'absolute' and 'intentional' will be further considered in the section 'Some criticisms . . .').

The killing of someone simply for advantage or convenience is inconsistent with recognition of that person's dignity, for the person is thereby treated as a mere means to the ends of others. Much advocacy of non-voluntary euthanasia is motivated by the thought that it is advantageous to others, in relieving them of the burdens of care for the handicapped and senile.

Before assessing justifications which seek to present killing as in some circumstances good *for the patient*, we should remind ourselves of the condition such justifications need to meet: they must be consistent with recognizing the dignity of every human being. This means that the justification must not take a form which in effect purports to show that no positive value attaches to a human life, so that to end that life cannot be to deprive a person of something of positive value, but rather terminates a condition of negative value and thereby 'benefits' the patient. Justifications of that type, if they have any place at all for recognizing a value attaching to our humanity (and many do not), in effect treat it as a commensurable and therefore eliminable value in calculating the overall 'worth' of a life. But to treat the basic human dignity of some human beings as an eliminable value is to proceed by denying to those human beings their status as subjects of justice and other moral duties.

All standard justifications of voluntary euthanasia, in so far as they represent it as a benefit to the patient killed, do so in a way which is inconsistent with recognition of the basic dignity of every human being.

One justification (4) represents human existence as no more than the possibility of enjoying goods. A human life is a benefit just in so far as it comes up to a standard of normality in the goods available in it. But if it sinks below that standard and is overtaken by evils it is overall an evil (4, p. 43). Deliberately to end a life in that condition (if the patient asks to have it ended) is to benefit the patient.

Clearly this justification of voluntary euthanasia as a beneficial choice begins from the premise that our mere existence as human beings has no value as such. So the justification is not consistent with recognizing the dignity of every human being.

Sometimes an attempted justification of voluntary euthanasia will concede that human life has value, but then argue that this value can be eliminated by the realities of suffering (5). But if one treats the value attaching to our humanity as eliminable by countervailing disvalues one denies that basic dignity belongs to every human being whatever his or her condition.

Some justifications of voluntary euthanasia start from the premise that human lives do not possess a basic objective dignity and value. What gives a life value, it is claimed, is the ability of the person whose life it is to find value in projects, activities and relationships. Without a felt, *subjective* sense of worth and value a life lacks value. If a person is competent he is the only possible authority on whether he enjoys a subjective sense of value. And those who lack presently exercisable abilities for finding value in their lives thereby lack lives of value. If so, there is no *objective* value essential to the lives either of those with or those without the abilities required to invest their lives with value.

A justification of euthanasia which proceeds from these background assumptions is clearly inconsistent with recognition of the basic dignity of every human being.

Some proponents of voluntary euthanasia purport to recognize the dignity of the persons to be killed. One such attempt finds expression in the formula 'continued life is not in the interests of some valued persons' (6). But this is mystificatory rhetoric. If one says that someone's continued existence is not in the interests of that person one means that person would be better off dead, that the non-existence of that bodily person is of less disvalue than continued bodily existence. This could be true only if continued existence is reckoned to have a negative value, for death as such can hardly be reckoned to have positive value (7,8). So this form of justification is inconsistent with recognition of the basic dignity of every human being.

To speak of the continued existence of some *'valued* persons' not being in their interests merely gives an appearance of evading the logic of the position espoused. For a human person is not something other than a living human body. If one does not value certain living human bodies one does not value the persons they are.

AUTONOMY AND THE JUSTIFICATION OF EUTHANASIA

Are the radical defects in standard justifications of voluntary euthanasia remedied by the fact that at least some part of a doctor's reason for killing is the patient's request? The mere fact of a request in itself provides little reason for a doctor to kill a patient. Doctors of every shade of opinion about the ethics of euthanasia would reject many requests for euthanasia, either because they believed the patient had a false view of his prognosis or because he was suffering from a relievable depression or because the prospects for the patient were otherwise good. Even a doctor who subscribed to the view that the value of any particular human life consisted exclusively in the value the person concerned found in his life may be thought to have reason to reject a patient's request to be killed, when he suspects the patient is capable of retrieving a sense of subjective value in his life.

What doctors who favour euthanasiast killing look for beyond the request to be killed is reason to think that killing would be a benefit to a particular patient. And the characteristic reasons offered for thinking it a benefit reduce to versions of the ones reviewed in the previous section.

So it is these reasons which bear the onus of justifying even voluntary euthanasia. If one thinks the value of a human life is reducible to some calculus of the goods and evils which compose it, one may have reason to take seriously the competent patient's own view of the value of his life, but will have little reason to refrain from denying to incompetent patients the 'benefits' of killing them. In other words, those who buy into the justification of voluntary euthanasia as beneficial and morally acceptable find that, willy-nilly, they have little or no reason for rejecting the proposal that non-voluntary euthanasia is beneficial and morally acceptable. Sometimes it is only tactical considerations which inhibit the clear-headed advocate of voluntary euthanasia from open advocacy of non-voluntary euthanasia (9,10).

SOME CRITICISMS OF AN ABSOLUTE MORAL NORM EXCLUDING EUTHANASIAST KILLING

Intentional and Foreseen Causation of Death

A number of writers have argued that there is no morally significant distinction between intentional and foreseen causation of someone's death. If, for that reason, an absolute prohibition were to include both intentional and foreseen causation of death people would be prevented from doing things which it is quite generally thought reasonable to do (engaging in high-risk sports, performing high-risk surgery, giving analgesics for pain control with the likelihood of hastening death).

It is important to be clear that the idea of the 'intentional' as it is employed in the moral norm ('It is absolutely impermissible *intentionally* to take innocent human life') is an idea refined by philosophical reflection: it refers to what one does, identified by reference to one's *chosen purpose* in acting and *the means* which are *chosen* precisely because of their relevance to the achievement of one's purpose. Both of these must feature in any adequate statement of why one is acting, i.e. in any adequate statement of one's *reasons* for doing precisely what one is doing. Now the rationale for the prohibition on intentionally killing which has been presented in this chapter is that we are forbidden to kill for *reasons* incompatible with recognition of human dignity. But when death is foreseen its causation does not standardly feature among the reasons one has for acting.

Why claim crucial moral significance for the distinction between intentional and foreseen causation of death? For two related reasons. First, many worthwhile activities, entirely consistent with recognition of human dignity, would be made impossible if all foreseeable causation of death was forbidden (examples already mentioned: high-risk surgery, or the giving of opiates to control pain in doses likely to hasten death). Indeed, one of the evident motives of those seeking to show there is no morally significant difference between intention and foresight is to make a prohibition of intentional causation of death seem as unreasonable as an absolute prohibition of foreseen causation of death would evidently be. But to permit a person to act on reasons incompatible with recognizing the basic dignity of others would be to permit that person to treat those others as though their dignity were irrelevant to how one chose to act towards them.

Secondly, our intentional acts, such as deliberate killing or lying, do not merely bring about effects external to us, they also shape our dispositions. If I choose to lie then I damage in myself the disposition to respect the truth. If I kill someone because I judge he no longer has a worthwhile life I make myself to be a person disposed to kill people for that kind of reason (11–14) (see also Chapter 4 in this book). That is why a certain kind of argument for the legalization of voluntary euthanasia is radically mistaken about what is at issue. The argument goes roughly as follows. A society should seek to prohibit only those practices which do harm to those who do not consent to the practices. But in voluntary euthanasia no party who has *not* consented to the practice is harmed. It is a purely private transaction between consenting doctor and consenting patient, the effects of which are contained within the confines of that relationship.

One reason that picture is false is that a doctor's character is very significantly shaped by killing patients on the grounds that their lives are now without value. A doctor disposed to think that some of his patients may lack inherent worth, and that he may therefore be justified in killing them, has seriously undermined in himself a disposition indispensable to the practice of medicine: the willingness to give what is owing to patients just in virtue of their possession of basic human dignity. The absence of that willingness is likely to be fateful for other patients, including patients who never consented to be killed or to be denied what they are owed in virtue of their basic human dignity.

Omitting Treatment and the Causation of Death

A person's reasons for action commit him not merely to a particular purpose but to a specific course of conduct chosen precisely for its relevance to achieving that particular purpose. When a doctor withholds or withdraws life-prolonging treatment and death results earlier than it otherwise would have done, bringing about that earlier death is often no part of the doctor's reason for his chosen conduct: in these cases it belongs neither to his precise purpose nor to the means necessary to achieve his purpose. But some try to assimilate omitting treatment, when doing so foreseeably results in a patient's earlier death, to killing that patient intentionally, by arguing that the underlying reasons for the omission of treatment are ones in which the very existence of the patient features as not worth preserving, and therefore disposable.

In considering the reasons for withholding treatment which are traditionally held to be morally acceptable, one needs to bear in mind the background assumption of traditional medical ethics that prolongation of life is not a separate goal of medical practice and doctors are not obliged to seek to prolong life in all circumstances (15). It is a convenient travesty of a sanctity of life ethic to represent it (as some authors do (16,17)) as committing doctors to maximal prolongation of life. The core of a sanctity of life ethic is a *negative* norm (defended in the present chapter) excluding intentional attacks on innocent human lives. Some part of the explanation for why doctors do not have an obligation to prolong life in all circumstances is implicit in the standard reasons why life-prolonging treatment may be withheld (18):

1. At some point in everyone's life death becomes inevitable and, if there is an opportunity to do so, it is important to compose oneself to die well, a need which can be frustrated by strenuous efforts at prolonging life.
2. While one should value the gift of life one may not be obliged to seek to prolong it at the cost of great pain consequent on the effort to prolong it, or at the cost of other burdens consequent on that effort such as excessive psychological strain, excessive restriction on physical liberty, excessive disruption of activities centrally important to one, and excessive expenditure which may be financially crippling to one's family (19).

Now it is true that whether or not the consequences of treatment are likely to prove very burdensome to a patient will depend upon the circumstances and condition of the patient, and these circumstances and his condition sometimes may be compendiously referred to as a patient's 'quality of life'. So in assessing a patient's prognosis with some life-prolonging treatment a doctor may take a view of the patient's 'quality of life'. But a 'quality of life' judgement of that kind is *categorically different from* a judgement that someone's life lacks (net, overall) value and so *for that reason* may justifiably be ended. As we have seen, the latter judgement is incompatible with recognition of the dignity and value inherent in our humanity. That value is something which perdures independently of our quality of life.

If a doctor decides to discontinue a particular treatment *in order to avoid imposing burdens on a patient*, even if in consequence death is likely to result earlier than it otherwise would have done, bringing about that death is neither his purpose in making that decision nor his chosen means to avoid the burdens. Such a decision to omit treatment cannot reasonably be conflated with a decision aimed at bringing about death because one now judges the patient's life to be on balance an evil. The conflation saddles the doctor with a view which need not be—and should not be—part of his reasoning: the view that human dignity depends on one's quality of life.

Absoluteness and the Scope of Intention

The difference between intending-and-causing and foreseeing-and-causing is not always plainly obvious. The fact that there can be disputes about precisely how to draw the distinction is sometimes thought to show the unreasonableness of holding there is an absolute prohibition of intentional killing (20). But uncertainty about the precise *scope* of a prohibition has no tendency to show that what clearly falls within its scope admits of exceptions. And dispute about borderline cases is not an exercise in identifying possible exceptions to the prohibition but an exercise in seeking to identify just what it applies to.

For the most part what is intentional is not in doubt. And if the person to be killed is 'innocent', then indubitably intentional killing should be recognized as absolutely impermissible.

The Absolute Prohibition and Intolerable Suffering

It is widely felt that certain admittedly rare situations of intractable and intolerable suffering make untenable the claim that there is an absolute (i.e. exceptionless) prohibition of intentional killing of the innocent. The authors of the British Medical Association Working Party Report on *Euthanasia* hold such a view. They believe that where there is unavoidable suffering before what is certainly an unavoidable death, 'a mercy killing can be condoned . . . when the strongest humanitarian motives act in accord with an incontestable factual prediction' (21).

If one allows such exceptions what in logic is conceded? First, that there are circumstances in which it is reasonable to treat the human dignity of the person to be killed as a value which can be nullified by the entirely predictable evils which are about to overtake a life. But as we have seen, human dignity is not a value which can be rendered nugatory in some overall calculation of the worth of a life to yield a judgement which justifies killing. If it were allowed that it can be, then reason would provide no sure way of containing the exceptions as narrowly as the BMA Working Party propose. A strong case would be made— indeed it is the standard case for voluntary euthanasia—that incontestably predictable evils of suffering and loss of faculties rob so many human lives of dignity and value that the proposal to end those lives has 'the strongest humanitarian motives'.

Absolute norms do confront us with hard cases where pressures of sympathy and compassion can make the norm seem intolerable. Those are moments when we are particularly prone to the illusion that the intolerable can be eliminated by a little 'rational management'. But clear-headed reflection can recognize and agree that the implications of such management go far wider than the relief of hard cases, and extend to the introduction, willy-nilly, of very great evils. When, in face of a patient's suffering, carers find they are unable to bring the *positive* relief called for by genuine compassion, then, out of respect for human dignity, they have to endure the pains of sympathy while adhering to the true moral norm which unconditionally excludes killing the innocent.

AGAINST THE LEGALIZATION OF VOLUNTARY EUTHANASIA

Having explained the wrongness of any choice intentionally to kill a patient for euthanasiast reasons, we may conclude with a brief statement of five reasons why voluntary euthanasia should not be legalized.

1. Precisely in so far as euthanasia is reckoned *beneficent* to patients it involves killing on the basis of judgements about the value of their lives which are inconsistent with recognition of the dignity of the patients. Since recognition of the dignity of every human being is fundamental to justice *and so to the criminal law*, it would be incompatible with what is basic to the criminal law to allow euthanasiast killing.
2. Killing, the fundamental justification of which is that the patient would be better off dead (because of the disvalue of his continued existence), comprehends non-voluntary euthanasia. As clear-headed advocates of euthanasia recognize, if euthanasia is at all justified, there can be no good reason for denying the 'benefit' of killing to a patient because he is incapable of consent. The evidence from Holland is that doctors are *aiming* to kill many more incompetent than competent patients (22,23).
3. Propaganda for the legalization of euthanasia in the past heavily emphasized its desirability to deal with intractable terminal pain. But developments in pain control associated with the hospice movement have provided a solution, at least in principle, to the large majority of cases of intolerable pain. In consequence, the case for legalizing euthanasia has significantly shifted from drawing attention to intractable pain to emphasizing 'intractable suffering'. But 'intractable suffering' is a very capacious category. One leading practitioner of euthanasia in Holland has said he would be prepared to treat as grounds

for killing a patient the 'intractable suffering' which arose from the patient's knowledge that his children would dearly love to be rid of him (Keown (23), p. 79). If 'intractable suffering' is a reason for euthanasia, there is an open invitation to children to make the lives of their dependent and debilitated parents such a misery that the 'burdensome' parents will be queueing up for euthanasia. But this in truth would be involuntary euthanasia masquerading as 'voluntary'.

4. In so far as legalization of voluntary euthanasia made doctors the authorized agents of euthanasiast killing, such legislation would profoundly corrupt the practice of medicine by corrupting the character of doctors (see p. 769–770 above). For the sake of all its citizens, who at one time or another are likely to become patients, civil society has a basic interest in maintaining a legal framework for the practice of medicine which is conducive to respect on the part of doctors for the basic dignity of all their patients.

5. Once legalized, euthanasia would become a quick and facile technical 'fix' to dispose of certain difficult patients (whether or not at their own request) in response to the heavy demands they made on care. Medicine would thereby be robbed of the incentive to find genuinely compassionate solutions to the difficulties presented by such patients. The kind of humane impulses which have sustained the development of hospice medicine and care would be undermined, because too many would think euthanasia a cheaper and less personally demanding solution (24). It is widely recognized that the country in which the practice of euthanasia has become widespread is a country in which palliative care medicine is very inadequately developed.

Those who protest that they advocate no more than the legalization of *voluntary* euthanasia are at best naive, though more often, it is to be feared, disingenuous (10). It is characteristic of certain advocates of legal reform to believe that they can remain in control of the reforms they propose once they are on the statute book. That is an illusion, as legalization of abortion has shown. What legalization of voluntary euthanasia would enshrine is the novel principle that one may be justified in killing people because, since they lack worthwhile lives, to do so is to benefit them. In enshrining such a principle in our laws we would have to contend with what Judge Cardozo described as 'the tendency of a principle to expand itself to the limit of its logic' (Kamisar (10), p. 474). We were given a clear picture of that logic in Germany in the middle years of this century. It would be hubristic folly for contemporary doctors to think themselves incapable of the inhumanity displayed at that time by so many 'respectable' and eminent German doctors.

ACKNOWLEDGEMENTS

I am grateful to Professor Elizabeth Anscombe, Professor John Finnis, Dr Mary Geach and my colleague Mrs Agneta Sutton for generously giving me, at very short notice, critical comments on an earlier draft of this chapter. Limitations of space prevented me from taking advantage of some of their suggestions.

REFERENCES

1. Kass, L. 1985. *Toward a more natural science*, pp. 157–246. Free Press, New York.
2. Finnis, J. 1980. *Natural law and natural rights*, pp. 161–197. Clarendon Press, Oxford.
3. Zahn, G. C. 1964. *In solitary witness. The life and death of Franz Jägerstätter*. Holt, Rinehart & Winston, New York.
4. Foot, P. 1978. Euthanasia. Pp. 33–61, *in* Foot, P. *Virtues and vices*. Basil Blackwell, Oxford, at p. 34.
5. Rachels, J. 1980. Euthanasia. Pp. 28–66, *in* Regan, T. (Ed.) *Matters of life and death*. Random House, New York, at p. 46.
6. Cahill, L. S. 1991. Notes on moral theology. Bioethical decisions to end life. *Theological Studies* **52**: 107–127, at p. 123.
7. Devine, P. E. 1978. *The ethics of homicide*, pp. 23–31. Cornell University Press, Ithaca, NY.
8. Wreen, M. 1987. The logical opaqueness of death. *Bioethics* **1**: 366–371.
9. Smoker, B. 1991. Remember the non-terminally ill and disabled. *VES Newsletter*, September, p. 10.
10. Kamisar, Y. 1958. Some non-religious views against proposed 'mercy-killing' legislation. *Minnesota Law Review* **42**: 969–1042; reprinted in Horan, D. J. and Mall, D. (Eds) *Death, dying and euthanasia*, pp. 406–479. University Publications of America, Washington, DC, at pp. 451–467.
11. Gormally, L. 1978. *The principle of respect for human life*, pp. 8–13. Linacre Centre Paper 1. Linacre Centre, London.
12. Müller, A. 1977. Radical subjectivity: morality versus utilitarianism. *Ratio* **19**: 115–132.
13. Finnis, J. 1983. *Fundamentals of ethics*, pp. 138–142. Clarendon Press, Oxford.
14. Gormally, L. 1989. Euthanasia: some points in a philosophical polemic. *Linacre quarterly (USA)*, **57** (2): 14–25, at 20–22.
15. Gormally, L. 1987. A response [to Roy Fox. Palliative care and aggressive therapy], Pp. 177–198, *in* Elford, R. J. (Ed.) *Medical ethics and elderly people*. Churchill Livingstone, Edinburgh.
16. Kuhse, H. 1987. *The sanctity of life doctrine in medicine*. Clarendon Press, Oxford.
17. Age Concern Institute of Gerontology and Centre of Medical Law and Ethics, London. 1988. *The living will. Consent to treatment at the end of life: a Working Party report*, p. 2. Edward Arnold, London.
18. Linacre Centre Working Party. 1982. *Euthanasia and clinical practice: trends, principles and alternatives*, pp. 49, 52. Linacre Centre, London.
19. Gormally, L. 1987. A Response. Pp. 193–196, *in* Elford, R. J. (Ed.) *Medical ethics and elderly people*. Churchill Livingstone, Edinburgh.
20. Byrne, P. 1990. Homicide, medical ethics and the principle of double effect. Pp. 131–159, *in* Byrne, P. (Ed.) *Ethics and law in health care and research*. John Wiley, Chichester, at p. 157.
21. British Medical Association. 1988. *Euthanasia*. Report of the Working Party to review the British Medical Association's Guidance on Euthanasia, p. 28. British Medical Association, London.
22. Fenigsen, R. 1991. The report of the Dutch Governmental Committee on Euthanasia. *Issues in Law and Medicine* **7**: 339–344.
23. Keown, J. 1992. Some reflections on euthanasia in The Netherlands. Pp. 70–100, *in* Gormally, L. (Ed.) *The dependent elderly: autonomy, justice and quality of care*. Cambridge University Press, Cambridge, at p. 84.
24. Twycross, R. G. 1990. Assisted death: a reply. *Lancet* **336**: 796–798.

66

The Dying Patient

DAME CICELY SAUNDERS, OM, DBE, FRCP

Chairman, St Christopher's Hospice, London, UK

The moment when trauma or disease moves a patient inexorably towards death may never be identified and the change from attempts at rehabilitation or cure to palliative and supportive care and treatment does not take place. This chapter presupposes that such a decision has been made, though even now it is with the knowledge that it may yet prove to be provisional. A change of condition must be recognized and responded to with appropriate measures that are ethically indicated for that particular patient.

Mrs C.E., a lady of 56 from West Africa, had lived and worked as a personal assistant in southeast London for many years before she discovered a lump in her breast in 1984. Mastectomy was followed by radiotherapy. Five years later she developed the first of what eventually became widespread bone metastases. Hormone treatment, followed by oophorectomy and adrenalectomy produced no improvement and she had several courses of radiotherapy, working and continuing a remarkably normal life whenever she could. By late 1991 she had pathological fractures of femur and pelvis but the bone destruction both there and in her cervical spine precluded surgery. Each phase of disease and treatment was discussed by the multi-disciplinary team with the patient, a determined and dominant lady with great ambition to fight her disease, but often unrealistic expectations of her possibilities. Giving her sufficient information to make an informed choice was not straightforward and took much time.

At this stage she was in too much pain in her leg to remain at home and was admitted to a hospice at which her oncologist/radiotherapist was a regular consultant. Relief of pain was quickly achieved with a psoas catheter inserted by the visiting anaesthetist from the regular consulting pain clinic and Mrs C.E. was able to sit out in a chair in comfort. However, at a clinical meeting the precarious state of her cervical spine and its management was debated at length. How serious was the danger of quadriplegia, how fully should the patient, still talking with some bravado of a return to work, be warned of this and how could the resentments and demands on the nursing staff of her two daughters be helped? Family meetings were held but cultural differences made real communication and support difficult. They only partially understood and accepted that surgery was no longer a feasible option, and that their mother could no longer expect to return home. Mrs C.E. herself seemed equally dissatisfied with her treatment. With some doubts as to the advisability of the journey, further radiotherapy to her cervical spine was arranged.

Principles of Health Care Ethics. Edited by Raanan Gillon.
© 1994 John Wiley & Sons Ltd

Before this took place, however, the feared quadriplegia developed over the course of a few days, high-dose steroids having little effect. Telephone discussion with her oncologist was duly reported to Mrs C.E. and she finally seemed to accept the situation with greater equanimity, especially after the doctor on duty for the weekend had spent a considerable time explaining it both to her and her daughters.

She lived a further nine days, her general condition deteriorating slowly. Increase of analgesia was needed for intermittent pain but this was effective. She did not share her feelings fully with the staff, who respected her privacy and continued meticulous care until she died peacefully with her daughters beside her. They, too, had appeared to accept finally what was happening, and that nothing further could be done and that their mother was peaceful. Bereavement counselling was readily accepted.

Care for dying people should enable them to exercise as much autonomy as they can, and to live as fully as possible until they die. This takes time—but one long interview with careful communication should be attempted and may require many short visits for further explanations. Choices about possible treatments may need discussion as often patients have decided that they no longer want to fight for recovery or even for an extension of living, by now much impaired. It is not unusual to hear requests that are sometimes taken to be an asking for release but they need to be carefully elucidated and discussed.

LET ME DIE

'Let me die' is a request that any treatment that is designed to prolong life should now be discontinued. The patient is afraid of a continued existence with a quality of life that can no longer be faced. Many people today fear that they will inevitably find themselves involved with all the procedures of an intensive care unit with little or no choice in the matter. Decisions concerning appropriate as compared with possible treatments need to be discussed with the patient and the family after due consideration by the professional team. They may also need reassurance that the medications or procedures being given are designed solely for symptom control and will make the time remaining easier but not longer. A competent patient can refuse any or all treatments but needs to be suitably informed and choices respected. Not every patient understands this. Any decision should be open to review, for people must also know that they are free to change their minds. Family members can only make decisions for an incompetent patient in their best interests (1). A team may need to consider this issue at length both with and apart from the family. Much treatment can be offered in symptom control and support, and this may need to be spelled out more than once to the patient, the family and the staff.

There are other matters to be considered. The team need to discover what it is that makes continued life so grievous, and this may emerge in a series of conversations with different team members. Patients ask different questions and discuss different issues with the various professions. It often helps to give some idea of the likely time span for, while we must recognize how difficult it is to be at all certain in this area, some people are contemplating living on for months when the reality may more likely be weeks or days only. To explain this may be sufficient to ease the weary expectations.

Pain, weakness and the humiliations of dependence can all be tackled. The first is obviously the easiest to obliterate but the nursing team can lift much dependence by the way they carry out all their caring. Someone who can no longer turn over in bed without help may find the procedure has happened almost unnoticed because of the way it has been done and the attentive listening that has accompanied it. Unrealistic encouragements should not be given as a means of answering difficult questions but reassurance and explanation about the likely nature of the final coming of death may well be needed if anxious fears are to be eased. Hospice patients in a bay may be helped by seeing how others have died, 'I just want to go off peaceful like that old lady over there', said one elderly woman with confidence that she, too, would have her last symptoms controlled and that she would not be left alone.

I WANT TO DIE

'I want to die' expresses anguish that demands attentive and experienced listening. Once again, the team member must try to disentangle the reasons for this wish. It often arises when past treatment for distress has been inept and listening cursory. There is likely to be much past emotional pain that can only be guessed at. The doctor must analyse and treat symptoms and the nurse monitor the treatment, but here the social worker or chaplain member of the team, both well used to negative feelings and even despair, may help the expression of such feelings. Much of their power to hurt may be dispelled as they are voiced, but the worker may need help from discussion with other members of the team in handling what has been said. Sometimes it reveals a treatable depression and a trial of medication may be appropriate. More often, the realization that there is a consistent readiness to go on visiting, whatever is said, will gradually bring a conviction of personal value to the patient. It is not possible to give a sense of purpose in the living out of their time to another person. They must, and frequently do, find this for themselves, but we can often help to ease the sense of worthlessness. A grossly changed body image, the anguish of leaving unfulfilled responsibilities, the hatred of a passive role after an active life, can be recognized for the burdens that they are, and the amazing endurance and ability to come to terms with adversity possessed by most people can be fostered by a team member who is able to sit alongside with no answers to give. But that member will need support in his/her own search for meaning from the rest of the team afterwards. To keep coming in this way may be extremely difficult in the isolation of home care, and some team discussion from time to time is essential if the professional is to continue to give real presence as they go alone to the home visit.

KILL ME

The specific request 'Kill me' or 'My father should not wake up again' is still extremely uncommon in spite of all the (often confusing) attention of the media to this subject. The person concerned almost certainly knows that we cannot do this, but may not be sure. We need to give a clear answer and a definite stance of this kind gives it own security. Once again, the team member concerned must listen, showing that he/she recognizes the desperation that has led to the stark request and which may stem from much past fear or a need to control. It may also come, very understandably, from a person in poorly treated pain. Once again, all that can be done in palliative treatment must be presented and the promise given that in no way will that come to an end or the patient be abandoned. Some people need reassuring that death itself comes easily when good care is available, and the relief of pain frequently means that the request fades away forgotten. It is surely largely because of this that the workers in palliative care speak out against direct and intended killing.

The doctor (or nurse) may not embark on any conduct with the primary intention of causing the patient's death (1). They may, however, if the patient wishes, help the patient to be more sleepy, though not to the point of permanent coma. This must be clearly explained and discussed with the patient, the family and the team. The latter must be clear what they are doing and why, time the offer of drinks and nursing care to wakeful moments and be ready to review the situation at any time. Some of the few who make a request for active killing will refuse the help to be more sleepy but they must know the offer remains and that they are free to change their minds.

Very occasionally there will be a series of confrontational requests from one or more members of a family. It must be clear that while their expressions of anger may help towards the resolution of differences, this may not come about, and the team as a whole will need to share their feelings and experience the strength of a cohesive group, greater than the simple sum of its parts. In one recent episode that stands out for its rarity, the difference between individual and institutional ethics was clearly spelled out by the social worker as the group as a whole, meeting in a crowded room as an emergency, recognized the strength that a previously undiscussed consensus had given them. There was no question of argument or blame for the person making the demand (the patient, though emotionally distressed, was more ambivalent). Discharge and home care were arranged, but after a short time at home the patient wished to return to the hospice and died without physical distress three weeks after the first confrontation. She did not come to terms with what was happening and the small nursing team who carried out all her care needed all the support of the rest of the team. Unable either legally or ethically to give her what she still requested from time to time, no-one withdrew from the caring and listening that they could offer.

At no time did Mrs C.E. make any of these statements. Having fought for normal living and then for a time at home for as long as her physical condition made possible, the hospice home care team identified the moment when a specific manoeuvre for pain control was essential, explained it fully and found her ready to accept hospice admission. Although cultural differences led to problems in the ward and initial unhappiness for patient, family and staff, quiet but determined efforts at communication eventually helped to a comparatively peaceful resolution. Many ethical dilemmas in deciding on appropriate treatment at this stage can be resolved in this way, and avoid recriminations and even litigation later.

Autonomy has to be seen in such a context. Control over treatment has to be tailored to what is feasible. Mrs C.E. asked for surgery but was able finally to accept the risks attached to any fixation of her cervical spine. There was little if any bone left to fix, but to find a way of explaining this to her in an acceptable fashion was not easy. The alternatives, however, were disaster or dissatisfaction and the effort was successfully made. To carry out inappropriate treatment in what can be an almost automatic commitment to active treatment aimed at what has become an illusory cure, is surely not ethically indicated. Neither, however, is the nihilistic statement still sadly heard 'There is nothing more I can do.' This is at the least unkind, and the progress in palliative medicine has shown that it is hardly ever true. Symptom control is a developing science as well as compassionate caring and at the least we can stand by those who find helplessness intolerable. Having at all times 'something to do' helps greatly in the often debated topic of answering the question 'Am I going to die?' It also gives a basis for day-to-day meetings with those who never ask such a question and wish either not to look at the matter or to keep their own counsel. Once open communication is seen as a possibility the patient will lead in this area.

Autonomy has to be considered not only in what is feasible but also in the context of family, of society as a whole and with what the carers and professionals concerned can reasonably offer. Many of the calls for the legalization of a doctor (or otherwise) assisted suicide, are based on the premise that autonomy is completely individualistic. But people belong to each other, they are persons in relation. Independence was denoted by the playwright George Bernard Shaw in *Pygmalion* as 'Middle class blasphemy' and he added, 'We are all of us dependent on one another, every soul of us on earth' (2). Any legalized 'right to die' would inevitably give the message to many vulnerable people that they have a duty to relieve others of the burden of caring for them.

Justice, fairness and proper duty to all concerned, with the dying patient and family as the unit of care, balances autonomy. It must, however, be seen at the deep level of the nature of persons, however impaired their capacity may seem to be. This is a time for them to search out their most important inner values, to find reconciliations and make farewells. Much anger and anguish may need to be expressed and in such expression move towards resolution. People move fast in a crisis, and all those experienced in care at the end of life see constantly how families, as well as patients, come to resolutions and find strengths they did not realize they possessed.

Justice also demands all the competence that can be mustered on the part of the caring team. It is surely unethical to fail to acquire the skills or to use those of others in order to fulfil a commitment to completing a patient's treatment and care if deteriorating illness reaches the stage described above in the case of Mrs C.E. No legal consideration of hastening death should take place until all the avenues of relief have been explored.

In some sense the issues of non-maleficence and beneficence have already been addressed. During the years when intensive care and ever more major surgery have been developing, many patients have received treatment so inappropriate as to merit the former classification. Making the decision as to what is ethically indicated for a newly admitted patient, at least temporarily incompetent, may be extremely difficult. Advance directives, more common in the United States than the United Kingdom, may be an important aid for professionals and family alike, but there surely needs to be a degree of flexibility available. A designated proxy could address the problem in part and help to elucidate what is now right in the current situation. Many years of experience in interpreting law in relation to the need for attendance in complex clinical and psychological conditions have given an awareness of its difficulty and gratitude that such decisions could be reviewed and were not irrevocable. But many dying patients are fearful that life may be prolonged regardless of its quality or their own wishes. Interpreting what these are may demand as much skill and effort as the technically complex treatment that might have been offered.

The omission of treatment itself raises ethical questions. Kennedy considers that the distinction sometimes made between a commission deliberately to bring about a patient's death which is at present unlawful (and the writer would consider unethical) and an omission, which may not be, is not helpful. It has certainly been disputed widely. He writes, however,

> the real argument is not how a doctor's conduct can be characterised but whether in the circumstances he has fulfilled his duty to the patient in good faith. The principles of good faith reflect professional ethics and general social morality. Neither at present condones euthanasia, so that to cause a patient's death, whether by omission or commission, would be a breach of the duty to care for the patient in good faith and hence unlawful. Both, however, contemplate allowing the patient to die, if, in the circumstances, the illness is terminal and any other form of treatment, other than treatment for dying, would not be ethically indicated (1).

There are misconceptions concerning the balance between pain and symptom control and side-effects. Contrary to much that has been taught, if a patient's pain is carefully analysed and treated specifically wherever possible (as was Mrs C.E.'s) there need rarely be the occasion to use doses of opiates that depress consciousness and respiration. If they are carefully titrated to an individual patient's optimum effective level, given on a regular basis according to the duration of effect with suitable adjuvants and orally for as long as possible, tolerance will not be a clinical problem. The fear of respiratory depression has denied many essential relief, and is largely unfounded. Mrs C.E. never needed a dose that brought this danger, and nor do most patients. The idea that doses need continued escalation has been shown repeatedly to be erroneous (3).

There are occasions, however, more often with patients who develop agitated confusion and terminal restlessness, when the essential sedation may indeed produce a chest infection by virtue of sleep and inactivity. Managing these patients and their families can stretch a team to its limits. In most other situations it is possible to involve the patient in the decision-making. Confusion is different. The caring team and the patient's family have together to decide the best, and ethically indicated, treatment (4). Careful explanation now, as is necessary when oral medication has perforce to change to injections or an infusion pump, should nearly always avoid misunderstanding and later recrimination. Devlin's summing up to the jury in the Bodkin Adams case gives ethical as well as legal guidelines for such situations:

If the first purpose of medicine, the restoration of health, can no longer be achieved, there is still much for a doctor to do, and he is entitled to do all that is proper and necessary to relieve pain and suffering, even if the measures he takes may incidentally shorten life. This is not because there is a special defence for medical men but because no act is murder which does not cause death. We are not dealing here with the philosophical or technical cause, but with the commonsense cause. The cause of death is the illness or the injury, and the proper medical treatment that is administered and that has an incidental effect on determining the exact moment of death is not the cause of death in any sensible use of the term. But . . . no doctor, nor any man, no more in the case of the dying than of the healthy, has the right deliberately to cut the thread of life (5).

Like Kennedy, Devlin does not use the term 'passive euthanasia', which the present writer considers confusing and unhelpful. We are discussing competent and compassionate clinical care unrelated to an act of deliberate killing with which it should not be classed.

The whole problem of a professional team's tendency to paternalism may be considered under the heading of beneficence. People have the right to question treatment and full discussion should help towards their understanding of what are realistic demands and what is now no longer feasible. This is illustrated in Mrs C.E.'s case and took considerable but, finally, well-spent time.

Not all families, however, are in agreement with each other, and great care and wisdom may be needed in deciding when and how to intervene when there is conflict. A patient has rights, but so has the caring family, and they may not see their way to a resolution. Each situation is different but time taken to ease tensions with open discussion is rarely ill spent.

This may be particularly acute when a patient is dying at home and may be compounded when dangerous drugs are needed for symptom relief. The great majority of families take careful responsibility once the professionals visiting the home or prescribing from an outpatient clinic have explained and written out adequate instructions. It is most important to explain ahead how help can be obtained in a crisis and adequate plans discussed, but there is no disputing the burdens handled by some families.

Much of the above has considered the treatment and care as given by a multi-disciplinary team. To give ethically appropriate treatment to a dying patient and family without the involvement of more than one profession will scarcely be adequate. New questions arise, however. Is this the best use of sometimes limited resources; how is true confidentiality to be maintained and how are differing points of view concerning ethics to be resolved?

Resources must be properly allocated, and some at least are being inappropri-ately used where the decision that treatment aimed at cure is no longer feasible and surely no longer ethically indicated. The WHO publications concerning palliative care are an attempt to address this point (6,7).

Confidentiality can be balanced with adequate team sharing where respect for the patient's wishes is coupled with due regard for what other colleagues may have to offer. Experience in team-working and in record-keeping should help solve most problems in this area. Disagreements over treatment, for example in questions of sedation, can similarly be tackled and are usually resolved.

Mrs C.E.'s demands and attitude to her nurses brought all these issues to the fore. Open and frank discussion and patience as she found her own way helped to a final peace that at one time seemed unlikely.

The last part of life can be of immense importance and value. A determination to keep the patient and family in their circumstances, common to all mankind and yet unique to them, central to the situation can resolve many dilemmas. Readiness to accept that all of us will eventually die, and a recognition that this time has come, will mean that the first steps in addressing the ethical issues have been faced.

REFERENCES

1. Kennedy, I. McC. 1984. The law relating to the treatment of the terminally ill. Pp. 227–231, *in* Saunders, C. (Ed.). *The management of terminal malignant disease*, 2nd edn. Edward Arnold, London.
2. Shaw, B. 1931. Pygmalion in Androcles and the Lion Overruled. *Pygmalion*. Constable & Co., London, standard edn, p. 278.
3. Hanks, G. W. and Hoskin, P. J. 1987. Opioid analgesics in the management of pain in patients with cancer. *Palliative Medicine* 1: 1–25.
4. Murphy, M. 1990. Confusion and sedation. Pp. 93–101, *in* Saunders, C. (Ed.) *Hospice and palliative care—an interdisciplinary approach*. Edward Arnold, London.
5. Devlin, P. 1985. *Easing the passing—the trial of Dr John Bodkin Adams*, pp. 171–172. Bodley Head, London.
6. World Health Organization. 1986. *Cancer pain relief*. WHO, Geneva.
7. World Health Organization. 1990. *Report of Expert Committee* (Technical Report Series 804); a review. WHO, Geneva.

67

The Ethics of Medical Publishing and the Four Principles

MAGNE NYLENNA, MD

Editor-in-Chief of the Journal of the Norwegian Medical Association, Lagåsen, Norway

POVL RIIS, MD

Former Editor-in-Chief, Journal of the Danish Medical Association; Professor of Medicine, University of Copenhagen; Chairman, Central Scientific–Ethical Commitee of Denmark; Herlev University Hospital, Herlev, Denmark

To publish is to bring information from the private to the public sphere. Medical publishing consequently comprises both printed and oral presentations. Oral presentations are important because of their inherent speed, the opportunity that they provide for psychological judgement of the speaker and the access to immediate discussion of a paper which they offer. Despite these important additional gains from oral presentations, the cornerstone of the international network for exchanging scientific information is still the printed version of research results. Besides, the ethics of both printed and oral versions are to a large extent the same. Thus 'publishing', in the following text, will mean printed publishing primarily in scientific journals.

THE AIMS AND EXTENT OF MEDICAL PUBLISHING

To understand the ethics of publishing one has first to analyse the aims of this widespread exercise. Throughout the history of modern medicine two major aims have evolved:

1. To constitute the dominating channel for intra- and extranational dissemination of scientific knowledge, clinical experience, health system problems and medical ethics.

Principles of Health Care Ethics. Edited by Raanan Gillon.
© 1994 John Wiley & Sons Ltd

2. To serve as an (often over-played and misused) indicator of doctors' individual scientific education and experience.

In addition it serves as the most important forum for the drug and equipment industry, enabling it to reach its target groups.

These aims reflect the mixture of motives represented in the process of medical publishing: curiosity, academic self-promotion, vanity, profit-seeking, altruism, social responsibility, etc. Further, this spectrum of motives explains how complicated an ethical analysis of medical publishing will prove to be.

In our view medical publishing ought first and foremost to serve as a way of communicating medical knowledge between clinicians, researchers and other groups involved, and only to a much lesser, if any, extent to serve as a mechanism for personal merit rating.

Medical publishing forms the basis for professional development, both for the medical society as a whole and for the individual clinician. The extent of professional reading and writing activities among doctors shows that these activities are by far the most important educational means in medicine.

There has been a steady increase in the number of scientific journals over the last 300 years at a rate of 6–7% per year. There are now around 20 000–25 000 biomedical journals, of which approximately 3000 are indexed in *Index Medicus/ MEDLINE*. The vast majority of journals are specialized rather than general, and as a result of the specialization of modern medicine new journals are covering ever narrower subspecialties.

No single doctor can keep up with the hundreds of thousands of medical papers published every year, not even within his or her own specialty. An average clinician reads medical literature for three to four hours per week, and most of this time is devoted to medical journals (1). The selection of what is to be read, and what is not, is an important part of the advancement of each doctor's practice, and the decision to read and what to read represents in itself an ethical challenge.

KEY PERSONS AND INTERACTIONS

Publishing involves a chain of key persons and key groups, each to be considered in the ethical analysis: author, editor, referee, publisher/owner, reader, trial patient/healthy volunteer, society. The number of interactions between these seven amount to 21 combinations. If both rights and duties are to be analysed for each actor, and if a further four or five principles are used as analytical angles, then the presentation would be very long and full of indirect repetitions. Consequently, the analysis must be very selective. It should also be centred around the editor, because he or she possesses the strongest influence on the ethical norms and sanctions within the publishing system. This arrangement does not necessarily place the full responsibility with the editor, but emphasizes the important observation post, for the ethics of publishing, at which he is placed.

THE FOUR PRINCIPLES

In Chapter 25 one of us (P.R.) discussed the four principles, their applicability and their ranking. Briefly to sum up, the four principles do not seem to fulfil the demand for groupings, that they are mutually exclusive, and that they are exhaustive, judged in relation to the conceptual universe. Thus the principles may conflict with each other and they are insufficient to cover all ethical considerations. In the present context at least one principle needs to be added to the four: the principle of *freedom*. Here freedom is defined as the sum of known personal options, plus the right to include new options, based, for instance, on innovative activity within arts and sciences, given that the options are legal.

The *right to autonomy, beneficence, non-maleficence* and *justice* cannot be ranked meaningfully in all societal and political universes. This counts especially for autonomy and justice. The right to autonomy within the health system of a democratic welfare state will be limited to options *within* the public health system (possibly with a few, marginal exceptions to serve the principle of justice). On the other hand, the right to autonomy in a very libertarian society might extend this right to include a high degree of personal responsibility for a citizen's own health service (a kind of service-for-fee/fee-for-service principle) at a cost of reduced justice.

In the following analyses we will apply the five principles without any other ranking than the one deducible from the context.

PUBLISHING ETHICS AND THE AWARENESS OF KEY PERSONS

Chapter 25 discussed whether 'the principles' came first, and the awareness of authors, editors etc. evolved from the ethical analyses. The conclusion was that complex ethical judgements often arose from watching serious practical events, without formally applying four or five fundamental principles, one at a time. The principles have rather emerged from repeated judgements, and then secondarily have been applied to new complex situations as a test technique. Again, the principles are not without practical value, but they have to be applied in educational situations, during conferences on ethically complicated cases, etc., instead of being considered a set of universal tools, well suited for ethical nut-cracking.

Despite the analyses resulting from application of the principles, which are later to be demonstrated, more important than introducing the analytical principles would be to open the eyes of all key persons as a first step. This could be done in practical teaching, based on contemporary cases or selected synopses, the overall analysis being primary, and the premises being encompassed secondarily, with or without the four or five principles. To sensitize the publishing profession within the health services in this way is a pressing task. This vast and influential sector has for too long slumbered during the ethical awakening experienced by medicine as a whole.

FRAUD AND MISCONDUCT IN MEDICAL PUBLISHING

Presentation of scientific misconduct is perhaps the most obvious and topical ethical issue in medical publication today. It applies to all key persons mentioned, and concerns all ethical principles.

Honesty is one of the basic norms of science, and science is an enterprise that, more than any other, is supposed to be devoted to truth. This means that scientists must pursue absolute truthfulness and objectivity in their publications and consequently must report only honest data. Unfortunately, this is not always so. Over recent years a number of cases of scientific fraud have been disclosed. In addition to the sad consequences for the authors, referees, editors and readers involved in each proven case of misconduct or fraud, this has also challenged the integrity of scientists in general and of science itself. The extent of deception in medical research is, for obvious reasons, unknown, but it has been stated that the problem is increasing.

Misconduct in medical publication covers a whole spectrum from minor 'adjustments' of data, through plagiarism to conscious falsifications and real fraud. Even widely accepted statistical and methodological practices may be recognized as potentially deceptive (2), and a decision not to publish scientifically valid medical results can in itself be seen as a form of scientific misconduct (3). Unjustified authorship, divided publications (so-called salami publication) and repetitive publication are other offences closely related to misconduct (4).

The pressure to publish has been seen as one of the major forces leading to these problems. Promotion and funding of doctors in academic medicine have been closely linked to the number of their publications, and limiting the number of publications that are to be considered in evaluating a candidate for promotion could be a way to reduce the pressure to publish, and thereby the temptation to undertake dishonest efforts (5). A ceiling has even, more or less seriously, been proposed for the number of papers that an individual researcher is allowed to publish during his lifetime, and if this limit (of for example 50) is reached, an earlier article should be retracted (6).

There is no simple way of dealing with misconduct and fraud in medical science. The main responsibility for preventing such breaches of ethical standards rests on the scientists themselves, and their supervisors within the academic society—i.e. on the *authors*.

Medical journal editors and referees can never act as detectives treating every manuscript with suspicion. Editors have, however, an important role in dealing with the more benign forms of deception such as fragmentation, overinterpretation and duplication, while it is harder for them to recognize plagiarism and fabrication of data (7). Good peer reviewing, and standards set for authorship, multiple publication and other formalities as done by the International Committee of Medical Journal Editors (8) may be helpful in preventing the minor sorts of misconduct, but deliberate fraud can hardly be avoided by such means. Here only active efforts to increase the ethical standards of scientists are effective (9).

THE AUTHOR

For all authors the principle of intellectual *freedom* is indispensable. This principle, additional to the four of the title, is often linked to political freedom of speech. It is, however, fundamental in science, too, as reflected in the many contemporary examples of repression exerted by authoritarian regimes against scientists, whose research fields and results did not suit well the dominating political forces. Repression takes different forms, preventing scientists from doing their work, removing financial support or detaining them from visiting international scientific meetings. In the context of publishing, freedom means the right to publish uncensored. The scientist must have a freedom to publish the results of his research, independent of the interests of funding agencies, governmental authorities and other bodies involved.

Unfortunately some authors mix up *censoring* and *editing,* considering demanded changes or rejection to be signs of a resuscitated tradition of censorship. They thereby forget that rejection of a manuscript will not prevent the author from submitting it to another medical journal, whereas censorship centrally closes *all* publication channels within a country.

The right to *autonomy* is important for the author because he or she preserves the right to withdraw his manuscript if the suggested changes are unacceptable. The author's autonomy is, however, sometimes insulted on a lesser scale, when it comes to editorial changes of the author's personal style. He might find his own peculiar wordings signs of good personal style, whereas the editor finds them incorrect or even misleading. But on many other occasions the condition for accepting an article seems to be invalidating, and scientifically unnecessary, changes of personal style, leading to a dull and dry final result.

The editor's *beneficence* towards authors shows itself on several practical levels. Authors benefit greatly from up-to-date instructions to authors, if the journal has not chosen the even more helpful solution of accepting the Uniform Requirements for Manuscripts Submitted to Biomedical Journals, with a few special additions (8).

Brief evaluation and publication times are considered very beneficent by all authors. The same holds true for openness in the editor's contact with authors, for instance when he rejects a paper and shows the courage to give the grounds for not accepting the paper, instead of just referring to 'our target group of readers' or 'the overwhelming number of manuscripts received during the last month'. Specific beneficence is demonstrated when editors try to educate young authors, despite rejectory their papers, by informing them in detail of their methodological shortcomings, and by showing them a better way of examining scientific problems in future projects.

By insisting on a strict definition of what constitutes a scientific author, editors can counteract the *maleficence* of unrightful authorship. This unfortunately rather common perversion of the authorship concept is a burden to those authors who actually did the work and who wrote the article, and at the same time constitutes misinformation for readers.

The Uniform Requirements for Manuscripts Submitted to Biomedical Journals (8) state that each author should have participated sufficiently in the work to take public responsibility for the content. Authorship credit should be based only on substantial contributions (a) to conception and design, or analysis and interpretation of data; and (b) to drafting the article or revising it critically for important intellectual content; and (c) on final approval of the version to be published. Conditions (a), (b) and (c) must all be met.

Editors may require authors to justify the assignment of authorship. It is an ethical obligation for authors on the one hand to avoid unrightful authorship, and on the other hand to secure that all co-authors that fulfil the requirements for authorship are included. The order of authorship should be a joint decision of the co-authors.

Breaking the author's confidentiality is another kind of maleficence. The International Committee of Medical Journal Editors has consequently issued a set of guidelines for respecting confidentiality (10). Important aspects are 'not disclosing of the author's ideas before publication or by revelation of the confidential details of the review of their manuscript'. It is further stated that 'editors should not disclose information about manuscripts, including their receipt, their content, their status in the reviewing process, their criticism by reviewers, or their ultimate fate. Such information should be provided only to authors themselves and reviewers'. The statement further emphasizes that manuscripts are privileged communications and are the private property of the authors. The authors' rights include protection against public discussion or disclosure of their ideas before publication. Even an internal dissemination within reviewers' institutions through photocopying of unpublished manuscripts is considered unethical. The same is true for reviewers' photocopying of manuscripts for their own files, and for editors' filing of rejected manuscripts. If reviewers wish to seek a secondary opinion from one of their staff members, this can be accepted only with the permission of the editor.

Maleficence by reviewers can be further counteracted by avoiding the anonymity of reviewers. Some journals now demand the signatures of reviewers; others make such open reviewing an option. Undoubtedly an international development is moving towards greater openness.

Securing reviewers' non-maleficence has a complementary concept in the *justice* of this quality-assuring activity. The same is true for the fairness of editors and reviewers. If an author consider a reviewer's or an editor's decision to be unjust, it is important that the journal accepts a mechanism of appeal. Such a procedure could involve the appointment of a new set of reviewers, to give the manuscript a second chance. This is a resource-consuming but fair procedure. Even editors should be ready to reconsider a rejection, if the author brings forward new evidence in favour of acceptance. Such appeal mechanisms can, of course, not go on for ever in the name of justice, but at least the possibility of one further run is a tribute to justice.

THE EDITOR

Editorial *freedom* is of paramount importance to editors and consequently to readers of medical journals (11). Such freedom in relation to the owners is rarely threatened in editorial offices of highly specialized journals, except for the financial aspects of the journal's life. And even such financial barriers to the editor's freedom rarely enter the sphere of contents, but rather the overall editorial line and practice. For editors of general medical journals, for instance owned by medical associations, the editorial freedom can be threatened by political forces and by the indirect influence of advertisers or the national drug industry. Rarely is the freedom to edit and publish pure scientific articles threatened (just as scientific editors show no inclination to interfere with pure announcements of an association). Editorial freedom to write and publish articles and comments within the grey zone of ethical problems, societal aspects of general health policies, etc., is sometimes more in danger. Here a living and readable journal needs room for active scientific journalism and for handling general topics that need not wait for the discussions and decisions of association boards, etc. These editorial degrees of freedom vary with the memberships and chairmanships of the boards involved. Generally speaking editorial freedom is never a static state, but an ideal to be watched and protected as a part of daily editorial work.

Instead of applying a principle of freedom one can consider the principle of *autonomy* as the operational correlate to the concept of editorial freedom. For editors the existence of a contract, clearly stating their rights and duties, besides mechanisms for resolving conflicts, will be an important safety measure. Further support to the editor's right to autonomy can be provided by an independent editorial advisory board. The editor should have direct access to the highest level of ownership, not only to a delegated manager (11). If an editor's right to autonomy is seriously threatened despite these measures, or if major transgressions have taken place, it is important that the international medical community reacts, primarily through the voices of other international editors. As in all cases of threatened intellectual freedom such moral support is often insufficient to turn a given case, whereas it undoubtedly always has some preventive effect towards future transgressions. Hugh Clegg, former editor of the *British Medical Journal*, has said that a medical editor has to be a keeper of the conscience of a profession; if he tries to live up to this ideal he will always be getting into trouble.

It is of great *beneficence* to editors if other key persons within the 'publication game' stick to written and unwritten rules for medical publishing, for instance authors respecting the rules for authorship, double publication and other requirements for manuscripts, referees following guidelines for peer review, publishers respecting editorial freedom, etc.

More than ever a just and unbiased judgement is needed when deciding on which papers to publish. *Justice* in this respect means keeping the ideals of medical publishing (i.e. the communication of sound medical knowledge) high and giving priority to high-quality work of relevance for the readers. The originality, scientific reliability and clinical importance of a paper must be crucial for its acceptance. The paper itself, not the names of its authors or the institution from where it originates, should be considered. On the other hand any pressure for newsy stuff or popular opinions from readers or publishers must also be balanced. The selection of manuscripts for publication has to be handled with special attention to avoid any preferences for 'positive' studies, which may lead to publication bias in a way that excludes important 'negative' studies from the medical literature.

In other words justice must be dominant as regards authors, referees, readers, publishers and society at large.

In relation to other editors a given editor has an obligation to respect the principle of *justice*. It is, for instance, unjust to try to prevent a manuscript from its planned publication by a conference organizer and editor by offering better conditions during a coffee break at the meeting, thus introducing conditions that otherwise are seen only in buying and selling professional football players.

THE REFEREE

The practice of editorial peer review in medical publishing did not become general until after World War II (12). Referring articles to outside experts, commonly two or three per paper, for their judgement is now seen as the normal means of securing the quality of published papers. Ensuring that peer review is as accurate, fair, and quick as possible is one of the principal tasks of most scientific editors (13). It must, however, be emphasized that the referee is an adviser to the editor, and not the final decision-maker.

The referees are selected among the author's peers (hence the term *peer* review). This way of recruiting sometimes raises the possibility of conflicts of interest and other ethical problems.

The question has been raised whether referees have a right to *autonomy* in choosing between anonymity and non-anonymity when reviewing a manuscript. Most journals employ reviewers who remain unknown to the author, while the identity of the author is known to the referee. The technique of blinding peer reviews has been tested, and has been shown to increase the quality of reviews (14). It is, however, still not commonly used.

Central for the reviewer is the principle of *beneficence*, expressed by the referee's key role in the editorial evaluation process. Despite the obvious shortcomings of the scientific referee system, no other way of securing quality of medical publishing has been invented (13). Beneficial to the referee himself is the existence of a set of guidelines for the refereeing process, linked to each journal. The editor's expectations and time limits should be stated clearly.

Risks of *maleficence*, and consequently a demand for explicit non-maleficence, are integrated in reviewers' work as anonymous advisers to journals. Problems may range from possible bias in their assessments, to theft of ideas and hasty duplications of the author's innovative work with priority-competing publications. Such serious transgressions are difficult to discover. A preventive effect can be obtained by issuing guidelines for reviewers. Most journals state in such guidelines that referees should adopt a positive, impartial attitude towards manuscripts. This means, for instance, that manuscripts should be returned immediately, if any conflicts of interest or other reasons preventing an impartial judgement appear. A further aspect of the non-maleficence of publication ethics, related to referees, is the demand that all comments intended for the author's eyes must be presented dispassionately, leaving out all abrasive remarks.

Justice is the overall principle behind the concept of fairness, and underpins that necessity, the appeal mechanism. The knowledge that such a mechanism exists undoubtedly helps to secure just treatment for authors.

THE PUBLISHERS AND THE OWNER

The people representing the political and commercial powers behind a medical journal have their ethical rights and duties too. They have the right to have *their* interests respected by the editor, i.e. a *freedom* to publish their points of view, on, for instance, agreements on appointments to medical associations, or for private publishing companies, to protect their economic interests against undue losses. In important business decisions the editor should, consequently, be involved to the fullest extent possible (11). The freedom of two parties meeting along a borderline, not marked in detail through the landscape, presupposes the presence on both sides of magnanimity and tolerance. If both parties constantly patrol their side of the frontier, both parties suffer, and most certainly so does the journal.

The *beneficence* demand that rests on publishers/owners is to create a sound financial base for the journal and its editorial freedom. A healthy economy is a necessary, but not sufficient, condition for a scientific quality journal. On the other hand, high scientific quality and readability are the editor's responsibility: he is the one who must effect the unnatural but necessary symbiosis between hard economic facts and soft scientific virtues that characterizes scientific publishing.

Non-maleficence for publishers/owners is the complementary principle to *beneficence* for editors: not to interfere with the quality judgements of the editor.

THE READER

This anonymous, paying and reading key person has his ethical concerns, which should be considered by the editor. He sometimes would like to possess the *freedom* to change the dialogue with the author from one-way to two-way. In other words he needs a correspondence column (15) which will enable him not only to raise his voice, but sometimes even to get an answer.

His *right to autonomy* is a right to choose in the last phase of the publishing process. Within his areas of interest he accepts the editor's quality control, but he does not want the editor to be his guardian in selecting the topics to be covered. He needs a *real* choice, i.e. to see a menu, and not just to be served the soup of today. To help him choose the right journal, and to enable him to read selectively, he prefers a journal whose editor has explicitly stated the journal's editorial policy, its target groups and level of approach: clinical, clinical–experimental or basic laboratory research. If editors signal such intentions clearly, the reader will certainly find it very *beneficent*. The same is true for an editorial line of scientific quality, readability and a coverage of topics comprising the entire field, at least within a time horizon of a few years.

Readers will consider themselves rather unprotected and innocent confronted with what later appear to be articles based on scientific fraud. Such *maleficence* must be counteracted by an ethical alliance between authors and editors.

Justice as a fundamental principle concerns the reader, as an underlying condition for editors' and referees' selection of manuscripts for publishing, among the many sent for consideration. It also means, however, such down-to-earth problems as subscription rates and practical access in geographically remote areas. Many readers, and potential readers, in the Third World must inevitably feel the First World price levels and postal cost standing between them and a subscription very unjust, and rightly so.

PATIENTS AND HEALTHY VOLUNTEERS

These in many ways altruistic and necessary co-workers in biomedical research represent important ethical aspects of both clinical and laboratory research. We have come a long way from the cruel transgressions of the Third Reich doctors, with the Geneva Declaration and the Helsinki Declaration, second version; constituting milestones in the protection of trial patients and healthy volunteers. Their *right to autonomy* and to *non-maleficence* are clearly expressed in the Second Helsinki Declaration, and are explicitly backed up by the International Committee of Medical Journal Editors (8), which demands that all manuscripts describing research on man, as a subject, state in the printed version that the underlying experiments were in accordance with the Second Helsinki Declaration and had been accepted by an independent research–ethical committee.

Further protection against *maleficence* is to be found in a statement by the International Committee of Medical Journal Editors on patients' right to anonymity (16,17). It stresses that detailed descriptions or photographs of individual patients, whether of their whole bodies or of body sections (including physiognomies) are sometimes central documentation in medical journal articles. Use of such material may lead to disclosure of a patient's identity, sometimes even indirectly by a combination of pieces of seemingly innocent information. The group strongly advocates that details that might identify patients should be deleted, unless essential for the understanding of the case. Authors and editors have sometimes changed factual information about patients in order to protect their privacy. Despite an obvious gain for patients, such a technique can be considered as deceiving readers, and consequently should be avoided. The group warns against masking of the eye region in clinical photographs as the only protection of anonymity. If in selected cases identification is unavoidable, the patient's informed consent is necessary. In order that these techniques be respected, medical journals are recommended to publish their editorial rules for publishing detailed descriptions of individual patients and photographs, stating that these rules insist that the patient's fully informed written consent to waive anonymity be sent to them.

Moving from individual patients to patient groups the *justice* principle applies to health economics which is being increasingly written about in clinical publications especially in the context of new and old diagnostic procedures, treatments, etc. In this way clinical research is directly linked to countries' health systems and their just distribution of scarce resources.

SOCIETY

The last group interested in the chain of publishing, seen from an ethical angle, is society as a whole. In contrast to prevalent opinions among biomedical scientists ('science is our business and none of society's'), the ethical perspectives of publishing are very important to society.

Society expects that the general freedom of speech also includes biomedical scientific literature.

The *beneficence* of medical publishing is its fundamental role as the main source of innovations to be applied in the health system, university teaching, etc. Without a quality-conscious network of authors and editors, the fast spread of new knowledge would not be possible. If medical journals did not exist, societies would have to invent them to secure a similar beneficent function, and that would be a formidable enterprise.

Some editors feel strongly about early disclosure of medical news to the media, at a time when the results await referee evaluation and detailed publication. Others tackle such problems with less rigour, but still find such disclosure a *maleficence*. Early disclosure directly to the media can be necessary in the case of warnings about new and serious side-effects of drugs in widespread use, in such cases being a beneficence, but in most others early disclosure does more harm than good, because such warnings circumvent the quality control of referees and editors, thereby often misleading the public; cf. the 'cold fusion' example.

THE GREY ZONES

All ethical rules have their neighbouring grey zones. Even if medical journals apply correctly the four or five principles in all central matters, there is still room for extra and outstanding ethical quality. This can be demonstrated in the fair distribution of delay (on a minimal level) between authors; in the eagerness to correct the mistakes that all (repeat: all) editors make; in the time spent educating the young author (unhappy because of his rejected manuscript) in order to help him progress further, etc. Also the ability and willingness to present the underlying reasons for editorial decisions are characteristics of a decent editorial office. Only time ought to set the limits here.

SUMMARY

The world of publishing within the health services has been a very closed one until recently. Authors were scattered, in the first phase anonymous and in the case of a rejected manuscript still so. Editors were autocrats with referees non-existent. Publishers or owners were anonymous plutocrats, and readers a group of grey consumers.

This picture has fortunately changed, and is still changing. Basic ethical principles have been set loose in this sector, with profound consequences for all stages of the publishing process.

When attempting ethical analysis the right to autonomy, beneficence, non-maleficence and justice, plus freedom as a fifth principle, can help us understand the essence of the many non-technical, non-scientific interactions between the many key persons involved. As in other practical fields of biomedicine, the principles are not the only set of tools for the complex judgements necessary. Psychology, health economics, lowered editorial thresholds for important new areas needing a lift, etc., are often complementary to the overall ethical judgement.

Irrespective of analytical techniques, however, the interest in ethics in medical publishing *per se* is a major step forward. Gone are the days when medical publishing was considered primarily an elitist value-free enterprise for the promotion of ambitious authors and prestigious editors.

REFERENCES

 1. Richards, R. K. 1986. Physicians' self-directed learning: a new perspective for continuing medical education. I. Reading. *Möbius* **6** (2): 1–13.
 2. Bailar, J. C. III. 1986. Science, statistics and deception. *Annals of Internal Medicine* **104**: 259–260.
 3. Chalmers, I. 1990. Underreporting research is scientific misconduct. *Journal of the American Medical Association* **263**: 1405–1408.
 4. Huth, E. J. 1986. Irresponsible authorship and wasteful publication. *Annals of Internal Medicine* **104**: 257–259.
 5. Angell, M. 1986. Publish or perish: a proposal. *Annals of Internal Medicine* **104**: 261–262.
 6. Durack, D.T. 1978. The weight of medical knowledge. *New England Journal of Medicine* **298**: 773–775.
 7. Angell, M. 1983. Editors and fraud. *CBE Views* **6** (2): 3–8.
 8. International Committee of Medical Journal Editors. 1991. Uniform requirements for manuscripts submitted to biomedical journals. *British Medical Journal* **302**: 338–341.
 9. Andersen, D., Axelsen, N., Riis, P. and Attrup, L. (Eds). 1992. *The trustworthiness of science* [in Danish]. Health Research Council, Copenhagen.
10. International Committee of Medical Journal Editors. Statements from the Vancouver Group: confidentiality. *British Medical Journal* **299**: 1394.
11. International Committee of Medical Journal Editors. 1988. Editorial freedom. *British Medical Journal* **297**: 1182.
12. Burnham, J. C. 1990. The evolution of editorial peer review. *Journal of the American Medical Association* **263**: 1323–1329.
13. Lock, S. 1991. *A difficult balance*. British Medical Journal, London.
14. McNutt, R. A., Evans, A. T., Fletcher, R. and Fletcher, S. 1990. The effects of blinding on the quality of peer review. *Journal of the American Medical Association* **263**: 1371–1376.
15. International Committee of Medical Journal Editors. 1989. Statements from the Vancouver Group: the role of the correspondence column. *British Medical Journal* **299**: 1394.
16. International Committee of Medical Journal Editors. 1991. Guidelines for the protection of patients' right to anonymity. *Journal of the American Medical Association* **265**: 2697.
17. Riis, P. and Nylenna, M. 1991. Patients have a right to privacy and anonymity in medical publication. *Journal of the American Medical Association* **265**: 2720.

PART IV

HEALTH CARE ETHICS AND SOCIETY

68

Health Care Ethics and Society—Introduction

Raanan Gillon

With the ever-increasing costs of health care, the ever-increasing concern to maintain and improve health as distinct from merely trying to restore good health when people become ill, and the ever-increasing concern of health care workers to carry out scientifically valid research, and the recurring potential tensions between the interests of individual patients and the interests of the community or society as a whole, societal aspects of health care ethics assume ever-increasing importance. In this section a variety of these social contexts are discussed.

In a reflective and stimulating chapter Boyd reminds us of the moral nature of the concepts of health and, less obviously, disease, the latter dependent on the former for its content; and of the danger to medicine if it ever allowed its scientific interest in 'diseases' to overwhelm its humanitarian interest in the wholeness of the people who have diseases (the very etymology of 'health' being an ever-present reminder that wholeness is at its heart).

HEALTH CARE MANAGERS AND ETHICS

Maxwell looks at the wide range of ethical obligations of health care managers, especially those in public health systems. Such managers are at an interface between society and its democratic representatives on the one hand, and patients and their health care workers on the other. Justice and efficiency are, claims Maxwell, their key moral guides. Efficiency (though he does not explicitly say so) is simply the injunction to achieve one's goal with minimal waste of resources, and is thus a way of increasing available resources and thus potential benefit in any context where such waste occurs. Justice for him, and he suspects managers generally, requires both allocation in proportion to need and a utilitarian concern that doing 'cheap and effective things well for many must take precedence over expensive things for a few'. This utilitarianism, however, is of the sort that requires respect for democratic processes, for honesty, and for personal integrity. Among the implications of the latter may be the readiness (and the toughness of character) to eschew the easy way out and instead make decisions in favour of fairer allocation of resources even when such decisions conflict with powerful entrenched interests; and a readiness to expose wrongs and to support those who do so ('Light in dark places—whether they are long-stay wards or children's homes—often depends on the few who have the courage to protest'). And while health care managers in a democracy 'have to be willing to serve under governments with which they disagree', and while Maxwell criticizes Clive Ponting, the civil servant who leaked anonymously criticisms of the government's handling of the Belgrano affair during the Falklands war, nonetheless 'there must in principle be issues on which civil servants and NHS managers should be willing to stand out against official policy to the point of resignation. Otherwise those who simply obeyed orders in Nazi Germany would have been guiltless'.

One of Maxwell's managerial ethical concerns is the strong tendency among clinicians 'to believe that because people definitely need help, the available technology must benefit them. To withhold treatment therefore seems unthinkable. Yet the historical evidence suggests that the therapeutic imperative is all too often misplaced with people often not being helped by the therapies of the day and sometimes being positively harmed.

NEED AND HEALTH CARE ETHICS

That theme has been taken up by Williams, who in his chapter implicitly argues that we should understand the term 'need' to mean 'capacity to benefit'. If we did that we should not waste so many health care resources trying to benefit people whose need is great, in the sense that their plight is severe (the more normal sense of need, which Williams implicitly rejects) but whose great need cannot in fact be met by existing treatments. In this context it seems worth suggesting a compromise position that tries to avoid the idiosyncratic re-definition of the ordinary word 'need' to mean 'capacity to benefit' (most of us can identify many ways in which we have a capacity to benefit, but which we would not dream of claiming as needs—more comfortable cars, holiday homes, more holiday homes, larger incomes, improved artistic sensibilities, the lists are potentially infinite). At the same time such a compromise would recognize the good point being made—notably that it is wrong to waste resources on treatments that we know cannot benefit people—cannot meet their *unmeetable* needs.

My own compromise position is to argue that need creates a presumptive claim in justice or fairness such that the greater the need the greater the presumptive claim on others who have fewer needs. This is consistent with normal humanitarian and medical assumptions that the most seriously ill or at risk take priority in claims upon our assistance, *even if giving them that priority entails that overall welfare is not maximized.* On the other hand to give them such priority should *not* involve giving them useless, non-beneficial treatment—for such treatment uses up resources in activities that by definition are useless and non-beneficial and therefore wastes those resources. What this compromise position does seem to require, however, is vigorous effort to respond to those of their needs that we *can* meet—i.e. to meet their meetable needs. To give an example, those who are inevitably dying may need a cure for their terminal condition, but that need cannot be met, and it would be unhelpful and useless and therefore wasteful to give them high-tech medical treatments if it were known (or extremely probable) that these could not benefit them. However, their needs for comfort, care, respect, concern, palliation of symptoms, *can* be met, and their greater overall needs give them priority over those whose needs are smaller (whose 'plight' is minor), even though the latter's needs could be met completely, more efficiently and more cheaply and with the production of more overall welfare, more quality adjusted life years (QALYs) per unit of resource. Of course this is not to argue that meeting meetable need in proportion to the extent of total need is the *only* relevant criterion for what Williams calls 'vertical equity' in the distribution of scarce health care resources; but it surely is a *necessary* member of any plausible group of relevant criteria. Nor is it clear that these competing criteria (which include Williams's widely shared desire to maximize benefit from a given resource) *can* be amalgamated into a unitary scale of the sort that his costed QALY approach attempts to provide. Instead the costed QALY approach seems more plausibly to be regarded as another of several potentially relevant but conflicting and incommensurable moral criteria, including need, and including respect for the autonomy of those who provide the resources to be distributed.

QALYs AND THE VEIL OF IGNORANCE

Williams is another contributor who proposes the use of the Rawlsian device of a 'veil of ignorance' in order to help us come to impartial decisions about just distribution of scarce health care resources. Yet it seems likely that this approach is highly unlikely to result in a costed QALY approach to distributive justice in health care. Why? Because it seems highly likely that all—or almost all—sick people would wish for their particular medical needs to be met; and that the worse their plight the greater priority they would want to be given to meeting their needs, including a greater priority for concern from their doctors and nurses. In order to maximize the likelihood that this would occur, rational people behind a veil of ignorance would surely propose that a wide spread of different types of health care should be made available to all, so as to maximize their chances of having their health needs met whatever those needs may turn out to be. Even if attempts to meet such needs must be rationed (as they must), people behind the veil of ignorance are surely likely to require at least a reasonable *chance* that any meetable health care need will be met—i.e. if not all kidney transplant needs can be met, they would want at least *some* provision for kidney transplants so as to provide some chance of having such needs met should they arise. It further seems plausible to argue that most people behind a veil of ignorance would prefer that if they were to be seriously ill their doctors and nurses should maintain their care and concern and palliation, even if not much else beneficial could be provided *and even if doing so would 'waste' medical and nursing time that could instead be producing more and cheaper QALYs among less sick patients who had more 'capacity to benefit' from that time and attention.* Yet this form of distribution of health care, plausibly likely to be recommended from behind a 'veil of ignorance', attempting to meet as broad a range of meetable health care needs as possible, and giving priority to those whose 'plights' or needs are more serious over those whose plight or needs are less serious, is not the sort of QALY-maximizing, cost-minimizing, outcome that Williams extols.

Whatever one's views about costed QALYs, there can be no doubt that health economists, and especially Williams and his colleagues at York University, are pushing forward discussion and analysis of both theory and practicalities in the sphere of fair distribution of scarce resources (a fascinating example is the York representation of Aristotle's formal theory of justice in chart form, with equals being treated equally represented as 'horizontal equity' and unequals being treated unequally in relation to some relevant inequality being represented as 'vertical equity'). While the clarity of Williams's proposals serves for many only to make their moral inadequacy pellucid, that very clarity demands equally clear alternatives, and such are few and far between. In their absence societies may, nonetheless, find it morally preferable to accept a variety of less precise, more clumsy, ways of attempting to respect the complexity and variety of the competing moral concerns of justice, than to settle for a simple and utterly clear approach that nonetheless seems to many to fail to respect some cherished values.

HEALTH PROMOTION

Tountas and colleagues look at the ethics of health promotion, analysing not only the standard interpersonal ethics of the doctor–patient relationship in the special context of healthy or apparently healthy patients, but also the societal and employment concerns and pressures that may impinge on that relationship. These include, as in ordinary therapeutic medicine, issues of major cost and thus of resource distribution—they contrast, for example, a low cost-per-life-saved anti-smoking campaign with a cervical screening campaign having a very high cost per life saved. In addition they discuss the socially divisive effects of differential benefits, when health promotion campaigns tend to favour the better-off groups in societies, thus exacerbating existing social inequalities in health status. And they warn about the potentially negative social effects of health promotion where it promotes not health but 'healthism' and its correlate 'medicalization', and of the dangers of 'victim blaming'. Nonetheless, they argue, awareness of such possible dangers, combined with sensible moral analysis of specific proposed projects, allows the potentially beneficial and autonomy respecting outcomes of good health promotion to be achieved, while minimizing its potential harms and wrongs.

PUBLIC HEALTH AND EPIDEMIOLOGY

Related themes are taken up later in the section by both Last and McCallum. In a wide-ranging discussion about ethics and epidemiology, one of Last's discussion points concerns the difference between epidemiological research and epidemiological practice. Just as ordinary medical practice does not need to go before research ethics committees, he implicitly argues, so, too, ordinary epidemiological practice should not have to go before such committees, and thus be subjected to delay. But might this distinction between work and research be inappropriate in the context of moral analysis of epidemiology and public health?

Its importance in clinical medicine is that it marks the distinction between the Hippocratic or therapeutic intent ('whatever I do and propose is primarily intended for your medical benefit') and the use of medical interventions for purposes not primarily intended for the particular patient's benefit. The importance of that distinction is that the patient can rely on doctors, in the therapeutic relationship, only to ask for personal and often extremely private information, only to propose interventions that may expose the patient to harm, risk or inconvenience, if the doctor believes that to do so is for the patient's medical benefit. Patients in the therapeutic relationship can with confidence 'drop their guard', trusting the doctor to act in their best interests. Research proposals, on the other hand, have to be monitored by ethics committees (Institutional Review Boards in the USA) precisely because that therapeutic or Hippocratic commitment to the individual patient is in doubt: either it is competing with an intent to acquire knowledge for the benefit of *other* potential patients of the future, as in therapeutic research, or it is entirely absent, as in non-therapeutic research. When medical researchers want access to patients' records in projects not intended to benefit the particular patients whose records they consult, they submit their projects to ethical scrutiny so as to ensure—and demonstrate to the public—that the interests of those individual patients are protected when doctors are intending to *use* them, and private information about them, in order to benefit others. Some argue that such ethics committee approval should not be granted unless individual consent is obtained from each patient whose notes are consulted; but few would accept that neither patient consent *nor* ethics committee review is needed.

If this rationale is appropriate for non-therapeutic research access to medical records it is difficult to see why non-therapeutic medical practice, whether in epidemiology or in public health or in any other discipline, should be exempt from ethics committee review. If access to the patient's confidential record is proposed not for the benefit of the patient but for some other purpose, then it seems that either direct consent from the patient is needed, or where that is impossible or impractical, approval by an appropriate ethics committee.

To set against this somewhat 'purist' approach, in which respect for the autonomy of the patient seems to many to weigh too heavily against the overall public interest, it may be worth considering ways in which presumed consent to such use of records, under the conditions of strict confidentiality described by Last, could be introduced so as to combine both respect for patients' autonomy and minimal impediments to medical research and the practice of epidemiology and public health medicine. One way might be to ask patients in advance for such consent, as part of the normal booking procedures (do you consent to your medical records being used for bona-fide medical research and public health activities under conditions of strict medical confidentiality?). Another approach might be for national health organizations, or indeed other health schemes, to state that, for the development of medical science and protection and promotion of public health, consent is presumed to such use of medical records unless the patient explicitly objects; and a third, more draconian approach would be to specify that it is a condition of treatment under the service that such use may be made of the records.

OCCUPATIONAL HEALTH CARE

While the ethical tension for public health doctors and epidemiologists is between the traditional Hippocratic obligation to the individual patient and their professional obligations to whole communities, occupational health physicians and nurses have several different roles simultaneously, the main ethical tension being between their role as personal practitioner and their role as employee or at least functionary of the company that employs their services. McCallum considers some of these dilemmas, describing solutions widely accepted within occupational health practice. For example in Britain occupational health practice has since the 1960s rejected arguments that because companies fund their occupational health services therefore they own their records and therefore they have a right of access to them. This professional stance does not stop companies sometimes trying on the argument, and, writes McCallum, 'NHS management has been one of the worst offenders in this respect, and in many cases very strong pressure is put on doctors to comply with requests for release of records.' Another ethical problem arises when managements try to use the occupational physician to get rid of an individual on medical grounds because they 'find it difficult to sack him on other grounds'. This of course 'has to be resisted by the physician on ethical grounds and it has to be made clear by the physician that he should not be asked to carry out what is essentially a function of company management'.

AIDS, DRUG ADDICTION, ETHICS AND SOCIETY

The moral tensions between obligations to society and to individual patients are nowhere more evident to many than in the contexts of both AIDS and drug addiction. Yet two contributors argue that the tension in both these contexts is largely illusory. Pinching, in an encouraging account 'from the front line', argues that this is because the only effective way of protecting the public health rests 'entirely on being able to influence positively the autonomous behaviour of the individual, whether infected or uninfected'. The more supportive both public and professional attitudes and behaviour are to the individual the more likely is such influence to be received and acted on. Similar reasoning leads Pinching to argue that for him, and in the context of AIDS at least, confidentiality is 'so near absolute as makes no difference'—and he cites the justification of an English judge; 'In the long run preservation of confidentiality is the only way of securing the public health . . . for unless those infected come forward they cannot be counselled and self treatment does not provide the best care.' Pinching also has some interesting observations about the role of the four principles in his own ethical approach to the management of the new disease, AIDS, and to medical ethics in general. It was not that he and his colleagues consciously used the principles in developing their policies of 'patient empowerment', the offering of potentially beneficial options, warnings about risks of these options, openness about the realities (including the reality of an earlier death) and a concern for the general good (for example via research)—rather that 'what has emerged seems also to embody—perhaps by good fortune, perhaps by subconscious design—the four principles of medical ethics . . . . That they emerge naturally in the response to the practical necessities of clinical care in this most tragic, complex and socially pervasive disease, encourages me—as a mere clinician—to think that the four principles do indeed have a powerful validity in the ultimate assay: the real world of clinical medicine.'

The theme that the perceived tension between the moral obligation to provide medical care for the individual patient and concern for the welfare of society is often illusory is also pursued by ten Have, writing about addiction to hard drugs. Too often, he believes, this tension is seen as stark—if the doctor treats the patient as having the illness of drug addiction, then terrible social consequences will follow, with the 'war against drugs' being undermined by ever more extensive a spread of the 'epidemic' of drug addiction and all the social evils that accompany it. Many of the social evils of drug addiction are the result of repressive social policies, he argues, and doctors and health care workers have been drawn into becoming part of the 'social supervision mechanism'. Instead society would itself benefit by re-establishment of the normal medical objective of helping the patient to 'relieve the drug abuse and ameliorate the primary problems of drug use'. Support and rehabilitation of the patient is the primary obligation of health care workers—and its pursuit—often requiring unconventional means—also benefits society by making it possible for health care workers to gain the trust of addicts and thus 'raise their health consciousness . . . change their injecting behaviour, and . . . distribute clean needles. These are public health benefits, easily lost in a repressive policy that makes no distinction between criminalization of drug users and drug traffickers'.

MEDICAL RESEARCH

The moral conflict between concern for the individual patient and concern for society is not so readily dissolved in the context of medical research, and several of the contributors to this section address it. Ackerman argues for what he calls 'the presumptive weighting strategy'. This gives presumptive priority to the interests of research subjects: 'However, this presumption may be overridden if it is necessary to undertake research activities that may prevent or remove important harms to others and there will be no more than minor compromises in protections for the interests of subjects.' This strategy, he argues, combines a respect for the priority of obligation to the research subject with a moral concern to promote the social good and a recognition that such social concerns must nonetheless not be allowed to override obligations to individuals in any substantially harmful ways (in an earlier strand of the argument he links such an approach to the widely recognized moral obligation to help others in severe danger where such help would cause the helper or rescuer only minor harm or inconvenience).

In a complementary paper, Lane, an American anthropologist with a nursing background, gives her perceptions of the development of research ethics guidelines in a developing country, Egypt. Until recently, she claims, lack of mechanisms for ethics review of research proposals had permitted instances of excessively risky human subject research. Contemporary developments within Egyptian medicine have led to the publication of *Ethical guidelines for human reproduction research in the Muslim world*, which include the recommendation that all such research is approved by a research ethics committee (1). Lane rightly warns that interpretation of general principles is likely to be highly culture-relative, and that this is as true of the Beauchamp and Childress four principles as of any others. However, her fears that the principle of respect for autonomy may not be acceptable within Egyptian (and other) cultures need careful unpacking. There are worries about how the principle would in fact be interpreted in a particular social and cultural context; worries about whether in practice people will allow the principle to guide their actions, even though they might in theory accept it; and worries about whether the principle is even in theory acceptable. So far as the first is concerned, I have argued in my introduction to the first section of this book that respect for autonomy not only permits but almost certainly in practice entails variable, culture-relative interpretation. So far as the second is concerned, rejection in practice of theoretically accepted moral values, this of course is a continual problem in all social contexts—the eternal battle between good on the one hand and evil, apathy, weakness and selfish self-interest on the other. However, it is not a specific problem for the principle of respect for people's autonomy, though its implementation in practice is likely, as Lane points out, to be more problematic in cultures whose traditions regularly override it in practice for certain groups, including women and sick people. So far as the third is concerned, suffice it to refer readers to the chapters in this volume by Serour and Hasan, who demonstrate that respect for autonomy is indeed an integral aspect of Islamic ethics, as are the other three principles.

MEDICAL TECHNOLOGY

Part of Jennett's chapter on medical technology also focuses on the social importance of research, not only in the context of drug research—its usual focus—but also in the contexts of technology and of surgery. Identifying two common faults in clinical attitudes to the use of technology, inadequately informed over-criticism and inadequately informed over-enthusiasm, he urges that technologies should be as rigorously subjected to quality assessment as are medications, preferably by controlled clinical trials but otherwise by accurate prospective audit. And he suggests that those responsible should make it a condition of funding and continuing support for any new technology that formal assessment both before and during use should be carried out. With the coalface understanding of an involved neurosurgeon Jennett dissects out various types of socially undesirable and inappropriate use of technologies (pithily characterized as unnecessary, unsuccessful, unkind, unsafe, unwise, and unwanted) and describes some of the motivations for these inappropriate uses. The desire to do or be seen to do *something* even for hopelessly ill patients (a recurring concern in this section); the 'excuse of uncertainty about prognosis' or of 'the possibility that intervention might help'; the 'cycle of commitment' in which one carer refers on to another, who thus feels committed to doing something; and having started then naturally tends to go on to the next stage along the line, regardless of probability of success; the paradoxical greater reluctance to stop unhelpful efforts to prolong life than not to start them in the first place; technical surgical 'dicta' such as 'arrest haemorrhage or relieve obstruction' (of the bowel); the fear, unfounded at least in Europe according to Jennett, of litigation if a doctor does not 'do everything possible'. Though understandable, such tendencies must be resisted where further intervention would be futile—for in such cases the medico-moral obligation to produce net benefit for the patient cannot be achieved; and continued intervention wastes resources that could otherwise be used for patients who *could* benefit from those resources.

A SOCIOLOGICAL ANOMALY

The chapter by Armstrong and Humphrey is an anomaly. In inviting a sociological contribution I had anticipated either sociological evidence that despite enormous variations in people's and cultures' actual behaviour certain common moral themes could be discerned, such as the four principles and or others: *or* sociological evidence that there were no such common moral themes, or that if there were any, they did not include one or more of the four principles. Alas, little such *evidence* appears. Instead the authors treat us to *ex-cathedra* assertions (e.g. 'Sociologists now recognize that the search for universal principles governing human behaviour is a futile one'); implied false antitheses ('The first question that a sociologist would ask about the four basic principles is whether they are genuine principles—in the sense of being universal attributes of human morality—or values that are socially derived'); and fanciful but unsupported hypotheses ('The function of medical ethics is neither to change nor study the world, but to reveal it as spectacle'). The authors imply that there could be no common moral principles shared by different societies because of 'the immense variation' of human behaviour. Yet it is clear that immensely variable moral behaviour *could* nonetheless share certain common themes, and indeed much of the material in this book suggests that it does. They reserve their strongest fire for the principle of autonomy, claiming that the very notion of personal autonomy emerged only some 200 years ago, that the 'ethical principle of autonomy, more than any of the others, celebrates western moral supremacy' and that 'there is no fundamental reason why the notion of autonomy, despite its widespread acceptance in western societies, should survive another two centuries into the future'. Yet one of the few positive things they have to say about contemporary medical ethics is to praise its 'emphasis on the legitimacy of different views'. Extrapolating from their implied moral relativism, this legitimacy presumably only applies in societies subject to 'western moral supremacy', and can be expected to evaporate even in those societies within a couple of centuries, as the principle of respect for autonomy, which I take morally to underpin this 'legitimacy', meets its quietus. Well, readers will make up their own minds about the usefulness, rigour and persuasiveness of this chapter: as an advocate of the transcultural value of the four principles, and as one who has experienced their acceptance in a variety of international and intercultural contexts, I intended, in commissioning and then not rejecting this somewhat contemptuous and dismissive chapter, to respect the autonomy both of its writers and of its readers!

REFERENCE

1. Serour, G. I. and Omran, A. R. (eds). 1992. *Ethical guidelines for human reproduction research in the Muslim world.* International Islamic Center for Population Studies and Research, Al-Azhar University. Cairo.

69

Health Care Ethics, Health and Disease

The Reverend Dr Kenneth M. Boyd

Is 'health' simply the absence of 'disease'? If we try to define these two terms, we find that they cannot be contrasted so easily, because while 'disease' is a *medical* category, 'health' is a *moral* one. The four principles of health care ethics provide a helpful framework for understanding some implications of this.

Alex Millar had a small business in a country town. He was a local councillor and church elder, and was popular in the community. He played golf with the local doctor, but rarely consulted him. In his 50s Mr Millar suffered from a duodenal ulcer and, after trying various ineffectual remedies, agreed to surgery which was successful. In his 60s he was again admitted to hospital, to investigate occasional vomiting: diverticulitis was diagnosed and he was reassured that this was not serious. Aged 79, feeling faint while out walking, he consulted a general practitioner, who explained that mild heart failure was not unusual at his age, and put him on appropriate drugs. The faintness did not recur and Mr Millar continued to lead an active life, bowling, fishing or gardening most days. In the July following his 86th birthday he and his wife went to see his older sister in Canada, whose Alzheimer's disease was much worse than on their last visit. Mr Millar fainted on the flight across, but quickly recovered without medical attention, and enjoyed his holiday, swimming in the lake, gardening and hill-climbing. Back home again, early in October, he had a sudden chest pain, lost consciousness and felt ill for some days. He was soon almost back to normal, but on his doctor's advice agreed to take things more easily. He continued to enjoy his pipe and whisky. In November, a little while after spending an afternoon clearing leaves from his garden, he collapsed and died within an hour. One of the last things he said was not to bother sending for the doctor.

Assume, for a moment, that health is the absence of disease. Draw a vertical line with 'health' at the top and 'disease' at the bottom, and at right angles to this a horizontal line with Mr Millar's 50th birthday at one end and his 86th at the other. Then plot the graph. If you are a doctor, dislike sophistry, and plot what you know about, a curve might emerge. But what if Mr Millar himself, a

---

Principles of Health Care Ethics. Edited by Raanan Gillon.
© 1994 John Wiley & Sons Ltd

member of his family or one of his friends had been asked to do this? Up to his last birthday, and probably until a month before he died, their graph would have looked very different. Everyone who knew him said how fit he looked, how young he was for his years; and when he died, friends of his own age found it difficult to believe that *they* had survived *him*. Even his death, in old age, with no suffering, was curiously in keeping with most people's idea of him as fit, young for his years, the picture of health.

Was that picture deceptive? Does the presence of disease, however slow its progress, exclude the possibility of health? That may sound like Solon's ancient paradox 'call no man happy until he is dead' (ref. 1, p. 47), or invite the modern rejoinder that 'life is a sexually-transmitted condition with 100% mortality' (Dr C. T. Currie, personal communication). But what we mean by 'disease' and 'health' is worth exploring in the context of health care ethics, since our answer can influence how we resolve moral conflicts.

This chapter will explore, in particular, the linguistic origins and implications of these two words, and especially the prolific metaphor of 'health'. But it may be useful to look first at another context where definitions of 'health' and 'disease' are needed—in relation to the goals of health education or promotion. In that context a number of definitions and models have recently been suggested, notably by Seedhouse (2), and by Downie *et al.* (3). The following outlines some aspects of the latter's perspective on disease and health.

DISEASE, ILL-HEALTH AND POSITIVE HEALTH

Disease, Downie *et al.* point out, is only one aspect of 'ill-health'. *Ill-health*, the 'negative' dimension of health, includes not only medically defined conditions, but also the experience of *illness*. The 'positive' dimension, or *'positive health'*, also involves more than one aspect—in this case both *'fitness '*and *'well-being'*. The goals of health promotion, therefore, are not only 'the prevention of physical, mental and social ill-health', but also 'the balanced enhancement of physical, mental and social facets of positive health' (ref. 3, p. 25).

This approach broadly accepts, but tries to refine, the 1946 World Health Organization definition of health as 'a state of complete physical, mental and social well-being, and not merely the absence of disease or infirmity'. An obvious criticism of that definition is that it is overambitious. 'Complete physical, mental and social well-being' is as difficult to measure as it is to achieve. Is not 'the absence of disease or infirmity', a simpler, more straightforward and more realistic goal?

Downie *et al.* doubt this, arguing that ill-health is more difficult to pin down than is often thought. It cannot be defined simply in terms of disease; people sometimes have a disease without feeling ill (a rash, for example); indeed their symptoms may be too minor to make much sense of saying that they are ill. On the other hand, some people may have unwanted symptoms (nausea, faintness, headaches, for example) when no disease or disorder appears to be present. But the fact that a condition is unwanted is not a sufficient reason to describe it as ill-health: it may be the normal infirmity of old age, for example. A condition's abnormality, however, is not sufficient either: a disability or deformity may be abnormal, but the person who has it may not be unhealthy; and much the same may apply to someone who has had an injury.

A complex combination of *'abnormal, unwanted,* or *incapacitating* states of a biological system' (ref. 3, p. 15), therefore, may have to be taken into consideration in order to assess whether or not physical ill-health is present. Things may be even more complicated when assessing *mental* ill-health: abnormal states of mind may reflect minority, immoral or illegal desires which are not sick desires; while a psychopath, for example, may neither regard his state as unwanted, nor experience it as incapacitating.

Positive health also is a complex concept, including the notions both of well-being and of fitness. A feeling of well-being alone is not sufficient to indicate positive health: 'it would be difficult', Downie *et al* (3) observe, 'to make a case for viewing an acute schizophrenic state with mood elevation and a blissful lack of insight as one of positive health' (p. 18). *'True' well-being,* rather, includes 'essential reference to some conception of the "good life" for a human being' and 'some conception of having a measure of control over one's life', including its social and political dimensions (p. 18). *Fitness* also requires further qualification; the 'specialist' fitness sought in athletic training, for example, sometimes is detrimental to physical health, and the desire to maximize physical fitness as an end in itself may become an unhealthy obsession. In many cases positive health requires only a 'minimalist' notion of fitness, age-related and geared to everyday activities.

In these authors' perspective then, health is 'the sum or product of all its components', both negative and positive. They also observe that 'the *precise* quantification of an individual's health is impossible' (ref. 3, p. 24)—not just because the sum is complex, but also because the components include value judgements. What this reference to value judgements suggests, in other words, is that while 'disease' is a *medical* category, 'health' is a *moral* one.

DIS-EASE, WHOLENESS, AND HUMAN WHOLENESS

A different route to the same conclusion—that 'disease' is a medical category and 'health' a moral one—can be found by examining the linguistic roots of 'disease' and 'health'. The medical category, for example, is a particular use of the more general *'dis-ease'*, or absence of ease; and the word 'ease' (when traced back through Romance to Latin origins—from 'aise' to 'adjaces' to 'adjacere') (4), appears to be essentially concerned with the idea of unimpeded movement through adjacent space. (The association of 'ease' with 'comfort' need not contradict this suggestion if one remembers that 'comfort' originally meant 'to make strong'.) At the most primitive level, therefore, a need for the notion eventually refined into that of disease, seems to arise from awareness of an obstacle to free movement. Thus the development from this simple idea of an obstacle to the medical category of disease, can be seen as a matter of defining the obstacle ever more precisely, with a view, where possible, to removing it.

'Health', by contrast, is derived (through 'heilida') from a Germanic root, related to the less simple and more elusive idea of being 'whole'. At the most primitive level the idea of *wholeness* seems to reflect an awareness, not of an

obstacle, but of empty space, which (by analogy with the more specific proverbial vacuum) human nature does not readily tolerate. One of the few things that can be said with much certainty about human nature, indeed, concerns our reaction to empty space—unknown territory, whether in the world around us, or in thought. Our natural tendency is towards movement rather than passivity; and although our initial reaction when confronted by the unknown may be to retract our tentacles and adopt a frozen posture, sooner or later we move, in an attempt either to get away from or to explore the latest empty external or mental space of which we have become aware.

The idea of wholeness seems to emerge from this movement to explore the unknown or empty space: if we can encircle and investigate the space (or some part of it) so that we comprehend it as somehow coherent, we regard that as a 'whole'. But it seems 'whole' only as long as our attention is fixed on what we have comprehended. When our attention shifts we become aware of further gaps or spaces in our understanding, and this relativizes or fragments the 'whole' we had encircled. Thus we have to begin exploring all over again, unless we choose to regard the unknown as itself a whole encircling us, to which (whether seen as threatening or as reassuring) stillness seems to be a more appropriate response.

'Wholeness', therefore, is an elusive idea; and it is even more elusive if we attempt to apply it to ourselves. We may speak of someone having a 'well-rounded character', or an 'integrated personality'. But any notion of *'human wholeness'* is culturally relative and provisional in the extreme. One reason for this is that our only tool for defining and measuring whatever 'human wholeness' might be, is the 'whole' of human knowledge. But that (like classical physics after relativity) is only approximately valid under defined circumstances, which clearly makes it inadequate for our purpose. In human beings, moreover, choice (albeit often hardened into habit) appears to take over at some point the place of instinct in other animals so that, beyond meeting the bare needs of mere survival, we have to determine our own cultural and personal goals. Thus, while we may have some agreed ideas about the specific characteristics which identify a 'good' member of another species, the question of a 'good' ('good for what?'), let alone a 'whole', human being has proved sufficiently difficult and controversial to have kept countless philosophers in employment for over 2000 years.

HEALTH AND METAPHOR

'Health', insofar as it derives from applying the notion of wholeness to human experience, also is likely to be an elusive idea. This need not cause problems if 'health' is regarded simply as a *metaphor*. That is how (like very many other words) it probably entered the language. Used with reference mainly to bodily wholeness (in practice, to feelings of well-being and the appearance of fitness), the metaphor covers sufficient common ground in the thinking of different individuals to serve its purpose: everyone has some idea of what 'health' means, and one person's ideas overlap sufficiently with those of another to reassure us that we are talking about the same thing.

Metaphors, however, are rarely as simple as they seem. Like human beings, they are both prolific and problematic. When we are exploring unknown territory in our thinking, a metaphor can suggest connections which we otherwise might not see, and in this way help us to orientate ourselves for practical purposes. But if a metaphor does this often and successfully enough, its implications and applications tend to proliferate.

'Health', for example, may have entered the language successfully because it helped us say something about the body, useful among other reasons, perhaps, for breeding purposes. But in doing so it did not shed the wider overtones of wholeness. The metaphor was readily extended (at least by the seventeenth century) both to spiritual health (for example in the Anglican General Confession: 'there is no health in us'), and to the body politic (for example in Shakespeare's reference [*Hamlet*, Act I, scene iii] to 'the safety and the health of the whole state'). In more recent times it has been extended further, to include not just the state, but society, groups within it, and states of affairs of various kinds.

Many of these extensions are generally acknowledged to be metaphorical. But they serve their purpose, which is to help orientate our action. These extended metaphors, moreover, normally modify, rather than radically change, action already orientated by other powerful metaphors. To call an accountant a 'company doctor', for example, may go a little way towards changing his balance sheet into the fever chart of a patient whose interests come first. But it is not likely to go very far; and even less mileage, of course, can be expected from 'doctoring the books', if that metaphor is offered as a mitigating plea to an authority aware that an accountant not only counts but also is accountable.

Extending a metaphor may have more significant practical consequences, however, if it is applied to spheres where there are no strongly competing metaphors already orienting action. Notions like 'healthy behaviour' and 'mental health' illustrate this. Since the Renaissance, the loosening grasp of traditional religion and morality on the popular imagination has weakened most potential rival metaphors, or at least limited their sphere of influence. The notion of mental health, in particular, goes back at least as far as Juvena's '*mens sana in corpore sano*', and so in this sense already seems familiar. Extending the metaphor of 'health' from the body to the mind is also given an easier passage, of course, when it is remembered that the functions of the brain cannot be dissociated from those of the body.

But the brain is not the same thing as the mind. Simply to allude to the vast amount of philosophical argument and scientific enquiry related to that fact, perhaps is sufficient to indicate the scale of the problems caused by extending the metaphor of 'health' in this direction. Extending the metaphor to mental health, that is, simply magnifies the problem of defining physical health with any precision.

One aspect of this problem is that a precise definition of 'health' may seem possible only by admitting exceptions which appear to empty the word of any meaning. Downie *et al.*, for example, argue very convincingly that 'true well-being' is a necessary condition of health, and that this entails 'some conception of having a measure of control over one's life'. But insofar as control over one's life is measured, ultimately, in terms of inner freedom, or psychological adjustment to one's circumstances, there are virtually no external circumstances or (at least physical) states of ill-health which of themselves prevent one having such a conception. The argument that 'positive' health need require only a 'minimalist' notion of fitness points in a similar direction. In other words, if someone has made his own psychological adjustment to the fact that he will shortly die in a state of total physical dependency, it may be difficult to deny that he lacks the minimum requirements of positive health.

This conclusion is not necessarily a criticism of the model proposed by Downie *et al.* for health promotion purposes (since they take disease and illness into account as well as positive health). But stretching the metaphor this far may well seem to evacuate 'health' of virtually any content. On the other hand, to recognise the possibility of 'health' in someone with an advanced terminal disease, is not entirely to deprive the word of its meaning. A physically dependent patient who has come to terms with his past life and his approaching death, for example, may well feel, and thus (because no-one else is better placed to judge) *be* nearer to 'wholeness' than ever before. Good terminal care will recognize and respond to this, however paradoxically, as a sign of health, whether or not the word 'health' actually is used to describe it. This recognition of and response to signs of health, indeed, is characteristic of all good health care of what is ambitiously called 'the whole person'.

OPEN SYSTEMS AND MORAL JUDGEMENT

It may now be clear why it is entirely appropriate that 'health' is so difficult to define. To 'define' something is to determine its limits (literally, 'to bring it to an end'). But a metaphor reaches its limits only when its power to generate new insights is exhausted, or when it is extended into an area where other metaphors have greater power to generate more fruitful insights. Neither of these conditions appears, as yet, to be true of 'health'.

The difference between 'disease' and 'health', it might be suggested, is reminiscent of the Aristotelian distinction between closed and open systems: 'closed systems degenerate' but 'non-degenerating systems are not closed' (5). 'Disease' belongs to the sphere of bodily systems which typically degenerate and are eventually 'closed' by death; and it is the object of systematic enquiry, seeking sufficient precision and certainty to 'close' debate on any particular question. The fact that medical science itself shows no sign of degenerating indicates that it has remained open to its inexhaustible subject matter. The only real risk of it becoming a closed, and hence degenerating system, is if it ignores the human subject in its subject matter, the person, in its preoccupation with the disease.

Medicine's dedication to 'health' safeguards it against this risk. The metaphor's openness invites extension into the notions of 'mental health', 'healthy behaviour' and 'public', or 'community health'; and this keeps both medicine and society open to the importance of many health-related factors which, because they are difficult to measure, might otherwise be ignored. This openness inevitably means that the metaphor will be extended to spheres in which its influence, and the insights it generates, may be thought inappropriate: the political, religious and moral spheres are obvious examples.

The influence and insights of health are inappropriate to these spheres, however, only if 'health' is allowed to dominate thinking in them. Health, obviously, is not the only thing to be valued, and for individuals or society to make it their primary goal would actually be counterproductive. The best defence against the undesirable (and it must be said, unlikely) possibility of 'health' becoming too dominant lies in the power and fruitfulness of other metaphors. But it is also important here to emphasize again that 'health' is not only a metaphor but also a *moral* category. Claims made in the name of 'health', that is, are essentially contestable and negotiable. This, in the end, is why 'health' cannot be compared in any simple or straightforward way with the largely uncontestable and non-negotiable medical category of 'disease'.

To determine how healthy someone or something is, therefore, is ultimately a matter not of scientific but of *moral judgement*. The essential features of moral judgement are summed up in Aristotle's definition of the human faculty which exercises it—'phronesis' or practical wisdom. This, he says (see ref. 1, p. 337), is 'a truth-attaining rational quality concerned with action in relation to things that are good or bad for human beings'. The fact that moral judgement is 'concerned with action' is crucial. As 'truth-attaining' and 'rational', it must take known and available facts into account. But because it is concerned with action, it must take responsibility for deciding which facts are relevant, and cannot afford to wait for the moral equivalent of a pathologist's report. As a result of this, particular moral judgements are always provisional, and in studying ethics we must be content with 'a broad outline of the truth' and 'generally valid conclusions' (see ref. 1, p. 9).

WHO MAKES THE MORAL JUDGEMENT?

This account of moral judgement may help to make sense of an apparent paradox noted earlier. Good terminal care, it was suggested, will recognize and respond to a sign of 'health' when a patient, however physically dependent, in his own eyes approaches 'wholeness' through coming to terms with his past life and approaching death. The apparent paradox here lies not in the patient's feeling of wholeness, but in the suggestion that his carers should see this as a sign of 'health'. His carers, after all, do not need to wait for a pathologist's report to know that he is dying; and it is morally as well as medically wrong to respond to this patient as other than gravely ill, as far as his physical condition is concerned. But as long as he remains or is kept lucid, his carers do not need to wait for a psychiatrist's report either, to make the moral judgement that he is healthy as far as his mental (and if they wish to extend the metaphor in this way, his spiritual) condition is concerned. The fact that he has only a short time to live provides no material evidence against that conclusion.

What is material, however, is *who* makes the moral judgement. Those who provide health care normally and naturally respond to someone whom they judge to be 'healthy' as a person rather than as a patient; and it is this particular patient's entitlement to be regarded as nothing less than a person, which requires moral recognition *by health carers* of nothing less than the 'health' that is in him. It is equally important for health carers to recognize such signs of 'health' when they are present in patients who are not dying, but whose 'disease or infirmity' again might make it seem that the metaphor is being stretched too far.

A much-discussed, if relatively rare, moral dilemma illustrates the importance of this in a patient who is not dying. The dilemma arises when a totally physically dependent patient makes a well-considered request for euthanasia. A crucial aspect of any morally appropriate response to this, is whether the carer to whom the request is addressed (who, if he is a doctor, has the technical means to grant it) judges that the patient is mentally healthy. In this case there is time, and there may be a responsibility, to seek first a psychiatric opinion. But again, the absence of disease is not sufficient reason for moral recognition of signs of 'health', which (provided there are no objections on other grounds) might justify granting the request. The responsibility for the moral judgement about signs of 'health' remains firmly on the shoulders of the carer to whom the request is addressed.

THE FOUR PRINCIPLES

The four principles, of beneficence, non-maleficence, respect for autonomy, and justice, provide a helpful framework for understanding the implications of this dilemma. Because euthanasia is discussed elsewhere in this book, only a few features of that framework need be mentioned here.

The principles of *beneficence* and *non-maleficence* require, first of all, clinical assessment of the patient's medical condition, including any psychiatric aspects, and the social background. This is needed to establish that there are no treatment (of clinical depression, for example) or other alternatives to the harm of killing, which the patient might be or become willing to accept. These two principles, however, also require the doctor to make a clinical assessment of potential physical or psychological harm which might result from not granting the patient's request (for example, the physical or psychological consequences of a failed suicide attempt).

If clinical assessment establishes no alternative to seriously considering the patient's request, the principle of *respect for autonomy* requires the doctor to provide good reasons for *not* judging the patient to be (at least mentally) 'healthy'. This requires the doctor seriously to consider, but not necessarily to grant, the request. He is not obliged to do so, for example, if this would infringe his own autonomy of conscience (although this is correlative to the patient's entitlement to a second opinion). He might also, more contestably, decide against granting the request by arguing from the view (6) that autonomy or

freedom presupposes the right to life. In the context of physical life, death is the exact opposite of freedom, the end of freedom. Freedom cannot negate itself: it is therefore not admissible to choose to become a slave. For that reason, in the event of a suicide attempt, a person who intervenes, even by force, to prevent this act . . . is not robbing but restoring that individual's freedom.

The requirements of *justice* also must be considered. It has been observed (7) that while 'all moral ideas interpenetrate each other', justice 'includes most of the others'. It includes, moreover, both the idea of weighing one thing against another, and the idea (from which the notion of rights derives) that some things are too valuable for anything to weigh against them. Thus, to consider the patient's request in the light of justice means, at the very least, to weigh up the possible consequences for other people whom it could indirectly as well as directly affect, in terms of how medicine and society are seen to value, respectively, human life, autonomy and the relief of suffering.

PRACTICAL WISDOM

All of this may sound as if making moral judgements is a matter of going through a checklist of ethical arguments. On the rare occasions when serious requests for euthanasia are made, that may be both possible and advisable. A moral algorithm may be useful and the four principles can help to structure thinking. But just as there is more to the moral recognition of signs of health than the absence of clinical indications of disease, so there is more to reaching a moral judgement than the absence of philosophical counter-arguments. One reason for this, of course, is that in practice there almost always are counter-arguments.

But in practice also, the need to act, if only by default, demands some conclusion to the argument. Weighing this up is ultimately a matter for what Aristotle called *practical wisdom*. How health carers deal with the most difficult moral dilemmas is largely determined by how much they have learned from making, reflecting on and discussing everyday moral choices, mostly in relatively unproblematic contexts. Learning how to put the principles of health care ethics into practice in these very ordinary contexts is one way of acquiring practical wisdom.

In order to drive home what he means by practical wisdom, Aristotle (see ref. 1, p. 339) describes it as the quality possessed by 'men like Pericles' (an example with which his hearers would agree). This, by implication, is a reminder of the part played in the acquisition of practical wisdom by role models and professional folklore, as well as listening to patients' own stories. These can supply the motivation which converts moral understanding, provided by the principles of health care ethics, into moral action. But equally, the principles provide a necessary critique of role models and stories, including those on which it would not be wise to act.

The principles of health care ethics can provide a framework for thinking about acute moral dilemmas. But they can also contribute to the acquisition of practical wisdom, mostly by being applied to relatively unproblematic everyday contexts. Some aspects of the case of Mr Millar, outlined at the beginning of this chapter, suggest how they might be applied.

Since the age of 16, Mr Millar (who took up a pipe only late in life) had smoked several packets of cigarettes a week. It is a reasonable assumption that smoking contributed to his cardiac condition, and perhaps also to some of his earlier troubles. Had his doctors known the risks, at the time of his first hospitalization, they might well have advised him to give it up, and he might well have agreed. Nowadays *beneficence* suggests that doctors at least offer this advice. The general practitioner who diagnosed the 79-year-old Mr Millar's cardiac condition did not. His practical wisdom, 'weighing-up' as *justice* requires, noted that his patient was not overweight, took regular exercise and was too well-informed not to know the risks of smoking. So, respecting his patient's *autonomy*, he made a moral judgement and acted accordingly. In the case of another patient, with a different prognosis, things might have been weighed up differently, and the advice offered. *Respect for autonomy* does not preclude gentle persuasion, especially if it might save the patient from the diminished autonomy of avoidable disablement. Another doctor might have decided that applied to Mr Millar. But if Mr Millar had declined his advice, *all four* principles would have precluded sanctions, or any less than the optimal medical treatment which he actually received.

In the light of *justice*, what the general practitioner judged right for Mr Millar has no wider implications for health education, except perhaps that there, too, practical wisdom is likely to achieve more than fanaticism. Its implications for the ethics of resource management are more debatable. Had Mr Millar been persuaded earlier to stop smoking, or later to see himself as diseased rather than healthy, or had he been resuscitated, he might have lived to develop some further condition requiring treatment, including long-term hospital care. His sister's Alzheimer's disease certainly was one condition which he had no wish to live for. But he had not mentioned that to his general practitioner—who in his wisdom had no reason to investigate it. This may have saved the patient suffering, and health care resources for someone who would benefit more from them. But in the end, it is impossible to say.

That 'it is impossible to say', may be the only conclusion which the wisdom of hindsight can reach about many moral decisions; and few, given sufficient retrospective scrutiny by a determined enough ethicist, are able entirely to 'scape whipping'. But there are also some, which most people with any experience and insight would agree were quite wrong. This chapter pointed earlier to what is probably at the root of a significant proportion of these in the health care context: namely failure to recognize and respond to signs of 'health' in patients whose disease or infirmity, or the mere fact that they are patients, persuade those making the decision that the metaphor of 'health' cannot be stretched so far.

Health carers are less likely to make this mistake if they have acquired practical wisdom. Learning to apply the principles of health care ethics to everyday choices is one way of acquiring it. The principle of respect for autonomy, in particular, requires good reasons for not recognizing these signs of 'health'. But sometimes there is no need to recognize them. Many 'healthy' patients, like Mr Millar, decide for themselves when to consult and when not to send for the doctor. In the end that is simply a salutary reminder that there is more to wholeness than health.

REFERENCES

1. Rackham, H. (transl.). 1926. *Aristotle; the Nichomachean ethics.* Heinemann (Loeb), London.
2. Seedhouse, D. 1986. *Health: the foundations for achievement.* John Wiley, Chichester.
3. Downie, R. S., Fyfe, C. and Tannahill, A. 1990. *Health promotion: models and values.* Oxford University Press, Oxford.
4. Onions, C. T. (ed.). *The shorter Oxford English dictionary,* 3rd edn. Clarendon Press, Oxford.
5. Hussey, E. (transl.). 1983. *Aristotle's physics,* Books III and IV, p. 169. Clarendon Press, Oxford.
6. Casini, C. 1991. Committee on Legal Affairs and Citizens' Rights Draft Opinion on the motion for a resolution on counselling for the terminally ill. European Parliament, 12 September. DOC EN PA 115232; 8f.
7. Bergson, H. 1956. *The two sources of morality and religion,* p. 69. Doubleday, New York.

70

Health Care Management: Are Ethics Relevant?

ROBERT J. MAXWELL

The King's Fund, London, UK

The ethics of medicine have an ancient and honourable lineage, to Hippocrates and no doubt beyond. Medicine is arguably the most respected of all the professions (at least in the UK) and this position rests in part upon a strong foundation of acknowledged duties, by which the physician must put the patient's interests above everything else and should always act with due skill, discretion and compassion. It is easy to see that several of the Beauchamp and Childress principles of ethical behaviour should underpin all clinical practice worth the name.

Health care management is another matter. It commands little public acclaim. Indeed it often receives a remarkably bad press, especially from the health care professions. Whether or not management of any kind qualifies to be classed as a profession is a matter for debate—as a manager myself, I would actually argue that management does not rest upon a body of established knowledge and practice of the kind that identifies a profession. Managers stand to be judged by the results of the organizations that they lead, not by their examinable skills. Nevertheless, management undoubtedly needs to be underpinned by a code of principled behaviour. Many recent examples, from banking, industry and commerce in many parts of the world, as much as from the public sector, demonstrate the appalling damage done by unprincipled acts on the part of managers and others in positions of authority and trust. This applies at least as much in health care as in any other human activity. It is high time that people began (as a matter of urgency) to devote to the broad field of health care management some of the attention to underlying principles that medical ethics (in a narrower sense) has long commanded.

In this chapter I will concentrate on four major management themes and then try to draw the threads together in terms of principles. The four themes are:

1. managing clinical activity,

Principles of Health Care Ethics. Edited by Raanan Gillon.
© 1994 John Wiley & Sons Ltd

2. allocating resources,
3. managing the politics of health,
4. rendering public account.

MANAGING CLINICAL ACTIVITY

The word 'managing' needs to be used with care. It does not (I hope) mean telling doctors, nurses and other therapists what to do in their professional roles. If that type of clinical direction were to be accepted—as at times it has been in, for example, the old-style regimes of Eastern Europe, or in some commercial, investor-owned systems—it would stamp out independent professional responsibility and remove the tension that should properly exist between the clinician's duty to the individual and a broader duty to the organization and the community. But it would be equally wrong to assume that individual clinicians should be able to do what they like, subject only to their professional codes. Managers cannot escape responsibility for what the clinicians do, even if they want to—which ought not to be the case. It is quite clear in UK law that the employing authority has a duty to ensure that acceptable standards of care are maintained, independent of the clinician's professional duty, and that the organization cannot simply shelter behind the latter. The Department of Health appears to take a similar line—that the health authority or trust board and its senior managers are accountable for standards within the services that they administer.

Nor is this solely a negative duty, to avoid abuse and negligence. It should also be positive. There are many ways in which managers can influence clinical standards for the better. For example, senior medical appointments offer a unique opportunity to draw talent into an institution and to match clinical activity to the needs of patients. The manager has a fundamental duty on behalf of the institution, to see the easy way out is not taken—which might be to allow a vacancy to be filled rather than the continuation of the post to be challenged, or to appoint someone because the candidate does not pose a threat to entrenched interests. Despite the legal requirements of equal opportunity there are all sorts of ways in which—often without an intention or consciousneses of wrongdoing—people will conspire to make a 'safe' appointment. The manager has to be satisfied that the processes in place have integrity: that the need for the post is scrutinized and that the appointment is open to all, and is made on merit.

To take a quite different example, junior medical and nursing staff do much of the 'hands-on' care in any institution. They often work long hours, face distressing situations in which they are only too conscious of their own inadequacies, and make mistakes. Of course there is a professional duty—which may be honoured in the breach—to support and supervise them. But the institution also has a duty, and can make a great difference to whether they feel valued, or whether they are stretched beyond their powers. All too often basic things such as junior staff accommodation seem to demonstrate that nobody knows and nobody cares. And management ought to have a shrewd and accurate idea of which junior staff positions are overstretched, exploited or undersupported and to be doing something to put the position right. After all, there is very little that the individual at the bottom of the professional heap can do except to endure, unless someone at a more senior level is willing to take an interest, find out what is going on and help to put it right.

It is not a question, then, of managing clinical activity in a dictatorial way, but of helping to create the conditions in which good clinical work will prosper and acting to eliminate the reverse. Although those of us who work in health often stress its uniqueness—and it is unique—its management also has many similarities to other professional fields and other human services. Someone who runs a university does not, if he or she has any sense, threaten individual independence of thought, enterprise or creativity. A successful vice-chancellor, principal or dean has a talent for collecting good people, giving them the backing and space that they need, and stimulating them to perform.

Successful organizations in the field of human services need a very clear idea of what it feels like to be on the receiving end of their activities, and to take pride in what they are doing and the way that they are doing it (1). At times these qualities are palpable, from the moment you are answered on the telephone or enter the building. It ought to be easier to achieve this in health than in most other services, because of the importance of the shared task, but it will almost never happen by accident. At a minimum, commitment to quality needs continually to be nourished.

ALLOCATING RESOURCES

Twenty years ago hospitals and other health institutions in the western developed world had become accustomed to sustained, cumulative expansion. The resource allocation task was largely about how best to use the extra money available for new developments. Even if (compared with the budget as a whole) this was a relatively modest amount in any one year, it was usually enough to enable managers with a taste for a quiet life to maintain peace. It could also be used to adjust an institution's pattern of services relatively painlessly, without too much direct challenge of established interests.

Of course it did not seem that easy at the time. Generally there were far more bids for new development than could possibly be met. But a manager could sleep easily at nights provided that the selection process for new developments was seen to be sensible and fair.

Nothing has changed the job of health service management more sharply in health than tighter resource constraints, combined with the continuing appetite for more sophisticated and expensive medical care. If the fair distribution of modest extra money for new development among competing bids was a relatively genteel administrative task, that is absolutely not the way to describe any serious attempt to make large institutions more efficient or to switch resources from one budget to another.

One popular metaphor for hospital administration used to be a sort of modular factory in which the institution provided workshop space for doctors (assisted respectfully by nurses) to pursue their honourable calling. It was up to the administration to see that the workshop was properly equipped, swept and maintained, but not to interfere unduly with what went on inside it.

Whatever the merits of that way of doing things—and, to be fair, it is not altogether as stupid as it may sound—it simply could not survive a much nastier financial world. It might be possible to govern a well-equipped conglomeration of workshops by consensus, but once you have to threaten or close some in order that others can survive, a much tougher and less consensual brand of management is going to be required.

Tougher, of course, does not necessarily mean principled, but in allocating limited public resources for health, principle is the only safe basis on which to act, and the principles must include efficiency and justice. That ought to be the managerial equivalent of motherhood, for nobody could possibly defend using limited health care resources inefficiently or unjustly. Nevertheless the fact is that we often do so use them, not because this is our individual or collective choice, but because inefficiency is often not obvious and justice does not always seem achievable. Take capitation funding as a case in point. The Resource Allocation Working Party concluded long ago, in 1976, that financial allocation among regional health authorities should be based on weighted resident populations adjusted for cross-boundary flows (2). The weightings took account of age and (through the proxy of standardized mortality ratios) morbidity. The result of implementing these recommendations, which were accepted by successive Secretaries of State, of each major party, would be a considerable diversion of money and manpower from the southeast of the country to the north and northwest. To most people (including me) the case did indeed seem overwhelming at the level of regional allocations—although the adjustment has not yet been fully completed, even now. At the next level down, however, within regions, the principle of relative justice remains just as strong, but how to achieve it in practice is much less clear. Was it necessarily right, for example, to switch money from deprived inner-city areas, which happen to have expensive teaching hospitals, towards the shires? How quickly is it right to do so? How can we be sure that the benefits achieved by budget increases will outweigh the harm done by dismantling existing institutions and services?

Efficiency is just as clear a principle to economists as justice is to philosophers. Inputs should be used to produce maximum output, or to produce a given output at least cost. The principle is uncontentious, even obvious. But in the context of resource allocation it can be even more elusive than the principle of justice. After all, justice can be translated into a mathematical formula for capitation-based funding. One may be queasy about some of the effects, but the device is quite robust, at least at the level of regional allocations. The same frequently cannot be said about the pursuit of efficiency, for the truth may well be counter-intuitive. In medicine there are immensely strong compulsions to believe that because people definitely need help, the available technology must benefit them. To withhold treatment therefore seems unthinkable. Yet the historical evidence suggests that the therapeutic imperative is all too often misplaced: people may not actually be much helped by the orthodox therapies of the day, however well-intentioned these may be. Even worse, on occasion they may actually be harmed, in the sense that medical intervention inflicts pain, discomfort and indignity without any compensating gain in the length or quality of their lives.

To sum up: resource allocation within a public health care system has to be a management responsibility. It cannot be left to the clinicians because they are by definition interested parties, advocates for their patients and their specialty. The tighter the expenditure constraints, the more onerous and unenviable the responsibility for choosing to put money and manpower in one direction rather than another. Such choices should be principled, not arbitrary, and the key principles are relatively clear. Putting these principles into practice is, however, entirely another thing.

MANAGING THE POLITICS OF HEALTH

Frequently UK physicians (and others) lament the fact that the governance of the National Health Service is subject to politics. 'Why cannot the NHS be taken out of politics?', they ask. The question is naive. Granted the importance and sensitivity of health care, and the fact that, in the UK, health services are for the most part paid for and provided publicly, there is absolutely no escaping politics. Health policy can only be bipartisan if (as happened in the UK between, say, 1950 and 1970) there is political consensus about both ends and means.

That currently is not the case in the UK. While there may be agreement about ends—such as optimizing the health of the British people—there certainly is no agreement about means. The Right prefers managed competition. The Left opts for some form of collective planning, based on need.

While managers may well have (and arguably ought to have), their own personal preferences between these two political philosophies, that is not the main point. What, as public sector managers, they must be able to do is to work constructively with people of diametrically differing political opinions. The issue is especially sharply posed when local political opinion and national government are at odds, as has been the case for some time in the inner cities and in much of Scotland and Wales. Then the senior manager has to try to keep faith with both points of view at once.

When Sir John Harvey Jones made his devastating television programme about Shropshire District Health Authority, he noted with sympathy and amazement the goldfish bowl in which NHS management was expected to work its miracles of expenditure reduction. Equally, and much more perceptively, he recognized that the managers concerned had no allies in what they were trying to do, and predicted that they would therefore fail. In due course they did. The job is so politically exposed (written with the small 'p' of professional, institutional and local opinion, as much as with the large 'P' of Party Politics) that managers will survive and achieve worthwhile ends only if they are politically attuned, and are skilled at building and maintaining alliances.

The tradition of the British civil service used to be that public administration was independent of party politics. Unlike the USA or France, even the most senior civil servants did not change when the party of government changed. It will be interesting to see what happens when the Conservatives ultimately lose office after their long period of power, from 1979 onwards, both in the civil service and in the National Health Service. For the chairs of health authorities have in most cases been filled by people who are clearly in sympathy with the Conservative Government's strategy for the NHS. Will they be swept away? If so, who will replace them, and will that confirm a pattern of political appointments for the future?

Against this background, what should an NHS manager do if the manager believes that what is required of her or him is dictated by political expedience and is not in the public interest? The classic civil service case study of this kind during the last decade was that of Clive Ponting, who believed (not without foundation) that his Minister was deliberately misleading the Commons over details of the Belgrano Affair during the Falklands war (3,4). In breach of the Official Secrets Act and of accepted civil service loyalty to ministers he leaked anonymously to Tom Dalyell, an MP savagely critical of government policy at the time, an official memorandum setting out what he believed to be the truth. When accused of the leak he at first denied it and only later admitted his action and resigned. Was he justified in what he did? On the facts, I believe that the answer has to be that he was not justified in that (a) he did not pursue a resolution of his dilemma first to the head of the civil service, as he was entitled to do, and (b) he resigned only after he was found out. Nevertheless, there must in principle be issues on which civil servants and NHS managers should be willing to stand out against official policy to the point of resignation. Otherwise those who simply obeyed orders in Nazi Germany would have been guiltless.

Of course many people will find that last statement so exaggerated and alarmist as to be offensive. In one sense they are right, since nothing nearly so dramatic or tyrannical is ever likely to occur within the NHS. Nevertheless the pressure to conform, or at least to keep silence, can be very strong and within the past decade has become stronger. Managerial performance is now judged and ranked, partly by objective measures, but inevitably also with elements of subjectivity, by people whose appointments border on the party political.

Fortunately most of the time people can work perfectly well together despite strongly held differences of opinion. It helps if the party in power is scrupulous to respect independence of thought and does not tamper with the truth, for example when asserting the success of its policies. Equally, those who enter public sector management in a democracy have to be willing to serve under governments with which they disagree. Provided that government policy is formed and implemented by due process, and that the individual manager believes it to be intended in the public interest, he or she may well find satisfaction in making it work to good effect. There must be NHS managers who have found themselves in that situation at some time in the past few years. It is even possible that some of them have altered their own opinion about specific proposals, as changes that they initially opposed have had a better impact than they feared. In an earlier generation I recall Sir Bruce Fraser, one of the most impressive Permanent Secretaries to serve in the Ministry of Health, remarking that it was the job of the politicians to bring the necessary irrational elements into public administration. There are times when that—in the sense of new, untried theories that open up new lines of attack on complex problems— is what moves us forward.

Nevertheless no manager should ever forget that opposition can be a personal duty, and that resignation is in some circumstances the only honourable course. They must also protect the autonomy of those who work under them and defend their right to speak out. Light in dark places—whether they are long-stay wards or children's homes—often depends on the few who have the courage to protest (5).

RENDERING PUBLIC ACCOUNT

The public has a fundamental right to know how massive sums of public money are spent in the NHS, and to be protected from fraud and waste. The Secretary of State for Health is therefore accountable to the electorate through parliament— at times in intimate and parochial detail as Nye Bevan pointed out (6,7)—and a range of institutions and procedures are in place to audit the way that the money is spent. These include the work of the National Audit Office, the Audit Commission, the Public Accounts Committee, and the Parliamentary Select Committees on Health and on Administration.

Necessary as these mechanisms are, they are not sufficient. For a start, there is a strong element of gaming about parliamentary accountability. In Churchill's words it is like ink to the cuttlefish—it often serves to conceal rather than to reveal. Protecting the Minister is near to the top of any senior civil servant's agenda. The parliamentary select committees, excellent as they are, are more like fencing matches (complete with ritual, chivalry, attack and evasion) than exercises in open government.

Second, local accountability is weak. For the most part health services are local: they serve mainly people in a particular area and affect the quality of their lives. It seems right that they should be locally accountable, at least for their local functions (regional and national tasks are another matter). Few would disagree with this proposition, yet the mechanisms for carrying it out are largely absent.

Obviously District Health Authorities and Family Health Service Authorities seek to represent the communities within their geographical boundaries, but their local legitimacy is not obvious and their accountability is upwards, via Regional Health Authorities and the Secretary of State. Community Health Councils can strengthen local accountability: their resources are meagre, however, and to have constructive impact they require a taxing mixture of tact, perseverance and analytical skills.

And then, of course, there is accountability to the individual. Largely this is a clinical matter, but not entirely, for the reasons given in the section on managing clinical activity. The institution and its management cannot duck responsibility. Hence managers are bound to be involved at least when something goes wrong, particularly if formal complaint systems come into play. They can also (as indicated earlier) help to create a climate that encourages individual accountability, for example by promoting intelligent audit and making it as easy as possible to translate audit findings into action.

So where do ethics come into this? The principle of autonomy helps, by underlining the rights of individuals and communities to take decisions for themselves, or at the very least to have a strong influence upon them. There is also, I suggest, an issue about truth-telling which stands in its own right, besides being a means towards autonomy. Individuals have a right to expect truth from their physicians, about their condition, their treatment, their chances and their progress. That does not mean the truth should be forced upon them, but that the physician has a presumptive duty to tell the truth. Similarly there is a management duty to tell the truth when rendering account to the public, its representatives and the media.

The truth, yes, but the whole truth? Is the manager of a public service entitled to be 'economical with the truth'? (8) (The phrase, which was not original, was made famous by its use by Sir Robert Armstrong on 18 November 1986 during the trial in Sydney, Australia, of an action by the UK Government to seek to block publication of *Spycatcher*, by Peter Wright.) This is a classic dilemma in ethics, dividing the deontologists like Kant from the teleologists, who would judge according to the balance of good or harm done by truth, half-truth or downright lie. There used to be—perhaps there still is—a tradition that Ministers may not lie to, or intentionally mislead, the House. That is perhaps a fair guide to where the public sector manager should also draw the line. He or she can avoid questions and decline to answer, and has no obligation to reveal weaknesses, but must not lie or deliberately mislead. This is not only because decent standards of personal behaviour call for this, but because, for a manager in the public sector, it is a public responsibility. When Sir Robert Armstrong admitted to economy with the truth it was perceived as a black mark for the British civil service, and rightly so. The British public is remarkably trusting and deserves better than the half-truth which is also a half-lie.

Managers in the NHS, and in similar organizations, will spend a considerable portion of their time on accountability—probably a larger portion than they recognize—in holding others to account and in rendering account themselves. If they cannot satisfy those above them they are unlikely to survive. In addition they need to be articulate on TV and radio and with the press, and in public and private meetings. They are more likely to survive these grillings if they see them not merely as personal performances, in which they may or may not have star quality, but also exercises in public accountability.

CONCLUSIONS

Although this is little recognized, the management of health care continually raises moral dilemmas where ethics has an important contribution to make. The field has been seriously neglected, and attention ought to be turned to it.

The issues are not precisely the same as in clinical medicine, where certain duties have long been recognized as fundamental. In the main the focus of clinical duties is the individual encounter, the relationship between physician and patient or between pupil and teacher. For management the focus is partly on supporting these relationships, but is also on broader public duties. No doubt this is one reason why a single set of principles seems even harder to identify, rank in order and apply than in clinical medicine. 'Above all, do no harm' is an unambiguous and useful commandment to a clinician. Managers unfortunately are much more likely to be dealing with balances of net good over net harm, although the reminder remains a useful guide to what clinical practice is about.

The Beauchamp and Childress principles of non-maleficence (do no harm) and beneficence (do the maximum good) have obvious force in clinical medicine. At the corporate level the idea of a 'constrained optimum' (9) is an important development of beneficence. When resources are limited, as they patently are in the NHS, it becomes important to meet needs at the highest level generalizable to the whole population. In other words individual patients will not get all that they and their physicians might like if (within the limits available) other patients with different needs have a higher claim. Doing cheap and effective things well for many must take precedence over expensive things for a few. This is, of course, a proposition that utilitarians will immediately recognize as their own: the greatest good of the greatest number.

This is also a very useful proposition in resource allocation, along with the Beauchamp and Childress principle of justice. The NHS has always been committed to meeting health care needs on the basis of need alone, without regard to ability to pay. Yet we have a long way to go before the least fortunate patient groups and the most deprived communities get their fair share of attention, which should be a basic feature of a just system (10). It ought to be the firm intent of the management of the NHS—and indeed of everyone who works in it—to shift the Service in the direction of greater justice.

Respect for autonomy is an important principle at the collective level, particularly in enhancing the (lamentably low) ability of communities to take decisions about their own health care and their own health. I have also suggested that truth-telling is an important principle in its own right, besides being a means of promoting autonomy. The public has a right to know what NHS management is doing on its behalf.

Overall the four Beauchamp and Childress principles stand up well, with the addition of truth-telling as a principle in its own right, but their application differs somewhat (naturally enough) at the management level compared with the clinical level. Management is very much about compromise, conflict resolution and pragmatism. In such circumstances operational principles need to be embedded in firm underlying values. For the public sector manager these are likely to include utilitarianism—if the ends in terms of maximum benefit for the greatest number do not always justify the means, they go a very long way towards doing so. Respect for democratic processes is another foundation stone. And a third has (I suggest) to be something about personal integrity, with a touch of the Kantian. If you cannot trust any individual public sector manager to stand up and be counted on certain issues, then he or she is unlikely, and probably does not deserve, to create anything substantial.

REFERENCES

1. Peters, T. J. and Waterman, R. H. 1982. *In search of excellence.* Harper & Row, New York.
2. Department of Health and Social Security. 1976. *Sharing resources for health in England.* Report of the Resource Allocation Working Party. HMSO, London.

3. *The Guardian*. 1985. Home News Report by Richard Norton-Taylor on Clive Ponting's trial under the Official Secrets Act. Tuesday 5 February.
4. Editorial. 1985. Official duties: before and after Ponting. *Public Administration* **63** (2): 125–131.
5. Beardshaw, V. 1981. Conscientious objectors at work: mental hospital nurses—a case study. *Social Audit*, London.
6. Foot, M. 1975. *Aneurin Bevan, 1945–1960*. Granada Publishing, St Albans.
7. Webster, C. (Ed.) 1991. *Aneurin Bevan on the National Health Service*. Wellcome Unit for the History of Medicine, Oxford.
8. Hall, R. V. 1987. *A Spy's Revenge*. Penguin, Harmondsworth.
9. Doyal, L. and Gough, I. 1991. *A theory of human need*. Macmillan Education, Basingstoke and London.
10. Rawls, J. 1972. *A theory of justice*. Harvard and OUP paperback.

71

Economics, Society and Health Care Ethics

ALAN WILLIAMS

Centre for Health Economics, University of York, UK

No society can afford to offer all its members all the health care that might possibly do them some good. Each society has therefore to establish priorities, i.e. it has to decide who will get what and, by implication, who will have to go without. Faced with such excruciating choices the general public may well try to run away from the ethical issues raised and delegate such decisions to politicians or to managers or to the health care professionals, who may find themselves facing these issues with very little guidance from society at large about what they are expected to do. Worse still, they may find themselves in the unenviable position of having to establish priorities in circumstances in which the rhetoric of public debate is dominated by those who say that it is unethical even to embark on the process of setting priorities!

It is therefore important to begin by establishing the inescapability of priority-setting, and to examine what guidance conventional medical ethics offers as to the elements that should influence such priority-setting. I will then consider how economists have approached these same issues, and argue that what they are advocating is perfectly compatible with conventional health care ethics. But conventional health care ethics are rather vague about certain key issues, and especially about what constitutes a 'fair' or 'equitable' system of health care provision, so an attempt will be made to sharpen up and clarify what is at stake here. We need to become more aware of the relative weights actually attached to the different ethical principles by the members of the society we serve, and what these weights imply for day-to-day priority-setting in health care. Here the economists have gone further than any other group of health care analysts in quantifying the implications of ethical positions, with predictably controversial results. But it will be argued that unless the participants in this ethical debate put their principles to the test in this practical way, ordinary members of society will be at risk of being misled into supporting fine-sounding rhetoric without realizing where its implementation would lead.

Principles of Health Care Ethics. Edited by Raanan Gillon.
© 1994 John Wiley & Sons Ltd

THE INEVITABILITY OF PRIORITY-SETTING

There seems no limit to the extent to which the health care system could expand if it pursued single-mindedly the objective of making everyone as healthy as possible. But whilst there are other beneficial things we could do with our limited resources (e.g. providing food and shelter for everybody, educating children, protecting ourselves from all sorts of hazards, etc.), we must acknowledge that expanding one good thing will always be at the expense of other good things. Obviously as societies grow richer they can afford more of everything if they so choose, and they may well choose to give the expansion of health care a higher priority than the expansion of other competing good things. But so long as there *are* other competing good things, then it will be necessary to limit the amount spent on health care to a level well short of satiation. Hence prioritization will be necessary.

In what follows it will be assumed that the broad prioritizing decision, about how much health care is affordable in our society, has already been made. The issue before us is then *on what principles should we choose what health care to provide and what health care not to provide, and for whom,* strictly *within* the predetermined budget. This restriction of scope carries with it the risk that we may forget that ensuring a high level of health in society depends on a great many things other than the provision of health care, but since the focus of attention here is health care, it is a risk we must take.

But even within the domain of resource-constrained health care provision there are those who argue that costs should not be a factor in decision-making about medical care (see for instance ref. 1). This conclusion stems from the belief that it is the doctor's duty to do everything possible for the patient who is in front of the doctor at the time, no matter what the costs. Quite apart from the fact that doctors have never actually behaved in that manner (they have always been jealous guardians of their own time and effort) (2), it is not clear on what ethical grounds the ignoring of costs is justified. In the face of resource limitations any resources used for one patient are denied to another. Thus 'costs' are health care activities denied to others, and hence are health benefits sacrificed by others. Can it be ethical to ignore the health sacrifices borne by others when making decisions about medical care? What guidance does conventional medical ethics offer us on this point?

CONVENTIONAL MEDICAL ETHICS

The central concern of 'medical ethics' has been to protect vulnerable patients from unscrupulous doctors. This has been approached by specifying the principles that should guide the behaviour of an ethical doctor. In summary these principles are: (a) preserve life, (b) alleviate suffering, (c) do no harm, (d) tell the truth, (e) respect the autonomy of the patient and (f) deal fairly with patients. It is acknowledged that none of these principles is absolute, that each may conflict with the others, and that the resolution of such conflicts is a matter for personal judgement (3). Different doctors may come to different conclusions in identical situations yet all may be behaving ethically within these general guidelines.

Note also that while items (a)–(e) could be interpreted as being directed only at the individual patient–doctor relationship, this cannot be said of the last item, which is essentially about distributive justice and refers to all patients (or, at the very least, to all the patients for whom that doctor is responsible). It is obviously this last item which undermines the assertion that it is a doctor's duty to do everything possible for the patient who is present at the time, no matter what the costs, for it might not be 'fair' to devote large amounts of resources to a patient who would gain only a small benefit, if it meant that many other patients would have to go without treatments that would benefit each of them a lot. An ethical doctor cannot simply ignore item (f) and hence must take these consequences into account when making a treatment decision.

Economists should have no difficulty whatever in seeing their own work in the health care field as being directed towards the fulfilment of those same six ethical principles. They would probably refer to them in different terms, however. For instance, the injunctions to preserve life and alleviate suffering would be seen as a definition of the objectives of health care, concentrating our attention on improving both the length and quality of people's lives. The injunction to do no harm would be seen to be about minimizing the risks of adverse effects from treatment. Telling the truth is a general duty accepted by all analysts, and respecting the autonomy of the patient would be seen as referring to the need to have the patients' values count rather than those of the practitioners when decisions about treatment are being made. But the final item on the list (about dealing fairly with patients) reminds us that we will seldom find ourselves dealing with situations in which only one patient's interests are affected, so that we will have to face the vexed question of how much weight to attach to the (possibly conflicting) values of *each* affected individual in such circumstances. And in any system in which the individual patient pays only part of the costs of care, the number of individuals who are affected in one way or another by a treatment decision may be very large indeed.

So the health economist, as an analyst, is seeking, through the use of appraisal techniques deriving from cost–benefit analysis, to help decision-makers to maximize the benefits of health care within the constraint of whatever level of resources society has chosen to devote to health care. These benefits are seen as improvements in people's length and quality of life (in probabilistic terms, since there are no certainties in these matters) in which the distribution of these benefits between individuals is a matter of some significance. Clearly there is nothing there that conflicts with conventional medical ethics. Even the stress laid by economists on the need to examine carefully the 'trade-offs' that are established at the margin between the competing good things that we seek in health care simply mirrors the relativity of ethical principles and the acknowledged need to strike a balance between them. The difficulties seem to arise because economists go further than others do in the quantification of these elements. We must now explore why they do so, and for this purpose adopt a somewhat different perspective, that of welfare economics.

CONVENTIONAL WELFARE ECONOMICS

Economists have sought to avoid making explicit interpersonal comparisons when judging whether one situation is better or worse than another, and a whole branch of the subject ('welfare economics') has grown from that ambitious objective. The basic idea is to separate 'efficiency' from 'equity', with 'efficiency' being kept free of interpersonal comparisons of welfare, all such judgements being encompassed in 'equity'. The definition of efficiency which achieves this separation is due to Pareto (and hence is often called Pareto-efficiency) and it declares a situation to be efficient if in that situation it is not possible to make anyone better off without making someone else worse off. If resources are being used 'wastefully' it should be possible to put them to some other use which will not harm the person from whom they are taken but will benefit those to whom they are given, thus the initial situation would have been 'inefficient'. The same would generally be true if resources are lying idle or are underutilized.

In the Paretian framework it is the individual's own judgement of whether he or she is better or worse off that counts, not the judgement of any third party; thus it observes very strictly the injunction to respect the autonomy of the individual. No judgements are made about the *status quo*, which is simply accepted as the starting point, our only concern being whether or not some change is an unambiguous improvement on it. The realm of application of this strict Paretian notion of 'efficiency' is, however, severely limited, since there are very few changes in real life that do not adversely affect the welfare of somebody or other. To ease this restriction on the applicability of the strict efficiency criterion, it was extended to cover situations in which the potential gainers from a change could fully compensate the potential losers, and still have some gains left over (compensation being paid in money terms, say). But identifying actual gainers and losers precisely, and setting up an incorruptible mechanism to enable such compensation actually to be paid, would in most cases be very costly. So this 'compensation principle' in turn got watered down to include cases where the compensation did not actually have to be paid, thus under the *potential* Pareto criterion' it has only to be shown that for a change to be declared 'efficient' the gains must on balance outweigh the losses (gains and losses generally being evaluated in money terms). To decide whether gains outweigh losses they must be measured in commensurable terms, so there has grown up a strong tradition of quantification and valuation, which has been applied to all kinds of gains and losses, including the value of life and safety (see for instance refs 4 and 5).

Calculating the 'efficiency' gains and losses in this way still leaves us with the distributional consequences to think about, and these are typically transferred to the 'equity' realm to be evaluated separately. In practice they are often ignored, however, in the hope that in the long run, over a multitude of different activities, they will all wash out. Thus the efficiency calculus as used in practice by economists does not really achieve the desired avoidance of all interpersonal comparisons of welfare. At best it says there are no losers, and it assumes that it does not matter who the gainers are. At worst it says that there are both gainers and losers, but it is up to somebody else to look at the equity implications.

In the health care field the general stance of economists has been that efficiency is about maximizing improvements in health, but this maximization process should be subject to some consideration of distributive justice. The precise meaning of 'an improvement in health' is not straightforward, but we will leave that matter on one side because a more pressing problem is that it is generally not clear exactly what any consideration of distributive justice should focus on, or what the actual equity rule should be. Is it to focus on outcome, or process, or resources? And is it to be a rule requiring strict equality of treatment, or one prescribing definite inequality of treatment? The possibilities are legion, and they carry us back to item (f) in the earlier list of items in conventional medical ethics, the one that requires that patients be dealt with fairly.

THE ANALYSIS OF EQUITY

When choosing the principles by which we would want our society to prioritize access to health care, we are naturally influenced by our own experiences and by how such principles would bear on us and on our nearest and dearest. In order to enhance our personal detachment when advocating ethical principles for adoption by society as a whole, we should imagine ourselves to be behind a 'veil of ignorance'. By this is meant that, although we know we are members of our particular society, we must imagine that we do not know which members of that society we are going to be. We must further imagine that *after* the priorization rules have been agreed, a ballot will be conducted to determine who will play which roles in the society. We may be fortunate and find ourselves in a role in which we do very well both for health and for access to health care, but we may be less fortunate and find ourselves in very adverse circumstances on both counts. In the latter case we need to feel that the rules applied to us as regards access to health care are at least 'fair', i.e. they are those we would have chosen from behind the 'veil of ignorance'. This thought experiment obviously calls for a great leap of the imagination, but it is essential to make that leap if we are to reflect systematically and empathetically upon the ethics of priority-setting in health care.

To help to clarify the tremendously complex situation which will face us in this enterprise, equity considerations have been divided into two groups, those concerned with *horizontal equity* (the equal treatment of equals), and those concerned with *vertical equity* (the unequal treatment of unequals). In each case we can distinguish three different sorts of element on which equity concerns may focus: structure (resources), process (activities), or outcome (benefits or effectiveness). If the focus is on outcome (e.g. improving the health of young people should have priority over improving the health of old people), this will constrain the distribution of activities and of resources, since these must be whatever is required for the outcome goal to be achieved. Similarly, if the focus is upon activities (e.g. everyone should have access to the same range of treatments), this will constrain the distribution of resources to be whatever is required to achieve the desired pattern of activities (which will be desired *per se*, not because of its outcomes, since in this case there is no equity interest in the outcomes themselves, which may be whatever they happen to be). Finally if the focus of equity concerns is resources (e.g. average expenditure per capita should vary by age in the same manner no matter where people live), then this has no particular equity implications for the distribution of treatments or for the distribution of outcomes (which will then be determined by the efficiency objective). So there is an asymmetric relationship between the elements in the columns of Table 71.1, those to the right constraining those to the left, but not vice-versa. For this reason it will generally not be possible to fulfil two equity concerns which are focused on two different columns in the same row. For instance it will not generally be possible *both* to have average expenditure per head varying in the same way by age wherever you happen to live, *and* for each person (irrespective of age) to have access to the same range of treatments. That combination would require (*inter alia*) an identical age-distribution of the population everywhere (so that total expenditure per capita were equal), and the costs of providing treatments to be the same everywhere (so that the same array of treatments could be provided out of the set amount of expenditure per head).

It will also be useful to distinguish between health and non-health characteristics of individuals, since either or both of these may be regarded as proper ethical bases for declaring people to be 'equal' or 'unequal', and a list of commonly adduced individual characteristics is given on the left-hand side of Table 71.1. In what follows it will be assumed that the efficiency objective is being pursued (i.e. the maximization of health benefits irrespective of who gets them), so that the equity issue concerns the extent to which the particular distribution of benefits which results from the pursuit of efficiency should be modified in some way or other. The reader might care to place an appropriate symbol in each cell in the table, to represent his or her own equity concerns (adding other relevant individual characteristics to the list on the left-hand side if necessary). The suggested symbols are 'H' to denote a horizontal equity concern, 'V' to denote a vertical equity concern. Leaving a blank means that the reader is content to let that item be distributed between people in whatever manner falls out from the pursuit of the efficiency objective and from any equity concerns that are expressed with the 'H' and 'V' symbols. Thus someone who is concerned only with the efficiency objective would leave all the cells in Table 71.1 blank. The discussion which follows should be used as an aid to reflection on the implications of holding whatever views the reader holds, bearing in mind that these views should be expressed as if from behind the 'veil of ignorance'.

VERTICAL EQUITY

We will concentrate first of all on the kinds of concern that people might express about vertical equity (denoted by the symbol 'V'). Down the left-hand side of Table 71.1 are listed various respects in which people are unequal, but about which there may be dispute as to whether they should be treated differently on that account (space has been left for others to be added should the reader wish to do so). Taking the health-related characteristics first of all, health care professionals are trained to distinguish between patients according to the first three items, and to vary treatments accordingly, so as to achieve the best feasible

TABLE 71.1 Table of equity concerns

Respect in which people are to be regarded as equal or unequal	Focus of equity concerns		
	Resources	Treatments	Benefits
1. *Health characteristics*			
1.1 Diagnosis			
1.2 Severity			
1.3 Prognosis			
1.4 Need			
1.5			
1.6			
1.7			
etc.			
2. *Other characteristics*			
2.01 Age			
2.02 Sex			
2.03 Family situation			
2.04 Race			
2.05 Beliefs			
2.06 Place of residence			
2.07 Citizenship			
2.08 Lifestyle			
2.09 Employment status			
2.10 Occupation			
2.11 Wealth			
2.12 Willingness to pay			
2.13 Past contribution to society			
2.14 Expected future contribution to society			
2.15			
2.16			
2.17			
etc.			

Additional individual characteristics may be added in the blank spaces. Columns may also be subdivided if the equity concerns relate only to *some* resources, or *some* treatments, or *some* benefits. For instance, a concern about resources may focus only on the initial distribution of money, or on the distribution of doctors, or hospital beds. With treatments, it may only be emergency treatments about which there is an equity concern, or perhaps initial access to GP consultations. With outcomes, equity concerns may concentrate on any of the possible objectives mentioned earlier in relation to the pursuit of efficiency (e.g. some aspect of life expectancy and/or quality of life).

outcomes. But that is to say no more than that they are pursuing the efficiency goal. An equity concern enters only when it is argued (say) that some people should get more resources devoted to them than would be justified on efficiency grounds. The equity argument here would be that certain diagnoses, or degrees of severity, or prognoses, justify the diversion of resources from the most efficient pattern, and hence justify the deterioration of other people's health which that diversion implies. For instance, it might be argued that in the last few weeks of a cancer patient's life we should do more for them—whether effective or not. But the implication of the assertion is that the last few weeks of a cancer patient's life are more important ethically than a cancer patient's life at other times, *and* than anyone else's life at *any* time! Giving especially high priority to one group always implies imposing additional sacrifices on all the other groups.

The last item on the list of 'health characteristics' ('need') requires rather more explanation of its role and implications. The term 'need' is much used in debates about priority-setting in health care, but its precise meaning is not always made clear (6). One common meaning is that need refers to the severity of someone's plight, whilst another is that need refers to the extent to which that plight can be ameliorated. In both cases it is usually assumed that judgements about need are to be made by third parties (not by the individuals themselves) since only third parties have the skill, experience and detachment to make such interpersonal judgements. For those who think need has the former meaning, the foregoing discussion about severity and prognosis (the cancer patient) is the relevant one. It then has to be acknowledged that giving extra resources to those in greatest need (in *this* sense) will reduce the overall level of health in the community. On the other hand, for those who think that need means capacity to benefit, and that resources should be distributed according to need (in *this* sense), there is no point in adducing this as an equity consideration, because the pursuit of efficiency alone will achieve this end. In this situation the demands of efficiency and equity coincide.

Turning next to the 'other characteristics' in Table 71.1, it is here that most of the contentious material lies. Should the young have priority over the old? Should a person's family responsibilities be taken into account? Or their race, religion, occupation, wealth, etc? Surveys conducted on the general public to elicit their beliefs on these matters (7,8) indicate a strong consensus favouring the young over the old (a view shared by the old themselves), and favouring the parents of young children over their childless contemporaries. There is less support for discrimination against smokers and heavy drinkers and others who are thought not to have cared for their own health, although many people believe that such behaviour weakens any moral claim such people may have on 'our' resources. There is a similar ambivalence about 'locals' versus 'outsiders' in tax-financed systems which offer care free (or at a nominal fee) at the point of use. Again there is frequently a feeling that only those who have contributed their 'fair share' should be entitled to claim the benefits, tempered by the fear that we may in turn find ourselves to be 'outsiders' in somebody else's system, and we wish to be treated generously in such circumstances. Such equity notions are a strong test either of the extent of people's fellow-feeling (love thy neighbour as thyself!) or of their risk aversion (there, but for the grace of God, go I!).

This is an appropriate point at which to note that the relative weight people attach to different equity principles can lead to radically different health care systems. This can be brought out most dramatically by considering items 2.11 and 2.12 on the list in Table 71.1, which refer to wealth and willingness to pay as possible foci for concerns about vertical equity. Here you will find strongly held views on both sides, with some people arguing that willingness and ability to pay should *not* influence access to health care, whilst others argue equally strongly that people should be free to spend their money as they wish, and that they are ethically entitled to spend some of it on health care if that is what they want most, and if they came by their money honestly. The differences may be encapsulated in two rival ideological positions, an egalitarian one in which access to health care is seen as a citizen's right, like access to the ballot box or to the courts of justice, which should not depend on willingness and ability to pay, and a libertarian one in which access to health care is seen as part of a society's reward system and should not be denied those who have earned their money honestly in the service of society at large (9). The first view leads to a public health care system where access is differentiated according to 'need'. The second view leads to a private health care system where access is differentiated according to willingness and ability to pay. Some people hold an intermediate position, namely that 'basic' needs should be met on the first basis, and the rest on the second basis. Others abhor a 'two-tier' system, and think it better for everyone to be in the same boat. The coexistence of public and private health care systems in the same society creates special ethical dilemmas for health care professionals. The viability of the private sector usually depends on it offering better health care than the public sector in some respect or other (e.g. standard of care, waiting time, amenity level). One way of ensuring this is not to strive too hard to improve the performance of the public system, and the temptation to go down that path will be strong when a practitioner's financial or professional interests lie significantly in the private sector.

Before leaving vertical equity it is worth noting that the justifications offered for the unequal treatment of unequals usually turn on notions of differential entitlement or desert, which might flow from a more fundamental analysis of rights and duties (see for instance ref. 10). Thus those who have knowingly risked their health for reasons which are not held to be ethically strong (e.g. simply for their own pleasure) are not regarded as 'deserving' (or 'being entitled to') care as strongly as someone who has done so for reasons that have strong ethical support (e.g. to save somebody else's life). Thus *how* a condition was acquired may carry moral implications which affect the behaviour and attitudes of health care professionals, even though it may be irrelevant to the 'health characteristics' (diagnosis, severity, prognosis) which on efficiency grounds would be their main concern when determining or carrying out treatment. It is also well known that even in health care systems which are imbued with a strong egalitarian ethic, people who are prominent because of their past and/or expected future contributions to society are likely to be treated differently from 'ordinary' people, with greater efforts being made on their behalf than would be usual (e.g. being treated only by the best professionals, never by the relatively inexperienced). Thus even where items 2.11 and 2.12 have been rejected, items 2.13 and 2.14 may still command support. For a discussion of the proper ethical attitude to output losses in the economic evaluation of health care, see ref. 11.

One final vertical equity consideration deserves some attention, namely that those individuals whose health is poor because life has treated them badly deserve especially favourable treatment from the health care system as some compensation for this misfortune. This argument typically focuses on items 2.08, 2.09, 2.10 and 2.11 (lifestyle, employment status, occupation and wealth, respectively), and suggests that people who have had little opportunity to get a decent job, and whose poverty has condemned them to a poor diet, poor housing and various other health hazards, deserve to be offered a better level of health care than would be offered to those on whom fortune has smiled more sweetly. Like all equity arguments it implies that it is right that others make health sacrifices that are larger than the health gains to this deserving group. The average level of health in society is reduced in order to improve its distribution between individuals.

HORIZONTAL EQUITY

Using Table 71.1 once more, our attention is now directed to the respects in which it might be held that equals should be treated equally, rather than unequals unequally. It should be noted that expressing a horizontal equity concern (denoted by 'H') is different from stating that an item is of no concern from the point of view of equity (denoted by leaving a cell blank). Consider again the case of a person's age in relation to the benefits of health care. We may say (apparently with the support of the majority of the public) that we want benefits to the young to be given priority over benefits to the old (a vertical equity concern). But other people might see it instead as a matter of horizontal equity, arguing that benefits should weigh equally whether they accrue to the old or the young. Yet others may say that the age of the beneficiary is not a matter of equity concern at all, what is important (say) is their family situation, and if that *happens* to favour people in a certain age range, so be it, but that is merely incidental and not a matter of equity concern in itself. All three positions are likely to be encountered in practice.

A further point to be noted here is that a concern for horizontal equity may be satisfied by ensuring that nobody with certain characteristics gets anything at all! The important thing is that if one person is denied treatment in a particular set of circumstances, *everybody* must be denied treatment in those circumstances. Whether treatment is offered or not would be determined through our concerns for efficiency and/or vertical equity. Thus it may be equitable to deny costly intensive care to people with a very poor prognosis, provided the criteria by which this decision is made are applied consistently.

As indicated earlier, an important horizontal equity concern regarding the provision of health care has been that it should not depend on wealth, position or willingness to pay, but it is often unclear whether those taking up that position see it as focusing on access to resources, treatments or benefits. The commonest expression of this view is probably 'equal treatment for equal need'. If need means capacity to benefit, and if personal characteristics such as age, sex, smoking and drinking habits, *and* wealth and position, affect capacity to benefit, they will thereby affect 'need'. So the ethically appropriate treatment will still indirectly depend on wealth and position, since they affect 'need'. If, on the other hand, 'need' means 'health plight' (i.e. the current severity of someone's condition, which may not be remediable) equal treatment of everyone in the same plight may have very heavy efficiency costs, since the effectiveness of treatment may depend on personal characteristics (including wealth and position). It is therefore essential to unpick fine-sounding slogans such as 'equal treatment for equal need' to see just where they lead on alternative plausible interpretations of what they might mean. As in this case, they may either add nothing to what we would achieve by the pursuit of efficiency alone, or they may disturb it and thereby impose health losses on some members of the community which will certainly outweigh those gained by whoever are the target group of the equity concern.

QALY LEAGUE TABLES

The time has come to turn to the economists' own distinctive contribution to the debate about priorities and health care ethics, which has centred on the quantification of the 'efficiency–equity trade-off'. The pursuit of efficiency has been interpreted as the maximization of improvements of health, where health is defined as improvements in the length and quality of people's lives. These two elements have been fused into the concept of the 'quality-adjusted life-year' or QALY, the basic idea being that if a year of *healthy* life-expectancy is worth 1, then a year of *unhealthy* life-expectancy will be worth less than 1, and will be worth less the more unhealthy it is (this is the 'quality-adjustment' element). The quantification of expected length of life creates no great problem of principle, though the practical difficulties in making such estimates are well known. The controversial step is the next one, in which an estimate is sought of the relative value that people attach to prospective improvements in the length of their lives as opposed to prospective improvements in the quality of their lives. People often face situations (e.g. when offered surgery) when they have to weigh a mortality risk against the prospect of a better quality of life, or ones (e.g. advice to change their preferred lifestyle) when they have to sacrifice quality of life to improve their survival prospects. By exploring these trade-offs empirically it is possible to assess the relative value people attach to different health states (see for instance ref. 12). In order to standardize these expressions of value, a common measurement convention is used in which it is assumed that being healthy is worth 1, and being dead is worth 0 (states rated worse than being dead attracting a negative score).

Unfortunately it is necessary to proceed beyond that stage in order to prioritize health care provision, because we need to come up with some set of *group* values that can be used on behalf of society generally. And if these group values are to be based on the values of the individuals who form the group, that means aggregating the (different) views of these individuals in some way or other. There are many ways of doing this, each of which has different implications for the weight given to each individual's views. The method most commonly utilized involves two steps: firstly assuming that one year of healthy life expectancy (i.e. 1 QALY) is of equal value for everybody (and so is being dead), and then, secondly, valuing each unhealthy state* according to the median value of the group.

---

* The manner in which health states should best be described for this purpose is itself a thriving and contentious field of research which cannot be explored further here. The interested reader is referred to refs 13–16, which collectively cover the ground well.

The first of these two assumptions is essentially a statement that *none of the individual characteristics set out in Table 71.1* should be regarded as a relevant equity concern. It is thus for those who wish to depart from that position to express whatever equity concern they think should be brought to bear on it. For instance, if it were held that, on vertical equity grounds, priority should be given to the young over the old, then the aggregation process could be amended accordingly, with extra weight being given to a QALY if it accrued to a young person rather than an old person. But people advocating such a substitution would need to specify *precisely what additional weight* they had in mind. If benefits to old people are still to count for something, what is the adjustment factor to look like? Is it to be 0.5 for over-60s and 1.4 for under-60s, or what? The great advantage of the quantification required in the QALY approach is that the vague arm-waving of fine-sounding rhetoric is no longer enough. The compromises required to accommodate equity concerns must be quantified, and their implications for health care provision explored systematically at an empirical level.

The second of the assumptions mentioned earlier (using the median values as the group values for the unhealthy states), also has important implications of both a political and an ethical nature. The political implication is that it mimics a system of group decision-making in which a simple majority is decisive. This is because the person with the median value has exactly the same number of people holding values higher than his or hers as holding values lower than his or hers. In a political system in which each person has one vote, the median voter is the focal person who will always be in the majority. The ethical implication therefore is that this is (implicitly) regarded as the ethically appropriate manner by which to come to a group value. Again there are other possibilities, like adopting the views of the one person who is deemed to be the ethically most appropriate person in the society (perhaps a religious leader, or an elected representative). In such circumstances we need only elicit that person's views, and the research task at an empirical level is greatly simplified. The point being stressed here is that even within the pursuit of efficiency there are important ethical issues that need to be brought into the open and examined, and if they are found to be unacceptable *some other explicit judgement needs to be put in their place*. There cannot be a vacuum, so objectors have to face up to their responsibilities, and state and justify an alternative position.

Having by this means, we suppose, developed a QALY measure that incorporates whatever ethical concerns are thought to be appropriate *as regards the measurement and valuation of outcomes*, we would still need to temper it with any independent equity concerns (vertical or horizontal) that we may have which focus explicitly on the distribution of *treatments* or *resources*. It may well be that we do not have any such concerns, however, and in that case we can pursue the broadened efficiency objective single-mindedly, and move directly to the comparison of the relative merits of different health care activities in terms of their benefits (in terms of equity-weighted QALYs) compared with their costs (i.e. in terms of their use of society's scarce resources). On this basis a 'league table' of health care activities could be drawn up, with those that deliver benefits (QALYs) at least cost at the top, and those which do so at greatest cost at the bottom. Efficiency dictates that we proceed down the list until we run out of resources, for only by that means will the (equity-weighted) health benefits to the community be maximized.*

However, if we do have equity concerns that focus directly on resources or treatments, we cannot stop there, and we must now work through the implications of each such concern in turn to see what it 'costs' in efficiency losses (i.e. in reduced QALYs, compared with the outcome from the unconstrained maximization process). This may or may not lead us to adjust our support for the equity principle in question, depending on what cost (in terms of health benefits forgone) we regard as acceptable in its pursuit.

CONCLUSIONS

The foregoing discussion has been conducted at a high level of abstraction, concentrating on issues of principle and setting aside the severe practical difficulties that confront us in implementing such a system. But it is important to have a sense of vision to guide our endeavours as professionals concerned on a day-to-day basis with improving the provision of health care in our respective societies. Economists working on the prioritization of health care have developed a framework of thought in which ethical issues can be considered in a practical manner. It would be a pity not to use it more widely as a means of clarifying our ideas and exploring their implications.

REFERENCES

1. Loewy, E. L. 1980. Cost should not be a factor in medical care. *New England Journal of Medicine* **302**: 697.
2. Williams, A. 1988. Health economics: the end of clinical freedom? *British Medical Journal* **297**: 1183–1186.
3. Ruark, J. E., Raffin, T. and The Stanford University Medical Center Committee on Ethics. 1988. Initiating and withdrawing life support. *New England Journal of Medicine* **318**: 25–30.
4. Mooney, G. H. 1977. *The valuation of human life*. Macmillan, London.
5. Jones, L. M. W. (Ed.). 1992. *The value of life and safety*. North-Holland, Amsterdam.
6. Williams, A. 1992. Priorities—not needs, Pp. 57–63, *in* Corden, A., Robertson, E. and Tolley, K. (Eds) *Meeting needs*. Avebury, Aldershot.
7. Williams, A. 1988. Economics and the rational use of medical technology. Esp. pp. 116/117, *in* Rutten, F. F. H. and Reiser, S. J. (Eds) *The economics of medical technology*. Springer Verlag, Berlin.
8. Lewis, P. A. and Charney, M. 1989. Which of two individuals do you treat when only their ages are different and you can't treat both? *Journal of Medical Ethics* **15**: 28–32.
9. Williams, A. 1988. Priority setting in private and public health care: a guide through the ideological jungle. *Journal of Health Economics* **7**: 173–183.
10. Gillon, R. 1986. *Philosophical medical ethics*, esp. Chapters 9, 14 and 15. Wiley, Chichester.

---

* There are some complications here about activities in course of development, or which have benefits in research or training terms, which will be ignored here. However, see ref. 17.

11. Williams, A. 1992. Cost effectiveness analysis: is it ethical? *Journal of Medical Ethics* **18**: 7–11.
12. Euroqol Group. 1990. Euroqol—a new facility for the measurement of health related quality of life. *Health Policy* **16**: 199–208.
13. Bowling, A. 1991. *Measuring health: a review of quality of life measurement scales.* Open University Press, Milton Keynes.
14. Spilker, B. (Ed.). 1990. *Quality of life assessments in clinical trials.* Raven Press, New York.
15. Spilker, B. *et al.* 1990. Quality of life: bibliography and indexes. *Medical Care,* suppl. 28 (12).
16. Teeling-Smith, G. (Ed.). 1988. *Measuring health: a practical approach.* Wiley, Chichester.
17. Williams, A. 1988. Economics and the rational use of medical technology. Esp. pp. 118–119, *in* Rutten, F. F. H. and Reiser, S. J. (Eds) *The economics of medical technology.* Springer Verlag, Berlin.

72

Health Promotion, Society and Health Care Ethics

YANNIS TOUNTAS, MD, MPH

*Assistant Professor of
Social Medicine, University of Athens, Medical School, Director of
the Institute of Social and Preventive Medicine, Athens, Greece*

TINA N. GARANIS

*Lawyer, MA in Medical Ethics and Law, Research and Teaching Fellow, Dept
of Public and Administrative Health, Athens School of Public Health, Athens,
Greece*

PANAGIOTA DALLA-VORGIA

*Lawyer, Dr Med.Sc, Assistant Professor, Dept of Hygiene and Epidemiology,
University of Athens, Medical School, Athens, Greece*

INTRODUCTION

When one refers to health care ethics one tends to think of the ethics of medical care rather than of the ethics of prevention or health promotion. Both medical practice and health promotion, however, constitute parts of the wider notion of health care which, as Dunstan puts it, 'presupposes a highly complex modern state, organizing *provision* for its citizens' health' (1). For a long time, medical practice has been considered as the principal component of health care. The concept of disease and, consequently, of the therapeutic role of medicine have dominated throughout the centuries. This phenomenon derives from the role that has almost always been attributed to medicine as the practice of absolute healing and to doctors as miracle workers. Historically, albeit heavily neglected, health promotion has not been an unknown concept. Its roots can be traced in

Principles of Health Care Ethics. Edited by Raanan Gillon.
© 1994 John Wiley & Sons Ltd

the theories of Hippocrates and Galen about the balance of the four humours of the human body (phlegm, blood, yellow and black bile), a balance which could be destroyed by an unhealthy way of living. Nevertheless, during the centuries that followed, and despite the emergence of various theories supporting the necessity and importance of health promotion, the curative role of medicine prevailed while health promotion was considered by the state to be a matter of lesser significance, and most activities concerning health concentrated on curing individuals rather than on preventing a certain disease or on trying to change life conditions of the population. It was only in the nineteenth century that this situation started to change when the movement of modern public health begun. This change was the result of the discovery that infectious diseases were largely attributable to environmental conditions and could often be prevented by control of the influences which led to them. The most significant advance in the twentieth century is the recognition that the same is true of many non-communicable diseases, including cardiovascular diseases and cancer, the two main killers of our days. Thus, it has been confirmed that the main determinants of health are related to living conditions, environmental factors, lifestyles and biological parameters such as age, sex and heredity (2).

This need for change in the ways and conditions of living in order to combat disease and promote health, has led in the last few decades to the formulation of the concept of health promotion. Health promotion represents a mediating strategy between people and their environment which synthesizes personal choice and social responsibility in order to create a healthier future (3).

The perspective of enabling people to increase control over, and to improve their health, derives from a conception of 'health' as the extent to which an individual or group is able, on the one hand to realize aspirations and satisfy needs, and on the other hand, to change the environment or cope with it. Health, therefore, is seen as a resource for everyday life, not as the objective of living; it is a positive concept, emphasizing social and personal resources as well as physical capacities.

THE ETHICAL DIMENSIONS OF HEALTH PROMOTION

The main principle of health promotion is the modification of people's lifestyles and life conditions through the involvement of the population as a whole in the context of their everyday life rather than a focus on people at risk for specific disease. The involvement of the population is defined as active participation in all health-related issues and activities in contrast to the patient-passive role of curative medicine.

This basic principle brings up a number of crucial ethical issues concerning:

1. The ideology of healthism and the medicalization of our societies.
2. The problem of victim blaming by locating the causes of illness more within the individual and less in social and environmental forces.
3. The balance between autonomy and justified paternalism in the process of changing lifestyle, of handling information and of collecting data.
4. The policy of resource allocation in relation to the limited resources and

conflicting interests, and to the preservation of justice whenever social or other differentiations and discriminations are involved.

5. The question of the effectiveness of health promotion.

HEALTHISM AND MEDICALIZATION

One of the main principles of health promotion is the active involvement of the population as a whole in the context of their everyday life. Thus, health promotion is directed to large target groups whose essential characteristic is that they consist of apparently healthy people, i.e. of people who consider themselves in good or even perfect health.

As a result of health promotion, these healthy people begin to observe their lifestyle and their various activities from a medical point of view. This 'medicalization' entails both positive and negative consequences. The former concern the actual utility to the person's health: better nutrition, more exercise, less smoking, etc. The latter include the additional stress and anxiety over health matters in general, or over knowledge about a particular health problem. Sometimes such knowledge can affect a person's private, professional and social life in many and possibly irreversible ways. Negative consequences also include the reinforcement of the tendency to define problems which do not have only a medical but a social dimension as well (e.g. alcoholism, drug abuse and mental illness) as medical ones requiring only medical treatment and not social intervention as well.

While such an attitude may present advantages both to individuals and society the medicalization of the latter has been attacked by many authors (4) and in some cases this attack has been quite radical (5). Medicalization may result in misattributing the causes of behaviour, affecting the appropriateness of our interventions and generating stress over health matters in general, or over knowledge about a particular health problem. Medicalization of life can also reinforce the ideology of healthism, which views health as the ultimate goal and not as a resource for everyday life. The main weapon against these problems is the preservation of the intersectoral character of health promotion; the participation of different sectors and professions can hinder the exclusive management of health by health services, which are mostly dominated by the medical profession.

VICTIM BLAMING

Another significant ethical question which arises from the practice of health promotion is that of 'victim blaming'. According to William Ryan, victim blaming is the locating of the causes of social or other problems in the individual rather than in social and environmental factors (6). In the field of health promotion victim blaming involves holding the individual responsible for his/her health problems and orientating action plans almost exclusively towards changing personal behaviour.

In order, however, to achieve their objectives, health promotion programmes should include behavioural changes alongside with social and environmental ones. If individuals are to reduce the risk of disease by modifying their behaviour, there must be a causal link between the behavioural risk factor(s) and the disease. It has been argued that in the case of some risk factors (above all obesity, exercise and cholesterol) the causal link is not as strong as it is in others such as smoking or the use of seat belts in cars (7). It has also been contended that the relationship between behaviour and health is a probabilistic rather than a deterministic one.

The plausibility of this line of argumentation depends on the extent to which we are capable of knowing certain things about protecting health on a population level. In the case of each individual, however, health is surrounded by much more uncertainty—which is why societies ought to be less enthusiastic about making the leap from the behaviour of ill people to conclusions about the causes of illness. Moreover, the fact that some health promotion programmes prefer to focus on risks chosen by the individuals, rather than on exogenous risks, is equally important. Environmentalists attack those who employ individual behaviour models of victim blaming, saying that poverty or underdevelopment present a greater risk to health than smoking. On the other hand the individualists accuse the environmentalists of using coercive methods. In the end, perhaps, the most important questions ought to focus on how to prevent each action plan from confining itself to the individual level, on what sort of society such an orientation would involve and on how the health professions can contribute to such a society—and not on whether health promotion ought to aim in changing individual behaviour. By maintaining and re-emphasizing the importance of individual choices, we can think about health promotion programmes as providing people with options, and health education as liberating (8).

AUTONOMY, INFORMATION AND DATA COLLECTION

The basic aim of health promotion, that of modifying human behaviour and living conditions, involves the manner in which people live, think and act. This aim can never be separated from its ethical consequences, even though it is motivated by the idea of human good. Health is a value-laden concept but the values it encompasses are not the same for all individuals. Every person faces his health in a different way according to his aspirations, his educational, financial and social background, his potential. Health, therefore, can be described with as many different colours as the persons asked about it. On the other hand, health promotion consists of uniform strategies which, after having taken into consideration all these different values, come out with a programme addressed to large groups of population. Which are the values lying under the notion of health, on what principles they rely and how health promotion handles the existing conflicts are among the questions which lie at the centre of the ethical dilemmas involved in the battle for environmental and behavioural change.

One major ethical dilemma which arises during any effort to change behaviour concerns the manner in which this effort is being carried out: in other words, whether the change should be the product of a free choice or whether it should be imposed for the good of the individual or of society. This crucial question refers us directly to the issue of paternalism v. autonomy in the health promotion context. Social influence strategies can be divided into three basic categories: coercion, manipulation and persuasion. These categories impose a continuum from those which are most compatible with autonomous choice and action (persuasion) to those which are least compatible with autonomous choice and action (coercion) (9). Faden suggests that health promotion campaigns should be categorized on the criterion of their respect for individual autonomy (10). Persuasive campaigns which attempt to induce change through an appeal to reason, are the least coercive. Manipulative coercive campaigns, on the other hand, attempt to reduce individual options through the control of information, such as deception or emotional appeals, or psychological manipulation, such as subliminal suggestion, flattery, guilt or feelings of obligation.

Such attempts, consisting of different forms of paternalism, claim that health professionals are better equipped to take appropriate health protection measures than the individual (11). It has been argued that promotion of autonomy in the long run requires sometimes sacrificing autonomy in the short run. However, the general assumption that individual autonomy can be infringed under certain conditions, albeit plausible, does not solve the problem of where the line of interference and tolerance should be drawn. Benjamin and Curtis (12) describe three criteria for judging paternalism to be acceptable: situations in which the individual is not in a position to decide, situations in which the individual will suffer serious harm if there is no intervention and situations in which the individual will agree, with hindsight, that the intervention was correct. Wikler (13), on the other hand, dismisses paternalism completely, arguing that decision-makers are not always reliable: health care and medicine are undergoing constant change as part of a process of continuous evolution and all people have preferences and values which should not be subject to rational criticism. One manner of coping with the ethical questions involved in respect for individual autonomy is to do so by promoting the participation of the population concerned (or its representatives) in all stages of planning, implementing and evaluating health promotion programmes (14). Of course, participation is not a panacea in dealing with these problems. As Minkler (15) observes, the participation of community representatives may lead to problems of cooperation and to questioning of intentions in terms of the interests which those representatives are called upon to serve. It should be borne in mind, however, that whenever there is a clash of interests between individuals or groups of agencies health promotion's duty is to weigh all the factors together and orientate itself towards the action best compatible with the principle of self-determination and freedom of choice. Ethical concerns may exist to the extent to which health promotion messages and actions are manipulative or coercive—such as the use of deception or subliminal messages—and to the extent to which they withhold or distort information about the expected benefits, costs and side-effects. Given the limitations in the scientific knowledge on which health promotion is based (limitations which are due to its complex and multisectoral character) we should be cautious in our behavioural prescriptions. As has already been mentioned, whenever health promotion activities are not adequately evaluated, health promoters should inform the people involved that the intervention is essentially experimental. If they fail to do this, health promoters are in effect deceiving consumers, since people normally assume that any health service provided is for their benefit.

Through health promotion programmes people should also be informed about the possibilities and the consequences of the need for medical services. Health promotion activities include diagnostic procedures which increase diagnosis of disease among populations and the demand for medical services. Apart from the ethical responsibility of a health system to satisfy demand and provide such services and funds there are other important ethical implications concerning the iatrogenic risks which are likely to increase as consumption of medical services grows.

Finally, the confidentiality of data collected in any health promotion activity poses serious ethical problems, since such data are usually stored in different data banks and are often used for research purposes through different networks. These ethical problems are addressed by the ethics of medical information technology and data collection in order to protect individuals and populations, especially when disclosure of health information can have an adverse effect on their occupational status (16).

HEALTH PROMOTION, RESOURCE ALLOCATION AND JUSTICE

The task of allocating resources and simultaneously trying to safeguard justice presents some of the thorniest ethical issues in health promotion. Justice connotes an equal distribution of social benefits without regard to factors such as age, sex, race, contribution or productivity. The scarcity of resources, however, sharpens the conflict between demands made by health promotion and demands made by therapeutic medicine. Undoubtedly disease and death are part of the human lot; we can promote health, we can prevent some diseases or postpone others, and sometimes we can postpone death. Better health promotion, albeit within a fixed health budget, means that fewer people will eventually become ill and, thus, less money will be spent for their treatment. In other words, placing money in health promotion is a successful financial investment as, in the long run, the cost of preventive medicine is lower than that of therapeutic intervention. This is particularly true for health campaigns, where technological or regulatory approaches are either inapplicable or unacceptable (e.g. AIDS prevention). However, even for those health problems for which there is a preferable alternative solution, there may still be an appropriate role for health campaigns in creating a consensus for regulation or legislation; that is, in creating the public climate needed to make these options politically possible (10). This amounts indeed to a just resource allocation, since the notion of resources does not refer only to money but to values such as professional competence and ability of cooperation.

The example of a campaign in an industry whose aim was to advise workers against smoking proves that it may well have a very low cost per life saved (17). But other health promotion/disease prevention interventions may be very expensive indeed. According to one estimate, the cost of saving lives by the British system of cervical cytology screening was in 1987 between £270 000 and

£285 000 per life saved (18). Since part of the purpose of ethical analysis is to question the predominance of economic criteria, the argument that health promotion would waste scarce resources seems implausible.

Some authors have noted that, at least in industry, there is an inferred link between the growth of health promotion programmes and reductions in governmental and employer-sponsored health programmes (19). From 1980 to 1984, for example, the proportion of US companies with health insurance deductibles over $100 increased from 5% to 40% (20). This issue raises an important ethical problem concerning resource allocation. Whether health promotion intervention is a waste or not of scarce resources depends on whether such interventions are both beneficial and not harmful, and whether the interventions themselves have an adverse effect on scarce resources. The answers to such ethical questions therefore depend on the particular case.

Health promotion activities include programmes which, although addressed to the entire population, eventually benefit only certain individuals. In these cases the majority of the population shoulders the cost of caring for minority groups which are at risk. For example, when taxation on alcoholic beverages is raised in order to make them more expensive and reduce consumption, the majority of the population, although not at risk, has to pay the price through alcohol consumption. Another relevant example is that of the reduction in smoking which was achieved in Sweden after wide-ranging and costly health education and health promotion campaigns. However, the reduction achieved did not affect the entire population: the middle and upper classes cut down on smoking much more than did the less well-off, while the unemployed and young unmarried mothers did not change their smoking habits at all (21). These examples reveal another important ethical dilemma: the more prosperous classes in a society are able to modify their lifestyle patterns more easily than the less privileged classes, and it may be that health promotion interventions in populations exacerbate existing inequalities in the health sector (22).

Of course there is increasing awareness of the need for health promotion programmes to be developed for special target populations (23). Proponents of health promotion have also emphasized the need for health promotion to be seen as a complement to other governmental or social programmes for disadvantaged groups, rather than as a supplement for them.

THE EFFECTIVENESS OF HEALTH PROMOTION

The question of the effectiveness of health promotion as raised during the discussion of resource allocation also has important ethical dimensions. Each health promotion intervention ought to benefit the health of the population to which it is addressed but also balance the costs and the benefits. The term 'benefit', however, does not mean only quantifiable goods. Acting according to the principle of beneficence means that health promotion should be carried out in such a way that it is also ethically beneficent for the population. Respect for confidentiality, for example, may not have direct effects on the population's health but it safeguards the relationship of health professionals with target groups and public opinion. On the other hand, the terms 'harm' and 'cost' include, as Beauchamp and Childress put it, 'any negative value that detracts from human health and welfare' (24). It has also been reported that health promotion interventions have in the past been implemented without sufficient evidence of their benefits (25,26) and as part of the same line of argumentation, it has been proposed that all health promotion interventions which have not been sufficiently evaluated ought to be treated as medical research addressed to the population. They should also be subjected to the same ethical evaluation as clinical studies. In addition, there ought to be a forum where the ethical demands of health promotion can be discussed (27).

The most convincing objection to these arguments is that health promotion is such a beneficial and praiseworthy action that any attempt to investigate its ethics is absurd. If all interventions which are not beneficial are deemed not to be health promotion action then health promotion most certainly is beneficial, by definition. This, of course, underscores the need for a distinction to be made between the proposed interventions which are beneficial and those which are not. Until positive results appear, such interventions should be subjected to careful evaluation—and the fact that they are experimental in nature should be explained to the individuals to whom they are addressed.

Meanwhile, until health promotion has run its full course of development (to such an extent that its effectiveness is guaranteed) we should take particular care to ensure that the process does not degenerate into ethical speculation.

CASE STUDY: A HEALTH PROMOTION PROGRAMME AND ITS ETHICAL ASPECTS

Despite the various ethical problems, the results of the international experience in carrying out health promotion projects have been particularly encouraging. This is why the Institute of Social and Preventive Medicine (ISPM), which was founded in Athens in 1990, has proceeded in collaboration with the World Health Organization and the European Economic Community in the planning and realization of a health promotion project addressed to commercial shipping workers. The rest of the chapter consists of a brief description of this project and its ethical implications. The programme consisted of two stages. The first stage included the assessment of the health status of Greek seamen, as well as their knowledge and their attitude concerning health issues. It also included the study of broader social, environmental and cultural factors, the working environment, causes of sea accidents and Greek and international legislation on marine hygiene and safety. Finally, the given medical and medicinal care, as well as the general use of health services by Greek seamen, were registered and evaluated. Information concerning the first stage was collected by:

1. Reviewing of the relevant health data available through health marine services.
2. Studying Greek and international bibliography.
3. Completion of an appropriate health survey questionnaire addressed to Greek seamen.
4. Basic laboratory and clinical examinations.

The second stage was based on the conclusions of the first stage and consisted of an intervention (carried out by lectures, seminars, publications and distance learning by new technologies, etc.) aimed at reducing the morbidity of Greek seamen and the improvement of their health status (smoking limitation, hypertension reduction, obesity fighting, etc.). It must also be noted that, as this project was an innovative one, there existed no previous data about its effectiveness. Therefore, one of its main goals was also the investigation of the effectiveness *per se* of a project of such a nature. The ethical ramifications of the project were dealt with in a way which shows that the basic principles of medical ethics can serve as theoretical guidelines to every health professional working in a variety of contexts.

As far as the first stage of the project was concerned, the most important ethical problems referred to the issues of consent and confidentiality. Since this sort of project was carried out for the first time, marine companies showed a big interest in it by actively encouraging their employees to answer the questionnaires and submit themselves to the clinical tests. Thus, although the participation of the research subjects was the consequence of their informed consent, it was also the result of a certain persuasion exercised by the employers. That sort of persuasion did not render the consent given 'coerced', as the participants did have the freedom to abstain. But it does show a paternalistic attitude by the marine companies, motivated by their specific interests: better health of the workers means bigger productivity and bigger financial gains.

As far as confidentiality was concerned, the participants were assured that the results of the tests would be disclosed only to them. Therefore, when some marine companies demanded from the ISPM access to the results of the survey, the ISPM refused, respecting the participants' right of autonomy and confidentiality. Undoubtedly the disclosure of such data to the employers might affect the occupational status of the employees by enabling the company to fire or to refuse to hire a seaman because of his health condition. It must be mentioned that the results were also disclosed to the company's doctor. The ethical issue here concerns the occupational doctor's professional relationship with his employers, a relationship which defines the limits of respect for the confidential information regarding the employees: if the nature of the relationship established between the doctor and the company obliges him to disclose the information to the latter, an important ethical problem is created which, unfortunately, falls outside the researcher's competence to handle.

The main ethical problems of the second stage concerned the use and evaluation of the information obtained. Although during the first stage the encouragement of the project was in the best interests of both employers and employees, albeit for different reasons, the conflict of these interests arises in the stage of evaluation of the collected data and active intervention. As the project aimed not only to diagnose, but to help practically as well, the results were sent by mail to each participant separately, advising him to get to a doctor as soon as possible where a particular health problem had been diagnosed. In this way respect for the principle of autonomy (respect for the individual's right to choose a course of action according to his own beliefs and wishes) was combined with the principle of beneficence.

However, the project's aim, to offer practical help, raises another issue which concerns the 'second part' of the programme, i.e. the necessity to meet the target group's needs after these have been diagnosed during the 'first part' of the programme. This responsibility falls on the shoulders of the ISPM research team, of the relevant health agencies and of the state. In order to meet these needs the research team included in its intervention health education materials, education concerning health matters addressed to the captains of the ships, and improvements in the medical and pharmacological equipment of each ship.

The responsibility of the health agencies and the state concerns 'positive action': according to the preamble of the WHO's Constitution of 1946: 'the enjoyment of the highest attainable standard of health is one of the fundamental rights of every human being'. This right entails an obligation of the state to act for its citizens' benefit. This, of course, is not always possible due to the scarcity of financial resources. But beneficence can also be constrained by other, exogenous factors: in this case such factors were the seamen's inevitable isolation and their actual inability to reach health services. Failure, however, of the proper agencies to take into consideration the results of such a survey can amount to a violation of the state's responsibility to act positively, since a considerable part of Greek economic life has a lot to do with the sea.

Health promotion can be realized by, on the one hand, health education and behaviour control and, on the other hand, by the enactment of legislation. In this particular example the part of health education was realized by the lectures, the seminars, the publications, etc. carried out by the research team. But the state can intervene as far as regulations and legislation are concerned: rules and laws concerning the health care of seamen (rules on individual behaviour, hygiene, health services, etc.); new rules for shipbuilding, as various studies have shown that the construction of a commercial ship and the formation of its different compartments play a considerable role in the seaman's physical and mental health. Dormitories near the engine rooms, for example, where the noise is continuous, isolated cabins or unfriendly common rooms, etc., constitute important environmental factors influencing the everyday life of these people. Since this project was carried out for the first time in Greece, the results could be of great value to the planning of a strategy aiming to promote Greek seamen's health. Nevertheless, it should be observed that in Greece the procedure of changing the existing legislation, or of enacting new laws, is especially time-consuming and most often delayed by various bureaucratic obstacles.

Although health promotion has proved to be very valuable, it is often accused of being a paternalistic concept. It is true that by aiming to modify individual behaviour (a behaviour which is the result of values and beliefs inculcated into every person and descending from generation to generation) it has various ethical drawbacks. Most concepts, however, have a positive and a negative aspect. The way in which health promotion is carried out plays a crucial role in the formation of such a judgement. By following the line of analysis proposed by the four basic principles, the health professional can recognize the ethical parameters of each case, the underlying dilemmas, the inherent rights and obligations of each side, and can handle them effectively without infringing deontological rules. According to Beauchamp and Childress (24) the rules justify— or not—the actions; and the principles, which are more general, justify the rules.

Thus, the four basic principles of medical ethics can guide the health professional towards a more specific application of a moral judgement: it is a methodological pathway from the *'abstracto'* to the *'concreto'*; and, although the principles are not absolute but generate many conflicts, they do constitute a useful tool of analysis.

REFERENCES

1. Dunstan, G. R. 1987. Evolution and mutation in medical ethics. Pp. 3–14, *in* Doxiadis, S. (Ed.) *Ethical dilemmas in health promotion*. John Wiley & Sons, Chichester.
2. McKeown, T. 1976. *The modern rise of population*. Edward Arnold, London.
3. Ottawa Charter for Health Promotion. 1987. *Health Promotion: An International Journal* **1** (4): iii.
4. Fox, R. 1977. The medicalization and demedicalization of American society. *In* Knowles, J. (Ed.) *Doing better and feeling worse: health in the United States*. Norton, New York.
5. Illich, I. 1977. *Medical nemesis*. Bantam, New York.
6. Ryan, W. 1971. *Blaming the victim*. Random House, New York.
7. Hamburg, D. A., Elliott, G. R. and Parron, D. L. (Eds). 1982. *Health and behavior*. Academic Press, Washington, DC.
8. Freire, P. 1985. *Pedagogy of the oppressed*. Continuum, New York.
9. Faden, R. and Beauchamp, T. 1986. *A history and theory of informed consent*. Oxford University Press, New York.
10. Faden, R. 1987. Ethical issues in government sponsored public health campaigns. *Health Education Quarterly* **14** (1): 27.
11. O'Connell, J. and Price, J. 1983. Ethical theories for promoting health through behavioral change. *Journal of School Health* **53** (8): 476.
12. Benjamin, M. and Curtis, J. 1981. *Ethics in nursing*. Oxford University Press, New York.
13. Wikler, D. 1978. Coercive measures in health promotion: can they be justified? *Health Education Monographs* **6** (2): 223.
14. Nathan, P. 1984. Johnson and Johnson's Live for Life: A Comprehensive Positive Lifestyle Change Program. *In* Matarazzo, J., Weiss, S., Herd, J., Miller, N. and Weiss, S. (Eds) *Behavioral health: a handbook of health enhancement and disease prevention*. John Wiley & Sons, New York.
15. Minkler, M. 1978. Ethical issues in community organization. *Health Education Monographs*, **6** (2).
16. Opit, L. J. 1987. How should information on health care be generated and used? *World Health Forum* **8**: 409.
17. Teeling Smith, G. 1989. *Measurement and management in the NHS*. Office of Health Economics, London.
18. Charny, M. C., Farrow, S. C. and Roberts, C. J. 1987. The cost of saving a life through cervical cytology screening: implications for health policy. *Health Policy* **7**: 345.
19. Allegrante, J. and Sloan, R. 1986. Ethical dilemmas in workplace health promotion. *Preventive Medicine* **15**: 1.
20. The Wyatt Company. 1984. *1984 Group benefits survey*. Wyatt Company, New York.
21. Svensson, T. and Sandlund, M. 1990. Ethics and preventive medicine. *Scandinavian Journal of Social Medicine* **18**: 275.
22. Simonds, S. 1978. Health education: facing issues of policy, ethics and social justice. *Health Education Monographs* **6** (1): 18 (Suppl.).
23. Minkler, M. 1985. Building supportive ties and sense of community among the inner city elderly: the Tenderloin services outreach project. *Health Education Quarterly* **12** (4): 303.
24. Beauchamp, T. L. and Childress, J. F. 1983. *Principles of biomedical ethics*, 2nd edn. Oxford University Press, New York.

25. Skrabanek, P. 1990. Why is preventive medicine exempted from ethical constraints? *Journal of Medical Ethics* **16**: 187.
26. McLeroy, K. R., Gottlieb, N. H. and Burdine, J. N. 1987. The business of health promotion: Ethical issues and professional responsibilities. *Health Education Quarterly* **14** (1): 91.
27. Gillon, R. 1990. Ethics in health promotion and prevention of disease. *Journal of Medical Ethics* **16**: 171.

73

Health Care, Sociology and Medical Ethics

DAVID ARMSTRONG

Department of General Practice, UMDS, Guy's Hospital, London, UK

CHARLOTTE HUMPHREY

Department of Public Health and Primary Care, Royal Free School of Medicine, London, UK

In keeping with the rest of this book, this chapter discusses the four key principles of medical ethics, namely autonomy, justice, non-maleficence and beneficence. However, these principles are not the everyday currency of sociology and cannot therefore be discussed as part of the sociological lexicon. As with the concepts, so with the tools—the mode of analysis which centres on the case history as an instructive device for the elucidation of appropriate behaviour is also alien to the way in which sociologists work, although in itself this approach is of some sociological interest because of the way in which its use affects the selection of problems for study. This chapter will therefore not use autonomy, justice, non-maleficence and beneficence as criteria for analysing ethical dilemmas. Rather, it will explore the four principles themselves as sociological concepts and discuss the ways in which they colour the very problems that they are intended to clarify, as does the case history approach so widely employed in ethical analysis.

PRINCIPLES AND VALUES

Following from the successes of natural science, sociologists have often dreamed of discovering laws or principles which govern human behaviour. Their search has usually involved looking for aspects of behaviour which occur in all societies, both contemporary and historical, on the assumption that such common or universal behaviour might indicate an underlying pattern which could then be

Principles of Health Care Ethics. Edited by Raanan Gillon.
© 1994 John Wiley & Sons Ltd

regarded as a general principle. However, the main result of this search for common patterns has been the discovery of immense variation. The best that can be achieved is a list of the activities that any social group must engage in to ensure survival, such as the procurement of shelter and food, but these common ends can be achieved by any number of different means, and thus their identification does little to explain the rich variety of everyday behaviour.

Besides these survival criteria, there are also some commonalities such as ideas of good and bad, or right and wrong, that are everywhere to be found. But these, on their own, explain very little of human behaviour because it is the content of these concepts that is important, not the fact that they exist. Human behaviour is not explained by the fact that all societies have a notion of good and bad, but rather by what counts as good and bad in each particular society. To give a specific example, many religions have dietary proscriptions, but the varying content of those proscriptions may result in the avoidance of quite different foods in different cultures.

Sociologists now recognize that the search for universal principles governing human behaviour is a futile one. What has proved to be much more rewarding is the examination of the values which characterize particular social groupings, since values have been shown to offer a much better framework for understanding behaviour and for exploring the richness of variation between societies.

The first question that a sociologist would ask about the four basic principles is whether they are genuine principles—in the sense of being universal attributes of human morality—or values that are socially derived. Convention has it that the principles were first elucidated in the civilization of ancient Greece. By implication, at some point in the dim and distant past before that time there was a pre-moral state. However, ever since their original identification in ancient Greece, there is a tacit belief that these four principles have provided the benchmarks by which ethical behaviour in medical practice may be evaluated. The task of the sociologist is to explore the social origins of these principles and the extent to which their significance may be culturally or temporally specific. It soon becomes clear that, far from being universal, the interpretation of the four principles and the circumstances of their application are both firmly wedded to fairly recent western ideals of human conduct.

NON-MALEFICENCE AND BENEFICENCE

Ethicists have sometimes attempted to prioritize the four principles in such a way as to separate out those that are most 'basic'. In such a framework, non-maleficence and beneficence come together as the foundations upon which ethics is built. In other words, it is the imperative to do good and not to do harm which underpins moral behaviour. No sociologist would quarrel with the importance of these two features of social life. As we have already acknowledged, all societies have notions of good and harm, and views about promotion of the first and avoidance of the other. In this sense they are universal concepts; even so, they still may have a social origin and sociologists have advanced ideas about why these concepts characterize all societies. The great sociologist Emile Durkheim (1858–1917) argued that the basic feature of all societies was the primacy of social life itself (1). He argued that the division of reality into the social and the non-social is encoded in two fundamental symbolic representations, namely what is considered sacred, and what profane; and this duality of classification extends to all facets of social values. In this sense, doing good and not causing harm are universal features of all societies inasmuch as they are components of social reality itself.

However, while all societies have notions of doing good and avoiding harm, it is clear that the actual components of what is regarded as morally correct vary considerably across cultures and over time. A discussion about the rights and wrongs of sustaining the life of a severely handicapped baby occurs in a society whose values and material circumstances are far removed from those where infanticide was, and is, regularly carried out for various social purposes. Moreover, even the context in which such a debate is set reflects the dominant individualist values that pervade modern western society. Neonatal controversies about who should live and who should die tend only to address the life of the individual concerned (particularly as the argument is usually based around the unique case history) and ignore the wider context of health care provision. The social, political and economic reasons why one infant and not another lies in the neonatal care unit in the first place are rarely perceived as a legitimate subject of ethical disputation. In short, the contemporary ethical view of non-maleficence and beneficence not only reflects values particular to modern western societies, but in the very context of its application embodies and reflects those same values.

JUSTICE

It might seem that the third ethical principle, justice, would attend to the wider inequalities in health care provision. In its widest context, justice refers to the allocation and distribution of what might be called goods and harms in a society. Of course, it is therefore constrained by the particular notions of good and harm which happen to prevail. In addition, like non-maleficence and beneficence, justice is usually considered in a decontextualized manner in circumstances involving individuals; wider issues tend to be ignored. For example, it has been known for several decades that a major factor determining health status is the particular social group to which a person belongs: lower social classes have higher mortality and increased morbidity. This issue has been identified, explored, and publicized by sociologists as a major problem in health and health care in western countries. Given the magnitude of the inequalities exposed, this would seem an obvious area for attention by medical ethicists concerned about justice. In fact they have devoted remarkably little attention to it. This neglect again reflects medical ethics' primary preoccupation with decisions about particular patients. It also, however, points to the inability of a method of analysis dominated by a case-study approach to comprehend discussion about variations between groups rather than unique individuals.

AUTONOMY

Preoccupation with individual interaction ultimately reflects the centrality of the fourth ethical principle of autonomy. Whereas all societies can be said to have notions of good and harm—whatever the words may mean—and all have a system of justice, inasmuch as these goods and harms are variously distributed, the notion of autonomy is distinct in seeming peculiar to modern western societies.

There is now a considerable sociological literature exploring the emergence of autonomy as a core value of modern industrialized society. Briefly, the argument is that concomitant with industrialization and growth in the division of labour, differences between people also increased. Whereas in primarily agrarian or hunter–gatherer communities people were united by their similar roles, in societies characterized by a strong division of labour people become differentiated through their different work activities and are held together by their mutual interdependence. In other words, the notion of universal personal autonomy only emerged in western societies about two centuries ago with industrialization. It is at that time that ordinary individuality, 'the everyday individuality of everybody', emerged 'from below the threshold of description' (2). This development can be seen in the early nineteenth-century concerns with counting individuals (the first census took place in 1801); with treating them—in hospitals and prisons; with changing and moulding them through providing education; and through giving them civil rights. Indeed, the word 'individualism' only appeared for the first time at the beginning of the nineteenth century (3). Whether it is economic, political, artistic or romantic individualism, the roots of the concept seem firmly located in one particular cultural and historical moment (4). In sum, the many moral positions which pervade western societies on the rights of individuals have their origins in the social and economic changes which produced a sense of individual identity over the last 200 years.

Corroborative evidence can be found in those anthropological and historical studies which have examined the extent to which individualism is a feature of other societies (5). Summarized, their findings indicate that while various facets of certain particular individuals seem to be celebrated in all societies, the notion that all members of a population have an autonomous individual identity remains unique to western culture.

The centrality of individualism in modern western societies explains why autonomy is viewed as a cardinal ethical principle. It also explains why the problems perceived as ethical dilemmas are largely about individual states, decisions and interactions. But the designation of autonomy as a 'principle' is something of a misnomer. Certainly it is a key feature of our society, and a strongly held value, but it is not a value which is shared with equal force in non-western cultures, nor even with our own recent ancestors.

ETHICS AND SOCIETY

Where does this leave the four key ethical principles? The first two—non-maleficence and beneficence—embody notions which are common to all societies but which vary substantially in actual content. The framework of good and harm might stand as a general principle, but the content is clearly value-laden and also influenced by material conditions. In the pluralistic societies in which we live, it becomes increasingly difficult to identify shared notions of what is to be evaluated as a good and what as a harm. In this sense, ethical debate, which tries to weigh the balance of maleficence and beneficence in any particular situation, to a large extent simply reflects a dialogue between different values in the society. Inasmuch as there is no single agreed notion of good or harm, but a variety of competing views, such dilemmas admit of no solution. Nevertheless, rehearsal of the different arguments for the purpose of defining the dilemma does enable the diversity and richness of competing value systems to be acknowledged and publicly celebrated.

The idea that all societies have a principle of justice is something of a truism. Of course, all societies have different allocations of goods and harms, and the pattern of allocation can always be called that society's system of justice. But what is to count as just in any society will depend on the nature of the behaviours and states which count as good, as well as other values surrounding social organization. Thus, for example, western societies institute systems of justice to ensure individual freedoms, but these freedoms are largely concerned with 'freedom to' do certain things. What tend to be ignored are the other 'freedoms from' which were once held as important, at least by the faded 'communist' societies of Eastern Europe. While rights of free speech and assembly are vigorously maintained as a cornerstone of social justice, millions of people do not have freedom from unemployment, homelessness, ill-health, etc. The notions of justice applied in medical ethics in western countries tend simply to reproduce what those same societies consider to be fair.

The final ethical principle of autonomy, more than any of the others, celebrates western moral supremacy. It has also become the dominant principle to which the other three have been subordinated, inasmuch as what is to count as good or harm and what as just are all subsumed under the greater good of individual autonomy. Nevertheless, as we have argued, this one core value is not an inviolable feature of all social patterning. Indeed there is no fundamental reason why the notion of autonomy, despite its widespread acceptance in western societies, should survive another two centuries into the future.

Perhaps the core difference between sociology and ethics as academic disciplines is the fact that the former tends to work with descriptive theories and the latter with prescriptive. Sociology is concerned with describing and trying to understand the world, thus most of its studies have some empirical basis, seeking to explain what 'is'. In contrast, ethics is concerned to decide what 'ought to be' and is less interested in identifying the empirical roots for the values it holds up as principles. No doubt sociologists *qua* sociologists have their own views of what is good, or just, or respects autonomy, but these are derived from and embedded in empirical theories of the world. This means that the very questions asked by ethicists and sociologists about health care provision (as well as other things) are different in the form of the questions, the assumptions which lie behind them, and what are to count as acceptable answers.

IMPLICATIONS FOR HEALTH CARE

Because the sociologist's perspective is concerned with describing and understanding the (social) world the subject of medical ethics itself falls under that description. This means that ethics is another 'belief system' which needs social analysis. Where might this start?

Clearly in view of the plurality of modern society there is a place for mechanisms through which values can be expressed and negotiated. In the past such processes were more likely carried out through suppression of unorthodox or different values, but, in large part, this facility is not available in modern industrialized societies. We have to live with different and often conflicting views. It might be argued therefore that this gives ethics an important social role as a discourse through which dissent can be ritually contained through a formalized discussion of and reflection on social values. Ethicists may see themselves as concerned with finding solutions to difficulties of individual behaviour: in practice, and probably more important since such solutions are often either obvious or impossible to agree, ethical debate provides a forum for displaying and reinforcing some of the core social values of our society. In particular, the emphasis on the legitimacy of different views, together with the focus on situations of high social drama, allows a secular route for the celebration of the complex link between medicine, society and health care. The function of medical ethics is neither to change nor study the world, but to reveal it as spectacle.

REFERENCES

1. Durkheim, E. 1948. *Elementary forms of the religious life.* Free Press, Glencoe, IL.
2. Foucault, M. 1977. *Discipline and punish: the birth of the prison.* Allen Lane, London.
3. Williams, R. 1976. *Keywords.* Fontana, London.
4. Lukes, S. 1973. *Individualism.* Blackwell, Oxford.
5. Carrithers, M., Collins, S. and Lukes, S. (Eds). 1985. *The category of the person.* Cambridge University Press, Cambridge.

74

Medical Technology, Social and Health Care Issues

BRYAN JENNETT, CBE, MD, FRCS

*Professor, Department of Neurosurgery, Institute of Neurological Sciences,
University of Glasgow, Glasgow, UK*

Much of the burgeoning interest in health care ethics can be ascribed to the increasing use of technology in medicine. Medical technology can be defined as the use of tools to assist in the tasks of medicine. Diagnostic technologies extend the capacity of doctors to find out what is happening in a patient's body. Examples are X-rays and other imaging techniques, and various endoscopes for looking into internal organs; electronic monitoring of the activity of the heart, lungs, brain and nerves and of the flow of blood in various organs; and examining the chromosomes in cells to detect inherited abnormalities. In addition the use of computers for processing information about individual patients allows comparison with banks of data about previous patients with similar conditions. In place of doctors' opinions that this or that is likely to happen computer technology makes it possible to provide more accurate diagnosis and prognosis, with statistical probabilities. Therapeutic technologies mostly involve interventions to remove diseased parts or to substitute lost function. Surgery is the oldest technology but it is still evolving, with procedures that were believed impossible 25 years ago now commonplace. Functional technologies include ventilators, kidney machines, heart pacemakers and fertility techniques, as well as aids for the disabled.

Diagnosis can often be reached in less stressful and more accurate ways using technology, and prognosis more reliably estimated, while therapeutic technologies can often save and extend lives of good quality, and improve the quality of life when death is not a threat. It might therefore be expected that technology would be regarded as a welcome development in medicine. However, the benefits of technology have to be balanced against a variety of burdens (1). Inevitably technology needs teams of doctors in different disciplines, aided by specialized nurses, physicists and technicians. As a result the patient is no longer alone with his doctor on the stage, nor at times does he seem to be centre stage.

Principles of Health Care Ethics. Edited by Raanan Gillon.

Doctors are even sometimes accused of being wedded to technology for its own sake, rather than for the patient's benefit, particularly when the result is to prolong life that is of questionable quality. Technology is also often seen as distancing doctors from their patients, consequently replacing or reducing the touching and talking that used to be at the centre of the doctor–patient encounter. In this respect technology is sometimes suspected of having a dehumanizing effect on medical practice.

Issues about each of the four principles of medical ethics therefore frequently arise when technologies are used. The balance between beneficence and non-maleficence—doing good and avoiding harm—is of particular importance for technological medicine. Patient autonomy, the right to choose, must always be considered—remembering that doctors are the servants of their patients, not their masters. Has the patient had an opportunity to give informed consent for the initiation of each technology, or its continued use? Traditionally it is only surgery that has to be 'signed for', no matter how minor the procedure, while many other life-saving and life-sustaining technologies are of much more significance. The fourth ethical principle, justice, is more contentious. Most technologies are costly in terms of capital investment, consumables and specialized staff, making them limited in availability, as well as competing with non-technological activities in health care. Justice or fairness in the deployment of scarce resources therefore often focuses on technologies. This applies both at the level of macro-allocation and of selecting which individual patients should be given the opportunity to benefit.

It is therefore no surprise that more than a third of the chapters in section 2 of this book relate to technology, either directly or indirectly, as do more than half the titles in section 3, and two-thirds in section 5. The chapters on consent, harms and benefits, risks, non-treatment decisions, economics, rationing and medical research are each likely to be dominated by technology—in addition to those devoted to specific technologies.

In this chapter some of the general features of medical technology will be considered, with the focus on the therapeutic because these pose the starkest ethical dilemmas. These concern respect for patients, quality of life, the balance of benefits and burdens, the issues of cost and distributive justice. The question is seldom whether a given technology is good or bad, but rather whether its use in particular circumstances is worthwhile—in terms of the individual patient or the health service as a whole. Examples will be from surgery in general and from intensive care, because these common activities are not the subject of specific analysis elsewhere in this book.

ATTITUDES TO TECHNOLOGY

The variety and complexity of medical technologies are such that few people can be fully informed about all the aspects of even one of them. That does not prevent strong views being held, views that inevitably reflect the perspective of a particular observer. The debate may be either about the level of *provision* by health authorities of devices and supporting facilities, or about the *use* made by doctors of the technological resources at their disposal. Provision depends on reaching a balance between the claims of the product champions for a given technology, and the perceptions of those deploying the limited budgets of providers or purchasers of health care. Most product champions are clinicians acting as advocates for particular patient groups. With newly emerging technologies, however, some clinicians may themselves have been involved in some aspect of an innovation; or they may have been encouraged to adopt a new technique by colleagues associated with its development or, where manufactured devices are involved, by marketing men from industry. Where budgets are fixed, product champions and health authorities have hitherto often been regarded as representing opposing vested interests—the one promoting and other tending to resist increased provision. Where market forces influence health care provision, however, managers may wish to acquire a certain technology in order to attract patients from competing providers, as commonly occurs in the USA.

The main influence upon the use of technologies that have already been provided has hitherto been the aggregated decisions of clinicians who treat individual patients. As increased attention is paid to the autonomy of patients, their role as the ultimate consumers will likely become more important. Neither doctors nor patients can, however, make rational decisions unless there are good data available about the efficacy and effectiveness of a technology in specified circumstances. In practice such data about technology assessment are often lacking, as explained later. As a consequence decisions are often unduly influenced by beliefs or prejudices. Evidence of the extent of professional uncertainty about the value of many technologies comes from the wide variations observed between their rate of use by different practitioners, particularly surgeons and intensivists (2).

Apart from those who are themselves involved in the provision and use of medical technologies, there are observers at a distance who may not hesitate to comment. The public as a whole, which can be regarded as made up entirely of patients past, present or future, is ambivalent about technology. Most often people seem to be calling for greater provision and use of certain technologies, usually because of unrealistic expectations of benefit. Yet some do seem increasingly aware that technology has the capacity for harm or at best for limited benefit. Public opinion may find expression in the patient advocate groups for certain diseases, or in organizations associated with hospitals. Either of these groups may raise money for the purchase of technological machines that they consider to be under-provided, and they may be encouraged in this by clinicians. Pressures may also come from politicians anxious to attract additional provision for their local hospital, or for some patient group which has lobbied them. The media also have an important role in informing the public about medical technologies. Whilst journalists are sometimes uncritical in raising false expectations, both broadcast and print media on the whole do good by increasing public awareness of the pros and cons of various technologies. This knowledge enhances the power of patients who wish to question their doctors when asked to consent to various procedures.

Also influential are the views of doctors in low-technology specialties, who commonly hold that too much of the health budget goes to their technological colleagues. Not only do they draw attention to the relative allocations between different specialties, they highlight the limited value of some technologies as they are often used. Psychiatrists, geriatricians, and others concerned with the care of chronic disabilities, are frequently supported in this by public health doctors, who frequently express concern about more equitable balance of resource allocation between the acute and chronic sectors of health care. These various doctors seem sometimes to be unaware of the capacity that some technologies have for reducing the dependency and improving the quality of life of chronically disabled people, and of the extent to which they are used to benefit the elderly (3). Implicit in the criticisms of these doctors is the belief that technological medicine is unduly expensive. It is therefore important to analyse the components of cost involved in technologies in general.

COSTS OF TECHNOLOGY

A few technologies entail large capital investment (> £0.5m), such as imaging machines, radiation therapy equipment and the lithotripter (for pulverizing stones). Many more cost several thousand pounds each, such as dialysis machines, monitoring apparatus, ventilators and endoscopes. Expensive consumables are a feature of some technologies (e.g. heart valves, pacemakers, implanted monitoring devices and chemical solutions for dialysis). But the major revenue cost for most technologies is the salary bill for skilled staff. On the credit side, however, apart from patient benefit many diagnostic and therapeutic technologies reduce the need for, or the duration of, admission to hospital, with significant cost savings. In calculating unit cost (per patient, test or treatment), an important factor is whether expensive machines are used sufficiently often to justify the fixed costs of investment and staffing. But it is not only bad economics to have a machine that is idle much of the time. A certain volume throughput is needed to develop and maintain the skills of operators (doctors, nurses and technicians). Appeals to provide expensive technology at a local level on grounds of greater convenience for patients, or for the prestige of a smaller hospital, seldom take account of this important aspect of quality.

What really matters in estimating whether a given technology is judged to be economically 'worthwhile' for certain patients is the cost per unit of health gain—usually expressed as quality life year (see Chapter 71). Even when these calculations are made it is all too easy to include the costs only of those patients who were successfully diagnosed or treated by a given technology. It is, however, often important to consider also the expenditure on the many patients who had negative investigations or unsuccessful treatment for each one that was counted as a success. For diagnostic technologies allowance must be made for the benefits of reassurance resulting from negative tests. When the outcome of life-saving treatment is prolonged survival with severe disability, much larger costs may be incurred over subsequent years of dependence than would have resulted from death. An estimate of these post-treatment costs for unsuccessful cases should also enter the equation for the cost of success. Likewise technological prolongation of the process of dying, for example by intensive care, may incur much greater expenditure than less active intervention and earlier death. These are all relevant factors when considering the ethical principle of justice in the allocation of resources. It is, however, important to remember that when rationing is rational the dictates of other ethical principles and those of economics often coincide, and it is often a false antithesis to assume a tension between ethics and economics (4,5).

INAPPROPRIATE USE OF TECHNOLOGIES

There are few technologies that are never of benefit, but even the best can do good only for selected patients. Most criticisms of technologies prove to be of their inappropriate use, which is surprisingly common even in countries where resources for technology are very restricted. Five types of inappropriate use have been identified (6). Use might be *unnecessary*, because the patient's condition is insufficiently serious to justify it. This applies to many diagnostic procedures as well as much of the monitoring in coronary and intensive care units and in labour wards and delivery rooms. The use of a technology may be *unsuccessful*, because the patient's condition is too far advanced to respond to that intervention. This applies to much rescue surgery for advanced cancer and to much intensive care for the terminally ill. A less absolute type of inappropriate use is when a technology's use is *unkind*, because it prolongs life of poor quality; or when it is *unsafe*, because the expected complications outweigh the anticipated benefits. Lastly the use of a technology may be deemed *unwise*, because it diverts resources from alternative health care activities that would bring more benefit to other patients. The first four of these inappropriate uses are to be regarded as offending the ethical principle of disproportion between the probability of beneficence and of non-maleficence. A sixth type of inappropriate use might be that it is *unwanted* because it is against the wishes of the patient, and fails to respect his autonomy.

Inappropriate use of technologies is widespread in a variety of countries with differing levels of health care provision and socioeconomic cultures. There are several reasons why doctors manage to ignore the claims of both ethics and economics when they coincide, and often indulge in inappropriate use of technologies in hospital (7). The most important is lack of knowledge about the benefits and burdens of applying a given technology in particular circumstances, often described as professional uncertainty. There may be no data available about what to expect from intervention; or the data may not be known to the decision-maker at the time. More often, however, that doctor chooses to ignore the data either because he does not think that they apply to this particular patient, or because he suspects the validity of the data. In desperate situations it may be reasonable to use treatment that has only a small probability of success.

However, due account should be paid to the difficult situation of clinicians confronted with patients who are critically ill or who have distressing symptoms or a dreaded diagnosis. The natural wish to respond positively in such circumstances certainly can contribute to the lack of rationality that sometimes appears to inform decisions to employ technologies, especially in emergency situations. Partly this may be a response to the perceived or supposed expectation of the patient and the family, and also of other doctors and nurses—both those who may have referred the patient and those sharing their care now. Decision-making in acute hospitals is today carried out in the presence of a host of witnesses, who may hold a variety of opinions and prejudices. To state the principle that it is bad medicine to persist with futile treatment, and that no patient has a right to futile treatment, is not difficult. Confronted with a seriously ill patient, however, some doctors are reluctant to make a decision to limit treatment. They will then often fall back on the excuse of uncertainty about the prognosis, or on the possibility that intervention might help, even when there is little or no evidence for either of these assertions.

Another factor that accounts for excessive (or unduly prolonged) use of technologies when dealing with hopelessly ill patients is what I have called the 'cycle of commitment' (6). Consider a severely head-injured patient who is transferred to a regional neurosurgical unit, perhaps with nurses and doctors in the ambulance and even police outriders. On arrival at the unit it is clear that the patient is irrecoverably injured, having regard to the responsiveness of the patient and his age. The correct decision would be to accept this situation and not to embark on any further investigation or treatment. In practice such a patient is often submitted to a CT scan, and this may reveal a large intracranial haematoma, causing cerebral compression. This discovery should make no difference, if it has already been decided that the patient's clinical state and age makes recovery impossible. Once this lesion has been found, however, it can be difficult to resist the 'imperative' to operate to remove the compressing clot, perhaps because of concern that those involved in transferring the patient might feel that insufficient response had been made. There may also be a worry about what the coroner might say if a pathologist reported an untreated haematoma. If, however, the doctor can give good reasons to believe that intervention would have been futile, it is highly unlikely that any coroner would challenge these. However, because of these doubts the patient may be subjected to surgery. If at the end of the operation the anaesthetist finds that the patient cannot breathe on his own, the choice is to let him die on the table, or to send him to intensive care for several days of futile ventilation—and too often this latter course is chosen.

It is easy to understand how the clinician finds it more difficult to resist further action once decisions to intervene have already been taken, and the cycle of commitment has begun. Reasons for justifying each decision at the time may be understandable, but in retrospect none of the decisions can be said to have met the crucial criterion of a reasonable expectation of net benefit. Indeed each intervention could be considered to have been inappropriate and even unethical, because the result was an unnecessarily protracted and undignified death for the patient, and an extended period of distress for his family and friends. The failure to withhold or withdraw treatment from a hopeless patient soon after arrival may also deny treatment to another who could have benefited— an example of distributive injustice in the use of resources. Similar clinical situations are not uncommon in other surgical specialties and in intensive care. Indeed the most frequent criticism in confidential enquiries of peri-operative deaths is of operations that were unjustified because the disease was too far advanced to benefit from surgery; many of these patients were also elderly.

It would be ingenuous not to include among the reasons (or excuses) for over-treatment of patients the fear of subsequent legal proceedings, whether this is real or apparent. In the United States so-called defensive medicine may be inevitable, but there is little excuse in Europe, where litigiousness is much less apparent and where the widespread availability of adequate medical care makes large legal claims for medically dependent survivors unjustified. A useful defence against such concern is the development of agreed guidelines or consensus statements that indicate the general circumstances in which a decision may properly be made to limit treatment (see Chapter 26).

TOWARDS MORE APPROPRIATE USE OF TECHNOLOGIES

There is little prospect of more rational and effective use of technologies until more data are available concerning their effects in various circumstances. But there is need also for wider recognition that good practice requires doctors to take account of such data when making decisions. A strategy of technology assessment should identify effective technologies and determine the limits of appropriate use based on a sliding scale of benefits and burdens for different types of patients (1). The next stage is to appraise effective technologies economically and then to consider the affordable level of provision.

The process of assessment begins with establishing that the technology is feasible and safe, at the technical level. Then it is necessary to discover whether or not its use improves patient outcome significantly, as compared with that predicted to occur with alternative methods. It also needs to be shown that this benefit does occur in a significant number of the patients treated. It is generally agreed that the most reliable way to demonstrate such efficacy is by a randomized control trial (see Chapter 40). Such trials are the rule for drugs, not only because there are strict regulations limiting the licensing of drugs unless adequate trials have been carried out, but because the considerable expense of controlled trials is commonly met by the pharmaceutical industry.

The problem with technologies is that there is no restriction on their introduction, particularly those that involve no more than a rearrangement or extension of existing practices—as is the rule with surgical innovations and new techniques in intensive care. Moreover there is no financial backer, and only a few such procedures have been submitted to controlled trials. Where these have been done the usual result has been to find that the technology is of value in a much more limited group of patients than had originally been claimed. Those responsible for the provision of expensive new technologies could make it a condition of providing capital and revenue funds that formal assessment was carried out. They might also make continued support contingent on satisfactory results from evaluation.

It is unrealistic to expect that all technologies will be submitted to randomized trials, particularly those many technologies that are already in common use but that have not yet been adequately assessed. The next best approach to their more appropriate application is to maintain accurate prospective audit of the use of such technologies, including the types of patients treated and the outcome. It is easier to determine the value of interventions when the outcome is evident within a short time, such as averting an immediate threat to life, or the relief of pain. It is much more difficult when the issue is increased survival many years after surgery for cancer. However, it was the collection of limited data in cancer registers that first cast serious doubt on the value of radical mastectomy for carcinoma of the breast. That in turn led to prospective trials which confirmed that this mutilating procedure, which had been advocated for many years as obviously the best treatment, gave no better results than more conservative measures that were much less burdensome for the patient.

The availability of computerized data collection and analysis to acquire better data concerning the prognosis of disease with alternative treatments, and to quantify the balance between the probability of benefits and complications, should make it possible to assess the value of therapeutic technologies, new and old, much more rapidly and less expensively than hitherto. There will, however, still be a need for randomized trials to resolve outstanding questions about some technologies, and the ethical questions that these trials raise are discussed elsewhere (see Chapter 40).

FEATURES OF SURGERY AND INTENSIVE CARE

Surgery is a technology that has been accepted for centuries as sometimes necessary, sometimes successful but always one that exacts a price from the patient. Before the development of anaesthesia, that price was high, and it was obvious both to the patients and to everyone within earshot. Yet legs were amputated, bladder stones removed and wounds repaired, and some patients lived long lives after the experience. Surgical patients today still face some pain and discomfort, and the risk of complications from the surgery or the anaesthesia (which can occasionally result in severe or fatal brain damage). Even if all goes well some operations inevitably result in some degree of scarring, mutilation or functional loss. Medical regimens, including technologies such as dialysis, can be altered or abandoned if they seem to be doing no good, or to be disproportionately burdensome. But surgery is irreversible, and this puts a particular responsibility on surgeons to balance the expected benefits and burdens for a particular patient. In doing so he needs to take account of the surgical skill of whoever will actually be operating. This factor is seldom given the weight it deserves, and decisions may be unrealistically based on the results reported from a distant specialist unit that has exceptional results. Local audit of outcome is the only way to monitor this factor. In general such personal skill factors do not affect outcome from non-surgical therapies so critically, although special units may have better than average results for some complex treatment such as cancer chemotherapy.

Surgeons need therefore to put the pros and cons of the operations they propose to their patients (see Chapters 39 and 40). Although written consent for surgery and anaesthesia has long been customary, until recently this was limited to signing what was almost a blank cheque. The form authorized the surgeon not only to carry out a specified named procedure ('the nature of which has been explained to me'), but also to do whatever else was found necessary. How much explanation the patients received varied widely from one surgeon to another. Many patients now expect a reasonable account not only of the proposed procedure but of its risks and the likelihood of success; and also of the natural history of their condition with alternative treatment, or with no treatment at all.

Surgeons need to become more sensitive to the wishes of patients, whose priorities and perceptions of risk and benefit may be quite different from those of their surgeon. Not only are the perspectives of the surgeon and his patient quite different, but so may be their ages and their backgrounds. Even among much more similar people there is a wide variation in attitude to risk-taking in respect of health decisions and other activities, and also about concepts of quality of life. When there is a marked divergence between the opinion of a patient and his surgeon about what to do, the patient's preferences should prevail—provided that the surgeon is satisfied that the patient realizes the implications of his choice.

That is all very well for elective surgery, when there is time for discussion with the patient and his family, perhaps even before coming into hospital. In some surgical specialties, however, many patients present as emergencies, as do most patients admitted to intensive care units—including those who have had emergency resuscitation elsewhere in the hospital after cardiorespiratory arrest, major trauma or another crisis. The exceptions in intensive care are patients who are having routine postoperative support and observation after major surgery, which would probably have been explained to the patient when seeking consent for operation. But if serious complications have occurred either during or soon after surgery or anaesthesia, the patient may unexpectedly find himself reliant on life-support technologies, and he may be in no condition to question their continuation, let alone have been able to consent to their initiation.

DILEMMAS IN RESCUE MEDICINE

Decision-making is often difficult in rescue medicine (emergency surgery, resuscitation and unplanned intensive care), and consent is not the only ethical issue. Such patients fall into three groups. Some have suffered sudden illness or accident and for them everything possible must be done initially in the way of life-saving and life-sustaining measures, unless or until it is certain that the situation is hopeless. There will often be some delay before relatives can be consulted in order to expand on information gained from the patient about his previous medical history and his attitude to rescue procedures. The second group are those undergoing surgery or other procedures in hospital who have developed an unexpected complication. Much is already known about these patients, and it may be that the possibility of such a crisis will already have been discussed with them. Thirdly are the patients with chronic, progressive conditions who suffer a crisis or relapse which may have been predictable. The probability of such an eventuality may already have been discussed with the patient and the family, and the possibility raised that it may be better not to intervene with rescue measures.

The problem is that the critical events that call for rescue can occur at any time of any day of the week. Even when there is background information about a patient this may be unknown to the doctor who has to decide what to do. Moreover he may be relatively junior, and senior advice may not be immediately available. These various factors contribute to the tendency to inappropriate over-treatment of some of these patients, which may begin a cycle of commitment as already described. Many doctors and nurses find it more difficult to withdraw treatment that has been started than to withhold it in the first place. Yet in patients without progressive disease it may not be clear that no immediate or lasting benefit is possible until after a trial period of resuscitation or intensive care. The majority of patients subjected to unjustified emergency surgery have advanced cancer, and they are also often elderly. Common presentations are obstruction of the colon or oesophagus, or massive bleeding from bowel or bladder. Even though such patients are terminally ill, surgery may sometimes be justified because it truly is the most effective form of immediate palliation. However, surgeons may not always consider as carefully as they should the alternatives of adequate doses of analgesic or sedative drugs. Partly this is because they are accustomed to surgical dicta about relieving obstruction of the gut or arresting haemorrhage. But it may also be because they are less familiar with the practicalities of terminal care than with a technological response. It is one thing to refer patients to a hospice a few months before they die, another to deal appropriately with a terminal crisis in the middle of the night when there is expectation of surgery.

Intensive care units offer a range of technological rescue options, both to save and to sustain life. These include ventilators, drugs to maintain blood pressure and cardiac action, transfusion of blood, other fluids and nutrition, and haemodialysis. Then there are many monitoring techniques necessary to identify the needs of a patient and his response to treatment. None of these is free of risk, with numerous possibilities for mistakes to be made—e.g. in connecting ventilators, manipulating invasive monitoring devices, withdrawing body fluids and injecting substances. There is also the high risk of cross-infection in intensive care units. Inevitably the continued activity around the patient, the lights on all night, the witnessing or overhearing of crises affecting nearby patients, all contrive to make the intensive care unit a disturbing environment for the patient who is conscious as well as for his relatives. Unless there is definite benefit to be derived from being there, it is no place to be.

Nursing staff in intensive care units are geared to making all efforts to save and sustain life, and it is their numbers and high level of training that make daily costs about five times greater than in an ordinary ward. It is, however, often difficult for the staff to scale down the level of care when this becomes appropriate because there is no longer any prospect of a favourable outcome. Whilst intensive care staff are naturally primarily devoted to saving life, this is because this is a means towards regaining good-quality life. Preserving life for its own sake, regardless of what that life makes possible, is sometimes referred to as vitalism—or the principle of sanctity of life. It is often easier when hopelessness becomes certain after several days to discharge the patient to another ward or hospital, which has the added advantage of signalling to the relatives that a decision has been made to limit treatment. Unless they have been kept fully informed of how this decision has been reached, however, the family may consider that care is being withdrawn and that the therapeutic team has lost interest. Both humanity and economics dictate that the decision to withdraw intensive care should be made as soon as possible. To do so only after a week or more of expensive futile treatment, when death is already imminent, is hardly a decision at all. Made earlier the patient and family can be spared days of useless technological intervention, whilst there may be the opportunity for one or more other less severely affected patients to benefit from treatment there. However reluctant they may be to accept the role of gatekeepers to the health care resources of society, doctors in these expensive high-technology fields should regard the fair and effective use of these as one of their duties or responsibilities.

GUIDELINES FOR MORE APPROPRIATE USE OF TECHNOLOGY

The theme of this chapter so far has been the frequency with which technologies that can be of undoubted benefit are often used inappropriately, often offending one or more of the principles of medical ethics without proportionate compensatory gain for another of these principles. Improvement might come from the availability of better data from technology assessment. But some decision-makers would still probably often ignore this if they felt it conflicted with some vague concept of what they considered (or believed others might consider) to be good ethical medical practice. They might appeal to the sanctity of life principle—that it is unethical to limit or stop treatment as long as there is any prospect of prolonging life. There may also be a reluctance to choose between patients on the basis of the relative benefits that treatment might confer on each.

Whether it is selecting patients for elective surgery or dialysis, or for admission or discharge from intensive care, it is helpful to have written guidelines or policies. These will have added authority if their principles have been stated by some national body (e.g. Royal College, professional society or consensus conference). This will reassure staff that such policies are in accord with good practice in the medical and nursing professions. However, what really matters is to have agreement on the guidelines between the doctors and nurses locally.

The value of guidelines stems from their having resulted from thoughtful and critical discussion outside the emotional context of an individual case, and of representing a group judgement. Perhaps their main contribution is an indication to everyone concerned that decisions about the use of technology should depend on explicit policies, rather than on the intuition or prejudice of individual clinicians. Declaring what these policies are makes it possible for them to be debated, and if necessary changed from time to time. Those who are reluctant to have guidelines may voice concern that insufficient account may be taken of the needs of individual patients. The reality is that without guidelines there are wide variations in practice, with many patients receiving suboptimal treatment that could be considered to offend the principles of medical ethics. Guidelines are particularly useful for decisions about rescue, which have often to be made without an opportunity for wide discussion at the time.

CONCLUSION

Technologies have great potential for reducing avoidable death and disability, for improving the quality of life, and for prolonging lives of good quality. To fulfil that potential requires more knowledge about the effects of technology, and greater willingness to reach agreement about optimal practice—in the present state of knowledge, however incomplete this is. This holds out the best hope for more rational, more humane, and more economic use of medical technologies, in accordance with ethical principles.

REFERENCES

1. Jennett, B. 1986. *High technology medicine—benefits and burdens.* Oxford University Press, Oxford and New York.
2. Jennett, B. 1988. Variations in surgical practice: welcome diversity or disturbing differences. *British Journal of Surgery* 75: 630–631.
3. Jennett, B. 1988. The elderly and high technology therapies. Pp. 177–190, *in* Wells, N. and Freer, C. (Eds) *Health problems of an ageing population.* Macmillan, London.
4. Jennett, B. 1987. Are ethics and economics incompatible in health care? *Proceedings of the Royal College of Physicians, Edinburgh* 17: 190–195.
5. Mooney, G. and McGuire, H. (Eds). 1988. *Medical ethics and economics in health care.* Oxford University Press, Oxford.
6. Jennett, B. 1984. Inappropriate use of intensive care. *British Medical Journal* **289**: 1709–1711.
7. Jennett, B. 1990. Decisions to limit the use of technologies that save or sustain life. *Proceedings of the Royal College of Physicians, Edinburgh* **20**: 407–415.

75

Medical Research, Society and Health Care Ethics

Terrence F. Ackerman, PhD

Professor and Chairman, Department of Human Values and Ethics, College of Medicine, University of Tennessee, Memphis, Tennessee, USA

Medical research involves systematic design and analysis of interventions involving human subjects in order to develop generalizable knowledge regarding the prevention and treatment of disease. The moral issues that it generates reflect the diverse consequences of these interventions. On the one hand, we may enhance the welfare of society by expanding generalizable medical knowledge. On the other hand, the design, procedures or circumstances involved in research studies may engender compromises in the interests of human subjects.

A pertinent illustration is provided by pediatric cancer research (1). Increased rates of survival for metastatic cancer at diagnosis require improvements in the safety and efficacy of multiple drug chemotherapy. This undertaking would be enhanced by a theory about how tumor cells proliferate and how chemotherapy can be optimally employed to destroy them, i.e., a theory of cell kinetics. The information would suggest what anti-tumor drugs to combine and what interval to allow between their administration. For example, drug A may block tumor cells at one stage of the cell division process for 48 hours, causing a build-up of cells in that stage. If drug B kills tumor cells in the next stage, it might be given 48 hours after the first drug to destroy maximally the synchronized group of cells entering that stage. In addition, an understanding of cell kinetics might be useful in predicting which patients will respond to therapy. That is, cancer drugs might not have their usual cell kinetic effects during the initial course in patients who will eventually fail to respond. This determination would allow a timely change to other drugs.

However, protocols investigating cell kinetics have troublesome features. They require that accessible tumor cells be obtained at frequent intervals after administration of chemotherapy. Invasive procedures must be employed, such as bone marrow aspirations, needle biopsies of solid tumor, lumbar punctures,

Principles of Health Care Ethics. Edited by Raanan Gillon.
© 1994 John Wiley & Sons Ltd

or venipunctures. Repetition of these procedures is not necessary to the treatment process. Moreover, the study populations usually include children who are not yet capable of providing consent. Thus cell kinetic studies raise the issue of whether non-consenting subjects may be exposed to risk of harm presented by non-therapeutic procedures.

Another helpful illustration of the diverse consequences of research activities involves offer of payment in recruiting subjects (1). In one case, investigators sought to evaluate a new therapy for polycystic ovarian disease and to improve knowledge about hormonal changes caused by the disease and its treatment. The study included three phases: an initial three-day clinical assessment in hospital; two months of treatment; and a repeat of the initial assessment following therapy. In-hospital testing included a complete physical, pelvic examination, and ultrasound of the ovaries. It also involved drawing blood from an indwelling catheter every 10 minutes for 24 hours, as well as other briefer tests, to chart hormone production. During the treatment period, subjects were to take the drug daily by nasal spray. Side-effects of drug-induced hormonal changes included vaginal bleeding, changes in menstrual cycle, hot flashes, breast tenderness and mood changes.

The study had considerable merit. Preliminary evidence suggested that the drug might prove effective in reducing hormonal abnormalities and symptoms associated with the disease. Moreover, the procedures for monitoring baseline and treatment-induced hormonal changes were carefully fashioned to overcome design weaknesses that had vitiated the results of previous studies.

However, the design also required recruitment of normal control subjects in order to clarify the hormonal abnormalities of the disease and the differential impact of treatment. Control subjects would be paid $750 and recruited from among patients at the university's gynecology clinic. Many of these women were poor or unemployed. Concerns arose about whether the amount of payment might constitute an undue inducement for control subjects to participate in a trial involving a series of rigorous, although not seriously risky, interventions.

MORAL ISSUES IN MEDICAL RESEARCH

These examples suggest that the key moral issues arising in medical research concern the extent to which the interests of subjects may be compromised, if at all, in pursuing the social good of expanded medical knowledge. The first step in addressing these issues is to clarify the interests at stake and the moral obligations generated by them.

The relevant interests of subjects fall into three categories: exercising autonomous choice, protecting and promoting personal welfare, and securing fair treatment. These interests reflect the distinctive capacities of persons and the role of social relationships in their recognition. In pursuing cherished activities, persons engage in deliberative, self-directed actions, and therefore have an interest in the protection of the capacity for autonomous behavior. Moreover, when engaging in these activities, interaction with physical and social environment results in consequences that satisfy needs or produce suffering and deprivation. As a result, persons have an interest in satisfaction of their welfare needs. Finally, exercise of personal autonomy and provision for welfare needs may be differentially affected by social arrangements that determine the distribution of autonomy rights and welfare goods. Thus, persons have an interest in the existence of distributive arrangements that treat them fairly *vis-à-vis* others.

The importance of these interests is reflected in norms of interpersonal conduct. The interest in exercising autonomy is reflected in the obligation to respect the capacity of persons to deliberate about and act on their life plans. In the research setting this obligation involves several specific requirements, such as duties to secure informed consent, to respect the privacy of subjects, and to protect the confidentiality of data linked to identifiable subjects.

The interest of persons in protecting and promoting their welfare is reflected in several categories of obligations directed toward individuals. These might be called obligations of individual beneficence. They include obligations to avoid harming, prevent harm to, remove harm from, and promote the welfare of persons (2). Each category is relevant in the context of medical research. The obligation to avoid causing harm to others suggests that subjects who are unable to consent should not be exposed to interventions involving serious risk not intended for their own benefit. The obligation to prevent harm generates the duty to minimize risks to subjects consistent with sound research design. Obligations to prevent and remove harms suggest that a therapeutic procedure evaluated in medical research should have a harm/benefit ratio that is thought to be at least as advantageous as any alternative treatment acceptable to the subject.

The interest in fair treatment is reflected in obligations of justice. Justice requires that the benefits and burdens of cooperative social endeavors be distributed in ways that provide persons with an equal opportunity to pursue their life plans. In the research setting this obligation requires that the selection of subjects not impose special burdens on specific classes of persons rendering them less able to pursue their life plans. It also requires that subjects with special vulnerabilities be accorded stronger protections for their interests than less vulnerable subjects.

Finally, research activities are sustained by the interest in promoting the general welfare of society. This interest is reflected in categories of obligations similar to those of individual beneficence, although focused on the welfare of groups of persons. Thus, they might be called obligations of social beneficence. Controversy exists about whether this interest generates duties in the context of medical research, and this question will be examined subsequently. However, if such duties are posited, they will fall into categories similar to that of individual beneficence. For example, the obligation to avoid causing harm to groups of persons would generate a duty to assess the safety and efficacy of standard medical procedures whose value is uncertain. Similarly, the obligations to prevent and remove harms would generate duties to test new therapies for curing or ameliorating disease.

Resolution of moral issues in medical research involves two separate critical tasks. First, we must specify the content of duties generated by our general obligations that are applicable in the research setting. Second, we must formulate a defensible strategy for weighting duties to subjects against pursuit of expanded medical knowledge when these factors conflict with one another.

SPECIFICATION OF DUTIES TO SUBJECTS

Specification of duties to subjects includes two aspects. The first involves formulation of the general conditions whose moral importance is acknowledged in the statement of general obligations. For example, paying research subjects creates concerns about compromising autonomy through the offer of undue inducements. An initial step in specifying our duties in this regard involves clarification of the relevant feature of autonomy, *viz.*, voluntariness of choice, and the manner in which it may be protected or compromised. Similarly, the use of non-therapeutic research procedures with sick children raises issues about causing harm. Specification of the relevant duty must begin with the formulation of the precise limits the general obligation to avoid causing harm places on activities involving non-consenting persons.

The second aspect of specifying duties to subjects is the determination of how the conditions whose moral importance is acknowledged in general obligations can be satisfied in the research setting. For example, duties of investigators in offering payments will consist in those conditions that assure voluntary choices of prospective subjects. Similarly, duties involving the use of non-therapeutic procedures with non-consenting subjects will consist in those conditions that circumscribe risk of harm as specified in the general obligation to avoid causing harm.

There are aspects of research ethics in which there is substantial agreement regarding the content of duties to subjects. An illustration is provided by the duty to secure informed consent. Some of the conditions captured in the general obligation to respect personal autonomy have been well defined. They include facilitating the efforts of persons to make thoughtful choices. Moreover, the means for satisfying this requirement in the research setting have been carefully identified. They include the provision of information prospective subjects might need to decide about participation in research, such as a description of the purpose of the study, the procedures used, the benefits and risks, and alternative treatments, if any, that might be appropriate.

However, the specification of other duties to subjects remains unsettled. For example, controversy persists about the limit of risk permissible in the use of non-therapeutic procedures with subjects unable to consent. This dispute is rooted in differing interpretations of the general obligation to avoid causing harm. According to one view it prohibits exposing non-consenting persons to any risk of harm unrelated to their own welfare. This interpretation would permit non-therapeutic research procedures with subjects unable to consent only if they carry 'no risk' or 'no discernible risk'. According to a less restrictive view the general obligation prohibits activities that expose non-consenting persons to increments of risk beyond the minimal level unavoidable in daily life. Underlying this interpretation is the assumption that daily living exposes all persons to a certain minimal level of risk that is unavoidable no matter what their activities. On this interpretation, the relevant research norm should circumscribe non-therapeutic procedures that expose non-consenting subjects to an increment of risk beyond the unavoidable daily minimum.

In other cases, disputes about the specification of duties to subjects focus on determining what means would serve to realize the requirements of general obligations. For example, it is generally agreed that respect for personal autonomy includes protection of voluntary choice. Moreover, it is agreed that choice is voluntary only when the capacity of persons to make choices reflecting their own values is not compromised by outside influences. However, there is disagreement about how to assure that offer of payment to prospective subjects does not compromise voluntary choice. Some commentators insist that voluntariness can be assured only if we enjoin all payments except reimbursements for subjects' expenses. Some maintain that voluntary choice is reasonably protected if payments do not exceed the standard of minimum wage. Others claim that no restrictions on payment are necessary, provided that subjects are not exposed to more than minimal risk of harm. These conflicting specifications of our duty reflect different assessments of how voluntariness of choice can be preserved in recruiting subjects.

Resolution of disagreements about the content of duties to subjects proceeds by assessment of several types of considerations. These include delineation of the human capacities and interests whose protection is sustained by the general obligations. They also include examination of the content of duties derived from the general obligations that are applicable in other contexts of human interaction relevantly similar to the research setting. Proposed specifications of duties to subjects can also be evaluated relative to their implications for paradigm cases in which there is general agreement about how subjects ought to be treated. Finally, alternative specifications can be assessed by clarifying the factual features of research practices and the resulting consequences of proposed norms for protection of the interests of subjects.

SOCIAL BENEFICENCE AND MEDICAL RESEARCH

Although there are disputes about the content of duties to subjects, their existence as grounded in general obligations is firmly established. By contrast, fundamental disagreement exists about whether general obligations of social beneficence impose duties on society to conduct medical research.

This disagreement reflects differing assumptions about the role of society and the impact of medical research. On one view the primary role of society is to institute norms of conduct that assure the preservation of society and protect its members from violation of their interests by others. Moreover, it is maintained that, although medical research may produce significant improvements in the welfare of society, these goods are not necessary for the preservation of society or for the protection of the interests of its members. Therefore, there are no duties of social beneficence incumbent on society to conduct medical research.

An opposing view claims that society has a broader function of providing essential conditions its members need to pursue their life plans. These include protection against harm by others, but also involve provision of basic goods such as adequate housing, nutrition and education. Moreover, adequate medical care is considered a basic good and medical research an essential component in providing adequate medical care for the members of society. Thus, society is viewed as possessing duties of social beneficence to conduct medical research.

In evaluating this controversy, it is useful to examine the logic of Hans Jonas's defense of the former view (3). Jonas admits that 'Progress is an acknowledged interest of society' and that 'in medical science experimentation on human subjects is a necessary instrument . . .' of progress. However, he asserts that 'Unless the present state is intolerable, the melioristic goal is in a sense gratuitous . . . . Our descendants have a right to be left an unplundered planet; they do not have a right to new miracle cures'.

Two mistaken assumptions undergird Jonas's argument. One is that the obligation of society to protect persons from the harm-causing activities of others does not require the conduct of medical research. In making the contrasting claim that society has an obligation to limit environmental damage that may deplete the resources of future generations, Jonas implicitly acknowledges that society has a role in controlling harm-causing practices. However, he fails to see how this role might be implemented through medical research.

The relevance of medical research relates to harm-causing medical practices. The history of medicine is replete with examples of widely accepted treatments later shown to be injurious. The widespread use of harm-causing medical practices reflects the extreme difficulties of identifying their inadequacies through uncontrolled observations. Minimization of their use requires the controlled interventions and observations that characterize medical research. Thus, even if we accept only the limited obligation of society to restrict harm-causing practices, these considerations suggest that society has a duty to conduct medical research (4).

The other key assumption of Jonas's argument is that there is a crucial moral difference between not causing harm and preventing or removing harms. While we can demand that persons refrain from harm-causing activities, we cannot morally require that they undertake positive actions to prevent or remove harm to others. Accordingly, Jonas concludes that we have a duty to our descendants not to plunder the planet, but are not obligated to develop effective therapies for relieving or curing diseases to which they will succumb.

However, it is difficult to sustain the claim that society should minimize harm-causing practices, but that similar obligations do not exist to prevent or remove harms. Not causing harm, and preventing or removing harm, have precisely the same objective: minimizing the extent of harm that may occur to persons (5). Moreover, the amount and type of effort required to prevent or remove harms is often no different from that required to control harm-causing practices. These points are illustrated in the context of medical research. Protocols that result in new medical treatments and studies designed to evaluate controversial standard therapies are both intended to minimize the extent of harm that might occur to patients. Furthermore, the same process must be undertaken to identify improved treatments or to expose current harm-causing therapies—their formal evaluation in well-designed clinical trials. Thus, if society has a role in reducing harm-causing practices, it has obligations to prevent and remove harms as well.

Moreover, medical research has an important role in satisfying the latter obligations. Seriously disabling or life-threatening diseases substantially compromise the ability of persons to pursue their life plans. Adequate medical care serves to prevent and remove the harms that might thereby be caused. When safe and effective therapy is not available, the societal obligation to prevent and remove harms requires that research be undertaken to develop the generalizable knowledge essential for improving treatment.

Thus, there are strong grounds for claiming that society has obligations to restrict harm-causing practices, as well as to prevent and remove harms, and that duties to conduct medical research are generated by these societal functions.

ASSESSMENT OF ALTERNATIVE WEIGHTING STRATEGIES

The second critical task in resolving moral issues in medical research is to formulate a defensible strategy for weighting duties to subjects against duties to conduct research. The nature of these duties suggests several points regarding the kinds of weighting strategies that merit consideration.

First, recognition of obligations to conduct medical research prevents us from viewing the weighting issue as a matter of balancing duties to subjects against merely desirable gains in medical knowledge. If the latter view were accepted, optional research goals would be properly constrained by full satisfaction of duties to subjects. Once we admit duties to conduct research, a weighting strategy other than one assigning absolute priority to full satisfaction of duties to subjects becomes a viable option.

Second, some commentators incorrectly assume that the only conceptual alternatives are to require complete satisfaction of subject-related duties *or* to permit their total subjugation to duties of social beneficence (6). However, the interests and duties at stake allow compromises of degree. For example, payment of subjects may compromise more or less the voluntariness of their choices. Similarly, a study using non-consenting subjects may employ non-therapeutic procedures whose degree of risk exceeds the level permitted by the duty to avoid causing harm to a greater or lesser extent. Thus, a weighting strategy may be considered that allows degrees of compromise in the fulfillment of duties to subjects and duties to promote the general welfare.

Third, subject-related duties and duties to conduct research need not be assigned equal weight in resolving conflicts between them. Resolution of a conflict of duties often involves setting priorities. One way of doing this is to specify unequal degrees of compromise in conflicting duties. For example, we might accept a weighting strategy that allows minor compromises of degree in the fulfillment of duties to subjects, without embracing wholesale violations. In this case the priority of duties to subjects is a matter of degree rather than absolute.

Three prominent weighting strategies merit examination: duties to subjects should assume absolute priority; the respective sets of duties should be balanced or equally weighted against one another; or each of the competing sets of duties should be assigned some degree of weight in the resolution of issues, but not in equal amounts.

The first approach is favored by numerous commentators. It assigns absolute priority to the fulfillment of duties to subjects. The clearest interpretation of 'absolute priority' is Rawls's lexical ordering strategy: the requirements of duties assigned higher priority must be fully satisfied before meeting the requirements of duties possessing lower priority (7). Applied to human research this means that pursuit of the general welfare must be constrained by full satisfaction of duties to subjects. The basic rationale for this approach involves two points. It offers firmly grounded protection for the rights and welfare of subjects. In addition, it assures that 'No amount of good consequences can overwhelm the inherent moral requirements' of duties to subjects (6).

Despite its initial attractiveness this approach has a fundamental flaw. It is widely agreed that individuals have limited general obligations of beneficence to prevent or remove significant harms to other specific persons when doing so will involve no more than minor costs to their own interests (5). A stock example is the case of a drowning child who can be easily plucked from the water by a stranger standing at the poolside. Positing this duty seems reasonable, despite the absence of a special relationship between the parties, because a great harm can be prevented to a person possessing basic moral worth at little more than the cost of wet clothes. More generally, 'duties of rescue' provide a 'social safety net' to protect the key interests of individuals when the usual mechanisms installed by society (e.g. lifeguards at pools) are unavoidably ineffective.

Similarly, when persons organized collectively can prevent or remove significant harms to groups of persons at modest costs to their own interests, it is reasonable to posit collective duties of rescue (8). The logical basis for this extension is the principle underlying the paradigm cases of duties of rescue. Harms that deprive persons of basic goods needed to pursue their life plans have sufficient moral importance to justify obligatory minor compromises in the interests of individuals who are able to prevent or remove them. This general principle forms the basis for a large variety of social programs, involving obligatory sacrifices by individuals (mainly through taxation), that provide other persons with basic goods of which they would otherwise be deprived.

Finally, it is reasonable to maintain that collective duties of rescue apply in the context of medical research. Preventing deprivation of the basic good of physical well-being for persons suffering from disease or injury sometimes requires medical research whose goal is the development of effective and safe treatment. Moreover, the design, procedures or circumstances of these studies may unavoidably require some compromise in the interests of subjects. If these compromises represent only a modest cost to the interests of subjects, the analogy with duties of rescue suggests that they are morally justified. The weighting strategy that assigns absolute priority to the interests of subjects fails to recognize these duties in the research setting.

Nevertheless, most agree that careful limits must be placed on compromises in the interests of subjects. This point is neglected by the weighting strategy which assigns equal weight to subject-related duties and duties to conduct medical research. According to this approach, resolution of particular issues involves striking a balance between competing duties (9). This weighting strategy encounters a fatal dilemma. On one hand, its most obvious interpretation results in inadequate protection for the interests of subjects. If we begin with competing duties possessing equal weight, striking a balance should involve compromising each to an equal degree. However, it is generally agreed that the interests of subjects should be broadly protected, while pursuit of the general welfare must be narrowly constrained. Thus, the idea of an evenly balanced compromise is not tenable. On the other hand, we might interpret this weighting strategy as assigning equal moral force to competing duties only in the abstract, with the resolution of conflicts proceeding by compromises of unequal degree in their respective requirements (10). Although this revision avoids the prior unacceptable result, it engenders a loss of clarity. The metaphor of striking a balance between duties of equal weight loses its directive power, providing no guidance regarding the extent to which competing duties should be compromised in resolving conflicts (11). Thus, this second weighting strategy either leads to clearly unacceptable results for protecting the interests of subjects or must be assigned an interpretation that lacks prescriptive clarity.

The last weighting strategy involves some degree of recognition for each set of competing duties, but not in equal proportion (12). One species of this approach might be called the presumptive weighting strategy. Presumptive priority is assigned to duties to subjects, requiring their full satisfaction in most circumstances. However, this presumption may be overridden if it is necessary to undertake research activities that may prevent or remove important harms to others and there will be no more than minor compromises in protections for the interests of subjects.

This position possesses several advantages. First, it recognizes the preeminent importance of protecting the interests of subjects. Full satisfaction of duties to subjects is normally required. Moreover, compromises in their fulfillment may involve only minor infringements of subjects' interests. This avoids the laxness or lack of clarity regarding subject-related protections inherent in the second weighting strategy.

Second, the presumptive weighting strategy acknowledges the pertinence of duties of rescue in the research context. It recognizes that important harms to groups of persons can sometimes only be prevented or removed through research that involves modest costs to the interests of subjects. Insofar as subjects acting collectively can mitigate these harms, duties are engendered to accept minor compromises of their interests. Thus, this weighting strategy takes better account of duties of rescue than the approach that assigns absolute priority to subject-related duties.

Third, while the presumptive weighting strategy allows pursuit of the general welfare to partly constrain fulfillment of duties to subjects, it does not permit substantial undermining of subject-related protections. Compromises are permitted only when practically necessary in the conduct of medical research. They must also involve no more than minor infringements of duties to subjects, and are permitted only when the research may generate knowledge that mitigates important harms to others. Thus, concern for the welfare of others is assigned limited weight in the resolution of issues, without functioning as the predominant factor.

This approach involves exercise of judgement in determining exceptions to the presumption favoring full satisfaction of duties to subjects. Key phrases, such as 'minor compromises in the requirements of duties to subjects', 'prevention of important harms to others' and 'necessary for the conduct of research' require interpretation. Concern may arise about excessive latitude in determining compromises in the interests of subjects. However, a more rigid approach prevents proper recognition of duties of rescue in the research setting. Thus, this latitude is inescapable if our weighting strategy is to acknowledge fully all dimensions of the moral landscape.

RESOLUTION OF MORAL ISSUES

Formulation of a defensible weighting strategy suggests the format for analysis of moral issues raised by specific research practices. First, there is a general presumption in favor of full satisfaction of duties to subjects. Accordingly, the initial focus in assessing a research practice involves specification of the relevant duties to subjects. If the practice fully satisfies these requirements, then it can be deemed morally acceptable.

For example, assessment of the use of non-therapeutic procedures with children unable to consent involves specification of the duty of individual beneficence to avoid causing harm. In delineating its requirements it seems reasonable to admit that activities of daily living carry a certain minimum degree of risk of harm, whether or not persons are involved in research activities. One function of this duty seems to be restriction of the involvement of non-consenting persons in any activities that would expose them to an increment of risk beyond the unavoidable minimum. Thus, the duty might be specified as requiring that non-consenting child subjects not be exposed to risk of harm from non-therapeutic procedures that exceed this level of minimal risk. This standard would allow procedures such as venipuncture, but arguably precludes other interventions, such as bone marrow aspirations, that might be used in cell kinetic studies.

Similarly, assessment of the practice of paying subjects involves specification of the duty to protect the voluntariness of consent. Consent is voluntary only when the subject's capacity to make a choice that reflects his or her own values is not compromised by outside influences. The relevant component of this system of values might be called a person's 'risk budget', which represents the risks a person is willing to undergo to achieve various goals (13). Thus, the duty to avoid undue influence might be specified as requiring that the amount of payment not compromise the capacity of prospective subjects to act according to the terms of their 'risk budget'. In the example considered, an offer of $750 would be likely to induce some control subjects to act contrary to restrictions on risk exposure to which they would normally adhere.

The second component of the weighting strategy becomes relevant if a research practice does not fully satisfy the requirements of duties to subjects. A practice may be morally permissible if it involves only a minor compromise in the fulfillment of subject-related norms and is necessary to the development of generalizable knowledge needed to prevent or remove important harms to other persons. For example, non-therapeutic procedures involving only a minor increase over minimal risk would be permissible in pediatric cell kinetic studies, if the studies were genuinely necessary for improving the efficacy and/or safety of treatments for pediatric cancer. This standard might allow procedures such as pelvic crest bone marrow aspirations or needle biopsies of easily accessible solid tumor masses, but only in children who do not experience substantial anxiety or discomfort from these procedures. Similarly, offer of payment in an amount that causes some prospective subjects to make minor compromises in their 'risk budgets' might be permissible provided that such an offer was necessary in order to carry out studies whose results might prevent or remove important harms to others. One practical way of implementing the standard is to allow payment amounts to be guided by 'market forces', provided that the interventions involved in the study do not exceed a minor increase over minimal risk. This assures that subjects choosing participation would not seriously compromise their 'risk budgets', no matter how conservative the latter might be.

However, these norms for using non-therapeutic procedures and for paying subjects would be acceptable only if practicably necessary in securing generalizable knowledge needed to prevent or remove important harms. Determination that this condition is satisfied involves assessment of various factors, such as the availability of alternative procedures for securing the same knowledge, the feasibility of using different subject groups, and the possibility of timely completion of the research using alternative means. These assessments demand attention to the circumstances of particular studies.

The foregoing approach does not assure easy resolution of moral issues in medical research. The requirements of general obligations must be clarified. Important disagreements may arise about the specification of duties to subjects and duties to conduct research generated by these general obligations. Moreover, application of the presumptive weighting strategy requires careful interpretation of its component terms. Nevertheless, the approach offers a useful conceptual framework for identifying and addressing the key moral issues posed by medical research.

REFERENCES

1. Ackerman, T. F. and Strong, C. 1989. *A casebook of medical ethics.* Oxford University Press, New York.
2. Frankena, W. K. 1973. *Ethics,* 2nd edn. Prentice-Hall, Englewood Cliffs, NJ.
3. Jonas, H. 1969. Philosophical reflections on human experimentation. Pp. 1–31, *in* Freund, P. (Ed.) *Experimentation with human subjects.* George Braziller, New York.
4. Engelhardt, Jr. H. T. 1988. Diagnosing well and treating prudently: randomized clinical trials and the problem of knowing truly. Pp. 123–141, in Spicker, S. F., Alon, I., de Vries, A. and Engelhardt, Jr., H. T. (Eds) *The use of human beings in research.* Kluwer, Dordrecht.
5. Feinberg, J. 1984. *The moral limits of the criminal law: harm to others.* Oxford University Press, New York.
6. Veatch, R. M. 1981. *A theory of medical ethics.* Basic Books, New York.
7. Rawls, J. 1971. *A theory of justice.* Harvard University Press, Cambridge, MA.
8. Goodin, R. E. 1985. *Protecting the vulnerable.* University of Chicago Press, Chicago, IL.
9. Beauchamp, T. L. and Childress, J. F. 1989. *Principles of biomedical ethics,* 3rd edn. Oxford University Press, New York.

10. Levine, R. J. 1986. *Ethics and regulation of clinical research*, 2nd edn. Urban & Schwarzenburg, Baltimore, MD.
11. Marshall, E. 1986. Does the moral philosophy of the Belmont Report rest on a mistake? *IRB: A Review of Human Subjects Research* **8** (6): 5–6.
12. Ackerman, T. F. 1992. The balancing of moral principles in federal regulations on human research. *IRB: A Review of Human Subjects Research* **14** (1): 1–6.
13. Fried, C. 1974. *Medical experimentation: personal integrity and social policy*. American Elsevier, New York.

76

Research Bioethics in Egypt

SANDRA D. LANE, RN, PHD, MPH

Assistant Professor, Department of Anthropology, Case Western Reserve
University, Cleveland, Ohio, USA

A small but growing body of literature examines bioethics from cross-cultural perspectives (1–5). Much of this literature explores the contrasts between the cultural specificity of value systems and the search for universal guidelines that can apply in diverse cultural settings. It is an anthropological given that ethical values cannot be separated from the cultural, social and political contexts in which they are embedded. Yet the formulation of the four bioethical principles upon which international codes of bioethics are based—respect for autonomy, beneficence, non-maleficence and justice—is an effort to identify standards that might transcend this specificity. Renee Fox and Judith Swazey (1), in their discussion of culture and bioethics in China, caution about the distortion of vision that can occur when scholars ignore the cultural contexts of bioethics:

> using biology and medicine as metaphorical language and a symbolic medium, bioethics deals in public spheres and in more private domains with nothing less than beliefs, values, and norms that are basic to our society, its cultural tradition, and its collective conscience. If this is indeed the case, we have reason to be concerned when bioethicists ignore or misperceive the social and cultural matrices of their ideas (p. 338).

I would like to add to this evolving discussion by describing the initial efforts to develop a code of research bioethics for Egypt. I first relate an incident that illustrates the need for such a code of research ethics, then describe the current efforts to develop an Egyptian code. Next I discuss the social and cultural context of Egyptian research, and finally address how the four principles that guide such codes around the world might be applied in the Egyptian context. I argue that the social and cultural contexts of the production of biomedical research in Egypt will influence the interpretation and application of the principles of autonomy, beneficence, non-maleficence and justice in the Egyptian code. Indeed, while internationally accepted principles can be applied in diverse settings, they will be perceived and applied differently in each context.

Principles of Health Care Ethics. Edited by Raanan Gillon.
© 1994 John Wiley & Sons Ltd

As a program officer for the Ford Foundation, I administer the Foundation's grants in reproductive health for the Middle East. A Foundation grant provided partial support for a conference on tropical pediatrics held by the faculty of a pediatric department in an Egyptian medical school.* This conference showcased the best faculty research on diseases of public health significance for Egyptian children. My interest in learning about the research turned to dismay, however, when I realized that in two of the studies the child subjects were given medical treatment that is not standard and may be life-threatening.†

In the first study children were administered potentially fatal drugs, when a recommended and safe drug was available. The second study administered intravenous fluids to premature infants in a manner that diverged greatly from generally accepted guidelines for parenteral therapy and endangered their lives. I wondered how such research could be conducted by the staff of a teaching hospital, and also how it could be prominently presented at a conference.

Joan Cassell (6) has cautioned anthropologists against the tendency, when faced with unethical biomedical practice, of becoming righteously indignant in the fashion of Old Testament prophets. I must admit that this attitude characterized my initial reaction to the two studies. I wrote to the faculty outlining my reservations about the research and then visited them to discuss the studies further. Upon meeting with the faculty, including the researchers who had conducted the two studies, I was struck by how sincere and enthusiastic they were about the care of their patients. Where I had expected insensitivity or worse, I found basically well-intentioned practitioners. Upon speaking with the researchers I realized that one of the main factors that allowed such unethical research to be conducted was the absence of an Egyptian code of research bioethics and the lack of formal bioethical review.

---

* The grant provided partial funding for the conference, but the research presented was chosen by the conference organizers and was not pre-screened by the Foundation.
† The first study compared the antipyretic activity of acetaminophen, salicylates, dipyrone, ibuprofen, tepid water sponging and placebo on 166 children ages six months to 10 years. In a clinical trial such as this one would need a much larger sample than 166. Nevertheless, the authors produced p-values to three decimal places, perhaps not realizing that the study's lack of statistical power made these calculations meaningless.
Much more troubling, however, was the administration of dipyrone and salicylates to children. Dipyrone, known as Novalgin in Egypt, can cause fatal agranulocytosis in some individuals. Salicylates, or aspirin, are contraindicated in childhood because of the risk of Reye's syndrome. The researchers stated that they were aware of the risk of agranulocytosis with dipyrone. They were not aware of the risk of Reye's syndrome with salicylates, which indicated that they had not conducted a thorough review of the international literature prior to conducting their study.
The second study compared three types of intravenous regimens administered to 30 very-low-birthweight infants. The researchers stated that the infants were not able to tolerate oral feedings or nasogastric feedings given in bolus amounts. They did not attempt nasogastric feedings by drip or in very small amounts. The researchers divided the infants into three treatment groups and gave them mixtures of dextrose and water, with the third group being given lipids as well, for an average of five days.
In pediatric and clinical nutrition texts there are standard protocols for parenteral nutrition for infants. The goal of this nutritional support for infants is growth and not simply fluid balance. None of the three treatment regimes in the study would allow growth, because they lacked amino acids, electrolytes, vitamins and minerals.

AN EGYPTIAN CODE OF RESEARCH BIOETHICS

Many Egyptian doctors are concerned about the problem of unethical research and would like to do something to remedy it. Following the pediatric conference in which two studies were presented that violated the protection of the child subjects, I spoke with a number of Egyptian scientists who not only agreed with my concern, but also privately shared with me other instances of unethical practice that had troubled them. I found that a consensus was developing among members of the Egyptian research community that something should be done to ensure the ethical nature of research. In particular, researchers at the Al Azhar University International Islamic Center for Population Studies and Research had longstanding interests in the intersection of medicine and religion and in the bioethics of reproductive technology. In conversations with the Center's director, Dr Gamal Serour, and other staff members, a plan was established for the Center to bring together a working group of research doctors and theologians from several leading institutes to write a research code of bioethics in the context of reproduction for Egypt and to plan a strategy for its implementation.* Such a code of ethics was to be based on internationally accepted principles regarding the protection of human subjects, but would be written in Arabic and would express these principles in a manner consistent with Egyptian culture and values. Since Al Azhar University, one of the oldest universities in the world, is the center for Islamic learning for the Muslim world, a code developed by its scholars could potentially be used throughout the Arab world and possibly in many non-Arab Muslim countries. The development of this code involved an Egyptian working group meeting over several months, followed by an international conference involving all Egyptian universities and research institutes and the Egyptian government as well as governments from a wide variety of other Islamic nations and other organisations. The result was an agreed set of ethics guidelines for research in the context of human reproduction (16).

THE EGYPTIAN CULTURAL CONTEXT OF RESEARCH BIOETHICS

A number of factors influence the ethical nature of research in Egypt, including the high value of scientific research, the regard for high-technology medicine, social inequality, and the lack of self-regulation in the medical profession.

Value of Scientific Research

In the pediatric research described at the beginning of this chapter the essence of the problem was not that the doctors did not care about their patients, but that they had placed the value of 'scientific knowledge' and the pursuit of high-technology medicine above the welfare of the research subjects. A number of factors led to this situation. First, Egypt is a highly medicalized society in which research assumes considerable importance, and where a great deal of it is

---

* The development of this code and the conference at which it was presented were funded by the Ford Foundation, the World Health Organization and the Population Council.

conducted. With a population of 56 million, latest estimates indicate that Egypt has one doctor for every 770 people (7). There are 11 medical schools, with over 2900 faculty members and 7900 doctors studying for advanced degrees, and at least 15 governmental and private research institutes that carry out health-related research (8). In addition to meeting the nation's needs for health information, such research is essential for doctors and other scientists to obtain advanced degrees and for academic promotion.

Despite this plethora of research there are no institutional review boards mandated to examine research protocols to ensure that they protect the welfare of human subjects. Research protocols written by students in Egyptian universities and research institutes are usually reviewed by the concerned departmental and faculty councils before implementation. The reviewers may consider the protection of the research subjects, but are mostly concerned instead with issues of research design and whether the research qualifies for the degree sought. Responsibility for maintaining ethical research standards is generally left to the faculty advisors who supervise the student. Often, however, one or more faculty members have helped the student to design the research and thus have a personal interest in it being conducted, so that this review may be biased in favor of approving the study. Once a doctor obtains the doctorate in medicine, his or her research is no longer automatically subject to university review.

Certain categories of research require governmental approval, including studies involving more than 250 research subjects, studies funded by foreign agencies, studies conducted by expatriate researchers and those conducted by private, non-governmental agencies. The governmental review may take into consideration the protection of research subjects, but is not specifically conducted for that purpose.

International agencies that fund research, such as the World Health Organization, and joint projects with western universities, often require investigators to adhere to internationally accepted guidelines regarding the treatment of human subjects. Very little of the total research conducted in Egypt, however, is either funded by such agencies or conducted in concert with the faculty of western universities.

An expatriate researcher working in a joint Egyptian–American research team that has had a longstanding collaboration described a situation in which, with each new study, the United States' principal investigator, in order to meet his university's requirements, requests the Egyptian university to provide certification that the research meets Egyptian criteria for the protection of human subjects. The Egyptian researchers that he works with view this request as a bothersome but necessary bureaucratic hurdle to which they must respond in order to secure funding and get on with the study. No standing committee for bioethical review has been established. Rather, an *ad hoc* review committee is set up each time. In setting up the committees, the Egyptian researchers seek to choose committee members who have specific characteristics. For example, one of the Egyptian researchers in the Egyptian–American collaborative team argued that the members should represent every powerful sector of local society, including professors of religious law and the security forces. A second investigator insisted that the committee members be chosen for their prestige. Neither of these individuals suggested choosing committee members for their knowledge of bioethical issues or their potential contribution to the protection of the research subjects, because there are as yet very few Egyptian scholars specializing in bioethics and no university programs devoted to the subject. Instead, their choices stemmed from their perception that the committee's purpose was to protect the researchers from potential criticism.

Even when externally funded research is subject to bioethical review, in practice the research may still violate the rights of the research subjects. Soheir Morsy (9) describes such a situation, which occurred in a clinical study of long-term contraceptive implants, conducted by the faculty of an Egyptian university. During a visit to the study site Morsy found that many of the female subjects had repeatedly requested that the contraceptives be removed, only to be refused by the research doctors because it would have increased the drop-out rate of women in their study.

In both of these situations where protection of human subjects guidelines were imposed from abroad, or were tied to funding, their purpose was either misperceived or disregarded. These examples illustrate the potential pitfalls of a foreign agency imposing what is essentially a set of values in a language and manner of expression that is not part of the culture in which the research is to take place.

High-technology Medicine

A second factor that impedes the protection of research subjects is the high value placed on medical technology, without an equal emphasis on the potential iatrogenic consequences of treatment. Since the establishment of Egypt's biomedical system in the last century, doctors have been inspired by technological developments in Europe and the United States. Sophisticated, hospital-based care, including organ transplants and *in vitro* fertilization, exist in the same society where the majority of rural women give birth at home with untrained traditional birth attendants (10,11). While some of this advanced medical technology is appropriately employed by highly trained specialists, in other cases poorly trained practitioners risk disability and death in their patients because of overuse of invasive techniques that they have not mastered (11). In the research context, such as the pediatric studies discussed earlier, the testing of drugs or invasive treatments, when conducted by Egyptian doctors in clinic or hospital settings, may be viewed by some as acceptable, despite the potentially dangerous consequences for otherwise healthy research subjects.

Social Inequality

A third factor is that the pool of research subjects is drawn from public governmental hospitals and clinics, where the patients are largely poor and illiterate. Egypt's two-tier medical system includes both public and private medicine, and in most surveys analyzing sources of medical care the majority of people seek private medical care. Patients in governmental hospitals, therefore, represent the poorest members of the population; doctors, in contrast, enjoy very high status. While many doctors are compassionate towards their poor patients, this immense social distance between the researchers and their subjects may lead the researchers to take less seriously the welfare and the rights of the subjects.

Lack of Self-regulation in the Medical Profession

A final factor decreasing the protection of research subjects is the reluctance of doctors to speak about their colleagues' actions with which they disagree. Several aspects of Egyptian medical institutions and Egyptian culture present barriers to the frank discussion of possibly unethical treatment. Egyptian doctors are assigned by the government to a university or research institute while studying for postgraduate medical degrees and generally remain in the same institute for their entire career. Their colleagues in the institute are thus theirs for life. Any disagreement and open discussion of a colleague's misjudgement would have repercussions that could last 20 or 30 years. In addition to this structural factor, Egyptian culture places great value on face agreement and politeness. People may privately disagree intensely, but in public situations, and especially among people of unequal status, honest expressions of negative opinions or feelings are viewed as rude.

An Egyptian doctor who has grappled with these problems described to me his attempts to interest his colleagues in establishing a confidential inquiry procedure for maternal mortality in the hospital. His efforts were unsuccessful because, although they agreed that such a policy would be beneficial for medical care, the doctors were reluctant to speak out about the mistakes of their colleagues or to admit to their own mistakes in the treatment of patients. Furthermore, they had no confidence that such a report could remain confidential, and feared that it would be used against them at some future time. These factors create an environment in which unethical research, and indeed unethical medical treatment in general, may be carried on without regulation.

THE FOUR PRINCIPLES AND EGYPTIAN CULTURE

Beginning with the Nuremberg Code of 1947, a number of codes governing the treatment of human research subjects have been written, including the Helsinki Declarations of 1964 and 1975, and more recent efforts of the World Health Organization and the Council for International Organizations of Medical Sciences that deal with research in developing countries (12,13). Each of these codes embodies four basic principles: autonomy, beneficence, non-maleficence and justice. During 1991 I had a number of discussions with Egyptian medical and social scientists about these principles and how they might be perceived and applied in the Egyptian context. I have drawn some tentative conclusions about their fit within Egyptian values and social customs.

Autonomy

The principle of autonomy rests on respect for self-determination and demands that subjects enter into research voluntarily and with adequate information (ref. 12, pp. 5–6). In the research setting these criteria apply to the process of informed consent, in which the subject participates voluntarily with sufficient knowledge of the potential risks and benefits to make a free choice.

As Fox and Swazey argue (1) in their discussion of bioethics and medical morality in China, the concept of autonomy derives from the notion of the sovereignty of the individual (p. 352). In Egypt, as in China, however, individual wants and desires are often subordinated to the family and social group. In particular during illness, the sick person rarely makes decisions for himself or herself regarding treatment. Rather, the family decides if and when to consult a doctor or other practitioner. Once consulted, the doctor gives his or her recommendation regarding therapy. Doctors do not generally expect family members or the sick individual to participate in choosing the type of treatment. Equally, families do not expect to be consulted. If, however, the family does not agree with the doctor's prescription, they are likely to seek the advice of a second or third doctor without informing the primary doctor. Such doctor shopping is very common, and is the way that Egyptian patients exercise their options to choose therapy, without openly disagreeing with or questioning the doctor.

In their study of the health experiences of Arab immigrants to San Francisco, Lipson and Meleis (14) found that Middle Eastern patients were puzzled and often unhappy when their American doctors offered them choices regarding their treatment. The Middle Eastern patients regarded this choice as a sign that the doctors did not themselves know what to do, and began to question their doctors' competence.

An Egyptian anthropologist working with the World Health Organization, Dr Hind Khattab, described the two days of heated discussion she and her colleagues engaged in while trying to translate English-language AIDS materials into Arabic. In particular the group was stuck on the meaning and translation of the word 'counseling'. The concept of counseling embodies a respect for the autonomy and choice of the person being counseled. Dr Khattab explained that there was no colloquial Egyptian–Arabic word, that the group could agree on, meaning 'to counsel'. Finally, they agreed on *al-Irshaad*, which means guidance. While guidance may well be the best choice, it nevertheless implies a hierarchical relationship where one person knows what is best for another and seeks to lead.

An insightful Arab colleague placed the whole issue of autonomy in a wider context by explaining that it would be difficult for doctors to accept an open dialogue with their patients and the power of decision-making being given to patients, because they may not have experienced this type of give-and-take in their own lives. In perhaps the majority of traditional families the father holds decision-making power. In schools, from primary through doctoral study, the teacher's word is not openly questioned and encouraging student discussion is not a commonly employed teaching method. In professional settings the employer or supervisor does not generally seek the opinions of his or her employees. It is no surprise then, that in the clinic, hospital and research setting the concept of a patient's autonomy and choice may be misunderstood.

The principle of autonomy and the concept of informed choice are therefore likely to be the most difficult of the four principles to translate into Arabic and Egyptian values. As with the translation of the word 'counseling' subtle shifts in meaning and perception are likely to occur in the process.

Beneficence and Non-maleficence

The principles of beneficence and non-maleficence embody both a positive obligation to do good and the Hippocratic maxim, 'to do no harm' (ref. 12, p. 7). In the research context these principles encompass a weighing of the potential risks and benefits of the research for the individual and for the society. Beneficence and non-maleficence are likely to be readily understood within Egyptian culture because the country's two major religions, Islam and Coptic Christianity, contain numerous prescriptions to do good and to protect the vulnerable from harm. Because of their resonance with Egyptian values, the concepts of beneficence and non-maleficence are likely to be considered more important than that of autonomy and to take priority among the four principles.

Nevertheless, in light of the high value placed on research and on medical technology, a critical aspect that will need to be stressed in writing the Egyptian code is a clear statement that the protection of research subjects from harm takes precedence over the generation of scientific knowledge.

Justice

The principle of justice implies fairness, both in choice of research subjects and in determining who benefits from the research (ref. 12, p. 8). An infamous United States example of the breaching of this principle is provided by the Tuskegee Syphilis Study, which denied poor black men treatment for syphilis in order to study the natural history of the disease (15). As mentioned previously, research subjects are almost always drawn from the poorest, illiterate members of Egyptian society, and yet the research does not always benefit them. This unequal burden to serve as research subjects without a corresponding benefit of improved medical services will need to be addressed in writing the Egyptian code.

This issue of using poor women as research subjects was raised quite forcefully in a national Egyptian conference that presented the results of research on long-term contraceptive implants. An Egyptian professor not associated with the research* asked why no middle- and upper-class women had been selected to serve as research subjects. He further asked if the contraceptives, when they receive governmental approval and are released for sale, will be widely available to poor women or will be too expensive for them. The researchers vigorously defended their protocol, saying that they had not used the poor women as 'guinea pigs'. The audience, which consisted of Egyptian specialists in obstetrics and gynecology, responded with a lengthy and heated discussion, and the

---

* The professor was Dr Gamal Serour.

majority stated agreement with the professor who raised the question (personal communication, Serour, 1991).

The principle of justice is embodied in Egypt's constitution and legislation, largely written after the socialist revolution in 1952. The progressive ideas expressed in the constitution are based on respect for human beings and seek to ensure an equitable distribution of resources. While it is true that in some instances these progressive ideals are today circumvented or ignored, they are nevertheless part of Egyptian social history. Thus, the principle of justice is likely to translate smoothly into Arabic and Egyptian values. The implementation of this principle in day-to-day research settings, however, may present a greater challenge.

CONCLUSION

This chapter has described events leading to a plan to establish a research code of bioethics for Egypt and for other Islamic countries. At the time of writing, although a great deal of research is conducted, little of it is explicitly designed with the intent to protect the human subjects of the research. Consequently, in some instances the largely poor, illiterate research subjects are exposed to harm directly from the research.

The initiative of doctors at the Al Azhar University's International Islamic Center for Population Studies and Research has resulted in an Islamic code of ethics for research in the context of human reproduction (16). The four principles—autonomy, beneficence, non-maleficence and justice—provide an analytic framework for the code. As with all cultures, however, application of these internationally recognized principles will need to be sensitive to Egyptian and other Islamic cultural, social and political values if the code is to prove a truly useful document.

ACKNOWLEDGEMENTS

I would like to thank a number of colleagues and friends who read drafts of this paper and gave me helpful advice: Jose Barzelatto, Abdullah Lolo, Patricia Marshall, Cynthia Myntti, David Nygaard, Emma Playfair, Robert A. Rubinstein, Gamal Serour, and Necla Tschirgi.

REFERENCES

1. Fox, R. and Swazey, J. 1984. Medical morality is not bioethics—medical ethics in China and the United States. *Perspectives in Biology and Medicine* **27** (3): 336–360.
2. Kunstadter, P. 1980. Medical ethics in cross-cultural and multi-cultural perspectives. *Social Science and Medicine* **14B**: 289–296.
3. Coward, H., Lipner, J. and Young, K. 1989. *Hindu ethics: purity, abortion, and euthanasia.* State University of New York Press, Albany, NY.
4. Macklin, R. 1989. Perspectives of different cultural and religious settings. Pp. 68–85, in Bankowski, Z., Barzelatto, J. and Capron, A. M. (Eds) *Ethics and values in family planning.* CIOMS, Geneva.
5. Crigger, J., Campbell, C. and Homer, P. 1988. International perpectives on biomedical ethics. *Hastings Center Report, Special Supplement* **18** (4): 1–39.

6. Cassel, J. 1989. Moral problems in studying doctors' morality. Paper presented at the American Anthropological Association Conference, November.
7. World Bank. 1990. *World development report 1990: poverty,* p. 232. Oxford University Press, Oxford.
8. Wahab, Y. 1989. Egypt: Country report on the present status of health research for development. Unpublished manuscript.
9. Morsy, S. 1993. Biotechnology and the international politics of population control: long-term contraception in Egypt. *Signs: Journal of Women in Culture and Society* (in press).
10. El-Kady, A., Loza, S., Abdel-Tawab, N. and Potter, L. 1989. Daya's practices and maternal mortality in Giza, Egypt. Report to the National Population Council, Cairo, Egypt.
11. Serour, G., ElGhar, M. and Mansour, R. T. 1991. Infertility: a health problem in the Muslim world. *Population Sciences* **10**: 41–58.
12. National Commission for the Protection of Human Subjects of Biomedical and Behavioral Research. 1979. *The Belmont Report: ethical principles and guidelines for the protection of human subjects of research.* Washington: DHEW Publ. No. (OS) 78–0012.
13. Bankowski, Z., Levine, R. (Eds) 1993. Ethics and research on human subjects—international guidelines. CIOMS/WHO, Geneva.
14. Lipson, J. and Meleis, A. 1986. Methodological issues in research with immigrants. Paper presented at the Transcultural Nursing Society Conference. Edmonton, Alberta, May.
15. Brant, A. 1978. Racism and research: the case of the Tuskegee Syphilis study. *Hastings Center Report* **8** (6): 21–29.
16. Serour, G. (Ed.) 1992. Ethical guidelines for human reproduction research in the Muslim World. International Islamic Center for population studies and research, Al-Azhar University, Cairo, Egypt.

77

Drug Addiction, Society and Health Care Ethics

Henk A. M. J. ten Have, MD, PhD

Professor of Medical Ethics, Catholic University of Nijmegen, The Netherlands

INTRODUCTION

Drug addiction confronts the health care practitioner with a complex and ambivalent problem. On the micro-level of the doctor–patient interaction the addict may present himself as a person in need of help, as a victim of concomitant disease or complications of drug use, or as a client with specific pharmaceutical demands. On the macro-level of the health care system drug addiction is a social and legal policy issue, primarily because of the huge financial interests and criminal activities involved. The problem is that both levels are strongly interconnected. A doctor can hardly refuse to assist an individual addict if appealed to for help, but he knows that the results of his efforts depend very much on the social conditions leading to drug use. At the same time society, being unable effectively to influence those conditions, tends to refer the management of the problem to the health care system.

In this chapter I will discuss and compare the social and medical perspectives on drug addiction, and show how the medical treatment of drug addicts is in fact subordinated to the social approach of the addiction problem. I will argue that both perspectives should be disconnected as much as possible. Drug use is understood as the regular intake of so-called hard drugs (e.g. heroin and cocaine) since there is consensus concerning their addictive effect, risks and complications. The moral dimensions of drug addiction can only partly be analysed with the assistance of the four moral principles.

THE SOCIAL PERSPECTIVE ON DRUG ADDICTION

There is hardly an issue on which there seems to be so much agreement between developed countries as drugs. The 1961 New York Single Convention states that all nations are obliged to cooperate in reducing the availability of drugs within

Principles of Health Care Ethics. Edited by Raanan Gillon.
© 1994 John Wiley & Sons Ltd

their borders. Countries with a permissive policy have changed their laws in order to comply with this international repressive policy. Within the framework of the United Nations and the European Community legislation on drugs is harmonized (1).

The history of this political consensus is interesting since it reveals the political factors involved, as well as the relative newness of the world-wide condemnation of drug use. For instance, in The Netherlands the first law forbidding the possession and use of opiates was enacted in 1919. Before that time the only relevant law stated that selling *less* than 50 grams of opium was restricted to doctors and pharmacists; more than that amount apparently could be sold freely by anyone without legal restrictions. Similarly, the first legal steps in the United States (1875) were directed against the Chinese habit of *smoking* opium; the more fashionable practice of using opiate mixtures was not prohibited (2).

The conclusion from historical evidence is that the perception of drug use as a relevant social problem is quite recent. The origin of this perception can be dated back to the International Opium Treaties of Shanghai (1909) and Den Haag (1912). Since that time the pressure towards an international drug policy has become more and more effective. The emphasis of this approach is on prohibition, repression and criminalization. Drug use is considered a moral threat to society. The recent AIDS epidemic has turned this threat into a real and physical one. Intravenous drug use creates an HIV reservoir, potentially harmful to all members of society. Hard drugs is a topic that incites moral indignation about organized crime, drug dealing, robbery, prostitution, and the physical and mental deterioration of young adults. The problem and its control is usually described with a military metaphor. Heroin and cocaine are regarded as 'the enemy within', against which all national forces have to be mobilized. An enormous amount of money and manpower is spent on police forces and penitentiaries. The moral motivation towards this war on drugs is so strong that the repressive policy is not often critically evaluated.

THE MEDICAL PERSPECTIVE ON DRUG ADDICTION

Policies aimed at the repression and prohibition of drug use as a social problem have become popular because they linked up the military metaphor with the imagery of disease. Drugs are discussed in medical terminology: there is a heroin or cocaine 'epidemic', involving 'transmission' by direct contact and 'contamination' of young people with lower resistance. The vocabulary assumes the existence of a communicable disease, cause and effect relationships, and the need for prevention. From the medical perspective drug addiction is not a vice, requiring penalties and a strong effort of the will, but a 'disease' having little to do with free action. The consequence of the disease metaphor is that drug use is primarily seen as an individual problem, in the sense that it refers to a pathological condition of an individual; since addiction is not the result of voluntary choice, the sick person is not responsible for his disease; neither is he to blame for his condition. This view implies that addicts need treatment, not punishment; every addict should be treated energetically, and intervention for his own benefit is requested. Military and disease metaphors could therefore reinforce each other.

Redefining drug use from a medical perspective as a disease could justify and even call for vigorous action and coercive social policies. Introducing the language of medicine makes it more plausible to introduce severe drug controls than merely appeals to public morality.

In practice, medical and social perspectives thus converge in the fight against drug use. This is illustrated by the evolution of treatment programs. Initially, the primary aim of medical intervention was abstinence; it still is in some countries, where a user must be 'drug-free' even to begin a therapeutic program. But in many countries intervention is directed at secondary problems of drug use (infection, malnutrition, prostitution, crime) and less at the primary problem (the direct results of the pharmacological effects of the drug). Therapeutic and rehabilitative facilities are usually less well equipped and financed than criminal justice and law enforcement systems. Moreover, the emphasis on detection and punishment may discourage drug users from seeking medical help and treatment.

CRITICISM OF REPRESSIVE POLICIES

Upon careful consideration, current drug policies themselves seem to generate harmful consequences:

1. Their effectiveness is questionable. Repressive action does not really produce better control of the drug problem. In spite of all efforts, police and the law currently have little hold on the criminal subculture of drug users and dealers. Fighting drug use often has paradoxical effects. Intensified police action, for instance, may lead to a higher price for heroin and cocaine on the black market; this induces (more) criminal behavior of users, which in turn invokes extra efforts by police and law. Even dealers may have an interest in continuous police action; they benefit because it keeps up the prices. A repressive policy, therefore, does not have a substantial effect on the availability of drugs; in fact it may lead to more drug-related crime.

2. Criminalization of drug use has implications for the quality of the legal system and the administration of justice. Over the last two decades the penal system in many countries has got out of order: the number of convictions for possessing and selling drugs has multiplied; the increasing number of this category of convict takes up most prison capacity. In addition, these prisoners make special demands on the wardens. In practice it appears to be impossible to exclude drug use and drug traffic from prisons; a substantial number of prisoners even become addicted during detention (3).

   What is more important, with current political and judicial preoccupation with drugs comes a tendency towards a less sensible administration of justice: special narcotics divisions, special criminal investigation methods (undercover techniques), relatively severe penalties, and international cooperation modeled on measures against terrorism. What is at stake here is the moral quality of the legal system in a democratic community (4). The preoccupation with drugs puts a strain on the acceptability of the law, especially on the relationship of the agents of the state with lower social classes and ethnic minorities. Drug-dependent persons frequently have a weak socioeconomic status; they are primarily concentrated in poor, minority urban areas. A repressive policy may further marginalize vulnerable segments of the population.

3. The correlation of drug use and criminality is usually taken for granted. However, hard data are lacking. Not much is known about the nature of the drug–crime connection. Is criminality the result of the scarcity of the drug, so that the criminal activity is a type of instrumental behavior on the part of the addict, while programs for free distribution of drugs or methadone maintenance may eliminate the paucity of drugs and its associated criminality? Or is there no causal relation, and are criminality and drug use both manifestations of a deviant lifestyle and a marginal social status, so that the criminal activity of the drug user is a motivated behavior emanating from his chosen identity and related to the meaning-structure of his life (5)?

PUNISHMENT OR THERAPY?

Questioning drug policies also produces a moral debate on the nature of the problem and its preferred solution. The current policy of repression defines the problem primarily in normative terms. Drug users deviate from socially accepted and legally codified norms. They are considered as autonomous agents, understanding what they are doing and willing to use substances that are illegal, harmful to their health, and potentially deleterious to public health. Because they are autonomous agents, users are held accountable for the drug use itself, its consequences and associated activities. Emphasis therefore is on punishment. Enforcement of legal sanctions against users is justified through the intention to deter (possible) other users, as well as to deter those punished from continuation of their use. Given this normative characterization of the problem, medicine is expected to contribute to the elimination or neutralization of the social consequences of drug use. The aim of medical intervention has gradually shifted from therapy to containment. Doctors are performing drug tests for companies and government agencies; they are involved in methadone maintenance programs; or they are reporting drug use of patients to colleagues, authorities or employers. Instead of helping the drug user to get rid of his or her addiction, doctors are more and more involved in fighting the expansion of drug use, restricting public nuisance and crime, and maintaining law and order as much as possible. The intertwining of the military and disease metaphors has produced a startling ambivalence regarding the nature as well as the goals of medical intervention (6).

A NEW APPROACH: NORMALIZATION AND INTEGRATION

Critical assessment of current drug policies is leading to a growing awareness that a new approach is needed, particularly since intravenous drug use is associated with HIV infection (7). Policy-makers realize that the effects of drug use should not be confused with the effects of drug policy (8). Repressive policies, criminalizing drug users and making possession of and trafficking in all drugs illegal, create secondary problems that might be worse than the primary problems, *viz.* the harmful effects of the drug on the user. Once such a distinction between primary and secondary problems has been made, a pragmatic instead of moralizing characterization of the drug problem is the next step. It implies that the interconnection between social and medical perspectives must be broken, and priority given to the medical perspective, focusing on the primary effects of drug use. A pragmatic approach emphasizes rehabilitation. Attention is primarily given to reducing harm to the user. Through prevention, education, treatment and support helping agencies try to improve the user's physical well-being and social functioning. Inherent in the medical perspective, now given priority, is that no normative judgement is made on the user or his condition. He is approached and treated as any other patient, although he may be in certain respects a more problematic patient. The aims of medical intervention are redefined as normalization and integration (9,10). The physical risks of drug use are minimized as well as complications medically treated, so that the drug user can retain relations with society as long as possible. Many drug-dependent persons are in fact capable of living a 'normal life' without criminal behavior or serious physical harm (11,12).

MORAL EVALUATION

What can be concluded so far is that drug addiction and drug policy are intimately connected. Specific drug policies are associated with specific perceptions of drug use; they are thereby producing different conceptions of what is the major problem. That conclusion is ethically relevant since a moral debate on drug addiction could start from at least two types of normative characterizations of the problem: drug use as a vice or as a disease. Moral norms and values determine what we take as the relevant moral issue. This illustrates one of the difficulties with the principles approach in health care ethics: principles and problems are not independent variables. Particularly in the context of drug addiction, with coexisting social and medical perspectives on what constitutes the primary problem, it is confusing to ask what principles may be applied on the problem of drug use; *implication* rather than application is the case.

It follows that a moral evaluation of drug addiction and drug policy should proceed from a comparison of the medical and social perspectives on drug use. At least three issues are ethically relevant: (a) the balance of harms and benefits, (b) the autonomy of the patient, (c) the duties of the doctor.

Harms versus Benefits

The potential physical harm which the addiction induces in the drug user himself justifies a primarily medical approach. It follows that treatment must be aimed at counteracting the drug dependency and its consequences. Abstinence, however, is difficult to accomplish. This indicates that apart from somatic factors, psychosocial determinants are involved; a transformation of the addict's lifestyle is necessary to obtain results in the long run. Thus detoxification must be followed by psychosocial rehabilitation. To achieve this, a wide range of health care services has been developed: differentiated treatment facilities, counseling, prevention, health education, rehabilitation services. Since drug addicts are not inclined to contact health facilities, unconventional methods are used to contact them: e.g. street corner work, open-door centers, methadone bus. Apart from reducing harm for individual users, this approach also has the advantage that helping agencies are keeping close contact with addicts, and can therefore reduce harm to others. This is especially important for AIDS prevention. If most addicts can be reached by (conventional as well as unconventional) health care agencies, it is effective to try to raise their health consciousness, to change their injecting behavior, and to distribute clean needles. These are public health benefits, easily lost in a repressive policy that makes no distinction between criminalization of drug users and drug traffickers. A legal climate with a low enforcement priority for possession and use of small quantities of drugs, at least makes the distribution and use of drugs to some extent visible, thus partly manageable. From a moral point of view the balance of (individual and public) harms and benefits seems therefore in favor of a pragmatic, medical approach.

Autonomy of the Addict

A repressive drug policy seems to consider drug users as autonomous agents, responsible and accountable for drug use as well as their drug-related criminal activities. Autonomy apparently justifies the goals of punishment and deterrence through legal sanctions.

A pragmatic drug policy makes a distinction: the drug user, like other citizens, is held responsible for criminal acts and other behaviors related to drug use, but as regards the drug use itself, his autonomy is diminished. If autonomy is subdivided into autonomy of action, autonomy of will, and autonomy of thought (13), what is impaired is autonomy of will (and perhaps, in some cases, autonomy of thought). Drug users have a compulsion to take drugs, associated with a physically based dependency. Many of them intend many times to stop drug use, but many are unable to execute that intention. However, it is not clear what the restricted autonomy of will implies. In some cases the *efficacy* of will is diminished: some drug users are unable to do what they will; they are characterized by 'weakness of will' (the Aristotelian *acrasia*), viz. they fail to do what they believe to be in their best interest. In other cases the *deliberateness* of will is impaired: what drug users will is not the fruit of deliberate choice but determined by their immediate desires and impulses (14).

But in both cases a pragmatic policy aims at normalization. Drug users are treated as if they are normal persons with the same responsibilities as other people. The difference from other persons is that they act in accord with their appetite for immediate pleasure. However, in this respect there is no rationale for treating the users of drugs in a different way than the users of other potentially harmful substances such as tobacco or alcohol. In fact, many more people die as a result of smoking or alcohol abuse than as a result of drug use. A pragmatic policy, recognizing diminished autonomy of will, tries to reduce immediate harm for the drug user, and assists the user, with a variety of services, to increase his autonomy of will. It can in principle be discovered what the patient actually wants and what he thinks is in his best interest in the long run, so that present interactions can be focused on regaining control of his own life in the not-too-distant future. Such policy implies a different way of respecting autonomy than the repressive policy. The latter wrongly assumes that autonomy is not diminished, but it also operates with a different notion of autonomy. Usually, autonomy is understood as self-determination. The autonomous person determines his own ends and sets his own course of conduct; his actions spring from values he has in some sense decided upon. But a repressive policy cannot in the end accept that the drug user has his own notion of what is right and best. His lifestyle is an affront to the basic values of our culture; he drops out of community life and makes a parasitical use of societal relationships. So his autonomous choice should be morally condemned. Paradoxically, the repressive policy cannot accept the autonomy of the drug user (and his affirmation of particular values), precisely because it assumes that his lifestyle results from a voluntary choice of an autonomous person (being free to choose his own values).

Duties of the Doctor

The different perspectives on both the nature of the problem and the autonomy of the drug user also create uncertainties regarding the duties of doctors, and health care workers in general. Should they focus on the interests of the addict or those of society? Broader moral questions are involved. How to balance the requirements of social order, safety, and public health against the need for individual freedom and diversity of experience? How to weigh societal norms and an individual's norms?

In a repressive policy the intervention of the treatment staff is primarily aimed at controlling drug use as a social problem. Treatment of drug users is part of a series of strategies to control, repress and prohibit drug use, trafficking and related crime. Medical intervention is regarded as a component of a social supervision mechanism. When the medical perspective on drug use is subordinated to the social perspective, then the duties of the doctor are primarily in the interests of society. Protecting societal norms is in that case more important than accommodating the individual patient's preferences.

On the other hand, in a pragmatic policy medical intervention is distinguished from sociocultural strategies. Here the health care worker has two separate sets of duties: duties as an agent of the individual patient, and duties as an agent of society. Normally, his *prima facie* duty is to the individual patient, overriding those to society. But given a pragmatic policy, this situation is more complex: it is defined to be in the interest of society to focus intervention primarily on the individual drug user, supporting and rehabilitating his physical and social functioning. Within this policy framework the primary obligation is in the interest of the patient (15). The principle of beneficence does require that a serious and unconditional attempt is made to relieve the drug abuse and ameliorate the primary problems of drug use. Mere reinforcement of legal and social norms is undesirable.

REFERENCES

1. Diez-Ripolles, J. L. 1989. Current trends on the works of the European Parliament with regard to narcotic drugs. Pp. 21–28, *in* Albrecht, H. J. and Van Kalmthout, A. (Eds) *Drug policies in Western Europe.* Max Planck Institute, Freiburg.
2. Bakalar, J. B. and Grinspoon, L. 1984. *Drug control in a free society.* Cambridge University Press, Cambridge.
3. Van Kalmthout, A. 1989. Characteristics of drug policy in the Netherlands. Pp. 259–291, *in* Albrecht, H. J. and Van Kalmthout, A. (Eds) *Drug policies in Western Europe.* Max Planck Institute, Freiburg.
4. Levinson, S. 1982. Under cover: the hidden costs of infiltration. *Hastings Center Report* **12**: 29–37.
5. Meyer, R. E. and Mirin, S. M. 1979. *The heroin stimulus: implications for a theory of addiction.* Plenum, New York.
6. Ten Have, H. and Sporken, P. 1985. Heroin addiction, ethics and philosophy of medicine. *Journal of Medical Ethics* **11**: 173–177.
7. Gostin, L. 1990. Waging a war on drug users: an alternative public health vision. *Law, Medicine & Health Care* **18**: 385–394.
8. Engelsman, E. L. 1991. Drug misuse and the Dutch. *British Medical Journal* **302**: 484–485.
9. Baanders, A. P. 1989. *De Hollandse aanpak. Opvoedingscultuur, druggebruik en het Nederlandse overheidsbeleid.* Van Gorcum, Assen.
10. Van de Wijngaart, G. F. 1990. *Competing perspectives on drug use. The Dutch experience.* Utrecht: thesis.
11. Cohen, P. 1987. Cocaine en cannabis. Een gelijk beleid voor verschillende drugs? *Tijdschrift voor Criminologie* **29**: 244–268.
12. Reinarman, C., Waldorf, D. and Murphy, S. B. 1988. Scapegoating and social control in the construction of a public problem: Empirical and critical findings on cocaine and work. *Research in Law, Deviance and Social Control* **9**: 37–62.
13. Gillon, R. 1986. *Philosophical medical ethics.* John Wiley & Sons, Chichester.
14. Kupfer, J. H. 1990. *Autonomy and social interaction.* State University of New York Press, Albany.
15. Gillon, R. Editorial. 1985. Heroin, health and disease. *Journal of Medical Ethics* **11**: 171–172.

78

AIDS: Health Care Ethics and Society

ANTHONY J. PINCHING, DPHIL, FRCP

Professor of Immunology, St Bartholomew's Hospital Medical College, London

INTRODUCTION

As a clinical scientist working on the clinical features and biological basis of immunosuppression when AIDS was first described, I felt that this novel disease was likely to teach us something about the nature and mechanisms of immunosuppression and, by implication, about the normal function of the immune system. So it has. But little did I realize how it was going to affect my approach to clinical practice and to widen my understanding of the practical expression of medical ethics.

My involvement in patient care and scientific enquiry early in the HIV pandemic drew me, both formally and informally, into the development of public policy in response to the issues raised by AIDS and HIV. Quite apart from professional knowledge, it rapidly became evident that insights gained by work with individuals affected by HIV and AIDS were a valuable resource in advising on the priorities and the practicalities of policy development for the public health and the individual good.

There was much to be done, especially in the early years, and the development of a response to AIDS in health care and public policy was done in the hothouse atmosphere of crisis management. While this may have seemed less than the ideal approach, we did not have the luxury of time for strategic planning. Subsequent reflection and observation has suggested that, on occasion, strategic planning can be a luxury of dubious benefit that is more often liable to produce paper solutions, which tend to be remote from the realities of the individual or the social problem.

Given this context, there was a need for the practical and the policy response to be guided by certain basic principles. The numerous and diverse issues raised by AIDS required that the response be guided by internally consistent principles

---

Principles of Health Care Ethics. Edited by Raanan Gillon.

that were relevant to the needs of the individual good and the public health. Whence came these principles?

In reality, at least from my own perspective—and I suspect of many others at the front line—they were expressions of implicit views on medical ethics, many of which had not been formally articulated, still less taught, but rather represented an ethos derived from experience and example. AIDS became the anvil on which these ideas were forged and honed. Indeed, it was through an almost instinctive response to the issues raised that one's philosophy and ethical stance were revealed to oneself. With the benefit of hindsight, and in particular of discussions with those trained in philosophical medical ethics, one became aware that the central guiding principles were in fact the 'four principles' of medical ethics— respect for autonomy, beneficence, non-maleficence and justice. I find it somewhat encouraging that these principles emerged as they did—as a practically appropriate response in the context of individual and public health—rather than being set out, in tablets of stone, as the templates against which we were obliged to respond. Thus I would argue, as a practising clinician, that the four principles are essentially descriptors of contemporary medical ethics, as expressed in clinical practice and public health medicine, rather than its determinants.

In this chapter I will not therefore attempt to set out the principles as an explicit formulation of the response to AIDS, but rather to see them as the implicit framework for that response. However, others may find that they are a useful basis for determining which of a number of possible responses to ethical dilemmas is most appropriate. While HIV and AIDS probably raise under one head more ethical issues than any other medical problem, I shall focus almost entirely on the issues central to treatment of the individual and to prevention of the further spread of HIV, as they encapsulate the perceived dichotomy and tension between the needs of the individual and the needs of society—a dichotomy which I would argue is more apparent than real.

PREVENTION AND TREATMENT

Superficial analysis of the issues at hand in a pandemic human infectious disease, such as HIV, would separate treatment (for the individual good) and prevention (for the public good) as discrete issues. It could be argued that treatment encompasses the need to respect autonomy and to show beneficence in the clinical response to a person's needs arising from disease, while prevention is more concerned with non-maleficence and justice in ensuring that those who are not infected are given maximal protection from infection.

However, this is evidently too simplistic: those needing and receiving treatment are central in prevention of further spread of a human-to-human infection. If their help is to be enlisted in preventive efforts, they too will need to be protected from any, even unintentional, maleficence in the process; i.e. alienation and discrimination must be avoided not only on general moral grounds but also on pragmatic ones, to ensure participation. Equally, they need to be assured that justice and equity underlie our approach to them in the context of prevention. By the same token, those we wish to protect from infection are autonomous individuals who may or may not share our sense of priorities and must be allowed to exercise choice in behaviours on which the preventive effort bears. They must be the judges, against the backcloth of accurate and personally relevant information of how the risks of acquiring HIV infection relate to other risks, whether medical or other, that they consciously take.

HIV INFECTION AND ITS NATURAL HISTORY

These issues assume even greater force in the light of some key characteristics of HIV transmission and the natural history of the infection. Once HIV is acquired, infection is life-long; infectiousness is also effectively life-long, albeit with evidence of greater risk as disease advances. This contrasts with many other infectious diseases where the period of infectiousness is time-limited, often to a matter of days or weeks. Furthermore, the natural history is such that infected individuals may remain well for very many years; because the early period after infection is usually clinically silent, people may be unaware that they are infected. Thus preventive efforts directed towards people who are not attending for treatment—i.e. the 'general public'—must recognize that these include infected as well as uninfected individuals, and have to encompass the needs of both groups.

ROUTES OF TRANSMISSION

The particular routes of HIV transmission are also crucial. Sexual transmission requires that preventive efforts must recognize the generally consensual nature of sexual relations and also the fact that they are very private, even clandestine—especially if a person has multiple partners or is bisexual. Transmission during intercourse necessarily involves conjunction of an infected and uninfected partner. Does consent to intercourse imply consent to acquisition of sexually transmitted infections, especially if one partner is unaware of the sexual behaviour of the other that would put them at risk for such infections? In the past the issue may have been regarded as less important, since most such infections were readily treatable anyway. HIV brings new imperatives of honesty and/or caution to consensual intercourse.

Moreover, sexual intercourse results from very basic drives that are not entirely under rational control, ranging from the sexual urge itself through to the wish to bear children. Alcohol and other drugs may further affect the effectiveness of rational control on sexual behaviour. Amongst those who have sex for money, there may be additional factors—poverty and the need to provide for immediate needs of self or children, or the need to finance the imperatives of drug addiction—that can influence the willingness to accept the infectious risks entailed in sexual behaviour.

Injecting drug use is almost always illegal, and takes place in contexts that are remote from most social restraints. Drug-using activity is driven by irrational urges, reflecting physiological or psychological dependency in regular users and by the desire to experiment and the response to subtle or overt peer pressure in the new user. Illicit behaviour is conducive to the emergence of a subculture with its own norms and peer pressures. Risk-taking may be seen as an essential ingredient of drug-using behaviour and the long-term risk of HIV disease may seem remote from the imperatives of drug use. Again alcohol or other non-injected drugs may affect judgement and ease of risk-taking.

The third major route of transmission, from infected mother to her infant *in utero* or possibly at delivery, is also subject to very powerful and not always simply rational drives. The desire to have children is driven by strong instinctive needs, and by social and cultural pressures. That drive may even be enhanced by the knowledge that one or both parents are at risk of early death from HIV disease.

Thus, the major routes of transmission of HIV worldwide represent human behaviours that are amongst the most inaccessible to direct intervention in preventive effort, both literally and metaphorically. Ultimately, the implementation of prevention rests with the individual, whether infected or uninfected, and in contexts that are least amenable to rationally based intervention.

ALIENATION OF AFFECTED GROUPS

An important background to intervention in the HIV pandemic has been the prior social alienation, isolation and disempowerment of many of the individuals or groups most affected in the early phase of the pandemic—whether homosexual men, injecting drug users, prostitutes (especially in developing countries), the poor, recent migrants—whether from one country to another, or from rural areas to townships and urban slums—and populations affected by regional military conflict. Many of these groups were explicitly or implicitly seen to be outside the main stream of their societies. Analogous processes can be perceived in developing countries in the early years of the pandemic—especially in Africa and the Caribbean—who viewed with hostility the suggestions from people in the developed world that AIDS was a major issue for them.

Injunctions for members of such groups to respond to the needs of HIV prevention for the benefit of society in general, let alone their own peers, were readily misconstrued and misunderstood. In some instances, exhortations about HIV prevention seemed to be thinly veiled expressions of prior social prejudice and served to enhance their sense of rejection from society at large. Whether or not these implications were intended—and in some cases there is little doubt that they were—they served as powerful forces to demotivate such individuals from acting for the general good. In many instances they also led to early denial of the reality of HIV, seeing it merely as further propaganda against them, explicitly or implicitly blaming them for the current ills of society.

Thus, the context in which HIV emerged was one where preceding social injustice was readily exacerbated, yet where the only viable solution for either individual or public good was its resolution, that is to say, the explicit and implicit recognition of people in marginalized groups as being full members of a community and of society at large. In many areas, however, this fundamental injustice has not been addressed adequately and thus constantly serves to undermine preventive efforts.

THE PIVOTAL ROLE OF THE INDIVIDUAL

It is a self-evident consequence of the routes of transmission outlined above that the behaviour of individuals, both infected and uninfected, is at the heart of any preventive effort. Transmission events are in essence an expression of the autonomy of two individuals, and approaches to the public health in HIV prevention can only be mediated through such individuals. In reality, the individuals concerned—infected and uninfected but at risk—comprise virtually every member of society. There is perhaps no more explicit example of how the integrity of society depends upon the participation of its individual members. Even if wider social injustices cannot immediately be rectified, preventive efforts rest entirely on being able to influence positively the autonomous behaviour of the individual, whether infected or uninfected. Given the powerful irrational forces at play in the activities that allow transmission, the fact that both potential participants in a transmission event are accessible to behavioural change can offset the effect of these forces to some degree.

PUBLIC EDUCATION AND INDIVIDUAL COUNSELLING

How can this be achieved? Firstly, one has to be able to inform and to motivate all those who might be at risk of transmission in the future, as well as those who are already infected but who are unaware of it and who could pass on the infection. Since this encompasses little short of the whole population—though some evidently will be at greater risk than others—the central tool must be public education, together with explicit or implicit means for effecting or enhancing behavioural change, including changing social attitudes and novel peer pressures.

Secondly, at least a proportion of those who are infected and those who are at risk can be reached on a one-to-one basis in the setting of individual health care. Those already infected will increasingly need personal health care and support for the many aspects of HIV infection and disease. Moreover, others who may have been at risk may come forward to determine whether or not they are infected; even if found to be uninfected they can be accessed at an individual level towards personal behavioural change. The size of this latter group can be influenced by the public educational process in encouraging them to come forward to seek assistance, by the removal of any social penalties that may otherwise discourage them from so doing, and by the effectiveness and accessibility of the individual health care offered to them and their peers. Through individual counselling, people can be helped to relate the generalities about HIV infection to their own personal situation and can be empowered, through support and the acquisition of life skills, to reduce risk of HIV transmission to or from others in the future.

The effectiveness of both of these means in HIV prevention will be determined by the social milieu and attitudes conveyed in public education and public policy on the one hand, and by the responsiveness of individual health care and counselling to their personal needs on the other. This is the nub of the issue: if social or personal disadvantage is seen to result from accessing individual care and advice, it will either not be sought or the advice not followed. If such individual provision is inaccessible or unavailable, public education and exhortation may at best be unhelpful, or at worst may enhance isolation and demotivate the individual from behavioural change. If individuals are not empowered to reflect on and to change behaviour in relation to their own actual and likely future personal behaviour, the opportunity to reduce the frequency of potential transmission events will be missed.

One-to-one counselling and advice provides that opportunity against the backcloth of general advice. It can make the issues more personally relevant, as well as providing a person with the means with which to translate knowledge about risks in general into more appropriate specific behaviour that can reduce risk. Counselling, when properly done, empowers individuals and provides them with the means for behavioural change and for coping with their personal and medical situation. However, this empowerment needs to be fostered in the type of counselling provided.

Non-directive counselling can raise the public health as well as the personal issues, but enables people to reach their own conclusions and then supports them in effecting these; common sense, enlightened self-interest (reduced risk behaviour not only reduces risk of acquiring HIV for the HIV-uninfected person, but also reduces risk of acquiring other infections that may enhance progression of HIV disease in the HIV-infected person), and a degree of altruism typically ensures that the personal goals are shared with the public health objectives. Directive counselling, into which it is all too easy to slip if the counsellor allows his/her own strongly held views to impinge on the process, can readily become counterproductive; this is because the counsellor comes to be seen not as a personal guide but as an agent of public health enforcement.

In this way it can be seen that the care and support of the individual—and how these are perceived generally by potential users—are a vital springboard for HIV prevention. Only if we respond fully to the needs of the individual can we access the only tool for prevention—the individual, with or without HIV infection, who may later engage in risk activity and who, appropriately informed, empowered and motivated can reduce or eliminate the risks of such encounters. In other words, only if the individual is treated and is seen to be treated with express respect for autonomy and with a beneficent approach that lacks any explicit or maleficent consequences for that individual can we effect non-maleficence to those we wish to protect from infection. Justice means that all, irrespective of HIV infection status, must have their autonomy respected.

ACHIEVING THE OBJECTIVES

What are the prerequisites for implementing these realistic ideals? Firstly, the development of public policy and societal response must be informed by an understanding of these complex but tightly interrelated issues and must unambiguously recognize the realities of the pandemic and of those affected. Secondly, health care provision must be accessible, user-friendly and confidential; it must also be seen to be acting primarily with the interests of the individual at heart. While this does not exclude also serving the needs of the public health, individuals must see that the latter in no way undermines their own rights and needs. Since the arguments deployed above will be by no means self-evident to the public and to affected individuals in particular before they make contact, individual health care must be seen from outside very explicitly to respect the individual's autonomy.

Once individuals are in contact, and are comfortable with the ground rules of their own care and the high level of confidentiality that must necessarily apply, the opportunities for involving them in prevention will more naturally and comfortably follow. If they have confidence in their carers they will reveal most, if not all, of the relevant behavioural background to their own risk of HIV infection. Hence they will identify the issues that are most relevant in helping them to reduce future risks to themselves or others; for those already infected it will also raise the issues relating to previous and current contacts. People are more likely to respond to advice and to accept support from those whom they respect as being interested in their health and well-being.

People with HIV infection will also learn that continuing HIV risk behaviour may be detrimental to their own health, through the acquisition of intercurrent infections that may speed HIV disease progression. Furthermore, in my experience, the overwhelming majority of patients with HIV infection are all too keen to ensure the protection of others from the formidable problems they themselves are facing. The idea of 'revenge' sex and the like belong more to the realms of fiction and tabloid headlines than to reality; yet if any setting is conducive to the emergence of such attitudes, then it is where people with HIV are personally alienated by their status, being regarded as outside society, or where they are not personally counselled and supported through the painful transition of addressing their HIV status.

CONFIDENTIALITY

A person approaching a carer or counsellor for the first time to address the issues raised by HIV may be wrestling with many competing concerns and emotions. The sensitivity of the issues, the prevalent social attitudes and, not infrequently, the person's own ambivalence to the risk behaviour or to knowing his/her HIV status all conspire to inhibit that person from attending or from revealing all the material background. In addition such people are meeting a stranger whose professional code of conduct may only be dimly understood and only partially trusted (from lack of previous contact or from earlier bad experiences). It is therefore wholly unsurprising that, apart from getting to know the carer and their approach along the lines indicated above, they will often want some explicit reassurance on the ground rules of confidentiality.

Medical confidentiality, like that of the priest or the lawyer, is widely known in principle. However, there is, among both the public and the medical and allied professions, a recognition that it is relative or conditional, and that differing degrees of confidentiality operate in different clinical settings. Ethical standards, embodied in professional guidance such as that of the UK General Medical Council, specify certain settings (including explicit reference to HIV) in which risk to third parties *may* override the duty of confidentiality.

The extent to which confidentiality is applied is thus a matter of judgement for clinicians, in part determined by their own ethos and in part by the nature of the specific confidence. Clearly the latter is only apparent after a patient has revealed information within the context of the confidential professional relationship. Thus the tone of that relationship, and the limits that a particular clinician will set, will need to be identified by the patient from an avowed ethos by the clinician in advance of sharing specific confidences. It is apparent that some clinicians are approached specifically because of their publicly stated or personally known attitude to confidentiality—which serves to emphasize the signal importance attached to the issue. It also shows how there is a conditionality imposed on the information provided by the degree to which confidentiality is assured.

If patients perceive that certain confidences will jeopardize the overall duty of confidentiality, such patients will not reveal them; if so, they exclude from the clinical discussions the very information that may be essential if clinicians are to be able to help them act on behalf of the public health, let alone in respect of their personal health. If this happens there are few, if any, other settings in which a person can receive such help. Therefore any general or individual breaches of confidentiality—or perceptions that they would be breached—will in the end serve to undermine the public health.

Legal protection to confidentiality is only explicitly set out in the UK Statute on Venereal Diseases. Notably, the first case-law in England to cover medical confidentiality specifically related to a case occurring in the setting of HIV ('X vs Y', 1988/2 AER 479). While this related to an intended revelation by a national newspaper of medical information obtained within a confidential relationship, it carries strong implicit reference to more restricted breaches of confidentiality. Justice Rose, the trial judge, eloquently set out the general concern, stating: 'In the long run, preservation of confidentiality is the only way of securing the public health; otherwise doctors will be discredited as a source of education, for future patients will not come forward if doctors are going to squeal on them. Consequently, confidentiality is vital to secure public as well as private health, for unless those infected come forward they cannot be counselled and self-treatment does not provide the best care.'

Many have expressed concern about what clinicians should do when they become aware of a patient who continues to put another person or persons at risk of HIV infection; should the clinician inform the other party? As indicated above, such instances are unusual. In many instances the clinician can enable the index case to find a way of either informing the contact or avoiding putting that person at risk. Sometimes, when both individuals are under the care of the same clinician, the contact can be given advice that protects without explicitly or implicitly revealing confidences.

In the rare instances where such approaches fail, should the clinician breach confidence, with all that that implies? The wider danger is evident from the above. If the clinician 'comes on heavily', pressuring the individual with implied or actual threats to breach confidence, the patient may simply disappear and hence be lost to the one setting in which he or she can be helped to reduce the risk to others. I am painfully aware of such a case where the patient assumed (wrongly) that I would seek out and inform the partner; now no-one is advising the patient about how he could protect the partner, let alone providing care. We are all losers from such dissonances.

Another angle is that the clinician, in giving an assurance of complete confidentiality, can emphasize that this imposes a consequent duty on the patient to pick up the social and medical consequences, painful though they may be, of previous or current behaviour. It does seem unreasonable for clinicians to be expected to carry the full weight of the consequences of their patients' social behaviour; this would seem to be one of many adverse consequences of old-fashioned medical paternalism. In the same sense that clinicians will encourage the patients to make their own decisions regarding treatment, as discussed below, so the patients are given, or rather retain, responsibility for their own actions. This approach seems to put responsibilities where they properly belong and, while empowering the patient, allows the clinician to take on the more appropriate role of help and support in picking up the consequences.

Ultimately, confidentiality—which I personally would see as so near absolute as makes no difference—embodies, as outlined here, one of the most complete conjunctions of the four principles of respect for autonomy, beneficence, non-maleficence and justice to be found in clinical practice.

PATIENT EMPOWERMENT IN CLINICAL CARE

When we turn to the clinical management of people with HIV infection, we encounter further ways in which the pandemic has served to influence our thinking on the practical applications of the four principles of philosophical medical ethics. AIDS and HIV have caused a major acceleration in the previously gradual shift from an outmoded medical paternalism to a more contemporary model in which patients are empowered to take a central role in determining their own treatment.

The context is one where large numbers of young people face a chronic disease with a high likelihood of a premature death, and are brought into contact with health care providers, many of whose patients hitherto had increasingly been, at least in developed countries, among older people. As well as their predominant youth, which I would see as the most critical factor, many of these patients are articulate and well used to expressing their views, most notably as members of marginalized social groups such as gay men. Another factor was the fact that, when AIDS first appeared and little was known about it, AIDS care tended to attract clinicians who were prepared to be challenged and to face the unknown; such clinicians were least likely to be railroaded into dealing with AIDS according to pre-existing formulations and to be threatened by change itself or by patients who wished it. It was in this setting that patients demanded, and clinicians willingly provided, models of care based on patient empowerment.

THE PATERNALISTIC MODEL OF CARE

To caricature the old model somewhat, clinicians used to assess the patients, decide what and how much they should be told (generally less than everything) and tell them what treatment would be given. Sometimes the 'relatives' would be told more than the patient, would be given the opportunity to determine what the patient should be told, and would be expected to collude in varying degrees of secrecy about the actual state of the patient. In other words the patient's autonomy would be unceremoniously wrested away, completing the process already started by the disease itself. This approach was taken by undoubtedly conscientious and caring clinicians who took on the mantle of beneficence ('don't worry, we'll look after everything') and non-maleficence ('he couldn't cope with knowing he had cancer') for all the best of motives.

However, there were severe consequences from such a model for the clinical relationship and the patients themselves. Above all, it undermined trust; the patient confided everything in the clinician, only to be told partial truths about what the conclusions were. While patients may even, as part of the self-protective instinct of denial, have colluded with the clinician to some degree, they all too often ended up in a rather bizarre gavotte, where the patients didn't know whether good news was just jollying them along or was really good news; increasingly aware of the realities of their disease as it affected them directly, they were increasingly alienated from the people who were most able to explain what was actually going on, and what could and could not be done.

Relatives were often placed in an invidious position: they were being expected to make decisions about what a person should know and how that person would wish to be treated without necessarily being in a position to do so; indeed their own perspective might have conflicted with assumed or actual preferences of the patient. Also, they were having to keep secrets from the patient at a time when they most needed to be close; such secrets, often imposed on them without their appreciating the consequences, could undermine trust within the personal relationship.

Even more seriously, patients were not offered choices of treatment approaches from which they could determine their preferred option. Disease was starting to take over control of their lives, and the clinician was completing that removal of control. Yet one of the most powerful tools a clinician has is the ability to reinforce the fact that, within the inevitable constraints that disease imposes, the patient can retain a personal control over the disease and its management, and hence on his or her destiny. That control can and does greatly outweigh the losses involved in acknowledging the realities imposed by disease, which often worries the clinician and the relatives more than the patients themselves.

Another consequence of the paternalistic approach is that the clinician, having taken on responsibility for decision-making, was often obliged to make arbitrary judgements on crucial, literally life-or-death, matters. These painfully difficult decisions would involve much soul-searching amongst benevolent clinicians who adopted the paternalistic approach. Most of the difficulties arose from the fact that the decision did not properly belong to the clinician but to the patient— the only person who had the appropriate frame of reference with which to make it. While judgements were undoubtedly made in good faith according to sound ethical principles, the fact remains that the locus of control was in the wrong place.

THE PATIENT EMPOWERMENT MODEL

According to this model, the dominant one in HIV practice, patients are provided with all the information about their clinical state and about current evidence regarding prognosis and possible approaches to treatment. This is given at a level of detail and complexity commensurate with the person's prior knowledge and level of education, without that implying any selectivity—rather the manner of its explanation. The clinician should very explicitly indicate at an early stage that the decision-making rests ultimately with the patient. Where, as is frequently the case, there are a number of possible approaches, the clinician will indicate these and allow the patient to decide. In this model the clinician is acting as a guide, outlining the terrain ahead and the possible ways through it, but enabling the travellers (patients) to choose the route that suits them best (1).

Patients often show considerable reassurance and relief that they are being told the truth, and it helps to cement a sound clinical relationship. This is, from my own experience, often particularly so for people whom others had deemed to need to be 'protected' from the truth; they also have often coped rather better than those who, at least superficially, conveyed an overtly coping veneer.

It is sometimes argued that this approach prevents people who would genuinely prefer not to know from having that option. But how are we or they to know who they are, unless they are put in the actual situation and given the chance to express their preference? Yet in doing so, don't we undermine that choice? The answer is not as self-evident as it seems. We have seen elsewhere in the AIDS pandemic just how powerful is the human capacity for denial. It seems that denial serves an important protective function, especially in the process of adjustment to unpleasant realities; it becomes pathological only where it prevents a person from dealing with those realities.

Patients who have been told the truth about their situation can indeed choose to deny or 'forget' what they have been told, using the form of denial known as positive avoidance. This is itself a legitimate coping mechanism and can be very effective. Nonetheless, in my experience of several hundred people with AIDS, all of whom have had their disease explained to them, this strategy is extremely rare—particularly when set against what many would have expected, and against what relatives and partners have expressly warned. The handful of patients exercising positive avoidance have shown that, at other levels, they are assimilating and dealing with the specific issues very adequately. The approach thus provides people with the choice as to whether or not they themselves in the actual setting of, say, AIDS, wish not to know. In such rare instances this must be carefully and consistently respected, as to remove their coping strategy would be dangerously counterproductive.

Again it may be argued that patients do not want to have a series of choices of treatment offered to them, and would find such decisions burdensome. I have not found this a problem. Clearly, having had the issues displayed before him/her, a patient may decide to ask the clinician for advice. The patient is thus granting permission for the clinician to act as a proxy; it is a positive transfer of decision-making and itself represents a clear choice. It may be offered for some decisions and not others and should never be assumed. Even if the patient has not made the decision, at least he/she will understand the context in which it was made.

In such instances it is not for the clinician to impose a personal choice but to advise or act based on an understanding of patients and their approach. In the same way as patients who wish to decide may make a range of choices according to who they are and how they approach things, so clinicians must respect the nature of the person for whom they are proxy. In some relationships and cultures the patient may wish to give the proxy to a relative or partner; here again, the patients retain control by determining to whom, among many potential others, they prefer to entrust this vital role, rather than a clinician making an arbitrary choice, based on 'next-of-kin' or other concepts.

In other words the clinician does not remove control or autonomy from the patient without permission and, even when control is given to the clinician, there is still further room for the respecting of autonomy. By recognizing autonomy more than in the paternalistic model, the clinician is achieving thereby a greater exercise of beneficence (enhancing well-being by reinforcing control against the disease) and avoidance of maleficence (undermining of trust in clinicians or loved ones).

A significant benefit from this approach is that patients understand the essentially dynamic state of knowledge about their disease and indeed of their own expression of it. The clinician can share current scientific uncertainty with the patient, enabling him or her to determine, knowing what is established and what remains uncertain, how he or she will act. Patients can decide what is a sufficiency of information to take a particular course of action. A common example is the decision whether or not to take zidovudine during asymptomatic HIV infection on current, admittedly incomplete, evidence. The approach avoids the clinician being obliged to behave as though all the information needed is available, and that such and such is the only course open—which is rarely, if ever, the case in clinical practice—only to have that overtaken by subsequent data.

Another substantial advantage of addressing the uncertainties and imperfections of current knowledge is that patients can better understand why clinical trials are being done—to resolve these uncertainties. By the same token clinicians can better understand how the uncertainties are viewed by the people in the real front line, and can use this to inform the design and conduct of such trials.

One of the issues that is particularly affected by the application of this model is death. From the earliest stages of the pandemic, AIDS was recognized as carrying a near-certainty of premature death. It has therefore always had to be addressed, as not to do so would imply lack of truthfulness or an inability on the part of the clinician to deal with it, each of which would undermine the clinical relationship. By opening up the discussion, explaining what happens in the final phase and what can be done about it in symptom control, the clinician empowers the patient to address the issue; this can prevent it from persisting unresolved as a spectre that hangs over the patient's remaining health and life. By demystifying death and removing much, though not all, of the taboo surrounding it, one can render it manageable. It also avoids the reverse paternalism where the patient, seeing death as perhaps representing 'failure' to the clinician, protects him or her by not raising the issue. Again the bizarre gavotte, which in this case prevents the patient from articulating fears and the clinician from engaging effectively in the palliative mode of care.

If patients know in advance that the issue is discussable, agreement can be reached about how it is to be managed and where. Above all, patient and clinician can discuss, and the patient decide, when it is appropriate to transfer from active treatment mode ('getting better medicine') to the palliative mode ('going well care'). My experience has been that raising this issue at an early stage greatly assists later management. Virtually all the obstacles are on the clinician's side and, with a will, can be surmounted. This strategy removes the need for the clinician to agonize over such issues, which is the inevitable consequence of the paternalistic model mentioned above. While not the primary intent, it does make the clinician's role easier too!

Another consequence of dealing explicitly with the issue of dying and how it will be managed has been that it has largely removed the pressure to offer euthanasia. Much of that pressure seems to derive from fear of the process of dying: that it will not be effectively managed, that the patient will lose control, and that he or she will be left to cope with it alone. All these perceptions typically derive from a failure to address the issues in advance within the clinical relationship. Patients who are offered the prospect of effective palliative care, and a say in when it is introduced, well understand and respect the constraints on clinicians regarding euthanasia.

CONCLUSIONS

It will not have escaped attention that the patient empowerment model of clinical care applies with equal force to the care of patients with other diseases. Indeed it has been evolving in parallel, albeit at different rates, in several other areas of medicine. AIDS has provided, for a variety of contextual reasons, a catalyst for the transition to a model of care that is evidently more in tune with the expectations and aspirations of contemporary individuals and society.

What has emerged seems also to embody—perhaps by good fortune, perhaps by subconscious design—the four principles of medical ethics. Similarly, in the earlier consideration of the perceived tension between individual care and public health, the principles serve as excellent descriptors of the pragmatic approaches that have been forged in response to HIV infection. Furthermore, the many other practical responses to the complex web of clinical and social problems resulting from HIV and AIDS that have not been considered here have conformed remarkably well to these four principles. That they emerge naturally in the response to the practical necessities of clinical care in this most tragic, complex and socially pervasive disease, encourages me—as a clinician—to think that the four principles do indeed have a powerful validity in the ultimate assay: the real world of clinical medicine.

REFERENCE

1. Pinching, A. J. 1991. AIDS—Therapeutic strategies and models of care. *Journal of the Royal College of Physicians* **25**: 332–338.

79

Epidemiology, Society, and Ethics

John M. Last

Professor Emeritus of Epidemiology and Community Medicine, University of Ottawa, Canada

INTRODUCTION

Three ways to study health and disease are clinical observation, laboratory investigation, and measuring the effects on populations. The third method is called epidemiology, which is defined as the study of the distribution and determinants of health-related states or events in specified populations, and the application of this study to control of health problems (1). Epidemiology is the basic science of public health, and is also an essential part of good clinical medical practice.

Epidemiology has been responsible for great improvements in the human condition during the past 100 years. This method of studying health and disease has clarified our understanding of many physical, biological, and behavioural dangers to health. Much of the knowledge obtained through epidemiological studies has been applied to the control of physical and biological hazards to health, such as diseases due to drinking polluted water. Other epidemiological knowledge has become part of general knowledge and popular culture, leading to changes in attitudes and behaviour, and thus has led to improved health. Examples include attitudes towards personal hygiene, tobacco smoking, diet and exercise in relation to heart disease, use of safety equipment in the workplace, seat-belts in cars, and, most recently, prudence and precautions in sexual relationships.

THE ETHICAL CONTEXT OF EPIDEMIOLOGY

Epidemiologists usually work in direct contact with people, the subjects of their studies, so the same basic principles of biomedical ethics that apply in clinical medicine and clinical research are relevant in epidemiology. These principles are respect for autonomy, non-maleficence, beneficence, and justice.

Principles of Health Care Ethics. Edited by Raanan Gillon.
© 1994 John Wiley & Sons Ltd

There are however, some important ways in which the ethical issues encountered in epidemiology differ from those faced by doctors who deal with individual patients. The differences arise because of some unique features of epidemiological methods and because of the aims or purposes of epidemiology.

As the basic science of public health, epidemiology is concerned with study and control of health problems that threaten populations rather than individual patients. Epidemiologists and public health practitioners work with, and are concerned about, the well-being of groups of people. Sometimes they may be obliged to give higher priority to the needs of the group or the community than to the rights of the individual. The term 'macro-ethics' has been used to describe the ethical approach to groups (2), in contrast to 'micro-ethics' which is concerned with interactions among individuals.

Epidemiologists usually must be able to identify precisely each individual person in populations they study, and although identities are obliterated in the aggregated tables that result from statistical analysis, guardians of privacy are sometimes concerned about the process of identifying people and the implied threat that intimate personal information might fall into unauthorized hands. There is, however, no record of this ever having happened in either the United Kingdom or the United States (3). In this respect epidemiology has an enviable track record which is in sharp contrast with the published record of clinical research: for example, case reports in widely circulating journals often contain photographs in which only the most perfunctory attempts are made to conceal the identity of patients, who by no means always have given their consent for such revealing information to be published; a recent policy decision by the International Committee of Medical Journal Editors (4) should, however, put a stop to this practice.

Epidemiologists often interact not only with individual subjects but with special-interest groups—public advocates and activists, labour unions, industrialists, stockholders in commercial corporations, politicians, the media. These interactions have the potential for producing conflicts of interest, a topic further discussed later.

Epidemiologists often make general statements about risks to health that are associated with such factors as ethnic origin, social background, occupation, place of residence. These statements are intended to reduce or eliminate remediable risks to health, but they can sometimes inadvertently cause embarrassment or harm to an identifiable community or group by stigmatizing them.

Epidemiology, drawing on its close relationship to public health, is regarded by those who practise it as an entirely beneficent activity. Sometimes, however, the actions and statements of epidemiologists are perceived as paternalist. This subject also is further discussed later.

EPIDEMIOLOGICAL PRACTICE AND RESEARCH

The distinction between practice and research in epidemiology is ill-defined. For example, epidemiologists working in a cancer registry are primarily concerned with surveillance of cancer incidence and survival rates in relation to methods of treatment among members of a defined population; this is routine epidemiological practice. But the epidemiologists in a cancer registry commonly conduct original hypothesis-testing research that requires independent financial support from a research-granting agency, and this research normally undergoes ethical review. There can be problems trying to determine which activities of the cancer registry should be subjected to ethical review and which activities it would be unethical to impede by imposing a delay for scrutiny by an ethical review committee. Similar questions arise in studies of infectious disease, when routine epidemic or outbreak investigation does not yield an answer, and special research projects with independent funding by a research-granting agency have to be conducted to elucidate the problem. This happened, for example, in the studies that clarified the cause of legionnaires' disease: the initial epidemic investigation did not identify a causal organism, and further studies supported by expensive research grants were required (5). Should these have undergone ethical review? Perhaps they should, but epidemic outbreak investigations are often public health emergencies that cannot be held up to await the next meeting of an ethics review committee: this could expose large numbers of people to the risk of death or serious illness that could be prevented by identifying and controlling the source of the epidemic.

Ill-defined boundaries also exist between health services research and routine health care evaluation which is an essential component of audit in the practice of medicine in an institution such as a hospital or community clinic. It would be professional misconduct not to carry out routine quality control procedures on all aspects of medical care; but it is not easy to define the difference between routine quality control and special studies that could be described as health services research—which ought to be submitted to ethical review like other forms of research involving human subjects.

INDIVIDUAL RIGHTS AND COMMUNITY NEEDS

In public health practice there can be some ambiguity about the precedence of individual human rights and dignity over the needs of the community. This ambiguity is best illustrated by features of communicable disease control, but it occurs also in environmental health, food handling, prevention of injury in the workplace and on the roads, and in many other settings.

Communicable Disease

Ever since the origins of the concept of contagion, communities have taken action to identify and sometimes to restrict the free movement of persons suffering from certain kinds of disease. The practice of identifying victims of infectious disease is as ancient as the leper's bell and distinctive clothing; identification often stigmatized the victims and sometimes still does. Restricting freedom of movement dates back to the lazaretto and to quarantine, which was established in European city-states around the end of the fourteenth century.

The practice of restricting the freedom to move of persons suffering from conditions that are known or thought to be infectious is called isolation.

Restricting free movement of those in contact with them, such as members of their families, is called quarantine. These practices were codified in the eighteenth century by Johann Peter Frank (6), and have been written into laws or regulations in almost all nations in the world.

It has long been customary to isolate patients suffering from such conditions as typhoid, diphtheria, poliomyelitis, tuberculosis, measles and hepatitis. At times it has also been usual to quarantine the close contacts such as family members of patients with these and other conditions, and these methods of controlling the spread of infection have usually been reinforced by laws or regulations. Many infectious diseases previously subject to these control measures are now rare in western industrial nations, and in some instances modern methods of antibiotic treatment have made isolation and quarantine obsolete.

Sexually Transmitted Diseases

The ethical (and legal) issues remain acutely sensitive in relation to some infections, notably sexually transmitted diseases, and especially in relation to human immunodeficiency virus (HIV) infection.

When persons are diagnosed as suffering from sexually transmitted diseases such as syphilis or gonorrhoea, it is necessary not only to treat them, but also to treat those with whom they have had sexual contact—who must first be traced, identified, and notified, with appropriate counselling, that their sexual partner has a sexually transmitted disease. This is often a highly sensitive, emotionally charged matter. Ideally, contact-tracing, partner notification and counselling should be preceded by obtaining the informed consent of the index case. (Informed consent in relation to epidemiological research is further discussed below.) These procedures of contact tracing and partner notification are standard practice in public clinics for the treatment of sexually transmitted diseases, but in private medical practice they are sometimes ignored. Not infrequently a male patient with gonorrhoea will attempt to prevail upon his doctor to obtain treatment for his wife without informing her about the nature of the condition for which she is being treated. This, of course, is not merely unethical but in many jurisdictions it is illegal; it is professional misconduct for a doctor to comply with such a request by a patient.

HIV Infection

The practices and procedures of identification, contact tracing and partner notification in cases of HIV infection often differ from those that have long prevailed for other sexually transmitted diseases. This has happened because of the unique features of the acquired immunodeficiency syndrome (AIDS): it is a lethal disease; and especially in the first wave of the epidemic in the industrialized nations, considerable stigma was attached to the diagnosis. Moreover, the principal victims of the early phase of the epidemic, homosexual men and haemophiliac children, had eloquent and aggressive advocates who promoted their interests in ways that led to some variations in the rules, regulations, and laws that governed the control measures customarily applied to control of sexually transmitted diseases.

There are important variations in procedures for testing, reporting, and notifying cases of HIV infection and AIDS, and in subsequent actions. Mandatory testing is conducted by blood banks, organ and tissue donation agencies and the like, and by life insurance companies which will not issue life insurance policies until they have verified the freedom from HIV infection of the aspiring policy-holder. In some settings, HIV testing of health care workers is in effect mandatory. In 1991 the US Senate approved legislation that would make HIV testing of health care workers compulsory—though whether this would violate the US Constitution if enacted into law is debatable.

Persons who suspect they may have HIV infection can obtain an anonymous HIV antibody test in some jurisdictions. The argument in favour of this is that access to facilities for anonymous testing encourages persons to attend for testing; the argument against is that public health authorities have no way of controlling subsequent events, in particular the notification and counselling of sexual partners of persons who test positive.

For surveillance of HIV infection rates in populations, the procedure which is now routine in almost all industrial nations, except The Netherlands, is anonymous unlinked HIV testing of aliquots of blood, e.g. heel-prick samples collected from newborn infants to test for inborn errors of metabolism such as phenylketonuria. This test is done after the samples have been stripped of all personal identifying information. Initially many doctors had misgivings about this method of surveillance, which of course makes it impossible to identify and counsel persons who have a positive HIV antibody test result; but almost all now agree with the expert committee of the WHO Global Programme on AIDS (7), that the advantage of anonymous unlinked HIV antibody testing, in providing valid ongoing surveillance data, outweighs this small and mainly theoretical disadvantage. This is an example of a situation in which the ethical principle of distributive justice is given greater weight than the principle of beneficence: while no individual benefits, anonymous unlinked HIV tests benefit society as a whole by providing facts to follow the course of a life-threatening epidemic disease.

There are important and often unpleasant consequences for the individual who publicly acknowledges a positive HIV antibody test. Almost everywhere there are penalties, such as restrictions on employment, on eligibility for life insurance policies, and on freedom of movement; although it makes no epidemiological sense, many nations restrict the entry of persons with a positive HIV antibody test, even, in some countries, if they are returning nationals (8).

Other Aspects of Epidemiological Surveillance

Surveillance is defined as ongoing scrutiny, generally using methods distinguished by their practicability, uniformity, and frequently their rapidity, rather than by complete accuracy. Its main purpose is to detect changes in trend or distribution in order to initiate investigative or control measures.

Cancer and Other Registries

Other than notifiable infectious diseases, the principal conditions under surveillance in many communities are malignant diseases. Cancer registries gather information comprehensively about all newly identified cases of cancer, using routinely reported pathological examination results, records of other investigations such as diagnostic imaging, surgical operations for malignant diseases, autopsy results, etc. The process of reporting to a cancer registry is routine and automatic: patients with cancer have no say in the matter and may remain unaware of the fact that information about them and their condition is on file in a regional or national cancer registry. In some jurisdictions, cancer registration requires informed consent, i.e. it becomes voluntary. It therefore is no longer comprehensive in relation to the population at risk of getting cancer, and becomes much less useful; indeed for epidemiological research on cancer it becomes almost useless. Proposed regulations (as of 1992) threaten to impose this constraint on cancer registries throughout the European Community.

The information on file in a cancer registry is personal and often quite intimate. Does collection of such information invade privacy? Does it violate confidentiality? Privacy is respected and confidentiality is safeguarded because staff in cancer registries, like staff in government information-gathering departments, are sworn to secrecy. Moreover, no personal identifying information is ever released; only aggregate statistics are published. In this regard, cancer registries, like epidemiology in general, have an impeccable record of respect for autonomy or personal dignity. Records in a cancer registry are analogous to records maintained in a hospital—accessible only to authorized users.

EPIDEMIOLOGICAL RESEARCH*

Epidemiological research is observational or experimental. Three varieties of observational research are distinguished: cross-sectional studies (also known as surveys), case–control studies, and cohort (or longitudinal) studies. These types of study involve no risk to study subjects; they require no intervention other than asking questions, conducting medical examinations, occasionally laboratory tests, X-rays, etc. The informed consent of study subjects is normally required, but there are some exceptions to this, for example very large cohort studies that are conducted solely by analysing information contained in medical records.

A cross-sectional study is commonly done on a random sample of the population. Study subjects are asked questions, medically examined, or asked to undergo laboratory tests. The aim is to assess aspects of the health of a population, sometimes to test hypotheses about possible causes of disease or suspected risk factors.

A case–control study compares the past history of exposure to risk among

---

* Parts of this section are reproduced from *International guidelines for ethical review of epidemiological studies* (CIOMS, Geneva, 1991); the descriptions and commentary on epidemiological research methods in these *Guidelines* were drafted by the author of this chapter.

patients who have a specified condition (cases) with the past history of exposure to this risk among persons who resemble the cases in such respects as age and sex, but do not have the specified condition (controls). Differing frequency of past exposure among cases and controls can be statistically analysed to test hypotheses about causes or risk factors. Case–control studies are useful in investigating rare conditions, because they can be done with small numbers of cases. They usually do not involve invasion of privacy, although sometimes investigators must ask intimate personal questions, for instance about aspects of sexual behaviour. In all case–control studies there are rigorous safeguards of individual and sometimes of group confidentiality. If direct contact between research workers and study subjects occurs, the subjects' informed consent is necessary; if the study is done solely by examination of records, informed consent is not necessary and indeed may not be feasible, for instance if the subjects are deceased.

In a cohort study, individuals with differing levels of exposure to suspected risk factors are identified and observed over a period, commonly years, and the rates of occurrence of the condition of interest are measured and compared in relation to exposure levels. This is a more robust research method than a cross-sectional or case–control study, but it requires study of large numbers for a long time, and is costly. Usually it requires only asking questions and routine medical examinations, sometimes more elaborate procedures such as laboratory tests or X-rays. Informed consent is normally a requirement, but an exception to this rule is a retrospective cohort study that uses linked medical records. In a retrospective cohort study the initial or baseline observations relate to exposure many years earlier to a potentially harmful agent such as a drug, ionizing radiation or occupational hazard about which details are known for all members of the population; the final or end-point observations may be certified causes of death or the occurrence of specified disease. The numbers of subjects may be very large, perhaps millions, and at the time the study is done all or some subjects may be deceased, so obtaining informed consent may be neither feasible not practicable. The essential requirement is a method to identify precisely all members of the population being studied; this is achieved by methods of matching that are built into record linkage systems (9). After identities have been established to compile the statistical tables, all personal identifying information is obliterated, and therefore privacy and confidentiality are safeguarded—autonomy is respected.

An experiment is a study in which the investigator intentionally alters one or more factors under controlled conditions to study the effects of doing so. The usual form of epidemiological experiment is the randomized controlled trial, which is done to test the efficacy or effectiveness of a preventive or therapeutic regimen or diagnostic procedure. In accord with the Nuremberg Code (reprinted in ref. 10) and the Declaration of Helsinki (11), such experiments on human subjects are unethical unless there is genuine uncertainty about the regimen or procedure. Usually, in this form of experiment, subjects are allocated at random to groups, one group to receive, the other not to receive, the experimental regimen or procedure. The experiment compares the outcomes in the two groups.

Random allocation removes the effects of bias, which would destroy the validity of comparisons between the groups. Since it is always possible that harm may be caused to at least some of the subjects, their informed consent is essential.

Informed Consent

Informed consent is a mark of respect for the autonomy and dignity of research subjects; it has been discussed in detail in monographs (12,13) and in many learned articles in journals of ethics and the law. It is both a legal requirement and an ethical imperative in medical interventions. It is normally an absolute requirement in research involving human subjects although, as noted above, there are occasional exceptions in some forms of epidemiological research conducted solely by examination of the medical records of the study subjects.

The process includes informing subjects of all essential details about what is to be done to and for them, what the consequences are expected to be, what will happen if anything goes wrong, and ensuring that the subjects not only know but also understand essential aspects of what is happening. Subjects may give their consent orally or be asked to sign a consent form. In randomized controlled trials the information communicated to subjects must include the fact that there is uncertainty about best methods of dealing with the problem under investigation.

Knowledge of this uncertainty can arouse anxiety among persons who may already be anxious about their condition, so communication about it has to be made with sympathy and tact. Persons may be intimidated by those they regard as having power or influence over them, so although it is inappropriate to delegate the task of obtaining informed consent to a junior nurse or medical student, it may also be inappropriate for a senior clinician to be the principal in the process if that clinician is identified by subjects as the decision-maker about subsequent management. Subjects may not be autonomous—children, the mentally impaired, prison inmates, personnel in armed services, all have diminished or absent autonomy; consent then must be obtained from a proxy. This also applies in cultures in which people defer to a tribal headman or religious leader, or in which women are chattels of their husbands—although in these situations it is customary for investigators to ask individuals for consent, as well as to obtain the consent of the person who speaks for the group.

In some epidemiological studies, full disclosure of aims, methods, and procedures would jeopardize the outcome, for example by leading study subjects to respond in ways that they believe are expected or hoped of them. In this situation it is ethically acceptable to practise conscientious non-disclosure, i.e. informing study subjects only that they are subjects of an investigation, but not giving details that might influence their behaviour or responses to questions.

Random Allocation

The process of random allocation can arouse anxiety among study subjects; persons chosen for or excluded from investigation may become anxious or concerned about the reasons for choosing or excluding them. Investigators may have to communicate to members of the study population some elementary ideas about operation of the laws of chance, and provide reassurance that the process of random allocation is not discriminatory.

The above account of epidemiological research methods refers to some ethical issues associated with research design. Other ethical dilemmas may arise in the work of epidemiologists.

THE EPIDEMIOLOGIST AT WORK

Modern epidemiology often requires a multidisciplinary team that includes persons without training or traditions associated with medicine or other health-related professions. Statisticians, data analysts, computer programmers, trained interviewers, may become members of a team doing an epidemiological study, for example using community-based household interview surveys to study determinants of long-term disability. Along with briefing about the research project itself, those members of the team who come from professions entirely unrelated to any that are involved in health care may need some introduction to health care ethics, to ensure that they know how to conduct themselves.

For example, household interviewers doing a health survey are often asked for advice about respondents' health problems. Interviewer training should include sessions that deal with ways to cope with such requests. Interviewers should always remain impartial and non-judgemental; must emphasize the confidentiality of the information they are gathering, and they should not become involved as care-givers to the persons they are interviewing. Interviewers and other team members in contact with the public may encounter situations that severely challenge their equanimity. Suppose an interviewer is in a household in a confidential relationship with a respondent in a survey, and witnesses criminal behaviour; what is the proper course of action for the interviewer? Child abuse is an indictable offence in Canada, and anyone observing it is required by law to report it to child welfare authorities. Intent to commit robbery with violence is also a criminal offence punishable by law. Is there a difference in the way a household interviewer should react on becoming aware of either of these forms of criminal behaviour? In epidemiological studies of health care, investigators sometimes become aware of professional misconduct—but may do so as a result of discovering facts elicited in response to a promise of confidentiality. How should a health services research worker react to the discovery of professional misconduct?

There is a legal precedent for disclosure of confidentially obtained medical information when disclosure could save lives that might otherwise be endangered (14). This precedent is a useful guide to appropriate conduct by members of the epidemiological team: child abuse, for instance, ought to be reported even if this means breaking a promise of confidentiality. Intent to commit robbery, on the other hand, might not be reported, depending upon other circumstances that would enter into the decision. Whether professional misconduct should be reported by a research worker when it is revealed while bound by a promise of confidentiality depends upon the nature of the misconduct;

if lives of patients are endangered, or there is serious risk of other harm, the situation and circumstances would justify breaking a promise of confidentiality.

Processing and Analysing Research Results

Consider the distributions of data in Table 79.1. The distributions in Part A just reach 'statistical significance' at the 5 per cent level; the distributions in Part B do not. It would be easy to yield to the temptation to discard an observation on the grounds that it is an outlier, or to repeat an observation until a desired result is obtained. Such behaviour on the part of a research worker (in epidemiology or in any other field) might seem a venial sin, and perhaps is not uncommon. Nonetheless, it is professional misconduct.

TABLE 79.1 Data distributions

	A. 'Significant' differences		B. 'Not significant' differences	
	+	−	+	−
+	20	31	20	30
−	30	19	30	20
Total	50	50	50	50
	$p < 0.05$ (= 0.045)		$p > 0.05$ (= 0.072)	
+	5	14	6	14
−	45	36	44	36
Total	50	50	50	50
	$p < 0.05$ (= 0.041)		$p > 0.05$ (= 0.080)	

It is difficult to detect such behaviour unless log-books giving full details of all steps in research procedure are rigorously maintained. Biomedical journal editors and research grant administrators have become concerned in recent years about more gross forms of professional misconduct such as fraud and misrepresentation. Several conferences of editors have discussed ways to detect and prevent such behaviour (15,16). The Institute of Medicine of the National Academy of Sciences in the USA has developed a set of policies and procedures (17) which include the requirement to compile and retain detailed log-books of research protocols and procedures so that work can be reassessed if there is a subsequent suggestion of professional misconduct on the part of the investigators. The National Institutes of Health requires its grant award-holders to comply with this practice.

APPLIED EPIDEMIOLOGY—SCREENING FOR DISEASE

Screening is the presumptive identification of unrecognized disease by means of tests or other procedures that can be applied easily and cheaply to populations (18); individuals whose screening test is positive can then be given further tests to confirm or refute the presumptive diagnosis. The use of population screening tests is preceded by epidemiological studies and analysis of the evidence for the efficacy, effectiveness, and efficiency of the test, and accompanied by further epidemiological studies to evaluate the use of screening in the field. These studies enable health planners to determine whether population screening is an ethical policy; it would not be if the test were too costly, or if nothing could be done to treat or cure persons whose screening test were positive.

There would be fewer problems associated with screening populations for presumptive evidence of diseases such as cancer of the breast or cervix if the screening test could discriminate with absolute certainty between all those who have the disease and all those who do not. Alas, in the real world there is often uncertainty: tests can give false-positive or false-negative results. A false-positive screening test exposes the individual to the worry and expense of confirmatory investigations; a false-negative test can have disastrous consequences if the individual is wrongly told that she does not have cancer when in fact she does. Persons who thought themselves to be healthy can become worried and needlessly assume a 'sick role' when told that the screening test has disclosed the fact that they have high blood pressure. Mass screening of populations is usually conducted by a special team, often directed by public health authorities who may not always be diligent in informing personal doctors that their patients have been found to have a health problem; such people can get caught in the cross-fire between public health and personal health care services if there is disagreement between these about the best method of managing the problem. This too can cause needless worry and expense for individuals. Perhaps these problems fall more in the realm of medical etiquette than medical ethics, but they can be troublesome, and can be avoided easily by education and good lines of communication among all parties to the situation.

EPIDEMIOLOGISTS AND SOCIETY

Much of the work of epidemiologists is aimed at identifying risks to health, and implicitly if not explicitly at correcting, controlling, and preferably eliminating these risks. When the risks are associated with environmental problems such as polluted air or water, few people object to actions that lead to elimination of the problem, save perhaps industrial or commercial interest groups who may be required to pay for the corrective measures.

Many risks to health, however, are associated with activities that are pleasurable or profitable or both. Examples include tobacco smoking, use of alcohol and recreational drugs, high-calorie diets, indolent behaviour such as habitual television viewing, violent body-contact sports. Epidemiologists who study these aspects of behaviour have identified and measured the associated risks to health. In a similar manner, epidemiologists, often working with toxicologists and other environmental scientists, have identified and measured risks to health of working in or living close to a polluting industrial plant such as a coke oven or asbestos factory.

Epidemiology and Advocacy

Epidemiologists who have gathered evidence of the harmful effects on health of such behaviours or environmental conditions naturally seek to ameliorate the situation. But the people who are at risk may not want to give up behaviours that are pleasurable, may not want to risk unemployment consequent upon closure or relocation of a polluting industry in their neighbourhood. Moreover, the epidemiologist who marshalls the scientific evidence is acting as a scientist; the epidemiologist who uses the evidence to support the case for intervention is acting as an advocate—certainly as an advocate for what most of us would agree is a good cause, but an advocate nevertheless. It is not possible for an advocate to remain impartial, whereas a scientist objectively gathering and analysing data must necessarily be impartial. Thus there can develop a conflict between reason and emotion. This conflict must be resolved according to the conscience of each individual epidemiologist.

Perhaps the most telling example of this situation is control of the tobacco addiction epidemic. There is unassailable evidence that tobacco addiction is responsible for huge numbers of premature deaths (19). While many believe it is possible to reconcile the roles of scientist and advocate in relation to this epidemic, others, among them some of the most eminent epidemiologists in the world, have asserted that their role is to assemble the evidence, and it is up to others to advocate actions that will lead to control, eventually to elimination of the epidemic.

Paternalism in Epidemiology

It can sometimes be only a small step from advocacy to paternalism. By definition, paternalism means diminishing the autonomy of those at whom the paternalist measures are directed, and it can therefore be argued that it is not a justifiable approach for public health specialists or epidemiologists to adopt. However, most public health practitioners and many epidemiologists can cite examples of situations in which some degree of paternalism is or might be justifiable. One example is the mandatory use of safety equipment in industrial settings, another is mandatory use of seat-belts in automobiles, and crash helmets by motor cyclists. Epidemiological evidence has convincingly demonstrated reductions in mortality and irreversible morbidity (e.g. spinal cord injury, permanent brain damage) among populations where such safety measures are mandatory; and this has not only saved lives but has reduced costs of long-term care that would otherwise have to be borne by society, i.e. the taxpayers who are obliged to pay for lifetime care of permanently brain-damaged young adults injured in traffic crashes. Some advocates of smoking control measures assert that the evidence now is strong enough to justify action against habitual exposure of infants to cigarette smoke because of their parents' failure to control their tobacco addiction, but many would argue that punitive measures against habitual smokers would be counterproductive.

Fluoridation of municipal drinking water supplies presents a more difficult dilemma. The epidemiological evidence for efficacy and safety of fluoridation is unassailable; fluoridation protects against dental caries, and perhaps osteoporosis, and it carries no health risks—suggestions that it increases cancer risk have been refuted (20). It does, however, diminish autonomy and it could therefore be argued that this form of mass medication is ethically unjustifiable.

Conflicts of Interest

Studies of environmental or occupational health problems, and studies of the effects of prescribed medication (a field known as pharmaco-epidemiology) may be of interest to any of several parties that can be in an adversarial relationship to one another: industrialists, stockholders in corporations, consumer advocates, social activists, labour unions, the media, government regulatory agencies, political parties in or out of power. Studies of these problems may be conducted by epidemiologists who are employed by one or other of these adversarial parties, commonly by industrial corporations. Sometimes such corporations have been accused of applying pressure to epidemiologists in their employ, with the aim of encouraging production of results that favour the commercial interests of the corporation. Government agencies have similarly been accused of applying pressure to encourage research results that favour the political position of the government.

At times, epidemiologists have been influenced by pay, promotion, or recognition, to present a carefully contrived conclusion based on manipulation of the evidence, inadequate study design, or inappropriate methods of analysis. Sometimes when doing so they have failed to declare a conflict of interest. Conflict of interest is often considered to be a particular problem for epidemiologists who provide services to industry, but it is a broader issue. The government scientist who falsifies or selectively uses data in pursuit of official policy, or the academician who behaves similarly to enhance the prospects of publication (and promotion or tenure) are all victims of conflict of interest. Conflict occurs 'whenever a personal interest or a role obligation conflicts with an obligation to uphold another party's interest, thereby threatening to compromise normal expectations of reasonable objectivity and impartiality in regard to the other party' (21).

Causing Harm and Doing Wrong

One common outcome of epidemiological studies is identification of risk factors. Results are often presented in the form of generalizations, for example smokers are many times more likely than non-smokers to get and die of lung cancer, indolent and overweight people are more likely than active and lean people to get and die of ischaemic heart disease; prostitutes, long-distance truck-drivers in Africa and promiscuous homosexual men are more likely than chaste or monogamous people to be HIV antibody positive, capable of transmitting their infection to others. It is easy to make such generalizations, easy to make them in a manner that can lead to stigmatizing of whole sections of society, or at least to blaming victims. This is both harmful and wrong. Epidemiologists have an obligation to avoid causing harm and doing wrong to groups in society who have been identified as 'high risks' for conditions that have been the subject of study. Avoiding stigmatization requires a rigorously non-judgemental approach, careful communication, and painstaking explanations to representatives of the media who so easily can misquote or can themselves make sweeping and harmful generalizations which it is the epidemiologist's obligation to correct.

CODES AND GUIDELINES FOR EPIDEMIOLOGISTS

Like many other professional groups, epidemiologists have been concerned about standards of conduct. Several societies and associations of epidemiologists have discussed at length the way their members should behave in relation to individual persons who are the subjects of their studies, to the community, to employers, to each other, to clients, governments, and to health workers in other fields. Several professional associations have developed codes of conduct or guidelines (22). These guidelines have evolved along similar lines to those in related professional disciplines such as official statistics (23). The process of developing guidelines is leisurely and requires open discussion among as many members of the professional discipline as possible (24). Guidelines include a preamble, definition of the field, a statement about the values or beliefs of epidemiologists, and clauses dealing serially with the responsibilities and obligations of epidemiologists to science, to society, to individuals, to each other, to employers, etc. Members of the medical, nursing or other health-related professions who practise or do research in epidemiology of course adhere to the code of conduct of their profession. On the other hand, epidemiologists whose prior education has been exclusively in biology or statistics have come into the field without a background in or traditions of a health profession such as medicine or nursing; some of them have felt keenly the need for guidelines to define acceptable limits of professional conduct.

Ethical review committees also require help in formulating a consistent response when they review research proposals for epidemiological studies. Some guidance has existed in the handbooks published by national research councils in several countries (25,26). The Council for International Organizations of the Medical Sciences (CIOMS) convened a working group in 1990 to develop guidelines for the ethical review of epidemiological studies; guidelines (27) were published in 1991 and approved by the advisory committee on health research of WHO in 1992. These describe the nature of epidemiology, including ways in which epidemiological studies differ from other forms of biomedical research, give advice about ethical responses to situations that arise in epidemiological studies, and conclude with a checklist of items that members of ethical review committees are entitled to expect in research proposals.

CONCLUSION

Epidemiology is a fundamental science that can enrich our understanding of the natural world. It has been described as a liberal art or one of the humanities (28) because it can be an instrument of social justice. It is the basis for health planning and policy-making. Like other sciences, it is not 'value-free', but coloured by and reflective of culture, custom, and tradition. Wherever and however it is practised, epidemiology involves people and therefore must abide by the same rules of conduct that govern other aspects of human intercourse.

REFERENCES

1. Last, J. M. 1987. *A dictionary of epidemiology*, 2nd edn, p. 42. Oxford University Press, New York and Oxford.
2. Gostin, L. O. 1991. Macro-ethical principles for the conduct of research on human subjects: Population-based research and ethics. Pp. 29–46, *in* Bankowski, Z., Bryant, J. H. and Last, J. M. (Eds) *Ethics and epidemiology: International guidelines*. CIOMS, Geneva.
3. McCarthy, C. R. 1991. Confidentiality: The protection of personal data in epidemiological and clinical research trials. Pp. 59–63, *in* Bankowski, Z., Bryant, J. H. and Last, J. M. (Eds) *Ethics and epidemiology: International guidelines*, CIOMS, Geneva.
4. International Committee of Medical Journal Editors. 1991. Statement on protection of patient anonymity. *British Medical Journal* **302**: 1194.
5. McDade, J. E., Shepard, C. C., Fraser, D. W. *et al.* 1977. Legionnaires' disease; Isolation of a bacterium and demonstration of its role in other respiratory disease. *New England Journal of Medicine* **297**: 1197–1203.
6. Frank, J. P. 1976. *A system of complete medical police* (translated by Erna Lesky). Johns Hopkins University Press, Baltimore, MD.
7. Global Programme on AIDS. 1989. *Guidelines for monitoring HIV infection in populations (anonymous unlinked HIV antibody testing)*. World Health Organization, Geneva.
8. Duckett, M. and Orkin, A. J. 1989. AIDS-related migration and travel policies and restrictions; a global survey. *AIDS* **3** (Suppl.): S231–S252.
9. Newcombe, H. B. 1988. *Handbook of record linkage*. Oxford Medical Publications, Oxford.
10. *Trials of the war criminals before the Nuremberg military tribunals under Control Council Law.* 1949. No. 10, Vol. 12, pp. 81–82. US Government Printing Office, Washington, DC.
11. World Medical Association. Declaration of Helsinki, adopted by the 18th World Medical Assembly, Helsinki, Finland, June 1964; amended by the 29th World Medical Assembly, Tokyo, Japan, October 1975, the 35th World Medical Assembly, Venice, Italy, October 1983, and the 41st World Medical Assembly, Hong Kong, September 1989.
12. Faden, R.R. and Beauchamp, T. L. 1986. *A history and theory of informed consent*. Oxford University Press, New York and Oxford.
13. Applebaum, P. S., Lidz, C. W. and Meisel, A. 1987. *Informed consent; legal theory and clinical practice*. Oxford University Press, New York and Oxford.
14. *Tarasoff* v. *Regents of the University of California*. California Supreme Court. 17 California Reports, 3rd Series, 425. Decided 1 July 1976.
15. Council of Biology Editors. 1990. *Ethics and policy in scientific publication*. CBE, Bethesda, MD.
16. *Guarding the guardians.* 1990. Proceedings of the First International Conference on Peer Review in Biomedical Publication. *Journal of the American Medical Association* **263**: 1317–1441.
17. Institute of Medicine, National Academy of Sciences. 1989. Report of a study on the responsible conduct of research in the health sciences (Chairman: A. H. Rubenstein). National Academy, Washington, DC (reprinted in part in *Clinical Research* **37** (2): 179–191).
18. Wilson, J. M. G. and Jungner, F. 1968. *Principles and practice of screening for disease* (Public Health Papers No. 34). World Health Organization, Geneva.
19. US Department of Health and Human Services, Office of the Surgeon General. 1964. *Smoking and health.* Annual Reports, 1964 and subsequent years. Government Printing Office, Washington, DC.
20. Rozier, G. 1991. Dental public health. Pp. 1008–1011, *in* Last, J. M. and Wallace, R. B. (Eds) *Maxcy–Rosenau–Last Public health and preventive medicine*, 13th edn. Appleton and Lange, Norwalk, CT.
21. Beauchamp, T. L., Cook, R. R., Fayerweather, W. E., Raabe, G. K., Thar, W. E., Cowles,

S. R. and Spivey, G. H. 1991. Ethical Guidelines for Epidemiologists. *Journal of Clinical Epidemiology* **44**, 5 (Suppl.): 151S–169S.

22. Last, J. M. 1990. Guidelines on ethics for epidemiologists. *International Journal of Epidemiology* **19**: 226–229.

23. Jowell, R. 1986. The codification of statistical ethics. *Journal of Official Statistics*, **2**: 217–253.

24. Herman, A. A., Soskolne, C. L., Malcoe, L. and Lilienfeld, D. E. 1991. Guidelines on ethics for epidemiologists. *International Journal of Epidemiology* **20**: 571–572.

25. Commonwealth of Australia, National Health and Medical Research Council, Medical Research Ethics Committee. 1985. *Report on ethics in epidemiological research*. Canberra.

26. Medical Research Council of Canada. 1987. *Guidelines on research involving human subjects*. Ottawa.

27. Bankowski, Z., Bryant, J., Last, J. (Eds) 1991. *Ethics and epidemiology: international guidelines*. CIOMS, Geneva.

28. Fraser, D. W. 1987. Epidemiology as a liberal art. *New England Journal of Medicine* **316**: 309–314.

80

Ethics in Occupational Health

R. I. McCallum, CBE, MD, DSc, FRCP, FRCP(E), FFOM

Emeritus Professor of Occupational Health and Hygiene, University of Newcastle upon Tyne; Honorary Consultant in Occupational Medicine, Institute of Occupational Medicine, Edinburgh, Scotland

INTRODUCTION

Occupational health is a multidisciplinary activity which includes medical and non-medical specialisms. Although its origins extend back to the sixteenth or seventeenth centuries, it has emerged since World War II as an important influence in developed and developing countries alike. In addition to medically qualified practitioners there are nurses, occupational hygienists, safety specialists, health physicists in radiation protection, and first-aiders.

In the UK, concern over the effects of work on health has its roots in the early part of the nineteenth century when a combination of some enlightened politicians and employers gradually introduced legislation covering the conduct of work in factories and mines, a process which has continued to the present day (1). A series of acts and regulations have spelt out changes in working practices and in the work environment which were necessary to improve the health and welfare of workers, and incidentally their efficiency.

The mass of legislation introduced since the 1830s has culminated in the broad provisions of the Health and Safety at Work etc. Act of 1974 (2) and its regulations, which embrace virtually every work activity and are having far-reaching consequences for industry in the UK.

World War II required healthy munitions workers, and Ernest Bevin, the then Minister of Labour, introduced medical supervision and welfare services for them. The postwar nationalization of large industries helped this process on, and academic bases were established by the Nuffield Foundation in 1945 in Glasgow, Manchester and Newcastle. In the 1960s interest in this field intensified, and the report of the Robens Committee of 1970–72 led to the setting up of the Health and Safety Commission and the Health and Safety Executive in 1974. This added to it a medical branch (Employment Medical Advisory Service) which had been instituted in 1972.

Principles of Health Care Ethics. Edited by Raanan Gillon.
© 1994 John Wiley & Sons Ltd

In 1983 the report of a Select Committee of the House of Lords on Science and Technology, chaired by Lord Gregson, described occupational health as an integral part of primary care and underlined the need for provision of occupational health services in industry funded by employers. The Select Committee particularly recognized the need for appropriately trained doctors, nurses and hygienists for work in industry.

There have been parallel developments in other countries such as the USA. In addition international bodies such as the International Labour Organisation, the World Health Organization and in particular the European Economic Community can all influence or change the practice of occupational health in Britain.

The development of professionals in the occupational health field has been piecemeal, beginning with medical practitioners and then nurses in the nineteenth century, and increasingly involving non-medical scientists in this century.

OCCUPATIONAL MEDICINE

Early legislation (1847) covering the employment of young people required certification of their age, and led to the involvement of the medical profession in industry. This, however, was limited in scope but gradually extended so that by 1935 there were sufficient numbers of medical practitioners to form an Association of Industrial Medical Officers (AIMO).

As industries began to recruit their own medical advisers the AIMO became the Society of Occupational Medicine. Dropping the quasi-military term used previously is significant in reflecting a different view of the function of the doctor in industry.

Since 1978 occupational physicians have had their own faculty, within the Royal College of Physicians of London. It is now responsible for the main specialist qualifications (Associateship and Membership; and Fellow of the Faculty of Occupational Medicine). The faculty has over 1700 members.

At present, however, there are still many physicians employed in industry and in occupational health services who do not hold these qualifications, although it is becoming more common to have at least an AFOM as a requirement for appointments.

PROFESSIONAL ETHICS AND OCCUPATIONAL MEDICINE

Ethics in occupational medicine cannot be seen in isolation from other branches of medicine; the responsibilities of the occupational physician are those of any other medical practitioner. The General Medical Council, the British Medical Association, and the Royal College of Physicians of London have brought out reports on ethics since 1984, which are all relevant to the doctor working in industry.

Ethical problems related to the clinical trials which have been carried out extensively since the postwar period have been a major concern, and the Royal College of Physicians has published guidelines on medical research on human subjects (3). However, there are other types of ethical problems besides those raised by research. Those pertaining to medical practice are rather different, and may refer predominantly to relationships between professionals, being aspects of medical etiquette, or come into the purview of the General Medical Council's disciplinary committee.

Research ethics committees are now easily accessible through hospitals, research institutes, National Health Service Regions, Health Boards, etc. There are fewer practice ethics committees, and the Ethics Committee of the Faculty of Occupational Medicine is an example.

Occupational medicine has its own ethical problems which arise out of the dual relationship which a doctor who works in or for industry must face. The occupational physician (industrial medical officer, medical adviser, etc.) is usually employed by a company. This may be done in several different ways; it may be a direct relationship with the owner or manager or through a personnel department, or by contract for specific purposes. The doctor may be part-time, usually in conjunction with general practice, or full-time with a company. In the past when the functions of a doctor in industry were less clearly and closely defined, it was often an appointment made between friends, manager and doctor, on the golf course.

Sieghart (4) has pointed out that serving more than one master, as opposed to the simple traditional two-party model of doctor and patient, has come into medicine with the advent of a third party, the NHS, with which, at least in hospitals, the doctor has a contract, and not with the patient. The problem of dual responsibility has also been perceived in general practice (5), especially in relation to life assurance and consent to releasing medical information to third parties.

A recurrent problem is where an employer, or a solicitor acting for an employer, takes the view that as the doctor is paid by the company the medical records are therefore company property and available to personnel departments and managers, and where litigation is threatened, to lawyers without consent of the patient.

NHS management has been one of the worst offenders in this respect, and in many cases very strong pressure is put on doctors to comply with requests for release of records. In Sieghart's view serving more than one master at a time can lead to two or more moral principles coming into conflict, a sphere to which the study of ethics can contribute.

Pressure for access to records can be especially strong in hospitals in respect of health service employees who have attended a hospital occupational health service because of an accident at work. It is interesting that as long ago as 1968 the Tunbridge Report (6) was most emphatic that all records relating to the health of individual staff in a hospital should be accessible only to the medical and nursing staff of the occupational health service, and express permission of the employee concerned should be given before records were made available, save in exceptional circumstances (these were not defined).

Where there are quite clear-cut dangers to an individual or for those working with him, or where the employer would be at fault in employing someone with a disability which might pose some unnecessary risk, it is not unreasonable for the employer to specify for new employees that certain medical criteria must be met, and for the doctor to go along with this. In such a case the medical advice would presumably be that the person was unsuitable on medical grounds, but with no need to disclose why.

It has to be pointed out to an employer that as there is no way in which, for example, epilepsy and some other common conditions can be diagnosed in these circumstances, other than by the candidate giving the information in his medical history, neither doctor nor management will necessarily find this out; but the doctor is much more likely to find it out or to be given confidential information on the understanding that the information is privileged and will be kept confidential.

A candidate who is already an employee may have strong reasons not to have medical details disclosed. If, however, the candidate is willing to give formal consent to disclosure it is difficult to contest. But in these circumstances, even if candidates give consent to disclosure of medical records, there may be serious concern about the possibility of coercion and undue pressure being applied in relation to their wish for promotion. This point is one which an occupational physician should put to management.

CONFIDENTIALITY

The ethic in which doctors are trained demands a primary commitment to the patient, whose medical interests are paramount, and whose medical history is confidential between doctor and patient. It is not surprising that conflicts between the interests of the employer and those of the patient/employee can and do occur from time to time.

The conflict of duties arising from the multiple roles of the occupational physician is quite different from the therapeutic role in which the doctor is in the usual one-to-one relationship with the patient, to whom he is solely responsible. The occupational physician may be an impartial medical examiner reporting to a third party (the employer); an adviser to management and to workers' representatives; a research worker; a manager in relation to his own staff; a guardian of commercial secrets relating to materials or processes; and in relationships with other doctors (general practitioners and consultants), occupational health nurses, occupational hygienists, safety specialists and first-aiders. Under recent legislation in the UK (Data Protection Act 1984; Access to Medical Reports Act 1988; Access to Health Records Act 1990) employees have the right of access to medical reports and records on them.

Each employee in a company will also have his own general practitioner in the National Health Service, who carries the main responsibility for his primary care. Any action by the occupational physician must take this into account especially if any question of therapy is involved. In practice in the UK occupational physicians avoid therapeutic intervention very largely, but there are situations where it helps to keep a person at his/her job if treatment prescribed by the general practitioner can be given in a suitably equipped works medical centre. But it is unusual and generally unwise for an occupational physician to initiate treatment without very close liaison with the patient's general practitioner, unless it is to deal with an acute condition arising at and out of the employment: appropriate first aid for injuries; emergency medical care for illnesses/injuries arising in the course of work, and rehabilitation.

On the other hand in some circumstances, particularly in developing countries and in eastern European countries, occupational medical services have provided complete general practitioner care and specialist hospital care for the workers and their families.

Furthermore there is not only confidentiality in relation to the employee's medical condition, but sometimes the question of commercial secrets relating to industrial processes becomes relevant in the task of maintaining the health of workers.

HAZARDS AT WORK

The use of hazardous materials at work may be perceived as a special ethical problem for the occupational physician (7). The argument about the degree of risk in a job and its acceptability to society or to legislators, or more importantly to the people who are exposed to the risk, has been widely debated. One problem is that there may be no easily definable boundary between what is safe and what is hazardous.

Under the Health and Safety at Work etc. Act 1974 (2) among an employer's general duties is the provision of such information, instruction, training, and supervision as is necessary to ensure, so far as is reasonably practicable, the health and safety at work of his employees (section 2(2)c); and in the design and supplying of any article for use at work he must take such steps as are necessary to secure that there will be available in connection with the use of the article at work adequate information about the use for which it is designed and has been tested, and about any conditions necessary to ensure that, when put to that use, it will be safe and without risks to health (section 6c).

Thus the responsibility for the prevention of hazards at work is primarily that of the employer who now, under the Control of Substances Hazardous to Health Regulations (1988), has the clear duty to assess and control potential risks to health from dangerous substances. This will involve a complex approach including assessment of the hazard, monitoring of the environment, control practices as necessary and at some point may require medical surveillance.

Where the worker is in some way particularly susceptible to harm from the work methods or materials, or is judged to be physically unfit for a particular task, there may be ethical considerations for the physician in making a decision on what he recommends. There is, for example, the possibility of the physician operating a system which discriminates unfairly against some individuals (8).

This situation is similar to that in which there is an attempt to use the physician to get rid of individuals on medical grounds because management do not like them, or consider them inefficient or a liability, and find it difficult to sack them. This has to be resisted by the physician on ethical grounds, and it has to be made clear by the physician that he should not be asked to carry out what is essentially a function of company management.

The view that the workers and the public should decide what are acceptable risks in the workplace (9) is probably realistic.

TESTING FOR DRUGS AND ALCOHOL

There is considerable concern about the involvement of occupational health staff in 'policing procedures', and that there might be a risk of conflict of interest, and an ethical dilemma. Safety of nursing staff might be a problem; in one company at least it is the security staff who carry out breathalyser tests. One opinion is that occupational health personnel do not need to be involved in the tests, on the analogy of police practice in not using doctors unless a blood test is required. This is an interesting point of view, especially in the light of the historical use of the term 'medical police' in the eighteenth century in connection with preventive medicine and public health.

One might argue about the way in which detection of drugs in urine differs from the detection of sugar in the search for diabetes, in both cases in an effort to improve health and safety. Much depends on the attitude of society to the different problems.

RESEARCH

Research projects are often carried out with factory or other occupational populations as subjects. While the ethics of these investigations are in principle no different from those involving hospital patients (3), most are epidemiological and few of them require the administration of drugs. The main concerns are those of confidentiality of information. As in tests which have a statutory basis, individual confidentiality must be observed, full explanations must be given to subjects and results given to individuals personally.

HIV INFECTION IN WORKERS

'It is perhaps the general public's perception of human immunodeficiency virus (HIV) which causes the greatest problem for the HIV-infected employees in a workplace' (10). Fellow-workers may express concern if they become aware that a colleague is HIV-positive, and the doctor is likely to be asked to intervene. Managers will sometimes put pressure on an occupational physician over the screening of new employees for HIV infection as a condition of employment, but this is not ethically acceptable and would raise unnecessarily difficult issues of confidentiality.

CODES OF ETHICS IN OCCUPATIONAL HEALTH

These have been drawn up in several of the disciplines concerned with occupational health, particularly in the USA. For example the American Occupational Medical Association (1976), the American Association of Occupational Health Nurses (1977) and the American Academy of Industrial Hygiene (1979) (8). Here consideration will be given only to codes which have been formulated in the UK.

In 1937 the British Medical Association brought out 'Duties of and Ethical Rules for Industrial Medical Officers', but in 1980 the Faculty of Occupational

Medicine of the Royal College of Physicians of London, through its Ethics Committee, responded to current concerns about ethics by preparing a guidance statement on ethics (11). The Ethics Committee, which has two lay members, is a source of advice on ethical matters for occupational physicians, but it has been little involved in the ethics of research projects, preferring where there is a clinical content to have these monitored by local research ethics committees. However, the chairman of the Faculty Ethics Committee sits *ex officio* on the College Committee on Ethical Issues in Medicine.

'GUIDANCE ON ETHICS FOR OCCUPATIONAL PHYSICIANS'

This document has been well received and widely read and quoted. It has been periodically revised in the light of experience and other relevant publications. In the Faculty's Lucas Lecture for 1981 (4) the late Paul Sieghart pointed out weaknesses in it, and made some constructive criticisms which were largely incorporated in a further edition. This also took into account recent changes in emphasis in medicine, and the problems which had been referred to the Ethics Committee by occupational physicians. The text of the latest edition (11) was widely circulated in draft form to the Royal Colleges, the British Medical Association, the General Medical Council, the Confederation of British Industry (CBI) and the Law Society, for their comments.

The points are made that, although the underlying ethical principles in the practice of occupational medicine change very little, they are not static and are affected by changes in the attitudes of society, in the law and in technology, which lead to the need for changes in emphasis in the *Guidelines* from time to time; and there are no universally applicable answers to ethical problems and often no single correct action.

Ethical behaviour is seen as a self-imposed duty, and often a matter of conscience related to individual circumstances. This differentiates ethics from its near relative, best practice. The occupational physician's differing roles in being an impartial medical examiner reporting to a third party (the employer), on occasion a research worker, advising on the health/work interface to managers, employees and their representatives and on occasions in a more traditional relationship involving general medical advice, must be clearly expressed to the patients. The need for impartiality of the occupational physician is stressed.

The question of access to clinical records is dealt with in detail, and indeed this is one of the most difficult areas for the medical staff of an occupational health service. The confidentiality of such records must be rigorously guarded and they must be only released, particularly where litigation is involved, with the explicit consent of the individual to whom they refer. Any relaxation of this principle is seen as seriously undermining the impartiality of the medical staff and the confidence of the employees in them.

It is prudent for the doctor to record separately personal clinical information which is elicited during the course of a medical examination, from that which relates specifically to the job, such as the results of tests, some of which are done as a statutory requirement under regulations.

CONFLICTS OF INTEREST

While doctors may be employees of a particular organization they have an ethical duty to put their patients' interests first. The Faculty has formulated a clause for inclusion in the contract of employment of an occupational physician spelling out the distinction between responsibility to an employer and ethical obligations. Where problems still remain the *Guidelines* suggest discussion and consultation with appropriate senior colleagues. It is emphasized that informed and formal consent of a patient must be insisted upon before any clinical information is passed on.

The Australian College of Occupational Physicians has published *Ethics for occupational physicians* which, although it differs in scope, is very similar in content.

ROYAL COLLEGE OF NURSING SOCIETY OF OCCUPATIONAL HEALTH NURSING

Nursing services in industry began in a limited way in 1878 with the appointment of a nurse to Colman's mustard factory. World War II provided a stimulus to the more general introduction of nursing services to industry and as they developed the Royal College of Nursing formed a Section of Occupational Health Nursing in 1953.

Factory nurses have now become occupational health nurses, with their own post-registration training and qualification (the Occupational Health Nursing Certificate). The occupational health nurse may often be in sole charge of a works health service with either no medical cover at all or only intermittent cover.

The Royal College of Nursing Society of Occupational Health Nursing has published a *Code of Professional Practice in Occupational Health Nursing* (1987). There is little on purely ethical issues, and much of the code is concerned with ideal organization from the nurse's point of view, and with rules of good practice, as the title of the code makes clear.

The nurse's primary responsibility is to the workers, to safeguard their health and well-being. The nurse is obliged to disclose results of health assessments and medical examinations to an employer only in general terms to enable him to judge fitness for employment. Confidentiality of information on personal problems is to be respected. There is a duty to safeguard records, and to allow disclosure only with informed and specific consent of the employee concerned. The responsibility for transfer or destruction of records, other than statutory ones, rejecting employer's attempts to get access to records of individual workers, dealing with computerized records on leaving the job, are covered. The code deals less than adequately with the question of screening employees for alcohol or drugs.

The occupational health nurse is also required to work in accordance with the *Code of Professional Conduct of the United Kingdom Central Council for Nursing, Midwifery and Health Visiting*.

THE INSTITUTE OF OCCUPATIONAL HYGIENE

This has been a well-developed scientific discipline for a long time in the USA, but came to the UK in the late 1940s. It is now difficult or impossible for the occupational physician to practise occupational medicine without the collaboration of occupational hygienists as colleagues. The multidisciplinary British Occupational Hygiene Society was formed in 1956, and has a substantial medical membership.

Occupational hygienists themselves have had an Institute of Occupational Hygienists since 1975, which runs an examining board and serves to register its practitioners. The Institute describes occupational hygiene as a multidisciplinary profession whose concern is the recognition, evaluation and control of potential health hazards in the working environment. It seeks to define and maintain standards in occupational hygiene, and of conduct, which 'are as rigorous as those demanded by other professional groups such as medicine and the law'. This statement suggests that a clear understanding of the constraints on the two latter professions is lacking.

Other matters dealt with include: confidentiality regarding not only the hygienists' findings but also their client's business operations or manufacturing processes; giving advice which is honest and responsible; drawing attention to contraventions of statutory regulations; ensuring that information is used for legitimate purposes, and for the benefit of the workforce; duties to the general public. There is provision for the investigation of complaints against a member, and for penalties such as a reprimand or expulsion.

These are largely matters of good professional practice, rather than dilemmas requiring application of ethical principles.

THE INSTITUTION OF OCCUPATIONAL SAFETY AND HEALTH

This large non-medical professional group, who used to be called safety officers, set up an Examination Board in 1979. Their *Code of Professional Conduct* (1991) also emphasizes the primary responsibility to the worker, and to the community they serve. Again this code relates mainly to good professional practice and competence, the range of professional activities, etc. There is the possibility of disciplinary action under the Articles of Association.

INTERNATIONAL COMMISSION ON OCCUPATIONAL HEALTH AND SAFETY

The Commission is a non-governmental society founded in 1906, having both individual and collective members. Many occupational health professionals in the UK belong to it. The Commission has not hitherto given formal guidance on ethical matters, but a draft *Code of Ethics* was circulated as a working document in August 1990.

In its present form it has a number of defects. There is insufficient distinction between different professional codes, and between those professions which are already covered by formal ethical codes of practice and those which are not.

The document combines disciplines such as medicine, which have had for a long time structured codes of practice, both for medicine in general and now for occupational medicine, with other disciplines which have not traditionally had such codes. It would be preferable for it to include some general statements relating to the common ethical ground for all the disciplines, and then to separate in the text those aspects relating to actions by medical and those by non-medical personnel.

Its main defect is that what is best practice is not distinguished from what are strictly ethical problems. Guidance on issues such as the ethics of testing for alcohol, drugs and HIV positivity would be valuable. Reference to WHO standards and those of professional bodies in the various countries is lacking. The document makes no mention of the physician's duty to an employer, who is legally responsible for the health of the worker in the first place. The potential conflict between the interests of the worker and those of the employer, and the ethical problems this may pose, requires mention.

When this document emerges from discussion, and has absorbed comments from a variety of countries and their professional bodies, it will not have any legal status, but it could be a useful international contribution to ethics in occupational health.

THE FUTURE

In each case where a professional body has been set up, training and examination systems have followed so that it is now possible to define experts and those specially qualified in various aspects of occupational health, although official recognition of some of them has been slow. Each of them has also in due course set out rules of conduct for their profession which more or less deal with ethical matters—that of the Faculty of Occupational Medicine being the most developed and comprehensive.

The whole field of occupational health has changed over the past two decades, and further changes may be on the way. The emphasis has shifted from the individual with occupational disease or accident at work to prevention of these tragedies by the control of the environment, use of biological indices of exposure, and appropriate design of machinery and processes. The medical practitioner, as the leader of the occupational health team, has been challenged by others and may be further assailed in future. If some of what is now carried out by occupational physicians is seen to be better and more cost-effective when performed by others, it is best to concede this. However, biological changes in humans are the ultimate yardstick, and the position of the medical practitioner with privileges derived from long and demanding training and experience, a high degree of responsibility and accountability, plus legal standing derived from statutory recognition, mean that he is essential at some point.

The doctor in industry can take ultimate responsibility for individuals or groups, but standards and training of occupational physicians must match the position which they seek to occupy, and the ethical problems which they face will continue to be highly demanding.

REFERENCES

1. Raffle, P. A. B., Lee, W. R., McCallum, R. I. and Murray, R. (Eds). 1987. *Hunter's diseases of occupations.* Hodder & Stoughton, London.
2. Health and Safety at Work etc. Act. 1974. Chapter 37. HMSO, London, 1975.
3. Royal College of Physicians of London. 1988. *Guidelines on the practice of ethics committees in medical research involving human subjects,* 2nd edn. Royal College of Physicians, London.
4. Sieghart, P. 1982. Professional ethics—for whose benefit? The Lucas Lecture 1981. *Journal of the Society of Occupational Medicine* **32**: 4–14.
5. Toon, P. D. and Jones, E. J. 1986. Serving two masters: a dilemma in general practice. *Lancet* **1**: 1196–1198.
6. Joint Committee. Ministry of Health. Scottish Home and Health Department. 1968. *The care of the health of hospital staff.* Central and Scottish Health Services Council Report. HMSO, London.
7. Lee, W. R. 1977. Some ethical problems of hazardous substances in the working environment. *British Journal of Industrial Medicine* **34**: 274–280.
8. Derr, P.G. 1988. Ethical considerations in fitness and risk evaluations. Pp. 193–208, *in* Himmelstein, J. S. and Pransky, G. S. (Eds) *Occupational medicine: worker fitness and risk evaluations,* Vol. 3, No. 2. Hanley & Belfuss, Philadelphia.
9. Watterson, A. 1984. Occupational medicine and medical ethics. *Journal of the Society of Occupational Medicine* **34**: 41–45.
10. Baylis, P. J. and Gallwey, J. M. 1988. Acquired immune deficiency syndrome. Pp. 424–441, *in* Edwards, F. C., McCallum, R. I. and Taylor, P. J. (Eds) *Fitness for work: the medical aspects.* Oxford University Press, Oxford.
11. Faculty of Occupational Medicine, Royal College of Physicians of London. 1986. *Guidance on ethics for occupational physicians.* 3rd edn. Faculty of Occupational Medicine, 6 St Andrews Place, Regents Park, London NW1 4LE.

PART V

ETHICAL PROBLEMS OF SCIENTIFIC
ADVANCE

81

Ethical Problems of Scientific Advance—Introduction

RAANAN GILLON

Many of the preceding chapters in the last three sections have included discussion about ethical issues arising from scientific advances—but this section concerns itself primarily with ethical issues that have emerged directly from three major scientific advances that have impinged on medical practice, genetics, *in vitro* fertilization and transplantation. In addition papers in this section concern themselves with the ethical and other philosophical issues involved in our concept of death (issues that have resulted from the development of resuscitative technology but which have been given additional practical import by scientific developments in transplantation medicine), and with the ethical issues arising from the use of animals in scientific research.

GENETIC COUNSELLING

In her chapter on genetic counselling Seller highlights the importance of giving impartial, autonomy-respecting, information. But she also points out that in some circumstances patients will wish not to be told certain sorts of information (for example while some patients will wish to be told that they have a genetic predisposition to develop a nasty and/or fatal genetic disease such as Huntington's chorea, others will wish *not* to be told); and she argues that in some circumstances genetic counsellors may properly wish to withhold certain items of information on the grounds that it would be uselessly damaging to pass them on; beneficence and non-maleficence would override respect for autonomy in such cases, she argues. Two examples are discovery of non-paternity in pre-natal genetic diagnosis (found in some 2 per cent of cases screened in a series referred to by Weatherall in his chapter); and 'androgen insensitivity', in which genetic males with internal testes develop and are brought up as apparently normal females and quite often are only discovered to have the condition in their teens when being investigated for their failure to menstruate. In the former case both Seller

Principles of Health Care Ethics. Edited by Raanan Gillon.

and Weatherall argue that there is no moral point in potentially threatening disaster to a marriage by revealing such information to the couple, who are told simply that the tests have been uninformative about the genetic abnormality— but in a later discussion with the mother alone Seller would explain the situation and its implications for genetic counselling in relation to a future pregnancy.

In the case of androgen insensitivity Seller would normally not tell the patient the details of the finding, saying rather that a (genetic) medical problem had been discovered to account for the infertility and that (alas) there was nothing that could be done to remedy it. However the extent of the information divulged would, she adds, depend on the particular case and especially on the extent of the benefits and harms likely to result from alternative courses of action.

Another dilemma described by Seller concerns the maintaining of confidentiality in cases where divulging of genetic information about the index patient may be of crucial, perhaps life-saving, importance to other members of the patient's family. Normally patients are keen to be of help to their relations in this way but sometimes, perhaps because they are ashamed of their condition, they utterly refuse to allow any medical information about themselves to be passed on. Apparently the majority of genetic counsellors are likely to respect such patients' confidentiality, but some would override it if they thought that doing so would prevent serious harm to others. Perhaps one way to avoid the dilemma would be to make it clear before taking on a patient or couple for genetic counselling what the 'moral norms' of the clinic or counsellor are, in relation to such dilemmas—in the same way that, as Seller advises, patients should be warned that often genetic studies on an individual may require tests of his or her entire family, with any information relevant to the health of those other members likely to be passed on to them.

Further potential moral dilemmas for the genetic counsellor may arise if information is requested by insurance companies and by prospective employers. While, as Seller points out, there is normally no moral obligation to either, problems might arise, as in other branches of medicine, if a patient is discovered to have a condition that threatens the safety of other people; as, for example, if the patient is a pilot or train driver and is found to have a condition that produces a substantial risk of sudden unconsciousness. Here, as in other branches of medicine, a genetic counsellor may feel obliged to override confidentiality to protect others. In addition there may be a further problem if an insurance company has obtained the patient's permission to seek genetic information from the genetic counsellor: as Weatherall points out, it is already regarded as acceptable, given such permission, to pass on other aspects of a patient's medical condition; why should genetic information that may predict a patient's health status be excluded? Weatherall calls for urgent public debate on this issue.

Both authors also discuss the moral issues of the new genetics that arise in the context of possible abortion of genetically abnormal fetuses. Recognizing that for some patients the very possibility of abortion is morally unacceptable, they both argue that the issue should be primarily one for the prospective mother to determine, though the degree of abnormality that might in any case be allowed to justify abortion should be socially determined. Weatherall points out that most biologists feel it wrong to allow selective abortion on grounds of fetal sex merely to satisfy parental preference for a child of one sex rather than the other, and Seller, while accepting termination on the grounds of sex in cases of severe sex-linked genetic disorders, rejects it for mere satisfaction of parental sexual preference: 'To be male or female is not a genetic defect, rather it is part of the normal condition of life and is therefore not to be interfered with by geneticists.'

GENE THERAPY, SOMATIC AND GERM LINE

Weatherall considers additional ethical problems arising from actual or predictable advances in genetic manipulation techniques. One of the most debated of these is gene therapy, and in particular gene therapy that would be passed on to subsequent generations through the reproductive process—so-called 'germ line' gene therapy. Weatherall sees no new moral problems with somatic gene therapy, in which the adverse effects of a deleterious gene are corrected by insertion of genetic material into cells other than the germ line, so that the new genetic material is not passed on to the patient's offspring. He, like the majority of contemporary geneticists, opposes—at least 'at the present time'—germ line therapy, in which the new genetic material (and any beneficial or harmful effects that it brings) is transmissible to the patient's offspring. First, he argues, parents at risk of serious genetic disease can be helped to avoid having affected offspring without such risky activity, by diagnosis at *in vitro* fertilization. Second, we know too little about the stability over successive generations of inserted genetic material, and about any potential long-term deleterious effects. Furthermore 'we will undoubtedly be playing with the evolution of our species and taking decisions on behalf of future generations'. He does not rule out the possibility that future generations may decide differently, but for the time being he is firmly opposed to germ line genetic therapy.

While such caution seems morally highly desirable, the possibility that it might in particular contexts be morally appropriate to permit germ line therapy must also be borne in mind. If, for example, it became possible to offer parents germ line genetic treatment that would protect their offspring (and theirs, recursively) against retroviruses such as the AIDS virus, or against certain sorts of cancer, and if animal experiments had given no cause to anticipate deleterious effects of such therapy, then it seems at least morally plausible to argue that long-term clinical trials of such therapy might be permissible. Weatherall suggests that it is better not to dwell on what at present are science fiction possibilities, and simply exclude them by fiat for the time being, concentrating instead on what is currently possible, beneficial and unlikely to be harmful, leaving succeeding generations to deal with the science fiction possibilities when and if they become even remotely probable.

As against that view, however, are two considerations; first it can help to make our moral positions clearer to explore hypothetical morally complex situations in 'thought experiments'; second, the speed of scientific advance is so great that today's science fiction has an increasing tendency to metamorphose into tomorrow's—or just later today's—science.

Weatherall also considers the developing contemporary problem of ownership of human genetic components, and the associated issues of commercial exploitation of human recombinant DNA technology. 'It should be self-evident', he declares, 'that no part of the human genome can be the sole property of anybody. Equally there is little doubt that a particular method designed to isolate, analyse or express a particular DNA sequence can be patented; there is no reason for concern if companies wish to patent methods, but not individual sequences.' He urges that commercialization of human genome science must not be allowed to cause deterioration of normal standards of medical practice, or to interfere with medical research or dissemination of its results.

IN VITRO FERTILIZATION

Braude considers many of the ethical problems arising in the context of *in vitro* fertilization (IVF). He warns of the negative side of the process both when it is unsuccessful (he cites a 'take-home baby rate of about 15 per cent per attempted cycle' and writes of patients' profound sense of disappointment and loss when the procedure fails); and even when it is successful, including the risks of multiple pregnancy, and the invasion of a couple's reproductive privacy by the whole procedure. Discussing questions of distributive justice in the context of IVF, he points to common inconsistencies of approach, with public purchasers of health care being prepared to buy from the public purse surgical treatments for infertility such as tubal surgery, yet refusing to purchase IVF from the public purse. This seems unjust given the better cumulative pregnancy rates of IVF— he cites a 50 per cent 'take-home baby' rate for five cycles of IVF, and contrasts this with a 2-year conception rate of less than 15 per cent for tubal surgery. Leaving the general argument about abortion—which is as relevant to IVF as it is to genetic counselling—to others (see the four relevant chapters in Part III of this volume), Braude notes one specific argument that he claims is anomalous in the context of IVF, notably the argument from potential. Unlike the embryos and fetuses considered in the abortion debate, the potential of *in vitro* human embryos, precisely because of their *in vitro* environment, is very limited 'unless transferred to a suitable uterus'. Furthermore, and paradoxically, the older the *in vitro* human embryo becomes, especially after some 6 days of development, the *less* likely is it to produce a pregnancy even if it is transferred. 'Thus perversely, the older the embryo *in vitro*, the less its potential for further development.' Braude also rejects the moral relevance of arguments claiming that the embryo is genetically unique and of arguments that because IVF embryos are 'human' therefore they necessarily have special status. 'Human' in this context of IVF, he argues, simply distinguishes the type of species to which the embryo belongs, rather than specifying the morally special properties characteristic of 'a human being', which in his view pre-implantation embryos do not possess.

BUYING AND SELLING HUMAN ORGANS

Transplantation of organs and tissues has provoked major moral debate on a variety of fronts, and many of the issues are addressed by Brecher and Sells. In a philosophically reflective paper Brecher analyses what might be wrong with the selling and buying of human organs and tissues. Focusing on a notorious English case heard by the General Medical Council, in which a patient obtained a renal transplant as a result of the selling of a kidney by a poor Turkish peasant, Brecher analyses what might be wrong with the selling and buying involved. Using the four-principle approach he finds it difficult to fault—autonomy is respected, good is done, harm is minimal for the donor/seller, and there is benefit for the recipient not to mention the entrepreneur, the surgeon, and even the beneficiaries of the Turkish peasant's newly acquired relative wealth (which was allegedly used to buy medical care for a close relative). Nor does justice seem to have been transgressed—resources were efficiently used by mutual agreement, no rights were transgressed, and at the time no law was transgressed (I have added slightly to Brecher's analysis). Yet, he argues, this principle-based analysis fails to satisfy a strong moral sense that what happened *was* wrong, which, he concludes, demonstrates the inadequacy of the four principles as an analytic method. Instead, he argues, the moral problem lies in the 'social vision' within which these principles function and from which they take at least part of their very meaning. 'It is not some formal or theoretical notions of justice, or for that matter, of beneficence, let alone autonomy [and he could of course have added "or non-maleficence"]—which shape our vision of a good society: rather our ideas of what justice, etc. amount to are in considerable part a function of such a vision.' And he goes on to imply, though not explicitly to state, that a society in which the practice of buying and selling of organs is *necessary*, either for recipient or seller, and in which such a practice is morally acceptable, is a society with a morally corrupt vision of the good communal life, a corrupt vision of what constitutes a good society. My interest is doubly pricked by this sensitive and evocative paper. First it is pricked by the claim that the use of the four principles cannot in principle do justice to his moral analysis of the issue. Secondly it is pricked because I personally would argue that the buying and selling of organs and tissues—under carefully controlled conditions—is morally justified in societies that, for whatever reason, would otherwise allow the potential recipients to die.

So far as the moral analysis of the issue is concerned it seems, *pace* Brecher, that his argument, if I have construed it correctly above, *can* be presented in terms of the four principles. Essentially his argument is based on a vision of the good society in which people accept far more of an obligation of beneficence to others than currently pertains in our own (and I suspect any other) society, correlated with a theory of justice in which pursuit of one's own autonomous interests, and respect by others for that pursuit, is given far less moral weight than is given currently in our own society and other libertarian societies (and would be more like the weight that socialist or communist societies allocate to respect for autonomy relative to beneficence). Thus in Brecher's implicit vision of the good society, benefiting others, and doubtless especially those in greatest need, would be given greater moral priority over respect for autonomy. Within such a conception of the good society the buying and selling of organs would be morally unacceptable because, though the practice respected individuals' autonomy, it would undermine the primary objective in such a society of doing

each other good altruistically rather than doing good only, or mainly, as a means
to our own ends.

The buying and selling of organs would undermine the priority of the principle
of beneficence as morally required in such a society; moreover it would reduce
the *scope* of (altruistic) beneficence in such a society. And maybe too, if there
were an element of utilitarian welfare maximization integral to this vision of
the good society, the practice of selling and buying organs would be condemned
as tending to undermine the maximization of beneficence, by perverting people's
sense of altruistic obligation to benefit others (manifested by, for example, their
giving their tissues and organs to others) and degrading it into a selfish pursuit
of their own ends. And of course Brecher could add, as his early approving
reference to Titmuss suggests he might be inclined to do, that the practice of
selling and buying tissues and organs is likely to be maleficent, by increasing
the harmful effects of transplantation; the argument here would be that because
the poor members of society would differentially tend to become providers of
organs and tissues, and because they are in general more likely to be unhealthy,
this would result in increased dangers both to themselves and to recipients. The
point of all this is to show, in the context of Brecher's particular case, what I
argued for in more general terms at the end of Part I of this book—namely that
the four principles plus scope approach is neutral between particular conceptions
of what the proper balance of these principles should be—it is neutral between
particular philosophical or moral or political or religious theories or visions of
the good life. But it is *compatible* with any such approach, and *can* be used for
descriptive and analytic purposes by adherents of any approach. And above all
it allows people with conflicting moral visions nonetheless to remain part of a
community of moral agents who share moral values, even if they combine those
moral values differently, and even if they justify them from entirely different
theoretical bases.

As for my second concern with Brecher's argument, I think it simply boils
down to a conception of the good society that gives more moral weight to the
importance of respect for people's autonomy at the expense of less moral weight
to egalitarian theories of justice. In *such* a social context (and as he implies, it
is within such a social context that we actually live) I *suspect* that more
beneficence—more overall benefit to people—can be achieved by carefully
controlled practices of paying for donations of human tissues and organs than
can be achieved by rather self-righteously (as I see it) refusing to countenance
such payments while preferring instead to let people die unnecessarily; and
while at the same time preventing at least some of the poor and oppressed from
gaining a substantial financial benefit from selling some tissue or organ under
social controls that prevented such selling from being more than minimally
risky. But my conception of the good society demands and deserves no more
weight than Brecher's. The point is that it depends on the same sort of moral
values as does his, but proposes a different approach to their relative weighting,
or harmonization. When it comes to conflicting prioritization of these shared
values I believe all we can do is reflect on the alternatives, choose, and then
try, through an adequately autonomy-respecting mechanism, to persuade others

of the acceptability—and when we are threatened with markedly inferior visions, the superiority—of the vision we prefer.

OTHER MORAL PROBLEMS WITH TRANSPLANTATION

After Brecher's somewhat philosophically theoretical analysis, Sells offers a comprehensive and knowledgeable account of the ethical issues evoked by transplantation, from the perspective of a transplant surgeon. He too addresses the question of selling and buying of organs, analysing the variety of arguments offered on each side of this controversy and even discussing proposals for a 'futures market' in organs, in which people would undertake to make their organs available at their death, in return for payment either to themselves in life or after their death to their beneficiaries. (He argues that, apart from any other faults, such an idea is unlikely to be workable in practice.) Among the many ethical issues he discusses are brain death; the acceptance of living relatives as organ donors; different systems of buying and selling organs, including the carefully controlled method used in some parts of India known as 'rewarded gifting'; legal proposals to presume the consent of a deceased person to donate organs; or, as in many parts of America, to require doctors to ask relatives for permission to transplant organs—'required request' legislation; social reluctance in some countries to use corpses for transplantation; use of animals for transplantation and the genetic manipulation of animals, notably pigs, so as to minimize problems of rejection; and the development of 'elective ventilation' of mortally ill patients in order to ensure that their organs will be maintained in optimal condition for transplantation after they die.

PHILOSOPHICAL SUPPORT FOR 'BRAINSTEM DEATH'

Sells's discussion of brain death, approached from the perspective of an expert clinician who like the vast majority of doctors in Britain and America accepts brainstem death as death, is followed by two contrasting philosophical contributions on the matter, one by Lamb, giving philosophical support to the consensus approach, the other by Evans rejecting it. Lamb's account explains that while in ordinary human contexts that do not involve intensive medical care the age-old criteria of cessation of breathing and of heartbeat for a reasonable length of time (for of course they recurrently and frequently cease throughout our lives only to restart soon afterwards) are reliable criteria for the death of human beings (as of other mammals), in the context of intensive care units such reliability is lost. For in ICUs the breathing and heart beat can be maintained by medical intervention not only for long after a person *would* have died without such intervention (especially mechanical ventilation) but also for a substantial duration after the patient has *actually* died. Death in Lamb's account is taken to mean the end of the patient's life *both* as a person *and* as an integrated biological organism.

The basis for his assertion is the strong neurological evidence, overwhelmingly accepted by medical opinion and by contemporary law, that life in this sense is dependent on life of the brain, and that life of the brain is in turn dependent on life of a small part of itself, the brainstem. The brainstem is so crucial because it contains two vital types of control centre. One is the reticular activating system, functioning of which is necessary for the having of experiences, for the possibility of consciousness. The other type comprises those control centres or transmission neurones necessary for integrating the biological functions of the human body; without this type of brainstem function individual biological processes such as breathing, heart beat and blood pressure control, temperature control, hormonal control, kidney function, either will not occur at all (as with breathing, the control centre for which resides in the brainstem) or they will occur, but in an unintegrated way; the biological life of the human and indeed mammalian body cannot continue as an integrated whole without function of the brainstem.

Because of the coincidence of these two different types of control centre in the brainstem, brainstem death provides both necessary and sufficient conditions for death of the human being. This is because people on the whole want an account of human death and its diagnosis that satisfies *both* the concept of death of a human person (permanent cessation of existence of a human person) *and* the concept of death of a human being seen as an integrated biological organism (permanent cessation of existence of the integrated biological organism, human being). Only an account combining these two different concepts of human death, personal and biological, will satisfy most people in contemporary cultures. If biological death alone is considered this leaves open the (science fictional) possibility of a conscious human brain shorn of its body and much of its brainstem except the reticular activating system, but nonetheless having the capacity for conscious and self-conscious experiences, and thus of continued existence as a (sort of) human person. People would want, on obvious moral grounds, not to count any such living brain as dead, and to give it the moral respect due to human persons (even if in such a context that respect amounted to sedating or killing the brain-only person—though one could also imagine, again counterfactually, communication with such a brain-only person through electrical sensory and motor links, and a possible desire to continue to live and perhaps contribute to brain research—and speculate about the ensuing bioethical battle about whether respect for such views would be ethically acceptable!).

On the other hand most people would also be unhappy with a working account of human death that was concerned only with death of a human person and which did not incorporate biological death, death of a human being as an integrated biological organism. This is because such an account would entail that humans who were permanently unconscious, and thus dead as persons, would be classed as dead even if they remained alive as integrated biological human organisms. Thus patients in permanent coma and those in persistent vegetative state would, under such a definition, be dead even though they remain biologically alive as functioning human organisms. The contemporary brain death definition of death defended by Lamb accommodates both of these social concerns, by stating in effect that for a human being to be dead he or she must be dead both as a person and as an integrated biological organism.

PHILOSOPHICAL OPPOSITION TO BRAINSTEM DEATH—AND AN EDITORIAL RIPOSTE

Evans, also a philosopher, rejects this definition, on the grounds, essentially, that people tend not to be happy with the idea that a human being on a ventilator who is pink and warm, and whose heart is beating, *could* be dead. Implicitly—though not quite explicitly—having a beating heart (and being pink and warm?) are part of the everyday *concept* of being alive; and conversely cessation of heart beat (and of warmth and pinkness?) are part of the everyday *concept* of death. This, he argues, is simply part of what people mean by these words, and it is not for scientists to tell ordinary people that they are wrong about what their ordinary words *mean*.

There is much to disagree with in Evans's paper, but suffice it here to argue against this main theme, first by denying that 'people' in general do have these views—rather I believe they quite properly *associate* prolonged absence of heartbeat, coldness and lack of pinkness in normally pink tissues, with death— for it is a fact that normally these are signs of death; they just do not happen to be signs of death in certain circumstances of medical intervention. Conversely there is no evidence that people in general believe that if a person's heart is pumping, and if he or she is warm and pink, then the person *must* be alive; again this is normally the case, and it is a good working rule in non-medical contexts to assume that it is the case; but in certain medical contexts it is not the case. Secondly I argue that people who do hold such views are simply mistaken, as the implications of such mistaken views make clear to most of us. Thirdly I argue that views avowedly dependent *merely* on strong feelings, emotional responses, 'convictions', or intuitions, and unsupported by reasoning, are inadequate for moral argument. Fourthly I argue that these particular views would, if widely accepted, be very harmful, indeed life-threatening, to many people. We thus need very good reason indeed to accept them, and in the absence of very good reasons we should reject them as unjustifiably harmful.

Readers will check my interpretation, but in summary Evans claims that people feel very strongly that if a human being has a beating heart he or she must be alive; and because such feelings—part of 'the way we react to and describe what we see'—are 'determined by values rooted in our cultural and moral traditions'; and because such values 'stand beyond theoretical explanation', therefore scientific explanations that we are *wrong* in certain such cases to rely on our strong feelings are unacceptable; 'the question of the *human meaning* of the beating heart is not of course a scientific question'.

It is always dangerous to make generalizations about what 'people' believe. Suffice it to say that I know of only very few people who hold the conceptual views ascribed by Evans to ordinary people; I have been unable to find support for his conceptual claims in any dictionaries I have consulted (dictionaries do not settle philosophical disputes—but they do give good indications of what people may actually mean by the words they use); and if the views that Evans alleges to be rooted in our cultural and moral tradition were widely held, I would have expected widespread public disquiet with now well-established laws which accept medical accounts of brain death and by implication reject the claims made by Evans.

People who accept Evans's *conceptual* view of the role of heartbeat in their concepts of life and death would seem to be committed to the claim that a person *could not* be alive who has an absent heartbeat nor be dead with a beating heart; for a beating heart, he seems to claim, is a *necessary* component of our concept of being alive (hence the horror at burying a body with a beating heart, for we should only bury the dead, and a body with a beating heart must be alive and therefore not dead); and a non-beating heart is a *necessary* component of our concept of death (hence our horror at calling dead anyone whose heart is still beating).

While in most ordinary circumstances people are quite right to believe that if a person's heart is beating the person is alive, and conversely that if a person's heart has stopped for any substantial time that person must be dead, they would be simply mistaken if they insisted on extrapolating this belief to the special context of resuscitative medical intervention. Perhaps the most obvious example of the fact that cessation of a beating heart is *not necessary* for, nor necessarily evidence of, human death (and therefore not part of the meaning or concept of human death) are two items of surgical fact. The first is that the heart is deliberately stopped for certain surgical operations on the heart: a cooled 'poison fluid' based on potassium is injected into the heart after the aorta has been clamped off so that it gets pumped into the coronary blood vessels and stops the heart, which can then be operated on. Alternatively the heart can be stopped from pumping by giving it an electric shock using a 'fibrillator'. Both techniques are used to try to *prevent* the patient from dying by stopping the heart in order that it can be repaired, while maintaining oxygenation of the brain using a mechanical system that oxygenates and circulates the blood. For certain sorts of operation on the brain itself, where arterial pulsation in the brain would endanger the patient's life during the operation, the heart is either very considerably slowed or on occasion totally stopped by cooling the blood from the normal 37 degrees centigrade down to about 15–18 degrees (information obtained in personal communication with a cardiothoracic anaesthetist, Dr Angela Cullum).

Anyone who believed that a person whose heart has stopped *must* be dead would be committed to believing that the medical profession is wrong to say that the heart is stopped in such operations in order to increase the chances of *saving* the patient's life; instead doctors should, according to such a view, say that they kill the patient in order to do the operation, and then bring the patient back to life, after the operation on the corpse is over. Presumably under such an account doctors should also be charged with murder if they fail to 'bring the patient back to life' in such operations, having deliberately killed the patient. I think most people would accept that such examples show that it is simply a mistake to believe that if the heart has stopped beating the patient must be dead, by virtue of that fact and the meaning of the word 'dead'.

What about the converse alleged 'common-sense' view, that if the heart is beating the patient the person must be alive? This is the view that Evans is most concerned to promote, and he offers some pen pictures that are supposed to convince us. They are all based on human bodies to be buried; body one really is dead even by Evans's account but is dumped in a lime pit—and he points out that we feel disgusted when we see such behaviour. Body two is similar but found to have a beating heart and pink warm flesh. Body three is similar to body two but is also found to be breathing, despite a massive head injury. Very few people, even doctors, would be prepared to declare body three as dead: yet if they would be prepared to accept body two as dead this is irrational, says Evans, for why should breathing be any more important than heart beat? Now according to his own arguments irrationality should be irrelevant, since it is feelings that are determinative.

However, as he points out, for opponents of such arguments good reasons are crucial—and there are perfectly good reasons for distinguishing between the two cases. Body two is dead by the double criterion defended by Lamb and most contemporary doctors and western laws: notably it is dead as a person *and* dead as an integrated biological human organism. Body three is only dead as a person—but it continues to be alive as an integrated biological human organism. Given the requirement of a working concept of human death that combines both personal and biological death, thus acknowledging widespread societal rejection of the notion that death of a person is sufficient for death of a human being, body three is not dead because the biological integration functions of the brainstem persist, as demonstrated by spontaneous respiration. Body two is dead both as a person and as a biological organism (assuming brainstem death); even though the heart of body two is still beating this is not evidence of brainstem life and thus of the biological integration necessary for continuation of a biological human life (and by implication Evans's body two has been diagnosed as brainstem dead).

As for the repugnance that Evans continues to feel, it is a perfectly reasonable repugnance if it is treated as the appropriate response in cases such as he so vividly imagines; for in most such cases there would be good reason to suspect that bodies whose hearts are beating, let alone bodies whose hearts are beating and whose lungs are breathing, are live humans. But in the real context of medical resuscitation, and given the reasons for accepting the concept of brain death outlined above, the repugnance in the case of body two is, however understandable as a human reaction, nonetheless inappropriate if it leads people to regard the body as *necessarily* not dead but alive. As argued, such a reaction does not stand up to reason, for body two is dead, is indeed a beating heart cadaver. While it would be pointlessly and cruelly shocking to *bury* such cadavers before their hearts stopped, the understandable shock and repugnance at such an idea is simply irrelevant to the question of whether or not death has occurred, and utterly inadequate as a justification for preventing totally different and potentially beneficial actions such as transplantation of organs from such bodies.

Such an outcome cannot be justified by reason, and because it would lead to harm to others without good reason, it would be *wrong*. Emotions, convictions and intuitions, especially those perceived as moral, are very important indicators of areas of potential moral importance. But if those emotions, convictions or intuitions lead to harm to others then they should only be accepted as valid action guides if supported by sufficiently strong reasons to *justify* the harm caused by doing so. Some people feel deeply convinced intuitive and emotional repugnance when they see people who are very ugly, or mutilated, or simply who have a different skin colour from themselves; some might even attempt to dignify such repugnance by calling it moral repugnance. But unless good reasons can be adduced to show that such repugnance is morally justified—and they cannot be—reasonable people *ought* to teach themselves to cease feeling such emotions if they can, and if they cannot they can and ought to avoid encouraging such emotions in others; and at the very least they should not allow such emotions to lead them to actions which actually impair the lives of others. Undermining the concept of brain death on the basis of negative emotional reactions that have no reasoned justifications actually endangers the lives of others—notably by discouraging social acceptance of organ transplantation from beating-heart cadavers. Readers will ask themselves if Evans's arguments provide any reason, any *justification*, for accepting such potentially harmful consequences.

THE USE OF ANIMALS IN MEDICAL RESEARCH

The final pair of chapters offer arguments for and against the use of animals in medical research. Although Sprigge opposes all harmful use of animals, including for food, his main concern in his chapter is to argue in support of his 'urge that people of good will should support policy by which all painful experimentation will be banned from some given date in the future'—he later suggests within 10 years. He also urges the legal abolition of use of or research on animals 'whose living conditions do not give them a reasonable environment for the performance of their normal behavioural patterns'. Mammalian research animals are, argues Sprigge, 'fellow conscious subjects' and 'individual subjects of experience'—they should be respected as such, rather than treated 'as mere objects with whom any kind of empathy is mere sentimentality'. Basing his moral claims on a utilitarian premise, Sprigge acknowledges that calculations of overall welfare are notoriously difficult; nonetheless he is clear that 'readiness to treat animals as mere objects at the complete disposal of human beings goes with a general attitude to other life forms which is deeply damaging to the human condition'; and that people cannot be happy in the knowledge that their health depends on 'massive suffering to other creatures' unless they have developed 'a generally callous attitude to other living creatures the prevalence of which would certainly be detrimental to the welfare of sentient life on this planet as a whole'.

Frey argues for a position that supports animal experimentation and which he describes as intermediate between the two opposite extremes of totally rejecting animal experimentation on the one hand and, on the other, justifying animal research in any circumstances where human advantage, no matter how minimal, can be claimed. Like Sprigge he argues as a utilitarian, but for a different substantive position, much more sympathetic to animal research. However, he too condemns a careless or dismissive approach to animals— animals 'are members of the moral community' and what we do to them is thus of moral concern. Moreover in his view pain is 'as much an evil for an animal as for a human, and I agree with animal liberationists that it is a form of speciesism or discrimination to pretend otherwise'. Nonetheless, he argues, in the majority of cases the richness of human life gives it a greater value than that of animal life, and it is this difference that can justify certain sorts of experimentation on animals. However, like Singer before him, he argues that this view provides no general argument always to prefer to use animals rather than humans as research subjects. In principle, at least, it would be morally better to use as research subjects certain greatly impaired human lives than to kill healthy normal non-human mammals. However, such a practice would currently, he acknowledges, produce sufficient adverse side-effects to make him refrain from advocating it!

The thrust of both authors' contributions is to urge that, whether one sees animals as moral equals or as having a lower moral status than humans (or most humans, for neither author accords all humans higher moral status than all other animals) they must be accorded considerable moral weight. Thus *any* use of animals that causes them to suffer must be justified by proportionate likely benefit to humans; and Sprigge leaves us with a challenging argument for a social policy that aims to abolish, within a specified time span, preferably 10 years, *all* experiments on animals that cause them suffering.

82

Genetic Counselling

MARY J. SELLER, PhD, DSc

Reader in Developmental Genetics, The United Medical and Dental Schools of Guy's and St Thomas' Hospitals, London, UK

Genetics is concerned with heredity and variation. From time immemorial, people have realized that certain characteristics vary between individuals, and that some of these traits tend to run in families. Such characters include both normal variation, for example 'red' hair rather than brown or black; and abnormal variation, which may produce illness: for example, a defect of the normal blood clotting mechanism resulting in a bleeding disorder, haemophilia. Until well into this century the application of genetics to medicine was largely restricted to its being this type of observational science; but recently there has been an enormous expansion in understanding: the nature of the hereditary material itself is known down to the molecular level, and with advances in parallel fields such as biochemistry, cytogenetics and obstetrics, powerful tools are now available for the diagnosis, and the analysis and elucidation, of genetic disease. An accurate estimate of the total number of diseases with a genetic component is not possible, but the burden on both individual and society is great; they account for around one-third of childhood admissions to hospital [1]. A common feature of genetic disorders is that they are often severe, sometimes lethal, and even to this day most often incurable and even untreatable. With advances in the treatment of infectious diseases and other childhood complaints, and improved general health care, there has been a significant decline in perinatal mortality and morbidity; the exception is when genetic disease is involved. This means that genetic disease is apparently more important nowadays than hitherto.

Genetic counselling is the process which imparts to individuals at risk for a specific genetic disease, in themselves or their offspring, the often complex information about the disease, its inheritance, its implications, and the options open to them to deal with it in the absence of a cure. Communication and information-giving, including truth-telling, therefore, are essential elements of genetic counselling. The aim of genetic counselling is to provide those seeking advice with all the facts and possibilities surrounding the genetic problem that affects them, so that they may comprehend and appraise their situation, and

Principles of Health Care Ethics. Edited by Raanan Gillon.
© 1994 John Wiley & Sons Ltd

make up their own minds as to their actions in the future—usually concerning whether or not they will procreate. Genetic counselling is therefore non-directive, and as such is relatively unusual in medicine, which is most often directive.

The most common situation causing people to seek genetic counselling is when a couple have either had a child with a genetic disease, or they themselves, or another family member, are affected, and they want to know what their risks are of having a future affected child. When such a couple presents, it is fundamental that there is an accurate diagnosis of the particular genetic disorder which concerns them, and that a correct family tree is constructed for them. A precise diagnosis may appear obvious, but some genetic diseases have similar symptoms but different inheritance patterns, and there are some environmentally induced disorders which mimic genetic disease and thus are not inherited at all. So precision is needed—the starting point for genetic counselling must be the correct information on the disease, then accurate risk figures on future occurrence and recurrence of it can be given.

Whilst it is relatively easy to explain how inheritance contributes to a particular disease, some people have difficulty in grasping the idea of risk, and ways must be found to ensure that this is understood. Also, notions of 'risk' vary amongst people: to some a 10% risk is low, while to others a 4% risk is high, and it has been known for individuals to consider a 1% risk high. The counsellor usually puts the risk figure in the perspective of the fact that around 3% of all newborn babies have a disorder of some sort. All aspects of the disease in question are gone into: its symptoms and extent, the likely course it will take, palliative measures that can be offered and support available. In addition, all options regarding a future pregnancy are offered, such as possibilities for prenatal diagnosis, and termination of pregnancy should a fetus be found to be affected, or the continuation of the pregnancy with this knowledge. Other alternatives are artificial insemination by donor or *in vitro* fertilization with a donor ovum, or no pregnancy at all, whereupon contraceptive measures need to be discussed, and possibilities for adoption. All these options are complex, and involve moral, as well as medical, issues, the resolution of which can be undertaken only by the individuals actually involved, as only they know their own cultural and moral framework, religious beliefs, economic and social background which will influence their decision. Also only they know how they perceive the seriousness of the disease and the extent of the risk, which may be affected by personal factors such as whether they have a close experience of someone with the disease. This is why the counsellor is completely unable to decide what is right for a particular patient, and why genetic counselling seeks first and foremost to promote patient autonomy. Patients will often ask the counsellor to make their decision: 'what would you do if you were me?'—they are often understandably overwhelmed by the complexities of what they have heard, and also may believe they are unable to make the decision. Often, too, they may wish to avoid making such a responsible and often far-reaching decision about their future. But the counsellor is patently not that patient, and should not oblige; there is no correct objective answer, only a subjective one. Instead, the counsellor should try to make the information given even clearer, to facilitate their decision. This obviously consumes time, and it can be difficult. Despite all efforts it must be noted that no-one can always be totally impartial, for very subtly and quite unintentionally some things may be emphasized more than others. Also, there are often different ways of saying the same thing. For example, it can be stated 'your risk in a future pregnancy is one chance in ten of having an abnormal baby'; or it can be said 'your risk in a future pregnancy is nine chances out of ten of having a normal baby'. Both give the same piece of genetic advice, but the former mentions abnormality while the latter does not: it is only implied, and the statements can be seen to carry different moral weight.

Once a decision has been made by the patient, the final role for the counsellor is to support the family in whatever course they have chosen, to help them live through it and come to terms with it; and, if necessary, enlist ancillary help. Support may be needed at other stages of the counselling process too, for talking about an affected child who has died may bring to light unresolved grief, and the discovery that one carries 'harmful' genes which one has passed on, though unwittingly, to one's child can cause intense feelings of guilt even though that person is in no way responsible or at fault. Affirmation is needed at all times. Thus, genetic counselling is more than simply diagnosis and information-giving: great sensitivity and empathy are needed, and it involves support which may be wide-ranging.

The role of the genetic counsellor as presented so far would appear to be relatively clear-cut and straightforward, so long as its non-directiveness and respect for the patient's autonomy are borne in mind. But moral dilemmas do, in fact, not infrequently occur, because genetics and its implications are often not always straightforward. One area is whether all the genetic information obtained concerning a patient is divulged to him/her. An instance of this has long been a dilemma in prenatal diagnosis in older women who are at risk for a child with Down's syndrome, and for whom the karyotype of the fetus is examined to see if an extra chromosome 21 is present. Every so often, chromosome abnormalities other than Down's syndrome are found, some of which, particularly those involving extra sex chromosomes, have relatively minor effects on individuals. Should the parents be told of these findings, or only that Down's syndrome is not present, which is the truth?

At this juncture, consideration will be given to the part played by the four *prima facie* moral principles of biomedical ethics—autonomy, beneficence, non-maleficence and justice in moral discourse. In genetic counselling the principle of respect for autonomy is overwhelming and supreme; it is central to its practice. Encompassed within this is truth-telling, which is of cardinal importance. In many ways genetic counselling is the art of not being prescriptive; it is also the art of being impartial. A consequence of this is that, in one sense, it is difficult to apply the other three principles because, in order to do so, one has to act partially. For, to secure beneficence, one is to act positively on the patient's behalf; for non-maleficence, one must specifically minimize the harm; for justice, one should distribute the benefits and risks fairly. To act preferentially in favour of the patient one is dealing with is the antithesis of genetic counselling. In the sphere of the genetic constitution, and its determinant for health and disease, the only person who can ensure the greater good of a patient and minimize any harm is the patient him/herself. For example, a couple whose second child has

Tay–Sachs disease seek genetic counselling because they want to embark on another pregnancy. The child is extremely sick and handicapped and needs continuous day and night care; their first child is normal and is an active 4-year-old. The genetic counsellor seeing an exhausted couple before him might think that, with a 25% risk of recurrence, then under the principle of beneficence their greater good might be secured by avoiding another pregnancy for the moment, and under the principle of non-maleficence, harm would be minimized if contraceptive advice were given, for to have another child, whether normal or abnormal, might be more than they could cope with at this time. But the principle of autonomy overrides everything else. The genetic counsellor cannot know all the personal factors which contribute to the couple wanting another pregnancy now: they alone know what is for their own good. The genetic counsellor thus has a responsibility to them to provide them with the genetic information, so that they can act autonomously; not to decide what is for their greater good and what might minimize harm to them.

It is in some senses easier to understand genetic counselling more in terms of this responsibility. In the sphere of reproduction, in western society people are considered to have an inviolable right not to be prevented from having children. In those people where genetic disease is a factor, genetic counselling aims to enable people to make an informed and free decision as to whether to exercise that right or, instead, to exercise the right not to procreate. In this respect, in terms of morality, the genetic counsellor has obligations and duties to ensure that people can exercise these rights. Indeed, genetic counsellors have a responsibility to do so; their responsibility lies in an obligation to give clear, comprehensive, pertinent and impartial information. It is their duty, wrought by their professional capacity, in response to the needs of a patient.

This perspective fits well with the findings of Fletcher (1989) (2), who made an analysis of the moral reasoning of genetic counsellors in terms of their work, and found that they did not apply the four basic ethical principles. He believes this is because the principles are too abstract and general. Instead, he devised a more applicable system, which he called 'the ethics of relationships' to compensate for these deficiencies. This takes into account the experiential nature of genetic counselling in which there is reciprocity between the counsellor and patient. The patient has needs and the counsellor has a responsibility to fulfil these needs; also the patient has rights and the counsellor an obligation to ensure that the patient can exercise those rights.

That is not to say that the four principles are not applied to some extent in genetic counselling; they are, and they may carry some weight, but often other moral imperatives seem to supervene. This may be seen in dilemmas about disclosure of genetic information to a patient. In the case already mentioned, of prenatal diagnosis for Down's syndrome in the older mother, when an abnormal karyotype is discovered, but the fetus does not have Down's syndrome, this extra information is usually given to the mother. This is because it is considered that truth-telling is important, and also so that she can have autonomy to act on this knowledge if she wishes. But it is certainly true that it is also disclosed to her because it is considered to be for her greater good to know everything, and also because it is thought that any harm will be minimized: for instance, the hurt she may feel should the abnormality be inadvertently revealed as the child grows up. It is difficult to say which principle really takes precedence: they all play a part in the decision-making process.

There are perhaps only a few instances where these principles play a more major role. One such is the case of androgen insensitivity, a rare condition where, due to lack of end-organ sensitivity to androgens, a genetic male, with internal testes, is phenotypically a normal female. The diagnosis is often only made in the teens when the patient presents with primary amenorrhoea. For a person brought up as a female, and regarded by both herself and society fully so, and possibly even already married, the news that in fact, genetically, she is a male may be psychologically harmful to her, and it is for her greater well-being that truth-telling may be partially or totally suspended. Usually, however, it is considered she is best served by disclosing some of the facts: for instance, that a medical reason for her infertility has been discovered and that it is not treatable. This is, however, not a cardinal rule: in some cases it may judged that it is for her greater good that the entire truth is told. Thus beneficence is an important guiding principle.

With the now widespread application of molecular genetics to diagnosis, a genetic counselling problem which has always been known to exist, but was rarely provable, is now often made obvious and definite. This is non-paternity. Analysis of the DNA itself means that the genetic counsellor will often know almost certainly that the putative father is not the real father. Here again, beneficence and non-maleficence carry the day as to whether, and to what extent, this information is divulged, for the information could ruin the marriage. If it is of no consequence to diagnosis, then it will not even be mentioned, but it may well make prenatal diagnosis in a fetus impossible. To minimize the harm it seems prudent to advise the couple that a diagnosis has not been possible because the tests have been uninformative in their case, which is the truth. For genetic counselling for a future pregnancy beneficence dictates that the mother should be seen alone on a separate occasion and the actual situation explained to her, and she can decide to what extent it will be divulged further afield—her autonomy has therefore been preserved.

Thus it would seem that, when the dilemma involves the disclosure of very sensitive information, the principles of beneficence and non-maleficence are decisive. In the two examples given, the genetic counsellor has made an exceptional decision to withhold information. The more general rule is that patients should have access to all information about themselves. But there are situations where patients themselves do not wish to know, and autonomy directs that this too must be respected. This applies especially to severe, non-treatable dominant disorders of late onset. The most common of these—Huntington's chorea—is a severely debilitating and progressive dementia with uncontrollable movements of the body which has an inexorable course, the symptoms of which first appear in the fourth decade. Probable carriers of this disease can often now be identified. Some individuals from at-risk families wish to know whether they carry the gene; others do not—such knowledge has on occasion driven people to suicide. In this situation, not giving patients information because it is their choice preserves their autonomy as much as giving complete information, and it avoids possible harm in the form of depression and suicide. In the rare instance of a patient not wanting to know about a severe disease which is treatable, then both beneficence and non-maleficence impel the genetic counsellor to spend time in trying to show the patient how the information would be beneficial.

Confidentiality is one of the cardinal rules of the practice of medicine. This has often presented problems in genetic counselling, especially when a dominant disorder is involved. Once a firm diagnosis has been made in the consulting patient, and the family tree has been constructed, it becomes obvious that certain other family members may be at risk for the disease. But to approach them would mean divulging confidential information about that individual, and should not be done without his/her consent. The patient may be unwilling to give this, as he may feel he will lose the esteem of other family members if they know of his condition. In some cases their lives might be at risk, and could even be saved if they could be approached and examined. There can be no single rule directing the resolution of such dilemmas, especially in the case of autosomal dominant conditions of late onset. Confidentiality ensures the autonomy of the patient, and this is respected because of beneficence and non-maleficence. Any reluctance on the patient's part to disclose the condition to relatives who are at risk of having the gene for the condition too, can be acceded to in diseases such as Huntington's chorea which, at present, are untreatable. For no benefit is achieved for the relatives, and harm might be done to not only the individual, in revealing the condition, but also to relatives, in hearing that they may be at risk for a serious, untreatable disorder of which they were blissfully unaware. But when the condition is treatable, a different case is sometimes made. An example is polyposis coli. If this disease is diagnosed at an early stage, which is usually pre-symptomatic, appropriate operative treatment can be instituted, then subsequent preventive care, so that the lethal cancerous phase of the disease is avoided. The benefits to relatives are so great that there are some who would submit that a case can be made for the autonomy and beneficence of the original patient to be superseded by the principles of beneficence and non-maleficence to the relatives. The justification for breaking the confidentiality rule is that it will allow serious harm to be prevented in one or more other people. Those who adhere to this point of view also couch the justification in terms of a genetic counsellor's duty, a duty to the relatives. For the patient has opted out of his/her own duty to tell relatives, and the counsellor alone now carries this possibly life-saving information. The counsellor's duty which exists to the patient in terms of confidentiality has been over-ridden by the duty to save the lives of others. The reason it has been over-ridden is because of consideration of beneficence and non-maleficence. However, this is probably a minority view; usually autonomy and confidentiality are respected, but in this difficult situation pressure would be applied to divulge the relevant information with permission.

The advent of molecular genetics, and the possibilities this has given for the genetic testing of individuals for all manner of genetic diseases hitherto resistant to diagnosis, has focused problems of confidentiality most acutely. For such testing can often only be undertaken if most family members contribute a sample of tissue, for the method necessitates comparison of patterns of the DNA between the individuals in several generations, and then interpretation, to determine whether a particular person is a carrier of that disease, during which, of course, not only must all family members be approached, but also information about all family members tested comes to light. Since it appears that, increasingly, genetic studies on an individual will require the testing of entire families, for the greater good of all, it would seem wise to warn people of this fact before the studies are begun. This will of course not avoid the occasional situation of a person demanding complete privacy of information, but it should pave the way for a more open attitude.

There are other instances when a third party might want confidential information about a patient. This relates not only to those diseases already mentioned, inherited in an autosomal dominant manner and which can be detected in a pre-symptomatic stage, but also to carrier detection of autosomal recessive conditions such as cystic fibrosis, where carriers are themselves unaffected but can have affected children if their partner is also a carrier. With molecular genetics an increasing number of diseases are becoming testable, and additionally, another dimension is on the horizon: genetic markers will soon become available for some of the diseases of adulthood with a more diffuse genetic component, such as cardiovascular disease and diabetes mellitus, so that 'susceptible' individuals may be identified in childhood or even *in utero*. This has medical advantages because the various environmental components which also contribute to the development of the disease can be avoided at an early stage of life, and so prevention may be possible. But such genetic information would be of inestimable use to insurance companies and future employers. Here it seems clear that the genetic counsellor has no obligation at all to the third party comprising corporate interests; there is no duty to protect such bodies from harm. To divulge genetic information about a person would do him harm, in terms of perhaps being refused a job for which he was qualified and the inability to get adequate insurance protection. There is, however, one exception, and that is if there was the threat to the safety of other people by a person with a specific genetic condition having a particular job—for example, as a pilot or train driver. But this is an already accepted example in medicine where confidentiality may be breached, and there is no case for genetics being an exception to this.

A dilemma which arises more indirectly out of genetic counselling is whether the abortion of a genetically abnormal fetus is justified. Of course, for some people it is not a dilemma because they consider abortion totally wrong and never justified. When prenatal tests indicate that a woman is carrying a fetus with a genetic abnormality, there are two main objects of concern: the mother and the fetus. If the mother chooses to continue with the pregnancy (and most genetic counsellors believe that it is within their remit to ensure that it is possible for her to do this) then she has preserved her autonomy. This is a decision which she believes is best for her and for her fetus, even though they may well both later suffer in different ways from the effects of the genetic disorder. If she selects the option to abort, then clearly this is harmful to the fetus, and she herself may suffer both discomfort and psychological trauma, but she believes it is in her long-term interest, and that it is better for the fetus never to be born alive and face the possibly intense suffering which may be wrought by the genetic disease.

Thus, autonomy, non-maleficence and beneficence contribute significantly to the decision-making process. But the fact that there is a decision to be made, that abortion is allowed for cases of genetic disease, is dependent on something else and that is the moral status of the fetus. The fetus is considered to have less moral significance than the mother. Basically it is the immaturity of the fetus which renders it so. The mother as an adult has responsibilities and ties, including probably being a wife, and possibly a mother to other existing children. The fetus has none of these things, and also 'officially' does not even yet exist, so it has less moral weight than the mother. Whilst its claim to life is respected, this claim, or right, to life may have to be surrendered if there are strong reasons which compel such an action. In the case of genetic disease this is often stated to be that the mother's right to life supersedes that of the fetus— her life being defined in its fullest sense as a wife and mother, and encompassing the life of the family, which might be jeopardized by having to care for a severely handicapped child, and later, if he survives, adult. This consideration seems to weigh the equation more than the quality of life which the fetus would have when born. For severely handicapping disorders such as spina bifida this is often nominally mentioned—that children may suffer intensely with many operations, possibly being confined to a wheelchair and perhaps doubly incontinent. But children with Down's syndrome seem not to 'suffer' in life, and indeed are regarded by many as 'happy children'. Yet most fetuses diagnosed with Down's syndrome are aborted, just as spina bifida ones are.

Those who oppose abortion for genetic disease (or any other reason) consider that the fetus has the same moral status as its mother, and the principle of non-maleficence with respect to the life of the fetus, and justice to the fetus, are the prime considerations: the mother is not a factor. It is believed that it is a matter of injustice, that simply because a fetus has been diagnosed as having a genetic disease, it is condemned as unworthy of life, and not given the same chance of either life or medical treatment and care as others not so diagnosed.

Within the context of abortion, further dilemmas may arise in specific circumstances, such as in the case of twins, where one is abnormal but the other is normal. As usual, autonomy should operate: it is important for the mother to make the decision herself as to whether to sacrifice the life of a normal fetus in order not to have an abnormal one. Individuals will make different decisions, and often this is governed by extraneous factors, such as particular family circumstances or experience of the disease in question, rather than on grounds of beneficence and non-maleficence. With advances in the field, however, this particular dilemma is receding, because selective termination of the affected twin is now often possible.

Every so often a genetic counsellor is approached for prenatal diagnosis to find out the sex of the fetus with a view to termination of pregnancy if the fetus is not of the desired sex. Certain severe genetic diseases are sex-linked and occur only in one sex, usually males. In such cases this procedure is warranted, and termination of a particular sex is justifiable on medical grounds, just as in the case of other genetic diseases. But in a recent survey (2) it was found that a surprising (to some) number of genetic counsellors would refer patients to obstetricians for fetal sex diagnosis solely on grounds of parental whim. Such counsellors justify it as preserving patient autonomy and on grounds of beneficence, enabling the parents to organize their lives and families as they see fit, believing it is for their good to have children of the preferred sex. Others view it differently, believing that the matter of the sex of the fetus is not the concern of the geneticist. In the case of genetic disease, geneticists are intervening in the processes of life by doing prenatal diagnosis and condoning abortion when indicated, as an attempt to manage a grave genetic problem, in the absence of the availability of successful treatment of the condition. To be male or female is not a genetic defect; rather it is part of the normal condition of life and is therefore not something properly to be interfered with by geneticists. Further, many believe that children are 'given', rather than ordered according to specification, and if one accepts the responsibility of parenthood, one should accept the givenness of gender along with all the other characteristics of the child. Thus, none of the four principles is involved in this view. However, another approach does incorporate the principle of justice—and that is that sex selection is unjust to the undesired sex. It also implies a concept of sexual inequality, which is also unjust. Not to permit such sex selection could be construed as beneficence—to the good of the parent—in the following way: if a person believes he/she has a dislike of one sex, actually to have to bring up a child of that sex may lead that person to discover that the dislike is unfounded. But these considerations would seem to be secondary to the main argument.

The principle of justice has not figured largely in this discussion of the ethical principles governing the practice of genetic counselling. An individual suffering the effects of a severe genetic disease may be perceived as being the victim of a grave injustice. Injustice implies a source which can select one course or another, giving benefit to some and detriment to others. One's genetic make-up is not meted out in this way; equally, no individual has a choice concerning his/her genetic inheritance. We all carry several mutant genes, but most people go through life oblivious of the fact. In those people suffering genetic disease, a particular deleterious gene has identified itself, because the gene involved is vital to well-being.

The genetic counsellor may encounter injustice, however, in terms of the availability of medical services to help people with genetic disease, both in diagnosis and care. Genetic and other services are not necessarily universally or equally provided. For instance, the United Kingdom is divided geographically into separate health regions. There is provision for genetic services in each, but the fine details of the actual policy are determined locally. In some areas all women over the age of 35 years are tested for Down's syndrome, while in others the cut-off point may be 37, or even, 38 years. *In vitro* fertilization services are available in some regions but not others. There is patently injustice in the situation if a genetic counsellor decides a patient needs a particular service but finds it is not available because of where the patient lives. This form of injustice is something which society as a whole needs to rectify.

Justice does, however, play a part in the whole ethos of genetic counselling, in terms of the approach which a genetic counsellor makes to the patient, the aim of which is to meet the needs of the individual. Viewed more globally, however, the burden of genetic disease is not only on the individual, but also on society. For the costs of caring for people with genetic disease, many of whom are severely handicapped, are enormous. It would be in the interests of society if genetic disease could be eliminated, or at least reduced to the level which new spontaneous mutations produce. This, of course, conflicts with the interests of patients affected directly or indirectly with genetic disease who wish to have families. Justice to such people dictates that the genetic counsellor is primarily concerned with individual interests and their rights to reproduce if they so wish, and also with their right to bring into the world a child with a handicap if they so wish. In genetic counselling the needs of the individual take precedence over the needs of society, and this is determined by justice.

The attraction of the idea of having basic ethical principles to guide one's approach to moral problems is that in whatever situation one finds oneself, they will be helpful in the resolution of how one should act. In medicine these principles should apply both to normal practice, and to the more difficult dilemmas encountered within it. In genetic counselling, although the four principles are all implicit in the routine practice of genetic counselling, the preservation of patient autonomy is supreme. This is because of the nature of this branch of medicine which demands that impartial information is given. Another necessity for proper practice is truth-telling. However, when dilemmas occur, then the principles of beneficence and non-maleficence have increasing power and often determine a course of action. Considerations of justice are fairly subsidiary. Thus it would appear that in the moral reasoning surrounding genetic counselling, the four principles are not universal and general: they are more specifically applicable, and other criteria for moral reasoning are often employed.

REFERENCES

1. Weatherall, D. J. 1991. *The new genetics and clinical practice.* Oxford University Press, Oxford. See also Chapter 83, this volume.
2. Fletcher, J. C. 1989. Ethics and human genetics: a cross-cultural perspective. Pp. 457–490, *in* Wertz, D. C. and Fletcher, J. C. (Eds) *Ethics and human genetics.* Springer-Verlag, Berlin.

83

Human Genetic Manipulation

DAVID WEATHERALL

University of Oxford, Oxford, UK

Advances in the basic sciences, particularly molecular and cell biology, over the past 15 years will have important implications for clinical practice. In the short term the developments that will stem from this work should raise few fundamentally new ethical issues. However, because it is difficult to predict the long-term outcome of our increasing ability to manipulate human DNA it is important that research workers in this field establish and maintain a dialogue between practising clinicians and the public about what is, or might be in the future, acceptable in the name of medical progress and the advancement of knowledge of human biology (1).

In this short chapter I will try to anticipate what medical advances are likely to stem from the manipulation of human genetic material, and then discuss the ethical issues which have already been highlighted by work in this field and those that might be posed in the longer term.

THE SCOPE OF HUMAN MOLECULAR GENETICS

Before discussing the ethical issues which might arise from the manipulation of human DNA it is important to appreciate what is possible now and where this field might take us in the future.

What is Possible Now?

Human beings have between 50 000 and 100 000 genes which make up their genome. Until recently, inherited diseases could be studied only by tracing different defects through families and attempting to define their biochemical basis and hence making a guess at the function of the particular gene involved. The advent of recombinant DNA technology has changed all this (2). It is now possible to isolate individual genes and to pinpoint the precise defect that underlies a particular disease at the molecular level. Furthermore, now that the structure of our DNA has been characterized in more detail it is apparent that

Principles of Health Care Ethics. Edited by Raanan Gillon.
© 1994 John Wiley & Sons Ltd

there is a remarkable degree of individual variation. This has provided numerous markers so that it is now possible to trace and localize defective genes by linkage studies, isolate them, and, by a process called reverse genetics, to determine the nature of their products. The development of these new techniques has made it possible to provide extremely accurate diagnoses of carrier states for different genetic disorders and to identify genetic disease very early in fetal life or even in fertilized ova (2).

In the 1990 edition of McKusick's *Mendelian inheritance in man* (3) over 4000 diseases are listed which seem to result from the action of single gene defects. Although many of them are rare, overall they produce a major burden of illness on society; about one per cent of all newborn babies have some kind of genetic defect. Already the molecular pathology of many of the common inherited diseases has been worked out and they can be identified both in symptomless carriers and in fetal life.

The ability to isolate human genes has also made it possible to insert them into bacterial cells or other foreign environments where they can be expressed and produce large quantities of their products for therapeutic purposes or for generating diagnostic agents. The commercial exploitation of human recombinant DNA technology is still in its infancy, but there have already been enough successes to suggest that this new field may revolutionize medical treatment in the future.

Since it is possible to isolate and clone genes attempts are being made to replace defective genes as a form of therapy. It is also possible to insert human genes into the fertilized eggs of animals and to encourage them to be expressed in the progeny. Already this approach has been used for producing human therapeutic agents, in the milk of animals for example. It also has enormous potential for helping us to understand the function of human genes and how these may be defective in various diseases.

Thus it is already clear that recombinant DNA technology will revolutionize clinical genetics and the pharmaceutical industry. But as we shall see this is only the starting point of what may be a major revolution in clinical research and practice.

What May be Possible in the Future?

Single gene disorders are inherited according to simple Mendelian laws, and the environment is usually of little consequence in their clinical outcome. Other diseases are due directly to environmental factors such as malnutrition, infection, exposure to toxic chemicals, and so on. However, it is becoming increasingly clear that many of the common killers of western society—such as heart disease, stroke, major psychiatric disease, rheumatism, and others—result from complex interactions of environmental factors with our genetic constitution which render us either more or less likely to develop these conditions after a similar environmental exposure (2). The development of recombinant DNA technology should enable us to dissect the complex interactions between our environment and our genetic make-up which underlie these common diseases. In other words it seems very likely that in the future we will be able to define individuals as being particularly prone or resistant to noxious environmental agents. And as we start to understand the agents which cause these common diseases we may be able to prevent some of them much more effectively, by concentrating our public health activities on subsets of particularly susceptible individuals for example.

Another major area in which recombinant DNA technology should advance medical practice is in the understanding of the complex series of events that leads to cells losing their normal regulatory mechanisms and becoming cancerous. Indeed, it is already clear that the development of malignant transformation involves the acquisition of mutations in a number of key genes which are involved in the regulation of the growth and proliferation of different types of cells. It is also becoming apparent that some of these genetic changes may be inherited while others may result from environmental agents. Thus we are likely to understand the genesis of cancer very much better and, hopefully, how to prevent or treat it.

Recombinant DNA technology also has the potential for helping us to tackle broader biological questions including the causes of ageing, how we develop into a human being from a fertilized egg, and how we have reached our present place in the evolutionary tree. Furthermore there is already sufficient progress in the molecular neurosciences to suggest that we may start to make some progress in understanding the molecular and chemical basis of behaviour and other higher functions.

It is mainly because of these broader applications of recombinant DNA technology that there is so much current interest in what has been called the human genome project, that is in constructing a linkage map or, ultimately, in determining the complete sequence of the DNA that makes up all our chromosomes. It has been argued that once we know the position of most of our key genes we will be able to move much more quickly to define the major players in the common diseases of western society and in understanding many other complex issues including the control of behaviour and other important aspects of neurobiology. Work has already started on mapping the human genome in many countries, and it seems very likely that we will have a linkage map within the next 10 years.

It is against this brief background of what is or might be possible following the advent of recombinant DNA technology that we must examine the ethical issues which it may pose. Readers who wish to learn more about this complex and rapidly advancing field are referred to several recent reviews and monographs written for the non-specialist (1,2,4).

ETHICAL ISSUES ARISING FROM HUMAN RECOMBINANT DNA TECHNOLOGY

There is no doubt that our new-found ability to tinker with human genes is causing a considerable amount of public anxiety. This is not always helped by the media which, for obvious reasons, tend to exploit only the more sensational aspects of this extraordinary new field. However, the present applications of human genetic engineering do not pose many fundamentally new ethical issues, but rather they highlight those which have been with us for some time. In the following account I shall try to describe those which seem to be of genuine concern because they reflect what is actually possible at the present time. In a later section I will outline briefly some of the broader concerns which arise from human genetic manipulation, and suggest how we might best approach them from an ethical standpoint.

Genetic Screening and Counselling

The ethical issues arising during genetic counselling are described in the previous chapter. Here I shall simply outline those which seem to have been highlighted by our increasing ability to identify individuals at risk for genetic disease or those who are already affected.

Genetic counselling and prenatal diagnosis of disease has been possible for some time but until recently its scope was limited. The advent of DNA technology and the ability to identify single gene disorders is greatly expanding the number of diseases that can be avoided in this way. Hence there will be a major temptation to extend the scope of genetic screening. Already women of appropriate racial backgrounds are screened routinely for inherited blood disorders such as sickle cell anaemia and thalassaemia, and it seems very likely that screening for cystic fibrosis will become generally available within the near future; many other rare genetic diseases are already amenable to screening by DNA analysis. As we come to understand more about the major gene loci that are involved in susceptibility or resistance to common disorders such as coronary artery disease, the major psychoses, diabetes, hypertension, rheumatic disease, some forms of cancer, and so on, it may be possible to extend the process of screening to offer individuals an estimate of their risk of developing these diseases. This kind of advice will be of value only if it is possible to take steps to prevent these disorders occurring in those who are at a particularly high risk. Currently this type of screening is not possible, but rapid progress is being made in defining the genetic component of some of our common killers, and this is a problem that we will have to face over the next few years.

Currently, genetic screening follows two paths. Where a disease is very common in a particular society, thalassaemia or sickle cell disease in individuals of tropical origin or cystic fibrosis in north Europeans, it may be considered cost-effective to offer screening to entire populations. This may be done in the antenatal clinic or, occasionally, as part of a population screening programme, concentrating on school-leavers or similar groups, for example. More commonly, however, screening is restricted to those families in which there is a history of a particular genetic disease and a couple want to know the risk of their children being affected.

Recombinant DNA technology has raised no fundamentally new ethical issues for screening but has simply widened its scope. Some well-defined principles must be applied (5–7). First, of course, screening must be carried out only with the permission of the family or population involved. Second, professional counselling must be available to explain why the screening is being carried out, and to provide information about the results of the screening tests.

The importance of educating a community about genetic disease is emphasized by experiences of screening programmes for sickle cell anaemia or thalassaemia in the UK and in the USA (2). For example, there is a major difference between Cypriot and Asian immigrant populations with respect to their response to screening and prenatal diagnosis for thalassaemia in the United Kingdom. The London Cypriot population have taken up the programme with great enthusiasm and it has been extremely successful, whereas the same does not apply to the Asian populations in the UK. The reasons are complex, and religious and ethnic factors undoubtedly have played a role. However, the major difference is the limited extent to which the Asian communities in the UK have been educated in preparation for screening and prenatal diagnosis of thalassaemia. The disastrous results with their associated racial overtones of screening for sickle cell disease in the US, where a large programme was set up without adequate facilities for counselling or explanation, should act as a constant reminder of the potential dangers of introducing this type of activity into an ill-prepared society. Ethnic minority groups are particularly sensitive. The success of the introduction of prenatal diagnosis of thalassaemia in the London Cypriot population is largely the result of the major effort that was put into educating the community by an enthusiastic clinician and her colleagues (2).

It goes without saying that any screening programme should ensure complete confidentiality about the results (6). There is considerable current concern about who should be provided with information about an individual's genetic make-up. For example, in the United States doubts have been expressed about whether it is correct for information of this type to be given to agencies such as insurance companies or employers. This is a very difficult question which needs urgent debate by society. After all, we already provide information about our height and weight, blood pressure, exposure to AIDS, and so on. It is difficult to understand why if, in a few years' time we are able to predict with some accuracy whether somebody is highly likely to have a heart attack in early middle age, this information should be kept from an insurance company. Similarly, if our genetic make-up makes us particularly prone to accidents at work this information should be made available. But how far should we go? Obviously there are situations in which genetic information must be provided to potential employers; a colour-blind individual should not drive a high-speed train, and a person with a genetic susceptibility to particular toxins should not have an occupation which involves exposure to these agents. But the more subtle question of whether somebody with a 20 per cent increased likelihood of developing maturity-onset diabetes should have to tell a future employer or insurance company is much more difficult.

Because DNA analysis has the potential to provide so much information it poses ethical problems about what types of genetic disability should be considered as candidates for screening and prenatal diagnosis with termination of pregnancy. What is a serious genetic disability? Here I believe that much depends on the perception of the particular society in which a family live. It is difficult not to respect the wishes of parents who feel that it is wrong to bring a child into the world with a crippling genetic disease, perhaps associated with serious mental retardation or the necessity for life-long painful treatment. But what about milder genetic disorders? For example, it is current practice in China to offer prenatal diagnosis for a mild form of thalassaemia which is compatible with a normal lifespan. However, the argument that is used is that if the state has decreed a one-child family policy the child has to be as perfect as possible. The ethical norms for a rural worker in China may be different from those of a family with a potential for a similarly affected child living in a western industrialized society.

The recombinant DNA era has also raised a number of new ethical problems in relationship to genetic screening and counselling (2). First, there is the question of the additional information which may be obtained as part of a genetic screening procedure. A particularly important example is non-paternity. When carrying out prenatal diagnosis by DNA analysis, particularly if genetic linkage is used, it is absolutely vital to determine the biological parentage of a fetus. This can be done by DNA fingerprinting on the same fetal DNA sample that is being used for detecting a disease. What are we to do if we find that the 'father' is not a biological parent of the child? In screening DNA from the prenatal diagnosis programme for thalassaemia and other haemoglobin disorders which is run in Oxford for the whole of the UK we have found that this occurs in about 2 per cent of all cases referred to us. Since non-paternity of this type may lead to a mistaken prenatal diagnosis result it is important to tell mothers as part of the counselling procedure that these tests will be valid only if parents are the true biological parents of the child. If, as has occurred on several occasions, we find that the putative father is not the biological parent it has been our practice to say that we cannot give a result for technical reasons. We have not specifically told the mother the reasons why we are not able to provide a diagnosis. Curiously, on some occasions in which there has been a problem of this type the mother has offered this information. But the ethical dilemma still remains; should this information be disclosed in such cases, given its potential for catastrophic effects on a family or marriage. While it is this author's view that in most cases it should not, this approach is, in effect, breaking our general rule that all information found during genetic analysis should be disclosed.

A second ethical issue which has arisen from advances in DNA technology is the possibility of identifying diseases early in life which are not manifest clinically until much later (8). While the identification of disorders that require immediate treatment or possible termination of pregnancy raises no new ethical problems, the growing list of conditions that appear in middle age, such as adult polycystic disease of the kidneys, Huntington's disease, colon cancer due to familial polyposis coli, myotonic dystrophy, retinitis pigmentosa, and so on, together with the idea that we may be able to identify individuals at particular risk for common polygenic disorders, poses new ethical issues for those who look after children.

While there may be a very good case for identifying some of these conditions in childhood, decisions of this type will have to be made with extreme care and after long discussion with parents. In some cases there may be a good argument for trying to exclude a particular disease. For example, ruling out the possibility of adult polycystic kidney disease might prevent children having to be closely followed up with regular blood pressure estimations over many years. Similarly, if familial polyposis coli can be excluded, children of affected families will not require regular surveillance with colonoscopy in case they develop adenomas and subsequent cancer of the colon.

On the other hand, it may be much too difficult to make a decision about screening for Huntington's disease. This may necessitate other family members discovering that they will develop Huntington's disease when they get older. If patients who are at risk for this disease wish to know whether they have inherited the gene and are at risk of passing it on to their children it is difficult to deny them this information. Some at-risk individuals simply wish to know one way or the other for their own peace of mind, and the question of whether it is ethically justified to refuse to obtain this type of information for them will arise. Can they cope with this knowledge? How far should doctors withhold such information in a paternalistic effort to protect them from a life marred by the prospect that they will develop an unpleasant disease in middle life?

Counsellors who deal with these problems will have to act with particular sensitivity, often bridging the difficult decision of whether to go along with the parents' wishes, and yet on the other hand trying to protect the child from living with the information that he or she has the gene for a particularly distressing disease which will only affect that person later in life.

Genetic Manipulation to Cure Inherited Diseases—Gene Therapy

In considering the potential ethical problems that may arise from the application of genetic manipulation designed to control or cure a genetic disease it is very important to distinguish quite clearly between somatic and germ-line gene therapy (2). In somatic gene therapy the objective is to insert a gene into a cell line other than germ cells to correct a genetic disease. This may be achieved in a variety of ways, including the insertion of a gene directly or attached to a virus, or by trying to correct the genetic defect by using nature's way of exchanging genetic material, that is by site-directed recombination. But whatever technique is used in somatic gene therapy the idea is to correct a genetic defect in a particular tissue, bone marrow cells for example, for the lifespan of the affected individual. The change in genetic make-up would not, therefore, be passed on to future generations.

On the other hand, germ-line gene therapy follows quite a different principle. Here, the idea would be to insert a gene into fertilized ova so that it would be incorporated throughout the genome of the individual. The inserted gene would be expressed in the appropriate tissues to correct the genetic disease but would also be incorporated into the germ cells and hence be passed on to future generations. Hopefully, the disease would be eradicated in the progeny of the individual that was treated. The insertion of genes into fertilized ova and their expression in later generations has been carried out successfully on many occasions in mice and other animals; it is technically feasible to use this method in human beings.

While somatic gene therapy raises a number of practical problems similar to those encountered in any new form of medical treatment, it does not differ in any important way from any other form of organ transplantation. The inserted genes will, if the treatment has been successful, function during the lifetime of an individual to correct a genetic disease. Obviously there will be important issues regarding consent, the appropriate time to start this form of treatment, and others, but none of them are fundamentally new or differ in any way from decisions about organ transplantation. For the successful treatment of some genetic diseases it may be essential to transfer genes very early during development, and this will raise important issues regarding consent and the responsibility of parents, and similar questions. Otherwise there are no major new ethical problems that will arise from attempts at somatic gene therapy.

Germ-line therapy is fundamentally different from somatic gene therapy in that the inserted genes will undoubtedly be passed on to future generations and therefore we would be embarking on a completely new road. If we decided that we wished to develop this approach we would, in effect, be altering the genomes of our great grandchildren who would have had no possibility in taking part in the decision. Here we will undoubtedly be playing with the evolution of our species and taking decisions on behalf of future generations. For this reason germ-line gene therapy is not being contemplated, and in fact has been forbidden in many countries.

As well as these completely new ethical issues there are several reasons why it seems quite inappropriate to consider germ-line gene therapy at the present time. First, it is now possible to identify genetic diseases in fertilized human ova. Thus all we need to do to help parents who are at risk of producing children with a serious genetic disease is to obtain ova after *in vitro* fertilization, determine which of them carry the genetic defect, and then replace only those that do not. In this way a family can be assured of having normal children, and there is no need to tamper with the genetic make-up of future individuals.

Furthermore, there are a number of even more pragmatic reasons for not indulging in germ-line gene therapy. For example, we have no idea about the stability over successive generations of genes inserted into fertilized eggs, or about any potential long-term deleterious effects that they might have. Thus for the moment there seems no reason to consider this approach in humans. Whether there ever will must remain for future generations to decide, but currently the majority of human geneticists are convinced that experiments in human germ-line gene transfer should not be carried out.

Who Owns the Human Genome?

A few years ago a picture appeared in a leading scientific journal showing a businessman looking rather self-satisfied and carrying the caption 'my company owns chromosome 7'. Although it is self-evident that nobody 'owns' the human genome, or any part of it, there is increasing concern about the potential for commercial exploitation of human recombinant DNA technology. Attempts are being made to patent different sequences of human DNA which might be used for commercial gain, and there is the broader concern that as human genetics becomes increasingly attractive to commerce even more pressures will be put on individuals to undergo screening procedures.

The patent problems that are developing as the result of recombinant DNA technology are still ill-defined. It is to be hoped that common sense will prevail. It should be self-evident that no part of the human genome can be the sole property of anybody. Equally, there is little doubt that a particular method designed to isolate, analyse or express a particular DNA sequence can be patented; there is no reason for concern if companies wish to patent methods, but not individual sequences.

It will be important to monitor the exploitation of the human genome and to make sure that commercial pressures do not push human genetic manipulation into directions that are anyway foreign to the normal standards of medical practice, or that interfere with medical research or the dissemination of its results (2).

Crossing Genetic and Evolutionary Boundaries

Evolution can be depicted in the form of a tree with diverging branches, representing increasing diversity and the way in which species have developed by mutation and natural selection. It is a general rule that reproduction between different species is impossible in that it leads to infertility or fetal death. Although there may be some horizontal passage of genes, by retroviruses for example, nature's way seems to be the vertical transmission of genetic material with a major accent on continuous diversification of the species.

Our new-found ability to transfer genes between species by genetic engineering is posing the question of how far we are justified in changing evolution in this way. So far there has been no major concern about placing human genes into bacteria for the production of human protein products. Furthermore, a great deal is being learnt about normal and abnormal gene action by inserting human genes into mice by the transgenic route (2). But attempts are being made to generate human gene products by inserting genes into large animals by the same route; proteins that are secreted into milk for example. Where do we draw the line? For example, by suitable manipulation of oncogenes, or by inserting the genes for specific growth factors into transgenic animals, it is possible to create breeds of mice with high probability of producing cancer, or a clinical picture reminiscent of leukaemia. On the one hand such experiments may well be justified in helping us to understand human cancers. On the other, however, the commercial exploitation of mice that are guaranteed to develop cancer in a fixed time, complete with a lurid trade name, seems to reflect a lack of sensitivity on the part of the scientific community and industry.

Of course, animal and plant breeders have been doing this kind of thing for centuries. However, we need to monitor these activities with extreme care. If the insertion of genes from one species into another is being carried out for a specific purpose, with a view to learning more about how genes function in health and disease, and if the experiments are carefully designed with minimum discomfort to the recipient animal, there may be a genuine justification for carrying out work of this type. But there is certainly no reason to carry out this type of experiment just for curiosity to see 'what turns up'; on reviewing some of the current scientific literature in this field it is hard to believe that some of the reported experiments had a more rational basis. This is a highly sensitive area and one that must be monitored very carefully by both scientists and public.

Dysgenic Effects

It is often asked whether the widespread use of genetic screening, prenatal diagnosis and selective abortion will encourage reproduction in families with genetic disease and thus help to maintain or increase the frequency of these conditions in populations. This subject has been discussed in detail by a number of geneticists (2,9). Clearly it needs watching, but there is no evidence that a programme of avoidance of serious genetic disease will have a major effect on the size of the pool of our less attractive genes. We may, in the long term, provide more work for our genetic counselling clinics, but it is to be hoped that by the time these effects are mediated we will have learnt how to treat the more important genetic disorders.

Avoidance or Treatment

In recent years several respected geneticists and individuals with genetic diseases have written expressing the view that society has no right to decide on such delicate issues as the quality of life of those with congenital or genetic disabilities (2). Wider objections are sometimes raised when the topic of selective termination of pregnancy is aired. They centre round questions about whether it is appropriate for society to decide that physical disability is always a bad thing. Surely, it is argued, some of our greatest creative artists suffered from such afflictions. Can we be sure that their talents were not expressed as the result of their physical or mental disadvantages? Do we, it is asked, want to terminate a pregnancy and lose a Beethoven?

It does not seem helpful to base our attitude on the avoidance of genetic disease on the lives of unusually creative individuals. After all, there are numerous examples of outstandingly original people who have remained in rude health throughout their working lives. It is difficult to substantiate the argument that unusual talent, or even genius, is seen only in the context of serious disability.

These are problems which have to be examined in the context of the moral stance of particular societies at a given time. As mentioned earlier, when describing attitudes to the avoidance of mild genetic disease in China with its one-child rule, it is impossible to draw any hard-and-fast conclusions about what is desirable or acceptable in terms of genetic fitness. But although it seems reasonable to give individual parents the right to decide on what kind of children they wish to bring into the world, we will have to watch the situation carefully and maintain a constant debate between the medical profession and society. Most biologists feel that it would be wrong, for example, to allow parents to choose the sex of their children. The simple pragmatic reason is, of course, that this might cause a major imbalance of the sex ratio within a particular population. Indeed there is some evidence that this type of practice is going on in parts of India today. Thus individual societies will have to decide on how far they want to go in the regulation of the genetic make-up of their population, and make value judgements on the quality of life, difficult though this may be. In particular they will have to consider the particularly difficult question of the rights of individual parents compared with those of the communities in which they live.

Similarly, it will be very important that in our efforts to screen and avoid serious genetic disease we do not forget to pay enough attention to developing methods to treat these conditions. It is unlikely that we will be able to develop screening programmes to cover all genetic diseases, and in any case the widespread use of selective abortion should surely not be the ultimate goal of clinical genetics.

FUTURE CONCERNS FOR HUMAN MOLECULAR GENETICS

Although most of the ethical issues that have been raised in this chapter are already with us there are other issues which are causing a good deal of public concern. Most of them are based on the 'slippery slope' argument; where might human genetic manipulation take us in the longer term (10,11).

These concerns are based on the following argument. Supposing that in the future we can replace defective genes, and that somatic gene therapy becomes as routine as organ transplantation, surely it might be tempting to indulge in germ-line therapy for a few serious diseases. And where might this all end? Once we understand the genetic basis of musical talent, athleticism and other desirable traits wouldn't it be tempting to indulge in gene transfer for enhancing our offspring? Of course such arguments are based on highly speculative assumptions about how far we will be able to understand the physical basis of human attributes in the future. Considering that we do not even understand much about the regulation of single genes in higher organisms such fears will remain in the realm of science fiction, at least for the foreseeable future.

There are also concerns about the resurgence of eugenics. This word, which literally means well-born, was invented by Francis Galton, a talented English eccentric who was born in the same year as Mendel (12). Eugenics is concerned with the improvement of the species by selective breeding. Galton had observed that distinguished people tend to come from distinguished families and thought, therefore, that heredity must determine not only physical features but also talent and character.

The eugenics movement was developed at the beginning of this century and was initiated with great success both in this country and in the United States. It subsequently spread rapidly throughout Europe and as far afield as Japan and South America. It had major political repercussions in the USA, where it underpinned several immigration laws and Acts to prevent marriage of subnormal individuals. Although it never had a great impact in the United Kingdom it undoubtedly attracted many of the founders of human genetics and remained active until the onset of World War II.

Because of the perceived results of eugenics in Nazi Germany, and the mistaken genetic concepts on which much of it was based, the movement declined after World War II but reared its head again in the 1960s when new eugenic questions were raised. In 1969 the problem of racial differences in IQ became a major issue, and it was suggested that the lack of performance among the American Black population might reflect a genetically determined lack of intelligence. Although it is not active at the present time the development of socio-biology and the resulting debate on biological determinism, again with strong political overtones, has revived memories of its earlier successes (13). It has been claimed by a number of prominent molecular biologists that once we have sequenced the human genome we shall know all that there is to know about Man. Such pronouncements have done little to reassure a public that is increasingly concerned about what might be going on in the field of human biology.

The truth is that we have no idea how far it will be possible to go in modifying human beings by changing their DNA. But it would be a tragedy if slippery slope arguments of this kind, or misconceptions about the genome project, were to set back progress in a field which has so much potential for human well-being. It is not possible for one generation to set ethical norms for their great-grandchildren. However, as the potential for human molecular biology is so great it is essential that scientists are completely open about their activities and are willing to develop and maintain a continuous debate with the public about the way their field is moving.

In this context it is interesting to reflect on whether, had physicists attempted to educate the public about the future potential of the extraordinary developments in their field earlier this century, the catastrophes of Hiroshima and Nagasaki could have been prevented. The assumption that it would have made no difference is no reason for biologists and doctors not to do their best to ensure that the equally extraordinary developments in molecular genetics are not misused by future generations.

Much of the confusion and public alarm about the genome project has been generated by debates on issues of this type, many of which seem almost irrelevant to the present state of human molecular genetics. The issues that I outlined earlier in this chapter, and that are already with us, are complex enough, and they should not be clouded by vague concerns about the slippery slope of human genetic manipulation. The latter is surely for future generations to sort out.

REFERENCES

1. Weatherall, D. J. 1991. Manipulating human nature. *Science and Public Affairs*, 25–31.
2. Weatherall, D. J. 1991. *The new genetics and clinical practice*. Oxford University Press, Oxford.
3. McKusick, V. A. 1990. *Mendelian inheritance in man*, 9th edn. Johns Hopkins University Press, Baltimore MD.
4. Emery, A. E. H. and Mueller, R. F. 1987. *Elements of medical genetics*, 7th edn. Churchill Livingstone, London.
5. Holtzman, N. A. 1989. *Proceed with caution. Preventing genetic risks in the recombinant DNA era*. Johns Hopkins University Press, Baltimore, MD.
6. President's Commission for the Study of Ethical Problems in Medicine and Biomedical and Behavioural Research. 1983. *Screening and counselling for genetic conditions. A*

report on the ethical, social and legal implications of genetic screening. Counselling and education programs. Government Printing Office, Washington, DC.

7. Fletcher, J. C. 1982. *Coping with genetic disease.* Harper & Row, San Francisco, CA.

8. Harper, P. S. and Clarke, A. 1991. Should we test children for 'adult' genetic diseases? *Lancet* **335**: 1205–1206.

9. Motulsky, A. 1983. Impact of genetic manipulation on society and medicine. *Science* **219**: 135–140.

10. Suzuki, D. and Knudson, P. *Genethics.* Harvard University Press, Cambridge, MA.

11. Yoxen, E. 1986. *Unnatural selection. Coming to terms with the new genetics.* Heinemann, London.

12. Kelves, D. J. 1985. *In the name of eugenics.* Alfred A. Knopf, New York.

13. Rose, S., Kamin, L. J. and Lewontin, R. C. 1984. *Not in our genes. Biology, ideology and human nature.* Penguin Books, Harmondsworth.

84

Fertilization In Vitro

PETER R. BRAUDE, BSc, MB, BCH, MA, PHD, MRCOG,
DPMSA

Professor and Chairman, Department of Obstetrics and Gynaecology, United Medical and Dental Schools of Guy's and St Thomas', St Thomas' Hospital, London, UK

On 25 July 1978 the birth of Louise Brown in the United Kingdom permanently altered the prospects of fertility for many childless couples (1). However, with this same event many of the worst fears of the scientific nihilists had been realized (2). Scientific advance had plunged society into Aldous Huxley's Brave New World, where sex and love would no longer have any relevance to reproduction, and where babies would be produced in factories on demand and to order.

Despite the hysterical reception of this major innovation in medical technology, for the first time there were realistic hopes of conception for women with severely damaged fallopian tubes not amenable to surgery, for men with reduced sperm numbers and reduced sperm quality, and for those couples with protracted unexplained infertility. Indeed the recent advent of microsurgically assisted fertilization, where a single sperm can be placed under the zona pellucida (3,4) or injected directly into the cytoplasm of the oocyte (5), will mean that men with so few sperm that they would usually have been advised to consider donor insemination, now have the possibility of having their own child.

Nor are *in vitro* fertilization techniques now limited to the alleviation of infertility. The advent of single-cell DNA technology has made it possible to analyse the genetic material from a single embryonic cell removed during the early stages of *in vitro* development in order to examine for the presence of significant genetic disease in the embryo (6,7). Couples at substantial risk of transmitting a life-threatening genetic disease to their progeny can now opt to undergo IVF and to have replaced only those embryos which have been shown to be free of the specific genetic disease for which they were at risk (8,9).

Although some of these scenarios may give some credence to the fears originally voiced against IVF, most of the difficult ethical and moral questions have been debated vigorously, and decisions reached as to their acceptability

Principles of Health Care Ethics. Edited by Raanan Gillon.
© 1994 John Wiley & Sons Ltd

in current society. In general the response has been the introduction of guidelines, and in some countries the introduction of law, to ensure good clinical and laboratory practice, to clarify family relationships in order to protect the children born as a result of this technology, and to control and limit research using human preimplantation embryos (10).

The principle of beneficence is at the root of all treatment by IVF (11). The theoretical possibility of helping women with damaged fallopian tubes to conceive by bypassing the tubes was first discussed in the 1930s (12), but it took until 1969 before the practice of human extracorporeal fertilization was achieved in the laboratory (13), and a further nine years before it became a clinical reality. Despite major improvements to the technique of IVF, the chances of implantation and that conception proceeding to live birth are still not high, about 15% per attempted cycle (14). Thus although beneficence is intended, the reality of disappointment and loss may be more profound than failure to conceive. Furthermore it is clear that IVF treatment itself brings with it a number of medical, social and psychological hazards and dilemmas which are difficult for an infertile couple to appreciate fully before embarking on treatment.

The therapeutic procedure of *in vitro* fertilization requires oocytes to be retrieved from the woman's ovaries and fertilized in the laboratory with a sample of sperm prepared from a masturbated ejaculate from her partner (15). The oocytes are aspirated from the egg-bearing follicles in the ovaries either during a laparoscopy procedure performed under general anaesthetic, or now more frequently, using a transvaginal approach under ultrasound guidance and heavy sedation. As the proportion of oocytes (eggs) which will be fertilized by the spermatozoa is unpredictable, and not all follicles may yield an oocyte, the woman's ovaries are primed with superovulatory hormones to stimulate the development of a number of follicles (usually in the order of 6 to 10). However, the individual response to the stimulation regime is variable, and some women may be idiosyncratically sensitive to it, resulting in the production of many more follicles than expected (say over 20 per ovary), which may put the woman at risk of ovarian hyperstimulation syndrome (16). In this condition the ovaries become excessively large and painful, fluid may be extruded into the peritoneal and sometimes the pleural cavities, and in its most severe form can result in haemoconcentration, renal impairment and, if not appropriately treated, the demise of the patient. This condition can usually be avoided by close monitoring of hormone levels and withdrawal of hormonal stimulation should the process seem likely. The severity of the syndrome is also ameliorated if pregnancy does not ensue. Thus when there is a substantial risk it may be safer not to replace fertilized oocytes into the uterus. One option which may be available is to have them all cryopreserved for later transfer once the condition has settled.

Normally all the retrieved oocytes are placed with the partner's sperm and examined after 20–24 hours in culture for the presence of fertilization. Those oocytes that have fertilized are placed into culture for a further 24 hours, during which period they should have undergone two rounds of cell division to the four-cell stage, a stage of development suitable for transfer to the woman's uterus in order to try and establish a pregnancy. Pregnancy is far from inevitable once cleaving embryos are transferred. It is clear that not all embryos have the same likelihood of implantation. The odds are in part related to the quality of the embryos to be transferred, and in part due to the receptivity of the uterus (17). Since the likelihood of implantation is in the order of 10% per embryo replaced, the more embryos which are returned to the uterus in a treatment cycle, the more likely it is that pregnancy will ensue. However, it also follows that the more embryos that are replaced the higher the risk that multiple pregnancy and often higher-order multiple pregnancy (triplets and above) may result. For many couples this stage of the treatment cycle presents an intolerable dilemma; whether to maximize their chance of pregnancy by having all or many embryos replaced, but in so doing to risk a high-order multiple pregnancy with its attendant risks to both mother and fetuses of miscarriage, prematurity, neonatal death and handicap (18), or to have a lower number replaced and reduce the likelihood of pregnancy. In some countries assistance is given by law or by guidelines which limit the number of embryos that may be replaced (10,19). Nevertheless, even with the replacement of only three embryos, triplet pregnancies will ensue in about 4% of cases and twins in more than a quarter (20). Couples thus embark on embryo replacement in the uncertainty of any pregnancy, and in the fear that if successful the pregnancy may be multiple with its attendant risks and hazards of morbidity and loss.

Cryopreservation of embryos and replacement of single frozen–thawed embryos provides one means by which some of the problems which can be engendered by the establishment of multiple pregnancy or ovarian hyperstimulation syndrome may be avoided. Preimplantation embryos can be frozen most successfully at early cleavage stages (on day 2 or 3, when the embryo contains four to eight cells) or at the two-pronucleate or zygote stage (on day 1—immediately after fertilization has been confirmed) (21,22). However, the potential benefits of cryostorage of embryos present further dilemmas for the couple. If freezing is to be carried out at the pronucleate stage then the two or three embryos for fresh replacement in that cycle must be selected at this stage to be cultured for a further day, and the rest are cryostored. There is no guarantee that those which are selected for continued culture will cleave normally and be suitable for replacement. On the other hand those selected to be frozen may not survive the freezing–thawing process. Thus, although freezing pronucleate zygotes appears to be more successful than freezing cleavage stage embryos, many clinics and couples prefer to wait until the 'best three' embryos have divided and been replaced into the woman before freezing the remainder at cleavage stages. By so doing, the number of embryos that are suitable for freezing will be reduced as the quality of embryos deteriorates with increasing time in culture.

Despite the potential advantages of single frozen–thawed embryo replacements, because of the substantial financial cost which may be incurred in having a frozen replacement cycle, many couples still opt to have three embryos replaced in a therapeutic cycle and then, if unsuccessful, to have three frozen embryos replaced rather than one, in order to maximize the chances of pregnancy once again despite the recurring risk of multiple pregnancy. Thus although beneficence may underlie the provision of service, and non-maleficence is intended, there are very real hazards and stressful decisions which a couple will face in opting for IVF as a treatment modality.

Besides the grief that a couple may feel for the inability to have a child, they are further compromised by the loss of their reproductive liberty, their autonomy to procreate naturally and in privacy (23). In no other aspect of infertility treatment is this invasion of the intimacy of a couple's relationship more profound than in IVF. Instead of being able to pursue a basic human function and need as part of a natural loving union, IVF requires dependence on third parties, on the physician and team of scientists to conceive. It is not surprising that couples may feel that they have 'relinquished their gametes to the doctors', and that many of the choices about their future and family are no longer theirs. This loss of control and autonomy has now been exaggerated in some countries, as in the UK, where there is now the need by law for the treating doctor to ascertain information as to whether the couple are suitable for IVF therapy in the interests of any child so resulting, before he may offer such treatment (10).

Choices which face a couple at all stages of their treatment are profound and difficult for them to make objectively under the stress of their predicament of protracted subfertility. Many, having been infertile for many years, will be seeking a resolution to a long struggle without necessarily re-evaluating their position with advancing age or ever stopping to question whether treatment by IVF is appropriate in their current circumstances. The very availability of new reproductive technologies, such as IVF, is coercive, and infertile couples are vulnerable to new offers whether substantiated or not. Although it behoves the clinician to explain to the couple the hazards and risks of therapy as objectively and as sympathetically as possible, it would be presumptuous and paternalistic for him/her to make the choices for them. However, because of the complexity of social and legal relationships between the potential parents and the embryos to be replaced or cryostored, there are often strict rules and guidelines with which practitioners have to comply and, in some countries, laws within whose framework practice must take place. These laws, guidelines and rules mean that patients lose their autonomy in dealing with their problem in the way that they feel best fits their social and emotional circumstances. For example, in the United Kingdom where no more than three embryos may be replaced into the uterus during any therapeutic cycle, cryostorage facilities may not always be available within a therapeutic programme. Thus embryos surplus to immediate therapeutic needs are either discarded or requested for use in research (24). Each of these options restricts the couple's autonomy either by limiting success or further complicating their treatment by the risk of multiple pregnancy. In Germany; where the law does not allow more oocytes to be fertilized than there is the intention to replace (19), the likelihood of pregnancy may be compromised beyond the couple's control, especially where the man has spermatozoa of poor quality and the likelihood of fertilization is reduced.

Perhaps the most stressful of all issues facing couples needing IVF in order to conceive is the issue of whether this treatment is provided as a legitimate part of routine health care, whether state-funded or whether underwritten by health insurance schemes. In many countries there has been a reluctance to provide money for the provision of fertility services, but this reluctance seems to have been exaggerated in the case of IVF. In part this may be because IVF is still regarded as experimental and having a very low success rate, and in part because it involves ethical, legal and social issues in which health providers may not want to become embroiled. There are also those who believe that with the intense pressures on primary health care funding today, infertility services in general deserve a low priority. In considering the justice of this provision it should be borne in mind that many providers of medical care do pay for alternative and often less efficacious forms of therapy as long as they do not involve IVF (25). Although pregnancy rates of around 25–30% per embryo transfer procedure are achievable, IVF still rarely results in much more than a 17% 'take home baby' rate. However, when a cumulative pregnancy rate of over 50% for five cycles of IVF treatment (14) is compared with alternative therapies such as tubal surgery, which has a two-year conception rate of less than 15% (25), it is clear that IVF deserves a substantive place in mainstream treatment for subfertility (26). Even if funding were to be provided for this type of treatment, there would still be difficult decisions about provision. How many cycles should be provided? Since success rates for live births following IVF reduce with age, and dramatically so over the age of 40 years (14), should provision be limited to younger women and over what age should the service be limited? Should provision be restricted if there is already a child (children) in the family? After how many children should the restrictions apply and do they apply if the children are of a previous union?

Why have the law and ethics become more involved in the provision of IVF than other treatments for infertility which may raise many similar issues about cost–benefit of provision, risk of multiple pregnancy, altered family relationships and loss of autonomy? The crucial difference in the provision of treatment service by IVF is the extracorporeal presence of a preimplantation embryo (see refs 27 and 28 for discussion of the term pre-embryo). The relevance of the principles of autonomy, beneficence, non-maleficence and justice to the embryo *in vitro*, depends on the status accorded to the preimplantation embryo *in vitro*, which is usually argued on its properties of potentiality, genetic uniqueness and being human (29).

Although many of the ethical constraints and concerns about potentiality of preimplantation embryos are common to those which have been raised in the abortion debate, and thus will not be discussed here, some are specific to preimplantation stages created *in vitro* and maintained in culture in the laboratory (28). The preimplantation embryo *in vitro* occupies a special status in the potentiality argument. In the abortion debate, embryos at all stages are in their appropriate environment and thus, unless prevented from implanting (e.g. by an intrauterine contraceptive device) or removed from that environment, may have the capacity to develop completely. The older and more developed the embryo, the more likely its potential to reach viability. The preimplantation embryo *in vitro* does not conform to this model. Firstly, fertilization and early cleavage occur outside of a natural environment. Since complete ectogenesis is not possible, nor does it seem feasible, in this environment the embryo has no potential for appropriate further development unless transferred to a suitable uterus. Secondly, the longer that a preimplantation embryo is maintained *in vitro*, especially beyond the blastocyst stage (six days) the less structured is development and the less likely transfer to a uterus is to result in a pregnancy.

Thus perversely, the older the embryo *in vitro*, the less its potential for further development.

Uniqueness of the egg after fertilization is another property which is deemed to confer upon it a special status. On completion of the process of fertilization with cleavage to the two-cell stage, the cleavage stage embryo has a genetic constitution unique to itself derived from the paternal and maternal genetic contributions. During further development over the next week the genetically unique cells of the preimplantation embryo continue dividing, giving rise to some cells which will constitute the true embryo and others which will constitute the placenta. Thus the specific genetic constitution is not 'unique' to the developing embryo, but is shared with a tissue developing in the uterus which will be discarded at birth. Indeed if a monozygotic twin pregnancy, then the 'unique genetic identity' will be shared not only with the placenta but with the sibling. Thus uniqueness of genetic material *per se* should not confer any special status on the embryo *in vitro*.

Nor indeed ought the title of 'human' necessarily confer special status. Human is simply a generic term to distinguish members of the species *Homo sapiens* from other species. All cells of the body of man (or woman) are human and those of the embryo, whether in culture or *in utero* are no different. Unfortunately, human is often used synonymously with 'human being', a term intended to describe a state requiring the presence not only of a genetic constitution of human chromosomes specific to *Homo sapiens*, but also requiring properties of sentience, cognizance and physical characters equated with being human. None of these are relevant during preimplantation embryonic stages where the only property that can be defined is a genetic one.

Despite these caveats many countries worldwide have set restraints and restrictions on what may be done with or to a human preimplantation embryo *in vitro*, according to it a special status based primarily on properties of potential and humanness, and a fear of uncontrolled manipulation in the laboratory. Most of these protect the embryo by limiting the time for which it may be kept in culture (after which it must be destroyed!) and by defining what manipulation may or may not be performed on the cells which constitute the embryo; e.g. banning cloning by gene injection but not preimplantation biopsy for the purposes of genetic diagnosis. Thus implementation of the four principles of beneficence, non-maleficence, justice and autonomy for the preimplantation embryo seems not to be the predominant sentiments in determining guidelines and legislation for the practice of IVF, but rather an attempt to adhere to some of these principles for the benefit of the woman, the couple and society which rightly are given precedence.

REFERENCES

1. Edwards, R. G., Steptoe, P. C. and Purdy, J. M. 1980. Establishing full-term human pregnancies using cleaving embryos grown in vitro. *British Journal of Obstetrics and Gynaecology* **87**: 737–756.
2. Kass, L. R. 1971. Babies by means of *in vitro* fertilization: unethical experiments on the unborn. *New England Journal of Medicine* **285**: 1174–1179.
3. Cohen, J., Talansky, B., Malter, H., Alikani, M., Adler, A., Reing, A., Berleley, A.,

Graf, M., Davis, O., Liu, H., Bedford, J. M. and Rosenwaks, Z. 1991. Microsurgical fertilization and teratozoospermia. *Human Reproduction* **6**: 118–123.

4. Cohen, J., Malter, H. E., Talansky, B. E. and Grifo, J. 1992. *Micromanipulation of human gametes and embryos*. Raven Press, New York.

5. Palermo, G., Joris, H., Devroey, P. and Van Steirteghem, A. C. 1992. Pregnancies after intracytoplasmic injection of single spermatozoon into an oocyte. *Lancet* **340**: 17–18.

6. Handyside, A. H., Pattinson, J. K., Penketh, R. J. A., Delhanty, J. D. A., Winston, R. M. L. and Tuddenham, E. G. D. 1989. Biopsy of human pre-embryos and sexing by DNA amplification. *Lancet* **1**: 347–349.

7. Navidi, W. and Arnheim, N. 1991. Using PCR in preimplantation diagnosis. *Human Reproduction* **6**: 836–849.

8. Handyside, A. H., Kontogianni, E. H., Hardy, K. and Winston, R. M. L. 1990. Pregnancies from human preimplantation embryos sexed by Y-specific DNA amplification. *Nature* **344**: 768–770.

9. Braude, P. R. 1992. Embryo therapy: What can be done? Pp. 1–9, *in* Bromham, D. R., Dalton, M. E., Jackson, J. C. and Millican, J. R. (Eds) *Ethics in reproductive medicine*. Springer-Verlag, London.

10. HMSO. 1990. *Human fertilisation and embryology act*. HMSO, London.

11. Braude, P. R., Johnson, M. H. and Aitken, J. 1989. Benefits of *in vitro* fertilization. *Lancet* **2**: 1327–1328.

12. Editorial. 1937. Conception in a watch glass. *New England Journal of Medicine* **217**: 678–679.

13. Edwards, R. G., Steptoe, P. C. and Purdy, J. M. 1970. Fertilization and cleavage *in vitro* of preovulatory human oocytes. *Nature* **227**: 1307–1309.

14. Tan, S. L., Royston, P., Campbell, S., Jacobs, H. S., Betts, J., Mason, B. and Edwards, R. G. 1992. Cumulative conception and livebirth rates after *in vitro* fertilisation. Lancet **339**: 1390–1394.

15. Fishel, S. and Symonds, E. M. 1986. *In vitro fertilization: past present and future*. Oxford: IRL Press, Oxford.

16. Forman, R., Frydman, R., Egan, D., Ross, C. and Barlow, D. 1990. Severe ovarian hyperstimulation syndrome using agonists of gonadotrophin-releasing hormone for in vitro fertilization: a European series and a proposal for prevention. *Fertility and Sterility* **53**: 502–509.

17. Walters, D. E., Edwards, R. G. and Meistrich, M. L. 1985. A statistical evaluation of implantation after replacing one or more human embryos. *Journal of Reproduction and Fertility* **74**: 557–563.

18. Botting, B. J., Macfarlane, A. J. and Price, F. V. 1990. *Three, four and more: A study of triplet and higher order births*. HMSO, London.

19. Diedrich, K. 1991. The embryo protection law after the unification of Germany. *Focus on Reproduction* **1**: 7.

20. HFEA. 1992. *Annual report of the Human Fertilisation and Embryology Authority*. HFEA, Paxton House, 30 Artillery Lane, London E1 7LS.

21. Trounson, A. O. and Mohr, L. 1983. Human pregnancy following cryopreservation, thawing and transfer of an eight-cell embryo. *Nature* **305**: 707–709.

22. Cohen, J., De Vane, G. W., Elsner, C. W., Fehilly, C. B., Kort, H. I., Massey, J. B., Turner, T. G. Jr. 1988. Cryopreservation of zygotes and early cleaved human embryos. *Fertility and Sterility* **49**: 283–289.

23. Lauritzen, P. 1992. What price parenthood? Pp. 75–83, *in* Campbell, C. S. (Ed.) *What price parenthood? Ethics of assisted reproduction*. Dartmouth Publishing Co., Aldershot, Hants.

24. Braude, P. R. 1989. Research on early human embryos *in vitro*. Pp. 35–44, *in* Shinebourne, E. A. and Dunstan, G. R. (Eds) *The process of decision: ethics in practice*. Oxford University Press, Oxford.

25. Watson, A. J. S., Gupta, J. K., O'Donovan, P., Dalton, M. E. and Lilford, R. J. 1990. The results of tubal surgery in the treatment of infertility in two non-specialist hospitals. *British Journal of Obstetrics and Gynaecology* **97**: 561–568.

26. Lilford, R. J. and Watson, A. J. 1990: Has *in vitro* fertilization made salpingostomy obsolete? *British Journal of Obstetrics and Gynaecology* **97**: 557–560.

27. Braude, P. R., Monk, M., Pickering, S. J., Cant, A. and Johnson, M. H. 1989. Measurement of HPRT activity in the human unfertilized oocyte and pre-embryo. *Prenatal Diagnosis* **9**: 839–850.

28. Braude, P. R. and Johnson, M. H. 1990. The embryo in contemporary medical science. Pp. 208–221, *in* Dunstan, G. R. (Ed.) *The human embryo*. University of Exeter Press, Exeter.

29. Warnock, M. 1985. A question of life. *in The Warnock Report on Human Fertilisation and Embryology*, p. 128. Basil Blackwell, Oxford.

Editor's note For a chapter complementary to this one, see also Chapter 52 in this volume.

85

Organs for Transplant: Donation or Payment?

BOB BRECHER, BA, PHD

Principal Lecturer in Philosophy, University of Brighton, UK

INTRODUCTION

Is payment for an organ morally acceptable? Is the buying and selling of, for example, kidneys for transplant something we should accept with (comparative) equanimity, or should we insist on donation as the only permissible form of transaction?

In 1989 a major scandal occurred when it was revealed that a human kidney transplanted into a private patient at the Humana Wellington Hospital in London had not been donated, but rather had been sold by an impecunious Turkish peasant (see ref. 1, n. 1). The doctors involved were eventually found guilty of serious professional misconduct by the General Medical Council (ref. 1, n. 2, n. 8), despite their protestations of unwittingness; a budding entrepreneur's business was rapidly closed down (ref. 1, n. 4); and little has been heard of 'the kidney trade' since. But just how are we properly to understand and morally evaluate such a transaction? Was the peasant concerned earning money illegitimately? Was the recipient wrong to jump the queue by paying? Were the doctors concerned acting improperly? Was the dealer who wished to act as a broker between potential sellers and buyers of kidneys conducting a business significantly different from those dealing in other commodities (1–3)?

Bearing in mind some recent treatments of the matter which focus particularly sharply on the fundamental issues underlying the question of the moral status of a market in bodily parts, I shall begin with a brief comparative discussion of the buying and selling of blood; consider whether or not there might be something morally special about selling (irreplaceable) *parts of one's body* and/or *buying and selling* bodily organs; go on to suggest why the traditionally overarching moral concepts of autonomy, beneficence, non-maleficence and justice *tout court* are inadequate to the issue; and finally return to Titmuss's salutary emphasis on social effect.

Principles of Health Care Ethics. Edited by Raanan Gillon.

TITMUSS'S ARGUMENT

With all too acute prescience, Titmuss wrote in 1970 (4):

> If blood is considered in theory, in law, and is treated in practice as a trading commodity then ultimately human hearts, kidneys, eyes and other organs of the body may also come to be treated as commodities to be bought and sold in the marketplace (p. 158).

Quite so: for if the buying and selling of blood for transfusion were morally unacceptable, then so would be the buying and selling of kidneys and other irreplaceable organs. (While one kidney is normally sufficient for satisfactory human functioning, voluntarily to give one up is clearly a far greater step than giving a pint of blood, not least because of the risk incurred should the remaining kidney malfunction—and this is of course also the case with eyes, fingers and patches of skin, but not with hearts or livers.) But is it unacceptable? Aside from contingent questions of price, administration and safety—all important, but all manipulable—Titmuss's argument (4), however laudably old-fashioned, amounts to little more than distaste for the market. What he assumes to be an almost unaskable question—'Should men be free to sell their blood?' (p. 13)—is one which perhaps the majority in Britain, and certainly the majority in the USA, would readily answer in the affirmative. His concern for those 'fundamental distinguishing marks of social policy which differentiate it from economic policy' and with 'the question "who is my stranger"' lead him ultimately to rely on an emphasis on 'the unquantifiable and unmethodical aspects of man' (pp. 223–224), a reliance which, 20 years on, would require to be justified in considerable detail. (Michael Ignatieff's is an interesting recent attempt to think about such issues (5).) Blood may well be a basic need, such as air and water: but these are bought and sold, the former implicitly, the latter by private water companies. It may, as Titmuss argued, be objectionable that health should depend on wealth. But it clearly does so depend right across the board, even under the aegis of a National Health Service: from the availability at all of specific treatments; to the time it takes to obtain them; to the likelihood of one's need for them (ref. 4, pp. 240 ff.; see also refs 6 and 7)—a situation which shows no sign of changing, but rather of increasingly becoming the norm. It remains to be shown, however, whether or not blood should be an exception here: and thus, by extension, whether or not organ transplants should be. The question is indeed one about different conceptions of society, as Titmuss rightly emphasizes in his final chapter: but that, as I shall suggest later, is the beginning, and not the end of the argument.

PARTS OF THE BODY

Perhaps, however, the buying and selling of organs is morally different from that of treating blood as a commodity, precisely because they are *organs*, so that the discussion above is hardly to the point. The classic statement of the view that one has a moral duty to specific parts of one's own body, such that parts are not to be bought and sold, is Kant's (p. 124): '[A] human being is not entitled to sell his limbs for money, even if he were offered ten thousand thalers for a single finger' (8). Fundamentally, the argument concerns the alleged intrinsic degradation of treating one's own (or another's) body in this way, and it is a view which I readily imagine one might share whether or not one agrees with Kant's intricate notions either of duty or of one's relation to one's body. (Chadwick is the best guide and critic here (9).) Given that some people feel distaste for a prostitute or a surrogate child-bearer renting out their body for others' use; or models selling images of (parts of) their body for others' consumption in pornographic magazines, etc., it is likely that they will feel even greater distaste for the practice of literally selling parts of one's actual body. But the fact of such distaste constitutes of itself no argument to the effect that there is anything morally reprehensible about such a practice. For, as Chadwick shows, the insistence that there is something intrinsically degrading about it remains just that, an insistence: 'If I can have my foot amputated to save my life, why not sell my kidney to pacify the loan sharks from whom I am in fear of my life?' (ref. 9, p. 134). There is nothing *prima facie* special about my foot, such that under no circumstances is it to be sacrificed for my own good: and, given that it is perfectly permissible to sell my labour (ref. 9, p. 133) it is difficult to see how selling part of my body for my own good should be intrinsically degrading. There would have indeed to be something special about parts of my body, such as to differentiate them in this regard from, among other things, my labour. But what might this be? Kant's reliance on the idea that there is something intrinsic at issue will not do, and neither, I think, will Harré's restatement of his argument (10): for to say that parts of one's body are intrinsic to one's identity as a person, for example, leaves open the very question at issue. *What* is intrinsic about them if I may legitimately divest myself of some among them for my own good or even survival? Chadwick's example of the medically necessary amputation of a foot seems decisive.

What remains is the question of buying and selling. How, for instance, might my agreeing either to *sell* or to *buy* a kidney differ morally from my agreeing to enter a society-wide 'spare part' lottery in which I have a minuscule chance of being killed for my body in return for the security of knowing that any spare part I might one day need is definitely going to be available (11)? (For subsequent debate see refs 12–17.) Whatever objections there might be to the latter, and there are of course many, they focus upon questions of the sort of society such a practice would require and/or foster, problems of individuals' psychological security, abuse of the system by a 'nomenklatura' etc., rather than upon the commercial nature of the transactions in question. As Tadd insists in his response to Chadwick, people *are* paid for voluntarily undergoing drug tests, undertaking surrogate child-bearing and working as prostitutes, let alone merely selling their labour in more ordinary ways (18): and if bodily organs such as kidneys have no special status as compared with the nervous system, uterus or genitalia, then to argue that buying or selling a kidney is wrong, because in some way a *commercial* transaction, must imply that these practices are similarly wrong, which, Tadd and many others would argue, they are clearly not. Thus it would appear that focusing on buying and selling also fails to offer any obvious solution to the question of just what, if anything, might be wrong with a commercial market in kidneys.

But before leaving this train of thought it might be helpful to consider an extreme example. Margaret has Alzheimer's disease. She knows this, and knows what the consequences will be. She decides that, rather than endure the pain and indignity of gradually succumbing to this fatal disease, she would rather, while her mind is still clear, combine two deeply and sincerely held moral beliefs about what it is right to do in such circumstances. The first is that suicide is an appropriate response: and the second that one should offer one's organs to others for transplant after one's death. Now, whatever one's views about suicide, I think it is pretty clear that her second conviction would meet with general approval, Jehovah's Witnesses and certain others apart: and for present purposes I shall simply assume that suicide is not morally impermissible, while recognizing that this is highly contentious. Nevertheless, given that Margaret *is* going to commit suicide, there seems to be no obvious reason why her doing so should constitute any sort of reason for her not donating her organs for transplant, or for potential recipients not to accept them (either in ignorance, because anonymously donated; or despite being told of their provenance, just in case a recipient might have qualms in this case, qualms which of course might count as a good reason for some people not to accept a suicidee's organ. Such people I shall simply exclude as not central for the example, but note in passing that their possible responses raise interesting questions about confidentiality and individual conscience.) So far, so good: I imagine one might well do rather more than merely condone Margaret's action, since it is clearly, among other things, altruistic. Certainly a number of people will be saved from death and/or considerable handicap by her generous donation. However, suppose now that her decision were somewhat different. She still decides to commit suicide: but instead of *donating* her kidneys, heart, lungs, eyes, etc., she determines to *sell* them, leaving the proceeds, of course, to a beneficiary of her will—say an impecunious brother. The good she has done would appear to be even greater in this second case, for she also helps yet another person, and considerably: imagine, if you like, that the money her brother obtains in this way enables him to have a private operation without which he would otherwise die, and which he otherwise cannot possibly afford. And yet there seems to be at least something worrying here, a worry in respect of the brother's penury summed up by Chadwick's citing of 'the social conditions in which these sorts of situation arise' (ref. 9, p. 137). *If* the sale of organs is wrong, then the proceeds of such a sale being put to good use fails to cancel the wrong, because the wrong in question is of a quite different order. It might well explain, mitigate or even perhaps excuse an individual's action in such circumstances: but that is another matter. Consider, for example, differences between moral objections to slavery and making a moral judgement about a particular Athenian slave-owner. To condemn Margaret for her action in selling some of her organs so that her brother might benefit would be to demand of her something like either sainthood or callousness—I am not sure which. Of course, this does not of itself show that such action is in general not wrong.

But the whole problem arises only *if* selling one's organs is indeed wrong: its arising does not show that such acts are wrong, only that the agents concerned do not necessarily deserve moral censure even if selling one's organs is morally wrong. And we are still no nearer showing that it is wrong.

RELATIONS BETWEEN SELLER AND BUYER

What, however, the above has succeeded in doing, I hope, is to drive a small wedge between making a moral judgement about the practice of selling an organ for transplant and making such a judgement about, on the one hand, the person who sells it, and on the other the buyer. I shall henceforth distinguish, therefore, between both practice and participants: and, in the latter case, between the seller and the buyer in such a transaction, for I think that the differences between their relative positions deserve emphasis—just as does the difference between, say, people who sell their sexual services and people who buy them. If there is anything morally objectionable about such a practice, then there are important issues hanging on the relative moral censure properly accruing to customer and prostitute respectively (1–3). I have in mind as an example the terms in which a Parliamentary Commission reported on the workings of the Contagious Diseases Act in the 1860s: whereas men who used prostitutes did so merely in fun, the women concerned were obviously morally depraved.

Now, let us see whether or not the central moral notions of autonomy, beneficence and/or non-maleficence and justice might help, in light of our distinguishing between buyers and sellers, to settle, or at least to clarify, the moral issue of a market in bodily organs, and then relate the discussion to the practice that this would constitute.

Clearly the seller's act in offering a kidney to someone who needs it is in some sense a beneficent one, for without the kidney the latter will die. Of course, to offer a kidney as a gift would be an act of considerably greater beneficence: but on what grounds should anyone be expected to help a stranger in this way? Surely acts of supererogation cannot be advocated as the moral norm, on grounds of logic as well as practicality. And given that an act need not be at all supererogatory to be beneficent, would not the number of such beneficent acts be considerably increased if those people who might consider selling a kidney were offered payment, partly as an incentive to undertake so beneficent an act, and partly as reasonable compensation for the pain, risk, etc., involved—just as, for example, North Sea oil workers might reasonably expect higher than average pay for their more dangerous than average, but highly beneficial, work? Turning to the buyer, there is certainly no question of maleficence towards the seller. Indeed, the more money buyers were willing to offer, the more beneficent their acts of purchase: so long, of course, as they did not thereby force prices up so much that other potential buyers suffered. But even this would hardly count as maleficence, giving rise instead to quite general questions of justice in relation to just any market arrangements—a matter to which I shall briefly allude later.

For the moment let us consider questions of autonomy. One possible reason why I ought not to sell one of my kidneys might be that in doing so I in some

way act against myself, a view which recalls the earlier Kantian worry. Yet if I
freely choose to do so, and, far from harming anyone else, thereby help another
individual, it is a commonplace that it is interference with my voluntarily
undertaken action that would be morally wrong, and not my own action:
'Individuals may freely choose to engage in these practices, so that they may
express a person's autonomy' (ref. 2, p. 97). Any deleterious impact my selling
one of my kidneys might possibly have is outweighed by the fact of my having
freely chosen to do so. Attempts to prevent me from exercising my autonomy
in this way amount to a wholly unacceptable paternalism. Of course, if I wished
to sell, say, my heart and lungs—that is, in effect, to sell my life—that might be
another matter, one susceptible to the same sort of argument as Mill's (19)
against permitting people to sell themselves, however, autonomously, into
slavery:

> By selling himself for a slave [a man] abdicates his liberty: he forgoes any future
> use of it beyond that single act. He therefore defeats, in his own case, the very
> purpose which is the justification of allowing him to dispose of himself ... (p. 103).

Slavery, that is to say, is seen as a sort of non-physical suicide, logically negating
the essential autonomy of human beings on which is based any argument
against permitting people to sell themselves as slaves: safeguarding autonomy,
therefore, does not entail that such transactions be permitted. However, merely
to sell a kidney, or an eye, is of course quite unlike selling myself into slavery
in just this respect, among others: it does not deprive me of the opportunity of
exercising that very autonomy, respect for which is at issue. But now suppose
that either what I intend selling is my heart and lungs, or that there is some
sense, my argument above notwithstanding, in which even selling one of my
kidneys would at least in some way and to some extent interfere with my
(future) autonomy; so that, however much I may wish to strike the bargain, and
recognizing that no-one would be morally justified in preventing me from doing
so, on grounds of interference with my autonomy, there were nevertheless
grounds why no-one should assist me in the matter. The argument is of course
analogous to that around my not preventing, but also not assisting in, a person's
suicide. In the case of organ transplants, the role analogous to that of such an
assistant falls to the buyer of the organ concerned: that is to say, it might be
argued that even though I ought not to be prevented from selling a kidney
(since that is an exercise of my rightful autonomy), nevertheless, because there
is something morally wrong about doing so other people are under a moral
obligation not to assist me, in this case by agreeing to buy the kidney. And
what might be wrong is that, while exercising my autonomy in selling a kidney,
I am in some way acting against the exercise of that same autonomy in future,
on account, perhaps, of the increased risk to my health: on your own head be
it, but I'm not going to be party to it. Now, I am not at all clear how plausible
this might be, because I am not at all sure about the notion of autonomy. Am
I morally justified in autonomously depriving myself of (some of?) my autonomy?
But let us suppose that it is at least sufficiently plausible to continue the
argument. Is then the buyer in a position analogous to that of the properly

unwilling assistant in the suicide case? If so, then the argument would have to be something to the effect that the buyer damages the 'real' interests of the seller. But such an argument would tell also against all sorts of practices we accept: wage labour, for instance. As before, the problem is that selling an inessential organ seems no different from selling labour or time—which everyday state of affairs, far from being morally problematic, constitutes the bedrock of our way of life.

Turning now to the idea of justice, it is difficult to see how questions *specific to this particular case* of the justice or otherwise of the transaction even arise in respect of the seller. For if there is some place for qualms, then they are no different from those—if any—properly attendant upon virtually any use of one's endowments to advantage. If it were unjust for me to sell a kidney, a course of action open to very many, then it would certainly be similarly unjust for me to sell the fruits of my intellect; or entrepreneurs to profit from their risk-taking expertise and capacity; or models from the size and shape of parts of their bodies; or tennis-players from their capacity for physical co-ordination, and so on. As the would-be dealer in the case cited at the beginning of the chapter commented: 'My clients are businessmen who have a certain standard of living which they wish to improve and they are willing to sell a kidney to achieve it' (20) (see also ref. 21).

Congratulations on imaginative enterprise would seem to be called for, rather than any strictures about taking allegedly unjust advantage of being born with two kidneys. Certainly one of the central objections to an obvious alternative to a market in bodily parts, the sort of 'conscripted donor' lottery described by Harris (11), concerns the injustice which might be done to those identified by lot to be killed for their organs.

Turning to the buyer, however, the case is very different. In a context where kidneys are available for sale, and where there is *any* shortage of donated kidneys, a person who can afford a life-saving kidney is clearly in a very different position from someone who cannot. Nor is it difficult to see how questions of injustice arise: is wealth not an unjust determinant of whether or not one lives? Would not desert—whether in the shape of quality-adjusted life years (QALYs) or in some other form—be at the very least less unjust a criterion? Or, if that is taken to pose unfathomable difficulties, then simply chance, rather along the lines of actually existing arrangements? The difficulty here is that, if one does suppose wealth to be an unjust determinant of health in this case, then one has either to show how it differs from many other, all-too-familiar, cases concerning the distribution of limited health care resources, or similarly condemn all the latter in the name of justice. For on what grounds might access to organs be an *exception* to the injustices accepted in other areas of treatment? If, for example, hip replacements are readily and easily available for those able and willing to pay for them, but not for National Health Service patients; or if spectacles are readily available in the 'first', but far less so in the 'third' world; then why should their availability not be governed according to similar economic principles? Remembering Margaret, however, it is important to remind ourselves that, even if one holds such arrangements and states of affairs to be unjust, this is not to say that a particular potential beneficiary, whether of a well-functioning kidney, an artificial hip joint or a pair of glasses, is necessarily acting unjustly as an individual. For to act unjustly towards other people, whether the owner of the kidney or other potential beneficiaries of it, is different from, and more than, failing to act with the greatest possible altruism. Even if, however, one does regard the buying of a human kidney as unjust—on grounds, roughly, of inequity—and is willing—on grounds of consistency—to accept concomitant judgements about other areas of health care, a focus on the justice or otherwise of the acts of those individuals concerned, in this case the buyers or sellers of kidneys, is inadequate.

It is inadequate in the same way and for the same reasons as we found earlier when thinking about similar foci in respect of the notions of autonomy and of beneficence and/or non-maleficence. So long as we concentrate on individuals, the moral import of these notions remains indecisive, inasmuch as we have failed thus far to resolve the question of the morality of a market in bodily organs. In the case of 'autonomy', this seems to me to be inevitable, because the notion is fundamentally individualistic, taking as it does the individual as its point both of reference and of departure. 'Justice', 'beneficence' and 'non-maleficence', however, might fare rather differently when thought of as considerations to do with social and moral climate, rather than with the characters of individuals' actions. For what is really at issue behind all this, and what should still give us pause before we condone the buying and selling of bodily organs because we cannot put our finger on just what exactly is morally objectionable about the practice, is characteristically, if simplistically, summed up in what its author apparently takes as a statement of the obvious:

> Since the time that primitive man [*sic*] bartered a goodly hen for a sack of grain the market place has flourished. Indeed without the concept of trade the world as we know it could not exist. Whether we like it or not the ethic of the market is here to stay (ref. 18, p. 100).

MORAL PRACTICES AND THE MARKET

One cannot make a final judgement about the morality of buying and selling bodily organs for transplant before coming to terms with the moral and political vision of human life encompassed in Tadd's final sentence. One cannot invoke the concepts of justice or of beneficence *tout court*, for—even if it makes sense to speak of 'the same' concepts in different contexts—what they mean and imply is a function of the social structure under discussion. One example will suffice here. In Rawls's famous discussion in *A theory of justice* (22) he asks what degree of inequality is compatible with justice, and derives an answer based on what people behind a theoretical veil of ignorance (so that they did not know where on the scale of inequality they would find themselves) would prefer in this respect. He urges that they would want society to be ordered in such a way that the only inequalities in the distribution of wealth would be those which were necessary conditions of those who were going to be least well-off being better-off than they would be under any other arrangement:

All social primary goods—liberty and opportunity, income and wealth, and the bases of self-respect—are to be distributed equally unless an unequal distribution of any or all of these goods is to the advantage of the least favored (p. 303; cf. p. 83).

But *is* it simply obvious either that this is what most people would prefer, or that, even if it were, that it constitutes the basis of a *just* distribution of inequality? Certainly it does so within the context of liberal social structures and convictions: but that is just a restatement of the problem. It is not some formal or theoretical notions of justice, or for that matter, of beneficence—let alone autonomy—which shape our vision of a good society: rather, our ideas of what justice, etc., amount to are in considerable part a function of such a vision. Consider differences between, for example, Rawls's notion of justice and that of communitarian Christians; or between a utilitarian conception and a Socratic one. The exact nature of the dialectical relationship between ideas and their contexts is of course an enormous issue, and one which I am glad to say I cannot pursue here: Alasdair McIntyre's work is especially stimulating on this (23,24).

If this is roughly right, then an answer to the question of how morally to assess a market in bodily parts must await what justification can be given to the social vision within which it might be offered. What *can* be said here, however, is this. The practice of buying and selling bodily organs needs to be morally evaluated *as a practice*, and not as a set of isolated acts with no connection to anything else in the world in which they are undertaken. And this is the case not simply because the categories of moral judgement such as justice, autonomy or beneficence have otherwise no purchase but, just as importantly, because the practices of a society cannot but themselves be a factor in that society's character. To put it very briefly and baldly: a society in which commercial practices come increasingly to constitute the norm across the whole spectrum of life is one in which the values and attitudes underpinning just such a development will themselves be strengthened. What we do has consequences not only for other individuals and for ourselves, but also for the value-system of the society in which we live. This is not the place either to argue this structural point or to attempt to justify any particular moral and political vision of society on the basis of which buying and selling bodily organs for transplant could be understood and evaluated (I attempt to deal with this structural point in ref. 25). All I will say here by way of conclusion is this. Unless the sort of society and relationships within it suggested by the sort of obeisance to the commercial values of the free market apparent in the sorts of view epitomized by the quotation above is to be welcomed, then, to the extent that the practice of selling organs for transplant, or blood for transfusion for that matter, helps to institutionalize, encourage and justify just those values, then to that extent such a practice is morally objectionable. Thus, however much the Turkish peasant who sold a kidney may have needed the money he was paid; however genuinely he may have wished to exercise his autonomy in this enterprising venture (as a means, perhaps, of avoiding the particularly fruitless, grinding drudgery which was the sole alternative); however sincere his wish to benefit his family with the proceeds, and however great their need; nevertheless what he did was wrong: understandable, doubtless, even in many ways laudable, and certainly not worthy of censure—but wrong. However much the anonymous recipient of the kidney may have needed it, and whether or not we are inclined to censure such a person for buying it, s/he ought not to have done so. However genuinely altruistic and/or ignorant the doctors involved, what they did was wrong—and far more so, of course, if they were neither. What was carried out was wrong, whatever one makes of the motives and morality of the individuals concerned: and the fact that there are doubtless far worse forms of exploitation than that either constituted or encouraged—or both—by such transactions is no reason for not opposing them.

REFERENCES

1. Brecher, B. 1990. The kidney trade: or, the customer is always wrong. *Journal of Medical Ethics* **16**: 123, n. 1.
2. Buttle, N. 1991. Prostitutes, workers and kidneys: Brecher on the kidney trade. *Journal of Medical Ethics* **17**: 97–98.
3. Brecher, B. 1991. Buying human kidneys: autonomy, commodity and power. *Journal of Medical Ethics* **17**: 99.
4. Titmuss, R. M. 1970. *The gift relationship—from human blood to social policy*. George Allen & Unwin, London.
5. Ignatieff, M. 1984. *The needs of strangers*. Chatto & Windus, London.
6. Townsend, P. and Davidson, N. (Eds). 1982. *Inequalities in health: the Black Report*. Penguin, Harmondsworth.
7. Mitchell, J. 1984. *What is to be done about illness and health?* Penguin, Harmondsworth.
8. Kant, I. Transl. 1963. *Lectures on ethics*, p. 124 (transl. Louis Infield). Harper & Row, New York (quoted on p. 132 of ref. 9).
9. Chadwick, R. F. 1989. The market for bodily parts: Kant and duties to oneself. *Journal of Applied Philosophy* **6** (2): 129–140.
10. Harré, R. 1987. Body obligations. *Cogito* **1**: 15–19.
11. Harris, J. 1975. The survival lottery. *Philosophy* **50**: 81–87.
12. Morillo, C. R. 1976. As sure as shooting. *Philosophy* **51**: 80–89.
13. Hanink, J. G. 1976. On the survival lottery. *Philosophy* **51**: 223–225.
14. Singer, P. 1977. Utility and the survival lottery. *Philosophy* **52**: 218–222.
15. Trammell, R. L. and Wren, T. E. 1977. Fairness, utility and survival. *Philosophy* **52**: 331–337.
16. Harris, J. 1978. Hanink on the survival lottery. *Philosophy* **53**: 100–101.
17. Green, M. B. 1979. Harris's modest proposal. *Philosophy* **54**: 400–406.
18. Tadd, G. V. 1991. The market for bodily parts: a response to Ruth Chadwick. *Journal of Applied Philosophy* **8** (1): 95–102.
19. Mill, J. S. (Collini, S. (Ed.)). 1989. *On liberty*. Cambridge University Press, Cambridge.
20. Adlemann zu Adelmannsfelden, Graf, R. R. (quoted in Hoyland, P.). 1989. £20,000 offer by German dealer in kidneys. *Guardian* 30 January, p. 20 (col. 5).
21. Boseley, S. and Tomforde, A. 1989. A kidney dealer's baby trade is shut down. *Guardian* 31 January, p. 2 (cols 1–3).
22. Rawls, J. 1973. *A theory of justice*. Oxford University Press, Oxford.
23. McIntyre, A. 1985. *After virtue*, 2nd edn. Duckworth, London.
24. McIntyre, A. 1988. *Whose justice? Which rationality?* Duckworth, London.
25. Brecher, B. 1987. Surrogacy, liberalism and the moral climate. Pp. 183–197, *in* Evans, J. D. G. (Ed.) *Moral philosophy and contemporary problems*. Cambridge University Press, Cambridge.

86

Transplants

ROBERT A. SELLS

Director, Renal Transplant Unit, Royal Liverpool University Hospital, Prescot Street, Liverpool, UK

INTRODUCTION

Clinical organ transplantation started in 1954 with the first successful human kidney transplant which was carried out at the Peter Bent Brigham Hospital by Dr Joseph Murray (1). Its evolution through the early stages of experimentation, to its present successful application in the treatment of terminal diseases of vital organs, exemplifies what is best in surgical research: the speed of scientific innovation has been rapid, and in few other fields in medicine have the results of laboratory studies and clinical trials proceeded so quickly to routine clinical application. Progress in renal transplantation provides an excellent example: in 1970 there were 300 renal transplants performed in the United Kingdom with a mortality at one year of approximately 15 per cent and a success rate of no more than 50 per cent. Twenty years later, 1900 grafts were performed in the United Kingdom with a mortality at one year after the operation of around 2 per cent and an expectation of normal life with a functioning transplant after five years at around 80 per cent. With improvement in immunosuppression and a better understanding of the nature and prevention of rejection, the field has expanded to include other organs: nearly 75 per cent of terminally ill patients receiving heart transplants expect to survive to at least three years, recipients of heart–lung transplants 60 per cent at two years, and 60 per cent of liver transplant recipients at four years. Transplantation of the pancreas for diabetes, complicated by renal failure, offers 80 per cent graft survival at two years in some centres in the United States of America; the expectation of sight in a blind patient receiving a corneal graft is approximately 85 per cent (2).

The pursuit of success in organ transplantation was, and is, carried forward by a humanitarian imperative: to replace the single failing organ with a healthy one from a dead or living donor and thereby to relieve the patient from inevitable death due to organ failure, and/or to restore him or her to a normal life; and

Principles of Health Care Ethics. Edited by Raanan Gillon.
© 1994 John Wiley & Sons Ltd

(in the case of renal disease) to release limited and expensive dialysis spaces so that new patients can have dialysis who would otherwise be denied treatment.

THE EVOLUTION OF TRANSPLANT ETHICS

The ethical justification for transplanting cadaveric and living relative donor organs has been based largely on intuition. The ethical reasoning in the early days of transplantation went something like this: if a technique exists to rescue a patient from a lingering and distressing death, with a reasonable chance of a good outcome, then the moral duty of the doctor is to obtain an organ for that patient, provided that the circumstances of organ removal did not transgress 'normal ethical standards of care'. Thus, it was reasoned that, if a person had been certified dead, where the body was maintained on a ventilator and vital organs were functioning normally, where the person had not objected during life to the removal of organs, and if the close relatives had no objection to their removal, then the transplantation of organs from that cadaver seems to be ethically quite straightforward. Clearly the dead person had no further use for the organs, and the fact that they would be given to save the life of a patient in dire need seemed to be an act of such overwhelming goodness that emotional, aesthetic, or logistic problems were overcome, or at least subjugated, by the dire need of the recipient. In the interests of the greater good, cultural objections to cadaveric organ donation in the west have gradually receded, although they have not completely disappeared; the act of altruistic donation has also attracted approval from religious authorities (3).

Where cadaver organs have been scarce, other sources have been used. When close relatives of sick patients with end-stage renal disease have offered to donate a kidney, the ethical principles of giving and self-determination fully justify, in many surgeons' view, the removal of a healthy kidney from a normal individual, provided that every attempt is made to reduce the short- and long-term risks of the procedure to the minimum, and that those risks are accepted by the donor and his related recipient. In the 1960s, before the brain death criteria had been formally accepted by the profession and when cadaveric vital organs for transplantation were in very short supply, and when a living related donor was not forthcoming, surgeons turned to other sources of transplants: living unrelated donor volunteers, some of them prisoners, provided kidneys for transplantation; the 'greater good' done to the recipient seemed at that time sufficient justification. Since then, concern has been voiced and doubt expressed about the validity of informed consent in these cases. At that time the shortage of cadaver organs even impelled other workers to use non-human primates (baboons) as donors of transplants (4). This small series of pioneering heterografts was performed within the legal and ethical framework of animal experimentation, the donor animals being treated as humanely and considerately as was required by the legal and moral standards of the time.

These examples illustrate the basic utilitarian, benefit-maximizing, view of organ transplants which provided the framework for progress. As in many other areas of bioethics, the technical advances and their clinical application developed a momentum of their own, sustained by the successful treatment of more and more patients who would otherwise have died. And inevitably the new medical concepts in transplant practice attracted interest from the public through the press, and from lawyers, clerics and moral philosophers, all of whom recognized the special issues thrown up by transplantation which merited, even demanded, their comment and influence.

It is—or has been—a tradition in western society to let the scientists develop, reveal, and apply their innovations free of interference from ethical watchdogs. Detailed hypothetical debate on their ethical implications usually follows publication of their results. Transplant surgeons have never had a 'watchdog' committee to which they were obliged to report any nascent developments which might have an ethical impact. Rather, and true to the form of other sciences, the ethical discussions have followed the publication of clinical results. And the momentum of progress has not been significantly held up by the legislature: enabling laws have been passed in almost every western country practising transplantation, which allow the removal of organs from dead people provided that the diagnosis of death is certain, and that due regard is paid to the donor's objection in life (or lack of it), and/or the wishes of his family. Laws relating to living related organ donation by living relatives have been largely accommodated within pre-existing legislation concerning informed consent.

The dominant influence on transplant practice has always been societal attitudes to the rights of the individuals to donate, as well as to receive an organ transplant. The ethical approach to organ donation is conditioned principally by those rules which seek to confer benefit while preserving autonomy; what is and is not 'ethical' will be determined by the balance between clinical utilitarian demand (saving lives in a cost-effective way) and respect for the individual's right to donate or not to donate, in life or after death. Unsurprisingly, the level at which this balance is set varies between cultures and countries. For example, attitudes to the use of executed criminals as organ donors varies widely between countries. In the UK executed criminals have never been donors, and the majority of donors are cadavers who die while receiving intensive care, death being confirmed using the standard clinical criteria for brain death adopted by the profession (5). In the People's Republic of China, religious and other constraints are not conducive to cadaver donation from people who cannot be resuscitated following brain injury, and the major source of organ donors is executed criminals, over 2000 of whom 'donated' their organs in 1986. These two examples illustrate the polarity of opinion and practice regarding what is ethically allowable in transplant surgery; that polarity originates directly from the essential (cultural) differences in attitude of those two countries to religious belief about death, the nature of consent, the ability to provide secondary and tertiary health care facilities (intensive-care units), the co-symbolization of clinical transplantation with the act of execution, as well as the attitudes to capital punishment itself.

THE HOPE FOR 'A UNIVERSAL TRANSPLANT ETHICS'

Given the variation in cultures in different countries, and in attitudes to these and other issues related to organ transplantation, is a universal code of practice desirable or attainable? And if attainable, would it be useful as a code which could be accepted by all national medical and government bodies as a basis for action and prescription? That question is actively being considered by transplant surgeons and others, in the west (where the demand for organs has prompted a re-examination of the ethics of organ sale) and in some Third World countries (where doctors and governments seek to promote cadaveric organ donation).

In posing this question we are challenging our profession, in all its variegated cultural forms, to provide a commonly agreed fundamental code of medical *principles* on which rules for ethical and non-ethical *practice* can be built. Straight away we have to consider whether our hitherto utilitarian approach is a sufficiently sensitive indicator of ethically acceptable practice. I would argue that through the primacy of consideration for our recipients of organs, the sheer usefulness of the transplant operation has biased our system of ethical evaluation beyond the limits of equitability and justice demanded by those (for instance) who represent the interests of the donor. Perhaps a better 'balance of representation' is needed. To take further the philosophical analysis of our position on transplant-related issues in a way which allows consideration equally of all interests and parties, we should perhaps apply the two analytical techniques of deontology and consequentialism.

Deontology

Ethical judgement is deontological when the good that ought to guide actions is summarized as principles that must be followed, either without exception (absolutist deontology), or '*prima facie*' (where they do not conflict, they ought to guide actions). Deontological principles are stated ahead of the time when the decision is to be made (7). The four principles of moral decision-making—autonomy (self-determination), beneficence (the obligation to help others), non-maleficence (the obligation not to harm others) and justice (the obligation to deal fairly with competing claims) (8), provide a useful *prima facie* deontological framework for medical and moral assessment of the ethics of transplantation (9). But the problems arise when the principles *do* conflict: a very simple example of such a conflict would be the act of making a surgical incision to perform an operation: the harm (of the incision) is a necessary step towards the beneficent objective (a successful operation). Here, as so often in biomedical ethics, coexisting yet ethically divergent acts can be justified by a consideration of net gain to the person compared with the net cost in terms of personal risk to life and comfort. An absolutist deontological analysis results in an intrinsic paradox; a *prime facie* deontological approach does not tell us how to act; but a utilitarian, 'consequentialist', approach may allow us to decide on the basis of optimizing the consequences.

Consequentialism

Ethical judgement is consequentialist when it asks whether the effects of a particular action are likely to produce beneficial states of being. Here we focus on the intended and foreseeable effects of a new surgical procedure, and we ask ourselves about possible abuse. For example a consequentialist question would be: how likely is gene therapy to be misused in order to alter human gene structure in potentially harmful ways? Is the net gain to patients worth the risk of potential injury to society?

The ethics of transplant practice, perceived from several different viewpoints, can be analysed by either method with a good chance of at least achieving a systematic basis for discussion, if not a universally accepted 'book of rules'.

What follows in this chapter is a description of some ethical issues in transplantation which currently cause debate by doctors, lawyers and philosophers. They have in common intrinsic conflicts of principle which, if the principles are regarded as absolute, will defy logical reconciliation. Some issues would be solved, or at least relieved, by making good existing deficiences of resource, or by appropriate legislation (e.g. the sale of organs).

These issues, and the scenarios which illustrate them, are not presented in a way which 'answers the problem'. At the time of writing, transplant ethics is in the process of differentiating into its own ethical sub-specialty, and we are still at the stage of defining the problems and learning how to approach them. The luxury of a researched, well-argued and globally accepted answer to any particular problem is not yet available: it is debatable whether it ever will be. In the meantime, these examples will, or should, enable the reader to imagine the doctor's dilemma and to seek the best way through to a solution which least injures the participants and which most benefits the subject. And, please note, the 'subject' is not always 'the patient'.

ALTRUISTIC CADAVER DONATION

Who Should Get the Organ?

The ethical bedrock of clinical transplantation has always been the notion that an organ, taken from a dead body for no charge, may be transplanted into a recipient who has a reasonable chance of benefit; where there are two or more potential recipients, the clinical urgency of the need for a transplant, and the degree of compatibility of the donor (blood group and HLA antigen matching) are major determinants of the survival of renal transplants; these and other medical factors should determine the choice of recipient. The ability to pay, racial origins, religious convictions, political behaviour, and nepotistic or other personal preferences of doctors are unacceptable reasons for steering a precious commodity such as a transplant towards, or away from, any individual who needs it. We perceive it as wrong for a transplant co-ordinator to hold a telephone auction in order to sell (e.g.) a liver graft to the highest bidding recipient. It would on the other hand be perfectly right (and desirable) for a duty officer of an organ distribution service to choose the best-matched recipient from a national pool and to offer a cadaver kidney graft to the person who will benefit the most from it. Here the principles of justice in choosing, and utility in outcome, are satisfied and work to achieve the same goal. Patients, in enrolling on a national waiting list, agree to forgo an early transplant if another patient is better matched; and surgeons, out of respect for their patients' consideration for their own and for others' prognoses, are duty bound to avoid commercial gain from the process of choosing a recipient (10).

The Certainty of Death

The decision by the medical profession to accept the brain-related criteria for death was the product of a deep examination of the effect of new technology in resuscitation, and prognosis, of brain-injured patints. Permanent cardiac standstill unambiguously signals and causes the end of an organism's life because, without an effective circulation, irreversible injury from lack of oxygen rapidly destroys the brain, liver, kidneys and other vital organs. However, a patient, rescued from such injury by prompt ventilation at the time of respiratory arrest due to brain trauma, may still suffer brain death (if for instance a vessel bleeds within the rigid skull and squashes the delicate cerebral tissue) while the heart and other organs continue to function.

Guidelines for the clinical determination of death recommended by the *ad hoc* committee of the Harvard Medical School (11) and by the Conference of Medical Royal Colleges in the UK (5) have been published and accepted almost universally within the profession as a method of diagnosing brain death with certainty. In summary, the first step in determining brain death is to exclude metabolic (e.g. hypothermia, diabetes) or pharmacological (e.g. relaxants) causes of brain suppression; thereafter the viability of the brainstem (where the vital centres reside) is ascertained by attempting to elicit reflexes which involve central neuronal connections within the brainstem. If these tests are all negative, the final test of whether the person can breathe under normal physiological circumstances is carried out (the body is taken off the ventilator for 10 minutes whilst oxygen is delivered by passive diffusion through the trachea). Reliance on the electro-encephalogram has been discouraged because of the possibility of false positive results, and cerebral angiography—X-ray testing of blood flow in the brain—is not deemed to be necessary to demonstrate the absence of a circulation to the brain, if the brainstem reflexes are negative. However, in some countries angiographic demonstration of cessation of blood flow to the brain is taken, *per se*, as confirmation of brain death. Certain diagnosis of death derives from the absence of these reflexes, plus the patient's inability to breathe spontaneously; but because every opportunity must be taken to minimize human error and potential bias from this process additional safeguards are required. Thus the British and American codes of practice insist that two doctors independently carry out these tests on two separate occasions; both practitioners must be experienced in the technique, and neither must be associated with the care of a potential recipient of any organ taken from the corpse as a result of their diagnosis of brain death.

This protocol has stood the test of time: in no case has a patient been described in the medical literature who recovered any brain function following the diagnosis of brain death according to these criteria, even when the putative corpse was ventilated and the blood pressure supported to the point of cardiac arrest. There is now widespread (though not universal—see Chapter 88) agreement in medical and moral philosophical circles that nothing other than the destruction of the brain will meet the necessary and sufficient conditions for a biological definition of death, since the brain is the critical system of the human organism responsible for independent existence, integrated activity, and consciousness. Formal recognition of this principle was published in 1979 and has been widely accepted (12).

There are, of course, degrees of severe brain injury which cause coma but not brain death. It is critically important to be able to distinguish non-lethal causes of coma following brain injury from the coma of brain death: in the absence of death (as detected by tests described above) we must presume the presence of life, no matter what the quality of that life. Cadaveric organ removal cannot be considered until the brain death criteria are fulfilled. There are two clear-cut clinical conditions which approximate to the state of brain death, which are in fact examples of severely incapacitated life. On account of the very severe neurological injury in each case, and the inevitability of eventual death, there have been debates concerning their candidacy as organ donors:

1. The 'persistent vegetative state' may result from a temporary episode, e.g. a respiratory arrest, when the blood level of oxygen falls to a level which destroys most of the higher brain function. Restoration of normal oxygenation of the blood (perhaps by artificial ventilation) rescues the patient from brainstem death: in these rare and tragic cases, spontaneous breathing and blood pressure control may return but sensation, expression, coordinated movement and therefore self care and feeding are impossible.
2. Anencephaly, the condition when a child is born with a brainstem but without a higher brain, is also incompatible with independent life after birth without intensive physiological support being given.

In neither case can we categorize the patient as brain dead, since the fundamental attributes of respiration and cardiovascular control are present, and brainstem reflexes persist. These patients die naturally, often by intercurrent pneumonia; or the doctors may decide that physiological support should be withdrawn.

Can one use cases of the persistent vegetative state and anencephaly as cadaver organ donors? The question has to be asked if one pursues the consequentialist line of thought that if death is inevitable, the doctors ought to try and make that death as useful as possible. In the case of the persistent vegetative state, the answer is a universal 'no', since the termination of life under conditions which would allow cadaver organ donation would be a wilful, elective, putting to death of a patient. Lingering death by pneumonia usually prohibits successful organ retrieval for transplantation because of the general systemic deterioration which occurs towards the end of life under these conditions; so organ retrieval following natural death from a condition of a persistent vegetative state is not possible for practical reasons. Organs have, however, been removed from anencephalic neonatal children; a re-examination of this situation has led to the general view that although this grotesque and inevitably lethal abnormality is so severe as to exclude the existence of a personality or sentient being, capable of independent life, nevertheless, the presence of normal brainstem anatomy and function, together with our limited understanding of neurophysiology in the neonate, now causes us to exclude anencephalics as organ donors.

Most cadaver donors suffer rapid progression to a state of brain death from brain trauma, intracranial haemorrhage or stroke. After artificial ventilation is started, they are maintained in intensive care until brain death is diagnosed. If transplantation is not being considered, the ventilator may be turned off and the heart will stop beating within several minutes. If organ donation is possible, the heart-beating corpse can be transported to an operating theatre whilst ventilation is continued and organs may be removed for transplantation while ventilation and heart beat are maintained. It is important to realize that the certification of death will already have taken place after the second set of brain death criteria have been fulfilled. In preserving the heart beat during the dissection and removal of the organs for transplantation, the surgeon is doing his best to preserve the quality of transplantable organs, to maximize the benefit to the recipient; this is essential for successful transplantation of the liver, heart, or pancreas, and is also desirable to ensure viable kidneys which perform well in the new host.

LIVING ORGAN DONATION

Healthy relatives of patients suffering end-stage renal disease frequently come forward and offer one kidney to be transplanted into the recipient. The removal of such an organ from a living healthy donor differs from practically every other surgical procedure in that the operation will not be carried out to improve the health of the donor himself, but to benefit another, the recipient of the organ. Here the surgeon clearly has to weigh very carefully the risks of the procedure to the donors, against its benefits to the recipient, given that the clear-cut medical improvement in health derived from a 'normal' operation to the patient is absent. It is incumbent on the doctor to minimize risk, and this will normally be done by a very extensive evaluation of the health of the donor who must be demonstrated to be free of any significant disease which could either increase the donor's own risk or adversely affect the donor organ. The possibility of a complication-free recovery must be high. In addition, it is common in many centres to refer the donor to an independent doctor, perhaps a psychiatrist, who can establish that the person understands the risks, is intellectually and psychologically competent to give informed consent, and can warn the patient or the surgeon of any predictable psychological complication which might result from the procedure. HLA matching of donor and recipient is also an important consideration, since the better the match grade, the better will be the long-term chances of the graft surviving.

The risks of major surgery such as unilateral nephrectomy in a healthy person are those associated with the operation, and the early postoperative course, and the long-term effects of living with one kidney. The risk of dying from the operation and the anaesthetic in a fit person are probably of the order of 1 in 4000 (a figure derived by adding the risks of unpreventable and unexpected pulmonary embolism to that of the rare and unpredictable mortality associated with sensitivity to anaesthetic agents). Once the patient has recovered from the operation, there is no convincing evidence that life with one kidney is any more hazardous than life with two; insurance companies do not normally raise the premium on life insurance of individuals with one kidney. It is ethically imperative to ensure that the donor is fully aware of the operative risk before the procedure is undertaken.

There is wide acceptance in transplant medicine that donation of a kidney by a living relative is ethically acceptable. The attitude is well summarized by Schreiner (13):

> Man obviously has the right to maim himself; he can amputate his leg or cut off an infected area if it is for the good of his whole organism. If giving a kidney is for his spiritual or psychiatric good, and this is recognised as part of the total person, it seems to me that the particular mutilation becomes quite permissible under the extension of the principle of physical totality to the totality of a spiritual person.

The governing principles here are self-determination and informed consent, when the surgeon helps the donor to carry out a humanitarian act for a loved one. Provided that the essential safeguards to minimize morbidity and mortality are undertaken, and that the donor understands the risks, the procedure seems acceptable. It is up to the individual to make up his mind whether his love and concern for the recipient overrides his fear of the small risk of the operation. But altruistic motivation may take several forms in this situation. For example: a volunteer donor of a kidney to his ailing brother was asked by a surgeon whether he felt compelled to donate a kidney. The donor replied that he could not conceive of any stronger pressure than the obligation of a close brother to donate a kidney whatever the risks. Some might argue that the benefits to the recipient would be such that the demands imposed on the donor by his love for his brother amounted to compulsion. Should the doctor step in here and refuse to perform the procedure, having determined that the conflict in the potential donor's mind might be psychologically harmful? I think not: the brother still has the freedom to choose not to give, and, in my experience, other no less well-motivated relatives have decided not to donate when the hazards are pointed out to them, though their decision may only be taken after much agonizing thought and self-examination. So the organ can be withheld (at the cost of harming the recipient) or can be given (at the cost of hurting the donor). In these cases the recipient's plight has forced the dilemma on to the relative, and the degree of compulsion experienced by the relative is proportional to the strength of their relationship. In obeying the donor's wishes, the surgeon is acceding to the principle of self-determination so long as he is convinced that the donation is truly voluntary.

For the doctor to give a donor good advice about the likely risk and outcome, he must have a 'scale of risk' in his mind which he can use to advise the donor, as his patient. There will always be a threshold point on that scale, above which the doctor may consider the risk to be too serious to allow the operation to proceed, and below which the risk is not excessive, and is indeed 'acceptable'.

The use of the word 'scale' implies some sort of objective scoring system, each risk carrying a certain number of points, the threshold being exceeded when total aggregate exceeds a predetermined number of points, as in contract bridge. Nothing could be further from the truth: the doctor relies on his experience, his knowledge of the literature relevant to the operation, and his intuition. Unexpectedly, there has been little written about the risk of surgery to normal people in the medical literature to act as an objective guide in assessing the quantum of risk. Most surgeons would, however, advise the overweight, the hypertensive, the aged, and those suffering chronic infective, autoimmune, or vascular degenerative disease that the risks were too great to advise surgery.

We believe that altruistic living related kidney donation can be beneficial to the donor as well as to the recipient, and this has been measured by Roberta Simmons (14). She tested the state of mind of donors five to nine years after altruistic voluntary donation using standard psychological testing, and compared them with a group of non-donor controls. Few (8 per cent) regretted their act, and donors scored higher in self-esteem and low depressive effect after donation than before, irrespective of whether the transplant failed or not. There is much evidence in this case material of the act of donation having been psychologically beneficial and having improved family ties.

Occasionally the surgeon has to take account of risks to third parties of living donation. For instance, if the donor has young children who depend on him or her for their livelihood, the risk of death, though minute, can be considered to affect also the children of a bread-winning parent. A surgeon who performs a nephrectomy on a donor who subsequently dies has therefore caused not just the death of one person, but has possibly caused very serious harm to the bereaved children, and impoverishment of the family. As one might expect, opinions about taking organs from parents of young children vary considerably: in some units the surgeons are not prepared to take the risk, acknowledging their responsibility to the children to protect their mother or father from even that very small risk; other surgeons will proceed with such an operation; in doing so they 'enclose' the risk of family injury in the self-determined act of informed consent made by the donor himself or herself. This balance between concern for autonomy and paternalistic intervention seems to depend more on doctors' personal perceptions of their duties not to risk harm to families and society rather than to any prescribed set of rules.

EMOTIONALLY RELATED AND UNRELATED DONORS

Where no compatible living related donor comes forward, the spouse or close friend of a recipient may offer a kidney. Provided such donors are compatible, and where altruism is clearly the motive, such operations are generally thought to be ethically acceptable on the grounds that the motivation may be qualitatively no different from that of a living related donor.

Occasionally offers are made of kidneys from individuals who have no particular donor in mind but who altruistically wish to benefit 'someone'—a genuine gift of an unusually humanitarian nature, not evinced by the emotional pain of having a family member or friend suffering end-stage renal disease.

Surgeons are generally uneasy about such offers, and being sensitive to the growing debate on payment for organs, will be suspicious that, covertly, an organ is being offered for sale. Alternatively, the mental state of such a donor may come into question, such dispassionate humanitarianism being, at least statistically, 'abnormal'. Yet is it difficult to think of any deontological or indeed consequentialist moral principle which should prevent such a humanitarian act.

THE QUESTION OF PAYMENT

Cadaveric renal donation has developed in most western countries where there is a relatively high expenditure on health care and widespread availability of intensive care unit facilities, together with laws evolved to promote cadaveric donation; dialysis is generally available to those who request it. However, in many developing countries chronic dialysis cannot be provided outside the private sector, cadaver donors are infrequently available, and so patients who cannot pay for chronic dialysis and who do not have a compatible living related donor will usually die of renal failure. Since many surgeons in these countries are trained and are keen to carry out the potentially lifesaving transplant operation, markets in organs have developed, sparking a debate concerning the rectitude of payment which has spilled over into the west. Indeed, the prerequisite of altruism in living donation has been questioned during attempts to introduce commercialism in those countries, notably the USA, where there is still a shortage of cadaver organs. Doctors, in adhering to the time-honoured principle of altruism, have been accused of being too restrictive in their attitudes to this problem: 'The organ transplantation enterprise has indulged in an orgy of romanticism, mandating altrusim and communitarianism at the possible expense of saving lives' (26).

So transplant doctors and surgeons are now under pressure to justify their pro-altruism stance and their resistance to paid organ donation. In approaching this subject it is perhaps best to classify the different types of paid organ donation:

PAID ORGAN DONATION

Living donors		Cadaver donors
1. Blood-related	+/− Hidden payments	Futures market in organs
2. Emotionally related		Payments to families
3. Non-related		
4. 'Rewarded gifts'		
(a) Compensated donation	Open payments	
(b) Donation with incentive		
5. 'Rampant commercialism'		

THE ORIGINS OF THE DEBATE: 'RAMPANT COMMERCIALISM'

The first reports of a market in organs worldwide appeared in the international press in the early 1980s: western surgeons, knowingly or unknowingly, transplanted organs from supposedly related donors into private fee-paying recipients. It subsequently became clear that the recipients had paid the donors, who were actually unrelated. Revelations in the newspapers, notably the *Pittsburgh Press*, revealed that there were extensive networks of organ procurement agencies involving middlemen who scoured local indigent populations for fit potential donors. These people were tissue-typed and matched to recipients who were willing to pay exorbitant fees for these organs. Since HLA typing is one way of checking consanguinity of donor and recipient, it was difficult to prove that these well-matched pairs were not in fact related. The hallmarks of this 'rampant commercialism' were that middlemen were involved taking a large proportion of the fee, surgeons were alleged to be making a lot of money out of the trade, and in those centres where such procedures were performed 'underground' there was no proper medical screening of the donor. Informed consent rules were being ignored, no independent review of the procedures was conducted; the postoperative care of the donor was substandard, and often resulted in serious morbidity.

Western governments and professional transplantation societies reacted vigorously against what was perceived as a repugnant practice; legislation followed (15,16). The Council of Europe in resolution (78)29 concerning the harmonization of legislation of member states relating to removal, grafting and transplantation of human substances, resolved that 'no substance may be offered for profit'. The Transplantation Society condemned such practice (17) and the British Transplantation Society drew up guidelines and prescriptions for living donor transplantation, threatening with expulsion any member who willingly took a part in the sale of organs (18).

Despite the general outcry the practice persisted, and in 1991, Salahudeen *et al.* published the results of living unrelated organ transplants from Indian donors in Bombay into fee-paying Arab immigrants (19). Not only were the survival figures for the transplants very poor, but a significant number of patients suffered HIV infection from the unscreened donor tissue. At least some of the doctors conducting such practices appear to have abandoned normal professional and ethical standards of care, and operations conducted under these circumstances are now universally and roundly condemned.

'REWARDED GIFTING' (DONATION WITH INCENTIVE)

The subject of payment of living donors for transplants in public institutions, where proper medical facilities can be provided, is under constant re-examination. In India a mere 3.7 per cent of the total national budget is allocated to health and family welfare, and a negligible proportion of that is given for the treatment of renal failure. Dialysis care in such an economic environment is practically impossible in a country where the incidence of end-stage renal disease is high (20). In Madras a group of surgeons, faced with a seemingly unending stream of fatally ill renal patients for whom no care could be provided, decided purposely to accept healthy donors who wished to sell their kidneys and who were demonstrably fit and free of transmissible disease (21). These authors pleaded that the inevitable death of a recipient could be prevented by a safe operation in the donor, who would receive a solatium, a sum of money (not indecently substantial), to compensate for trouble, risk and pain. In a universal sense both parties would benefit: in addition to the restoration of life to the recipients (80% of whom were claimed to be well two years after the operation) the donor would be paid a sum (£1000), small by western standards but very large by Indian standards. In addition the donors were given three years' free medical insurance and the reported morbidity was negligible with a zero mortality. No offence was deemed to have been committed since:

1. The operation was done in good faith.
2. Proper informed consent was obtained from the donors.
3. The operations were done in order to save the life of the patient.
4. The payment of a solatium to the donor is within the framework of the law.

However, the majority of these patients were private fee-paying individuals. At that centre in Madras the 'rewarded gift' is therefore not available to the vast majority of non-paying recipients.

The medical responses to 'rewarded gifting' fall broadly into two categories:

1. In those countries where national health programmes exist to provide free care (including dialysis and transplantation) all forms of organ payment, including 'rewarded gifting', have been condemned.
2. However, in America were health care is provided on a fee-paying or an insurance basis, there is evidence that the united medical front against commercialization may be cracking: two notable figures in clinical transplantation have implied that, perhaps, under some conditions, financial incentives are acceptable. Francis D. Moore has stated that 'the selling of kidneys from living donors, evidently a common practice in India, finds a negative response in our society *unless* the recipients are chosen without respect to ability to pay, ie some form of government subsidy' (22). A. P. Monaco, noting that modern methods of immunosuppression would achieve superior success with living unrelated kidney donors, recommended that the use of such kidney donors should be encouraged and developed: 'consideration should be given to the development of appropriate motivational incentives ... which might include financial ones from government sources, particularly to cover the financial burden from the loss of work' (23). Some lawyers in America take a stronger view that altruistic donation is not a prerequisite of organ transplantation between living people, and lament the insistence on the exclusion of commercial incentives which could augment the supply of organs available for transplanation (24). In 1991 the World Health Organization issued guiding principles on human organ transplantation and recommended that 'in the light of the principles of distributive justice and equity, donated organs should be made available to patients on the basis of medical needs and not

on the basis of financial or other considerations'. The WHO also ruled against doctors engaging in organ transplantation if they have reason to believe that the organs concerned have been the subject of commercial transactions, that the human body and its parts cannot be the subject of commercial transactions and all giving or receiving of payments for organs should be prohibited, but that the payment of reasonable expenses incurred in donation by the donor should not prohibit reimbursement of these expenses (25).

PAYMENT FOR CADAVERIC ORGANS

A cadaveric organ has traditionally been regarded as a gift: the value of the new life endowed by the organ has not hitherto been measurable, and so the price of the donor family's recompense, relative to the value of the new life given, has been incalculable: and so since these organs are gifts, the cost to the donor's family has been ignored. However, as a result of pressure, mainly from the United States of America, we are under pressure to re-evaluate this concept as a 'sine qua non' in the practice of transplantation. To quote Blumstein again:

> [Medical] ideology has caused a romantic glorification of the symbolic act of next of kin donation of organs from family members, and dying relatives ... at the expense of a more rational (and compassionate) shifting of the timing of decision making to an earlier stage, when potential 'donors' in a more relaxed manner (and with the lure of financial [inducements] could confront their own mortality, self-interest, and altruistic desire to help others (26).

And Monaco, addressing the same topic; has said:

> One could argue that a trial programme should be initiated testing the effects of providing some type of additional incentive to the donor family. These might be in the form of federal fixed payment grants for deferral of burial expenses, tax deductions for the donor's estate, tax deductions for the immediate next of kin, and so on (23).

This brings into focus two aspects of payment for cadaver organs: firstly direct payment to families at the time of death of the bereaved donor (in addition, that is, to any expenses incurred in the act of donation which could be reimbursed under existing law and without much ethical objection), and secondly the idea of a futures market in organs.

1. Payment of donor families necessarily excludes altruism, and introduces the concept of commodification of body parts. We have to consider whether such implications are acceptable, given that the main stimulus for developing the idea of paying bereaved people is the economic imperative championed by some authorities who, in common with the insurance companies in the United States of America, wish to expand cadaveric organ donation for mainly monetary indications. We must consider, for instance, the warm satisfaction in the mind of the bereaved family which accompanies cadaveric donation,

which would necessarily be jeopardized if the family had received payment.

Also it has been asserted by Vining and Schwindt (27) that altruistic giving is not incompatible with payment, and that there is no reason why the two could not coexist. As a response to this we have to consider the possibility that knowledge by relatives of a deceased person that cadaver donation can be remunerated might tempt family members to seek reimbursement from the potential donor's institution before giving permission for organs to be removed. I personally find it difficult to defend this sort of payment, whereby we would encourage, indirectly, the incursion of greed in people suffering from grief. There is also another subtle attribute of the altruistically obtained cadaver organ which may well change with the introduction of a market: the gifting of an organ imposes a duty on the surgeon who uses that organ which is subtly different from the duty which a surgeon recognizes when he transplants a *purchased* organ. The bought kidney is truly a commodity, the effective use of which will be determined only by the surgeon's own standards of care. On the other hand, an altruistically given organ carries with it the hopes of the donor's family that the organ will be used to the best possible advantage, i.e. the sacrifice by the relatives imposes the highest ethical as well as medical standards of care on the surgeon. This extra obligation, though difficult to define, must influence the morally aware surgeon to put that organ to the very best possible use, perhaps by being even more careful than he would otherwise have been to ensure a good prognosis for the recipient. That pressure helps us to maintain ethical standards in our service (28).

Despite these possible objections the American Society of Transplant Surgeons has received and approved a report from its Ethics Committee (29), which has reviewed the concepts of financial incentives for organ donation and has suggested that this approach be considered for endorsement by the society. They recommend that a well-defined pilot study be set up to investigate the possibility of developing compensation to cadaver organ donor families, that compensation to be given only when actual donation has occurred; the pilot study being supervised and critiqued by a group to include an ethicist, a pro-active media representative, and a cross-section of socioeconomic groups. (The term 'compensation' in this report means not only reimbursement of extra expenses incurred by donation, but the giving of a solatium in addition to that sum.) No doubt this pilot study will illuminate the attitudes not only of the public but also the profession to payment for organs. Perhaps the results will enable us to rationalize, rather than speculate on, our ethical attitude to the payment of bereaved families.

2. The futures market is an ingenious notion put forward by economists as a way of significantly increasing organ donation (26,30); as an exercise in theoretical economics it is an innovative and thought-provoking idea. Schwindt and his co-authors ask us to consider a futures market in organs defined as 'an organized publicly operated future delivery market where an individual can contract for valuable consideration with a government agency for delivery of a specific organ upon death'. Payment would be made during the enrolled

donor's life, or to the donor's family at the time of death and organ delivery. The proposition rests partly on the issues of property rights: it is clear that the property rights of the organ donor and indeed of the recipient are at present weak compared with (for instance) the rights which an individual has over his own material property. In countries where opting out legislation does not operate, the decision for cadaveric organ donation depends not only on the permission of a donor *inter vivos* to donate an organ, but also on the lack of objection by his family to the removal of organs after death. A veto can thus be applied by the relatives and most surgeons will acquiesce to the donor family's wish. If the veto were ignored, that extra family grief would be inflicted by a surgeon who mistook the voluntary declaration of willingness to donate for a statement of obligation that the deceased *had* to donate. Therefore (28), a contract between the dead person and the insurance company drawn up in life, which legally requires donation after death, takes no account of the injurious effects on families caused by the removal of that protective veto. No evidence has yet been provided that objecting families would be less likely to object if the dead person had been paid for the organs during his life. Refusal by relatives for organ removal is high (30 per cent in the UK) (31). It is debatable that the practice of a futures market would significantly decrease the loss of organs by a family objection unless 'opting out' legislation were concurrently adopted (see below).

The right of a recipient to receive a supplied organ, or a 'contracted' organ from a pre-emptively paid donor, is also weak, much weaker indeed than the right of a donor to give his organ: the circumstances of the initial cadaver donation and the final transplant operation are so remote from each other (and for ethical reasons must remain remote) that proper representation of the recipient's interests at the scene of the death of the donor must be impracticable.

Perhaps the idea of a futures market in transplantable organs is also rather impractical: a futures delivery market will involve paying a large number of healthy people, only a small percentage of whom would die as suitable donors in intensive care units, and accessible to transplant teams. The obvious economic problems of such a system have not yet been properly worked out. Also, insurance companies will have to influence other health practitioners concerned with resuscitation of a 'contracted' donor in order to increase the likelihood of him or her completing his contract by delivering his organs after death: paramedics, doctors, nurses and ambulance drivers must be persuaded to work towards the completion of the contract by expeditiously resuscitating the donor and by creating space in an intensive care unit and operating room to facilitate organ donation. In my experience most members of staff would regard such a request on legal/monetary grounds as offensive, although currently such appeals to allow organ donation on purely altruistic grounds are rarely refused.

There are also problems of fixing a price for an organ. Schwindt (27) has pointed out that, as the transactor ages, the probability of death increases (which raises the values of the contract), but the quality of the organ declines (which lowers the value of the contract). As I have stated elsewhere (28), clerics and symphony orchestra conductors live notoriously long lives: contracts with these groups are unlikely to provide good value for money, whereas dangerous car drivers and motor cyclists would prove very good value for money since the chances of delivering quality organs are much higher. Computing differential payments by group is thus going to be very contentious and divisive; and in an acquisitive, profit-aware society it is conceivable that, if such schemes became popular, lifestyles might be altered by the introduction of a futures market.

I see more practical problems than ethical ones in the debate on the futures market. Deontological considerations cannot be said to raise many serious objections to the notion unless a strong or absolute 'deontological' rule against commerce in body parts were invoked; but the major criticism appears to be consequentialist, i.e. the introduction of market forces into the cadaver organ business will seriously threaten altruism both in cadaveric and living related transplantation. Any ethical justification of a market must take into account the likely extinction of altrusim which can be expected to follow the introduction and legislation for payment above compensation for expenses incurred.

ETHICAL ATTIUDES OF DOCTORS AND THE PUBLIC TO PAID ORGAN DONATION

In the extensive literature on this subject, the following attitudes recur as indicators of pro and con opinion:

1. Pro payment:
(a) A person has the right to use his body as he wishes (32).
(b) A free market in kidneys and other organs (both cadaveric and living donors) would abolish the deficits of grafts, and would save many lives as a result (30).
(c) Medical objection to marketing, and the insistence on the preservation of the principle of altruism by doctors amounts to squeamishness, and logical objections to it have not been provided (26).
2. Contra payment:
(a) Operations should be performed for therapeutic indications; it is debatable whether acquiring money is a therapeutic indication, no matter how humanely and unselfishly that sum of money could be used (32,33).
(b) Can a rewarded donor give voluntary consent? Under the conditions cited in the Third World, the reward of a relatively large sum of money can be perceived effectively to overwhelm or at least subjugate the notion of voluntary consent.
(c) Paid organ donation by a living person may predispose, ultimately, to the sale of *all* a person's transplantable organs; this is the 'slippery slope argument', a logical end-point of which could be a terrible scenario in which an impoverished father might sacrifice his whole body for a sum of money which would buy his family out of penury.

(d) Many doctors believe that traffic in organs divides society in that the donor will always be the relatively poor and the recipient the relatively rich (17).

(e) In a free market for organs, profit may become the first objective and there will be increased pressure to pursue monetary gain at the expense of medical standards (34).

(f) Financial gain seems to preclude or at least endanger altruistic organ donation: potential living related donors and bereaved relatives would be tempted to seek payment at an institution which offered payment (33).

These 'contra' objections confront and would deny the deontological principles of autonomy and justice—the self-determined act of selling part of one's body, or of agreeing to removal of a deceased family member's organ for gain. But these principles do not find favour universally in medical circles. Our objections are intrinsically consequentialist, deriving from concern for the negative impact which markets in organs would exert, a desire to conserve traditional attitudes to non-commercialization of the human body, and a worry that monetary gain could become a recognized state-approved indication for surgery.

ETHICAL SOLUTIONS TO THE SHORTAGE OF ORGANS FOR TRANSPLANTATION

The debate concerning payment for organs continues at the present time, and we must wait to see if legislation changes in the wake of the determination by society and by the medical profession whether buying and selling organs is acceptable or non-acceptable. In the meantime, however, legislation has been adopted throughout the west and Middle Eastern countries against the practice. Meanwhile the waiting lists for organs grow steadily: in the USA 200 people join the waiting list for an organ per month and currently 24 000 patients are awaiting organ transplantation, 19 000 of them for a kidney. It has been estimated that at least 30 000 patients per year could benefit from renal transplantation alone in that country, whereas at present only 8000–9000 patients receive a graft (36). This is 'a paradox of shortage in the face of plenty' (37), and if this is true our system of organ procurement is clearly failing. Can we say with certainty that altruistic organ donation, the traditional method of obtaining cadaveric and living donor organs, has failed and that the only alternative, marketing, should be favoured? Several countries in Europe have achieved transplant rates in excess of 45 transplants per million per year utilizing the principle of altruistic donation, and have not found it necessary to resort to paid organ donation. Furthermore there is a variety of ways in which slack in the present system can be identified and presently wasted resources can be utilized.

Changing Transplant Law

Legislation such as the Uniform Anatomical Gift Act, drafted over 20 years ago, recognizes the right of competent adults to will their organs for donation on death, and when no such directive has been made, the next of kin may grant permission to take organs at the time of death. The Human Tissue Act of 1961 in the United Kingdom is basically the same sort of law. Ways may be introduced to increase the enrolment of potential donors within this law by encouraging people to carry kidney donor cards, or by signing a statement on a driver's licence. There is little evidence, however, that such encouragement to increase cadaveric donation by 'willing' of organs after death has made any significant impact on the supply. In an attempt to rectify this problem, some form of 'required request' legislation has now been passed in most American states (38). In those states, legislation mandates that hospital personnel ask families of suitable patients who have died, about organ donation; the preliminary results of data from those areas where this law exists suggest that there has been little, if any, improvement in donation rates (39).

Laws have been changed in some countries in an attempt to relieve families of the burden of having to make a decision about organ donation after the death of a loved one, and at the same time to increase the number of donors available. These 'presumed consent' laws allow doctors to take organs for transplantation from cadavers without explicit relatives' consent, unless the potential donor had expressed an objection before death, or the donor's family objected at any time near the time of death. There are obvious attractions in such a system, although such legislation has had its critics (40). At least 13 European countries have adopted such legislation, and it is claimed that in Belgium there have been significant increases in the number of transplanted organs (41), and on the basis of these data the Council of Europe recommended that its members moved towards presumed consent. Not all countries have taken this advice, mainly because of lack of adequate methods of recording objections from members of the public in a way which makes such objection readily available to doctors. On the basis of this evidence it seems that changing the law to an opting-out type legislation is unlikely to remedy the deficit in organs.

Elective Ventilation

Recent evidence suggests that there is still a large number of stroke patients who die in hospitals in the UK who are not resuscitated for organ donation, but who may well be suitable. In these patients the inevitability of death is recognized at the time of admission, and because of resource limitations, or because of the risk of 'the persistent vegetative state' ensuing after resuscitation, these patients have conventionally been allowed to die peacefully on a medical ward behind closed curtains. Feest *et al.* have published the results of a policy of 'interventional ventilation' in these fatally ill patients at the Royal Devon and Exeter Hospital in the UK (42). In summary, the consultant in charge of the patient approached the relatives and asked permission for the patient's transfer to the intensive care unit, and for ventilatory support to be given so that organ donation could take place. This courageous experiment, requiring the introduction of a protocol throughout the hospital in an exceedingly sensitive field, was initially extremely successful: in 19 months, 11 patients were identified as potential organ donors and permission was refused in only two cases. It seems likely that if this protocol were repeated on a national scale in the UK, it would add 16 donors per million population per year to the donor pool, and thus more than satisfy the demand for transplantable organs.

Helping Developing Countries to Define and Accept Cadaver Organ Donation

There is agreement among western transplant surgeons and nephrologists working in developing countries such as India, that the long-term strategic aim of achieving cadaver organ donation is worth pursuing; indeed it is the only alternative to a free market in organs in these countries. It has been suggested (32) that doctors in India who are on the verge of starting cadaver programmes should be helped by western agencies who could finance or donate training programmes and tissue-typing reagents, support negotiations with authorities to introduce legislation to enable cadaver donation, and help provide publicity and educational material and computer software for the setting up of transplant registries. In India the majority of doctors are absolutely opposed to rampant commercialism, and to the role of middlemen and 'organ brokers'; but a substantial proportion of doctors think that rewarded gifting, with very strict controls, is currently acceptable in India as an alternative to death for their patients, although this is viewed as a temporary expedient until such time as cadaver donor transplantation is established and widely available.

Xenotransplantation

Rapid progress has recently been made towards the goal of transplanting animal kidneys into humans. Inseparable from this issue is the debate over whether or not animals have rights, and if so whether their rights are sufficient to preclude their use as transplant donors. In the absence of future legislation against animal research it is difficult to rationalize any objection to using animal tissues for transplantation of their organs into humans. For practical, physiological and immunological reasons it turns out that the pig is likely to be the most suitable species for organ donation to humans, and that genetic manipulation of pigs so that they might provide organs which are not immediately rejected is a distinct possibility (34). There are, however, formidable practical and technical obstacles to the routine deployment of such xenotransplants: even if the immunological and physiological barriers can be overcome there are formidable hazards concerning the transmission of viruses from animals to humans.

SUMMARY

Many ethical dilemmas have been thrown up by the science and clinical practice of organ transplantation both in technologically advanced and in developing societies and countries. Rules concerning ethical standards of behaviour, initially intuitive, have come under the bright light of legal and moral philosophical examination. In reviewing progress in this field in the past 20 years one is left with a degree of satisfaction that the initial intuitively derived decisions regarding clinical practice have to a large degree been accepted, and have received theoretical support from deontological and consequentialist analysis. Nevertheless, a re-examination of the principles of transplantation has been prompted by considerations of autonomy of the individual, particularly in the debate on the sale of organs, and by different forms of legislation which could aid transplantation. No certain developments can be predicted towards the solution to the deficit in the supply of organs; and doubtless technical innovation will generate new problems to tax bioethicists. One thing seems certain: that although the act of transplantation appears an act of outstanding and useful benevolence, specialists, and the public whom they seek to help, must recognize and reconcile those elements of freedom of choice, altruism and duty to society in determining the future of their art. And where these elements compete, and attempts at their reconciliation give rise to ethical discomfort, perhaps it is as well to remember that society is best served by doctors whose basis for professional standards is concern for the individual, rather than the dictats of the society in which they work. So long as we remain responsible for the consequences of our clinical action, concern for the individual will remain the cornerstone for transplantation ethics.

REFERENCES

1. Merrill, J. P., Murray, J. F., Harrison, J. H. and Guild, W. R. 1956. Sucessful homotransplantation of the human kidney between identical twins. *Journal of the American Medical Association* **160**: 277–282.
2. Various authors. 1989. Pp. 185–245, *in* Brent, L. and Sells, R. A. (Eds) *Organ transplantation, current clinical and immunological concepts*. Baillière Tindall, London.
3. Address of the Holy Father to the participants of the Society for Organ Sharing. 1991: *Transplantation Proceedings* **23**: xvii–xviii.
4. Reemtsma, K. 1969. Renal heterotransplantation from non-human primates to man. *Annals of New York Academy of Sciences* **162**: 412.
5. Conference of Medical Royal Colleges and their Faculties in the United KIngdom. 1976. Diagnosis of brain death. *British Medical Journal* **2**: 1187–1188.
6. *Chinese people's daily* (overseas edition) 28 March 1991, p. 68.
7. Keyes, C. D. 1991. Four ethical concerns. P. 10, *in* Keyes, C. D. (Ed.) *New harvest*. Humana Press, Clifton, N.J.
8. Beauchamp, T. and Childress, J. 1983. *Principles of biomedical ethics*, 2nd edn. Oxford University Press, New York.
9. Gillon, R. 1990. Transplantation: a framework for analysis of ethical issues. *Transplantation Proceedings* **22**: 902–903.
10. Council of the Transplantation Society. 1985. Commercialisation in transplantation: the problems and some guidelines for practice. *Lancet*, 28 September: 715–716.
11. Report of the Ad Hoc Committee of the Harvard Medical School to examine the definition of brain death. 1968. *Journal of the American Medical Association* **205**: 339–340.
12. Conference of Medical Royal Colleges and their Faculties in the United Kingdom. 1979. Diagnosis of death. *British Medical Journal* **1**: 3320.
13. Schreiner, G. E. 1968. Problems of ethics in relation to haemodialysis and transplantation. P. 130, *in* Wolstenholme, G. and O'Connor, M. (Eds) *Law and ethics of transplantation*. Churchill, London.
14. Simmons, R. 1983. Long term reactions of renal recipients and donors. Pp. 275–287, *in* Levy, N.B. (Ed.) *Psycho-nephrology*. Plenum, New York.
15. USA Public Law 98–507, 19 October 1984.
16. *The human organ transplant bill*. 1990. HMSO, London.

17. Council of the Transplantation Society. 1985. Commercialization in transplantation: the problems and some guidelines for practice. *Lancet*, 28 September: 715–716.
18. Sells, R. A., Johnson, R. W. G. and Hutchinson, I., on behalf of the British Transplantation Society. 1986. Recommendations on the use of living kidney donors in the United Kingdom. *British Medical Journal* **293**: 257–258.
19. Salahudeen, A. K., Woods, H. F., Pingle, A., Nur-El-Huda Suleyman, M., Shakuntala, K., Nandakumar, M. Yahya, T. M. and Daar, A. S. 1990. High mortality among recipients of bought living-unrelated donor kidneys. *Lancet* **336**: 725–728.
20. Yadav, R. V. S. 1990. Transplantation as a health priority in India. *Transplantation Proceedings* **22**: 908–909.
21. Reddy, K. C., Thiagarajan, C. M., Shunmugasundarm, D., Jayachandran, R., Nayar, P., Thomas, S. and Ramachandran, V. 1990. Unconventional renal transplantation in India. *Transplantation Proceedings* **22**: 910–911.
22. Moore, F. D. 1988. Three ethical revolutions: ancient assumptions remodelled under pressure of transplantation: *Transplantation Proceedings* **20**: 1061.
23. Monaco, A. P. 1989. A transplant surgeon's views on social factors in organ transplantation: *Transplantation Proceedings* **21**: 3403–3406.
24. Blumstein, J. F. 1992. The case of commerce in organ transplantation. *Transplantation Proceedings* **24**: 2190–2197.
25. World health organization. 1987–91. *Human organ transplantation.* Report on developments under the auspices of WHO.
26. Blumstein, J. F. 1989. Government's role in organ transplantation policy. *In* Blumstein, J. and Sloan, F. (Eds) *Organ transplantation policy issues and prospects.* Duke University Press, Durham and London.
27. Vining, A. R. and Schwindt, R. 1988. Have a heart: increasing the supply of transplant organs for infants and children. *Journal of Policy, Analysis and Management,* **VII**: 706–721.
28. Sells, R. A. 1992. The case against buying organs and a futures' market in transplantation. *Transplantation Proceedings* **24**: 2198–2202.
29. American Society of Transplant Surgeons. 1991. Ethics committee report. *Chimera,* no. 1, 22 January.
30. Rodgers, S. B., Reinbacher, L. Strengers, P. F. W. and Cohen, B. 1991. Legal and practical consequences of the commercial use of human cells and tissues. Pp. 218–224, *in* Land, W. and Dossiter, J. B. (Eds) *Organ replacement therapy: ethics, justice and commerce.* Springer Verlag, Berlin.
31. Gore, S. M., Taylor, R. M. R. and Wallwork, J. 1991. Availability of transplantable organs from brain stem dead donors in intensive care units. *British Medical Journal* **302**: 149–153.
32. Daar, A. S. and Sells, R. A. 1990. Living non-related donor renal transplantation—a reappraisal. *Transplantation Reviews* **4**: 128–140.
33. Sells, R. A. 1991. Voluntarism of consent in both related and unrelated living organ donors. Pp. 18–24, *in* Land, W. and Dossiter, J. B. (Eds) *Organ replacement therapy: ethics, justice and commerce.* Springer Verlag, Berlin.
34. Bach, F. H., Platt, J. and Cooper, D. K. C. 1991. Accommodation—the role of natural antibody and complement in discordant xenograft rejection. Pp. 81–101, *in* Cooper, D. K. C., Kemp, E. Reemtsma, K. and White, D. J. G. (Eds) *Xenotransplantation, the transplantation of organs and tissues between species.* Springer Verlag, Berlin.
35. Radcliffe-Richards, J. 1991. From him that hath not. Pp. 190–196, *in* Land, W. and Dossiter, J. (Eds) *Organ replacement therapy: ethics, justice and commerce.* Springer Verlag, Berlin.
36. Spital, A. 1991. The shortage of organs for transplantation—where do we go from here? *New England Journal of Medicine* **325**: 1243.
37. Matas, A. J. and Veith, F. J. 1984. Presumed consent for organ retrieval, *Theoretical Medicine* **5**: 155–166.
38. Caplan, A. L. and Welvang, P. 1989. Are required request laws working?. Altruism and the procurement of organs and tissues. *Clinical Transplantation* **3**: 172–176.

39. Jonasson, O. 1990. Obligations of the health care community in organ procurement. *Transplantation Proceedings* **22**: 1010–1011.
40. Sells, R. A. 1979. Let's not opt out: kidney donation and transplantation. *Journal of Medical Ethics* **5**: 165–169.
41. Roles, L., Vanrenterghem, Y., Waer, M., Gruwez, J. and Michielson, P. 1990. Effect of a presumed consent law on organ retrieval in Belgium. *Transplantation Proceedings* **22**: 2078–2079.
42. Feest, T. G., Riad, H. N., Collins, C. H., Golby, M. G. S., Nicholas, A. J. and Hamad, S. N. 1990 Protocol for increasing organ donation after cerebrovascular deaths in a district general hospital. *Lancet* **335**: 1133–1135.

87

What is Death?

DAVID LAMB, BA, PhD

Reader in Philosophy, University of Manchester, UK

CASE HISTORY

Mrs Cain was admitted to St Vincent's Medical Center in Jacksonville, Florida, on 18 November 1976, for a hysterectomy. The day after her operation she complained of a severe headache, developed breathing problems and lapsed into a coma. She was taken to intensive care and placed on a ventilator. Following extensive investigation a neurologist diagnosed brain death and recommended disconnection from the ventilator. At that time Florida did not have any law dealing with the concept of brain death but followed common law and practice, maintaining that a person is dead when his/her heart ceases to beat. Despite the death of Mrs Cain's brain, disconnection from the ventilator was a legally dubious course whilst ventilation (and hence heartbeat) were being mechanically sustained. Her husband was advised that there was no possibility of her ever emerging from the coma and that further delay in releasing the body might delay evidence of what caused her death. He petitioned the courts for the release of his wife's body for autopsy. At the hearing on 3 December 1976, doctors testified that her brain was dead and dissolving, that she would not be capable of breathing if removed from the ventilator. After hearing testimony the judge ruled: 'This lady is dead and has been dead since November 21, 1976 and she is being kept alive artificially through the use of supportive devices that not only from a medical but a humane standpoint should be discontinued.' He therefore ruled that she should be disconnected from the ventilator for 45 minutes at the end of which, if heartbeat persisted, she should be reconnected. The machine was disconnected at 12.25 pm on 4 December 1976 and her heartbeat ceased 13 minutes later (1). There is no reference to any necropsy ever being performed.

This case is typical of early attempts to come to terms with the phenomenon of 'the beating heart cadaver' before neurologically oriented concepts of death had been adequately assimilated. The judge's contradictory remarks—'this lady is dead' and 'is being kept alive'—reveal confusion over the concept and criteria for death. It is not difficult to see that among the ethical issues raised by such cases are the principles of beneficence and non-maleficence. Would further ventilation have been of any benefit to Mrs Cain? These cases reveal the moral need for precise guidelines to enable doctors to know when to recognize death as it may be encountered in an intensive care unit.

Principles of Health Care Ethics. Edited by Raanan Gillon.
© 1994 John Wiley & Sons Ltd

INTRODUCTION

From earliest records the traditional view, enshrined in commonsense beliefs, was that death occurred with the last breath of life. This view pre-dates modern scientific medicine. It is found in the Hellenic Judaeo-Christian and Islamic religions. Most religions see death in terms of the separation of soul and body, but it is recognized that this does not provide the basis for a practical diagnosis of death. The Roman Catholic and Protestant Churches do not appear to regard the manner of diagnosing death as a theological issue, nor do the Orthodox Church, Judaism, Hinduism, Buddhism, and various African religions. Although most religions advocate guidelines which express moral concern over the integrity of the body and its post-mortem disposal they have not addressed the practical issue of determining death.

Despite the importance of death in human culture discussion of the practical identification of death is not prominent in religious texts or early scientific literature; for the early theologians and philosophers what mattered most were the problems of coming to terms with death and of what happens after death.

Nevertheless, there are significant cultural and ethical beliefs surrounding the notion of death which have to be considered when formulating guidelines for determining death. Principles requiring respect for autonomy and beneficence support an ethical imperative to maintain a distinction between the living and the dead. It is as wrong to treat the living as dead as it is to treat the dead as alive. Many practical consequences are bound up with this imperative; there are legal and political requirements to maintain a distinction between the rights and obligations appropriate to the living and the duties to the deceased. There is a need for relatives to be spared unnecessary doubts, and there is a need for doctors to know when to cease treating a patient and issue a death certificate authorizing disposal of a corpse.

In view of alleged difficulties in determining the precise moment of death some philosophers have adopted a skeptical attitude, maintaining that a definition of death is an unnecessary requirement (2). Others (3) have argued that the determination of death should be based on a contractual agreement between doctors and patients. Against this 'skepticism' it is necessary to point out that such a policy flies in the face of cultural expectations. No society is prepared to tolerate a state of ignorance concerning the boundary between life and death, or situations where the fact of death is subject to barter.

DEFINING DEATH

The definition of death is primarily a philosophical and moral matter. This is because technical data alone cannot answer purely conceptual questions. An acceptable medical definition should not be incompatible with cultural and religious beliefs about life and death. The following guidelines specify cultural and moral aspects of a definition of death.

A Definition of Death Must Refer to a Recognizable and Irreversible Physical Transformation

Any valid concept of death must be linked to an irreversible physical change in the status of the individual which can be clearly and unambiguously determined by empirical means. It must follow that if a patient, declared dead according to a particular concept, were to recover, it should not be said that he or she was dead but is now alive again, but rather that he or she was alive all the time but mistakenly diagnosed as dead. The appeal to 'irreversibility' is only superficially at odds with accounts of miracles and Divine intervention. Cole (4) appeals to miraculous reversals to demonstrate the logical possibility of death-reversal as part of a critique of the concept of 'irreversibility' in medical concepts of death. If this merely means that one can speak of 'death-reversal' without implying a contradiction, nothing of any practical importance is at stake. Both the miraculous and the 'logically possible' fall outside the practical expectations of mortals who seek a definition which specifies an irreversible state based on acceptable and plausible scientific knowledge. The logical possibility of Divine intervention (or of doctors based on far-away planets who can reassemble and revitalize long-dead corpses) has no place in a definition of death and cannot be considered here. It should, however, be stressed that the medical requirement of irreversibility is perfectly compatible with religious beliefs in resurrection and afterlife. Religious beliefs concerning 'immortality' are unaffected by concepts and criteria which determine the cessation of *this* life, and the possibility of spending eternity in heaven or hell is not a repudiation of medical knowledge. Moreover, no religious authority would forbid proper disposal of a corpse on the grounds of a possible Divine (and beneficent) intervention.

A Definition of Death Must Be Selective

Strictly speaking, from a biological point of view, death is a process. It begins when one or more vital organs cease functioning and ends when the whole organism has decayed, when every single cell in the body is undergoing putrefaction. Definitions of death have been selective: they have referred to the loss of functions and not to the destruction of structures. Vital functions are often irreversibly lost *before* the cells dissolve into decay.

In practice, and throughout history, doctors have not sought to diagnose the death of the whole organism. They have sought to identify a stage in the ongoing course of events when the individual organism no longer functions as an integrated whole. It has long been recognized that residual functions may persist after death, that muscles may respond to percussion for several hours, and that tissues such as skin, bone or arterial wall, may remain viable for transplantation purposes for a day or more. In this important respect brain-related criteria of death do not mark a significant departure from the traditional cardio-centric approach. Spinal reflexes may persist beyond the death of a brain, and in fact do so when no cardiac activity can any longer be demonstrated.

It is therefore essential, when considering criteria of death, that a sharp distinction be maintained between (a) death (irreversible loss of function) of the whole organism (total destruction of every cell) and (b) death of the organism as a whole. The former has never operated in practice.

A Definition of Death Must Be Universal and Holistic

The requirement for universality implies that criteria must be unambiguous and the results of tests repeatable. It also implies that the mechanism of death be the same for all people whether in the backwoods or in the most sophisticated intensive care unit of a university hospital.

When cultural beliefs and values are considered it is clear that significance is attached to both mental and physical attributes of the dying person. A definition of death which disregards continuous mental functioning is morally unacceptable. The same might be said for a concept of death which disregards essential physical functions such as spontaneous respiration—although some formulations of the definition by Gervais (3) and Puccetti (5) have questioned the significance of this function. A holistic definition, in keeping with most theological and secular beliefs, should be non-reductionist and include both mental and physical functions, recognizing that among the important features of life are integration and organization (6). Thus death is not strictly equated with the loss of the vital function of any one or more organs, but with the loss of the capacity to *organize* and *integrate* vital functions. The claim that the elimination of certain functions— for example, those of the skin, liver, heart, and kidneys—may lead to death is not the same as saying that the loss of those functions *is* death. An individual undergoing dialysis is not dead, although she may well die if she forgoes dialysis. But she will then die—directly or indirectly—of the cerebral consequences of renal failure. The functioning of the organism as a whole will have been irreversibly compromised.

THE CONCEPT, CRITERIA, AND TESTS FOR DEATH

There are many concepts of death operating at different levels. There is the legal fiction, used in wartime, of 'missing presumed dead', the religious concept of separation of soul from body, and the Brahmin concept, implicit in the belief, that 'marriage outside the social group' is death, which even involved funeral ritual. These concepts may be significant to lawyers, theologians and anthropologists, but they do not yield criteria that can be used in a medical context. The missing person cannot be clinically examined, the soul cannot be anatomically located, and although married outside one's caste one can still pass a stringent clinical examination that would satisfy a life insurance office.

A definition of death should be specific as to its context. In a medical context an appropriate definition must refer to basic biological functions. The preference for a medically grounded concept of death is bound up with its universality. Poets and moralists employ numerous concepts of death which derive their meaning from the various issues they address. The expression 'cowards die a thousand deaths' makes a significant moral point about the psychology of fear, but in an intensive care unit there should be only one death which applies to all humankind.

Yet even in the medical context the borderline between life and death is not a matter to be determined exclusively by medical science. A definition of death involves a philosophical perspective. This will become apparent as soon as one perceives the distinction between the concept of death, and criteria and tests for death. A concept of death is primarily a philosophical matter, as is the decision that it is to rest purely on empirical considerations. Although pitched at a certain level of abstraction a definition of death must indicate its scope, exclude esoteric considerations, retain a sense of universality, and stress the practical relationship between the concept of death and certain functions of the body.

The criteria of death refer to specific functions which must be totally and irreversibly lost. The tests for death involve the examination procedures used to ascertain whether the criteria have been met. Both criteria and tests must be unambiguous, depending upon accepted medical and biological facts. The tests should be straightforward, reliable and repeatable; they should mutually support one another and produce a clear yes/no answer. Criteria and tests for death—and arguments about better criteria and tests—are meaningless unless related to some overall concept of what death means. Table 87.1 indicates the relationship between concept, criteria and tests in a number of contexts.

TABLE 87.1 Relationships between concept, criteria and tests

Concept	Criteria	Tests
1. Separation of soul from body	No criteria	No tests
2. Irreversible loss of function of the whole organism	Irreversible metabolic arrest in every cell of the body	Microscopic evidence of severe ultra-structural damage in every cell of the body
3. Irreversible loss of the capacity to maintain circulation	Irreversible cardiac standstill	No recordable pulse or blood pressure; asystole on ECG
4. Irreversible loss of personhood	Loss of higher brain function, mental function	'Isoelectric' EEG, PET scan abnormalities
5. Irreversible loss of integrated functioning of the organism as a whole	Irreversible loss of brainstem function (irreversible apnoea with loss of the capacity for consciousness)	Clinical signs of a non-functioning brainstem, in the context of specified preconditions and exclusions

COMMENTARY

The Separation of the Soul from the Body

This concept does not yield empirical criteria and tests.

The Irreversible Loss of Function of the Whole Organism (i.e. Every Cell in the Body)

This concept could not be seriously proposed in any medical context. Although it meets the requirement of irreversibility it does not meet the need for selectivity, and fails to rise to the requirement for a holistic view of humankind. The implication of this concept is that the function of each individual cell is as important as that of any other cell or of all cells functioning together. It reduces the characteristics of life to those of chemical metabolism. While chemical metabolism is clearly necessary to produce the energy that sustains life, there is clearly more to life than a series of chemical equations.

The Irreversible Loss of the Capacity to Maintain Circulation

It will be argued in the following section that failure to maintain circulation is not, strictly speaking, a concept of death. Whether they realize it or not, proponents of cardio-centric concepts of death are in fact arguing that irreversible cardiac standstill is part of the criteria of the death of the brain. Loss of cardiac function is a necessary but not a sufficient indicator of death, as an individual's heart may irreversibly cease, only to be replaced by an artefact or transplant. This concept therefore fails to meet the condition of irreversibility; it fails to capture important features of life, such as integration and organization, and is reductionist in that its key indicators of life—heartbeat and circulation—can be maintained by machines long after any semblance of integrated life has ceased. The fact that the elimination of circulatory functions *leads to* death does not justify the conclusion that the loss of those functions *is* death. The same might be said for the loss of the function of other organs and tissues such as the liver, kidneys, or skin. The requirement for selectivity is not met either, as the definition does not indicate why circulation is more important than any other function. A definition should capture some of the distinctive features of life; it is not sufficient simply to record the loss of certain physical functions.

Irreversible Loss of Personhood

This formulation of the concept of death is sometimes described as an 'ontological definition' (3). For personal identity theorists the loss of mental functions, capacity for speech, observation, abstract thought, and meaningful interaction with other beings and the environment are deemed to be necessary and sufficient indicators of death. Residual functions, such as spontaneous respiration, are not considered to be significant features of life. Criteria for loss of personhood are often bound up with loss of higher brain functions, such as the cerebral cortex (7). According to this formulation patients in persistent vegetative states and anencephalic infants could be diagnosed as dead. Personal identity theories of death have found popularity among philosophers, but so far no medical authority in the world has adopted them for diagnosing death, although Green and Wikler (8) have made a strong case for regarding loss of personhood as a condition where a being should be allowed to die. Critics (9,10) argue that the criterion is indeterminate, and that it conflicts with the holistic view of humankind which requires absence of both mental and integrated physical functions. The following objections have been made against ontological definitions.

1. The condition of irreversibility cannot be guaranteed. There are—mainly anecdotal—reports of reversals of persistent vegetative states. One widely reported case involved an American woman, Mrs Carrie Coons, who in 1989 regained consciousness following five and a half months in what was described as an 'irreversible vegetative state' (11, 12).
2. Because of the inherent vagueness of personal identity criteria it is believed that such a definition would introduce qualitative criteria to the diagnosis of death; in some cases obliterating the distinction between termination of therapy when the patient is dead and euthanasia.
3. Whereas definitions specifying loss of circulatory function are excessively concerned with physical functions, an ontological definition can be criticized on the opposite grounds; namely that it is excessively concerned with mental functions at the expense of the physical.
4. There are also problems in establishing an empirical connection between ontological definitions and functions of organs in the body. At the present state of knowledge it is not possible to identify the *exact* parts of the brain responsible for mental function. Whilst mental function requires a brain, it can nevertheless be maintained with an impaired brain. This leads to 'sorites' objections concerning the amount of impairment before mental function is deemed to have been sufficiently lost to warrant loss of personhood. There are, for example, problems involving borderline cases (such as profound dementia) where there is progressively impaired mental function.

Irreversible Loss of Integrated Function of the Organism as a Whole

This definition overcomes the shortcomings of previous definitions. Its starting point is the view that a living being is an integrated whole, and that death is the loss of that which is required to enable continuous function as an independent biological unit capable of responding to both its external and internal environment. This requires loss of *both* the mental and physical features of integrated life, including loss of respiration—and hence loss of heartbeat—and irreversible loss of the capacity for consciousness. This definition is selective in that it focuses on coordination between different functions rather than the totality of function. Life as an integrated whole is not measured by the ability of certain organs to go on functioning in a ventilated corpse, or mechanically animated in a laboratory detached from a body, or after transplantation in someone else's body. Hearts, lungs, kidneys and livers can all be replaced and the wholeness of an individual be retained. Certain limbs and non-vital organs can be excised and the wholeness of an individual be retained. But the brain, the critical system, which coordinates and integrates organic function, is irreplaceable. A definition of death in terms of the *'irreversible loss of integrated function of the organism as a whole'*, yields empirical criteria based on the function of the brain as a whole. The brain governs mental functions, such as consciousness, intellectual activity and memory.

From the brain autonomous physical functions, such as respiration, blood-pressure control, and thermostat are regulated. So are the vital functions performed by the heart and lungs. When the brain is dead the integration of mental and physical functions is terminated. Although respiration and circulation may be artificially maintained for a limited period, and spontaneous heartbeat may survive brain death for a few minutes, and some cells may metabolize for several days, these are isolated functions without cohesion.

The empirical criterion for this concept of death is the irreversible cessation of brain function as an integrated whole. This refers to the cessation of brain function, not to the dissolution of the brain's biological structures. It means that the death of the brain occurs *before* total necrosis. It should, however, be stressed that the definition is aimed at the death of the individual as a whole, not the death of a particular organ. In this respect the expression 'brain death'— suggestive of the death of a specific organ—has generated confusion, implying a special kind of death. This confusion has been compounded with reference to other anatomically specific 'deaths', such as 'neo-cortical death' and 'cerebral death'. Properly understood, criteria for the death of a brain are met only when the individual can no longer function as an integrated whole. The expression 'brain death' refers to the loss of a critical system which integrates and activates component systems.

THE EMERGENCE OF THE CONCEPT OF BRAIN DEATH

An acceptable definition of death, it has been argued, must specify an irreversible state. It must be selective, such that death can be recognized before total destruction of all cellular components. It must also reflect a holistic view of life, recognizing that life is essentially bound up with the capacity to organize and integrate essential functions. At a general level the concept of death can be formulated as 'the irreversible cessation of integrated functioning of the organism as a whole'; at a specific level the expression 'brain death' makes the empirical connection between the definition and the functions of the body. From this standpoint the challenge of a brain-related formulation to the traditional cardiorespiratory concept of death can be assessed.

During the 1950s and 1960s developments in the technology of intensive care undermined confidence in the traditional cardiorespiratory concept and redirected attention towards neurological criteria. Improvements in resuscitation technology meant that thousands of pulseless and apnoeic patients could be restored to fully conscious states. Although some at the time interpreted this as resurrection, the prevailing cultural view was that as the condition was reversible, temporary cardiorespiratory standstill was not equated with death. In recent years a sub-field of research has developed in which the experiences of patients undergoing temporary cardiorespiratory suspension have been described as 'near-death experiences' (13), thus implicitly recognizing that death had not occurred.

However, success in cardiorespiratory reversal generated a major scientific and ethical problem: the problem of the 'beating heart cadaver', where ventilation to asystole was becoming distressing to doctors and relatives as a clear boundary between life and death was no longer apparent. It later became obvious that the artificial continuation of cardiac and respiratory activity, in certain conditions where brain function had irreversibly ceased, was not equated with the maintenance of life, and was of no benefit to the patient. In cases of this kind conventional cardiorespiratory criteria had proven incapable of giving a clear and unambiguous answer to the question of the borderline between life and death, and a reassessment of traditional cardiorespiratory criteria was inevitable.

The way forward lay in considering the importance of the brain. Notwithstanding the emotional significance of the heart the significance of the brain as both the unit of consciousness and cognition, and as the organizing faculty of the body 'as a whole', has long been recognized. For centuries human beings have decapitated and hung or beaten the heads of their unfortunate fellows in the knowledge that a brain sufficiently damaged or separated from its body was equivalent to death. The connection between brain function and those of the respiratory and circulatory organs is straightforward. First, spontaneous respiration is dependent upon brain function. Second, the brain is dependent upon a supply of oxygenated blood. With total brain infarction spontaneous respiration is ruled out, although in certain circumstances respiration can be artificially maintained for a few hours or days. If the brain has been deprived of oxygen (for example, due to cardiac arrest) for about 15 to 20 minutes, then its functions will be totally and irreversibly lost, never to be replaced by surgery, medication or technical aids. These elementary facts are not new, and were known long before criteria for brain death were proposed. But resuscitation technology led to a re-assessment of the connection between brain function and the respiratory and circulatory organs. What did emerge from the 1950s was the awareness that intervention could make it possible to prevent the brain from succumbing to cardiac and respiratory arrest on the one hand, and make it possible, on the other hand, artificially to maintain the heartbeat and circulation of blood in a body whose brain had ceased to function as an integrated whole. In short: the natural link between the function of the brain and the heart and lungs had been severed.

During the 1960s and 1970s the majority of countries throughout the world adopted criteria which referred to the cessation of brain functions. None have returned to the traditional cardiorespiratory concept. However, during this time there was uncertainty regarding the legal status of neurological criteria for death, and in a minority of cases attempts were made to retain both the cardiorespiratory concept and brain-related concepts. During the early 1970s Kansas operated a dualistic standard, whereby a patient could be diagnosed as dead according to either cardiorespiratory criteria or brain-related criteria, thus introducing the ambiguous prospect of being alive in one hospital but dead in another (9,14).

In Sweden an attempt was made to adapt traditional criteria to the new circumstances, such that 'decisive importance was attached to the possibility of maintaining—spontaneously or artificially—a circulation of oxygenated blood in the human organism' (ref. 15, p. 25). Some philosophers still find this approach to be relevant (16), and whilst emotive appeals can be made to 'pink perfused bodies' there are significant problems with it, as indicated when the Swedish Royal Commission recommended a brain-oriented approach.

In 1984 the Report of the Swedish Royal Committee on Defining Death made the following criticisms of a definition based on absence of circulation. First, they argued that the idea of basing criteria for death on the sophisticated technology required, rather than on biological facts, is foreign to most medical personnel. Second, it was argued that circulatory criteria engender uncertainty with personnel unclear whether they were dealing with alive or dead patients. Doctors were unclear whether or not to discontinue treatment and unclear on what to communicate to the next of kin. The report concluded that the traditional criteria, even when 'adapted', were 'no longer compatible with the need for scientific tenability. Nor do they meet reasonable demands of unambiguity' (ref. 15, p. 25).

Given the potential reversibility of states associated with the traditional cardiorespiratory concept only a brain-related concept yields necessary and sufficient criteria for the death of the organism as an integrated whole. Although loss of circulation has for centuries been considered a 'point of no return', providing acceptable criteria for a diagnosis of death, it does not amount to a satisfactory concept of death. This is because cessation of heartbeat and circulation is lethal only if it lasts long enough to cause critical centres in the brainstem to die. If the heart function can be replaced in time then death will not occur. But the brain is irreplaceable in a way that the cardiac pump is not. This is not a newly discovered fact but simply a rearrangement of what has been long known. Strictly speaking, brain death is neither a new concept nor an alternative one. It is a reformulation of the traditional concept according to which loss of heartbeat and circulation is not a state of death itself, but an indication (in certain cases where ventilatory support is absent) of the imminence of death. That is to say, according to a brain-related concept of death, criteria such as loss of heartbeat, respiration and pulse, acquire a different status. They are indicators regarding the state of the brain; for the patient is alive until the brain is dead.

FROM BRAIN DEATH TO BRAINSTEM DEATH

Whilst the past 25 years have seen the gradual acceptance of the proposition that death of the brain yields both necessary and sufficient criteria for death of the organism as a whole, the past 15 years have seen a parallel development: the gradual realization that death of the brainstem is a necessary and sufficient condition for the death of the brain as a whole—and that brainstem death itself is therefore synonymous with death of the organism as a whole. The brain is the critical system of the living organism; the brainstem is the critical system of the brain. 'Death of the brain occurs when the organ irreversibly loses its capacity to maintain the vital integrative functions regulated by the vegetative and consciousness-mediating centres of the brainstem' (17). Brainstem death signifies the death of the brain as a whole, not death of the whole brain. It has been described as 'the physiological core of brain death' (18). From this standpoint residual cellular activity following irreversible cessation of brainstem function does not indicate the persistence of life.

Brainstem death is a clinical concept: 'It implies an irreversibly unconscious patient with irreversible apnoea and irreversible loss of brainstem reflexes' (ref. 19, p. 443). It must be stressed that the term 'brainstem death' does not refer to pathological changes which are confined to the brainstem. Although brainstem death may very occasionally occur as a primary event it is, in the vast majority of cases, the result of massive increase in intracranial pressure which produces the crucial clinical signs—apneoic coma and absent brainstem reflexes—which are detected in an intensive care unit when brain death is diagnosed.

The significance of brainstem criteria can be appreciated with reference to the brainstem's contribution to the continuous integrated function of the organism as a whole. In its upper part the brainstem contains crucial centres for generating the capacity for consciousness. Thus whilst extensive damage to the cortex, from trauma or anoxia, may not cause permanent unconsciousness, there is one functional unit without whose activity consciousness cannot exist. This is the ascending reticular activating system, or ARAS, which is a function of the upper part of the brainstem. Acute, strategically situated bilateral lesions in the paramedian tegmental area of the rostral brainstem entail loss of the capacity for consciousness. In the lower part of the brainstem are mechanisms which control the respiratory centre. Thus lesions of critical areas in the lower part of the brainstem are associated with the permanent cessation of the ability to breathe, which in turn deprives the heart and cerebral hemispheres of oxygen, causing them to cease functioning.

A brain starved of oxygen cannot function. Loss of heartbeat and circulation for between 15 and 20 minutes will therefore provide *indirect* criteria for brainstem death. For the majority of deaths outside an intensive-care unit cardiorespiratory criteria will provide adequate *indirect* criteria for death. On the other hand *direct* criteria and tests for brainstem death require neurological examination.

THE DIAGNOSIS OF DEATH IS A CONTEXT-RELATED ACTIVITY

The requirement for irreversibility is crucial to the employment of criteria and tests for brainstem death. Meeting this requirement is a context-related activity undertaken in the knowledge of what is plausible and practical. An unfettered imagination can quite easily manufacture scenarios where any pathological state can be reversed, but the determination of death in an intensive care unit must operate within the constraints of existing reality. To meet the requirement for irreversibility a battery of conditions have been formulated. 'There must be a known and sufficient "primary diagnosis" to account for the patient's condition, and all reversible causes of brain dysfunction must have been excluded' (ref. 19, p. 443). Satisfying the requirement for irreversibility may take time, appropriate to the particular context. Thus: 'The passage of sufficient time and resort to all relevant therapeutic measures are also essential components of irreversibility' (ref. 19, p. 443).

The essential criteria and tests for a dead brainstem have evolved over the past 20 years (18–22). Tests involving EEG measurements or angiographic tests for cerebral circulatory arrest are not considered essential to the determination of brainstem death, despite the popularity of high technology in the media. A flat, or more correctly, an isoelectric EEG reading is of no significance in the diagnosis of brainstem death. A recording taken from the scalp gives little information about brainstem activity; it only records the activity of a small proportion of cortical neurones. Patients with electro-cerebral silence have been known to recover and even walk out of hospital within 48 hours of the initial injury. On the other hand an EEG reading can be obtained from a decapitated head or a slice of brain tissue in a Petri dish, thus raising the question to what concept of death does the EEG relate?

Patients have also survived negative angiographic tests and 'no-flow situations' have—in some cases—been reversed (19). There are also clinical problems over the conducting of angiography tests, such as the problem of moving ventilator-dependent patients to X-ray departments, and there are problems of assessing the significance of reduced, but not totally absent, blood flow. In some instances angiographic tests are invasive and carry the risk of creating the very condition that they have been employed to diagnose.

The guidelines for the diagnosis of a dead brainstem have been documented by Pallis (18,19), who recommends a clinical rather than an instrumental approach, and are worth recapitulating. They involve three steps: (a) ascertaining that certain *preconditions* have been met; (b) ensuring that all reversible causes of a non-functioning brainstem have been *excluded*; and (c) establishing by clinical bedside *tests*, carried out at the right time, that the comatose patient is genuinely apnoeic and that brainstem reflexes are absent. The objective is to determine that the condition is irremediable. This can be achieved only with reference to the context. It is therefore crucial to make sure that the tests are carried out only on the right patients at the right time. Unless the patient has passed through this 'double filter' of *preconditions* and *exclusions* the tests are invalid. The three crucial stages are as follows:

Preconditions

Ascertaining that the patient is comatose and on a ventilator and that a diagnosis of the responsible condition is 'fully documented and unequivocally accurate' (17). There must also be irremediable structural brain damage. The judgement that there is irremediable damage should be made only after vigorous attempts to remedy it. This, again, will take time, involving repeated attempts at resuscitation.

Exclusions

The exclusion of reversible causes of a non-functioning brainstem, among which are hypothermia and drug intoxication. Both time and context are crucial. A boxer knocked out in a ring, later lapsing into a coma, may be easier and quicker to assess for exclusions than a drunk who has sustained head injury in a brawl, for it may take up to six or eight hours to exclude the sedative aspects of alcohol intoxication. If drug intoxication is suspected then access to a drug-screening centre will be significant. If it is not available: 'it is reasonable to allow 72 hours to elapse for matters to sort themselves out' (ref. 19, p. 472). By that time if the brainstem is dead then asystole may very well have developed.

Tests

The conducting of tests, at the right time, to ascertain that the comatose patient is genuinely apnoeic with absent brainstem reflexes. This entails an 'unhurried' approach with an attitude that ventilation of the comatose patient should continue 'for as long as it takes to ascertain that the preconditions have been met, and that all conditions that have to be excluded have in fact been properly excluded' (ref. 19, p. 472). This will vary from case to case and may take 24 hours or more. The objective of the tests is to ascertain absence of brainstem functions and rigorously document apnoea. This entails a battery of tests, such that the determination of death does not depend upon a single procedure or the assessment of a single function (ref. 19, p. 473). For this reason it is a mistake to perceive brainstem death as the loss of a particular organ, or to conduct arguments about the accuracy of the tests independent of the context.

INDEPENDENCE OF CRITERIA FOR DEATH

It is important, both scientifically and morally, to maintain a clear separation between the concept and criteria for death on the one hand and extraneous factors on the other hand. Matters relating to the cost of therapy, poor prognosis, quality of life, arguments for euthanasia, and the need to procure transplant organs, are all fundamentally distinct from criteria for death. Criteria for death must be related exclusively to the condition of the patient. Thus proposals to classify patients in persistent vegetative states, or anencephalic infants with functioning brainstems as dead, for the purpose of early organ removal, seriously confuse arguments about the definition of death with other extraneous needs. Too often proponents of brain-oriented definitions of death have spoken of the benefits of harvesting organs from brain-dead donors. Thus their opponents have gone on to accuse them of gerrymandering the definition of death in order to facilitate early organ removal. A common criticism of brainstem death is that an interest in organ procurement put pressure on neurologists and neurosurgeons to redefine death. This was not the case. In the 1950s, long before cardiac transplantation, when renal transplants were highly experimental, conducted only on genetically identical twins, with massive irradiation of the recipient, there were profound ethical discussions concerning the value of ventilation to asystole when treatment for patients in irreversible apnoeic coma was obviously hopeless and increasingly gruesome.

To maintain independence of brain-related criteria for death it is therefore important that statutes and guidelines for brain death should specify that the primary interest in formulating a definition of death is to recognize a morally significant boundary between the duties owed to a living patient and those which are appropriate to a corpse. Any baiting of the definition of death with extraneous benefits will only taint the scientific purity of the case for brainstem death, and introduce the notion that an individual's death can be determined by societal needs. In some cases to allay public anxiety about criteria for death it has been suggested that additional tests be conducted when organ transplantation is envisaged. This kind of public relations exercise should be resisted as it forges an unnecessary link between criteria for death and the requirement for organs. It is misleading to propose either looser or more stringent criteria for diagnosing the death of organ donors, as this would entail the absurd suggestion that there is a special kind of death awaiting them.

Sophisticated technology in intensive care units has confronted us with a need to understand and define death. If transplant surgery were outlawed, if a supply of artificial organs eliminated all need for human cadaver organs, if the costs of maintaining patients for prolonged periods in intensive care units were dramatically reduced, there would still be a need for precise guidelines on brain death. The need for a definition of death is a by-product of medical science, and objective criteria for death are essential for the cessation of therapy, but the primary reason in formulating objective criteria must be strictly limited to the interests of the dying individual.

REFERENCES

1. Fatteh, A. 1977. 'Dead' woman allowed to die: a unique case in Florida. *Journal of Legal Medicine*, January, p. 24.
2. Browne, A. 1991. Defining death. Pp. 312–321, *in* Almond, B. and Hill, D. (Eds) *Applied philosophy*. Routledge, London.
3. Gervais, K. G. 1987. *Redefining death*. Yale University Press, New Haven.
4. Cole, D. J. 1991. The reversibility of death. *Journal of Medical Ethics*, 3: 25–29.
5. Puccetti, R. 1988. Does anyone survive neocortical death? Pp. 75–90, *in* Zaner, R. M. (Ed.) *Death: beyond whole brain criteria*. Kluwer, Dordrecht.
6. Lamb, D. 1979. *Hegel: from foundation to system*. Kluwer, Dordrecht.
7. Zaner, R. M. 1988. Introduction. *Death: beyond whole brain criteria*, pp. 1–14. Kluwer, Dordrecht.
8. Green, M. B. and Wikler, D. 1981. Brain death and personal identity. Pp. 49–77, *in* Cohen, M., Nagel, T. and Scanlon, T. (Eds) *Medicine and moral philosophy* Princeton University Press, New Jersey.
9. Lamb, D. 1985. *Death, brain death and ethics*. Routledge, London.
10. Lamb, D. 1990. *Organ transplants and ethics*. Routledge, London.
11. Ackerman, F. 1991. The significance of a wish, *Hastings Center Report* 21 (4): 27–29.
12. Steinbock, B. 1989. Recovery from the persistent vegetative state? The case of Carrie Coons'. *Hastings Center report* 19 (4): 14–15.
13. Woodhouse, M. 1992. Philosophy and frontier science: is there a new paradigm in the making? Pp. 26–48 *in* Lamb, D. (Ed.). *New horizons in the philosophy of science*. Gower, Aldershot.
14. Kennedy, I. 1971. The Kansas Statute on Death: an appraisal. *New England Journal of Medicine* 285: 946–950.
15. Report of the Swedish Committee on Defining Death. 1984. *The concept of death: summary*. Swedish Ministry of Health and Social Affairs, Stockholm.
16. Evans, M. 1991. Death in Denmark. *Journal of Medical Ethics* 16: 191–194. (See also Chapter 88, this volume.)
17. Plum, F. and Posner, J. B. 1982. *The diagnosis of stupor and coma*, 3rd edn. F. A. Davies, Philadelphia, PA.
18. Pallis, C. 1983. *The ABC of brainstem death*. BMJ, London.
19. Pallis, C. 1990. Brainstem death. Pp. 441–496, *in* Vinken, P. J., Bruyn, G. W. and Klawans, H. L., (Eds) Coedited by Braakman, R., *Handbook of clinical neurology*, Volume 57, Revised Series 13, *Head injury*. Elsevier, Amsterdam.
20. Conference of Medical Royal Colleges and their Faculties in the UK. 1976. Diagnosis of brain death, *British Medical Journal*, 2: 1187–1188.
21. Conference of Medical Royal Colleges and their Faculties in the UK. 1979. Memorandum on the diagnosis of death, *British Medical Journal* 1: 322.
22. President's Commission for the study of Ethical Problems in Medicine and Biomedical and Behavioural Research. 1981. *Defining death*. US Government Printing Office, Washington, DC.

88

Against Brainstem Death

MARTYN EVANS, BA, PhD

University College Fellow, Centre for Philosophy and Health Care, University College of Swansea, Wales

A horse-drawn cart stands, in the streaming rain of a bitter morning, beside a gaping hole in the ground. Two men pull a crude wooden box from the cart and, holding it over the edge of the pit, tip out the coarse-woven sack it contains. The sack slides out and lands heavily in the pit, on a heap of other such sacks. A third man scatters a few shovelsful of quicklime over the heap, then all three rejoin the cart and the horses haul them and it away into the veiled morning. The pit yawns for its next delivery.

An unremarkable series of events except for two details: the sack contains the body of a man, and the man is Wolfgang Amadeus Mozart. The power of this, the penultimate scene of the film version of Peter Schaffer's *Amadeus*, is therefore two-fold: the horror of the final indignity of a pauper's death is compounded by the fact that the man who has suffered this indignity has given the world incomparable musical riches. Two hundred years on from the events portrayed, we recoil both at the moral injury which it seems is done to any man who is thus discarded in death—and at the moral injustice of this having happened to, of all people, Mozart. Anyone who has felt the power of this scene has experienced aesthetically what we know in fact and substance: the human body is worthy of moral concern and respect even in death; it matters morally how we treat the dead.

I have begun this chapter with a visual image, a picture. It is central to the view of human death which I shall set out here that what we *see* is both the key to many of our moral judgements, and also to a very large extent beyond the reach of either moral analysis or scientific explanation. To put this at its simplest, when we are confronted by human remains, we are confronted with something which most of us know we should *without question* treat with respect— be it the body of Mozart or the body of the humblest stranger. No moral theory or analysis can plausibly supply us with the foundations of this respect: moral theories must start by presupposing our holding of at least some moral values,

Principles of Health Care Ethics. Edited by Raanan Gillon.
© 1994 John Wiley & Sons Ltd

and the idea of respect for the human body seems too central and universal to permit explanation. It would be as odd as to ask for a theoretical account of why generosity (or beneficence or justice) is virtuous: the answer can be no more than 'this is just the sort of thing that a virtue *is*'. Equally science is powerless to account for moral values: although anthropology or neurology may be able to describe the role of a respect for the deceased in terms of social development or the mechanisms of emotional reaction, what makes the human body *in itself* worthy of respect is something that can be expressed only in moral terms. Thus the picture of the human body, trussed in a rough sack and tossed into a pit without ceremony or tenderness, claims our moral attention regardless of whether social utility, public hygiene, or the view that pity is a chemical phenomenon within our nervous systems, invite us to pass it by.

The view that I shall develop in this chapter—which is concerned with defining human death as well as with responding to it—is that the particular, the concrete, the *seen* can in certain contexts have decisive moral force over against what we are told about the abstract, the underlying, the theoretical, the causal, the unseen: and further that the definition of death places us in a context of precisely this kind. What we see—the way that we react to and describe what we see—is determined by values rooted in our cultural and moral traditions. Those values stand beyond theoretical explanation.

My first picture confronted us with our responses to a human body; my second picture confronts us with the question of whether we recognize that body as dead at all. The scene is as before; but a second sack, pitched onto the heap, bursts open as it lands. From the edge of the pit the body it contains can quite clearly be seen. The bloody gulf in the head marks the mortal wound. But enough of the unfortunate's flesh is visible to reveal the body as pink; the vapours rising from it in the chilly air suggest the warmth of the very-recently dead. Upon examination it is obvious that the man is not breathing, nor will again; but his flesh is warm and is perfused by a still-beating heart. This time we recoil in horror of a different sort: the man who is being buried is not dead!

Thus, at any rate, our reaction. The moral horror of this second scene is—according to our reaction—the treatment of the still-living as though already dead. Yet modern conceptions of death, available to us through the advances of medical science, challenge us to reconsider our reaction: not by questioning the proper treatment of the still-living, but by asking whether our classification of the living and the dead is adequate to the new knowledge that science has given us, and to the special and emergent circumstances which it can describe. In such a case, then, science challenges not so much our moral *judgements about* what we see as *what it is* that we think we see. The moral horror of treating the living as though they were dead is not in dispute; what is in dispute is that this is such a case, for science denies that what we see in the pit is a living human being. The death of the pauper was the death of his brain, beyond which any persistent heartbeat has no purpose, no function and no meaning. Our horror, says science, was misplaced: a relic of our ignorance about the heart's true role.

By contrast my own claim is that the information which science makes available to us regarding the beating heart's role is of merely secondary interest compared to the place which the beating heart has in our culture's conceptions of the life and death of a human being; our seeing this beating heart as counting for life is a commitment to a certain moral regard for the human being as a whole, a regard which it is beyond the reach of science to dispel. In stressing the heart's functional subordinance to the brain, science is describing a causal or mechanical role for the heart. Whereas in seeing the beating heart as 'counting for life'(1), I express a commitment to a certain kind of respect for the human body as a whole, in which the beating heart occupies a role recognized and understood by our culture as central.

How could this conflict of understandings be settled? Clearly appeals to further scientific information are unlikely to persuade where the existing—and vastly powerful—revelations of physiology and neurology are not already conclusive. For the question of the *human meaning* of the beating heart is not of course a scientific question. Equally clearly, I think, appeals to moral *principles* cannot settle the question either. To benefit someone or to avoid or remove harms on their behalf is possible only if they are capable of being harmed or benefited: invoking duties of welfare (or beneficence) and protection (or non-maleficence) on their behalf is already to presume that they are so capable. Principles such as these can therefore tell us that we ought not to harm the living or (in an attentuated sense) the dead; they can also make it clear that it matters, morally, a very great deal that we correctly distinguish the living from the dead: but they cannot tell us *how to make this distinction*.

Faced with this impasse, my own response is to look as clearly as I can at the concrete, particular, visible aspects of what both science and morals describe in more abstract, theoretical terms. To complete my opening triptych of pictures, let me describe a third sack which is flung into the pit: on examination it contains, quite simply, a man with two obvious characteristics: he has an overwhelming head injury; and he is breathing. Even today there are relatively few doctors who would openly declare that such a man could be regarded as dead, whatever the state of the victim's brain and no matter how final the loss of consciousness, even of the conceivable possibility of consciousness (as when someone suffers catastrophic destruction of the cortex). Yet I hope to show that there is no convincing reason why those who accept the idea of 'brainstem death' can distinguish—as they do—between the moral significance of the persistent heartbeat and the moral significance of persistent breathing. That is to say, I hope to show that those who are morally undisturbed by my second picture, above, have no good reason to recoil from the third picture. (And reasons, be it noted, are important to them.) The corollary of this is that those who simply cannot bring themselves to entertain the third picture have very good reasons to abhor the second. I shall be asking them, in effect, to embrace more fully the *logic* of their view of the 'beating-heart cadaver'; or alternatively to take more seriously their *moral* reaction to the 'breathing corpse'. If I succeed in this, it will be partly because I will after all have managed to show that our moral reactions to what we see are in key respects beyond the reach of science to dispel: indeed, that in this context a picture can be decisively more powerful than an explanation.

DOES THE HEARTBEAT MATTER?

Consider a 'brainstem-dead' patient, in the intensive-therapy unit, from whom the ventilator has been disconnected for the second and final time, allowing a confirmatory apnoea test to be carried out and the declaration of 'brainstem death' to be made. This patient has a massive and lethal insult to the brain, has not regained consciousness since that insult five days previously, and has irreversibly lost the possibility of ever regaining consciousness. Neither will the patient ever breathe again—that capacity, too, is judged irreversibly lost. The patient, then, is still. Death having been declared, the behaviour which is appropriate towards the dead may now legally be instituted. We may lawfully do any of the following things to the dead: we may send them for post-mortem examination; we may send them to be 'laid out' in a funeral parlour; we may place them in varying degrees of visible display at the centre of a rite, public or private according to our custom; we may embalm them; we may bury them in the ground; we may cremate them in a furnace; we may remove their vital organs for transplantation into others. Since the 'brainstem dead' patient has been declared dead, we may do any of these things to such a patient. One very temporary obstacle may, however, present itself in the case of the 'brainstem dead' patient. Her heart may still, for a while, beat of its own accord.

Of the various kinds of death behaviour I have mentioned, there is one kind—the removal of organs for transplantation—for which this obstacle seems not to apply. (Indeed, it is important that it does not, since the continued spontaneous heartbeat is necessary for the supply of certain organs in transplantable condition; to maintain the heartbeat, and the perfusion of the organs and tissues with oxygenated blood, it is necessary to revert to the position immediately before the tests for 'brainstem death', and to re-connect the ventilator.) But with this conspicuous exception, I believe that I am expressing no more than an intuitive and widely held *conviction* that the persistence of a spontaneous heartbeat would—while it lasted—stand in the way of our doing any of the other things which I listed as appropriately done to the dead. I do not believe we would display, embalm, bury or cremate someone until her heart had stopped beating—because we would not until then *see her* as dead.

Of course we would not have to wait very long for this to happen once her breathing (artificially supported or not) had finally stopped. The final loss of her heartbeat and circulation follows the loss of respiration in fairly short order. In this sense it may be misleading to think of us as actually *waiting* for asystole, since we are rarely in so much of a hurry to begin 'death-behaviour' of the kinds I mentioned. Grieving might be an exception, but most of us know from personal experience that grieving is something that can meaningfully begin long before there is any suggestion that someone is dead in a clinical sense. Of the other kinds of death-behaviour, there is only one where haste of this kind is usual—for the successful procurement of transplantable organs, time is of the essence. But this is somewhat beside the point; for the heartbeat *can* persist for an hour or more; and before that time certain questions of the seemly treatment of the deceased may well arise. In such circumstances, does not evidence of a heartbeat give us pause? Does not the heartbeat in some sense matter?

My claim, then, is this: that whilst a heartbeat persists we would not, in any usual circumstances other than those of organ procurement, think it right to *treat as dead* someone in whom the heart persists spontaneously in beating. Such is the conceptual importance of the beating heart, that we would think it inappropriate—*morally* inappropriate, moreover—to count it for nothing where it persisted, and to begin our death-behaviour regardless of its presence. In short, I claim, the heartbeat does matter, and matters morally. If I am right, this presents an enduring problem for the application of 'brainstem death' as a definition of human death.

TESTING OUR CONVICTIONS

The challenge of brain-centred conceptions of death in general, and of the 'brainstem death' standard in particular, is one of many challenges which have been presented to us by the spectacular advances in modern medical science. In part, the stringency of this particular challenge arises from the explanatory force and power which scientific knowledge and understanding possess. Medical science is able to show us the relationships between human physiology and neurology on the one hand and the possibility of conscious human experience on the other. It can demonstrate beyond reasonable doubt that certain clinical conditions are incompatible with the possibility of human consciousness, and hence—at least, presumably (and this side of the grave)—of the possibility of any meaningfully human experience whatever. I do not wish to dispute that the conditions described as brainstem death are conditions of this kind, nor to doubt that the 'brainstem dead' patient has irreversibly lost the possibility of conscious human experience.

Now, if we take human experience to be at the core of human life in any meaningful sense—and again I do not wish to dispute this further claim—we might say that the final loss of the possibility of human experience marks the final loss of meaningful life. The question then arises whether this point is also the final loss of human life *as such*. I should say right away that I do not believe that it is any such thing. (It is tragically true that there can be human life without meaning. But life without meaning is life nonetheless.) Furthermore, prominent advocates of 'brainstem death' agree on this point: one such advocate regards death as combining the loss of the capacity for consciousness with the loss of the capacity for 'bodily integration' (2), while another insists that the final loss of human life *as such* is marked by the loss of not one but *two* specific capacities: the capacity for consciousness (and hence for meaningful life) and the capacity for spontaneous respiration.

> I conceive of human death as a state in which there is irreversible loss of the capacity for consciousness combined with irreversible loss of the capacity to breathe (and hence to maintain a heartbeat). Alone, neither would be sufficient (ref. 3, p. 2).

The precise role of this second capacity, the capacity for respiration, in their conception of human death is I think puzzling, and this is something that I will presently challenge. But first we should notice that these proponents are able to point out with great authority and detail that a 'brainstem dead' patient is in such a condition that the persistence of her heartbeat says little about the underlying condition of her brain. In particular, the persistent heartbeat gives us no conceivable grounds for hoping that some possibility of consciousness might be retained or might re-emerge. That hope is dashed by the disastrous neurological and physiological conditions of the patient's brain—conditions which are in themselves a necessary part of the establishment of the diagnosis of brainstem death. No-one, they point out, who is declared 'brainstem dead' has any hope of reprieve since their underlying condition was known, before the declaration was made, to be irremediable. Thus severed from any role in meaningfully human life, the persistent heartbeat (they say) is a detachable, irrelevant, arbitrary phenomenon on the margins of a vanished life: the echo of laughter in a now-empty hall.

If their view is correct, they will of course have no *conceptual* objection to any over-hasty examples of the kinds of death-behaviour which I rehearsed above. Unlikely though we may be ever to find ourselves in such a hurry, at any rate the beating heart gives us no compelling reason to delay our death-behaviour if what counts is that the dead be dead. For the proponents of the 'brainstem-death' view, the dead are indeed dead, heartbeat and all (and they have coined the term 'beating-heart cadaver' to prove it). In particular, and although they may find the relevant circumstances unlikely to arise, they can have no *conceptual* objection to a hypothetical action which I would myself take as sufficiently abominable as to be a *reductio ad absurdum* of the brainstem definition of death: the cremation of a beating-heart cadaver, persistent spontaneous heartbeat and all. To object that the horrible result is unlikely actually to occur is of course to avoid the moral challenge of thinking about exactly *why* the result would indeed be horrible. But thinking about this is, I believe, instructive: let us then spend a short while doing so.

Few would dispute that the cremation of a body whilst its heart continued to beat was in some sense a horrible thing; however proponents of brainstem death may wish to account for the horror either as evidence of unseemly haste (after all who would need to act so swiftly?) and a haste moreover which bespeaks little respect for the due processes of grieving; or as doctrinaire insensitivity, liable to upset an unscientific public who are ignorant of the facts of brainstem death (compare ref. 4). Of course both accounts point to properly moral concerns; but both miss the significance of the offence given to the public. For why is it that an unscientific public would be thus offended?— precisely because the human meaning of death and of the body's visible and palpable vital functions is public property, a matter of shared reactions and unspoken knowledge deeply ingrained in our culture: a common coinage and a common conviction that within that individual's warm and perfused body the beating heart must in its own right count for life, independent of its subservient connection to the brain (a connection which can, as science has shown us, be sundered). Thus the common conviction would be that to burn a body in which the heart yet beats is to burn one who yet lives, however tenuously, failingly and briefly: this is *part of the meaning of human life and death* in daily language.

Whilst science can cumulatively influence our common understandings of the world—and can accompany changes in our moral tradition—it does not own them. Science is after all itself simply a point of view, one way of being interested in the world: the laws of acoustics and of the harmonic series are no more real than are the tensions and resolutions in a Schubert song. Ultimately those descriptions pervade our common consciousness which are the most powerful; sometimes these are scientific descriptions and sometimes they are not. Although the image of the brain may one day usurp the image of the heart, it has not done so yet; and until it does then the proper conception of human death is that which is generally held and not that which some doctors—be it for theoretical conformity or for practical purpose—prefer.

I do believe, moreover, that some doctors who hold to the brainstem conception of human death might abandon it in the face of being asked to regard unequivocally as dead their own loved ones prior to asystole. That is, some doctors might test their scientific convictions in this moral *aqua regia* and find them to fail. But some might not; some might genuinely persist with the conviction that the heartbeat doesn't matter, finding my intended *reductio ad absurdum* to give them no discomfort. Since in effect they are not yet appalled by the second of my opening three pictures I wish now to return to the third, which I hope will reveal the durability of either their scientific understanding or their moral reactions.

DOES BREATHING MATTER?

The image of the still-breathing body in the pit derives part of its horror, no doubt, from the pitiless circumstances which surround it. That is, someone may object, it is not the idea of a breathing corpse as such which offends, but merely the casual and scornful treatment of it. Since my claim is that it is indeed the idea as such which offends, let me replace those distracting circumstances with the benevolent and compassionate circumstances of the clinical intensive care unit. The unfortunate patient is regarded as almost certainly 'brainstem dead' and the battery of confirmatory tests is being conducted. On disconnection from the ventilator, the patient seems to make slight movements resembling the movements of breathing. This patient is immediately reconnected to the ventilator, whilst doctors discuss what they have seen. Let us eavesdrop on their discussion.* The generally orthodox Dr Thompson is concerned that the movements he has seen are spontaneous efforts to breathe.† If indeed they are, then his understanding is that the patient is still alive, albeit vestigially and without hope of recovery. For him, breathing is *in itself* a characteristic of life. His more radical colleague Dr Dickson, however, has doubts. He argues that the observed movements were not the coordinated or integrated actions of breathing but merely primitive reflexive movements in the muscle groups and nerve networks concerned. He regards the movements as initiated by the spinal

---

* I depict here in fictional form the discussion represented in (and by) Haun *et al.* (5).
† 'Schafer and Caronna . . . reported three patients with severe brain injury who had spontaneous respiratory efforts at levels of $Paco_2$ ranging from 6 to 7.4 kPa (45–56 mmHg)' (ref. 5, p. 183).

ganglia, and not by the brain: they are comparable with the twitching of limbs and other manifestations of spinal reflexes. As such, the movements offer for Dr Dickson no evidence that the patient's brain retains any function, hence no evidence that the patient is alive.* Dr Harrison, finally, disputes Dr Dickson's interpretation. He sees no reason why these albeit shallow movements should not be regarded as breathing efforts which are initiated or at least mediated by the brain.†

Superficially, Harrison and Thompson are in agreement, in that both find the patient to be not yet dead. But at a deeper level Harrison's rejection of Dickson's speculations, concerning the spinal origin of the movements, tends nonetheless to confirm the underlying view of human death which Dickson holds: it is the brain as such which is the locus of human life and death, and breathing which could not be in some sense *attributed to the brain* would lack interest, and would certainly not 'count for life': in itself it would neither characterize nor even indicate life. For both Dickson and Harrison, the importance of breathing lies in its *evidential value concerning the status of the brain*, and not in any significance it has as a phenomenon in itself. Dickson and Harrison therefore disagree merely over whether these particular 'ventilatory efforts' implicate brain function: they do not disagree over the merely forensic role to which breathing has now been relegated. It is not breathing as such, but what breathing shows, which is significant. For them, breathing as a phenomenon in itself does not, after all, matter.

BREATHING AND 'BRAINSTEM DEATH'

The declared role of breathing in the classical exposition of brainstem death is as a characteristic of life itself (3). But then the obvious question concerns *why* breathing as a phenomenon should be invested with a significance which is so categorically denied to persistent circulation and heartbeat.

If there is a difference between breathing and circulation it does not lie among our ordinary reactions to what we see exhibited in a human body. It does not lie in our ordinary view of the phenomena themselves. We could find the difference only in the scientific explanations of what these phenomena mean in biological terms, specifically in their different relationships to the brain. Circulation is only partly controlled by the brain, and the heartbeat can persist even when the brain is dysfunctional. But spontaneous breathing cannot. So spontaneous breathing tells us that the brain is still to some extent functioning. But this means only that breathing has an *evidential value* regarding brain function whereas the heart does not. But the evidence which breathing supplies is conclusive regarding only one regulatory function of the brainstem, namely

---

* 'Ropper *et al*... . argued that in Schafer and Caronna's report the patients who exhibited respiratory efforts at higher levels of $Paco_2$ demonstrated ineffective, primitive respiratory movements. They further proposed that these movements were spinal in origin' (ref. 5, p. 183).
† 'However there is no evidence to suggest that these "shallow" or "primitive" ventilatory efforts are mediated by neuronal pathways that do not require medullary input' (ref. 5, p. 183).

that controlling breathing itself. And now we want to know, why is *this* function important?

It seems there could be three alternative answers to this. First it could be that the respiratory function of the brainstem is no more important than any of its other functions. In this case 'brainstem death' ought logically to mean the final loss of *all* brainstem functions, and a diagnosis of 'brainstem death' would have to rest on showing this total loss of function. But 'brainstem death' rests on nothing of the kind (6) (see also ref. 3, pp. 10–17). Indeed some sources maintain that identifiable brainstem functions, controlling for instance blood pressure, or the movements of the oesophagus, may persist beyond the conventional point of 'brainstem death'.* It is likely that many other brainstem functions have not yet even been identified, hence as yet could not be tested. Thus it is obvious that the logical sequence of declaring the brain as crucial within the human body as a whole, and the brainstem as crucial within the brain as a whole (see ref. 2, p. 40; ref. 3, p. 2; and ref. 6) has a further step not made clear by proponents of 'brainstem death': *within* the brainstem lies a more restricted set of functions, namely those which are tested, and human death must be conceived in terms of losing precisely that set of functions. But since I doubt whether many would think that corneal reflexes or 'dolling' of the eyes had greater human meaning than a persistent heartbeat, it is hard to suppose that the proponents would want to accept this result of their logic.

A second and more plausible answer might be that the function controlling respiration is important because of what it implies about other brainstem functions. Perhaps it shares with other tested functions such as corneal reflexes a confirmatory role concerning the testing of that truly important function which really does carry the burden of human life and death. The obvious candidate would be the particular function of the brainstem which is said to generate the capacity for consciousness. But this answer faces grave difficulties. For the capacity for consciousness takes its importance from the importance which consciousness has as such: this at any rate *is* something we would all generally value for its own sake. But if the possibility of conscious experience is categorically destroyed by other means—by neocortical injury for instance—then the associated function in the brainstem has lost its meaning. If it is really the capacity for consciousness which interests us, then in the still-breathing but permanently comatose patient the continued *organic* functions of her brainstem are without value, and can count for no more than the persistent heartbeat.

The third and most intuitive answer—that the function controlling breathing is important just because it underlies breathing, and breathing is important—is of course circular, and throws us straight back to the question of why breathing is important when the beating heart is not. Both are organic functions which lie at the core of our everyday conception of human life and death. They are distinguished from each other only by their relationship to the brain.

Now on what does the importance of the brain itself rest? There seem two aspects to this. First, the importance of the brain's integrating role in the body

---

* Observations reported in refs 7 and 8 are attributed by Evans and Hill (9) to persistent brainstem function including vasoregulatory function.

derives from *the importance of the body itself.* Once we see this we can see also how arbitrary it is to dismiss, as of no significance, those of the body's functions which survive the 'death' of the brain. Alternatively the importance of the brain might be thought uniquely to rest on its authorship of human conscious experience. Yet if *this* were really what counted for human life, then we should have to regard the persistently comatose as dead.

In either case I regard it as mere stipulation to hold that breathing counts, and circulation does not count, for the life of the human being. Of course no-one should be denied the opportunity to put forward stipulations of this kind (see ref. 3, p. 6), but we ought not to mistake such stipulations for either science or morals.

This returns me to the third of my pictures, the still-breathing body, and the challenge it offers those who regard the still-beating heart with equanimity. I ask supporters of 'brainstem death' to provide a persuasive explanation of why they recoil from explanting vital organs from the merely comatose, when the persistence of a heartbeat gives them no discomfort. As things stand I think they want it both ways. They want to retain the importance of breathing *as such* in their conception of human death, yet they shrink from acknowledging the moral place of the beating heart alongside that of the swelling lung. They want to disregard those of the body's phenomena which can survive disconnection from the brainstem's controlling function, regarding these as so lacking in human meaning that they offer no barrier to the harvesting of vital organs. And yet they shrink from regarding the merely comatose as dead: they shrink, that is, from the third of my opening pictures, that of the 'breathing corpse'.

In effect they are bestowing *human meaning* on the underlying causal processes at the expense of the visible realities of the human body: they are subordinating the seen to the unseen. On this view none of the visible and tangible phenomena of the human body count for life, once sundered from the brainstem's regulating influence; thus, logically, breathing becomes important not as part of a *conception* of human life and death but merely as a *criterion* for the state of the brainstem. This may reflect the concerns of science, but it cannot explain the moral horror of burying someone whose heart still beats, and it is not necessary in order to explain the moral horror of burying the still-breathing. Few attitudes towards the human body seem more remote from, or harder to reconcile with, our ordinary and familiar moral reactions.

ACKNOWLEDGEMENTS

I am grateful to Donald Evans, Neil Pickering and Zbigniew Szawarski for their comments and suggestions regarding the preparation of this paper.

REFERENCES

1. Jonas, H. 1974. Against the stream: comments on the definition and redefinition of death. *Philosophical essays: from ancient creed to technological man*, pp. 132–140. Prentice Hall, Englewood Cliffs, N.J.
2. Lamb, D. 1985. *Death, brain death and ethics*. Croom Helm, London. (See also Chapter 87, this volume.)

3. Pallis, C. 1983. *ABC of brainstem death*. BMJ, London.
4. Gervaise, KG. 1986. *Redefining death*, p. 193. Yale University Press, New Haven.
5. Haun, S. E., Tobias, J. D. and Deshpande, J. K. 1991. Apnoea testing in the determination of brain death: is it reliable? *Clinical Intensive Care* 2(3): 182–184.
6. Evans, J. M. 1987. Lower oesophageal contractility as an indicator of brain death in paralysed and mechanically ventilated patients. *British Medical Journal* 295: 270.
7. Wetzel, R. C., Seltzer, N., Stiff, J. L. and Roberts, M. C. 1985. Hemodynamic responses in brain dead organ donor patients. *Anesthesia and Analgesia* 64: 125–128.
8. Hall, G. M., Mashiter, K., Lumley, J. and Robson, J. G. 1980. Hypothalamic–pituitary function in the 'brain-dead' patient. *Lancet* 2: 1259.
9. Evans, D. W. and Hill, D. J. 1990. Correspondence. *British Medical Journal* 301: 178.

89

Animal Experimentation in Biomedical Research: A Critique

T. L. S. Sprigge

University of Edinburgh, UK

Room after room was lined with small, bare cages, stacked one above the other, in which monkeys circled round and round and chimpanzees sat huddled, far gone in depression and despair.

Young chimpanzees, three or four years old, were crammed, two together, into tiny cages measuring 22 inches by 22 inches and only 24 inches high. They could hardly turn round. Not yet part of any experiment, they had been confined in these cages for more than three months.

The chimps had each other for comfort, but they would not remain together for long. Once they are infected, probably with hepatitis, they will be separated and placed in another cage. And there they will remain, living in conditions of severe sensory deprivation, for the next several years. During that time, they will become insane (1).*

THE NOBLE ASPECT OF MEDICAL RESEARCH

One of the noblest tasks an individual or society can set themselves is the relief of the suffering and premature death caused by disease. Medical science and medical practice would, therefore, seem to be among the highest human callings and so, in fact, they are. But the tragedy is that the knowledge medical science seeks, and medical practice applies, are deemed to require a type of research which is itself the source of massive suffering.

The use of animals† in painful and lethal research in biomedical science is

---

* Jane Goodall is describing a scene on a video film of an AIDS research laboratory in the US. Apes are not used in research in Britain, but monkeys are.
† In this chapter, 'animals' will refer to non-human animals, birds, reptiles, and such other creatures as may be deemed to have at least as full a form of sentience as is possessed by whichever of these has the least. In the 1986 legislation 'animal' means non-human vertebrate, and thus possibly has a narrower denotation.

Principles of Health Care Ethics. Edited by Raanan Gillon.
© 1994 John Wiley & Sons Ltd

the most difficult issue which confronts people who work or argue against what they conceive as the abuse of animals. Animals are made to suffer in the interest of many other goods (e.g. luxury goods and field sports) which are hardly vital to human welfare. Even pure scientific enquiry may be regarded as promoting an ultimately optional human interest. (It will be said that no-one can tell what kind of basic research will lead to what eventual benefits. But, apart from the fact that there may be disbenefits as well, a general belief that benefit may come from biological or psychological research involving animal suffering and not directed at any specific medical goal seems hardly to justify giving this research priority over all the other research projects which just might have eventual beneficial results. Moreover, the notion that no distinction can be made between research likely and unlikely to yield tangible benefit is open to criticism; see, for example, ref. 2, pp. 15–18). But medical research and the testing of drugs pose a more difficult moral dilemma. The benefits promised are very real, and arguably essential if many people are to be given tolerable lives. But are they sufficient, or could they in principle ever be sufficient, to justify treatment of animals which in other contexts would be immoral, indeed illegal?

PAINFUL EXPERIMENTATION

There is no doubt that many animals used for research, medical and otherwise (including under this head the safety testing of drugs) are subjected to treatment which in other contexts would be deemed grossly cruel and which would be against the law. That this was so in Britain in the past, and continues to be so in many countries, cannot be denied. Is it perhaps different in Britain now since the *Animals (Scientific Procedures) Act 1986*? One hopes that that has improved things. It does, at least, have the great advantage that the power now given to the Home Secretary and his advisory committee, the Animal Procedures Committee, means that things can be improved (though presumably also made worse) in response to current moral attitudes without the immense labour required to bring in fresh legislation. But much evidently still occurs which causes immense distress to research animals (see refs 3 and 4, and the film of Professor Feldberg's work cited in the footnote on p. 1048).

However, I shall not attempt a survey of the present situation, but shall examine the essential moral issues, letting the cap fit where it may.

The morality of killing animals is, on the face of it, different from that of making them suffer. It would be difficult for a non-vegetarian rationality to object to the mere killing of animals after or in the course of research (or for the extraction of products, etc.), for surely medical advances are more important than provision of an optional form of diet. This does not mean that the killing is justified, for perhaps killing animals for food is not justified. Or possibly the killing of some animals, e.g. fish, is more justifiable than that of others, e.g. pigs, in virtue of their fuller degree of 'personhood' in some morally relevant sense. But it does mean that the issue of killing and making suffer should be considered separately.

However, I shall concern myself in this chapter largely with the morality of such use of animals in the direct course of the procedures, or in the keeping them captive, and breeding them or capturing them in the wild. Personally I do think that there is a moral presumption against institutions which depend upon the routine killing of the higher animals (as opposed to killing them in special crises). However, that applies to killing them for food as much, or more, as in the course of medical research. And since this is a case which cannot in consistency be taken very seriously by those who are not vegetarians it is more important to make a case which may be acceptable to vegetarian and non-vegetarian alike.

Moreover, even the critics of all animal-based research would agree that if medical science could develop through the use of animals, who were given good lives, and were not subjected to painful experimentation, the situation would be extraordinarily improved, even if they suspected that the sensitivities which would lead to that improvement would point eventually to, at the very least, a minimal killing of animals in the interests of medical science.

We should remember, however, that as things stand the animals who are killed are often badly looked after in their lives, and sometimes killed callously. The notion of happy laboratory animals who are eventually killed for some medical purpose may not be too realistic. Moreover, the routine killing of animals, often merely because they have served their purpose and are of no more use, does not cohere well with any great concern with them as the fellow conscious subjects they are. Having their life and death completely in one's control for one's own purposes, and not theirs, seems psychologically incompatible with much respect for them as creatures with lives of their own to live.

I turn now to the morality of causing animals to suffer in the course of medical research, whether this arises simply from their being in captivity, or the particular conditions of their captivity, or from the nature of the actual research procedures themselves, or indeed from diseases they have been bred or engineered to develop.

It is just possible that someone will maintain that (a few criminal acts apart) medical research today does not involve suffering. There is much evidence pointing the other way.* Even the Research Defence Society only claims that 'a substantial proportion of animal research conducted in this country involves little or no suffering for the animals'.† Surely the non-human primates held for long periods in so-called primate chairs must suffer greatly, for example baboons forcibly restrained and exposed to strobe lights, causing them to have epileptic

---

* For the official statistics of recent research see ref. 5; see also Smith and Boyd (6). Further information can be found in the literature of any of the more reliable animal welfare or rights campaigning organizations. Those put out by Advocates for Animals are always carefully checked. A pioneering work of continuing interest was Ryder (7). The most famous and very well-argued work on animal welfare generally is Singer (8); Chapter 11 is on animal research. Evidently the only countries which collect and publish detailed statistics on animal research are Britain and The Netherlands, and The Netherlands gives the more precise details of the severity banding of procedures performed. 'The Dutch statistics record that 57 per cent of experiments registered in 1987 were assessed as being likely to involve minor discomfort for the animals, 21 per cent as likely to involve moderate discomfort, and the remaining 22 per cent as likely to involve severe discomfort.' See Smith and Boyd (6), p. 21 and also Rowan (2).

† *RDS Newsletter* (9), p. 7. In the modern world, it is worth remarking, no-one can properly confine their concern to what is going on in their own country.

fits. Or mice placed on hot plates or rabbits given herpes infections of the eye to develop anti-viral drugs? And can one deny that laboratory animals who have suffered the injection of cancer cells into their eyes, brains, muscles or abdomens have not suffered greatly as a result, for example? (10). But it would take up too much space to cite detailed examples.

Should there be anyone who seeks to defend animal research, or animal biomedical research, on the grounds that it never involves animal suffering (or never any of any seriousness) then they cannot object to the proposal for an explicit legal ban on all research involving animal suffering, for, by their own account, that would simply make explicit the satisfactory present situation. Since my main concern is with the issue of painful research, or, more broadly, research which involves suffering, either directly or through the conditions in which animals are kept, I can take it that those who would think a total ban on such research objectionable, agree that there is such (legally permitted) research at present.

EXAMPLE OF THE WITCH DOCTOR

One way to approach the subject is to consider the moral situation one would be in if one became convinced that some witch doctor could cure various diseases by torturing, or if you think that too emotive a word, hurting and distressing animals before the patient's eyes. Of which diseases would you be prepared to be cured yourself by such a method? And I do not so much mean what degree of suffering would actually make you call for the witch doctor (for I dread to think myself what degree of suffering might induce me to betray an associate into a gestapo-like police's clutches) as what degree of suffering to yourself would you think made it decent for you to call upon his services. I am not saying that it is an easy question to answer, but it seems to me morally on a par with the question of what amount of painful research you would think it proper to have been used on behalf of likely sufferers such as yourself.

It is easier to deal with the question how much suffering you ought to permit upon yourself until you call for the witch doctor, than with the question what degree of suffering on your children's part would make it proper to do so. But surely even this is a difficult question and again it is on a par with a corresponding question about medical research.

We should distinguish in this connection between one-off situations and institutions basic to our society. Sometimes an anti-vivisectionist is asked whether it would not be right to kill a tiger to save a human baby, whether a driver should not swerve to kill a dog rather than a child, or whether one should not prefer the life of a rat to that of a child which might be saved by 'sacrificing' the rat in medical research.

The answer is that one may well think that, in a crisis situation, of a type which one can do one's best to stop recurring, human interests should be preferred to animal interests, and take a different view of a settled practice of basing human welfare on injury to animals.

These are questions about killing, which are not my main concern, but similar questions about one-off situations could perhaps be devised where suffering was the main issue. My point then is that you may think it deplorable that we should base human welfare upon a settled practice involving massive animal suffering while admitting that, in an exceptional crisis situation, not part of anyone's regular form of life, humans should receive alleviation first. I do not say that they always should; only that these are different types of situation. For the one makes the deliberate infliction of suffering acceptable in a way that the other does not.

Another comparison one might make is the use of torture to extract information from subversives. Although animals are not subversives, one could say that painful experimentation is the use of torture to extract information considered of great use for human well-being.

Why would most of my likely readers think that condoning the use of torture by our police forces would be absolutely illegitimate—whatever might be said about some unique crisis situation one can dream up? Surely it is because we do not think our society should be based upon the deliberate infliction of pain as one of its regular procedures. There are many reasons for this. Once torture was used for one sort of case considered of supreme importance, one can be sure it would gradually spread. For it would encourage callousness in the authorities, and more and more cases would be said to justify it. The only way to prevent its massive use in cases that no disinterested person would justify is probably to prevent its use altogether. One may have to accept that in some one-off cases the use of torture would have prevented more distress than it would cause, so far as the more immediate consequences go. One may even accept that the same would be true of some broad classes of case. But human nature being what it is, the most effective way of preventing certain sorts of evil practice is to have a simply understood taboo against all activities of a certain kind. Is not the deliberate causing of serious pain or distress to sentient creatures an example of something which needs to be checked by just such a taboo?

THE ATTITUDES OF EXPERIMENTERS AND TECHNICIANS

It is doubtful how far the matter can be evaluated on the basis of individual analyses of gains and losses. Opponents of animal experimentation usually emphasize the extent to which the testing of drugs on animals has failed to discover unfortunate side-effects in humans, and the positive possibilities of research not involving animals, including the use of human volunteers. They rightly emphasize the limitations of non-human animals as models of the human body.

But proponents of animal research will list numerous benefits conferred on humanity by medical advances which, it is said, could not have been made without the use of animals. Thus Sir William Paton has claimed that if there had never been animal experimentation we would probably today have the physics of Newton and Einstein, but would not yet have reached the biology and biomedicine even of Galen, and that if animal experimentation stopped

now we would be stuck for ever at our present state of biological knowledge.*
On the other hand we have such anti-vivisectionists as H. Ruesch and R. Sharpe,
who minimize the extent to which animal work has been essential for the
development of biomedicine and are still more insistent that it is not required
in the future (14–16).

Probably both sides overstate their case. Indeed, so controversial must the
balance of argument always remain that it is doubtful if this is the way to settle
the matter. While some anti-vivisectionists are inclined, rather unrealistically,
to deny that any medical advances have been made by, or at any rate required,
animal research, defenders of animal experimentation are over-confident about
how things would have gone, and may go in the future, without it. It is difficult
enough to know how medical knowledge would have advanced if painful animal
research had been outlawed in the past, and it is still more difficult to predict
what the possibilities are for the future.

Professor Michael Balls has criticized both those who assume that the
discoveries made with animal experiments could not have been made otherwise,
and those who seek to minimize 'the significance of animal experiments in the
improvements of the quality and length of human life during the last hundred
years or so':

> I reject both these biased attempts to manipulate the contribution made by animal
> experiments in the past to support a particular viewpoint. . . . All historians are
> tempted to ask what would have happened if a particular event had not taken
> place. The answer is that they cannot know, and they can only guess whether the
> consequences would have been better or worse than those which actually followed.
> Thus I do not accept that insulin would not have been discovered without the
> work of Banting and Best.†

Granted these difficulties, perhaps it is better to think rather of the whole
quality of our way of life. To me it seems that this is lowered to the extent that
our welfare is based upon matters which we either do not like to look in the
face, or which we can look in the face only at the cost of our own moral

---

* See Paton (11) at p. 42 and *passim*. See also Smith and Boyd (6), Chapter 3. Similarly the Medical
Research Council's Annual Report for 1988/1991 says: 'Medical research still needs to use animals.
Animal work is essential, for example, to the search for a cure for such life-theatening diseases as
cancer and AIDS. However, there has been a constant reduction in the use of animals over the
years, and the biggest cut has been in the use of domestic species and primates; 98% of animals
used in MRC establishments in 1989 were rodents. . . . The Council requires all the scientists it
supports to observe the principle that animals should be used in their research only when necessary,
and then in the minimum number consistent with achieving a valid result in any experiment. MRC
managers have a specific responsibility to ensure high standards of animal care and compliance
with the Act' (quoted in ref. 12). This rosy view of the dedication to animal welfare of those financed
by the MRC was somewhat spoilt when videotapes became public in May 1990 showing 40 hours
of Professor Wilhelm Feldberg's work on cats and rabbits at the National Institute for Medical
Research, Mill Hill, London, which is operated and funded by the Medical Research Council. For
details see ref. 13, pp. 21–31. It was made by Mike Huskisson of the Animal Cruelty Investigation
Group, and Melody Macdonald, who had gained the Professor's confidence by offering to prepare
his bibliography under the pretext that it was for teaching American students about animal
experimentation.
† Balls (17), at pp. 228–229. Michael Balls is chairman of the FRAME trustees (Fund for the
Replacement of Animals in Medical Experiments).

deterioration. And it is a real question how far painful animal experimentation is in practice compatible with a continuing sense of their status as conscious beings whose lives can be good or bad for them just as ours can for us.

For one person's picture of the attitudes of those involved in animal research the reader might like to consult the observations of Sarah Kite, an animal rights campaigner mentioned above, who infiltrated the Huntingdon Research Centre in Cambridgeshire by working there as a weekend assistant for eight months.* If her observations are correct and representative, it seems that standard medical research encourages an attitude in the staff of considerable callousness. So in addition to the crude calculus of losses and gains, losses to the animals and gains to humans, we must consider its effects upon the human beings who conduct it. It seems doubtful whether the development of a more compassionate society, and one in which animals are properly recognized as individual subjects of experience, is compatible with people working in this way or being aware that others are doing so. The whole practice of animal experimentation encourages the belief that the animals are mere objects with whom any kind of empathy is mere sentimentality.

> I do not believe that much trust can be placed in the consciences of researchers. Conscience usually takes second place to the chance of a DPhil. Nor do I have any confidence in the Home Office Inspectorate, having seen the appalling conditions which they permit to exist at times in premises under their jurisdiction (18).

In a recent report on the use of non-human primates in medical and related research between 1984 and 1988, the authors express considerable doubts about the attitudes to their experimental subjects of those working on these animals (19).

High standards are unlikely to be achieved purely by external policing by Home Office inspectors, or by the 'named vets' now required at each research establishment (with special responsibility for the welfare of the animals there) unless the experimenters themselves have some real respect for the animals as conscious subjects. But can people with such an amount of control over their animal subjects, who become so used to working upon them for reasons which are opposed to, rather than consistent with, the pursuit of the animals' own good, really keep in mind the moral requirement of respect? Doubtless they do in some cases, but ordinary humane impulses must surely be blunted by the nature of much of their work.†

---

* See Kite (3), at p. 35. Naturally the accuracy of her report has been challenged, though mainly, I believe, on the question of whether the law was being broken (see ref. 20).

† 'However, our greatest concern in reviewing published accounts of their work, written by the researchers themselves, was their widespread failure to communicate any real depth of appreciation of the distress and suffering caused to the animals used, because of the procedures applied to them, the conditions under which they were housed and generally cared for, or their origins or eventual fates' (19).

Some of the work conducted recently in Britain on non-human primates seems calculated to rest on a voyeuristic curiosity as to how surgery and drugs can modify behaviour with no very obvious human good in view. For example, work has been carried out at the MRC Reproductive Biology Unit, Centre for Reproductive Biology, in Edinburgh on the response in female marmosets to their male partners after hormone changes have been artificially induced by estradiol.

'Measurements were divided into male and female. The female was introduced into the male's cage and they were watched through a one-way mirror. In the male frequency of attempted mounts,

ALLEGED SENTIMENTALITY ABOUT DOGS AND CATS

Sometimes it is considered sentimental of people to be especially distressed at the fate of dogs and cats in laboratories. Those who think so will not be too impressed when the Medical Research Council assures us that the animals most used are rodents (22). However, while it is true that a concern limited to companion animals, or to companion animals together with those whose mere looks make an especial appeal to us, is irrational, it is not unreasonable to be stirred in the first place by the fate of animals of a type with which one is familiar. No-one who has the slightest experience of dogs and cats, and that is almost all of us, can seriously doubt that they are capable of happiness and unhappiness, and can suffer from pain. Dogs running about exhibit as much joy in life as any humans, cats enjoy a lie in the sun or a tempting piece of food as much as we do, and distress, loneliness and frustration seem much the same in them as in us. It must be a serious question why it is more justifiable to use them for our benefit than to use humans. Granted we should not use humans in this way, surely we should not use these animals. As for other animals, if there is reason to believe that they enjoy life and can feel misery and pain in the same sense, consistency requires that we extend our concern to them equally.

The use of non-human primates is particularly questionable ethically. Monkeys, and still more apes, are clearly very near to us in their cognitive capacities, social practices, and psychology. The research done by Bowlby involving the famous or infamous pit of despair is based upon this premise. Non-human primates, though not apes, are currently used in Britain in a wide range of research projects of a medical or related nature. In 1990 a total of 5284 non-human primates were used in medical research in Britain.

BALANCING COSTS AND BENEFITS: THREE POSITIONS

But surely the benefits are so great that the evil of the animal suffering must be considered as outweighed by the greater evil it prevents?

To this there are several possible responses.

1. One may simply agree that, although animals may suffer a good deal in certain experiments, this is justified if the final result is that these diseases are eradicated or alleviated since the net result is total diminution of suffering. Such a reply is likely to be based upon the ethical theory of utilitarianism which contends that activities are justified if and only if they will probably produce a higher surplus of pleasurable (or otherwise desirable) experience over painful (or otherwise undesirable) experience for all sentient creatures affected than would any alternative.

2. One may hold that, even if there is a net reduction in suffering overall, this

---

mounts and ejaculations were recorded, in the female the amount of tongue flicking prior to acceptance of the male' (ref. 21 but based on a paper published in *Hormones and Behaviour*, 1989, **23**: 211–220).

essentially utilitarian approach to morality is unacceptable. There are certain things it is wrong to do to sentient individuals, whatever benefits it may bring. No innocent creature should be forced to suffer for the benefit of others.

We would almost all think it wrong to use some innocent humans in this way for the benefit of others, even if the suffering prevented was worse than that caused. For each human is an end in himself or herself, not appropriately made an involuntary means to the benefit of others. And if one carefully considers what makes each human an end in himself or herself one will see that it can only be that each is a distinct centre of will and consciousness, and this applies equally to every animal, at least to every mammal.

Thus if it would be wrong to experiment on humans for the sake of research which may ultimately be of benefit to others, it must be so in the case of animals. To suppose otherwise is to be simply speciesist.

The usual grounds for denying animal rights, in a sense in which human rights are proclaimed, is that animals cannot claim or waive any rights ascribed to them, that animals are not 'rational beings', that animals are not moral agents.* All these objections seem adequately met by pointing out that human infants and grossly subnormal adults, and perhaps the severely senile, must be denied rights by the same token. Certainly there is no well-grounded logical case for saying that only moral agents can have rights, in the sense of rights not to be treated in certain ways by others (as opposed to rights to do things oneself). This line of thought has been presented persuasively by Tom Regan and Richard Ryder (7,23).

It will, however, be met by the objection that to regard animals as ends in themselves in the sense that human beings are is absurd, thus leading to an impasse in which each side simply states his own case more and more passionately.†

The trouble is that, although appeal to rights, either human or animal, is often a good way of stating one's ethical views, it is rather question-begging as a way of justifying them. Some may say that this is true of all ethical positions equally, since none can be more than the expression of one's personal feelings incapable of proof. However, it seems to me that there is an undeniability about the badness of pain and suffering and the goodness of pleasure and happiness which puts utilitarian considerations on a different level.

3. One may accept the basic tenet of utilitarianism, or something close to it, but claim that total welfare would probably be increased by bringing painful

---

* Another reason sometimes given is that at least most animals, even if conscious, are not self-conscious in the sense of having a concern with the pattern of their lives as a whole (22). This, however, is very much a matter of degree and could only show that animals possess certain rights in a lesser degree than most humans.

† 'Any serious attempt to apply the philosophy of animal rights to our society would require such drastic changes that it would be tantamount to removing civilised society as we know it' (ref. 24, p. 4). This was doubtless the attitude of supporters of slavery in slave-owning societies, but civilization has managed to survive its abolition. Surely a society which takes seriously the claims of all sentient life upon our compassion can never be described as uncivilized.

animal experimentation to an end.

In defending this position myself, I would argue that minute calculations about costs and benefits in terms of pleasure and pain cannot realistically be made, but that what one can form a reasonable opinion about is the worthwhileness of alternative general lifestyles in terms of their short- and long-term implications for human happiness, and that of the animals who interact with us.

To show how difficult detailed cost/benefit calculations are, consider these various suggestions which a utilitarian critic of painful animal experimentation might make of our first position as listed above:

1. That research into and development of the best forms of social organization for making maximum use of existing medical knowledge might well do more for human welfare than the increase of that knowledge, and that until absolutely adequate resources are provided for the former they should not be provided for the latter insofar as that requires the infliction of suffering on animals.

2. That if all painful experimentation were banned (perhaps after allowing a few years for adjustment) the encouragement to alternative methods of research would be such that medical knowledge might well advance at least as effectively as before, without the cost in terms of pain and suffering. The methods available for discovering what is going on within the human body or brain are already so striking that it must be questionable whether there may now really be much which can never be discovered directly by painless work on humans rather than by extrapolation from painful work on animals.

   Professor Michael Balls (17), who does not recommend the total abolition of animal experimentation now, but sees it as a realistic goal to work for, refers to the way in which

   > biomedical research and clinical practice are being revolutionised by recent developments, such as monoclonal antibodies, NMR imaging, gene detection by RFLPs, gene cloning and gene transfer, computer graphics and drug design, to name but a few. Should we assume that there will not be equally surprising new developments, in the future? Also, there are already many substantial discoveries which *could only* have been found through the use of non-animal methods. I believe that the current reliance on animal experimentation will be steadily reduced, and that it will one day be possible to take drugs from the design stages via non-animal alternatives to the patient—without any use of animals. The only question is, how soon? (p. 229).

   If he is thinking along the right lines, may one not surmise that a total ban on animal experimentation might give the needed fillip to the development of such alternatives?

3. That such a ban might be combined with a switch of resources to the alleviation of world hunger by policies and research goals, and thus to the prevention of a greater evil than that of disease in the affluent parts of the world, and that resources for fighting human (and animal) suffering by means not thus tainted should always be given priority over those which certainly involve suffering.

4. That even within the realm of the promotion of health in the affluent west

there are plenty of jobs needing doing which could do with resources currently going into medical research involving painful experiments.
5. That so far as medical research is dedicated to the prolonging of life it may bring as many troubles as it is relieving.

I do not say that these propositions are true. What I do say is that it is very difficult to know whether they are so or not, and thus what the effects of a total ban on painful experimentation on animals would or could really be, when such things are taken into account. The one thing which is certain, in the very nature of the case, is that a great deal of suffering would be prevented.

But perhaps the most important two things that a utilitarian critic of animal experimentation like myself can say are these:

1. Readiness to treat animals as mere objects at the complete disposal of human beings goes with a general attitude to other life forms which is deeply damaging to the human condition.
2. In fact most people cannot be happy in the knowledge that their health is (or is supposed to be) dependent upon massive suffering to other creatures, or if they can, they can only be so by developing a generally callous attitude to other living creatures, the prevalence of which would certainly be detrimental to the welfare of sentient life on this planet as a whole.

The list of barbarities to which animals have been subjected in the interests of medical and pharmacological research is so striking that it is hard to avoid thinking that so long as painful experimentation is tolerated at all, they will continue.* There certainly seems to have been considerable densensitizing of those employed in such industries. One may surmise that either human densensitizing to the lot of animals must increase, so that they are ever more at our mercy, and ever more treated as mere objects for man to do with what he likes, or we must make a resolute stride in the opposite direction, with what precise results on human welfare we cannot quite know.

All in all, there is so much uncertainty as to the precise effects of a complete ban on painful animal experimentation, so far as the advance of human welfare goes, that it seems to me that the undoubted harm to the animals concerned, and the desensitizing of the researchers, should be taken as the decisive factors. We should at least conclude that it cannot be satisfactory to base human life for the indefinite future upon a readiness to treat other sentient beings as mere research tools.† I would therefore urge that people of good will should support a policy by which all painful experimentation will be banned from some given

---

* The work with monkeys of Robert J.R. White on head transplantation was a particularly dreadful example which first involved me in this issue. See Ryder (7), pp. 73–74.
† Genetic engineering and the production of patented transgenic animals risks encouraging this in a more extreme form than ever before. Some of the problems it poses are the same as in more 'traditional' animal experimentation, but it poses the fresh dilemma of how far life on the globe will be impoverished for humans themselves if too many of the creatures around us are designed in this 'mechanical' way. But genetic engineering raises a host of new problems I cannot discuss here.

date in the future (together with the prohibition of the use of research animals whose living conditions do not give them a reasonable environment for the performance of their normal behavioural patterns);* perhaps legislation should aim at its total ban within 10 years.† This would not mean that animals could not be used in research at all. If it were forbidden to do to research animals what it would be considered wrong to do to farm animals or pets, animals could still be used for a large area of medical research. At that point thought might be given to a still further reduction in the use of animals as mere research tools, but the lot of the non-human would be so much advanced by such a ban, that it is perhaps sufficient as a goal behind which it may be hoped a large number of people can rally.

REFERENCES

1. Goodall, J. *New Scientist*, 29 September 1988.
2. Rowan, A. N. 1984. *Of mice, models and men: a critical evaluation of animal research*. State University of New York Press, Albany.
3. Kite, S. 1990. *Secret suffering: inside a British laboratory*. British Union for the Abolition of Vivisection, Islington, London, p. 35.
4. *Vivisection in Britain*. Recently (undated, 1991?) published by the National Anti-Vivisection Society.
5. *Report of the Animal Procedures Committee for 1990*. HMSO, London, September 1991.
6. Smith, J. A. and Boyd, K. M. 1991. *Lives in the balance: the ethics of using animals in biomedical research*. Report of a Working Party of the Institute of Medical Ethics. Oxford University Press, Oxford.
7. Ryder, R. 1975. *Victims of science*. Davis-Poynter, London.
8. Singer, P. 1976. *Animal liberation: a new ethic for our treatment of animals*. Jonathan Cape, London.
9. *RDS Newsletter*, October 1990.
10. 'The use of animals in medical research', and 'Behind Closed Doors', pamphlets published by *Advocates for Animals*, 10 Queensferry Street, Edinburgh EH2 4PG.
11. Paton, W. 1984. *Man and mouse: animals in medical research*. Oxford University Press, Oxford, at p. 42 and *passim*.
12. *Research Defence Society's Newsletter* for January 1991.
13. *Advocates for animals: pictorial review*, 1991.
14. Ruesch, H. 1982. *Naked empress—or the great medical fraud*. CIVITAS, New York.
15. Sharpe, R. 1988. *The cruel deception*. Thorsons, Wellingborough.
16. Sharpe, R. 1989. Animal experiments: a failed technology. Pp. 88–117, *in* Langley, O (Ed.) *Animal experimentation: the consensus changes*. Macmillan, London.
17. Balls, M. 1990. Recent progress towards reducing the use of animal experimentation in biomedical research. Pp. 228–229, *in* Garratini, S. (Ed.) *The importance of animal*

---

* There certainly are some researchers who are concerned with the 'environmental and behavioural enrichment' of the lives of their laboratory animals. Professor David B. Morton, at Leicester, has been especially concerned with this. But where there is not substantial expenditure to this end, one may doubt the seriousness of the concern with animal welfare.
† The aim of a movement called Target 2000. Certainly the possibility of research merely being driven overseas is a problem. Perhaps it could only be realistic at an EEC level with barriers against products depending on animal research elsewhere. If this is unrealistic, it is at least an ethically respectable goal towards which to ask politicians to push so far as possible. This contrasts with the apparent view of the Research Defence Society, which sees animal experimentation, painful presumably included, as a fixture of the human condition (see ref. 12, p. 6).

experimentation for safety and biomedical research. Kluwer Academic Publishers, Dordrecht.

18. Letter from a research worker published in the *Guardian*, 3 July 1980, quoted in *Behind closed doors*, pamphlet published by Advocates for Animals.

19. Hampson, J., Southee, J., Howell, D. and Balls, M. 1990. *An RSPCA/FRAME survey of the use of non-human primates as laboratory animals in Great Britain 1984–1988*. FRAME, Nottingham and RSPCA, Horsham.

20. *Research Defence Society Newsletter*, July 1990, p. 2.

21. 'Non-human primate use in Great Britain; review of published research papers, 1987–1991. Prepared for Advocates for Animals, based on research papers published between 1987 and 1991.

22. *Medical Research Council's Annual Report* for 1990/1991 as quoted in *Research Defence Society's Newsletter* for January 1991.

23. Regan, T. 1983. *The case for animal rights*. Routledge & Kegan Paul, London, Chapters 8 and 9.

24. *Research Defence Society Newsletter*, October 1990.

90

The Ethics of the Search for Benefits: Animal Experimentation in Medicine

R. G. FREY

Department of Philosophy, Bowling Green State University, Ohio, USA

Very broadly, on the ethics of animal experimentation, we can identify three positions. The first is the abolitionist position, according to which all experiments upon animals must cease. This is certainly the view of Tom Regan, who believes that all such experiments, at whatever stage and however promising, must stop at once (1); it is also the view of Peter Singer (2,3) and Stephen Clark (4), provided due allowance is made for a more progressive or gradual cessation. As concerns human health care needs, this abolitionist position is uncompromising: it is indeed a *tragic* affair that some humans will be adversely affected by cessation of animal experiments and by the wait for alternative models and techniques to be fully developed and integrated into basic health care research;* but it is an *immoral* affair to persist with the use of animals (though exactly why it is immoral differs among the above three authors).

I find this abolitionist position far too extreme; it seems to me that a compelling argument can be made in favor of at least some animal research. It also seems to me that this argument can be made, without our having to go to the opposite extreme and embrace the second position, namely, that in the search for human health care benefits, virtually anything we might care to do to animals is justified, provided only that we can make out the case that the benefit to be achieved, actually or potentially, is significant enough to offset massive animal

---

* I do not deny, of course, that replacement of animals with tissue cultures, computer models, etc., has occurred in some areas, and I support attempts at replacement. But I am not optimistic about our ever achieving full replacement, over the entire range of human health care needs.

Principles of Health Care Ethics. Edited by Raanan Gillon.

suffering and deaths.* This 'anything-goes' position I find also too extreme. For to hold it on philosophical grounds that can withstand even the slightest pressure, it must be held in conjunction with the view that animals do not matter morally; that, in other words, they are not members of the moral community. I cannot accept this; the mere fact that, say, rats have unfolding series of experiences, some painful, some not, all of which carry the possibility of diminishing or improving their quality of life, suffices in my view to confer moral standing upon them.

Once one allows that animals are part of the moral community, however, then one's act of inflicting pain and suffering upon them or killing them must be justified. Nor will it then seem so obvious that such acts *are* justified, by the rather bold and excessive claim that the saving of even one human life can justify the slaughter of countless numbers of animals. *In the absence of argument,* this claim seems arbitrarily to peg the value of one part of the moral community far too high *vis-à-vis* the value of other parts.

My position, then, is the third one, which is a compromise between the other two: it justifies some but not all experiments on animals, while conceding and taking into account the fact that they are members of the moral community and that, therefore, what we do to them is of moral concern. The report of an Institute of Medical Ethics working party (of which I was a member), *Lives in the balance: animal experimentation,* (5), in effect adopts this approach. The problem is to articulate the philosophy behind it, to make sure that the various facets of that philosophy are internally consistent, and then to show what the implications of the philosophy are for animal experiments. These are not easy matters.

In the philosophical world, this third, more moderate, position is sometimes associated with myself, at least so far as philosophical underpinnings are concerned. In a series of articles,† I have attempted to develop and defend the position, and to defend it, moreover, in a way that, among the four principles displayed throughout this volume, involves the principle of beneficence within constraints very much favored by animal liberationists. For reasons of space I confine myself to one aspect of the third position, though one which carries us to the very center of the debate over animal experimentation.

The justification of experiments upon animals is not, fundamentally, about painful experiments. In my view pain is pain, as much an evil for an animal as for a human, and I agree with animal liberationists that it is a form of speciesism

---

* What counts as significant enough can vary from researcher to researcher and sometimes, to an outside but informed observer, it can appear to amount to something trivial, e.g. any health-care gain whatever, however minimal.
† As background, see my books *Interests and rights* (Clarendon Press, Oxford, 1980) and *Rights, killing, and suffering* (Basil Blackwell, Oxford, 1983). On animal experimentation see my articles: (i) 'Vivisection, medicine, and morals' (*Journal of Medical Ethics*, 1983); (ii) 'Animal parts, human wholes' (*Biomedical ethics reviews*, eds J. M. Humber and R. F. Almeder; Humana Press, New Jersey, 1987); (iii) 'The significance of agency and marginal cases' (*Philosophica*, 1987); (iv) 'Autonomy and the value of animal life' (*The Monist*, 1987); (v) 'Moral standing, the value of lives and speciesism' (*Between the Species*, 1988); (vi) 'Animals, science, and morality' (*Behavioral and Brain Sciences*, 1990); (vii) 'Ethics, medicine, and animal experimentation' (*American Journal of Ethics and Medicine*, forthcoming, 1992). The present paper draws upon these articles, especially numbers (ii) and (vii).

or discrimination to pretend otherwise. Where pain is concerned, I can see no difference between burning a rat alive and burning a child alive, and the deliberate infliction of pain on a feeling creature requires justification. Yet, what concerns us at the most fundamental level is not the painful use of animals for human benefit but their use at all for human benefit. Only if we can justify using them in the first place can we go on to ask after the justification of their painful use, and if we cannot first justify their use then we must, I think, if we are morally serious persons, give up animal research.

Accountability is paramount. We are accountable for what we intentionally do, and this is as true of medical researchers as of everyone else. What is done to animals in our laboratories is done deliberately, intentionally, and we are accountable for and must justify what we deliberately, intentionally do.

Nor can medical people shift this burden on to the law, by claiming that, with approved protocols and project licenses, the law permits them to do what they are doing. For the fact is that, morally, we often demand more of ourselves and others than this. In Anglo-American law there is no general legal duty of rescue: one may legally walk past a drowning man even when one could easily save him. But one does not trumpet the fact that one has done so, or expect the lavish praises of others for having left a man to drown; one rather, in the advertising jargon, adopts a low profile and slinks away. We often expect more of ourselves and others than merely what the law permits. Deliberately inflicting pain on animals, drastically impairing their lives, killing them: to say only that the law permits these things is not to go far enough; we need to see whether the medical researcher adopts a low profile or accepts accountability and proffers a moral defense of what has been done. It is the character of that defense that concerns us.

The researcher might, of course, seeing the problem, shift to the 'anything-goes' position by suggesting that animals do not warrant our moral concern. The problem now is evident. What is it about animals that does not warrant our concern? There are two chief candidates, their pain and suffering, their lives. It cannot be the former that the researcher is appealing to, since his whole behavior with the animal shows he takes its suffering seriously. Indeed, today, ethics review committees, journals' peer review policies, hospitals' research guidelines, and professional societies' guidelines all insist that animal suffering be controlled, limited, mitigated where feasible, and justified in the course of the experiment proposed or carried out. And where these things are not properly seen to by individuals, government oversight committees are now empowered to challenge the research.* As for the latter, animal lives, it seems very implausible to suggest that, if their suffering counts, their lives do not; for much of the point about their suffering is the blight this imposes on their lives, just as it does in the case of humans. Unless animal lives have *some* value, it is hard to

---

* I do not think that we can affirm yet that these laudable aims are always achieved in practice, nor am I overly sanguine about the degree to which researchers will always abide by guidelines, without external, independent (government?) inspection. I favor much more strict inspection, and over longer periods than on the whole has heretofore been the case, in Britain but especially in the United States.

see why we should care about ruining them or, rather tellingly, why researchers should go to such great lengths to cite the actual or potential benefits that justify sacrificing such lives. If one thinks that animal life has even some value, then its deliberate destruction or the intentional lowering of its quality is something in which morally serious people can and doubtless should take an interest.

The 'anything-goes' position has a problem, as we have seen; for it must hold that the animal and human cases are different, where pain and suffering or the destruction of valuable lives is involved. That is, it must hold that there is a moral difference between burning a rat and burning a child, or between infecting each with a debilitating disorder or between killing each, even though *in both individuals* suffering ensues, the quality of life is drastically lowered, and a killing takes place. Put differently, these things done to a child would be wrong; done to a member of a different species, according to the 'anything-goes' position, they are right (or at least not wrong). Members of the 'animal rights' lobby insist that, in the absence of argument, this is speciesist or discriminatory, and I agree with them. In the case of pain and suffering, I can see no difference between the human and animal cases; in the case of the destruction of valuable lives, of lives of at least some value, those who destroy these valuable things must explain how species can be a morally distinguishing feature between two relevantly similar acts of killing.

If we focus upon killing, the boundaries to discussion are clear: animals count, morally; their lives have some value; and we cannot hide or mask the fact that killing them represents the destruction of things of at least some value. In answer to the question of what justifies killing them in medical research, human benefit is the answer nearly always given*, and this answer raises all kinds of questions about (1) what counts as a benefit, (2) how we tell which benefits justify animal research, (3) how large a benefit must be to justify some particular level of sacrifice, (4) how the duplication of research involving sacrifice is a benefit, (5) whether there are some medical benefits that are not worth the massive sacrifice of valuable lives that they require.† These questions weigh in on the medical researcher and demand that the *case be argued*, e.g. of how even a small benefit can, as is sometimes suggested, justify destroying valuable lives. And they draw our attention to a serious question: should an experiment be permitted or continued, if it is very costly in suffering and loss of life, given that the researcher is not always entitled to assume circumstances in which what counts as 'very costly' always eludes general agreement?

Obviously, then, the 'anything-goes' view can come to appear very attractive to researchers: by excluding animals from the moral community one does not have to worry, morally, about their suffering or their slaughter, and one can

---

* Of course, some animal research in medicine does indeed benefit animals, but that is almost never the aim or purpose of *medical* research. It is a by-product of such research.

† The idea of involuntary, even ultimate, sacrifice, by one party to benefit another is neither unknown nor apparently anathema to us. With eminent domain we take people's private property; with taxation we take their material worth; and with conscription we sometimes take their lives. Nearly all local taxing authorities treat single people as resources for married people with children, so far as free public education is concerned. In principle, if not in fact, all these laws are coercive and so apply in the absence of the consent of the party involved.

possibly avoid having to address the issue of how benefit to one species can justify the destruction of another. As I say, I think this path must be resisted. However difficult the questions to be answered, nothing really is achieved by trying to pretend that the pains of animals do not count, or that their lives are utterly valueless.

So, are we to be denied all opportunity to benefit and enhance our lives? But this plea is beside the point: the issue is how far we may go in order to benefit and enhance our lives? May we kill willy-nilly, in order to achieve these ends? This question resonates in ordinary human life: may I sacrifice another person to save myself? May I sacrifice a multitude?

In short, there are undeniably ethical issues involved in using and killing animals, and the morality of these things must be argued for and not presumed or held simply to consist in paying attention to pain thresholds and following laboratory policies for the proper care and custody of animals. For the destruction of valuable lives, killing, always remains to be settled, whether the prospective benefit of the experiment is supposed to be great or small.

There is one more important boundary to the discussion that needs to be noted. Suppose through a very substantial use of animals a very substantial benefit, e.g. a breakthrough on some form of heart disease, were at hand: most of us might very well think that prevention and cure of this dreadful malady justified the use of animals. We must be careful, however, not to overlook a particularly worrisome issue. Researchers and the rest of us are apt to think that, in the absence of artificial models, etc., the researchers in question had no choice but to use animals. But this is not strictly true; they could have used humans. They had, moreover, a powerful reason to do so: all the evidence suggests that we can more accurately extrapolate from human models to humans than from animal models to humans.* (I shall not bother here with a discussion of codes of ethics for researchers and clinicians that forbid any such use of humans, at least without consent of the individual or his trustee.)

In medical experimentation, then, either humans or animals can be used, and I have remarked already that the destruction of valuable lives needs justification. Accordingly, the justificatory boundaries of using and destroying animal lives must include both an account of what makes lives valuable and, in order to deal with our refusal to use humans, a non-speciesist account of why human life is more valuable than animal life, a view of the comparative value of human and animal life, it is worth noting, that even some animal liberationists accept (see ref. 6).

I think a good many of us want to say that, if one can kill a man or kill a rat, that it is worse to kill the man. But what *makes* it worse cannot be species membership. What, then, is the explanation? Whatever the complete answer, a part of it seems to involve our implicit view that the man's life is more valuable than the rat's. This view does indeed allow that the rat's life is of value; its point is that the rat's life does not have the same value as the man's. Plainly,

---

* The thalidomide tragedy is the standard reference here. But it is as well not to exaggerate the difficulty of extrapolation from animals to humans; after all, it is their similarities to us in certain respects that makes their use often so desirable.

then, this view is not a version of the 'anything-goes' position. But it will nevertheless be speciesist in character, unless something other than species membership makes the man's life more valuable. If we can show what this something else is, then we can claim a genuine moral difference between killing a man and killing a rat, and we can then use this difference in the argument from benefit to justify some animal experimentation.

The central issue thus becomes: what makes a life valuable, and why is the man's life more valuable than the rat's? The answer, I have suggested on a number of occasions, is a version of a quality-of-life view (see the articles referred to in the footnote on p. 1058): the value of a life is a function of its quality, its quality of its richness, and its richness of its capacities or scope for enrichment. In medical ethics generally, quality-of-life views of the value of life are today quite prominent, and they make the value of a life turn upon its content or experiences. A rat has an unfolding life, an unfolding set of experiences, so it has a life of some quality or other and thus of some value. Nevertheless, science and observation tell us that the richness of its life is not comparable to ours precisely because its capacities for enrichment are severely truncated when compared to ours. Of course, just as rats, we eat, sleep, and reproduce; but such activities come nowhere near describing the richness of lives with friendship, romance, love, children, art, music, literature, science, and the joys of reflective endeavors. And even these things do not encompass the whole story, if we think only of how we can mould our lives to exemplify certain excellences, whether in the form of artists or athletes. These last are ways of living that are themselves the source of value to us. No rat has ever lived such a life, and everything we know about rats leads us to believe that no rat ever will. Hence, we judge the value of the two lives to be different.

The claim about greater richness to our lives must be seen in context. It is not a claim of absolute knowledge, but a claim based on what we have evidence to believe. For example, we have every reason to believe that many animals, including mice, have a much more acute sense of smell than we do, and it is always possible, I suppose, that though mice lack many of our capacities, their fine sense of smell can send them into such an ecstasy that the quality of their lives approaches that of our own. While this sort of thing is possible, I can see no reason to believe it the case. But should I not give the animal the benefit of the doubt? (In this regard, see ref. 7.) Perhaps, generally, I should; but surely I am only required to do this where there is not only evidence but also evidence beyond a certain degree? Mere possibility does not approach that degree, however it be set. Furthermore, my richness claim is not contending that what pertains to the quality of human lives is precisely what pertains to the quality of animal lives. By all means let there be differences. But what must be given me is some reason for thinking that such differences enable the animal's life to approach the richness of ours, given all of our additional capacities, and this reason must cohere with what science and observation enable us to know of the capacities present in animals of the kind in question. In sum, what we normally think is this: when, at death, we say of a person that he or she led a rich, full life, we take ourselves to be referring to something incomparably beyond that to which we would refer, were we to say the same of a rodent. If this is not the case, we need more than benefit-of-the-doubt arguments to shake our confidence.

It should be apparent now what the upshot of quality-of-life views of the value of life is for our discussion: normal adult human life is more valuable than animal life, and that is why it is worse to kill the human. To kill a human is to destroy something of greater value. And this is so, not because of species membership, but because of the comparative richness of lives; the view, therefore, is not speciesist. This difference between the human and animal cases we can in turn insert into the argument from benefit to support animal experimentation.

It should also be apparent, however, that not all human life is of the same quality and richness as normal adult human life. Any number of humans lead massively impoverished lives, lives, moreover, that not only lack much richness, but lack even the potentialities for enrichment of normal lives. The seriously brain-damaged, severely handicapped newborns, such as those born with no brain or with hypoplastic left heart syndrome, elderly people fully in the grip of Alzheimer's disease, people dying in the final stages of cardiomyopathy—all kinds of examples come to mind. Depending upon how severely impaired these unfortunate lives are, they can fall so far below the quality of ordinary human life as to become lives that we would not wish ourselves to live, and that we would not wish to compel anyone else to live, and so to become lives that at least some of us may come to think are not worth living.*

In fact, the quality of a human life can fall to a point that the life of a perfectly healthy experimental animal can seem readily to equal or exceed it, can seem, indeed, to be a life not worth sacrificing for the human life. Then, only if one invokes the dictum that a human life of any quality, however low, exceeds in value an animal life of any quality, however high, can one be sure that human life will always remain more valuable. I can see no reason whatever to accept any such dictum, which in my eyes is just that.

Our situation, then, is this: we can indeed find a genuine difference between killing a man and killing a rat, but this difference exists only in the cases of human lives whose quality approaches that of normal adult human life. In the cases of those human lives that are massively below this quality, so that their quality of life is equal to or exceeded by that of the healthy experimental subject, we face the ultimate question: what justifies our using the animal over the human, given that the benefit we seek can be obtained through using either? As I say, what is needed, to avoid experimenting upon the human, is something that ensures of any human life, however low its quality, that its value exceeds that of any animal life, however high its quality. I know of no such thing.

Again, consider the use of animals as a source of organs for human transplants,

---

* It would, I think, be false to suppose that it is only philosophers, never doctors, that make this judgement about a life worth living, at least given my experience in medical ethics over the past decade. Who is the doctor to decide this issue? The person overseeing the case, who is neither the Almighty nor Solomon, admittedly, but who is charged with making decisions about what is best for his patient. Physician-assisted suicide would appear to fall, in the eyes of an increasing number of doctors, under this heading.

a practice on the rise:* every defence of this practice, as best I can tell, acknowledges directly or indirectly the value of animal life. Consequently, I can see no way consistently to bar using some humans in this way, since I can find nothing compelling that always cedes human life greater value than animal life. Moreover, as I noted earlier in another context, we at present† seem much more likely to achieve the benefit of a renewed human life through intra-species rather than inter-species transplantation. To date, the history of xenografting is essentially a history of failure.

One must be careful, moreover, not to be put off the rational consideration of using humans, the rational consideration *of the argument*, by attempts to invoke the imagery of the medical practices in the German camps of World War II. Quality-of-life decisions involving life and death are made every day in our hospitals, without those who make them being forced down the slippery slope of killing to the level of monsters. We need reason to believe we will be forced down the slope. My grandmother once said to me, 'Take a drink, and you will become an alcoholic.' She was wrong. Of course, if I never take a drink, I cannot become an alcoholic; but then not to take a drink over dinner is to forgo one of the great pleasures of life and so to avoid one of the great glories of France. My worry, obviously, is that rational consideration of arguments is too easily pushed aside, by invoking fears of slippery slopes leading to perdition.

Am I, therefore, *advocating* experiments on unfortunate humans? No, I am not;‡ that is to miss the point. The point is that envisaging such experiments is inescapable, *if* one employs the argument from benefit to justify animal experimentation and relies upon the comparative value of human and animal life to show why the benefit may not be obtained through experimenting upon humans. And this is, I submit, the position in which many medical experimenters find themselves: benefit drives their animal research, and the comparative value of lives is, when they are pressed, the philosophical underpinning they resort to in order to justify their non-use of humans. The only way I can see to avoid envisaging experiments upon humans, given these factors, is to give up animal experiments altogether, a curious rear-door entry for anti-vivisectionism. But how likely are medical people and the rest of us to give up the search for benefits? That leaves the comparative value of lives to be disputed, and what is required to supplant this, as we have seen, is something that guarantees *in each and every case* that a human life, no matter how badly off, is always more valuable than an animal life.

I think animal experiments, therefore, can be justified, but that their justification comes at a certain price, at least if that justification, as it does for myself and countless others, runs through the argument from benefit and the comparative

---

* I suspect that, should cross-species transplantation prove successful in several instances, some people will argue for medical facilities keeping and rearing animals as living repositories of organs for humans.
† I here envisage the prospect of several successful cases of inter-species transplantation.
‡ At the moment I know for a fact that the side-effects of such experiments would be very negative indeed. People would be outraged by such experiments, would be reluctant to go into hospital and to be attended to by medical people, and would definitely view the doctor/patient relationship in a new, sceptical, untrusting light.

value of human and animal life. That price is the exposure to the prospect of experiments upon humans. Our options are three. We can pay the price and perform human experiments; we can avoid having to pay the price by giving up animal experiments and, thus, by giving up many of the benefits that medical science bestows upon us; or we can name that magical ingredient that so conveniently transforms the value of our lives beyond anything that might be true in the case of animals.

Finally, I have said nothing in this essay about religion, for its introduction raises far too many other issues for it to be considered here. But it might be thought by some to provide the magical ingredient. To others, it will seem a non-starter. For many medical and other people are no longer religious, do not think their moral views are grounded in some religion, and cannot see the need for further, endless, metaphysical debates about the existence and nature of God, or about the self-proclaimed merits or truth of this or that religion, in order to address moral and social issues. To believers this will appear harsh. What impresses *me* most, e.g. with respect to Christianity, is the striking convenience for humans of so many of the doctrines: *we* are given dominion, *we* are made in the image and likeness of God, *we* are given an immortal soul, and *we* are the beneficiaries of sanctity-of-life claims (I do not deny that some Christians want to change all this; see ref. 8). If I may put the matter slightly pejoratively, these assertions make it too easy for us to construe animals as health-care resources, where the morality of any such resource view is part of what we want to argue about.

REFERENCES

1. Regan, T. 1983. *The case for animal rights*: University of California Press, Berkeley, CA.
2. Singer, P. 1977. *Animal liberation* (Avon, NY
3. Singer, P. 1988. Comment. *Between the Species* 4: 202.
4. Clark, S. R. L. 1982. *The Nature of the beast*. Oxford University Press, Oxford.
5. Smith, J. and Boyd, K. (Eds). 1992. *Lives in the balance: animal experimentation*. Oxford University Press, Oxford.
6. Regan, T. 1985. The case for animal rights'. Pp. 13–26, *in* Singer, P. (Ed.) *In defence of animals*. Basil Blackwell, Oxford.
7. Sapontzis, S. F. 1987. *Morals, reason, and animals*. Temple University Press, Philadelphia, PA.
8. Linzey, A. 1978. *Animal rights*. SPCK, London.

Index

Note: Page numbers in *italics* refer to figures and tables